W9-CHO-688

PRINCIPLES OF ORTHOPAEDIC PRACTICE

PRINCIPLES OF ORTHOPAEDIC PRACTICE

Roger Dee, M.D.
Editor in Chief

Enrico Mango, M.D.   Lawrence C. Hurst, M.D.

With the editorial assistance of

Hormozan Aprin, M.D.   Allen P. Kaplan, M.D.

McGraw-Hill Book Company

New York   St. Louis   San Fancisco   Auckland   Bogotá   Caracas
Colorado Springs   Hamburg   Lisbon   London   Madrid   Mexico
Milan   Montreal   New Delhi   Oklahoma City   Panama   Paris   San Juan
São Paulo   Singapore   Sydney   Tokyo   Toronto

PRINCIPLES OF ORTHOPAEDIC PRACTICE

1 2 3 4 5 6 7 8 9 0   HALHAL   8 9 3 2 1 0 9 8

ISBN 0-07-016201-8 (Vol I), 016202-6 (Vol II), 079996-2 (set)

This book was set in Cheltenham Book by York Graphic Services, Inc.
The designer was José R. Fonfrias.
The editors were Ray Moloney, Stuart D. Boynton, and Julia White.
The production supervisors were Robert Laffler and Elaine Gardenier
Arcata Graphics/Halliday was printer and binder.

Library of Congress Cataloging-in-Publication Data
Principles of orthopaedic practice / Roger Dee, editor in chief . . . [et al.].
p. cm. Includes bibliographies and index.
ISBN 0-07-079996-2 (set).   ISBN 0-07-016201-8 (vol. 1).   ISBN 0-07-016202-6 (vol. 2)
1. Orthopedia.   I. Dee. Roger, date.
[DNLM: 1. Orthopedics.   WE 168 P957]
RD731.P92 1988
617'.3—dc19
DNLM/DLC
for Library of Congress   88-9123
                                              CIP

CONTENTS

CONTRIBUTORS

Herbert T. Abelson, M.D.
Professor and Chairman, Department of Pediatrics, University of Washington, Seattle, WA

Behrooz A. Akbarnia, M.D.
Professor and Vice Chairman, Department of Orthopaedic Surgery, St. Louis University; Director, Orthopaedic Surgery, Cardinal Glennon Children's Hospital, St. Louis, MO

Edward Akelman, M.D.
Assistant Professor of Orthopaedics, Brown University Program in Medicine; Surgeon-in-Charge, Division of Hand and Upper Extremity Surgery, Rhode Island Hospital, Providence, RI

John F. Aloia, M.D.
Professor of Medicine, State University of New York at Stony Brook; Chairman, Department of Medicine, Winthrop-University Hospital, Mineola, NY

Peter C. Amadio, M.D.
Consultant in Orthopaedics and Hand Surgery, Mayo Clinic, Mayo Medical School, Rochester, MN

Hormozan Aprin, M.D.
Assistant Professor of Orthopaedics, State University of New York at Stony Brook, Stony Brook, NY

Harold L. Atkins, M.D.
Professor of Radiology and Chief, Nuclear Medicine Division, Department of Radiology, State University of New York at Stony Brook, Stony Brook, NY

Douglas G. Avella, M.D.
Peabody Research Fellow in Pediatric Orthopaedics, Massachusetts General Hospital, Boston, MA

Marie A. Badalamente, Ph.D.
Research Associate Professor and Director, Cell Biology/Cell Structure Laboratory, Department of Orthopaedics, State University of New York at Stony Brook, Stony Brook, NY

George H. Belhobek, M.D.
Chairman, Department of Diagnostic Radiology, Clinic Head, Section of Bone and Joint Radiology, Cleveland Clinic Foundation, Cleveland, OH

Louis U. Bigliani, M.D.
Assistant Professor of Orthopaedic Surgery, Columbia University; Attending Orthopaedic Surgeon, Shoulder and Elbow Clinic, Columbia Presbyterian Medical Center, New York, NY

Nestor Blyznak, M.D.
Assistant Professor of Orthopaedic Surgery, State University of New York at Stony Brook, Stony Brook, NY

J. Richard Bowen, M.D.
Director of Orthopaedics, The Alfred I. DuPont Institute, Wilmington, DE

Ernest M. Burgess, M.D.
Clinical Professor of Orthopaedics and Director, Prosthetics Research Study, University of Washington, Seattle, WA

Donald K. Bynum Jr., M.D.
Assistant Professor of Orthopaedic Surgery, University of North Carolina, Chapel Hill, NC

Stuart Cherney, M.D.
Assistant Professor of Orthopaedics, State University of New York at Stony Brook, Stony Brook, NY

David T.W. Chiu, M.D.
Assistant Professor of Surgery, New York University, New York, NY

Stanley Chung, M.D.
Associate Professor of Surgery (Orthopaedics), University of Hawaii; Chief, Division of Pediatric Orthopaedics and Department of Surgery, Kapiolani Children's Medical Center, Honolulu, HI

Patricia Connolly, P.T., M.A.
Senior Physical Therapist, Sports Physical Therapist, University Hospital, Stony Brook, NY

Jerome M. Cotler, M.D.
Professor and Vice Chairman, Department of Orthopaedic Surgery, Thomas Jefferson University, Philadelphia, PA

Henry R. Cowell, M.D., Ph.D.
Lecturer, Harvard Medical School, Boston, MA

Michael P. Coyle, Jr., M.D.
Clinical Associate Professor of Orthopaedic Surgery, UMDNJ-Robert Wood Johnson Medical School, New Brunswick, NJ

Kennedy Daniels, M.D.
Clinical Assistant Instructor of Orthopaedics, State University of New York at Stony Brook, Stony Brook, NY

Raymond J. Dattwyler, M.D.
Assistant Professor of Immunology, State University of New York at Stony Brook, Stony Brook, NY

Roger Dee, B.M., B.ch, F.R.C.S., Ph.D.
Professor and Chairman, Department of Orthopaedics, State University of New York at Stony Brook; Chief of Orthopaedics, University Hospital, Stony Brook, NY

Harold M. Dick, M.D.
Frank E. Stinchfield Professor and Chairman, Department of Orthopaedic Surgery, Columbia University, New York, NY

Thomas Dowling, M.D.
Clinical Assistant Instructor of Orthopaedics, State University of New York at Stony Brook, Stony Brook, NY

Georges Y. El-Khoury, M.D.
Professor of Radiology and Orthopaedics, University of Iowa Hospitals and Clinics, Iowa City, IA

Jerry L. Ellstein, M.D.
Assistant Professor of Clinical Orthopaedics, State University of New York at Stony Brook; Hand Surgery Service, University Hospital, Stony Brook, NY

Joseph A. Epstein, M.D.
Professor of Clinical Neurosurgery, State University of New York at Stony Brook; Clinical Associate Professor in Surgery (Neurosurgery), Cornell University Medical College, New York, NY

Nancy E. Epstein, M.D.
Assistant Professor of Clinical Neurosurgery, State University of New York at Stony Brook; Attending Neurosurgery, Long Island Jewish/Hillside Medical Center; Adjunct Clinical Assistant Professor of Surgery (Neurosurgery), Cornell University Medical College, New York, NY

Stephen E. Feffer, M.D.
Assistant Professor of Medicine, State University of New York at Stony Brook; Chief, Division of Hematology and Medical Oncology, Nassau County Medical Center, East Meadow, NY

Earl Feiwell, M.D.
Associate Clinical Professor, University of Southern California; Orthopaedic Chief, Myelodysplasia Team, Rancho Los Amigos Hospital, Los Alamitos, CA

Meredith Cook Ferraro, P.T., M.S.
Chief, Department of Hand Therapy, University Hospital, Stony Brook, NY

Lonnie W. Frei, M.D.
Clinical Assistant Professor of Medicine and General Surgery, State University of New York at Stony Brook, Stony Brook, NY

Gary E. Friedlaender, M.D.
Professor and Chairman, Department of Orthopaedics and Rehabilitation, Yale University School of Medicine; Chief-of-Service, Department of Orthopaedics and Rehabilitation, Yale-New Haven Hospital, New Haven, CT

Robert Y. Garroway, M.D.
Assistant Professor of Clinical Orthopaedics, State University of New York at Stony Brook; Assistant Chief of Orthopaedics, South Nassau Communities Hospital, Oceanside, NY

Richard Ghillani, M.D.
Assistant Professor, Department of Orthopaedics and Rehabilitation Medicine, State University of New York Health Science Center at Brooklyn, New York, NY

Joan T. Gold, M.D.
Director of Pediatric Physiatry, Hospital for Joint Diseases, Orthopaedic Institute; Assistant Professor of Clinical Pediatrics and Physical Medicine and Rehabilitation, Mount Sinai School of Medicine, New York, NY

Marc G. Golightly, Ph.D.
Head of Immunology, Assistant Professor of Pathology, State University of New York at Stony Brook, Stony Brook, NY

Antoni B. Goral, LCDR, MC, USNR
Clinical Assistant Professor, Uniformed Services University of the Health Sciences; Department of Orthopaedics, Naval Hospital Bethesda, Bethesda, MD

Peter D. Gorevic, M.D.
Associate Professor of Medicine and Pathology and Head, Division of Allergy and Rheumatology, State University of New York at Stony Brook, Stony Brook, NY

Robert Greenwald, M.D.
Professor of Medicine, State University of New York at Stony Brook; Chief, Division of Rheumatology, Long Island Jewish Medical Center, New Hyde Park, NY

Martin A. Gruber, M.D.
Clinical Associate Professor of Orthopaedics, State University of New York at Stony Brook; Clinical Director, Pediatric Orthopaedics, Nassau County Medical Center, East Meadow, NY

James Gurtowski, M.D.
Clinical Assistant Instructor of Orthopaedics, State University of New York at Stony Brook, Stony Brook, NY

John J. Halperin, M.D.
Assistant Professor of Neurology, State University of New York at Stony Brook, Stony Brook, NY

Richard B. Hindes, M.D.
Assistant Professor of Clinical Orthopaedics, State University of New York at Stony Brook, Stony Brook, NY

Drew A. Hittenberger, C.P.
Chief Research Prosthetist, Prosthetics Research Study, University of Washington, Seattle, WA

M. Mark Hoffer, M.D.
Professor and Chief of Orthopaedics, University of California, Irvine, Orange, CA

Lawrence C. Hurst, M.D.
Associate Professor of Orthopaedics and Associate Chairman, Department of Orthopaedics, State University of New York at Stony Brook; Chief of Hand Service, University Hospital, Stony Brook, NY

Robert W. Hussey, M.D.
Associate Professor of Orthopaedics, Medical College of Virginia; Chief, Spinal Cord Injury Service, McGuire V.A. Medical Center, Richmond, VA

Marianne R. Jahnke, Ph.D.
Research Fellow, West Virginia University, School of Medicine, Morgantown, WVA

Ali Kalamchi, M.D.
Attending Orthopaedic Staff, Medical Center of Delaware, A.I. DuPont Institute, Wilmington, DE

Allen P. Kaplan, M.D.
Professor and Chairman, Department of Medicine, State University of New York at Stony Brook, Stony Brook, NY

Donald M. Kastenbaum, M.D.
Fellow in Orthopaedic Surgery, New York University, New York, NY

Lee D. Kaufman, M.D.
Assistant Professor of Clinical Medicine, Division of Allergy, Rheumatology, and Clinical Immunology, State University of New York at Stony Brook, Stony Brook, NY

Louis Keppler, M.D.
Chief of Orthopaedic Surgery, St. Vincent Charity Hospital; Staff, Cleveland Spine and Arthritis Center, Cleveland, OH

Michael J. Kramer, M.D.
Assistant Professor of Orthopaedics, State University of New York at Stony Brook, Stony Brook, NY

Richard S. Laskin, M.D.
Professor of Orthopaedic Surgery, State University of New York at Stony Brook; Chairman, Department of Orthopaedic Surgery, Long Island Jewish/Hillside Medical Center, New Hyde Park, NY

Joseph P. Leddy, M.D.
Clinical Associate Professor of Surgery and Chief of Hand Surgery, UMDNJ-Robert Wood Johnson Medical School, New Brunswick, NJ

Wallace B. Lehman, M.D.
Associate Professor, Mount Sinai School of Medicine, New York, NY; Chief, Pediatric Orthopaedic Surgery, Hospital for Joint Diseases, New York, NY

Joan Lehmann, O.T.R./L.
Senior Occupational Therapist, University Hospital, Stony Brook, NY

John J. Leppard, M.D.
Assistant Clinical Professor of Orthopaedics, State University of New York at Stony Brook; Assistant Clinical Professor, Columbia University, New York, NY

Paul E. Levin, M.D.
Assistant Professor of Orthopaedics, State University of New York at Stony Brook; Chief of Orthopaedic Trauma and Fracture Service, University Hospital, Stony Brook, NY

Roger Levy, M.D.
Clinical Professor of Orthopaedics and Chief of Arthritis Surgery, Mount Sinai School of Medicine, New York, NY

Esther Lipstein-Kresch, M.D.
Physician-in-Charge, Division of Rheumatology, Queens Hospital Center, Jamaica, NY

Martin M. Malawer, M.D.
Associate Professor of Orthopaedic Surgery, George Washington University School of Medicine and Health Sciences, Washington, DC; Chief, Orthopaedic Oncology, Children's Hospital National Medical Center; Consultant, Surgery Branch, National Cancer Institute, National Institutes of Health, Bethesda, MD

Enrico Mango, M.D.
Assistant Professor of Clinical Orthopaedics, State University of New York at Stony Brook, Stony Brook, NY

Steven W. Margles, M.D.
Clinical Instructor of Orthopaedic Surgery, Boston University School of Medicine; Chief, Section of Hand Surgery, Lahey Clinic Medical Center, Burlington, MA

Frank C. McCue, III, M.D.
Alfred R. Shands Professor of Orthopaedic Surgery and Plastic Surgery of the Hand; Director, Division of Sports Medicine and Hand Surgery, University of Virginia, Charlottesville, VA

Cahir A. McDevitt, Ph.D.
Head, Section of Biochemistry, Department of Musculoskeletal Research, Cleveland Clinic Foundation Research Institute, Cleveland, OH

Bruce P. Meinhard, M.D.
Assistant Professor, State University of New York at Stony Brook; Chief of Orthopaedic, Trauma Services, Nassau County Medical Center, East Meadow, NY

M. Ather Mirza, M.D.
Assistant Clinical Professor of Orthopaedics, State University of New York at Stony Brook; Hand Surgery Service St. John's Hospital, Smithtown, NY

Constantine Misoul, M.D.
Attending Surgeon, Franklin Square Hospital, Baltimore, MD

William J. Montgomery, M.D.
Assistant Professor of Radiology, The University of Iowa Hospitals, Iowa City, IA

Robert Moriarty, M.D.
Clinical Assistant Instructor of Orthopaedics, State University of New York at Stony Brook, Stony Brook, NY

David S. Morrison, M.D.
Clinical Instructor in Orthopaedics, University of California, Irvine; Director, Shoulder and Elbow Surgery, Southern California Center for Sports Medicine, Long Beach, CA

Colin F. Moseley, M.D., C.M.
Associate Clinical Professor of Orthopaedics, University of California, Los Angeles; Chief of Staff, Shriners Hospital, Los Angeles, CA

Jay Nathan, M.D.
Clinical Assistant Instructor of Orthopaedics, State University of New York at Stony Brook, Stony Brook, NY

Daniel Fulham O'Neill, M.D.
Clinical Assistant Instructor of Orthopaedics, State University of New York at Stony Brook, Stony Brook, NY

Craig B. Ordway, M.D.
Assistant Clinical Professor of Orthopaedic Surgery, State University of New York at Stony Brook, Stony Brook, NY

Seth Paul, M.D.
Clinical Assistant Instructor of Orthopaedics, State University of New York at Stony Brook, Stony Brook, NY

Stuart B. Polisner, M.D.
Assistant Professor of Clinical Pediatric Orthopaedics, State University of New York at Stony Brook; Consultant, Nassau County Medical Center, East Meadow, NY

James Pugh, Ph.D.
Professor of Material Science and Engineering, State University of New York at Stony Brook; Director of Biomedical Engineering, Metallurgy, and Materials Science, Inter-City Testing and Consulting Corporation, Mineola, NY

Suzanne Ray, M.D.
Clinical Associate Professor of Surgery, University of North Dakota; Pediatric Orthopaedic Surgeon, Dakota Clinic, Fargo, ND

Michael D. Ries, M.D.
Clinical Assistant Professor of Orthopaedics, State University of New York at Stony Brook, Stony Brook, NY

Samuel Rosenfeld, M.D.
Clinical Instructor of Orthopaedic Surgery, University of California, Irvine, Orange, CA

Alan D. Rosenthal, M.D.
Associate Professor of Clinical Neurosurgery, State University of New York at Stony Brook; Clinical Instructor in Surgery (Neurosurgery), Cornell University Medical College, New York, NY; Attending Physician, Department of Surgery, Long Island Jewish/Hillside Medical Center and North Shore University Hospital, Manhasset

Melvin Rosenwasser, M.D.
Assistant Clinical Professor of Orthopaedic Surgery, Columbia University, New York, NY

Avron Ross, M.D.
Professor of Clinical Pediatrics, State University of New York at Stony Brook, Stony Brook, NY

Clinton T. Rubin, Ph.D.
Research Associate Professor and Director, Musculo-Skeletal Research Laboratory, Department of Orthopaedics, State University of New York at Stony Brook, Stony Brook, NY

Steven Sampson, M.D.
Assistant Professor of Orthopaedics, State University of New York at Stony Brook; Attending Hand Surgeon, University Hospital, Stony Brook, NY

Mark Sanders, M.D.
Clinical Assistant Instructor of Orthopaedics, State University of New York at Stony Brook, Stony Brook, NY

Barry M. Shmookler, M.D.
Director of Surgical Pathology, The Washington Hospital Center, Washington, DC

Joseph A. Spadaro, Ph.D.
Associate Professor of Research, Department of Orthopaedic Surgery, State University of New York Health Science Center at Syracuse, Syracuse, NY

Donald P. Speer, M.D.
Professor of Surgery and Anatomy, University of Arizona College of Medicine, Tucson, AZ

William Thomas Stillwell, M.D.
Associate Professor of Clinical Orthopaedics, State University of New York at Stony Brook; Instructor in Clinical Orthopaedics, Columbia University, New York, NY; Chief of Orthopaedic Surgery, St. Johns Episcopal Hospital, Smithtown, NY

Eric D. Strauss, M.D.
Attending Surgeon, Garden State Medical Center, Marlton, NJ

James W. Strickland, M.D.
Clinical Professor of Orthopaedic Surgery, Indiana University; Chief, Hand Surgery Section, St. Vincent Hospital and Health Care Center, Indianapolis, IN

George H. Thompson, M.D.
Assistant Professor of Orthopaedic Surgery and Pediatrics, Case Western Reserve University, Cleveland, OH

Ashok N. Vaswani, M.D.
Assistant Professor of Medicine, State University of New York at Stony Brook; Associate Director of Endocrinology and Metabolism, Winthrop-University Hospital, Mineola, NY

David J. Weissberg, M.D.
Instructor of Clinical Orthopaedics, State University of New York at Stony Brook, Stony Brook, NY

David Westring, M.D.
Clinical Professor of Medicine, State University of New York at Stony Brook; Director, Academic Affairs, Nassau County Medical Center, East Meadow, NY

Ira Wolfe, B.A.
Consultant in Sports Medicine, Columbia Presbyterian Medical Center, New York, NY

Kenneth R. Zaslav, M.D.
Clinical Assistant Instructor of Orthopaedics, State University of New York at Stony Brook, Stony Brook, NY

Joseph, Zito, M.D.
Assistant Professor of Radiology, State University of New York at Stony Brook; Chief, Division of Neuroradiology, Long Island Jewish/Hillside Medical Center, New Hyde Park, NY

PREFACE

The student of orthopaedic surgery, advised that reading the orthopaedic literature will be the foundation of knowledge, is somewhat chastened when faced with the reality of implementing such advice. Indeed, all orthopaedic surgeons today are confronted by a torrent of articles in an ever increasing number of subspecialty journals. Many of these will be of considerable significance. Some will shed new light on long standing controversy or provide new information or data significant enough to alter well established patterns of treatment. Others may be worthy of perusal but be of lesser significance.

This book was produced in response to the perceived need for a single source text which may be used by the student as a companion during study of the orthopaedic literature. We have produced a highly factualized text which, it is hoped, will provide the necessary knowledge base, and suitable frame of reference to facilitate such study. The secondary purpose of this work is to provide a curriculum for such postgraduate examinations in orthopaedic surgery as the American Board Examination, the Intraining Examination, and the proposed Specialist Assessment in Orthopaedic Surgery in the United Kingdom.

Contributors have, for the most part, followed the editorial guidelines, and included a review of the current literature. There is, therefore, less emphasis on anecdotal experience in this book than in some others. However, the editors feel that the text is also well leavened by the clinical expertise of the contributing authors. Consequently, we hope it may be used as a practical manual in the management of individual patients.

We have not attempted to provide a technical atlas of operative orthopaedics, and detailed accounts of individual surgical procedures should be sought in specialized texts or manuals. The goals and basic principles of the various relevant surgical procedures are, however, described when appropriate.

Beginning each regional section are chapters illustrating some key anatomical concepts which we believe to be important during surgical exposure. We have also included in these sections important special anatomy such as femoral head and talar blood supply in the lower limb section, and neuroanatomy in the spinal anatomy section. These sections on important surgical anatomy are placed for convenient reference. We have consequently avoided repetitious accounts in the subsequent clinical text, which would otherwise have been unavoidable.

In producing a work of this size, we have relied heavily on the generosity of others. We cannot possibly itemize the many acts of kindness we have been shown, but would like to express our gratitude to publishers and authors for their permission to reproduce illustrations from original material. In many cases, they have sent slides or original prints for reproduction, and we wish to express our considerable gratitude. Some of the illustrations in the text may be familiar. This is because certain tables and figures are unique and cannot be improved upon. We have tried to bring such important data together in one text. This achieves one of the goals of this work, which is to reduce the time that students and surgeons otherwise must utilize searching among many specialized volumes, monographs, or clinical journals looking for that elusive figure, table, or reference. We hope that this work will be especially valuable in that regard. If so, we will have succeeded in following Osler's advice to teachers to " . . . mint and make current coin the ore so widely scattered in journals, transactions, and monographs." Readers, however, will be wise to heed another piece of advice from this great medical teacher that "To study the phenomena of disease without books is to sail an uncharted sea, while to study books without patients is not to go to sea at all."*

The editors have been extremely demanding of the contributing authors during the preparation of this textbook. In many cases text has been rewritten at our suggestion, to more appropriately achieve the goals of the overall work. We are grateful to all our contributors for the courtesy and good humor they have maintained during this process. We have been fortunate in having available to us the resources of a computerized literature retrieval system (Orthopaedic Index) whose proprietors have also given us unlimited access to their excellent collection of original orthopaedic articles. We wish to express our thanks to the Department of Audiovisual Services at the State University of New York at Stony Brook, and in particular Edward Joseph, from the Department of Photography, and Ms. Cathy Gebhart, who drew many of the important anatomical illustrations throughout the book. I would also like to express my personal thanks to Dr. Marvin Kuschner, Dean of the School of Medicine at the

Osler, Sir William. *Aequanimitas,* 3d ed. Philadelphia, Blakiston, 1943.

State University of New York at Stony Brook, for his support during the preparation of this book.

We owe a tremendous debt of gratitude to our department secretaries, Mrs. Catherine Gale and Mrs. Gail Trocchio, without whose timeless labor and endless patience nothing would have been possible. Finally, we would like to pay tribute to the magnificent work of the team at McGraw-Hill who have brought this work to fruition, that is, to Mr. Raymond Moloney, Mr. Stuart Boynton, and Ms. Julia White. Their support and tremendous hard work have been a continuing encouragement.

ROGER DEE, M.D.

PART I

Basic Sciences of the Musculoskeletal System

CHAPTER 1

Musculoskeletal Embryology

Stanley Chung and Roger Dee

DEVELOPMENT OF THE MUSCULOSKELETAL SYSTEM

A discrete yet overlapping series of biosynthetic and restructuring events regulates the development of the musculoskeletal system.[3] Programmed by the genes, one molecule or cell state is replaced by the next more complex state (called its *molecular,* or *cellular, isoform*). Next, replacement molecules or cells are programmed for still another stage of development. The process is particularly well illustrated in the development of adult muscle and cartilage (see below).

Most structures differentiate during the first 8 weeks of embryonic life and then grow and mature in the next 28 weeks to term.

General Embryological Features

The zygote (fertilized ovum) produces a ball of cells, called the *morula,* by a series of mitotic divisions termed *cleavage.* The morula enters the uterus approximately 3 days after fertilization. A cavity forms within it converting it to a *blastocyst,* which attaches to the endometrial epithelium about the fifth or sixth day.

The Bilaminar Stage

The *epiblast* and *hypoblast* are two layers which next form on the dorsal and ventral aspect of the inner cell mass within the blastocyst. The epiblast will produce all three germ layers of the embryo: the ectoderm, mesoderm, and endoderm. The hypoblast is probably displaced to extraembryonic regions. The amniotic cavity, yolk sac, connecting stalk, and chorion develop.

The outer layer of the blastocyst is termed the *trophoblast.* It differentiates into an inner cell layer, the cytotrophoblast, and an outer cell layer, the syncytiotrophoblast. When a lacunar network forms within the latter, the uteroplacental circulation is established. This stage of development is sometimes referred to as the *period of twos* because two embryonic layers derive from the inner cell mass (the epiblast and

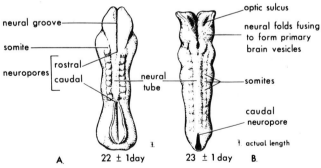

Figure 1-1 Four-week embryo. **A** and **B.** Dorsal views during stage 10 of development (22 to 23 days) showing 8 to 12 somites. **C** to **E.** Lateral views of embryos during stages 11, 12, and 13 of development (24 to 28 days) showing 16, 27, and 33 somites, respectively. *(From Moore, K.L.: The Developing Human: Clinically Oriented Embryology, 3d ed. Philadelphia, Saunders, 1982. Reprinted with permission.)*

the hypoblast), two cavities develop (the amniotic cavity and the primary yolk sac), and two cell layers are formed from the trophoblast.

The Trilaminar Stage

The third week is known as the *period of threes* because during this period the three germ layers develop and three important structures form: the primitive streak, the notochord, and the neural tube (Fig. 1-1).

The process by which the bilaminar embryo is changed into a trilaminar structure is termed *gastrulation.* Up to this point there has been little evidence of gene-controlled biosynthetic activity, such as the production of myosin or actin, and it is believed that the embryo is relatively immune to teratogenesis since the cells are unresponsive to embryonic inducer substances.[5] The *primitive streak* is a midline thickening of the epiblast from which mesenchymal cells migrate cranially, laterally, and ventrally between the epiblast and the hypoblast to form the intraembryonic mesoderm. The epiblast layer is then termed the *embryonic ectoderm,* the hypoblast becoming the *embryonic endoderm* (Fig. 1-2).

The *notochord* arises from a mass of rapidly proliferating cells at the cephalic end of the primitive streak termed *Hensen's node.* The ectoderm in the midbody region forms a thickening known as the *neural plate.* The neural plate becomes depressed centrally and elevated laterally, forming a groove. The lateral folds then approach each other, fuse, and form the *neural tube.*

Now the paraxial mesoderm starts to show evidence of the segmental plan of the embryo as it becomes organized into paired blocks of mesoderm visible externally as prominences termed *somites* (Fig. 1-1).

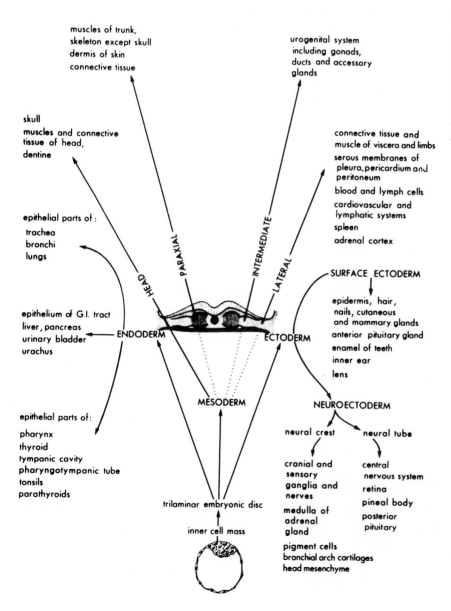

Figure 1-2 The origin and derivatives of the three germ layers. The cells of these layers make specific contributions to the formation of different tissues and organs. *(From Moore, K.L.: The Developing Human: Clinically Oriented Embryology, 3d ed. Philadelphia, Saunders, 1982. Reprinted with permission.)*

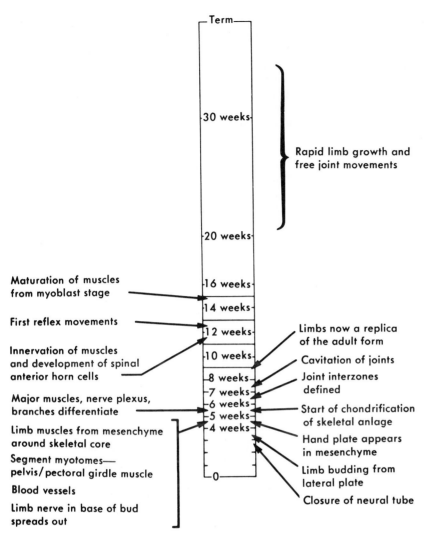

Figure 1-3 Timetable of musculoskeletal development. *(From Fuller, D., and Duthie, R., Instr Course Lect 23:1974. Reproduced with permission.)*

The Embryonic Period (Fourth to Eighth Weeks)

The neural tube begins to close in the region of the somites at the beginning of this period. The tube initially remains open at the rostral and caudal neuropores, but the former soon closes. At stage 12 (about 26 days) small upper limb buds appear as swellings on the ventrolateral body wall. The lower limb buds are present at about 28 days. Hand plates develop in the upper limbs during the fifth week. By the seventh week the limbs have become more defined, and the future digits take shape as notches develop between the digital rays in the hand plates. The fingers and toes become more distinct by the eighth week (Fig. 1-3).

The Fetal Period (Ninth Week to Birth)

The embryo now changes proportions as rapid growth occurs. At the ninth week the head accounts for almost half the body length. At 12 weeks the crown-to-rump length has more than doubled, whereas growth of the head has relatively slowed. The legs and thighs, which are short at first, gain proportionately in length and size. The upper limbs also reach their final relative length by the end of the twelfth week. Between the thirteenth and sixteenth weeks the skeleton shows clearly on radiographs, and ossification is proceeding rapidly. Between the seventeenth and twentieth weeks the final relative proportions of the lower limbs are attained.

The Articular and Skeletal Systems

Bone and joints develop from the mesoderm. A ventromedial sclerotome and a dorsolateral dermomyotome differentiate from each somite. Sclerotomal cells surround the notochord and neural tube and eventually form the vertebrae and their surrounding ligaments as well as the ribs. The dermomyotome develops into the dorsal musculature and the skin dermis.

DEVELOPMENT OF THE VERTEBRAL COLUMN

Vertebral Column

The sclerotome is composed of loosely arranged cells at the cephalic end and of densely packed cells more caudally. The intervertebral disc is formed from some of these densely packed cells which migrate cranially to lie opposite the center of the myotome (Fig. 1-4). The residual densely packed cells combine with the cephalic (loosely arranged) cells of the adjacent caudal sclerotome and form the mesenchymal vertebral centrum. The centrum is thus an intersegmental structure. The notochord forms the nucleus pulposus in the center of the intervertebral disc. It disappears in the region of the vertebral centrum. Mesenchymal cells, which surround the neural tube, form the vertebral arch.

During the sixth week two cartilaginous centers appear in the mesenchymal centrum and then fuse to form the cartilaginous centrum. Cartilaginous centers also appear in the vertebral arches, fuse with each other, and with the centrum form the cartilaginous model for the vertebra. Two primary ossification centers, one ventral and one dorsal, develop in each centrum, soon fusing to form a single ossification center. At about the eighth week an ossification center begins in each half of the vertebral arch. By the end of the embryonic period, three primary ossification centers are present in each vertebrae (one in the centrum and one in each half of the vertebral arch) (Fig. 1-5). The vertebral ring which encircles the rims of upper and lower surfaces of the vertebral body is an apophysis and does not contribute to growth.

Spinal Musculature

Each myotome separates into a smaller dorsal epaxial division and a larger ventral hypaxial division. Each spinal nerve divides, supplying a dorsal primary ramus to the epaxial division and a ventral primary ramus to the hypaxial division. Most myoblasts move away from the myotomes and form nonsegmented muscles, but some—like the intercostals—assume a segmental arrangement as seen with the somites. The myoblasts from the myotomes of the epaxial divisions give rise to the extensor neck muscles and the extensor muscles of the vertebral column. The sacral and coccygeal myo-

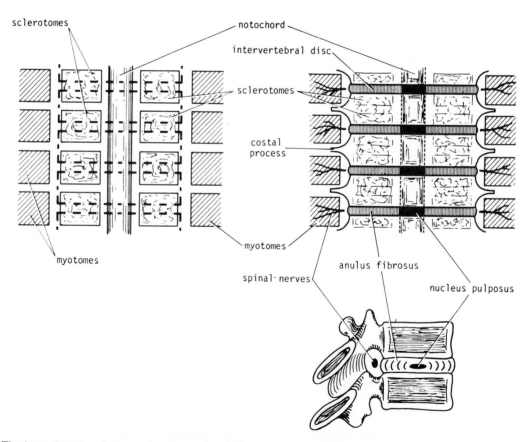

Figure 1-4 The formation of each mesenchymal vertebral body by the fusion of the caudal half of each sclerotome with the cephalic half of the immediately succeeding sclerotome. Each vertebral body, therefore, is an intersegmental structure. The costal processes grow out between adjacent myotomes. Also shown is the close relationship that exists between each spinal nerve and each intervertebral disc. *(From Snell, R.S.: in Clinical Embryology for Medical Students, 3d ed. Boston, Little, Brown, 1983. Reproduced with permission.)*

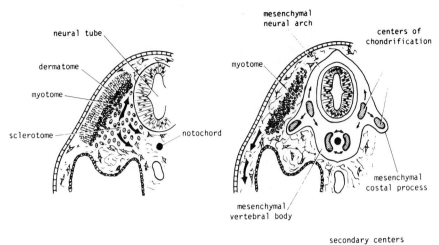

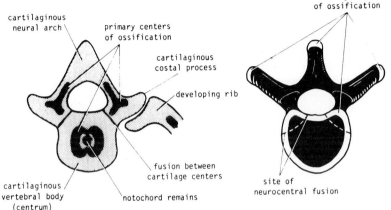

Figure 1-5 The stages in the formation of a thoracic vertebra. (*From Snell, R.S.: Clinical Embryology for Medical Students, 3d ed. Boston, Little, Brown, 1983. Reproduced with permission.*)

tomes degenerate; the dorsal sacrococcygeal ligaments are their derivatives.

The myoblasts from the myotomes of the hypaxial divisions give rise to the scalene, prevertebral, and hyoid muscles in the cervical region. In the thoracic region they form the lateral flexor muscles and in the lumbar region, the quadratus lumborum muscles.

LIMB DEVELOPMENT

The *limb bud* is a protrusion of the lateral nonsegmented body wall (somatopleure). This protrusion of somatic mesoderm occurs beneath a specialized layer of ectoderm that has important inductive influences on the developing limb mesenchyme. This ridge is known as the *apical ectodermal ridge (AER)*. The orderly pattern of limb development, from proximal to distal areas, in a defined temporal sequence requires the presence of the AER. The existence of a transmission factor necessary for the continuing activity of the AER and produced in turn by the limb mesoderm has been postulated. This apical ridge maintenance factor (ARMP) would appear to be a large molecule.[1,14] The limb mesoderm itself, however, contains inherently much of the responsibility of patterned

limb morphogenesis and may control regional specificity and distribution such as differentiation of limb appendages, whereas the AER may be primarily responsible for the anteroposterior orientation of such appendages.[1] The change from the paddlelike appendages to digital rays occurs by development of condensations in the hand plates by the end of the sixth week. It seems to occur by a process of "programmed cell death," which plays a significant role in limb bud shaping.[1] Sledge[14] has pointed out that this cell necrosis may occur by the release of lysosomal enzymes, and also notes that cortisone, which is capable of preventing the release of these enzymes, produces such embryological abnormalities as syndactyly. Rays also develop in the foot plates in the seventh week, and notches then form. The limb musculature develops in the mesenchyme to surround the bone elements.

In the seventh week the upper and lower limbs rotate into the positions found at birth. The upper limbs rotate 90 degrees laterally on the longitudinal axis. As a result, the elbows come to point posteriorly and the extensor muscles lie on the lateral and posterior aspects of the limb. The lower limbs rotate medially 90 degrees on the longitudinal axis. The knees come to face anteriorly, with the extensor muscles lying on the anterior aspect of the lower limbs.

Certain small areas of limb mesoderm can grow either a left hand or a right hand when transplanted into different positions of the developing limb bud of a host. Thus the areas from which such grafts have been taken have been called *zones of polarizing activity (ZPA).* It is thought that from these areas molecular material may diffuse over a distance of many cells controlling such events. A glycoprotein with a molecular weight in the region of 370,000 to 415,000 daltons, which has been found in this region may be implicated.[1] Much work remains to test the validity of these propositions and the relationship, if any, between the ZPA and the AER.

THE MUSCULAR SYSTEM

The myotomal mesoderm of the somites forms the striated skeletal muscle of the trunk. The mesenchyme in the limb buds develops into limb muscles. Limb muscle development is regulated by a fibronectin-containing matrix, along which myogenic cells migrate. The oriented fibronectin deposits are laid down by nonmyogenic cells as part of limb morphogenesis.[1] Produced in the mesenchyme, primitive cell myoblasts give rise to muscle tissue. The first myoblasts (myoblasts I) multiply and eventually fuse into myotubes, where contractile apparatus is produced. Myoblasts I fuse to form only small myotubes with four to six nuclei per cell. However, a myoblast II cell next appears which is capable of forming larger, multinucleated cells and is the isoformic replacement of the myoblast I cells. The motor axons are elaborated in the limb coincident with the appearance of the myoblast II population. These axons then sprout and innervate the entire length of the limb. At this time the last subgroup, the myoblast III, ap-

pears, whose arrival is nerve-dependent. If the neural phase is blocked by experimental manipulation, myoblast III does not appear. Both myoblast II and myoblast III form myotubes with 20 to 100 or more nuclei in each cell.

The development of the major muscle groups composed of muscle units with a complex contractile apparatus occurs when myoblast III units predominate (Fig. 1-6). The complexity of the interrelationship between muscle and nerve is shown by the fact that muscular branches fail to sprout from nerves invading limbs that despite their normal pattern of connective tissue are devoid of muscle fibers as a consequence of radiation.[1] Nevertheless, the pattern of tendon formation in the distal part of the limbs seems to be independent of the muscle development even when the muscle is ultimately destined to be attached to that tendon. The two seem to develop autonomously. It is interesting that the changes seen at the cellular level with these isoformic transformations during fetal development occur also at a molecular level. The myosin heavy chains seen in fetal muscle differ from those found in adult muscle, and there are also differences in the embryonic isoform of creatine kinase to the subsequently appearing muscle-specific form found in recognizable muscle cells.[1]

CARTILAGE DEVELOPMENT

Chondrogenesis is also preceded in the chick limb by a programmed pattern of fibronectin distribution, and collagen types 1 and 3 occur in the core mesenchyme. When chondro-

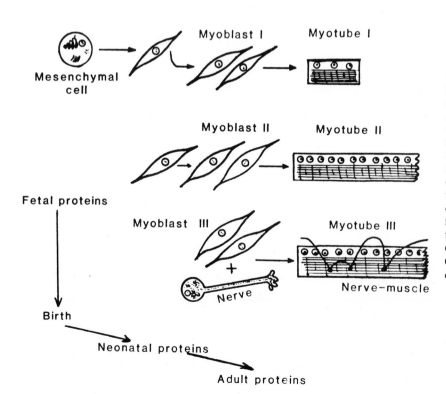

Figure 1-6 A schematic depiction of the isoformic transitions during muscle development. The first myoblasts (myoblast I) form only small myotubes (I). Myoblast II produced at a later stage forms large myotubes with many nuclei. Myoblast III arises in a nerve-dependent sequence of events in which numerous contacts are made between motor nerves and single muscle fibers but only one ultimately matures into the nerve muscle junction controlling that fiber. Similar isoformic transition of muscle-specific proteins occur with the appearance and replacement of fetal protein, then neonatal protein, and finally adult protein. *(From Caplan, A.I., et al, Science 221:922, 1983. Copyright 1983 by the A.A.A.S. Reproduced with permission.)*

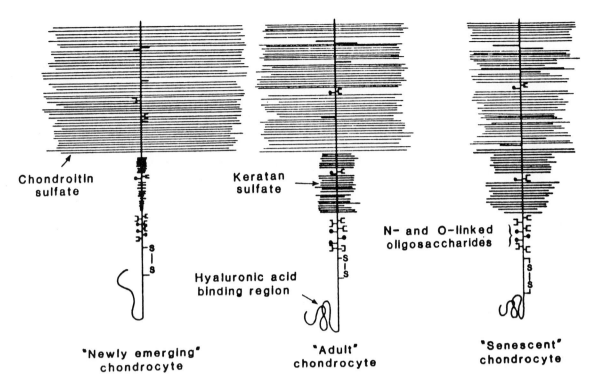

Chondroitin sulfate

Keratan sulfate

N- and O-linked oligosaccharides

Hyaluronic acid binding region

"Newly emerging" chondrocyte

"Adult" chondrocyte

"Senescent" chondrocyte

Figure 1-7 Schematic representation of the comparative structure of proteoglycans from cartilage during early development, maturity, and advanced age of chondrocytes. The chondroitin sulfate chains are larger since they are synthesized by young chondrocytes and are about one-half the size of those in senescent chondrocytes. The keratan sulfate chains are synthesized shorter in young chondrocytes, and longer in older cells. The ratio of chondroitin sulfate to keratan sulfate chain size is larger in younger cells, and this is another indicator of chondrocyte age. It is likely that these synthetic changes represent a natural developmental program which is programmed and irreversible. *(From Caplan, A.I., et al, Science 221:923. Copyright 1983 by A.A.A.S. Reproduced with permission.)*

blasts are formed, however, the fibronectin gradually disappears and type 2 collagen appears. Hyaluronic acid seems to be an important molecule involved in the process of cell condensation immediately preceding chondrogenesis.[1] There is thus a transformation of the extracellular environment, and it is significant that there is an increase in the hyaluronidase activity seen prior to transition of mesenchyme cells into the discrete phenotypes. As the isoforms change to type 2 collagen and cartilage-specific proteoglycan is produced, it may also be observed that the proteoglycan initially synthesized by the embryonic chondrocytes has larger chondroitin sulfate chains and smaller keratan sulfate chains than those synthesized by more adult cells (Fig. 1-7).

DEVELOPMENT OF BONE

In the limbs a cuff of perichondrially produced bone grows slowly by apposition and induces nutritional changes within the enclosed cartilaginous model. The cartilage becomes calcified; its constituent cells die. It is then invaded peripherally by vascular ingrowth and by osteoprogenitor cells which form bone within primary ossification centers. In most long bones, these changes occur in the diaphysis and spread toward the metaphyseal regions. Primary ossification centers are present in all bones of the limbs by the twelfth week. Most secondary centers of ossification develop after birth except the distal femur and proximal tibia which appear at the ninth month of intrauterine life and may be present at birth. The cartilaginous epiphysis at the articular ends of the bone continues to enlarge in a hemispheric fashion by interstitial growth. It remains separated from the primary ossification center in the diaphysis by the growth plate.

This endochondral process of ossification does not occur in the clavicle and the skull. In these bones the mesenchyme condenses and becomes vascular. Bone is produced without a cartilaginous intermediary stage by a process of intramembranous ossification beginning at the end of the embryonic period. In postnatal life, growth in these bones is by apposition until maturity since there is no proliferating layer of cartilage cells.

DEVELOPMENT OF JOINTS

Synovial joints form from interzonal mesenchyme between developing bones at around 6 weeks, upper limb joints devel-

TABLE 1-1 Causative Factors in Teratogenesis and the Most Susceptible Period, Measured in Weeks, for Their Actions

Teratogenic factors	Oogenesis and spermatogenesis		Embryo 0 1 5 F* I*	Fetus		Neonate	
	−8	−4		10 20 30		40 Birth	Lactation
Drugs	Hormones LSD	Phenytoin Thalidomide Methadone Estrogen	Hormones Contraceptives Abortifacients	Methylmercury Diethylstibestrol Thalidomide Phenytoin Trimethadione Alcohol Warfarin Aminopterin Estrogen Androgen Progestin Aminoglutethimide	Tetracyclines Quinine Chloroquine Goitrogens Thiouracil Teridax Salicylates Heavy metals Antibiotics Smoking	IV fluid Pitressin Salicylates Vitamin K Naphthalene Ganglionic blockers Reserpine Morphine Sedative analgesics Ammonium Cardiovascular drugs	Diazepam Lithium Mexachlorobenzene Methylmercury Sulfonamides Atropine Anticoagulants Antithyroids Antimetabolites Cathartics Dihydrotachysterol Iodides Tetracyclines Metronidazole
Microorganisms				Rubella Toxoplasmosis Varicella Syphilis Cytomegalovirus Herpes Herpes	Toxoplasmosis Varicella Syphilis Cytomegalovirus		Herpes Cytomegalovirus Varicella
Radiation	Chromosomal damage Death	Death Abortion Malformation Prematurity	Prematurity Abortion	Prematurity Abortion Death Malformation	Prematurity Abortion Organ damage Fetal morbidity	Neonatal morbidity	Infant morbidity
Maternal factors	Age Season Metabolism Emotions		Neural and endocrine states	Nutrition Maternal disease Crowding Social class Geography Season	Maternal disease		Maternal disease

*F = fertilization; I = implantation
Source: Modified from Goldman, A.S., in Schwartz, R.H., and Yaffee, S.J., eds: *Drugs and Chemical Risks to the Fetus and Newborn.* New York, Liss, 1980. Reprinted with permission.

oping a little earlier than those of the lower limb. The interzone region consists of a central loose layer of randomly arranged cells lying between two denser zones in which the cells are aligned parallel to the surface of the subjacent proliferating epiphyseal region.[14] Cavitation occurs in the central area as cells disappear under the action of mechanical stimu-

lation of joint movement and vascular invasion. Enzymatic factors may also be involved.[14] The denser zones form the articular cartilage caps of the articulating bones. Joint movement seems to be critical for the process, and immobility may have teratological significance in congenital deformity. Synovial membrane is formed from mesenchyme lining the primitive joint cavity. Capsule and ligaments arise separately from areas peripheral to the interzonal mesenchyme from adjacent cells. The interzone region may also form fibrocartilage (e.g., the symphysis pubis) or fibrous connective tissue (e.g., the skull sutures) when local morphogenesis require it.

TERATOLOGICAL IMPLICATIONS

It has already been mentioned that prior to gastrulation, cells may be relatively immune to teratogenesis since little tissue differentiation or specific morphogenesis has already occurred. Probably the most important factor that would determine the specific deleterious effects of a toxin is the *time* during development at which exposure to the toxin occurs (Table 1-1). Prior to gastrulation, although teratogenesis is unlikely, severe fetal damage and embryo death would be the probable outcome.

Fuller and Duthie have related the pathophysiology of certain common congenital anomalies with probable timetables for their development in embryo.[5] They point out (Fig. 1-8) that skeletal limb deficiencies occur between the fourth and the sixth week because of the predictability and consistency with which limb differentiation occurs. Since the upper limbs develop a few days ahead of the lower limbs, major upper limb deficiencies occur at about the twenty-eigth day and those of the lower limb at about the thirty-first day. For deficiencies affecting the distal end of the limbs, the timetable is a few days later. They also point out that the primary defect causing spina bifida occurs between the third and the fourth week which is the period of normal closure of the neural tube.

These authors have also indicated at what point during development such common congenital abnormalities as dislocation of the hip (Fig. 1-9), talipes equinovarus, and arthrogryposis multiplex congenita may develop, citing for each the chronological implications of the varying theories of the etiologies of these conditions. These chronologies are valuable in allowing experimental verification of new theories concerning teratogenesis and normal morphogenesis.

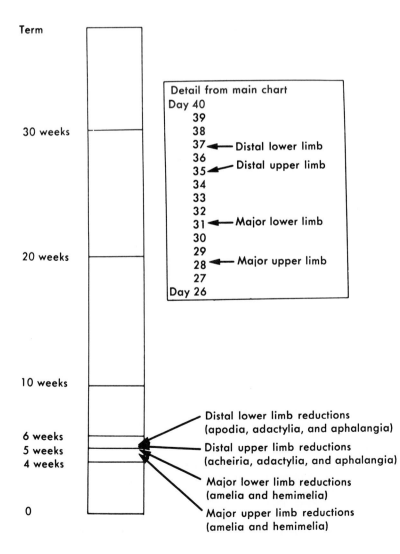

Figure 1-8 A timetable for development of congenital skeletal limb deficiencies. *(From Fuller, D., and Duthie, R., Instr Course Lect 23:53–61, 1974. Reproduced with permission.)*

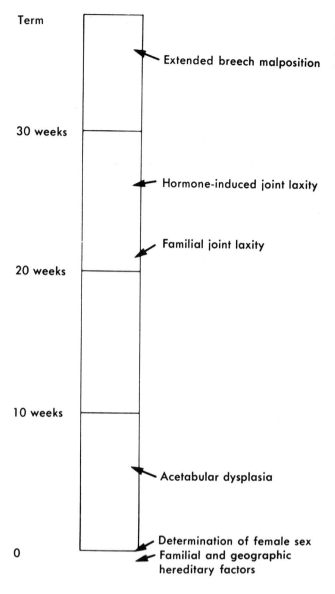

Figure 1-9 A chronology for development of congenital hip dislocation with major etiological factors. *(From Fuller, D., and Duthie, R., Instr Course Lect 23:53–61, 1974. Reproduced with permission.)*

REFERENCES

1. Amprino, R. The development of the vertebrate limb. Clin Orthop 188:263–284, 1984.
2. Austin, C.R., and Short, R.V. *Embryonic and Fetal Development,* book 2. Cambridge, University Press, 1972.
3. Caplan, A.I., Fiszman, M.Y., and Eppenberger, H.M. Molecular and cell isoforms during development. Science 221:921–927, September 2, 1983.
4. Crowley, L.V. *An Introduction to Clinical Embryology.* Chicago, Year Book Publishers, 1974.
5. Fuller, D.J., and Duthie, R.B. "The lined appearance of some congenital malformations and orthopaedic abnormalities," A.A.O.S. Instructional Course Lecture, 23:53–61, 1974.
6. Gasser, R. *Atlas of Human Embryos.* Hagerstown, Harper and Row, 1975.
7. Goldman, A.S. Critical periods of prenatal toxic insults, *Progress in Clinical and Biological Research,* vol 36. New York, Alan R. Liss, 1980, pp 9–31.
8. Gregg, N.M. Congenital cataract following german measles in the mother. Trans Ophthalmol Soc Aust 3:35, 1941.

9. Langman, J. *Medical Embryology.* Baltimore Williams and Wilkins, 1981.
10. Moore, K.L. *The Developing Human.* Philadelphia, Saunders, 1982.
11. O'Rahilly, R. *Developmental Stages in Human Embryos,* Part A: *Embryos of the first three weeks.* Washington, D.C., Carnegie Institution of Washington, 1973.
12. Rana, M.W. *Key Facts in Embryology.* New York, Churchill Livingstone, 1984.
13. Schwarz, R.H., and Yaffe, S.J. Drug and Chemical Risks to the Fetus and Newborn, *Progress in Clinical and Biological Research,* vol 36. New York, Alan R. Liss, 1980.
14. Sledge, C. B. Developmental anatomy of joints, in Resnick, D., and Niwaijama, G. (eds): *Diagnosis of Bone and Joint Disorders,* vol. 1. Philadelphia, Saunders, 1981, pp 2–20.
15. Streeter, G.L. Developmental horizons in human embryos. Contrib Embryol, Carnegie Institute 30:211, 1942.
16. Tuchmann-Duplessis, H. *Drug Effects on the Fetus.* Sydney, ADIS Press, 1975.
17. Widdowson, E.M. Nutrition, in Davis, J.A., and Dobbing, J. (eds): *Scientific Foundations of Paediatrics.* Philadelphia, Saunders, 1974, pp. 44–55.

CHAPTER 2

Connective Tissue: Structure and Function

Cahir A. McDevitt and Marianne R. Jahnke

The major macromolecules of connective tissues may be assigned to one of four broad families: (1) collagens;[6,22,26] (2) proteoglycans;[11,18,21] (3) noncollagenous nonproteoglycan glycoproteins;[27] and (4) elastin.[14] Cells can manufacture connective tissues which differ considerably in their material properties by varying the relative proportion of these four families and the relative proportion of the individual members within each family. The gellike nucleus pulposus or hard skeletal tissues, such as bone or cartilage, may result. Elastin is a trace constituent of cartilage and bone and will not be discussed here.

COLLAGEN

Collagen is a protein that contains a triple helix of three peptide chains (α chains), the amino acid sequence of which is the repeating tripeptide Gly-X-Y, where X is often proline and Y is often hydroxyproline.[1,6,22,26] The position of glycine at every third residue is a prerequisite for helix formation because glycine is the only amino acid small enough to fit into the interior of the helix. In contrast, the bulky amino acids proline and hydroxyproline are located on the exterior of the helix. The triple helix is stabilized by hydrogen bonding involving the hydroxyl groups of hydroxyproline.

Genetic Types of Collagen

The term collagen now represents a family of structurally similar proteins that are the products of different genes. In vertebrates there are at least 10 genetically distinct collagens, for which a minimum of 18 genes probably exist to code for their chains.[1,2,3,22,23,24] The different types of collagen have been assigned Roman numerals (e.g., type I, type II, etc.), and they differ in their amino acid sequence, in the length of their alpha chains, and in the presence or absence of globular domains in the molecule (Table 2-1). Type I collagen is by far

TABLE 2-1 Major Collagen Subtypes Found in Articular Cartilage and Other Connective Tissue Structures

Type	α Chains	Native Polymer	Distribution
Interstitial			
I	$[\alpha1(I)]_2\ \alpha2$	Fibril	Skin, tendon, bone, meniscus, annulus
II	$[\alpha1(II)]_3$	Fibril	Hyaline cartilage, nucleus pulposus, vitreous body
III	$[\alpha1(III)]_3$	Fibril	Skin, blood vessels, granulation tissue, reticulin fibers
Pericellular and basement membrane			
IV	$[\alpha1(IV)]_2$	Basement lamina	Kidney glomeruli, lens capsule
V	$\alpha A(\alpha B)_2$ $(\alpha A)_3$ $(\alpha B)_3$	Unknown	Cell surface, pericellular matrix

Source: From Buckwalter, J.A., in Evarts, C.M., ed, Instr Course Lect 32:349–369, 1983. Reproduced with permission.

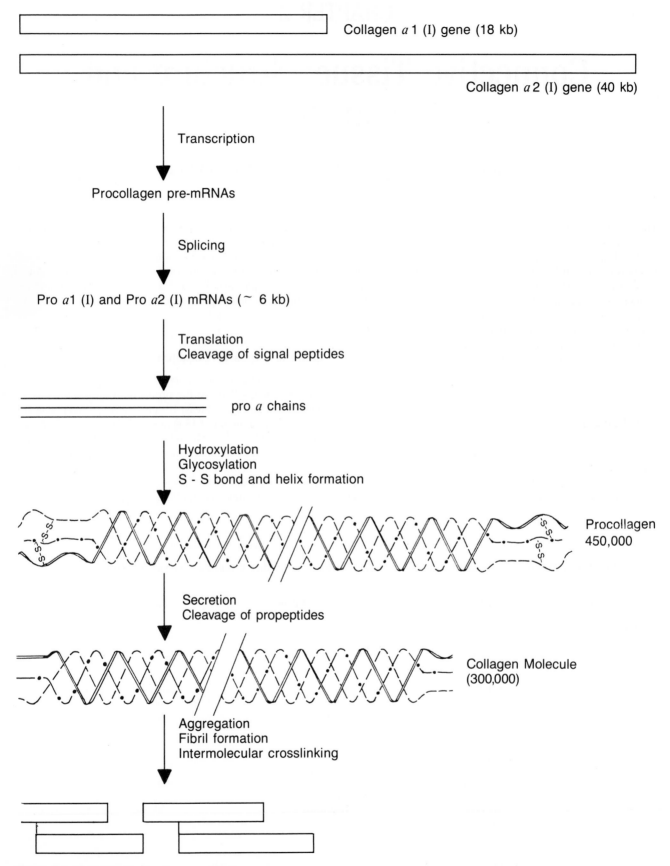

Figure 2-1 Biosynthesis of collagen molecule.

the most abundant type of collagen in vertebrates and is often considered the prototype of the others. It consists of two $\alpha1$ chains that are identical and an $\alpha2$ chain (Fig. 2-1). The molecular weight of each chain is about 100,000, and that of the composite three-chained molecule is about 300,000. About 95 percent of the molecule is in the form of a triple helix. Nonhelical peptide extensions (sometimes referred to as *telopeptides*) are located at both the N- and C-terminal ends of the molecule. The nonhelical extensions are important because they contain a lysine residue that participates in cross-linking. A striking feature of the triple helical domain of the collagen molecule is its relative resistance to enzymatic attack.

Type I is the major type of collagen in fibrous tissues[2,22,26] such as dermis, tendon, and the fibrous cartilage of the menisci in the knee joint.[4,6] It is the major collagen synthesized by fibroblasts.

Type II collagen is the major type contained in cartilage[5] and nucleus pulposus.[8] The type II collagen molecule is composed of three identical α chains (II). These chains have relatively high contents of hydroxylysine and carbohydrate. The carbohydrate consists of a galactose residue or a glucose-galactose disaccharide attached to the hydroxyl group of hydroxylysine.

Type III collagen usually coexists with type I, with the notable exception of bone where type III is absent. This type of collagen is present in significant amounts (35 to 45 percent) in the more distensible tissues such as the intestine, large blood vessels, and uterine wall.[22] The proportion of this type of collagen is generally higher in fetal tissues. Type III consists of three identical chains. It differs from types I and II in retaining a procollagen extension peptide with disulfide bonds when it is laid down in the extracellular space. This type of collagen gives rise to particularly thin fibrils.

Types I, II, and III are sometimes referred to as the interstitial collagens, as they are found in fibrillar form in the extracellular matrices. Other types of collagen, however, are associated with basement membranes, the specialized connective tissue lamina that underlie epithelia and endothelia. The best-characterized of the basement membrane collagens is type IV.

There are a number of minor collagens that normally coexist with the major types. In articular cartilage the minor

types so far identified include V and IX. Type V is found pericellularly, while type IX is probably distributed with type II in the extracellular space. Type IX has globular regions that are interspaced between the helical domains.[3]

Synthesis of the Collagen Molecule

A notable feature of the genes coding for the α chains of type I collagen is their enormous size: each gene is about ten times the size of the functional mRNA (Fig. 2-1). The gene coding for the $\alpha2(I)$ chains of type I collagen has 40 kilobases and contains 52 exons or coding regions that are separated from each other by large introns (intervening sequences) that range in size from 80 to 2000 kilobases. The RNAs are spliced after transcription to generate the specific mRNAs for each chain. These mRNA chains are translocated to the cytoplasm where translation occurs in the rough endoplasmic reticulum on membrane-bound polysomes.[3,26]

The α chains are synthesized in the form of larger precursors called pro α chains with extra procollagen extension peptides at both the N- and C-terminal residues. These chains then undergo an extensive array of posttranslational modifications before they are incorporated into the fully mature collagen fiber in the extracellular matrix. The enzymes prolyl and lysyl hydroxylase hydroxylate appropriate residues to hydroxyproline and hydroxylysine, respectively. Ascorbic acid is an essential cofactor for these enzymes. Glycosylation of specific hydroxylysine residues then occurs. Interchain disulfide bond formation occurs at the carboxy C terminal. The three pro α chains intertwine around one another to form the procollagen molecule. This is extruded into the extracellular space where N- and C-terminal peptidases cleave off the procollagen extension peptides. The collagen molecules thus generated can then assemble by aligning themselves laterally and longitudinally into a microfibril. The collagen molecule has all the information in its primary sequence for this assembly.

Genetic diseases due to a defective collagen molecule arise through deletions, additions, or substitutions of its

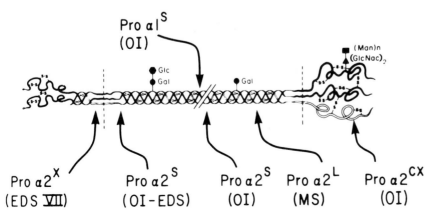

Figure 2-2 Approximate locations of molecular defects in the collagen molecule in Ehlers-Danlos (ED) and Marfans (MS) syndromes and in osteogenesis imperfecta (OI). *(From Prokop and Kivirikko, N Engl J Med 311:376–386, 1984. Reproduced with permission.)*

amino acids.[28] Figure 2-2 shows the approximate locations of the mutations responsible for some of the important diseases.

Cross-Linking of Collagen

The fibrils formed by spontaneous association of the individual collagen molecules have little or no tensile strength. Covalent cross-links are essential for the formation of the normal mature collagen fibril with its characteristic tensile properties. The detailed steps in the generation of the cross-links have been reviewed.[26] The process is initiated by the enzyme lysyl oxidase that oxidatively deaminates selective lysine residues on the collagen molecule with the formation of an aldehyde. Aldehydes are very reactive and will react spontaneously with free amino groups. The aldehyde generated by the lysyl oxidase reacts with neighboring amino groups on the triple helical portion or telopeptide of a neighboring collagen molecule to form a Schiff base (i.e., an N=C bond). These Schiff bases will then undergo a series of spontaneous chemical reactions to form temporary cross-links that are referred to as the reducible cross-links because they can be chemically reduced. These reducible cross-links will, in time, form chemically stable ("mature") cross-links. Stable cross-links composed of a pyridinium ring (i.e., a ring composed of five carbons and one nitrogen) have been identified. These pyridinium rings absorb light at about 330 nanometers (nm) and emit it as fluorescent light in the light blue region of the spectrum, at 400 nm. They are thus responsible for at least some of the autofluoresence of connective tissues.

PROTEOGLYCANS

A *proteoglycan* is a protein or peptide to which one or more chains of a specialized carbohydrate, termed glycosaminogly-

can (GAG), are attached.[21] The older term for a glycosaminoglycan was "mucopolysaccharide." A glycosaminoglycan is a highly negatively charged polysaccharide chain composed of a repeating disaccharide group. One sugar in the repeating disaccharide is an amino sugar, either galactosamine or glucosamine. These amino sugars are nearly always sulfated, the sole exception being the *N*-acetylglucosamine in hyaluronic acid. The other sugar in the repeating disaccharide is usually a uronic acid, which is a sugar residue containing a carboxyl group.

The distinctive feature of a glycosaminoglycan is its highly charged nature, with each sugar unit usually bearing a negative charge. These negative charges associate with positively charged sodium ions. The sodium counterions, in turn, will themselves envelop shells of water molecules because of the Donnan effect. Thus, the proteoglycan is a highly hydrophilic molecule with the capacity to entrain many times its weight of water. In articular cartilage, however, the molecule is somewhat underhydrated because the tensile strength of the collagen fibrils resists further inbibition of water by the proteoglycans.[15,16,17]

Structure

Figure 2-3 depicts the widely accepted model for the structure of the major type of proteoglycan found in hyaline cartilage.[21] It consists in part of an extended polypeptide (the protein core) that has little helical structure. One end of the protein core bears a globular region that is stabilized by disulfide bonds. The major portion of the protein core is richly substituted with chondroitin sulfate chains. There are about 100 of these chains per molecule, and the region is referred to as the chondroitin sulfate–rich region of the proteoglycan. Adjacent to this region is the keratan sulfate–rich region.

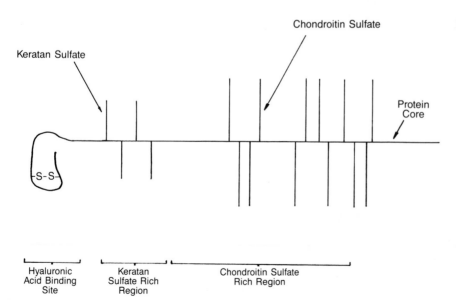

Figure 2-3 Proteoglycan molecule.

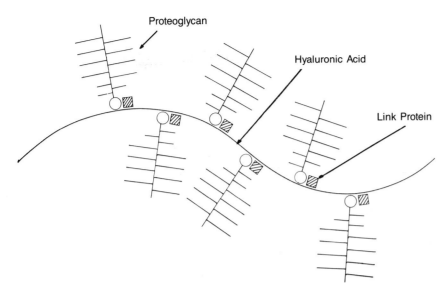

Figure 2-4 Proteoglycan aggregate.

Here is where the majority of keratan sulfate chains are located.

Proteoglycan Aggregation

The globular region next to the keratan sulfate–enriched region is referred to as the hyaluronic acid binding site. This binding site associates noncovalently, but very specifically, with chains of hyaluronic acid.[8,9,10,11] Many individual proteoglycan molecules can associate with a single hyaluronic acid chain to form a proteoglycan aggregate.[11] Figure 2-4 depicts such an aggregate. A family of moderately sized proteins, the link proteins, bind to both the hyaluronic acid chain and to the proteoglycan. The link protein serves to stabilize the interaction between hyaluronic acid and proteoglycan and to protect the binding site against enzymatic attack. Proteoglycan aggregation is thought to help entrap the proteoglycan molecules within the collagenous meshwork.

GLYCOPROTEINS

That cartilage and other connective tissues contain proteins other than the collagens, proteoglycans, and elastin has been known for some time. These proteins are mostly if not entirely glycoproteins and have been variously referred to as matrix glycoproteins, noncollagenous glycoproteins, etc. Their molecular forms and functions are largely unknown and are now the focus of active research.[27] Of particular interest is that subclass of matrix glycoproteins whose members participate in the attachment of cells to their extracellular matrices.[12,13,29]

Fibronectin

The most extensively studied of the cell attachment proteins is fibronectin (from the Latin: *fibra,* fiber, *nectere,* to blind).[13,29] This is the protein that mediates attachment of fibroblasts, as well as many other cells, to their type I and type III collagenous matrices. The molecular form of the fibronectin consists of two elongated protein subunits linked at one end by a disulfide bond. The structure of each subunit resembles that of a string of beads, with each bead representing a globular structure in which one or more binding sites are located for specific ligands. Domains exist for attachment to collagen, cell surface molecules, and heparin. A striking feature of fibronectin is that it is present in serum as a circulating soluble protein and in tissues as an insoluble extracellular matrix constituent. Because of its many domains that enable it to attach to a variety of different molecules and structures, fibronectin participates in a variety of biological processes other than cell attachment. These processes include coagulation and chemotaxis; they also serve as an opsonin for macrophages.

Chondronectin

Normal, fully differentiated chondrocytes may employ another protein, chondronectin, as their major attachment protein.[12] Chondronectin, in contrast to fibronectin, binds more strongly to type II collagen and cartilage proteoglycans.

FUNCTIONAL ADAPTATION IN CONNECTIVE TISSUE

The composition of articular cartilage varies with development and maturation. The articular cartilage of skeletally mature individuals is about 85 percent water. The residual dry weight is about 50 percent collagen, 45 percent proteoglycan, and 10 percent protein, with trace amounts of elastin and phospholipid.[19]

Articular Cartilage

The proteoglycan aggregates that occupy the spaces between the type II and (probably) type IX collagenous fibers in articular cartilage are somewhat collapsed and slighty underhydrated. The tensile strength of the collagenous fibers resists any further imbibition of water that would enlarge the spatial domains occupied by the proteoglycans. When load is applied to the cartilage, as in articulation of the joint, water is expressed into the synovial fluid. The proteoglycans, however, are retained within the collagenous network, presumably because of their enormous size as aggregates. The proteoglycans are now greatly underhydrated. On the removal of the load, water is reimbibed into the cartilage until the original shape of the tissue is regained.[15,16,17]

ARTICULAR CARTILAGE MACROMOLECULES AND OSTEOARTHRITIS

Osteoarthritis is characterized by a loss of articular cartilage from focal sites and by osteophyte formation at the articular margins.[30] Innovative work from Henry Mankin's group established that the chondrocytes in cartilage respond aggressively in osteoarthritis by increased synthesis of matrix components.[18] The development of animal models for osteoarthritis, notably from the research groups of Howell, Mankin, McDevitt, and Moskowitz, respectively, permitted a systematic approach to the study of disease processes.[18,24,25] McDevitt and co-workers established that an enhanced hydration and a disorganized collagen matrix were very early events in osteoarthritis.[19,20] An apparent consequence of the defective collagen meshwork is that the proteoglycan aggregates are less firmly entrapped within the matrix.[20] There is now almost universal agreement that the chondrocytes respond to the insult initiating the osteoarthritic process with an increased synthesis of collagen and proteoglycans.[7,18,19,20] These proteoglycans are similar in structure to those of immature tissues.[18,21] The newly synthesized collagen, at least in the very early phases of the disease, is type II.[7] With increasing severity in the disease, proteoglycan is progressively lost from the matrix and eventually the mechanical loss of cartilage is such that the underlying bone is exposed. The detailed molecular events in the degradative and repair processes in osteoarthritis are now the focus of much research.[18,21,25] There is also increased interest in the employment of biochemical markers in serum for diagnosis, management, and subclassification of the different types of osteoarthritis.

REFERENCES

1. Bornstein, P., and Traub, W. The chemistry and biology of collagen, in *The Proteins,* vol. 4. New York, Academic Press, 1979, pp. 411–605.
2. Bornstein, P., and Sage, H. Structurally distinct collagen types. Ann Rev Biochem 49:957–1003, 1980.
3. Cheah, K.S.E. Collagen, genes and inherited connective tissue disease. Biochem J 229:287–303, 1985.
4. Eyre, D.R., and Muir, H. The distribution of different molecular species of collagen in fibrous, elastic and hyaline cartilages of the pig. Biochem J 151:595–602, 1975.
5. Eyre, D.R., and Muir, H. Types I and II collagen in intervertebral disc: Interchanging radial distributions in annulus fibrosus. Biochem J 157:267–270, 1977.
6. Eyre, D.R.: Collagen: Molecular diversity in the body's protein scaffold. *Science* 207:1315–1322, 1980.
7. Eyre, D.R., McDevitt, C.A., Billingham, M.E.J., and Muir, H. Biosynthesis of collagen and other matrix proteins by articular cartilage in experimental osteoarthritis. Biochem J 188:823–837, 1980.
8. Hardingham, T.E., and Muir, H. The specific interaction of hyaluronic acid with cartilage proteoglycans. Biochem Biophys Acta 279:401–405, 1972.
9. Hardingham, T.E., and Muir, H. Hyaluronic acid in cartilage and proteoglycan aggregation. Biochem J 139:565–591, 1975.
10. Hascall, V.C., and Heingard, D. Aggregation of cartilage proteoglycans. I. The role of hyaluronic acid. J Biol Chem 249:4232–4241, 1974.
11. Hascall, V.C. Interaction of cartilage proteoglycans with hyaluronic acid. J Supramol Struct 7:101–120, 1977.
12. Hewitt, A.T., Varner, H.H., Silver, M.H., Dessau, W., Wilkes, C.M., and Martin, G.: The isolation and partial characterization of chondronectin, an attachment factor for chondrocytes. J Biol Chem 257:2330–2334, 1982.
13. Hynes, R.O.: Fibronectin and its relation to cellular structure and behavior, in Hay, E.D. (ed): *Cell Biology of Extracellular Matrix.* New York, Plenum, 1981, pp 295–334.
14. Keith, D.A., Paz, M.A., Gallop, P.M., and Glimcher, M.J.: Histologic and biochemical identification and characterization of an elastin in cartilage. J Histochem Cytochem 25:1154–1162, 1977.
15. Kempson, G.E., Muir, H., Swanson, S.A.V., and Freeman, M.A.R. Correlations between stiffness and the chemical constituents of cartilage on the human femoral head. Biochem Biophys Acta 215:70–77, 1970.
16. Kempson, G.E.: Mechanical properties of articular cartilage, in Freeman, M.A.R. (ed): *Adult Articular Cartilage,* London, Pitman Medical Publishing, 1979, pp 333–414.
17. Kempson, G.E.: The mechanical properties of articular cartilage, in Sokoloff, L. (ed): *The Joints and Synovial Fluid,* vol 2. New York, Academic Press, 1980, pp 177–238.
18. Mankin, H.J., and Brandt, K.D. Biochemistry and metabolism of cartilage in osteoarthritis, in Moskowitz, R.W., Howell, D.S., Goldbert, V.M., and Mankin, H.J. (eds): *Osteoarthritis: Diagnosis and Management.* Philadelphia, Saunders 1984, pp. 43–79.
19. McDevitt, C.A. Biochemistry of articular cartilage: Nature of proteoglycans and collagen in aging and osteoarthrosis. Ann Rheum Dis 32:364–378, 1973.
20. McDevitt, C.A., Gilbertson, E., and Muir, H. An experimental model of osteoarthritis: Early morphological biochemical changes. J Bone Joint Surg 59B:24–35, 1977.
21. McDevitt, C.A.: The proteoglycans of cartilage and the intervertebral disc in aging and osteoarthritis, in Glynn, L.E. (ed): *Handbook of Inflammation,* vol. 3: *Tissue Repair and Regeneration.* New York, Elsevier/North-Holland Biomedical Press, 1981, pp. 111–143.
22. Miller, E.J.: The collagens of joints, in Sokoloff, L. (ed): *The Joints and Synovial Fluids,* vol 1. Academic Press, New York, 1978, pp. 205–242.
23. Miller, E.J., and Gay, S. Collagen—An overview. Methods Enzymol 82:3–32, 1982.
24. Moskowitz, R.W. Experimental models of degenerative disease. Semin Arthritis Rheum 1:95–116, 1972.
25. Moskowitz, R.W. Experimental models of osteoarthritis, in Moskowitz, R.W., Howell, D.S., Goldberg, V.M., Mankin, H.J. (eds): *Oste-*

oarthritis Diagnosis and Management. Philadelphia, Saunders, 1984, pp 109–129.

26. Nimni, M.E. Collagen: Structure, function and metabolism in normal and fibrotic tissues. Semin Arthritis Rheum 13:1–86, 1983.

27. Paulsson, M., and Heinegard, D. Non-collagenous cartilage proteins: Current status of an emerging research field. Coll Relat Res 4:219–229, 1984.

28. Prokop, D.J., and Kivirikko, K.I. Inheritable diseases of collagen. N Engl J Med 311:376–386, 1984.

29. Ruoslahti, E., Engvall, E., and Hayman, E.G. Fibronectin: Current concepts of its structure and functions. Coll Relat Res 1:95–128, 1981.

30. Sokoloff, L. *The Biology of Degenerative Joint Disease.* Chicago, University of Chicago Press, 1969.

CHAPTER 3

Genetic Disorders

Henry R. Cowell

The science of genetics deals with the inheritance patterns of both normal and abnormal genes. The behavior of these genes alone, or in combination, and the manner in which they are modified by the environment will determine whether an individual will have the symptoms of a particular disease. Since genes act in defined patterns, this allows the possibility of predicting the chance of a particular individual having a specific disease. There are three different categories of patterns of inheritance, and although the rules that govern each category are similar, the result in each category may appear to be different. Mendelian disorders involve a single gene, whereas chromosomal abnormalities involve a portion of a chromosome containing many genes and multifactorial conditions involve the actions of several genes in combination with environmental factors.

Abnormalities of genes and chromosomes are inherited, but an individual who is affected with a particular condition may not have inherited it. When an individual has a known Mendelian condition and his or her parents neither have the condition nor carry the abnormal gene, the individual has developed the condition on a sporadic basis as a result of a new mutation. Once affected, the individual has the potential of passing the abnormal gene to one-half of all offspring. Similarly, an individual may have a chromosomal abnormality on the basis of nondysjunction of a pair of chromosomes. Although this event occurred in the sperm or the egg, the parents were normal. This error of cell division results in an inheritable condition.

Conditions that are inherited are not necessarily detectable at birth. For example, an individual may carry the abnormal gene for pseudohypertrophic muscular dystrophy at birth, but the condition may not be recognized until the patient is 3 years of age or older. Similarly, conditions that are present at birth, and therefore congenital, need not be inherited. Phocomelia is an example of this type of condition.

Orthopaedists should be aware of the many conditions they treat that are inherited since genetic counseling is indicated for these conditions. Although few orthopaedists will wish to offer genetic counseling, all should have a sufficient basic knowledge of genetics to recognize when counseling is indicated. In addition, the orthopaedist should be aware of the importance of making an accurate diagnosis when these inherited conditions are encountered as many orthopaedic conditions demonstrate heterogeneity, that is, a similar clinical condition may be seen in many syndromes. For example, clubfoot may be seen as part of many different syndromes such as arthrogryposis, diastrophic dwarfism, whistling face syndrome, and chromosomal abnormalities, or it may be an idiopathic condition.[5] The pattern of inheritance is different in each instance, and the counselor must be aware of this in order to give accurate information to the patient and family.

MENDELIAN DISORDERS

The basic unit of inheritance is the single gene. A number of genes joined together constitutes a chromosome. Humans have 46 chromosomes, which are divided into 22 pairs of autosomes and two chromosomes that determine the sex of the individual. A female has two X chromosomes, and a male has one X and one Y chromosome. Each pair of autosomes consists of a similar string of genes. Those genes at the same locus on each of a pair of chromosomes are known as *alleles.* If the Mendelian disorder is caused by inheritance of a single abnormal gene, the condition is said to be *dominant.* If both genes of the pair must be abnormal in order for the condition to be expressed, the disorder is referred to as a *recessive* condition. If the abnormal gene is located on one of the 22 pairs of autosomes, the condition is said to be *autosomal,* and if the

TABLE 3-1 Inherited Autosomal and X-linked Conditions

Autosomal		X-Linked	
Dominant	**Recessive**	**Dominant**	**Recessive**
Achondroplasia	Alkaptonuria	Pseudopseudohypoparathyroidism	Hemophilia
Brachydactyly	Cartilage hair hypoplasia	Vitamin D refractory rickets	Hunter syndrome
Calcaneonavicular coalition	Congenital insensitivity to pain		
Cleidocranial dysotosis	Diastrophic dwarfism		
Marfan disease	Gaucher disease		
Multiple epiphyseal dysplasia	Hurler syndrome		
Nail patellar syndrome	Hypophosphatasia		
Neurofibromatosis	Maroteaux-Lamy syndrome		
Polydactyly	Morquio syndrome		
Syndactyly	Phenylketonuria		
Triphalangeal thumb	Sanfilippo syndrome		
	Scheie syndrome		
	Smith-Lemli-Opitz syndrome		

Source: Adapted from McKusick, V.A.: *Mendelian Inheritance in Man,* 6th ed. Baltimore, Johns Hopkins, 1983.

gene is located on the X chromosome, the condition is said to be *X-linked,* or *sex-linked.*

Autosomal Dominant Conditions

Many orthopaedic conditions are inherited in an autosomal dominant fashion (Table 3-1). These conditions are determined by the abnormality of a single gene which is passed in the sperm or egg from one generation to the next. An individual who has such a condition has a fifty-fifty chance of passing this condition on to offspring. Since this is a random occurrence, the fifty-fifty chance applies to each offspring. The abnormal gene need be present on only one chromosome of the pair for an individual to have the condition. However, should an individual get a double dose of an abnormal gene by inheriting the abnormal gene from both parents, the condition may be more severe than it would have been in the presence of a single abnormal gene. Such increased severity may be seen in achondroplasia, for example.

When a normal child is produced by a parent who has a dominant disorder, the child may have failed to inherit the abnormal gene, has a normal genotype, and therefore cannot pass the abnormal gene on to an offspring.

Incomplete penetrance refers to the phenomenon of a normal-appearing individual carrying an abnormal gene. If this possibility is not considered, the counselor may not give accurate information to the patient. Some conditions, such as achondroplasia, are essentially completely penetrant, whereas other conditions such as polydactyly and syndactyly are not fully penetrant. Such incomplete penetrance gives rise to the phenomenon of "skipped generations."

Variable expressivity may be seen in these conditions. This term is applied to connote the different effect of the same gene in different individuals (Fig. 3-1). Thus, all individuals with Marfan syndrome have the same abnormal gene, but

this gene may give cardiac abnormalities in one individual, ocular changes in another, and scoliosis in a third.

Autosomal Recessive Conditions

In autosomal recessive conditions the same abnormal gene must be present on both chromosomes of a pair in order for the condition to be expressed. Thus, although both parents carry the same abnormal gene, they do not express the condition because the other allele of the abnormal gene that the parents are carrying is normal. These parents have one chance in four of producing a genotypically normal child, two chances in four of producing a normal-appearing child who carries an abnormal gene (as they do), and one chance in four of producing an affected individual. Several children in one generation may be affected, but both their parents and their children, if they have any, will be normal-appearing carriers of the abnormal gene. Even though affected siblings have the same two abnormal genes from their parents, they may have a variation in the severity of the condition. Orthopaedic conditions inherited in this fashion include cartilage hair hypoplasia, diastrophic dwarfism, and hypophosphatasia (Table 3-1).

X-Linked Dominant Conditions

The characteristics of this mode of inheritance depend on the fact that the gene is carried on the X chromosome. As the female carries two X chromosomes, affected mothers have the chance of having one-half of their sons and one-half of their daughters affected and the other half normal. Because the male carries one X and one Y chromosome, affected fathers must pass their X chromosome to a daughter (who is therefore affected) and their Y chromosome to a son (who is therefore not affected). In both situations it is assumed that

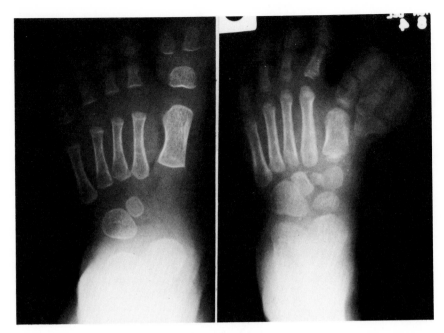

Figure 3-1 Variable expressivity is seen in many autosomal dominant conditions. **A.** This patient with polydactyly of the great toes demonstrates variable expressivity on the two sides of his body. The left foot (shown here) has duplication of the distal phalanx and enlargement of the proximal phalanx, whereas the right foot (not shown) has duplication of both the proximal and distal phalanges. **B.** A cousin demonstrates the variable expression of the gene in this family. He has triplication of the proximal and distal phalanges.

the mate is normal. These conditions, therefore, are seen in successive generations, and, as noted, either sex may be affected. Two orthopaedic conditions which are known to be inherited in this fashion are vitamin D refractory rickets and pseudopseudohypoparathyroidism. Idiopathic scoliosis has been reported to be inherited in this fashion,[4] but a multifactorial pattern of inheritance has also been suggested.[12]

X-Linked Recessive Inheritance

In X-linked recessive inheritance, males are affected with the disease but females are typically carriers. The only way for a female to express an X-linked recessive condition would be to have a father who had the condition and a mother who was a carrier. Carrier mothers produce normal or affected sons and daughters who are genotypically normal or who are clinically normal carriers. All daughters of affected males are carriers and all sons are normal.

The dosage effect of the gene may, on occasion, be seen in the female who is a carrier. The Lyon hypothesis[7] states that one X chromosome will become inactive during development. Thus some cells in a carrier female will have the abnormal X chromosome inactivated, whereas some cells will have the normal X chromosome inactivated. This principle may be of use in the detection of carriers of pseudohypertrophic muscular dystrophy. The creatinine phosphokinase may be elevated in such an individual if a large number of her cells contain the abnormal gene for this condition on the X chromosome that is active in those cells.

Conditions Exhibiting Various Forms of Inheritance

Some conditions may be inherited in more than one fashion. Although the family history may be helpful in establishing the general inheritance pattern, the history is absolutely essential in dealing with these conditions. Osteogenesis imperfecta, for example, may be inherited in either an autosomal dominant or autosomal recessive mode. The various forms of muscular dystrophy are also inherited in different modes. Becker muscular dystrophy is inherited as an autosomal dominant, whereas pseudohypertrophic muscular dystrophy is inherited as an X-linked recessive condition. Osteopetrosis, Charcot-Marie-Tooth disease, spondyloepiphyseal dysplasia, and Ehlers-Danlos syndrome may also be inherited in more than one fashion. Thus, counseling is extremely difficult for these conditions.

CHROMOSOMAL ABNORMALITIES

The correct number of chromosomes in humans was ascertained by Tjio and Levan[10] in 1956, but cytogenetic studies were not practical until a method to study the chromosomes in white blood cells was reported in 1959[9]. Down syndrome was found to be the result of a chromosome abnormality in the same year.[6] Accurate identification of individual chromosomes was made possible by the use of banding techniques in 1970[2] (Fig. 3-2). Clinical syndromes may result from the loss of a chromosome (monosomy) or a portion of a chromosome (deletion), from the addition of a whole chromosome (trisomy) or a portion of a chromosome (partial trisomy), from rearrangement of chromosome material (translocation), or from the occurrence of two cell lines in the same individual (mosaicism).[3,11]

Monosomy

Monosomy occurs when one chromosome of a pair is lost during cell division. Thus, the individual has only 45 chromosomes. While autosomal monosomy has been reported, the

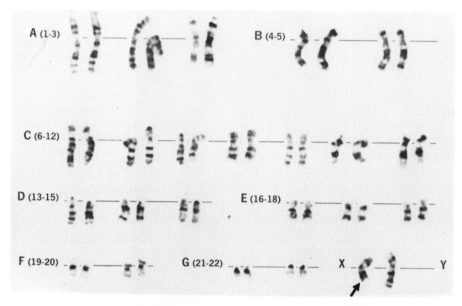

Figure 3-2 This karyotype illustrates how the 22 pairs of autosomes and the X chromosomes are grouped and individually banded. There is a loss of the distal portion (deletion) of the long arm of the X chromosome (arrow).

occurrence of this condition is rare and usually involves only smaller chromosomes since survival of the fetus is unlikely with the loss of the sizable amount of genetic material contained in one of the larger autosomes. However, survival of an individual with one X chromosome is not rare, thus producing an individual with Turner syndrome. These patients usually present to the orthopaedist for the evaluation of scoliosis.

Deletion

The deletion of a portion of a chromosome results in a *partial monosomy* (Fig. 3-2). A number of these syndromes have been reported, and clubfoot, for example, may be seen in conjunction with deletion of a portion of chromosome 9, 13, 14, or 18.

Trisomy

The addition of an entire chromosome was first reported by Lejeune[6] in Down syndrome. *Trisomy* occurs because of nondysjunction in the sperm or egg; the two chromosomes of a pair fail to divide properly during reduction division. Thus an individual is produced who has 3 chromosomes of a particular type instead of a pair and a total of 47 chromosomes. The orthopaedist may see this type of abnormality in a patient with a trisomy of chromosome 18 who may present with a vertical talus. As contrasted to the child who has a vertical talus but no other defects, these children fail to thrive; they have hernias, low-set ears, and micrognathia. Children with trisomy in the D group (of chromosome 13) have multiple anomalies including polydactyly and seldom survive. A common nondysjunction involves the X chromosome. Patients with two X chromosomes in addition to a Y chromosome have Klinefelter syndrome and may present to the orthopaedist for the treatment of scoliosis.

Translocation

This condition occurs when a whole chromosome or a portion of a chromosome becomes attached to another chromosome during cell division. If there is simply a rearrangement of genetic material, the translocation is a balanced one and the individual is normal. However, reduction division and subsequent fertilization may result in the addition or loss of genetic material. If an egg or sperm with additional material is fertilized, then an unbalanced translocation results and severe abnormalities are seen in such an individual. These may include severe scoliosis, genu valgum, clubfoot, vertical talus, dislocation of the radial head, and mental retardation.

Mosaicism

An individual who has two different cell lines— such as, for example, some cells with 46 chromosomes and others with 48 chromosomes—is said to have *mosaicism*. These patients may present with orthopaedic abnormalities including scoliosis.[1]

Indications for Chromosome Studies

Since the diagnosis of a chromosome abnormality allows for proper counseling and since amniocentesis can be used to detect an affected fetus, cytogenetic studies should be considered whenever the possibility of such an abnormality exists. Specific indications for chromosome studies include the finding of multiple orthopaedic abnormalities in an individual in whom no specific diagnosis can be made, the involvement of multiple organ systems with congenital anomalies, the involvement of two or more siblings with the same undiagnosed condition, a history of multiple miscarriages in the mother, or the presence of mental retardation in the patient. Since Mendelian disorders involve single gene defects which represent too small an abnormality to be detected by cytogenetic studies, such studies are not beneficial in analyzing patients with these disorder.

MULTIFACTORIAL CONDITIONS

Multifactorial, or polygenic, conditions are determined by the actions of multiple genes in conjunction with environmental factors. These conditions occur in families in a much higher incidence than they do in the general population, but they do not follow the Mendelian rules of inheritance. The overall risk of recurrence is about one in twenty for each subsequent pregnancy, but this risk varies from condition to condition and from one sex to the other. A different threshold is required for expression of the condition in each sex. Thus congenital dislocation of the hip is more common in females, and clubfoot is more common in males. If a male has a clubfoot, the chance of his sister having the condition is less than 40 to 1, but if a female has a clubfoot, the chance of her brother having the condition is as high as 16 to 1. Many other orthopaedic conditions including myelomeningocele, hallux valgus, femoral anteversion, and metatarsus adductus behave in similar fashion.

REFERENCES

1. Casey, P.A., Clark, C.E., and Cowell, H.R. 46,XY/48,XXY, + 8 in a male with clinical and dermatoglyphic features of mosaic trisomy 8 syndrome. Clin Genet 20:60–63, 1981.
2. Caspersson, T., Zech, L., Johansson, C., and Modest, E.J. Identification of human chromosomes by DNA-binding fluorescent agents. Chromosoma 30:215–227, 1970.
3. Cowell, H.R., and Clark, C.E. Cytogenetic abnormalities in orthopedic patients. Clin Orthop 135:4–14, 1978.
4. Cowell, H.R., Hall, J.N., and MacEwen, G.D. Genetic aspects of idiopathic scoliosis. Clin Orthop 86:121–131, 1972.
5. Cowell, H.R., and Wein, B.K. Genetic aspects of club foot. J bone Joint Surg 62-A:1381–1384, 1980.
6. Lejeune, J. Le Mongolisme. Premier Example d'Aberration autosomique Humaine. Ann Genet, Sem Hop Paris, 1:41–49, 1959.
7. Lyon, M.F. Sex chromatin and gene action in the mammalian X-chromosome. Am J Hum Genet 14:135–148, 1962.
8. McKusick, V.A. Mendelian inheritance in man, in *Catalogs of Autosomal Dominant, Autosomal Recessive,* and *X-Linked Phenotypes,* 6th ed. Baltimore, Johns Hopkins University Press, 1983.
9. Moorhead, P.S., Nowell, P.C., Mellman, W.J., Battips, D.M., and Hungerford, D.A. Chromosome preparations of leukocytes cultured from human peripheral blood. Exp Cell Res 20:613–616, 1960.
10. Tjio, J.H., and Levan, A. The chromosome number of man. Hereditas 42:1–6, 1956.
11. Valentine, G.H. *The Chromosome Disorders. An Introduction for Clinicians,* 3d ed. Philadelphia, Lippincott, 1975.
12. Wynne-Davies, R. Familial (indiopathic) scoliosis. A family survey. J Bone Joint Surg 50-B:24–30, 1968.

CHAPTER 4

Articular Cartilage

Roger Dee, Antoni Goral, and Nestor Blyznak

SECTION A

Structure, Function, and Repair

Roger Dee, Antoni Goral, and Nestor Blyznak

DEVELOPMENT OF ARTICULAR CARTILAGE

Immature articular cartilage has two zones of proliferating chondroblasts which provide additional cells required during growth.[82] A superficial zone just below the joint surface provides cells for the enlarging articular cartilage, whereas a deeper zone provides cells for the endochondral ossification of the ossific nucleus of the secondary ossification centers (Fig. 4-1). When the articular cartilage is thick enough during the first year of life, the superficial zone ceases to proliferate, and growth then only occurs at the deeper zone of dividing cells.[43,82]

Endochondral ossification associated with growth ceases with skeletal maturity, and a subchondral bony plate forms beneath the articular cartilage. Thereafter there is normally little growth or replication of cartilage cells. Some cell replication is, however, seen to occur in response to abnormal circumstances such as trauma and also in osteoarthritis and acromegaly.[84] Cartilage maturity is marked by the appearance of the *tidemark,* which separates the mineralization front (the zone of calcified cartilage) from the uncalcified articular cartilage. This hematoxyphilic line is not a continuous structure and occasionally shows small, periodically occurring gaps (Fig. 4-2).[6,18,117] Areas of reduplication of the tidemark indicate advance of the mineralization front into noncalcified areas; these are age-related changes but are also seen in fibrillated cartilage.[134]

Some endochondral ossification occurs simultaneously with these changes, the result being remodeling of the osteochondral junction occurring throughout life, probably in response to Wolff's law.[24] Present in the cells in the region of the calcified front are the calcium phospholipid complexes, glycoproteins, and extracellular matrix vesicles required for this process.[24] Changes in the proteoglycans occur in the region of the tidemark and indicate their role in the regulation of this process. Some chondrocytes are formed throughout life to regulate this activity and also to control synthesis and degradation of matrix.[24,69]

Structure

Light microscopy has demonstrated several layers, or *zones,* as one proceeds inward from the articular surface. These zones are not sharply demarcated but merge one into another showing differences in cellular activity and morphology and also in matrix components (Fig. 4-3). For description pur-

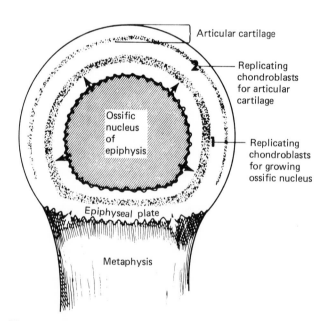

Figure 4-1 Long bone epiphysis within the first year of human life. A spherical growth plate surrounds the ossific nucleus (1). A more superficial zone of dividing chondroblasts contributes to the thickness of the articular cartilage (2). *(From Edwards, C., and Chrisman, O.D., in Albright, J.A., and Brand, R.A., eds: The Scientific Basis of Orthopaedics. New York, Appleton Century Crofts, 1979. Reproduced with permission.)*

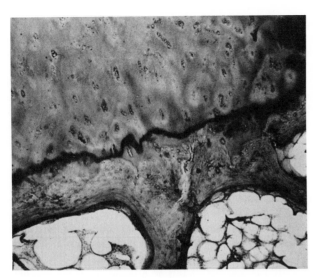

Figure 4-2 The osteochondral junction of articular cartilage with a well-defined tidemark. *(From Brower, T.D., and Hsu, W.Y., Clin Orthop 62:12, 1969. Reproduced with permission.)*

poses it is also useful to recognize within each zone the *pericellular region* (1 to 2 μm area around the cell), the region of the *territorial matrix* (within 7 to 9 μm), and the *interterritorial matrix.*

The *superficial zone,* sometimes known as the gliding zone, extends 40 μm deep.[114] According to Buckwalter, this zone represents the "lamina splendens" seen with phase contrast microscopy. It is the fine clear skin that can be mechanically stripped from articular cartilage. In this zone lie spindle-

shaped cells with a long axis parallel to the articular surface and a pericellular matrix encircling each cell.[20] The collagen fibrils in this "armor plate" layer are oriented in a tangential fashion, quite different from the pattern in deeper layers. These fibrils exhibit a pore size that admits most of the synovial fluid molecules but excludes larger molecules such as proteins and hyaluronic acid.[1] In the superficial zone the proteoglycans are also organized differently from those deeper in the cartilage. They have fewer glycosaminoglycans attached to each core protein, and some of the proteoglycans are unextractable and tightly enmeshed with the fine collagen fibers present in both the territorial and the interterritorial matrix, probably giving the strength necessary to resist shear.

The middle or *transitional zone* extends to 500 μm[114] beneath the articular surface. The cells in this layer are more metabolically active than they are in the superficial zone, but cells in both layers possess intracellular structures such as endoplasmic reticulum, mitochondria, and golgi complexes. Near the territorial matrix the collagen fibers are much larger in the transitional zone, lying obliquely relative to the articular surface.[20] The proteoglycan is more easily extractable in this layer.

The *deep zone* (sometimes called the *radial zone*) comprises the thickest portion of articular cartilage. The cartilage cells tend to lie in columns. The collagen fibers are more vertically arranged with some of them perforating through the tidemark and calcified cartilage to enter the subchondral bone layer, firmly anchoring the articular cartilage to the bone.[1] There is evidence that the proteoglycans in the territorial matrix and in the pericellular matrix are closely associated with collagen fibers, but there is a large proportion of monomer. Link protein is almost undetectable. However, in the interterritorial matrix, proteoglycan aggregation com-

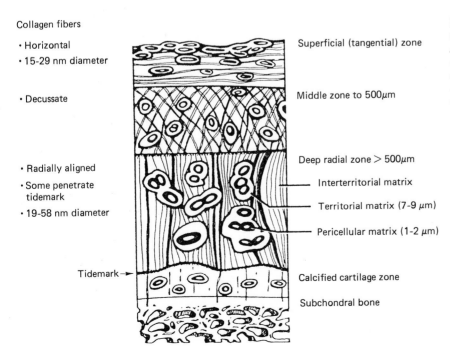

Figure 4-3 Schematic of the structure of articular cartilage. *(Modified from Poole, A.R., in Cruess, R.L. ed: The Musculoskeletal System, New York, Churchill Livingstone, 1982. Some data also from Buckwalter, J.A., in Evarts, C.M., ed: Instr Course Lect 32:349–369, 1983.)*

Collagen fibers
- Horizontal
- 15-29 nm diameter

- Decussate

- Radially aligned
- Some penetrate tidemark
- 19-58 nm diameter

Tidemark →

Superficial (tangential) zone

Middle zone to 500μm

Deep radial zone > 500μm
Interterritorial matrix
Territorial matrix (7-9 μm)
Pericellular matrix (1-2 μm)

Calcified cartilage zone

Subchondral bone

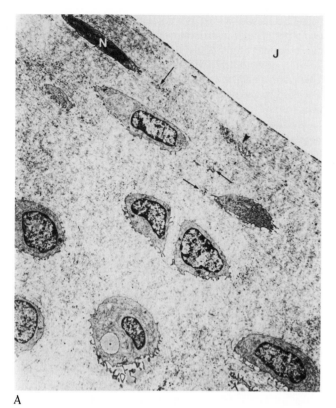

A

Figure 4-4 A. Superficial and transitional zones of articular cartilage from the femoral condyle of a 5-month-old rabbit. Note the elongated profiles of superficial chondrocytes. One of the chondrocytes is necrotic (N). Small foci of membranous and granular lipidic debris (arrows) derived from shedding of cell processes and a larger focus of debris (arrowhead) derived from in situ necrosis of a chondrocyte are seen in the matrix. Note the smooth articular surface adjacent to the joint space (J). ×4000. **B.** Autopsy specimen of adult human articular cartilage from the femoral condyle. In this routine H&E specimen, shrunken chondrocytes are seen lying in lacunae, as evidenced by the clear space between the chondrocyte and the wall of the lacuna. ×870. *(From Ghadially, F.N.: Fine Structure of Synovial Joints. London, Butterworth, 1983. Reproduced with permission.)*

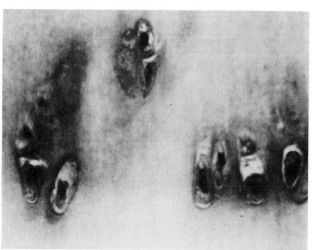

B

monly occurs and there are large aggregates on a hyaluronic acid backbone.[20,114] In this region the diameter of the collagen fibrils is at their greatest, possibly because they need to resist the swelling pressure of the proteoglycans.

The *zone of calcified cartilage* lies deep to the tidemark separating the hyaline cartilage from the subchondral bone. Before skeletal maturity, this layer shows the picture of endochondral ossification with degenerating chondrocytes. After maturity, the matrix is calcified and contains small chondrocytes that do not demonstrate much RNA synthesis.[2,49]

Buckwalter has speculated that the functional adaptation seen in the layers of articular cartilage reflect a change in the mechanical environment from predominantly shear forces at the joint surface to more compressive forces deeper in the cartilage. The radial and transitional zones primarily resist compressive loading, and the calcified cartilage anchors the articular surface to the subchondral bone.[20]

The surface topography of articular cartilage has been studied using both scanning and transmission electron microscopy. Whereas with light microscopy the surface of articular cartilage appears smooth, numerous studies employing scanning electron microscopy have revealed a surface resembling that of a golfball, with depressions measuring 8 to 15 μm in diameter separated by a distance upward of 300 μm.[11,54,55] More recently, studies using different preparative techniques suggest that such depressions may be artifactual. Normal articular cartilage may in fact be smooth. The undulating surface with ridges and depressions may represent desiccation prior to fixation.[11,30,141] Physical exercise does not significantly alter the surface topography of articular cartilage.[11] Joint overuse without a peak overload does not result in degeneration of surface cartilage as evidenced by scanning electron microscopy.[29]

Cellular Elements of Articular Cartilage

Cartilage is devoid of neural elements, blood vessels, and lymphatics.[20] The chondrocytes comprise 5 percent or less of the tissue volume.[38,60,67] The chondrocytes of articular cartilage are derived from undifferentiated mesenchyme. The mature cells vary in shape from round to flat, depending upon location, and occupy rounded lacunae (Fig. 4-4). The nucleus is often eccentric with ultrastructural characteristics varying with cell location and activity.[38,111] Cells of the transitional zone show a lobulated nucleus with one or more nucleoli. A prominent golgi apparatus is observed with a densely packed granular lamella as well as numerous adjacent vacuoles. The endoplasmic reticulum and mitochondria are well developed.[73] Cells in other regions may vary considerably in appearance. The more superficial cells show less endoplasmic reticulum and electron-dense vacuoles. The deeper cell layers show intracytoplasmic fibrils believed to be associated with cell degeneration. This finding is supported by tritiated label studies for RNA and protein synthesis.[54,85,86,111,141,153]

The metabolic activity of mature articular cartilage tissue occurs with a very low oxygen consumption, approximately one-fiftieth to one-hundredth of adult tissues by weight.[25] This reflects both a lower cell-to-volume ratio as well as a predominantly glycolytic metabolism.[89] Because cartilage is avascular, metabolism is generally anaerobic and a complement of the necessary enzymes is present. Articular chondrocytes produce matrix components and also synthesize and export the enzymes that degrade them. Cellular function is modified in turn by the matrix components and by their interrelationship with the cells and with influences such as the mechanical forces that affect them.[18,20,121]

Nutrition of articular cartilage occurs primarily by diffusion from synovial fluid. Intermittent loading of joint surfaces produces a pumping action that provides removal of waste products and nutrient penetration to deeper layers. Diffusion of nutrients across the osteochondral junction does not seem to occur.[18,86,121]

Matrix of Articular Cartilage

By virtue of its structure and volume, the matrix of articular cartilage provides for its functional properties.[21,70,71,87] Matrix consists of a dense organization of collagen fibers which comprises approximately 50 percent of its dry weight interconnected with aggregates of proteoglycan together with their bound water and cations. The collagen imparts tensile strength and the proteoglycan provides stiffness and compressive strength.[70,71] Both interact to stabilize the matrix and bind water (Fig. 4-5). Matrix water is attracted to the hydrophilic proteoglycan aggregates and exhibits compression-dependent flow. Matrix water contributes to the ability of car-

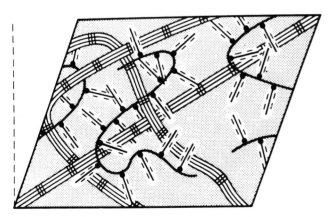

Figure 4-5 Schematic representation of the functional role of collagen fibril in resisting shear deformation in articular cartilage. The existence of a composite solid matrix is necessary for collagen fibrils to play an active role during shear. Proteoglycan aggregates alone do not provide significant shear resistance. *(From Mow, V.C., Holmes, M.H., and Lai, W.M., Biomechan 17:381, 1984. Reproduced with permission.)*

tilage to resist compression, to restore normal shape after deformation, and to maintain lubrication.[87]

The overwhelming majority of intracellular matrix collagen is type II, with fibers of varying thickness and size. In addition, type III collagen and other species have been isolated in the pericellular region of chondrocytes.[52] The tendency of type II collagen to swell with hydration may be related to its higher carbohydrate content compared with type I collagen.[20,47] Phenotypic variability has been described enabling articular chondrocytes to produce other collagen subtypes under different conditions.[47,93] Chondrocytes in culture in calf serum manufacture type II collagen unless *fibronectin* (a glycoprotein with molecular weight of 220,000 daltons) is added to the culture, in which case they will organize like fibroblasts and produce type I collagen.[151] *Chondronectin* (another glycoprotein of molecular weight 140,000 daltons) is cell-surface-related and is responsible for the adhesion of chondrocytes to the type II collagen with the help of proteoglycan.

In inflammatory conditions such as rheumatoid arthritis, vascular penetration of pannus is responsible for the synthesis of vascular-derived type III collagen and endothelial-based membrane-derived type IV collagen.[44]

Proteoglycan accounts for nearly 40 percent of the dry weight of articular cartilage matrix. It is this high concentration of proteoglycan that characterizes hyaline cartilage and differentiates it from such other forms of cartilage as fibrocartilage, which has far less proteoglycan relative to collagen.[21]

The synthesis of the protein core of proteoglycan is performed in the rough endoplasmic reticulum, but the glycosaminoglycans (GAG) are synthesized in smooth endoplasmic reticulum. Sulfation and assembly of the GAG onto the protein core occurs in the golgi complex with secretion into the matrix through large golgi vacuoles. Vacuole maturation to form matrix occurs in the extracellular space.[30] Generally speaking, the concentration of proteoglycans varies inversely with collagen concentration, and thus is lower superficially and higher in the deeper zones.[149] There is also an increase in chondroitin sulfate concentration toward the deeper zones in the cartilage, with a peak level in the radial zones.[149] Compression drives the chondroitin sulfate chains closer together, increasing their resistance to further compression and forcing tissue fluid out of their molecular domain. The varying concentration probably has functional significance. The glycosaminoglycan concentration varies with age, with keratan sulfate content increasing with age as the chondroitin sulfate content diminishes. There is also a gradual diminution in the water content of adult human articular cartilage from 75 to 65 percent with aging.[149]

It is believed that glycosaminoglycans play a role in the orientation of collagen fibers.[76] In certain circumstances proteoglycan monomers will bind to collagen and 1 proteoglycan molecule may bind as many as 30 collagen molecules. In cartilage the glycosaminoglycans and the proteoglycans interact with collagen type II, probably by electrostatic forces.

Additionally, proteoglycans at the surfaces of cells interact with fibronectin, providing points of interaction between collagen and proteoglycan.[73] The role of chondronectin has been discussed, and this glycoprotein may also be involved in the interaction between the various components of the matrix and the cells.

Matrix Degradation

Matrix synthesis occurs simultaneously with degradation in a controlled fashion in articular cartilage, but the mechanism of cellular control remains obscure. Thompson and Robinson have calculated that one-half of the matrix glycosaminoglycan in adult human cartilage is replaced annually whereas only one-half of the collagen matrix is replaced every 10 years.[149] These researchers point out that all the degradative enzymes needed are present in articular cartilage except hyaluronidase which is present in synovial membrane. They emphasize that the relationship between synthesis and degradation for individual cells is poorly understood.

Endogenous enzymes such as cathepsins B, D, and F are present within chondrocytes. *Cathepsin B* is active at neutral pH and may be more important in cartilage than *cathepsin D,* which is capable of degrading proteoglycan only at pH 4.5 to 5. The immediate pericellular area seems to be somewhat different from the rest of the territorial matrix. It is now known that the lacuna of each cartilage cell is an area where newly synthesized matrix components are present. It may be that the pH in this area is more acid, and cathepsin D is usually found in this region.[1] Cathepsin D cannot degrade collagen but can split the polypeptide backbone of the proteoglycan into small fragments suitable for degradation and attack by other enzymes.[1] The matrix cells are able to synthesize and degrade proteoglycan much more rapidly than collagen.

Collagenases are synthesized and exported from the cell by fibroblasts, synovial cells, and chondrocytes, but usually require activation by some other agent (e.g., plasmin).[114] Collagenase attacks the triple helix at neutral pH, causing a three-quarter to one-quarter split.[2] Newly synthesized collagen that has not developed cross-links is more susceptible than cross-linked collagen. Aging cartilage with more intermolecular cross-links may be more resistant to breakdown by these enzymes.

Some collagenolytic proteinases, e.g., those produced by polymorphonuclear leukocytes, cannot attack the triple helix of collagen, but they do degrade the nonhelical telopeptide regions by breaking the cross-links between individual tropocollagen molecules (e.g., the serine proteinases, *cathepsin G* and *elastase*).[14] Both these enzymes are absent from synovial fluid.

Proteinases, proteases, collagenase, and hyaluronidase may arise from lysosomes of both type A and type B lining cells of synovium and give rise to these exogenous enzymes in disease states, causing degradation of articular cartilage.

Tissues other than cartilage may secrete messengers that stimulate chondrocytes to degrade proteoglycan and collagen.[2] Such a substance is *catabolin*. This protein or family of proteins has no direct action on cartilage matrix. Only living cartilage, not dead cartilage, is affected. Catabolinlike factors have also been found to be produced by macrophages and monocytes.[2,58] Production of these factors can be increased substantially by adding lipopolysaccharides to macrophage cultures.[2]

PROPERTIES OF ARTICULAR CARTILAGE

Fluid transport within articular cartilage contributes to its physical properties. Matrix proteoglycan contains a high concentration of fixed negatively charged sulfate and carboxyl groups. These impart a swelling pressure in the aqueous matrix.[90,91] The interstitial fluid flow which governs the viscoelastic properties of articular cartilage is a function of cartilage permeability and of the fixed charged density of the proteoglycans. The proteoglycans impede the loss of water from the surface pores of loaded cartilage and also the resistance to fluid flow is proportional to proteoglycan concentration. A reduction of proteoglycan concentration will therefore increase the rate of creep in articular cartilage and reduce its compressive stiffness.[70,71] This action allows greater deformation to occur when the cartilage is loaded. Cartilage permeability is a nonlinear function and the tissue exhibits progressive "creep" during stress relaxation.[80]

Changes in the configuration of the proteoglycans occur with compression. These changes exclude water from the molecular domains of the proteoglycans but increase the amount of water which moves into the interfibrillar space of the collagen fibrils or which is lost from the surface. Decreasing pH or increasing salt concentration also collapses the stiff extended proteoglycan structure, and may cause water to be lost from its molecular domain.[150] The collapsing proteoglycan macromolecule relaxes the tension in the collagen fibers, allowing lateral expansion and increased intermolecular spacing. The water molecules have greater intermolecular access and mobility when the fibril is swollen, and this increases the freely exchangeable water in articular cartilage.[150] The collagen network within articular cartilage at rest is under a tensile strain.[90,106] The recovery of articular cartilage after stress experiments is not, strictly speaking, a physical property of the material since it depends on the size of the specimen and on any features of the experiment that determine which way the fluid can flow during the creeping process. Consequently, McCutchen states that *poroelastic* might be a better term than *viscoelastic* to explain its properties.[95]

Lubrication of Synovial Joints

Tribology is the study of interacting surfaces and relative motion under load.[8] Mechanical devices have usually been able to describe mechanisms of interacting surfaces and their lubrication in modes of rotational or oscillating motion. In biological systems where motion is often oscillatory and rotational at the same time, varying testing devices which tend to characterize joint motion and lubrication have been devised.[77,124] Unfortunately, where no accepted standard method for analyzing joint motion exists, there has been no great consensus regarding mechanisms of joint lubrication.[124] Resistance to joint motion is a function of the friction across the joint surfaces and the tension created in the enveloping soft tissues. Studies by Radin et al have shown that the energy required to overcome stretching of soft tissues is 100 times greater than frictional resistance of the joint.[109] Joint stiffness might then be more a function of increased tension in the soft

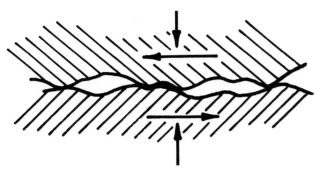

Figure 4-6 Dry friction. Representation of the two loaded unlubricated surfaces. The asperities of the surface are in contact and interact. *(From Radin, E.L., and Paul, I.L., J Bone Joint Surg 54A:607, 1972. Reproduced with permission.)*

tissues (muscle spasm, ligamentous contracture, or intraarticular adhesions) than of changes in joint surface lubrication.

Classic lubrication theories are derived from nonbiological systems in which friction and wear are the results of surface asperities (irregularities) making contact between two loaded surfaces (Fig. 4-6). The coefficient of friction that is generated depends upon the shear strength of the contact points. The presence of a fluid between two irregular surfaces functions to decrease the coefficient of friction in two ways. *Fluid film lubrication* implies a continuous, although thin, film of liquid between two loaded surfaces (Fig. 4-7). This fluid film may be maintained in three ways: by an externally applied pressure (hydrostatic lubrication), by an internally generated pressure upon the trapped fluid (squeeze film lubrication), or by continuous relative motion maintaining a wedge of lubrication at the leading edge of contacting surfaces (hydrodynamic).[94,118,121]

The second general mechanism in nonbiological systems for lubrication is that of *boundary lubrication*. Here a bearing surface is coated with a layer of adsorbed molecules that prevent contact of surface asperities. The nature of these adsorbed surface molecules is to slide more readily across one another rather than to shear off the adsorbed surface[118] (Fig. 4-8). In most lubricated surfaces, some combination of the two mechanisms exists depending upon the angle and velocity of contacting surfaces.[118] Elastohydrodynamic lubrication is an additional mechanism of action which may occur in a deformable surface consisting of elevation and depressions generating a fluid film squeezed out when a load is applied.

The investigation of biological systems of joint lubrication under different experimental testing and loading conditions has not yielded a clear single theory to explain the low coefficient of friction. Joint surfaces do not accurately mimic nonbiological contacting surfaces. Joint surfaces are usually viscoelastic and naturally moist; they frequently have multiple planes of noncontinuous sliding surface.[118]

There is no unaninmity among researchers concerning the function of synovial fluid in joint lubrication. The amount of synovial fluid in an noninflamed joint is usually less than 0.5 ml in the human knee. The film layer varies with the load applied.[39,40] The thicker the layer, the more the viscosity of the film contributes to a reduction in the coefficient of friction. It has been suggested that at low loads, the viscosity of synovial fluid may have an effect on joint lubrication, but it certainly does not behave solely as a viscous oil.[8,78,94,118]

Articular cartilage on compression "weeps" interstitial fluid into the joint surface, thus creating in effect a self-pressurizing form of hydrostatic lubrication.[118] This fluid is expressed through pores in the articular cartilage surface of upward of 100 nm in diameter. The hyaluronic acid content of synovial fluid directly affects its viscosity. However, this has little effect on joint lubrication. Although hyaluronic acid has been shown to be an effective lubricant for synovial membranes, it has not been shown to function as a lubricant in joints.[40,77,78,118] Another phenomenon, known as "boosted" lubrication, occurs when fluid trapped within the recesses of contacting asperities locally increases the concentration of lubricating molecules[78] (Fig. 4-9).

Radin, Swann et al have shown that the coefficient of friction in joints is not a function of the hyaluronic acid content alone. Digestion of synovial fluid with hyaluronidase, although changing the viscosity, does not affect the coefficient of friction. Proteolytic digestion, however, does markedly diminish the lubricating actions. Swann et al[5] identified a 2×10^5-molecular weight glycoprotein termed *lubricin,* which is felt to be an active agent in joint lubrication.[142–147] This glycoprotein is found in both normal and pathological synovial fluid of bovines and humans. It binds to articular cartilage surfaces and acts as a boundary lubricant.[142,143] Apparently an equilibrium exists between free[142,143] and bound lubricin molecules to the articular cartilage. Proteolytic digestion of synovial fluid as well as mechanical removal abolishes lubri-

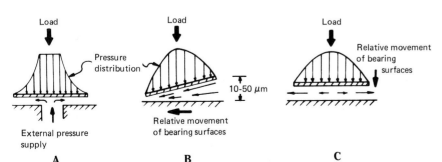

Figure 4-7 Fluid film lubrication illustrating load-carrying capacity of (**A**) hydrostatic lubrication, (**B**) hydrodynamic lubrication, and (**C**) squeeze film lubrication. *(From Armstrong, C.G., and Mow, V.C., in Owen, R., Goodfellow, J., Bullough, P., eds: Scientific Foundations of Orthopaedics and Traumatology. Philadelphia, Saunders, 1980, p 224. Reproduced with permission.)*

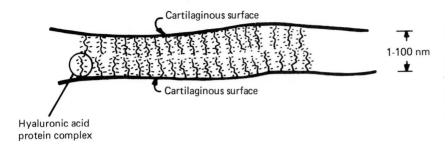

Figure 4-8 In boundary lubrication, the load is carried by a monolayer of adsorbed molecules, preventing cartilaginous wear. *(From Armstrong, C.G., and Mow, V.C., in Owen, R., et al, eds: Scientific Foundations of Orthopaedics and Traumatology. Philadelphia, Saunders, 1980.)*

cating activity. A turnover mechanism of lubricin molecules within the joint is suggested.[142,145,146]

In summary, joint motion is a function both of the tension within the soft tissues enveloping the joint and the frictional forces within the joint. Joint lubrication is a function of both fluid film and boundary film mechanics. Fluid viscosity plays little role in the lubrication of the synovial joints. Adsorbed lubricin contributes to joint boundary lubrication mechanics, although the specific mechanism of action is unknown. The compressible nature of articular surfaces with load and changes in surface characteristics suggest that the weeping of additional fluid into the joint at the time of loading may contribute additionally to joint lubrication. Boosted lubrication may similarly occur in areas of asperities.[8,94,124]

Repair of Articular Cartilage

The quality of the repair of articular cartilage after injury is dependent upon the particular structure of this tissue and the

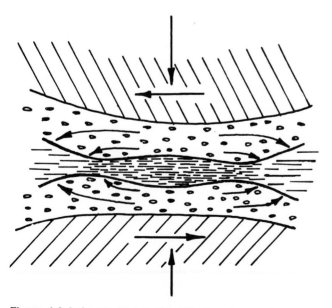

Figure 4-9 In boosted lubrication, filtering of water through cartilage concentrates the lubricant in the contact area. *(From Radin, E.L., and Paul, I.L., J Bone Joint Surg 54A:612, 1972. Reproduced with permission.)*

pattern of injury. The durability of that repair and the satisfactory maintenance of a load-bearing surface depends upon the properties of the healed tissue. Unfortunately, the repair process is often inadequate, predisposing a traumatized articular surface to later degenerative changes.[84,135]

Superficial damage depends for healing upon the metabolic activity of the articular chondrocyte, which is limited in its ability to restore the established structure accurately. Even if it can synthesize the proteoglycan and collagen molecules required and export them into the matrix, the incorporation of these newly synthesized molecules into the complex and established relationships may not be perfect. The functional characteristics of the repaired tissue, therefore, may not be adequate. The avascularity of the cartilage and the absence of chondrocyte replication limits the amount of repair possible. No inflammatory reaction develops. In addition, in vivo repair must occur in a functioning joint where loss of proteoglycans or a superficial laceration may expose the remaining collagen fiber network to further disruption.

By contrast, an injury produced either from infection or trauma that penetrates into the subchondral bone produces an outpouring of inflammatory products and mesenchymal cells, and a different mechanism of repair is triggered.[20,84,133,135] Ultimately, it is the type and amount of cartilaginous matrix produced which determines whether functional repair is adequate. The chondrocytes may replicate in a localized area of cartilaginous injury,[84,87] but the contribution that this makes to the repair process is not clear.[84,87] Clusters of chondrocytes which represent proliferated clones (shown by their uptake of radioactive thymidine) synthesize GAG, and are seen in degenerative joint disease.[134] Such proliferating chondrocytes may be active in digesting the pericellular matrix as part of the reparative process and may also be engaged in synthesis of new material.

In damage accompanied by inflammatory changes, numerous mediators of inflammation and protease activity have been isolated from joints (Table 4-1).[3,95,113] Prostaglandin E_2 (PGE_2) modifies the inflammatory process and has been shown to suppress the synthesis of GAG by rabbit chondrocytes.[80] Interleukin I has been isolated from degenerative human joints which exerts chemotactic and lymphocyte-activating activity and stimulates the production of neutral proteases from chondrocytes.[157] Messengers such as lymphocyte activating factor (LAF), mononuclear cell factor (MCF), and catabolin are also present in osteoarthritis.[3] These monokine factors do not have intrinsic degradative activity but serve as messengers to activate chondrocyte enzymes. Additional agents contributing to the pathological cartilage de-

TABLE 4-1 Examples of Cellular and Humoral Factors That Modulate Connective Tissue Destruction and Repair in Arthritic Diseases

Mediators	Sources	Target cells	Stimulatory effects
Osteoclast activating factor	T lymphocytes	Osteoclasts	Ca-release
PGE_2	Macrophages Synovial cells Chondrocytes	Osteoclasts	Ca-release
Macrophage activating factor	Lymphocytes	Macrophages (rodent)	Collagenase PGE_2
Immune complexes	Lymphocytes	Macrophages PMN leukocytes	Lysosomal enzymes
		Macrophages	PGE_2
Mononuclear cell factor or MCF-like	Monocyte-macrophages	Synovial cells Fibroblasts Chondrocytes	Collagenase PGE_2
MCF or MCF-like	Corneal epithelial cells	Corneal stroma cells	Collagenase
"Catabolin"	Synovium	Chondrocytes	Neutral proteases
Collagen	Fibroblasts Osteoblasts Chondrocytes	Synovial cells Fibroblasts	Collagenase PGE_2

Source: From Dayer, J.M., Krane, S.M., Goldring, Sr., Semin Arthritis Rheum 10:78, 1981. Reproduced with permission.

struction of osteoarthritis include the deposition of hydroxyapatite and calcium pyrophosphate crystals in the joint.

In septic arthritis, additional agents that may damage the joint include bacterial toxins. In rheumatic disease there is evidence that Ig and complement as well as immune complexes are found in more than 90 percent of articular collagenous tissues in involved joints contributing to the destructive change.[32,33]

In hemophilia, hemosiderin is found in chondrocytes as well as in the subchondral bone marrow. Extravasated erythrocytes are ingested and phagocytosed by the lining cells of the synovial membrane, which may then release enzymes that can damage the articular cartilage. Alternatively, the ferric ions may be directly toxic to the cartilage.[134]

Repair Following Mechanical Trauma

Blunt or impact injury to joints is a common occurrence. Articular cartilage loaded to less than 20 percent strain leads to no apparent damage[104] microscopically in vitro.[4,20,123] Long-term repetitive loading leads to matrix disruption, cell damage, and ultimately subchondral bone thickening in vivo.[20] Articulating regions of the hip repetitively loaded in vitro show reduction in the amount of proteoglycan matrix with increased synthetic activity of chondrocytes from the articulating regions.[152] Depending upon the rate of loading and the magnitude of load, cell death and collagen fibril disruption may occur.[123] A single blunt impact exceeding a critical threshold or multiple lesser insults of sufficient magnitude can produce irreversible cartilage damage. Lesser loads show matrix depletion but no chondrocyte necrosis. A repair process characterized by increased synthesis of matrix protein

follows.[20,122] The response is limited to the immediately adjacent chondrocyte population. It does not involve an inflammatory reaction or lead to the production of mediators and undifferentiated fibroblastic components.[20,84]

Lacerations disrupt the collagen fiber network, exposing fibers to degradative enzymes as well as to the possibility of local cell death. The defects do not, however, generally heal or extend.[20] Numerous animal models have shown a pattern of chondrocytic proliferation in clusters at sites of injury and increased matrix synthesis.[98] Although a burst of activity is seen upward of 6 weeks following injury, the repair process is incomplete and ceases shortly afterward.[28,43,84] Ghadially et al have shown on an ultrastructural level the progression of attempted healing of tangential injuries over a time course of 2 years.[53,54] As early as 1 week following injury, local cell necrosis and adjacent loss of proteoglycan are seen by light microscopy. Transmission electron microscopy of the remaining chondrocytes show evidence of increased metabolic activity. Six months following injury, defects are covered by a network of fine collagen fibrils oriented parallel to the surface. Irregularities in the surface, however, remain. Mankin et al suggest that the matrix proteoglycan of the damaged cartilage inhibits the adherence of platelets and the formation of a fibrous scaffolding required for fibroblasts to bridge the gap.[84] In experiments, intraarticular injection of proteoglycanolytic enzymes was shown to increase fibrous healing of superficial lacerations in experimental animals.[84] In one study, salicylates promoted healing of superficial defects.[132]

Injuries that penetrate subchondral bone result in a hematoma and fibrin clot that serves as a scaffold for a reparative process. Repair depends upon the restoration of symmetric surfaces and upon the type and quantity of reparative tissue. In contrast to superficial lacerations, osteochondral injuries have the capacity to heal with cartilaginous material. There is some difference of opinion regarding the nature of this material (whether it is fibrous or hyaline) and regarding the relative contribution of subchondral granulation tissue (metaplastic extrinsic cells) and adjacent chondrocytes.[20,27,28,42,43,53,54,103,104]

In immature dogs, DePalma observed that full-thickness articular defects are repaired with hyaline cartilage derived from subchondral granulation tissue.[43] Campbell noted that during the early stages of repair, collagen fibrils assumed orientations and distributions similar to fibrous tissue. The principal cells were similar to fibroblasts, and most of the collagen was type I, with only small amounts of type II. At 3 months however, type II collagen predominated in the repair.[27] The hyaline cartilage produced was irregular and showed sizable areas of matrix devoid of cells. The characteristic layered zonal organization of cartilage was not reproduced in sections through the injured area. Apparently, with time, the repair tissue becomes more like fibrocartilage, and is prone to degenerative fibrillation.[27] Loss of proteoglycan may accompany the gradual transformation from hyaline to fibrous cartilage.

Intraarticular fractures created in the distal end of adult rabbit femur that were inadequately reduced or reduced without compression healed by fibrocartilage alone. Fractures reduced and treated with compression and interfragmentary fixation healed with normal-appearing hyaline cartilage at the articular surface. Compression fixation may alter the mechanical microenvironment to enhance hyaline repair of the coapting articular surfaces, preventing ingrowth of granulation tissue, which interferes with superficial hyalinization.[104] Electric potentials can be recorded from mechanically loaded cartilage.[59] Articular as well as growth plate cartilage exhibit electric polarization, with actively growing sites being the more electronegative. It is possible that physical forces are transduced into electrical activity to which either the chondrocytes or the macromolecules may respond. Hall states that electronegativity is associated with growth, morphogenesis, and reparative and regenerative processes.[59] This may explain the improved results following compression fixation.

Certainly continual passive motion seems to promote improved hyaline cartilage repair of full-thickness articular defects in rabbits compared with immobilized or intermittently active mobilized controls.[129] Continuous passive motion can promote neochondrogenesis in free intraarticular periosteal autograft.[108,129] Joint immobilization causes damage to articular cartilage in experimental animals. In a rabbit, a cast does not completely immobilize the joint, yet microscopic evidence of cartilage damage was still visible 6 to 8 months after 6 weeks of such immobilization. In rats, rigid immobilization with a fixator gave irreversible changes up to 30 days after 30 days of immobilization.[2] Presumably not only is the normal mechanical stimulation of the matrix and its contained cells absent during immobilization, but the synovial pump mechanism required for nourishment of the chondrocytes is also impaired.

In summary, some generalizations may be made concerning the response of articular cartilage to injury. The physical structure and cellular physiology are so intimately related that any change in one alters the environment and function of the other. Enzymatic destruction changes the material properties of articular cartilage and will increase its susceptibility to structural damage. Superficial injuries that do not violate subchondral bone will not heal completely, but they will also not progress to degenerative joint disease. Deeper injuries penetrating the subchondral bone have the potential to heal with hyaline cartilage initially. There may occur subsequent transformation to fibrocartilaginous elements which structurally are not sufficient for repetitive load bearing.

SECTION B

Osteoarthritis

Roger Dee and Antoni Goral

NORMAL AGING OF ARTICULAR CARTILAGE

Normal age-related changes occur in articular cartilage. These changes have been well-characterized by Sokoloff.[126] This author points out that reduplication of the tidemark is a normal age-related change at the osteochondral junction and that some degeneration of articular cartilage occurs with normal aging. These time-related events include fibrillation of the surface of articular cartilage occurring focally and the formation of some bone spurs. Such changes do not therefore necessarily indicate osteoarthritis. The bone spurs seem to be related to vascular invasion of the calcified layer of the cartilage from the bone marrow followed by endochondral ossification in the affected region. These changes are clearly not secondary to fibrillation of the joint surface.[126] Normal aging also causes decreased protein synthesis with a decrease in the ratio of chondroitin sulfate to keratan sulfate in the matrix proteoglycan. There is also an increase in the collagen fiber diameter with aging but no change in the elastic properties of normal cartilage.[4,9,64,82,105,120]

OSTEOARTHRITIS

Osteoarthritis, rather than being a single disease entity, may be considered as a common pathway leading to a defined end point (Table 4-2). It is characterized by gross degeneration of articular cartilage, erosion and thickening of the subchondral bone, formation of marginal osteophytes and subarticular cysts, and eburnation and remodeling of bone.[63,68,95] More than 80 percent of the population over age 55 show radio-

TABLE 4-2   Some Causes of Osteoarthritis

Primary osteoarthritis
    Idiopathic
    Generalized
    Erosive
Secondary osteoarthritis
    Structural
        Malunited fractures with joint incongruity
        Joint instability
        Post-meniscectomy
        Genu valgum
        Genu varum
    Congenital or developmental
        Hip dysplasia
        Morquio syndrome
        Legg-Calvé-Perthes disease
        Slipped capital femoral epiphyses
        Multiple epiphyseal dysplasia
        Ehlers-Danlos syndrome
    Inflammatory
        Septic arthritis
        Psoriatic arthritis
        Reiter syndrome
    Endocrine
        Acromegaly
        Diabetes mellitus
        Hypothyroidism
        Hyperparathyroidism
        Estrogen excess
    Metabolic
        Hyperuricemia
        Hemochromatosis
        Ochronosis
        Chondrocalcinosis
        Paget disease
        Hemophilia
        Wilson disease
        Gaucher disease
    Miscellaneous
        Neuropathic
        Avascular necrosis
        Osteochondritis dissecans

graphic evidence of osteoarthritis, but only 25 percent of them will have clinically significant symptoms. There is thus a wide discrepancy between radiological signs of the disease and clinical symptoms.[63,75,125]

Pathophysiology of Osteoarthritis

Sokoloff[124,125] characterizes osteoarthritis as a noninflammatory remodeling of movable joints. He points to discrete pathological processes. The first of these is deterioration and loss of the bearing surface. The second is an exaggerated proliferation of new osteoarticular tissue at the joint margins similar to the changes seen with "normal" degeneration of cartilage but more severe and complex. There is also breakdown of the

osteochondral junction in osteoarthritis (Fig. 4-10). The combination of disintegration of the cartilage surface down to the bone plus subchondral microfracture exposes the joint surface to the proliferative activity of the subjacent bone marrow.[126]

The increased roughening of the articular surface with the appearance of surface erosions and irregularities is always focal with normal cartilage a few millimeters away.[13] Histologically, the cartilage becomes alternatively hypercellular and hypocellular with altered staining of the matrix in the region of the erosion. Diminished metachromasia parallels the loss of proteoglycan.[124] The tidemark at the junction of the calcified and uncalcified cartilage becomes irregular and reduplicates with expansion into the uncalcified cartilage.[124]

Antiangiogenesis factors and protease inhibitors normally prevent capillary ingrowth into normal cartilage (Fig. 4-11).[76] These inhibitors become defective or absent in osteoarthritis, and there is capillary ingrowth into the cartilage.[20] This ingrowth is an integral component of the endochondral ossification and bony remodeling of osteoarthritis. There is increased thickness of the calcified cartilage with extension into the uncalcified cartilage. Vertical clefts, or fissures, at the cartilage surface alter the normal arrangement of the collagen network and its physical properties.[42] The collagen interfibrillar distance is increased.[1]

The cartilage is eroded leaving denuded subchondral bone. Clusters of newly proliferative chondrocytes occur in clumps or clones near fibrillated areas. The overall cell population of chondrocytes decreases. There is a hyperemia along with venostasis in different areas of the subchondral bone.[99]

Later changes include thickening of the subchondral bone with cyst formation. Subchondral changes may show as either fibrous, fibrocartilaginous, cartilaginous, or sclerotic bone foci.[89,125]

Osteophyte formation involves proliferation with evolution of both bone and cartilage of cells at the chondrosynovial junction.[124] Inflammation of the peripheral synovial membrane may contribute to osteophyte formation by stimulation of vascularization peripherally.[51] The synovial membrane develops an inflammatory response with a mild lymphocytic infiltration. There is a fibrosis of the capsule and of the synovial tissues. Synovial fluid analysis may be normal. In association with inflammation, however, there is an increase of mononuclear cells, immunoglobulins, and protein and complement levels whereas viscosity declines.[103] Wear debris, with a number of discrete identifiable classes of particles, may be present (Table 4-3).[44]

Biochemical Changes in Osteoarthritis

Overall proteoglycan subunit synthesis is unchanged, but area-specific stimulation does occur.[118] Initially this may be localized to pericellular regions.[92] Proteoglycan subunit synthesis as well as glucosamine incorporation into hyaluronate increases, and these changes may occur prior to gross disruption of the cartilage surfaces.[117,130]

Overall proteoglycan content decreases in the specifically affected regions, and the proteoglycan aggregates tend

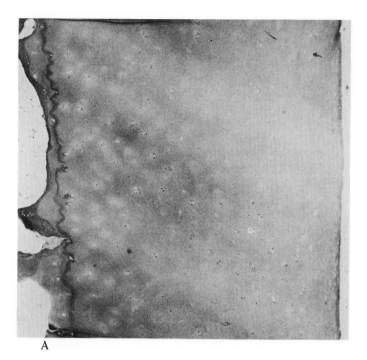

A

Figure 4-10 A. Coronal section through the articular cartilage of nonarthritic femoral head. The surface is smooth and chondrocytes are evenly spaced. The tidemark is singular and distinct. **B.** Coronal section through articular cartilage and subchondral bone of an arthritic femoral head. There is fissuring of the surface and interruption and duplication of the tidemark. *(From Einhorn, T.A., et al, Orthop Res 3:163, 1985. Reproduced with permission.)*

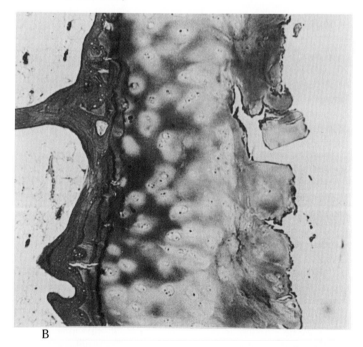

B

to appear as smaller and shorter chondroitin sulfate chains in osteoarthritic specimens.[16] This occurrence may represent changes in the production of link protein or increased degradation of GAG or the synthesis of immature forms.[16,41] Disparity exists in the literature with regard to these biochemical

changes. These difficulties can in part be attributable to the difficulties of tissue sampling in a disease which may be focal in some joints.[17,128] Differences however may occur from joint to joint.

In cartilage samples from human osteoarthritic knees showing surface fibrillation, there is a higher water content in the superficial layers that is characteristic of the disease, but no change in either the content or synthesis rate of glycosaminoglycan. Deeply fibrillated cartilage, however, shows an increased water content throughout its entire thickness and a loss of GAG. These results are at variance with those from the osteoarthritic hip where changes are more diffuse and where they are also found in cartilage not visually affected by the disease or demonstrating fibrillation.[17] This data supports a mechanical rather than a metabolic cause of certain kinds of osteoarthritis of the knee joint at least, which appears to be focal in origin unlike that of the hip. Further, studies of ^{35}S incorporation indicate that the cells are functioning normally until there is serious depletion of proteoglycans.[17]

ETIOLOGY OF OSTEOARTHRITIS

Attempts have been made in the past to attribute the development of osteoarthritis to wear and tear, aging, or mechanical derangement in joints. There is certainly no evidence to support an hypothesis that increased joint loading associated with athletic activity contributes to the disease.[8] Many experimental models for osteoarthritis have centered around situations of maximal joint loading, creation of joint instability, and articular damage with cyclic loading.[132] Clinical, histological, and biochemical studies have shown that a solely mechanical model for the development of osteoarthritis is untenable since inflammatory changes coexist with chemical factors to produce the disease entity.

Of additional interest is the inverse relationship that seems to exist between osteoarthritis and the presence of osteopenia. Although no significant differences in vitamin D or hormonal levels have been found between the two groups, they may be differentiated. Osteoarthritic patients tend to have above-normal bone mass, fat, and muscle strength but fewer fractures. Patients with osteopenia tend to be of slender body status with few degenerative joint changes. Primary osteoarthritic patients seem to have very slow loss of bone or no loss at all with age, or they may have started adult life with more bone than the osteopenic group.[30]

It is probable that the bone in osteoarthritis is stiffer, and therefore it absorbs impact loading poorly, transmitting it back to the cartilage, whereas the bone in osteoporosis, being more supple, spares the cartilage and protects against osteoarthritis. This is in keeping with the concept of Radin and co-workers that a primary defect in the subchondral bone is an important etiologic factor in primary osteoarthritis.[106,110] This defect, in turn, may be a result of some dysfunction in the normal coupled process of bony remodeling occurring at the osteochondral junction.

Osteoarthritis may be subdivided into two general classifications, primary (idiopathic) and secondary.

Primary Osteoarthritis

This condition may occur when there is no obvious predisposing cause for the disease.[125] In some cases there may be a genetic component.[83] This may be important in certain relatively homogeneous populations (for example, Denmark and China). Other factors such as the cultural habit of squatting in Asia may also be relevant.[59]

A generalized inflammatory form of primary osteoarthritis has been described with involvement of interphalangeal joints.[74] Commonly episodic, it is associated with a mildly elevated sedimentation rate. It is inherited as a dominant trait in women and a recessive in males.[27] The erosive subtype of primary osteoarthritis shows diffuse cartilage destruction with bony erosions and synovitis.[13] Though the synovium is histologically similar to rheumatoid arthritis, the sedimentation rate is normal and the rheumatoid factor nonreactive. More commonly affecting women, there may also be a predisposition for hand involvment in erosive primary osteoarthritis. A significant familial history is seen in 68 percent, and approximately 15 percent may go on later to develop rheumatoid arthritis.

Secondary Osteoarthritis

This condition may have multiple causes. Recent studies have shown a significant coexistence of inflammatory and crystalline deposition in some cases of secondary osteoarthritis.[29,32,33,34,103] In the main, mechanical factors appear to be the most prominent causative agent.[4,27] These may be related to static abnormalities in joint alignment or in joint geometry or stability as well as to dynamic forces created by motor imbalance or disrupted neurosensory feedback.[27,45,101] Animal studies utilizing joint mobilization, experimental joint instability, changes in contact loading through varying levels of amputation, osteotomy, and deafferentation have demonstrated histological changes of osteoarthritis.[7,12,56,63,101,111,131] Such models also suggest that developmental or congenital anomalies may influence the development of osteoarthritis.[54]

TABLE 4-3   Particles That May Be Found in Osteoarthritic Joints

Crystals sometimes seen in synovial fluid, cartilage, and synovium
    Calcium pyrophosphate dihydrate
    Basic calcium phosphates (e.g., hydroxyapatite)
    Monosodium urate monohydrate
    Cholesterol

Other particles sometimes seen in synovial fluid
    Fragments of bone and cartilage (wear particles)
    Fibrin/fibronectin aggregates ("rice bodies")

Source: Modified from Dieppe, P., and Watt, I., Clin Rheum Dis 11:367, 1985.

Crystal Deposition in Osteoarthritis

The etiologic significance of crystal deposition in osteoarthritis has been investigated because of its relative frequency in view of its age dependency.[32,33,34] It is likely that crystal deposition is an opportunistic event in osteoarthritis similar to the secondary infection of rheumatoid joints.[34] It is proposed that the disease produces the abnormal deposits which then contribute to and accelerate the disease process.[34] Intraarticular particles may consist of the fine crystals of calcium pyrophosphate dihydrate and hydroxyapatite as well as larger wear particles of articular cartilage and bone (Table 4-3).

Crystals have been identified in postmeniscectomy states, gout, chondrocalcinosis, ochronosis, hemochromatosis, and neuropathic joint conditions. Chondrocyte matrix vesicles act as nucleation sites for small aggregates of hydroxyapatite crystals, which suggest that these cells may have a role in the development of intraarticular crystals.[2] These crystals, however, may form only in the setting of altered proteoglycan matrix, since proteoglycan has been shown to be inhibitory to hydroxyapatite formation it is unclear whether pyrophosphate promotes or retards hydroxyapatite formation.

Hemophilia predisposes to osteoarthritic charges. The possible impact of erythrocyte destruction in joints and the effect of the ferric ion and synovial macrophages on articular cartilage have been outlined in the previous section. The arthropathy associated with hemochromatosis and other ion storage disease is uncommon and differs from hemophilia in that there is no intraarticular hemorrhage, so that another pathological mechanism seems probable. In hemochromatosis, chondrocalcinosis is seen in about one-third of cases; calcium pyrophosphate dihydrate is the predominant crystal found.[34] In ochronosis, cartilage damage follows the deposition of homogentisic acid in the matrix of the articular cartilage. This is often accompanied by calcification and deposition of apatite.

Role of Enzymes in Articular Cartilage Damage

The mechanisms available for articular cartilage damage following inflammatory processes have been described. Local enzyme activity shows significant changes in osteoarthritis. Chondrocyte-derived neutral proteases, latent proteoglycanases and latent collagenases are present in increased concentrations in areas of local erosion.[88,93] Activation by serine proteases of these latent enzymes responsible for cartilage matrix destruction has been proposed.[88] Unknown mechanisms in osteoarthritis lead to increased enzyme activity and also to crystal formation in the region of the tidemark.[42]

Secondary osteoarthritis can follow severe cartilage destruction. In joint sepsis large numbers of polymorphonuclear leukocytes, which engulf the bacterial agents with the release of lysosomal enzymes, obviously have the potential for injuring cartilage. The neutral serine proteinases, elastase and cathepsin G, are capable of degrading proteoglycans and then attacking the collagen of the matrix, and these agents plus plasmin are present in the synovial fluid. Additionally, messengers, such as catabolin, may induce the chondrocytes to produce destructive enzyme products. There exists then a

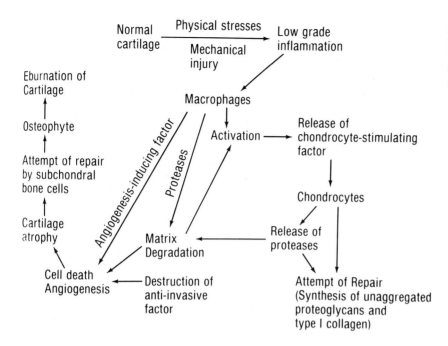

Figure 4-11 Hypothetical chain of events in osteoarthritis that may eventually lead to destruction of articular cartilage. *(From Phadke, K. J Rheum 10:857, 1983. Reproduced with permission.)*

cascadelike mechanism for sustaining an inflammatory response in osteoarthritis (Fig. 4-11).[104] Prostacyclin generation during the inflammatory reaction is inhibited by aspirin indomethacin and dexamethasone. This fact provides the basis for the use of anti-inflammatory agents.[25,31] Prolonged use of aspirin and nonsteroidal anti-inflammatory agents in experimental animals, however, have shown deleterious effects on proteoglycan synthesis in articular cartilage.[31]

Immune Complexes in Arthritis

Immune complex deposition probably occurs from time to time in polyarticular osteoarthritis, which is associated with a high frequency of Heberden's nodes and is commonly found in women. The pathological process is different, however, from rheumatoid arthritis where immune complex deposition may play an integral role in the inflammatory and destructive process. Immune complex deposition in osteoarthritis seems to be an infrequent and probably secondary event, following cartilage destruction rather than the cause of it.[26,27]

Local Injection of Steroids in Osteoarthritis

Structural and biochemical side effects of a harmful nature have been recognized following the local application of steroids into the joint space.[123] Although there are conflicting reports indicating that steroid does not always inflict damage upon the articular cartilage, chondrocyte degeneration in both the rabbit and the monkey has been noted by other authors together with fibrillation of the articular surface.[14,50,96,122] Frequent steroid injections should be avoided. A minimum interval between joint injections of 4 to 8 weeks is

advisable.[60] Intraarticular injection is particularly useful where secondary inflammation is prominent, e.g., where there is crystal deposition associated with the osteoarthritis.[34,65]

Endemic Osteoarthritis

Osteoarthritis also occurs in certain areas as an endemic disease, the cause of which is unknown. Kashin-Beck disease occurs primarily in mainland China, although originally described in nearby Siberia. No evidence of inflammation exists in this condition. Chondronecrosis is a pathological hallmark. At present various speculations about the cause include selenium deficiency or a mycotoxin.[127] Mseleni disease occurs in southeast Africa. Its principal manifestation is precocious coxarthrosis, which manifests itself usually during the first decade of life and may affect up to 42 percent of the women and 19 percent of the men in some communities.[127] The radiological appearances resemble those of spondyloepiphyseal dysplasia. In the Malnad region of southern India, a familial form of arthritis occurs. Some individuals have a genetic suseptibility to develop this disease, which characteristically commences with the development of painful hips in children between 5 and 15 years old. This progresses to arthritis of the hips and spine. The cause is unknown, but high-caste individuals who eat only vegetables are not affected. Much of the rest of the population glean food from the rice paddies, where environmental pollution may be an etiologic factor—particularly organic pesticides.[127]

Arthropathy in Endocrine Diseases

Arthropathy has been observed in certain endocrine disorders. In myxedema there is synovial thickening and effusion and deposition of hyaluronic acid in increased amounts in joint tissues. This reaction is thought to be caused by increased circulating thyrotropic hormones (TSH) found in primary hypothyroidism, which affects the properties of the ligamentous structures and the articular cartilage.[69] In hyperparathyroidism, arthropathy has been observed associated with erosive lesions in the subchondral bone.

In acromegaly, excess growth hormone results in accelerated chondrocytic and bony proliferation, leading to osteophytosis and secondary degenerative changes. Johanson points out that in this condition in the presence of elevated levels of somatomedin and growth hormone, unmodulated endochondal ossification will occur to a degree that is dependent on the relative concentrations of circulating thyroid hormone and estrogen.[69]

Neuropathic Joints

Diseases in which there is impairment of the efferent sensory input from joint receptors lead to characteristic changes. These neuropathic changes are seen in such diseases as congenital indifference to pain, tabes dorsalis, syringomyelia, and diabetes mellitus.[23,45,101] Fragmentation of the articular cartilage is a conspicuous feature, and portions of this tissue are displaced into the synovial lining.[126]

The massive destruction of the articular surface and the osteophytosis may be considered an extreme form of osteoarthritis. The neurological deficit may involve some component of the complicated sensory apparatus of joints. Such a deficit may include damage to the mechanoreceptors that relay information concerning static joint angle and also dynamic information during joint movement. Alternatively, it may be that the pain apparatus is impaired so that the protective sensation is lost. It is not uncommon, however, to find that, in a Charcot joint, pain is still discerned. Some authors believe on the basis of experiments in which the posterior nerve roots of cats have been sectioned that trauma in addition to deafferentation is necessary for the development of the neuropathic joint.[43] Others consider that neuropathy involving the sympathetic system leads to increased blood flow in the subchondral bone, which increases the osteoclastic activity and bone resorption, and that it is this lesion which underlies the changes in a Charcot joint.[18,19] It is possible that diabetic osteopathy is a separate condition from diabetic neuropathy. In the former, the joint destruction is secondary to bone destruction, whereas in the latter condition, the opposite is true. It may be that the pathological process is different if severe peripheral vascular disease associated with the neurological changes is present.[69]

SUMMARY

We may summarize this account by emphasizing the multifactorial nature of most forms of degenerative osteoarthritis. At the present time there is no satisfactory unifying theory to pinpoint the cause of the primary disease. Considering the considerable amount of research performed over the last decade, these complex processes are proving beyond simple solutions.

REFERENCES

Section A: Structure Function, and Repair

1. Akeson, W.H., and Gershuni, D.H. Articular cartilage physiology and metabolism in health and disease, in Resnick, D., and Niwayama, G. (eds): *Diagnosis of Bone and Joint Disorders,* vol, 1, no. 4. Philadelphia, Saunders, 1981, pp 175–194.
2. Albright, J.A., and Misra, R.P.M. Cartilage resorption and remodelling, in Hall, B.K. (ed): *Cartilage,* vol. III: *Biomedical Aspects.* New York, Academic Press, 1983, pp 59–86.
3. Altman, R.D., and Gray, R. Inflammation in osteoarthritis. Clin Rheum Dis 11:353–365, 1985.
4. Amiel, D., Coutts, A.D., Abel, R.D., Narwood, M., Stewart, W., and Akeson, W.H. Rib perichondrial grafts for the repair of full thickness articular cartilage defects: A morphological and biochemical assessment in rabbits. Trans Orthop Res Soc 262, 1985.
5. Anderson, C.E. The Structure and function of cartilage. J Bone Joint Surg 44A:777, 1962.
6. Anderson, C.E., Ludoweg, N.A., and Engleman, E.D. The composition of the orgainic component of human articular cartilage. J Bone Joint Surg 46A:1176, 1964.
7. Armstrong, C.G., and Mow, V.C. Variations in the intrinsic mechanical properties of human articular cartilage with age, degeneration and water content. J Bone Joint Surg 64A:88, 1982.
8. Armstrong, C.G., and Mow, V.C. Friction, lubrication and wear of synovial joints, in Owen, R., Goodfellow, J., Bullough, P. (eds): *Scientific Foundations of Orthopaedics and Traumatology.* Philadelphia, Saunders, 1980.
9. Aydelotte, M.D., and Kuettner, K.E. A comparative study of chondrocytes isolated from different depths of articular cartilage. Trans Orthop Res Soc 102 1985.
10. Benninghoff, A. Form und Bau der Gelenkknorpel in ihren Beziehungen zur Funktion. Z Anat Entwicklungsgesch 76:43, 1925.
11. Bloebaum, R.D., and Wilson, A.S. The morphology of the surface of articular cartilage in adult rats. J Anat 13:333, 1981.
12. Bloebaum, R.D., Wilson, A.S., and Clarke, I.C. Collagen fiber continuity and the radial fibrillar architecture in articular cartilage. Trans Orthop Res Soc 290, 1984.
13. Bloebaum, R.D., Jung, I., and Esposito, M. Macroscopic dissection of parallel fibers in human articular cartilage. Trans Orthop Res Soc 58, 1985.
14. Born, C.T. et al. The role of lysosomes in antigen induced arthritis. Trans Orthop Res Soc 7:216, 1982.
15. Bornstein, P., and Traub, W. The chemistry and biology of collagen, in Neurath, H., and Hill, R.L. (ed): *The Proteins,* 3d ed., vol IV. New York, Academic Press, 1979.
16. Broom, N.D., and Poole, C.A. A functional morphological study of the tidemark region of articular cartilage maintained in a nonviable physiological condition. J Anat 135:65, 1982.
17. Broom, N.D. Abnormal softening in articular cartilage. Arthritis Rheum 25:1209, 1982.
18. Brower, T.D., Akakoshi, Y., and Orlic, P. The diffusion of dyes through articular cartilage in vivo. J Bone Joint Surg 44A:456, 1967.
19. Brower, T.D., and Hsu, W. Normal articular cartilage. Clin Orthop 64:9, 1962.
20. Buckwalter, J.A. Articular cartilage, in Evarts, C.M. (ed): *Instructional Course Lecture Series,* vol 32, 1983, pp 349–369.

21. Buckwalter, J.A. Proteoglycan structures in calcifying cartilages. Clin orthop 172:207, 1983.

22. Bullough, P. Cartilage, in Owen, R., Goodfellow, J., and Bullough P. (eds): *Scientific Foundations of Orthopaedics and Traumatology.* Philadelphia, Saunders, 1980.

23. Bullough, P., and Goodfellow, J: The significance of the fine structure of articular cartilage. J Bone Joint Surg 50B:852, 1968.

24. Bullough, P.G., and Jagannath, A. The morphology of the calcified front in articular cartilage. J Bone Joint Surg 65B:72–78, 1983.

25. Bywaters, E.C.L. The metabolism of joint tissues. J Pathol Bactiol 44:277, 1937.

26. Calandruccio, R.A., and Gilmer, W.S. Proliferation, regeneration and repair of articular cartilage of immature animals. J Bone Joint Surg 44A:431, 1962.

27. Campbell, C. The healing of cartilage defects. Clin Orthop 64:45, 1969.

28. Cheung, H.S., Cottrell, W.H., Stephenson, K., and Nimni, M.E. In vitro collagen biosythesis in healing and normal articular rabbit articular cartilage. J Bone Joint Surg 60A:1076, 1978.

29. Clark, I.C. Human articular surface contours and related surface depressions frequency studies. Ann Rheum Dis 30:15, 1971.

30. Clarke, I.C. Articular cartilage: A review and scanning electron microscope study. Part I. The interterritorial fibrillar architecture. J Bone Joint Surg 53B:732, 1971.

31. Collins, D.H. *The Pathology of Articular and Spinal Disease.* London, E. Arnold, 1949.

32. Cooke, T.D.V. How does the mechanism of cartilage destruction influence surgical management of the rheumatoid joint. J Rheumatol 7:119–123, 1980.

33. Cooke, T.D.V. Pathogenetic mechanisms in polyarthicular osteoarthritis. Clin Rheum Dis 11:203–238, 1985.

34. Coventry, F.R., Akeson, W.H., and Keown, G.H. The repair of large osteochondral defects. Clin Orthop 82:253, 1972.

35. Curtiss, P.H. Cartilage damage in septic arthritis. Clin Orthop 64:87, 1969.

36. Curtiss, P.H., and Klein, L. Destruction of articular cartilage in septic arthritis I, in vitro study. J Bone Joint Surg 45A:797, 1963.

37. Curtiss, P.H., and Klein, L. Destruction of articular cartilage in septic arthritis II, in vivo study. J Bone Joint Surg 47A:1595, 1965.

38. Davies, D.V., Barnett, C.N., Cochran, W., and Palfrey, A.J. Electron microscopy of articular cartilage in the young adult rabbit. Ann Rheum Dis 21:11, 1962.

39. Davis, W.H., Lee, S.L., and Sokoloff, L. Boundary lubricating ability of synovial fluid in degenerative joint disease. Arthritis Rheum 21:754, 1978.

40. Davis, W.H., Lee, S.L., and Sokoloff, L.A. Proposed model of boundary lubrication by synovial fluid: Structuring of boundary water. J Biomech Eng 101:185, 1979.

41. DeBont, L.G.M., Boering, G., Havinga, D., and Liem, R.S. Spatial arrangement of collagen fibrils in the articular cartilage of mandibular condyles. J Oral Maxillofac Surg 24:306, 1984.

42. Denkel, S.L., and Weissman, R. Joint changes after overuse and peak overloading of rabbit knees in vivo. Acta Orthop Scand 49:519, 1978.

43. DePalma, A.F., McKeever, C.D., and Subin, D.K. Process of repair of articular cartilage demonstrated by histology and autoradiography with tritiated thymidine. Clin Orthop 48:299, 1966.

44. Dimitrovsky, E., Lane, L.B., and Bullough, P.B. The characterization of the tidemark in human articular cartilage. Metab Bone Dis Relat Res 1:115, 1978.

45. Edwards, C.C., and Chrisman, O.D. Articular cartilage, in Albright, J.A., and Brand, R.A., (eds): *The Scientific Basis of Orthopaedics.* New York, Appleton-Century-Crofts, 1979.

46. Eisenberg, S.R., and Grodzinsky, A.J. Swelling of articular cartilage and other connective tissues: Electromechanochemical forces. J Orthop Res 3:148, 1985.

47. Eyre, D.R. Collagen: Molecular diversity in the body's protein scaffold. Science 207:1314, 1980.

48. Fawns, N.T., and Landells, J.W. Histochemical studies of rheumatic conditions. I. Observations on the fine structure of the matrix of normal bone and cartilage. Ann Rheum Dis 12:105, 1953.

49. Freeman, M.A.R. *Adult Articular Cartilage.* New York, Grune and Stratton, 1974.

50. Fuller, J.A., and Ghadially, F.N. Ultrastructural observations on surgically produced partial thickness defects in articular cartilage. Clin Orthop 86:193, 1972.

51. Furkowa, T., Eyre, D.R., Koide, D., and Glimcher, M.J. Biochemical studies on repair of cartilage resurfacing experimental defects in the rabbit knee. J Bone Joint Surg 62A:79, 1980.

52. Gay, S., and Rhodes, P.K. Immunohistologic demonstrations of distinct collagens in normal and osteoarthritic joints. Semin Arthritis Rheum 11(suppl 1):43, 1981.

53. Ghadially, F.N. Fine structure of joints, in Sokoloff, L. (eds): *The Joints and Synovial Fluid,* vol I. New York, Academic Press, 1978.

54. Ghadially, F.N. *Fine Structure of Synovial Joints.* London, Butterworth, 1983.

55. Ghadially, F.N., Muschurchak, F.M., and Thomas, I. Humps on young human and rabbit articular cartilage. J Anat 124:425, 1977.

56. Grant, M.F., and Prockop, D.J. The biosynthesis of collagen, parts 1, 2, 3. *N Engl Med* 286:194, 242, 291, 1972.

57. Green, W.T., Martin, G.N., Eanes, E., and Sokoloff, L. Microradiographic study of the calcified layer of articular cartilage. *Arch Pathol* 90:151, 1970.

58. Hall, B.K. Tissue interactions and chondrogenesis, in Hall, B.K. (ed): *cartilage,* vol 2; *Development Differentiation and Growth.* New York, Academic Press, 1983, pp 309–338.

59. Hall, B.K. Bioelectricity and cartilage, in Hall, B.K. (ed): *Cartilage,* vol 3: *Biomedical Aspects.* New York, Academic Press, 1983, pp 309–338.

60. Hamerman, D., and Schubert, M. Diarthrodial joints: An essay. Am J Med 33:355, 1962.

61. Harris, E.D., Parker, H.G., Radin, E.L., and Drane, S.M. Effects of proteolytic enzymes on structural and mechanical properties of cartilage. Arthritis Rheum 15:497, 1972.

62. Hewitt, A.T. et al. The isolation and partial characterization of chondronectin in an attachment. J Biol Chem 257–2330–2334 1982.

63. Hough, A.J., Banfield, W.G., Mottrom, F., and Sokoloff, L. The osteochondral junction of mammalian joints. Lab Invest 31:685, 1974.

64. Hulth, A., Lindberg, L., and Telhag, H. Mitosis in human osteoarthritic cartilage. Clin Orthop 84:197, 1972.

65. Johanson, N., Vigorita, V.J., Goldam, and Salvati, E.A. Acromegalic arthropathy of the hip. Clin Orthop 173:130, 1983.

66. Jones, I.L., and Lemperg, R. The glycosaminoglycans of human articular cartilage. Clin Orthop 127:257, 1977.

67. Jurvelin, J., Kuvsela, T., Heikkila, R., Pelttari, A., Kivirenji, I., Tammi, M., and Heminen, H.J. Investigation of articular cartilage surface morphology with a semiquantitative scanning electron microscopy method. Acta Anat 116:302, 1983.

68. Keiser, H., Greenwald, R.A., Feinstein, G., and Janoff, A. Degradation of cartilage proteoglycan by human leukocyte granule neutral proteases: A model of joint injury, parts I and II. J Clin Invest 57:615, 5:625, 1976.

69. Kember, N.F. Cell kinetics of cartilage, in Hall, B.K. (ed): *Cartilage,* vol 1: *Structure and Function.* New York, Academic Press, 1983, pp 149–180.

70. Kempson, G.E. Mechanical properties of articular cartilage, in Freeman, M.A.R. (eds): *Adult Articular Cartilage.* Turnbridge, England, Pitman Medical, 1979.

71. Kempson, G.E. The mechanical properties of articular cartilage, in Sokoloff, L. (ed): *The Joints and Synovial Fluid,* vol II. New

York, Academic Press, 1980.

72. Kempson, G.E., et al. The effect of proteoglycolytic enzymes on the mechanical properties of adult human articular cartilage. Biochem Biophys Acta 428:741, 1976.

73. Kleinmann, H.K., et al. Role of collagenous matrices in the adhesion and growth of cells. J Cell Biol 88:473–485, 1981.

74. Kudic, J.A., and Blosser, J.A. Elasticity of articular cartilage. Clin Orthop 64:21, 1969.

75. Lane, J.M., and Weiss, C. Review of articular cartilage, collagen research. Arthritis Rheum 18:553, 1975.

76. Lash, J.W., and Vasan, M.S. Glycosaminoglycans, in Hall, B.K. (ed): *Cartilage,* vol 1: *Structure, Function and Biochemistry.* Academic Press, New York, 1983, p 237.

77. Linn, F.C. Lubrication of animal joints, I: The arthrotripsometer. J Bone Joint Surg 49A:1079, 1967.

78. Linn, F.C. Lubrication of animal joints, II: The mechanism. *J Biomech* 1:103, 1968.

79. Linn, F.C., and Radin, E.L. Lubrication of animal joints, III: Effect of chemical alterations of the cartilage and lubricant. Arthritis Rheum 11:5, 1968.

80. Linn, F.C., and Sokoloff, L. Movement and composition of interstitial fluid of cartilage. Arthritis Rheum 8:481, 1985.

81. Lyon, N.B., and Pottenger, L.A. Influence of type II collagen on the immobilization of proteoglycans within an artificial mesh. Trans Orthop Res Soc, 10:363, 1985.

82. MacConnai, M.A. The movements of bones and joints, 4. The mechanical structure of articulating cartilage. J Bone Joint Surg 33:251, 1951.

83. Malemud, C.J., and Sokoloff, L. The effect of prostaglandins on cultured laine articular chondrocytes. Prostaglandins 13:845–860, 1977.

84. Mankin, H.J. The response of articular cartilage to mechanical injury. J Bone Joint Surg 64A:460, 1982.

85. Mankin, H.J. Localization of tritiated thymidine in articular cartilage of rabbits. I. Growth in immature cartilage. J Bone Joint Surg 44A:682, 1962.

86. Mankin, H.J. Localization of tritiated thymidine in articular cartilage of rabbits. III. Mature articular cartilage. J Bone Joint Surg 45A:529, 1963.

87. Mankin, H.J. The articular cartilages: A review. Instr Course Lect 19:204, 1970.

88. Marchesi, V.T. Inflammation and healing, in Kissane, J.M. (ed): *Anderson's Pathology.* St Louis, Mosby, 1985.

89. Marcus, R.A. The effect of low oxygen concentration on growth, glycolysis and sulfate incorporation by articular chondrocytes in monolayer culture. Arthritis Rheum 16:646, 1973.

90. Maroudas, A. Balance between swelling pressure and collagen tension in normal and degenerate cartilage. Nature 260:808, 1976.

91. Maroudas, A., Bullough, P., Swanson, S.A.V., and Freeman, M.A.R. The permeability of articular cartilage. J Bone Joint Surg 50B:166, 1968.

92. Maroudas, A., and Evans H. Sulphate diffusion and incorporation into human articular cartilage. Biochem Biophys Acta 338:265 1977.

93. Mayne, R., and Vandermark, K. Collagens of cartilage, in Hall, B.K. (ed): *Cartilage,* vol 1. New York, Academic Press, 1983.

94. McCutchen, C.W. Lubrication of joints, in Sokoloff, L. (ed): *The Joints and Synovial Fluid,* vol I. New York, Academic Press, 1978.

95. McCutchen, C.W. Lubrication of and by articular cartilage, in Hall, B.K. (ed): *Cartilage,* vol 3: *Biomedical Aspects.* New York, Academic Press, 1983, pp 87–107.

96. McDevitt, C.A., and Muir, I.H.M. Biochemical changes in cartilage of the knee in experimental and natural osteoarthritis in the dog. J Bone Joint Surg 58B:94, 1976.

97. McKibbin, B., and Maroudas, A. Nutrition and metabolism, in Freeman, M.A.R. (ed): *Adult Articular Cartilage.* Turnbridge, Eng-

land, Pitman Medical, 1979.

98. Meachim, G. The Effect of scarification on articular cartilage in the rabbit. J Bone Joint Surg 45B:150, 1963.

99. Meachim, G. Age changes in articular cartilage. Clin Orthop 64:33, 1969.

100. Meachim, G. and Collins, D.H. Cell counts of normal and osteoarthritic articular cartilage in relation to the uptake of sulphate (S^{35}) in vitro. Ann Rheum Dis 2:15, 1967.

101. Meachim, G., and Stockwell, R.A. The matrix, in Freeman, M.A.R. (ed): *Adult Articular Cartilage.* Turnbridge, England, Pitman Medical 1979.

102. Miller, E.J. The collagen of joints, in Sokoloff, L. (ed): *The Joints and Synovial Fluid,* vol II. New York, Academic Press, 1978.

103. Mitchell, N., and Shepard, N. The resurfacing of adult rabbit articular cartilage by multiple perforations through the subchondral bone. J Bone Joint Surg 58A:230, 1976.

104. Mitchell, N., and Shepard, N. Healing of articular cartilage in intraarticular fracture in rabbits. J Bone Joint Surg 62A:628, 1980.

105. Mort, J.S., Poole, A.R., and Roughley, P.J. The molecular composition of cartilage link proteins following chemical deglycosylation. Trans Orthop Res Soc 226, 1984.

106. Mow, V.C., Holmes, M.H., and Lai, W.M. Fluid transport and mechanical properties of articular cartilage: A review. J Biomech 17:377, 1985.

107. Muir, H., Bullough, P., and Maroudas, A. The distribution of collagens in human articular cartilage with some of its physiologic implications. J Bone Joint Surg 52B:554, 1970.

108. Myers, E.R., and Mow, V.C. Biomechanics of cartilage and its response to biomechanical stimuli, in Hall, B.K. (ed). *Cartilage,* vol I. New York, Academic Press, 1983.

109. O'Driscoll, S.W., and Salter, R.B. The induction of neochondrogenesis in free intraarticular periosteal autografts under the influence of continuous passive motion. J Bone Joint Surg 66A:1248, 1984.

110. O'Driscoll, S.W., Kelley, F.W., and Salter, R.B. Regenerated articular cartilage produced by free periosteal grafts: The effect of CPM on its long term durability. Trans Orthop Res Soc 292, 1985.

111. Palfrey, A.J., and Davies, D.V. The fine structure of chondrocytes. J Anat 100:213, 1966.

112. Parsons, J.R., MacManus E., and Johnson, E. Time dependent histologic and mechanical alteration of articular cartilage with joint sepsis. Trans Orthop Res Soc 7:217, 1982.

113. Phadke, K. Regulation of metabolism of the chondrocyte in articular cartilage: An hypothesis. J Rheum 10:852, 1983.

114. Poole, A.R. Physiology of cartilage formation and destruction, in Cruess, R.L. (ed): *The Musculoskeletal System.* New York, Churchill Livingstone, 1982.

115. Prins, A.P.A., Lipman, J.M., and Sokoloff, L. Effect of purified growth factors on rabbit articular chondrocytes in monolayer culture. I. DNA synthesis. Arthritis Rheum 25:1217, 1982.

116. Prins, A.P.A., Lipman, J.M., McDevitt, C.A., and Sokoloff, L. The effect of purified growth factors in articular chondrocytes in monolayer culture, II: Sulfated proteoglycan synthesis. Arthritis Rheum 25:1228, 1982.

117. Radin, E.L., Ehrlich, M.G., Chernack, R., Abernathy, P., Paul, I.L., and Rose, R.M. Effect of repetitive impulsive loading on the knee joints of rabbits. Clin Orthop 131:228, 1978.

118. Radin, E.L., and Paul, I.L. Consolidated concept of joint lubrication. J Bone Joint Surg 54A:607, 1972.

119. Radin, E.L., Paul, I.L., and Lowy, M. A comparison of the dynamic force transmitting properties of subchondral bone and articular cartilage. J Bone Joint Surg 52A:444, 1970.

120. Ramachandran, G.N., and Am, H. *Biochemistry of Collagen.* New York, Plenum Press, 1976.

121. Redler, I., Mow, V.C., Zimni, M., and Mansell, J. The ultrastructure and biomechanical significance of the tidemark of articular cartilage. Clin Orthop 112:357, 1975.

122. Reimann, I., Christensen, S.B., and Diemer, N.H. Observations of reversibility of glycosaminoglycan depletion in articular cartilage. Clin Orthop 169:253, 1982.

123. Repo, R.U., and Finlay, J.B. Survival of articular cartilage after controlled impact. J Bone Joint Surg 59A:1068, 1977.

124. Roberts, B.J., Unsworth, A., and Mian, N. Modes of lubrication of human hip joints. Ann Rheum Dis 41:217, 1982.

125. Rodnan, G.P., and Schumacher, H.J. The connective tissues: Structure, functions, and metabolisms, in *Primer of the Rheumatic Diseases,* 8th ed. New York, Arthritis Foundation, 1983.

126. Rosenberg, L. Structure of cartilage proteoglycans, in Burleigh, P.M.C., and Poole, A.R. (eds): *Dynamics of Connective Tissue Macromolecules.* Amsterdam, North Holland Publishing 1975.

127. Roth, V., and Mow, V.C. The intrinsic tensile behavior of the matrix of bovine articular cartilage and its variation with age. J Bone Joint Surg 62A:1102, 1980.

128. Rothwell, A.G., and Bently, G. Chondrocyte multiplication in osteoarthritic articular cartilage. J Bone Joint Surg 55B:588, 1973.

129. Salter, R.B., Simmonds, D.F., Malcolm, B.W. Rumble, E.J., MacMichael, D., and Clements, N.D. The biological effect of continuous passive motion on the healing of full thickness defects in articular cartilage. J Bone Joint Surg 62A:1232, 1980.

130. Sheldon, H. Transmission electron microscopy of cartilage, in Hall, B.K. (ed): *Cartilage,* vol 1: *Structure, Function and Biochemistry.* New York, Academic Press, 1983, pp 87–194.

131. Silberg, R. Ultrastructure of articular cartilage in health and disease. Clin Orthop 57:233, 1968.

132. Simmons, D.P., and Chrisman, O.D. Salicylate inhibition of cartilage degeneration. Arthritis Rheum 8:960, 1965.

133. Smith, R.L., Gilkerson, E., Kajiyama, G., and Schurman, D.J. Differential proteoglycan loss from cartilage in staphylococcus infections. Trans Orthop Res Soc 338, 1984.

134. Sokoloff, L. Aging and degeneration of cartilage, in Hall, B.K. (ed): *Cartilage,* vol 3: *Biomedical Aspects.* New York, Academic Press, 1983, 109–141.

135. Sokoloff, L., personal communication.

136. Sokoloff, L., and Hough, A.J., Jr. Pathology of osteoarthritis, in McCarty, D.J. (ed): *Arthritis and Allied Conditions,* 10th ed. Philadelphia, Lea and Febiger, 1984.

137. Speer, D.P., and Kahners, L. The collagenous architecture of articular cartilage. Clin Orthop 139:257, 1979.

138. Stockwell, R.A. The cell density of human articular and costal cartilage. J Anat 101:753, 1967.

139. Stockwell, R.A. *Biology of Cartilage Cells.* Cambridge, Cambridge University Press, 1979.

140. Stockwell, R.A., and Scott J.E. Distributions of acid glycosaminoglycans in human articular cartilage. Nature 215:1376, 1967.

141. Stockwell, R.A., and Meachim, G. The chondrocytes, in Freeman, M.A.R. (ed): *Adult Articular Cartilage.* Turnbridge, England, Pitman Medical 1979.

142. Swann, D.A., Bloch, K.J., Sotman, S., Shipner, R., and Swindell, D. Isolation of a purified glycoprotein lubrication fraction from human synovial fluid. Arthritis Rheum

143. Swann, D.A., Bloch, K.J., Swindell, D., and Shore, E. The lubricating activity of human synovial fluids. Arthritis Rheum 27:552, 1984.

144. Swann, D.A., Henren, R.B., Radin, E.L., Sotman, S.L., and Duda, E.A. The lubricating activity of synovial fluid glycoproteins. Arthritis Rheum 24:22, 1981.

145. Swann, D.A., Radin, E.L., and Hendren, R.B. The lubrication of articular cartilage by synovial fluid glycoprotein. Arthritis Rheum 22:665, 1969.

146. Swann, D.A., Radin, E.L., Nazimiec, M., Weisser, P.A., Curran, N., and Lewinnek, G. Role of hyaluronic acid in joint lubrication. Ann Rheum Dis 33:318, 1974.

147. Swann, D.A., Slayter, H.S., and Silver, F.H. The molecular structure of lubricating glycoprotein, I: The boundary lubricant for articular cartilage. J Biol Chem 256:5921, 1981.

148. Thompson, R.C. An experimental study of the surface injury to articular cartilage and enzyme responses that weaken the joint. Clin Orthop 197:231, 1975.

149. Thompson, R.C., and Robinson, H.J., Jr. Current concepts review articular cartilage matrix metabolism. J Bone Joint Surg 63A:327–331, 1981.

150. Torzilli, P.A. Influence of cartilage conformation on its equilibrium water partition. J Orthop Res 3:473–482, 1985.

151. Urist, M.R. The origin of cartilage: Investigations in quest of chondrogenic DNA, in Hall, B.K. (ed): *Cartilage,* vol 2: *Development, Differentiation and Growth.* New York, Academic Press, 1983, pp 1–85.

152. Vasan, N. Effects of physical stress on the synthesis and degradation of cartilage matrix. Connect Tissue Res 12:49, 1983.

153. Weiss, C., Rosenberg, L., and Helfet, A. An ultrastructural study of normal young adult human articular cartilage. J Bone Joint Surg 50A:663, 1968.

154. Weiss, C., Shapiro, F., Trahan, C., and Altmann, K. The tangential zone of articular cartilage. J Bone Joint Surg 57A:584, 1975.

155. Whipple, R.R., Gobbs, M.C., Lai, W.M., Mow, V.C., Mak, A.F., and Wirth, C.R. Biphasic properties of repaired cartilage at the articular surface. Trans Orthop Res Soc, 1985.

156. Williams, P.L., and Warwick, R. (eds): *Gray's Anatomy,* 36th ed. Philadelphia, Saunders, 1980.

157. Wood, D.D., Ihrie, E.J., Dinarello, P.L.: Isolation of interleukin-l-like factor from human joint effusions. Arthritis Rheum 26:975–983, 1983.

Section B: Osteoarthritis

1. Adams, M.E., and Billingham, M.E.J. Animal model of degenerative joint disease. Curr Top Pathol 265, 1982.

2. Ali, S.Y., and Baylis, M.T. Cathepsin B and other proteases in human articular cartilage. Semin Arthritis Rheum 10(suppl 1):56, 1981.

3. Ali, S.Y. Crystal induced arthropathy, in Verbroggen, G., and Veys, E. (eds): *Degenerative Joints,* vol 2. New York, Excerpta Medica, 1985, p 357

4. Altman, R.D., and Gray R. Inflammation in osteoarthritis. Clin Rheum Dis 11:353, 1983.

5. Armstrong, C.G., and Mow, V.C. Variations in the intrinsic mechanical properties of human articular cartilage with age, degeneration and water content. J Bone Joint Surg 64A:88, 1982.

6. Barrett, A.J. Which proteases degrade cartilage matrix? Semin Arthritis Rheum 10(suppl 1):52, 1981.

7. Bentley, G. Papain induced degenerative arthritis of the hip in rabbits. J Bone Joint Surg 53A:32, 1971.

8. Bentley, G. Articular cartilage studies and osteoarthrosis. Ann R Coll Surg Engl 57:86, 1975.

9. Benya, P.D., Shaffer, J.D., and Nimni, M.E. Flexibility of the chondrocyte collagen phenotype. Semin Arthritis Rheum 19(suppl 1):43, 1981.

10. Bland, J.H., and Stulberg, S.D. Osteoarthritis: Pathology and clinical patterns, in Kelley, W.N. (ed): *Textbook of Rheumatology,* chap 89. Philadelphia, Saunders, 1981.

11. Blueston, R., et al. Acromegalic arthropathy. Ann Rheum Dis 30:258, 1971.

12. Bohr, H. Experimental osteoarthritis in the rabbit knee joint. Acta Orthop Scand 47:558, 1976.

13. Bollet, A.J. Connective tissue polysaccharide metabolism and pathogenesis of osteoarthritis. Adv Inter Med 13:33, 1967.

14. Bracker, W.D., and Martinique, R. An ultrastructural evaluation on the effect of hydrocortisone on rabbit cartilage. Clin Orthop 115:286–290, 1976.

15. Brandt, K.D. Pathogenesis of osteoarthritis, in Kelley, W.N. (ed): *Textbook of Rheumatology,* Philadelphia, Saunders, 1981.

16. Brandt, K.D., and Palmoski, M. Organization of ground substance proteoglycans in normal and osteoarthritic knee cartilage. Arthritis Rheum 19:209, 1976.

17. Brocklehurst, R., Baylis, M.T., Maroudas, A., Coysh, H.L., Obst, D., Freeman, M.A.R., Revell, P.A., and Ali, S.Y. The composition of normal and osteoarthritic articular cartilage from human knee joints: With special reference to unicompartmental replacement and osteotomy of the knee. J Bone Joint Surg 66A:95, 1984.

18. Brower, A.C., and Allman, R.M. The neuropathic joint in neurovascular bone disorder. Radiol Clin North Am 19:571–580, 1981.

19. Brower, A.C., and Allman, R.M. Pathogenesis of the neurotropic joint: Neurotropic vs. neurovascular. Radiology 139:349–354, 1981.

20. Bullough, P. Synovial and osseous inflammation in osteoarthritis. Semin Arthritis Rheum 10(suppl 1):146, 1981.

21. Bullough, P.G., Goodfellow, J., and O'Connor, J.J. The relationship between degenerative changes and load-bearing in the human hip. J Bone Joint Surg 55B:746, 1973.

22. Carney, S.L., Billingham, M.E.J., Muir, H., and Sandy, J.D. Structure of newly synthesized (^{35}S)-proteoglycans and (^{35}S)-proteoglycan turnover products of cartilage explant cultures from dogs with experimental osteoarthritis. J Orthop Res 3:140, 1985.

23. Caterson, B., et al. Diabetes and osteoarthritis. Ala J Med Sci 17:292, 1980.

24. Chrisman, O.D., et al. The relationship of mechanical trauma and the early biochemical reactions of osteoarthritic cartilage. Clin Orthop 161:38, 1981.

25. Chrisman, O.D., Ladenbauer-Bellis, I.M., and Fulkerson, J.D. The osteoarthritic cascade and associated drug actions. Semin Arthritis Rheum. 10(suppl 1):145, 1981.

26. Cooke, T.D.V. Immune deposits in osteoarthritic cartilage— Their relationships to synovitis, disease site and pattern. Semin Arthritis Rheum. 10(suppl 1):109, 1981.

27. Cooke, T.D.V. Pathogenetic mechanisms in polyarticular osteoarthritis. Clin Rheum Dis 11:203–238, 1985.

28. Dayer, J.M. Cellular and humoral factors modulate connective tissue destruction and repair in arthritic diseases. Semin Arthritis Rheum 10(suppl 1):77 1981.

29. Deshmukh-Phadke, K. Macrophage factor that induces neutral protease secretion by normal rabbit chondrocytes. Eur J Biochem 104:175, 1980.

30. Dequeker, J. Relationship between osteoporosis and osteoarthritis. Clin Rheum Dis 11:271–296 (1985).

31. DeVries, B.J., Van Denberg, W.B., and Van de Putte, L.B.A. Salicylate induced depletion of endogenous inorganic sulfate. Arthritis Rheum 28:922, 1985.

32. Dieppe, P.A. Inflammation in osteoarthritis and the role of microcrystals. Semin Arthritis Rheum 10(suppl 1):121, 1981.

33. Dieppe, P.A. Osteoarthritis, Are we asking the wrong question? Br J Rheum 23:161, 1984.

34. Dieppe, P.A., and Watt, T. Crystal deposition in osteoarthritis: An opportunistic event? Clin Rheum Dis 11:367–392, 1985.

35. Dingle, J.T. The role of catabolin in arthritic damage. Semin Arthritis Rheum 10(suppl 1):82, 1981.

36. Dingle, J.T. The role of cellular interactions in joint erosions. Clin Orthop 182:24, 1984.

37. Dingle, J.T., Saklatvala, J., Hembry, R., Tyler, J., Fell, H.B., Jubb, R. A cartilage catabolic factor from synovium. Biochem J 184:177, 1979.

38. Duncan, E. Cellular mechanisms of bone damage and repair in the arthritic joint. Rheumatology 4 (suppl):29, 1983.

39. Ehrlich, M.C. Patterns of proteoglycan degradation by a neutral protease from human growth-plate epiphyseal cartilage. J Bone Joint Surg 64A:1350, 1982.

40. Ehrlich M.C. Degradative enzymes in osteoarthritic cartilage. J Orthop Res 3:160, 1985.

41. Ehrlich, M.C. Mankin, H.J., Jones H., Grossman, A., Crispin, C., and Anacona, D. Biochemical confirmation of an experimental model of osteoarthritis. J Bone Joint Surg 57A:392, 1975.

42. Einhorn, T.A., Gordon, S., Siegel, S.A., Hummel, C., Avitable, M.J., and Carty, R.P. Matrix vesicle enzymes in human osteoarthritis. J Orthop Res 3:160, 1985.

43. Eloesser, L. On the nature of neuropathic affection of joints. Ann Surg 66:201–207, 1917.

44. Evans, C.H., Mears, D.A., and McKnight, J.L. A preliminary ferrographic survey of the wear particles in human synovial fluid. Arthritis Rheum 24:912, 1981.

45. Farfan, H.F. On the nature of osteoarthritis. Rheumatology 10(suppl 9):103, (1983).

46. Fell, H.B., and Jubb, R.W. The effect of synovial tissue on the breakdown of articular cartilage in organ culture. Arthritis Rheum 20:1359, 1977.

47. Gandner, D.L. The nature and causes of osteoarthritis. Br Med J 286:418, 1983.

48. Gay, S., and Rhodes, R.K. Immunohistologic demonstration of distinct collagens in normal and osteoarthritic joints. Semin Arthritis Rheum 10(suppl 1):43, 1981.

49. Gay, S., et al. Immunohistological study on collagen in cartilage-bone metamorphosis and degenerative osteoarthrosis. Klin Wochenschr 54:969, 1976.

50. Gibson, T., et al. Effect of intraarticular corticosteroid injections on primate cartilage. Ann Rheum Dis 36:74–79 1976.

51. Gilbertson, E.M.M. Development of periarticular osteophytes in experimentally induced osteoarthritis in the dog. Ann Rheum Dis 34:12, 1975.

52. Glyn, J.H. Heberden society. Ann Rheum Dis 32:387, 1973.

53. Grant, T., Mikecz, K., and Leva, G. The cell surface antigens of articular chondrocytes. Semin Arthritis Rheum 10(suppl 1):113, 1981.

54. Greisen, H.A., Lust G., and Summers, B.A. A morphological study of the synovial membrane and articular cartilage in the early stages of osteoarthritis in canine hip joints. Semin Arthritis Rheum 11(suppl 1):50–51, 1982.

55. Harris, E.D., Vater, C.A., Brinckerhoff, C.E., McMillan, R.M., and Hasselbacher, P. Patterns of regulation of collagen breakdown in articular cartilage. Semin Arthritis Rheum 10(suppl 1):69, 1981.

56. Havdrup, T., and Telhag, H. Papain-induced changes in the knee joints of adult rabbits. Acta Orthop Scand 48:143, 1977.

57. Hay, E.D. Origin and role of collagen in the embryo. Am Zool 13:1985, 1973.

58. Hoaglund, F.T. Experimental hemarthrosis. J Bone Joint Surg 49A:285, 1967.

59. Hoaglund, F.T. Osteoarthritis of the hip and other joints in southern Chinese in Hong Kong. J Bone Joint Surg 55A:545, 1973.

60. Hollander, J.L. Osteoarthritis perspectives on treatment. Postgrad Med 68:161–168, 1980.

61. Hough, A.J., Banfield, W.G., and Sokoloff, L: Cartilage in hemophilic arthopathy. Arch Pathol Lab Med 100:91, 1976.

62. Howell, D.S. The action of cathepsin D in human articular cartilage on proteoglycans. J Clin Invest 54:624, 1973.

63. Hulth, A., Linberg, L., and Telhag, H. Experimental osteoarthritis. Acta Orthop Scand 41:522, 1970.

64. Hulth, A. Experimental osteoarthritis. Acta Orthop Scand 53:1, 1982.

65. Huskisson, E.C., et al. Treatment of osteoarthritis. Clin Rheum Dis 11:421–431, 1985.

66. Inoue, H. Alterations in the collagen framework of osteoarthritic cartilage and subchondral bone. Int Orthop 5:147, 1981.

67. Jacobsen, K. Osteoarthrosis following insufficiency of the cruciate ligaments in man. Acta Orthop Scand 48:520, 1977.

68. Jimenez, S.A., Deiong, W.C., Bashey, R.I., and Brighton, C.T. Inhibition of proteoglycan degradation in rabbit articular cartilage organ cultures by superoxide dismutase and proteolytic enzyme inhibitors. Semin Arthritis Rheum 10(suppl 1):109, 1981.

69. Johanson, N.A. Endocrine arthropathies. Clin Rheum Dis 11:297–324, 1985.

70. Jukunen, I., Kiehela, J., and Julkunen, H. Etiological, social, and therapeutic aspects of osteoarthritis and soft tissue rheumatism in a Finnish health center material. Scand J Rheum 19:215, 1981.

71. Kellgren, J.H., and Lawrence, J.S. Rheumatism in minors. Br J Ind Med 9:197, 1952.

72. Kellgren, J.H., and Lawrence, J.S. Radiologic assessment of osteoarthrosis. Ann Rheum Dis 16:494, 1957.

73. Kellgren, J.H., and Lawrence, J.S. Osteo-arthrosis and disk degeneration in an urban population. Ann Rheum Dis 17:388, 1958.

74. Kellgren, J.H., and Moore, T. Generalized osteoarthritis and Heberden's nodes. Br Med J 1:181, 1952.

75. Kempson, G.E., Muir, H, et al. The tensile properties of the cartilage of human femoral condyles related to the content of collagen and glycosaminoglycans. Acta Biochem Biophys Acta 297:4561, 1973.

76. Kuettner, K., et al. Antiinvasion factor mediates avascularity of hyaline cartilage. Semin Arthritis Rheum 10(suppl 1):67, 1981.

77. Lane, J.M., Arnoczky, S.P., Savetsky, G.J., Warren, R., and Marshall, J.M. The effect of joint instability on periarticular matrix hexosamine and collagen content in rabbit and dog cruciate deficient osteoarthritic models. Semin Arthritis Rheum 10(suppl 1):49, 1981.

78. Lust, G., Hui-Chou, G.S., and Greisen, H.A. Collagen synthesis by cartilage from osteoarthritic canine joints. Semin Arthritis Rheum 10(suppl 1):47, 1981.

79. Malemud, C.J., Weitzman, G.A., Norby, D.P., Sapolsky, A.I., and Howell, D.S. Metal-dependent neutral proteoglycanase activity from monolayer cultured lapine articular chondrocytes. J Lab Clin Med 93:1018, 1979.

80. Malemud, C.J., Norby, D.P., Moskowitz, R.W., Goldberg, V.M., Sapolsky, A.I., and Howell, D.S. Neutral proteinases from articular cartilage chondrocytes in culture that degrade synthetic substrates and cartilage macromolecules. Semin Arthritis Rheum 1(suppl 1):61, 1981.

81. Mankes, C.J., Decraemera, W., Postel, M., and Forest, M. Chondrocalcinosis and rapid destruction of the hip. J Rheum 12:130, 1985.

82. Mankin, H.J. Current concepts review: The response of articular cartilage to mechanical injury. J Bone Joint Surg 64A:460, 1982.

83. Mankin, H.J. Biochemical and metabolic abnormalities in articular cartilage from osteoarthritic human hips. J Bone Joint Surg 63A:131, 1981.

84. Maroudas, A. Biophysical chemistry of cartilaginous tissue with special reference to solute and fluid transport. Biorheology 12:233, 1975.

85. Maroudas, A. Balance between swelling pressure and collagen tension in normal and degenerate cartilage. Nature 260:808, 1976.

86. Maroudas, A. Proteoglycan osmotic pressure and collagen tension in normal osteoarthritic human cartilage. Semin Arthritis Rheum 10(suppl 1):36, 1981.

87. Maroudas, A., and Venn, M. Chemical composition and swelling of normal and osteoarthritic femoral head cartilage. Ann Rheum Dis 36:399, 1977.

88. Martel-Pelletier, J., Pelletier, J.P., Cloutier, J.M., Howell, D.S., Ghandur-Mnaymheh, L, and Woessner, J.F. Neural processes capable of proteoglycan digesting activity in osteoarthritic and normal human articular cartilage. Arthritis Rheum 27:305, 1984.

89. Meachim, G. Cartilage breakdown, in Owen, R., Goodfellas, J., and Bullough, P. (eds): *Scientific Foundations of Orthopaedics and Traumatology.* Philadelphia, Saunders, 1980, pp 290–296.

90. Meachim, G., Whitehous, G.H., and Pedley, F.E., et al. An investigation of radiological, clinical and pathological correlations in osteoarthrosis of the hip. Clin Radiol 31:565, 1980.

91. Mikkelsen, W.M. Osteoarthritis: From the twenty-fourth rheumatism review. Arthritis Rheum 24:223, 1981.

92. Mitchell, N., and Shepard, N. Pericellular proteoglycan concentrations in early degenerative arthritis. Arthritis Rheum 24:958, 1981.

93. Morales, T.I., and Kuettner, K.E. Properties of the proteoglycan degrading enzyme released by the primary cultures of bovine articular chondrocyte. Semin Arthritis Rheum 10(suppl 1):59, 1981.

94. MoRetz, J.A., Goodrich, H.S., and Rod, J.W. Long-term followup of knee injuries in high school football players. Am J Sports Med 12:298, 1984.

95. Moskowitz, R. The biochemistry of osteoarthritis. Br J Reum 23:170, 1984.

96. Moskowitz et al. Experimentally induced corticosteriod arthropathy. Arthritis Rheum 13:236–243, 1970.

97. Mow, V.C., Myers, E.R., Roth, V., and Lalik, P. Implications for collagen-proteoglycan interactions from cartilage stress relaxation behavior in isometric tension. Semin Arthritis Rheum 10(suppl 1):41, 1981.

98. Muir, H. Structure and function of proteoglycans of cartilage and cell-matrix interactions, in Lash, J.W., and Berger, M.M. (eds): *Cell and Tissue Interaction.* New York, Raven Press, 1977, p 87.

99. Muir, H. Molecular approach to the understanding of osteoarthrosis. Ann Rheum Dis 36:199, 1977.

100. Muir, H. Proteoglycans: The state of the art. Semin Rheum 10(suppl 1):7, 1981.

101. O'Connor, B.L., Palmoski, M.J., and Brandt, K.D. Neurogenic acceleration of degenerative joint lesions. J Bone Joint Surg 67A:562, 1985.

102. Palmoski, M., and Brandt, K. Effect of joint disease and subsequent exercise on proteoglycan metabolism and aggregation in articular cartilage. Semin Arthritis Rheum 10:30, 1981.

103. Peyron, J. Inflammation in osteoarthritis: A review of its role in clinical picture, disease progress, subsets, and pathophysiology. Semin Arthritis Rheum 10(suppl 1):115, 1981.

104. Phadke, K. Regulation of metabolism of the chondrocytes in articular cartilage—An hypothesis. J Rheum 10:852, 1983.

105. Poole, A.R., et al. Extracellular localization of cathepsin D in ossifying cartilage. Calcif Tissue Int 12:313, 1973.

106. Radin, E.L. Role of mechanical factors in pathogenesis of osteoarthritis. Lancet 1:519, 1972.

107. Radin, E.L. Response of joints to impact loading. III: Relationship between trabecular microfractures and cartilage degeneration. J Biomech 6:51–57, 1973.

108. Radin, E.L., and Paul, I.L. Does cartilage compliance reduce skeletal impact loads. Arthritis Rheum 13:139–144, 1970.

109. Radin, E.L., and Paul, I.L. Response of joints to impact loading. In vitro wear. Arthritis Rheum 14:356, 1971.

110. Radin, E.L., Paul, I.L., and Lowy, M.A. Comparison of the dynamic force transmitting properties of subchondral bone and articular cartilage. J Bone Joint Surg 52A:444–448, 1970.

111. Reimann, I. Experimental osteoarthritis of the knee in rabbits induced by alteration of the load bearing. Acta Orthop Scand 44:496, 1973.

112. Ridge, S.C., Oronsky, A.L., and Kerwar, S.S. Induction of the synthesis of latent collagenase and latent neutral protease in chondrocytes by a factor synthesized by activated macrophages. Arthritis Rheum 23:448, 1980.

113. Rosenberg, I.C. Proteoglycans in developing cartilages. Semin Arthritis Rheum 10:25, 1981.

114. Rosner, F.A., Goldberg, V.M., Getzy, L., and Moskowitz, R.W. Ef-

fects of estrogens on cartilage and experimentally induced osteoarthritis. Arthritis Rheum 10(suppl 1):25, 1981.

115. Roughley, P.J., and Barrett, A.J. The degradation of cartilage proteoglycans by tissue proteinases. J Biochem 167:629, 1977.

116. Roughley, P.J. Age-related changes in the proteoglycan subunits isolated from human articular cartilage. Semin Arthritis Rheum 10(suppl 1):16, 1981.

117. Ryu, J., Treadwell, B.V., and Mankin, H.J. Biochemical and metabolic abnormalities in normal and osteoarthritic human articular cartilage. Arthritis Rheum 27:49, 1984.

118. Sandy, J.D., Adams, M.E., Billingham, M.E.J., Plaas, A., and Muir, H. In vitro and in vivo stimulation of chondrocyte biosynthetic activity in experimental osteoarthritis. Arthritis Rheum 27:388, 1984.

119. Sapolsky, A.I., Howell, D.S., and Woessner, J.F. Neutral proteases and cathepsin D in human articular cartilage. J Clin Invest 53:104, 1974.

120. Sapolsky, A.I. Neutral metalloproteases and their inhibitors from cultured articular chondrocytes. Semin Arthritis Rheum 10(suppl 1):71, 1981.

121. Saville, P.D., and Dickson, J. Age and weight in osteoarthritis of the hip. Arthritis Rheum 11:635, 1968.

122. Shaw, N.F., and Lacy, E. The influence of corticosteroid on the normal and papain treated epiphyseal growth plate in the rabbit. J Bone Joint Surg 55B:197–205, 1973.

123. Silfemann, M. Hormones and cartilage, in Hall, B.K. (ed): *Cartilage,* vol 2: *Development, Differentiation and Growth.* New York, Academic Press, 1983, pp 327–368.

124. Sokoloff, L. *The Biology of Degenerative Joint Disease.* Chicago, University of Chicago Press, 1969.

125. Sokoloff, L. The pathology of osteoarthritis. Semin Arthritis Rheum 10(suppl 1):3, 1981.

126. Sokoloff, L. Aging and degeneration of cartilage, in Hall, B.K. (ed): *Cartilage,* vol 3: *Biomedical Aspects.* New York, Academic Press, 1983, pp 109–141.

127. Sokoloff, L. Endemic forms of osteoarthritis. Clin Rheum Dis 11:187, 1985.

128. Sokoloff, L., personal communication, 1985.

129. Swann, D.A., Slayter, H.S., and Silver, F.M. The molecular structure of lubricating glycoprotein, I: The boundary lubricant of articular cartilage. J Biochem 256:5921, 1981.

130. Thompson, R.C., Jr. An experimental study of surface injury to articular cartilage and enzyme responses within the joint. Clin Orthop 107:239–248, 1975.

131. Thompson, R.C., Bassett, C., and Andrew, L. Histologic observations on experimentally induced degeneration of articular cartilage. J Bone Joint Surg 52A:435, 1970.

132. Troyer, H. Experimental models of osteoarthritis: A review. Semin Arthritis Rheum 11:362, 1982.

133. Walton, E.A. The role of serine protease inhibitors in normal and osteoarthritic human articular cartilage. Semin Arthritis Rheum 19(suppl 1):73, 1981.

134. Weiss, C. Ultrastructural study of aging articular cartilage. J Bone Joint Surg 53A:803, 1971.

135. Williams, J.M., and Brandt, K.D. Temporary immobilization facilitates repair of chemically induced articular cartilage injury. J Anat 138:435, 1984.

136. Woessner, J.F., Pelletier, J.P., Martel-Pelletier, J., Enis, J., and Howell, D.J. Direct measurement of cartilage collagenolytic activity in human osteoarthritis. Semin Arthritis Rheum 10(suppl 1):58, 1981.

CHAPTER 5

Synovial Membrane: Structure and Function

Thomas Dowling and Roger Dee

The synovial membrane lines all the intraarticular structures of the normal joint with the exception of articular cartilage and the main surfaces of the menisci[14] (though it may overlap their margins). Its surface is generally described as smooth and glistening, but villi occur in the region of the joint line and around the margins of the articular cartilage.[8]

It covers intraarticular ligaments, an important factor in ligament nutrition after injury. In large joints, such as the knee joint, it produces anatomically constant folds which may contribute to joint lubrication but which can also be a source of disease in the various "plica" syndromes.

SYNOVIAL MEMBRANE: STRUCTURE

The synovial membrane consists of two layers: the intimal, or cell lining, layer and the subintimal, or subsynovial, layer.

The Intimal Layer

This layer is located next to the joint cavity. It is very cellular, with a thickness varying from one to twelve cell layers but averaging about three or four cells thick.[4,9] This layer of synovial intimal cells is not continuous as in epithelium, and there may be gaps where cells are absent and the matrix is exposed to the joint space.[8] The cells sit in the matrix in a somewhat loose arrangement without either gap or tight junctions (but desmosomes may be seen in diseased synovium).[8] No basement membrane separates this intimal layer from the subsynovial layer, and there is a continual loss of cells and matrix at the surface, fresh matrix material being formed to replace it. Ghadially points out that this is in contrast to epithelia where only cells, not matrix, are shed.[8]

The normal synovial intima has two general cell types: A and B. The *type A* cell seems to be more numerous.[4,23] It has a prominent golgi complex and secretory vacuoles, and it is believed to have a secretory function in producing hyaluronic acid.[8] However it also has many features of a macrophage, and may play a part in phagocytosing debris from the joint space and in producing certain elements of synovial fluid.[4,9,12,23]

Type B cells in the synovial intima have a less prominent golgi complex, but there is more abundant, rough endoplasmic reticulum, which is consistent with the cell's function. It produces a protein-rich secretion that enriches the synovial fluid.[8,9,12,23] About 2 percent of the protein in the synovial fluid is of synovial origin firmly bound to hyaluronate.[8] In addition, a glycoprotein which represents about 0.5 percent of the total protein present in synovial fluid may be important in lubrication and is also probably synthesized by synovial intimal cells.[8,23,28] Much remains to be learned about the morphology of these cells in relation to their function. There is some evidence for the existence of a third *(type AB)* cell, and the possibility exists that there may be changes in morphology between one type or another according to functional needs[8,9] (Fig. 5-1).

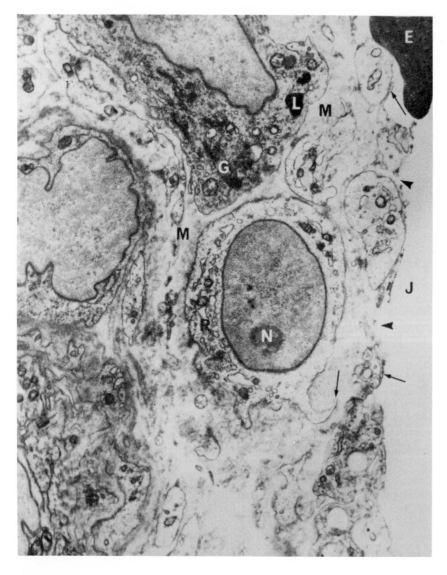

Figure 5-1 Synovial intima from a normal human knee joint. The synovial cells are set loosely in a matrix (M) which is exposed (arrowheads) to the joint space (J) in places. A type A cell with prominent golgi complex (G) and lysosome (L) is easily distinguished from a type B cell with some rough endoplasmic reticulum (R) even at this low magnification. Note nucleus containing a nucleolus (N), cell process (arrow), and an erythrocyte (E) lying in the adjoining space. Original ×9250. *(From Ghadially, F.N.: Fine Structure of Synovial Joints. London, Butterworth, 1983. Reproduced with permission.)*

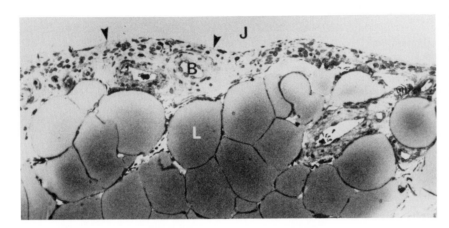

Figure 5-2 Adipose synovial membrane from a normal human knee joint. The synovial intima presents as a layer of cells (three or four cells deep) lying in a matrix that in some places is exposed (arrowheads) to the joint space (J). Blood vessels (B) and lipocytes containing large lipid (L) droplets are seen in the subintimal tissue. Original ×216. *(From Ghadially, F.N.: Fine Structure of Synovial Joints. London, Butterworth, 1983. Reproduced with permission.)*

The Subintimal (Subsynovial) Layer

Beneath the intimal layer lies the second layer of the synovial membrane known as the *subintimal*, or *subsynovial layer.* Most of the blood vessels of this more vascular layer lie just beneath the intima. This layer is also much more varied in structure than the intimal layer. Variation may take place in different places in the same joint as well as between different joints. In a fibrous type of synovial membrane, this layer contains numerous collagen fibers. The tissue may also be a more fatty (areolar) type with a sparser distribution of fibers. Here, the intervening space is occupied by lipid-containing cells. An intermediate fibroareolar subintimal tissue has also been described[8,9] (Fig. 5-2).

INNERVATION OF SYNOVIUM

Unlike the intimal layer, some nerve fibers are present which are associated with blood vessels.[7] Some free nerve endings and complex unencapsulated nerve endings have been described.[4,10,11] The synovial membrane is relatively insensate to painful stimulation. However, any mechanical deformation is transmitted to the deeper layer and to the richly innervated joint capsule, which is believed to mediate most pain sensation in the joint.[4]

The degree of vascularity of the synovium depends upon the morphology of the subintimal layer being less profuse in the fibrous type of tissue. Synovium is much more vascular than joint capsule.[4] At the articular margins the vessels of the synovial membrane surround the margins of the articular cartilage (circulus articuli vasculosus). This is the region where villi are seen and where both the degree of vascularity and the number of villi increase with age and in rheumatoid arthritis. Their location may be significant in the development of marginal erosions and pannus spreading over the articular surface from the margins.[4,23]

FUNCTION OF THE SYNOVIAL MEMBRANE

Paget and Bullough point out[23] that an important function of the synovial membrane is to regulate the movement of solutes, electrolytes, and proteins. The passage of these substances from the circulation into the synovial fluid may be controlled by macromolecules in the intracellular matrix of the synovial lining. The synovial lining cells may modify or catabolize certain plasma proteins during their passage through the synovial membrane.[28] The synovial lining cells, the intracellular matrix, and the capillaries each exert a regulative effect upon the type and amount of solute, electrolyte, and protein passing from the plasma to the synovial fluid.

Two other important functions of the synovial membrane are the production and enrichment of the synovial fluid and the clearance of various components (including phagocytosis of joint debris) accumulated within the joint space.

The synovial fluid is a viscous straw-colored filtrate of plasma to which hyaluronate is added by the synovial cells.[4] Hyaluronate is found in joint fluid bound to protein. It gives synovial fluid its viscosity and is sometimes termed *mucin.* It has a very large molecular size and molecular volume.[4] Enrichment of the synovial fluid with a glycoprotein that has lubricating properties has already been discussed. Fibronectin, which facilitates cell-to-cell adhesion and cell-to-collagen attachment, also appears to be secreted by synovial cells into the synovial fluid.[14]

The synovial fluid contains less protein than plasma, especially high-molecular-weight protein with asymmetrical shape. This observation supports the view that intracellular matrix may exclude such proteins from the synovial fluid.[4,33] Entirely absent from normal synovial fluid are proteins whose molecular weight is greater than 160,000 daltons including: fibrinogen, $alpha_2$ and $beta_2$ macroglobulin, and beta lipoprotein. This means that normal synovial fluid contains none of the blood clotting factors.[5] The ultrastructure of the subintimal capillaries, their fenestrations being similar to capillaries

TABLE 5-1 Classification of Synovial Effusions

	Normal	Noninflammatory (Group 1)	Inflammatory (Group 2)	Septic (Group 3)	Hemorrhagic
Viscosity	High	High	Low	Variable	Variable
Color	Pale yellow	Pale to dark yellow	Yellow to green	Variable	Bloody
Clarity	Transparent	Transparent	Translucent	Opaque	Opaque
WBS, mm^3	200	200–100	2000–75,000	Often 100,000	Same as blood
PMNs, %	25	25	50 (often)	75	Same as blood
Culture	Negative	Negative	Negative	Often positive	Negative
Mucin clot	Firm	Firm	Friable	Friable	Friable
Glucose	Nearly equal to blood	Nearly equal to blood	25 mg per 100 ml lower than blood	25 mg per 100 ml lower than blood	Same as blood

Source: Morrey, B.F.: *The Elbow and Its Disorders.* Philidelphia, Saunders, 1985. Reproduced with permission.

in organs where solute and water exchange occur, indicate that they are well-adapted for similar functions.[4,9,21,26] It is believed that the lymphatic system in synovium may also absorb colloidal particles from the synovial fluid.[4,8,14,15,23] Type A cells have been observed to phagocytose and pinocytose cellular debris from the joint.

Response to Injury

In general, synovial response to injury or irritation is an increase in vascularity, cellular content, and permeability. This, together with an increase in the number of villi, leads to an alteration in the amount and contents of the synovial fluid.[4,9,21,24] The changes seen in the synovial fluid as a response of this are shown in Tables 5-1 and 5-2. The constituents of synovial fluid in osteoarthritis resemble that of nonhemorrhagic trauma synovial fluid.[5] However, in rheumatoid arthritis there is considerable increase in the protein content of the fluid, which is accompanied by a low level of hyaluronate so that the mucin precipitate is poor. In addition, the glucose level is reduced, and there is a vigorous cellular response. With septic arthritis, the cellular response may be even more dramatic, but the culture will usually differentiate it from rheumatoid arthritis.

The synovial membrane has the ability to phagocytose whole erythrocytes and ingest hemoglobin. In hemarthrosis some erythrocytes may escape from the joint by passing between the synovial cells. Others, however, are phagocytosed by these cells leading to the formation of unicentric or multicentric whorled bodies called *siderosomes.*[24] Intimal cells can probably migrate into the subintimal matrix and continue to assimilate cells and debris.[8] There is a chronic inflammatory appearance of the subsynovial tissue due to cellular infiltration. There is cellular hyperplasia and some villus prolifera-

tion; these changes have been documented in experimental and human hemarthrosis.[3,16,19,24,25] Thickening and fibrosis of the synovium occur with chronic change, and the well-known yellow-to-brown tinge appears as well as adhesions.[3,25] Recurrent hemarthrosis alone is sufficient to produce a proliferative synovitis. In pigmented villonodular synovitis, the synovial fluid is usually not very viscous and generally does not clot. The mucin precipitate is fair, indicating a mild-to-moderate degree of inflammation.[5] The repeated hemorrhage seen in a blood dyscrasia such as hemophilia causes increased hemosiderosis so that the iron content of synovial tissue may approach 70 percent ash weight.[5]

The inflammatory response of the synovial membrane leads to an increased amount of plasma proteins, especially the large ones, passing into the synovial fluid because of its increased permeability.[23] The presence of collagenases has been noted in several types of arthritis,[13,19] and proteases and prostaglandins have been detected as part of the inflammatory response.[13] Resorption of cartilage matrix is considered to occur secondary to the production of extrinsic proteases from inflamed synovial tissue. A cartilage catabolic factor called *catabolin* has been identified and is thought to be produced in the synovium.[6]

In septic arthritis, a variety of enzymes have been isolated, mostly related to the polymorphonuclear leukocytes present in the synovial fluid and membrane. Lysosomal granules are also found in the synovial cells.[4] With septic arthritis, spontaneous fibrin clots are found, indicating that fibrinogen—not normally a constituent of synovial fluid—has escaped into the joint cavity.[4,23] It has been suggested that fibrin-heparin clots are produced which may interfere with phagocytosis and diminish absorption.[4] When deposited on articular cartilage, fibrin may also prevent the nutritional support of the chondrocyte normally derived from the synovial fluid.[2] Fibrin also neutralizes thrombin by absorption. However, sy-

TABLE 5-2 Conditions Associated with Types of Synovial Fluids

Group 1	Group 2	Group 3	Hemorrhagic
Acromegaly	Acute rheumatic fever	Acute tuberculosis	Anticoagulant therapy
Acute rheumatic fever	Ankylosing spondylitis	Bacterial infections	Hemophilia and other bleeding disorders
Aseptic necrosis	Arthritis of inflammatory bowel disease		Neuropathic joint disorders
Degenerative joint disease	Chronic infectious tuberculosis		Pigmented villonodular synovitis
Hypertrophic osteoarthropathy	Crystal-induced synovitis		Synovioma
Neuropathic arthropathy	Fungous arthritis		Thrombocytopenia
Osteochondritis dissecans	Psoriatic arthritis		Thrombocytosis
Osteochondromatosis	Reiter syndrome		Trauma
Systemic lupus erythematosus	Rheumatoid arthritis		
Trauma	Systemic lupus erythematosus		
	Viral arthritis		

Source: Morrey, B.F.: *The Elbow and Its Disorders.* Philadelphia, Saunders, 1985. Reproduced with permission.

novial fluid may have several anti-clotting mechanisms. Hyaluronate, being similar in structure to heparin, may have antithrombin activity in this situation. Antithrombin III has been documented in synovial fluid.

Recent studies of inflammatory synovitis have focused on the role of the mast cell in the pathophysiology of joint disease. It has multiple activators other than IgE antibodies.[18,31,32] The mast cell is now thought to have a part to play in many processes including vasoactive, chemotactic, and chemokinetic mechanisms and in immunoregulatory functions with far-reaching effects on connective tissue and bone.[1,10,15,31,32] These may affect blood flow and synovial permeability, regulate synovial inflammation, and perform homeostatic functions in the normal joint.[1,10,20,30,31]

REFERENCES

1. Azizkhan, R.G., et al. Mast cell heparin stimulates migration of capillary endothelial cells in vitro. J Exp Med 152:931–942, 1980.
2. Barnhart, M.I. Fibrin promotion and lysis in arthritic joints. Ann Rheum Dis 26:3:206, 1967.
3. Convery, F.R., et al. Experimental hemarthroses in the knee of the mature canine. Arthritis Rheum 19:59–67, January–February 1976.
4. Curtiss, P.H., Jr. The pathophysiology of joint infections. Clin Orthop 96:129–135, 1973.
5. Curtiss, P.H., Jr. Changes produced in synovial membrane and synovial fluid by disease. Instr Course Lect 18:11–23, 1973.
6. Dingle, J.T. Catabolin. A cartilage catabolic factor from synovium. Clin Orthop 156:219–231, 1981.
7. Freeman, M., et al. The innervation of the knee joint. An anatomical and histological study in the cat. J Anat 101:502–532, 1967.
8. Ghadially, F.N., et al. *Ultrastructure of Synovial Joint in Health and Disease.* New York, Appleton-Century-Crofts, 1969.
9. Ghadially, F.N. Fine structure of joints, in Sokoloff, L. (ed): *The Joints and Synovial Fluid.* New York, Academic Press, 1978, pp 132–150.
10. Goldhaber, P. Heparin enhancement of factors stimulating bone resorption in tissue culture. Science 147:407–408, 1965.
11. Goldie, I. The presence of nerves in original and regenerated synovial tissue in patients synovectomised for rheumatoid arthritis. Acta Orthop Scand 40:143–152, 1969.
12. Gross, A. *Arthritis,* sec 4, in *Orthopedic Knowledge, Update I,* Home Study Syllabus. Chicago, AAOS 1984, p 31.
13. Harris, E. Role of collagenases in joint destruction, in Sokoloff, L. (ed): *The Joints and Synovial Fluid.* New York, Academic Press, 1978, 243–272.
14. Harris, E. Biology of the joint, in Kelley, W.N. (ed): *Textbook of Rheumatology.* Philadelphia, Saunders, 1980, pp 255–276.
15. Hollingsworth, J.W. Cellular reaction to soluble foreign materials in the rabbit knee joint. Yale J Biol Med 37:360–412, 1965.
16. Hougland, F.T. Experimental hemarthrosis. J Bone Joint Surg 49A:285–298, 1967.
17. Italata, Z., et al. Innervation of the synovial membrane of the cat's joint capsule. Cell Tissue Res 169:410–415, 1976.
18. Lagunoff, D., et al. Cell biology of mast cells and basophils, in Glynns, L.E. (ed): *The Cell Biology of Inflammation.* Amsterdam, Elsevier/North-Holland Biomedical Press, 1980, 217–266.
19. Mainandi, C.L. Proliferative synovitis in hemophilia. Arthritis Rheum 21:137–144, 1978.
20. Marquardt, D.L., et al. Adenosine release from stimulated mast cells. J Allergy Clin Immunol 773:115A, 1984.
21. McCarty, D.J. The physiology of the normal synovium, in Sokoloff,

L. (ed): *The Joints and Synovial Fluid.* New York, Academic Press, 1980, pp 293–314.

22. McCutchen, C.W. Lubrication of joints, in Sokoloff, L. (ed): *The Joints and Synovial Fluid.* New York, Academic Press, 1978, pp 438–483.

23. Paget, S., and Bullough, P. Synovium and synovial fluid, in Owen, R. et al (eds): *Scientific Foundations of Orthopaedics and Traumatology.* Philadelphia, Saunders, 1980, pp 18–22.

24. Roy, S., et al. Ultrastructure of synovial membrane in human hemarthrosis. J Bone Joint Surgery 19A/B:1636–1646, 1967.

25. Roy, S., et al. Synovial membrane in experimentally produced chronic hemarthrosis. Ann Rheum Dis 28:402–413, 1969.

26. Schumacher, H.R. The microvasculature of synovial membranes of monkeys. Arthritis Rheum 12:387–404, 1969.

27. Sorew, A., et al. Microscopic comparison of the synovial changes in post traumatic synovitis and osteoarthritis. Clin Orthop 121:191–195, 1976.

28. Swann, D.A. Macromolecules of synovial fluid, in Sokoloff, L. (ed): *The Joints and Synovial Fluid.* New York, Academic Press, 1978, pp 407–437.

29. Trueta, J. *Studies of the Development and Decay of the Human Frame.* London, Pitman, 1968, pp 170–173.

30. Van Sickle, D.L., et al. Comparative arthrology, in Sokoloff, L. (ed): *The Joints and Synovial Fluid.* New York, Academic Press, 1978, pp 1–3.

31. Wasserman, S.I. Mediators of immediate hypersensitivity. J Allergy Clin Immunol 72:101–115, 1983.

32. Wasserman, S.I. The mast cell and synovial inflammation. Arthritis Rheum 27:841–844, 1984.

33. Zurifler, N.J. The immunopathology of joint inflammation in rheumatoid arthritis. Adv Immunol 116:265–336, 1970.

CHAPTER 6

Ligaments: Structure, Function, and Repair

Kennedy Daniels and Roger Dee

STRUCTURE AND FUNCTION OF LIGAMENTS

Ligaments represent a specialized form of dense connective tissue which connect bones or cartilages to one another, thus functioning to provide support for joints.[10] They have secondary functions as well, serving as transport media and storage areas for various nutrients and as a mechanical barrier to foreign proteins such as antigens, viruses, and bacteria.[46]

Ligaments are derived embryologically from pluripotential mesenchymal cells which are capable of differentiating into each of the cell types found in adult connective tissues. The predominant cell type found in ligaments is the *fibroblast.* The ultrastructure of the fibroblast includes a well-developed, rough endoplasmic reticulum and golgi apparatus which equips it for the production of large amounts of proteins.[23]

Ligaments consist primarily of acellular components produced by the fibroblasts. The acellular matrix surrounding the fibroblasts is composed of fibers and amorphous ground substance. The fibers in ligaments are predominantly (90 percent) type I collagen with a small percentage of type III collagen.[3] Reticular and elastic fibers are also present. The collagen fibers are generally oriented along the direction of the

tensile forces applied to the particular ligament, thereby contributing to the strength of the ligament, but the arrangement of the fibers is not nearly as uniform as that found in tendons and is probably ligament-specific. There is significant collagen turnover.[4]

Using polarized light, regular wavy undulations of cells and matrix have been described which are termed the "crimp" of the ligament and which may be different according to the particular structural needs of that individual ligament (Fig. 6-1). It has been proposed that crimp provides the safety mechanism that buffers ligament tension.[13] The elastic fibers are believed to be important in the recovery of the wavy configuration of the collagen fibers upon relaxation of strain within the ligament.[12] The ground substance is relatively scanty in ligaments and is composed of the mucopolysaccharides hyaluronic acid and chondroitin sulfate, which form a hydrophilic gel. Periarticular connective tissue levels of hyaluronic acid and chondroitin sulfate are diminished when joints are immobilized.[1] Glycosaminoglycans make up about 0.5 percent of the normal dry weight of ligaments. These substances are important in maintaining the molecular arrangement of the collagen fibers, water and electrolyte balance, and mechanical support of the tissue itself.[24,26] Collagen rep-

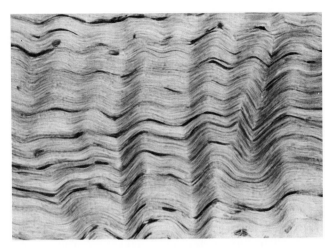

Figure 6-1 Histological appearance of relaxed collateral ligament using polarized light. Longitudinal arrangement of collagen and cellular components has undulating conformation called "crimp." *(From Frank, C.W., et al, Clin Orthop 196:15–23, 1985. Reproduced with permission.)*

resents three-quarters of the dry weight, but it should be remembered that the wet ligament is two-thirds water.

Ligaments make their attachments in the region of specialized structures histologically known as *Sharpey's fibers.* The perforating fibers of Sharpey, according to Frank, represent only collagen fibrils connecting adjacent lamellae in bone. The ligament actually inserts by a gradual transmission through layers of fibrocartilage into bone (Fig. 6-2).[9]

Response to Injury

In order for tissues to heal following injury, sufficient blood supply to the site of tissue repair is crucial. Ligaments are relatively avascular tissues. Several studies have shown with microangiographic and histological techniques that their predominant blood supply is not mediated by osseous structures but rather by the surrounding soft tissues. In the case of the anterior cruciate ligament, the infrapatellar fat pad and synovial membrane appear to be the major sources of vascular supply. Preservation and anatomic approximation of these tissues following surgical procedures may be clinically important.[3,7,47]

Biomechanical Considerations in Response to Injury

A stress-strain curve for a ligament shows an elastic region where deformation is reversible and then a "yield point" where it is irreversible. Failure of human anterior cruciate ligaments occur around 1500 newtons, at which time the ligament has elongated approximately 60 percent beyond its resting length.[30]

Species-related differences in ligamentous strength are difficult to quantitate since many other variables are in-

volved.[30] Primate anterior cruciate ligament when stressed in a direction parallel to its fibers fails at a slightly higher force than ligaments from cadavers of 48- to 86-year-old humans.[30] Specimens from younger humans exhibit twice the strength of primate ligaments.

Numerous studies have confirmed the finding that ligaments from younger subjects are stronger. However, there may also be a difference in the mode of failure. In Noyes's studies, ligaments from young subjects tended to fail within the substance of the ligament itself.[20,30,33] Specimens from cadavers of older humans tend to fail by avulsion fracture at the tibial insertion of the ligament, but histologically there was a decrease in cortical thickness and trabecular bone mass at the insertion of the ligament. The ligament itself was consequently not often stressed to failure, but subsequent stress-strain analysis revealed that the ligament itself still would have failed at lower maximum stress than those of specimens from younger humans.

When the rate of application of force was altered, anterior cruciate ligament preparations failed at a higher load and at greater elongation and they absorbed considerably more energy at a fast rate of deformation than at a slow rate. At a slow deformation rate the tibial insertion was the weakest point, tending to fail by avulsion fracture at that level. At a faster rate, more closely approximating physiological conditions, there was a more equal occurrence of failure by avulsion and by intraligamentous disruption. Avulsion fractures, as a consequence of rapid loading, usually produced larger osseous fragments than those produced by a slower rate of loading. This is in agreement with what is seen clinically in anterior cruciate ligament injuries with complete failure, the most common of which are accompanied by tibial avulsion and, in rare instances, femoral avulsion fractures.[29,30]

Considerable controversy exists as to whether the ligament, the ligament-bone interface, or the underlying bone is

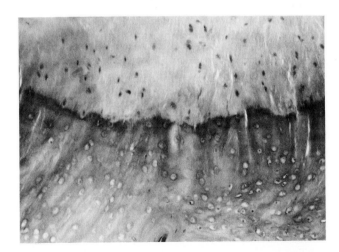

Figure 6-2 Rabbit medial collateral ligament insertion into bone. Note zones of transition from top to bottom of ligament to fibrocartilage, mineralized fibrocartilage, and bone. The horizontal dark line represents a calcification front. *(From Frank, C.W., et al, Clin Orthop 196:15–23, 1985. Reproduced with permission.)*

the weakest link in the complex. The answer is determined by many factors, including the species and specific ligament in question, loading rate, preparation process, age and level of activity of the subject, and the mechanism of injury.

The relative strength of different ligaments about the knee was measured by Kennedy et al.[20] The anterior cruciate ligament and tibial collateral ligaments were found to have roughly equal tensile strength at both fast and slow rates of deformation. The posterior cruciate ligament, however, was found to be almost twice as strong as the other two at both strain rates. This may explain the lower incidence of posterior cruciate ligament rupture, although obviously different mechanisms of injury are involved with different ligaments. Ligaments may be stressed to ultimate failure as confirmed by microscopic and rheologic studies and yet remain grossly intact.[20]

Effect of Conditioning

The effect of conditioning on ligamentous strength has been studied. Training significantly increased the amount of force necessary to avulse the anterior cruciate ligament from the tibia or femur, presumably by strengthening the bone at the site of attachment.[45] Tipton et al. showed that medial collateral ligaments of exercised dogs had a slightly higher collagen content than controls and an increased tensile strength.[40] In rats the increased strength was retained over an 8-week period of detraining.[45] Training resulted in heavier ligaments and in higher ligament weight-to-length ratios.[40,41]

Effects of Immobilization

Laros et al in 1971 studied the medial collateral ligament of dogs which had been subjected to various levels of inactivity for 6 to 12 weeks. They found that immobilization produced a histologically identifiable area of weakness manifested by bone resorption at the site of attachment of the ligament to the tibia.[28] In primate anterior cruciate ligament there is increased compliance, and a 39 percent decrease in maximum failure load following 8 weeks of immobilization. Isotonic exercises during the period of immobilization did not significantly alter these changes, and 20 weeks of resumed activity did not fully restore strength.[27]

A biochemical basis for these changes had been sought by several investigators. Akeson and his associates noted a marked reduction in concentrations of water, hyaluronic acid, and chondroitin-4 and -6 sulfate in the periarticular connective tissues about the knee in dogs and rabbits following 9 weeks of immobilization.[1,2] Klein et al reported increased collagen turnover in soft tissues of rat hind limbs resulting in immature cross-linking of collagen fibers. In further canine studies, however, they showed that loss of collagen was more significant in the bone and correlated this finding with increased mechanical failure by avulsion of the ligament from the weakened bone.[21]

Using calculations of ligamentous stiffness, Amiel et al felt that their studies showed the ligaments themselves to be more pliable when taken from immobilized joints. They pos-

tulated that increased collagen turnover resulted in collagen fibers being laid down in a haphazard fashion because of a loss of the usual control on orientation imposed by mechanical forces.[6] Further studies by this group indicated that up until 9 weeks of immobilization there was only increased turnover of collagen but that by 12 weeks there was significant loss of collagen mass.[6]

Effects of Steroid Injection

Single intracollagenous injections of steroids in clinical doses have resulted in significant lowering of ligament stiffness, failure load, and energy absorption which persisted up to 1 year.[32] Intraarticular injection, however, resulted in only minor alterations in mechanical properties. With higher doses (10 times the usual dose used clinically), mechanical compromise was demonstrated beginning at 15 weeks following intraarticular injection. Administering two injections in clinical doses 2 weeks apart had a statistically significant, although minor, effect on maximum failure load and energy absorption.[31] Oxlund believed that this decrease in strength of cruciate knee ligaments was due to weakening of the bony attachments, although Noyes still found that failure occurred by way of an intraligamentous mode.[31]

Effects of Immune Reactions

Immune synovitis induced in rabbit knees by Goldberg and associates reduced the strength of femur–anterior cruciate ligament–tibia complexes to one-third that of control specimens.[16] Many inflammatory processes (e.g., rheumatoid arthritis) compromise ligamentous integrity.

LIGAMENT HEALING

Miltner produced "sprains" by forcibly manipulating knee and ankle joints of rabbits.[25] At 1 week following a mild sprain, he found edema, fibroblastic proliferation, and lymphoid infiltration of the injured synovial tissue, ligaments, and joint capsule. These changes were found particularly near the bony attachments. Grossly, there was hemorrhage in the subcutaneous tissues. Two to three weeks after the sprain, the synovium was still inflamed and there was evidence of fibroblastic proliferation in the soft tissues surrounding the ligaments and capsule. At 4 weeks, there were no remaining gross external signs and the cellular response was subsiding. Healing by fibrous tissue was completed by 6 weeks. Severe sprains showed similar changes, but, in addition, the superficial layers of the local articular cartilage exhibited fibrillar degeneration, and the ligament repair process persisted for 8 to 10 weeks.[6]

Jack[18] observed histological changes in ruptured medial collateral ligaments of cats which were allowed to heal spontaneously following initial exploration to determine the site of rupture. The gap between the torn ends initially filled with blood. The clot was then converted to loose granulation tissue by invasion from the surrounding areolar tissue. The ligamentous ends became hypervascular, and at 4 days following rupture new collagen fibrils were formed by the proliferating fibroblasts penetrating the granulation tissue. The process continued, and at 2 weeks the gap was bridged by parallel collagenous fibers that were continuous with the original ligamentous fibers. At 3 weeks the vascular response was diminished and the collagenous fibers were larger and organized in bundles. The ligament appeared grossly normal at 7 weeks except for slight local thickening.

Clayton[9] and associates found that after 4 weeks of immobilization of canine medial collateral ligaments that had been transected and then either sutured or allowed to retract, the zone of weakness was still at the line of transection. However, after 6 weeks the suture line could not be disrupted and the ligaments parted through the ligamentous-osseous junction. The unsutured ligaments healed with lengthening, but the area of the incision continued to be the weakest link up to 9 weeks later. Exercise seemed to compensate for this difference. In subsequent studies, sutured and unsutured ligaments healed with approximately equal length when measured at rest. Stressing them, however, revealed differences since the sutured ligaments produced less elongation and joint laxity.

Frank et al[15] proposed that the seemingly normal strength exhibited by the repaired ligaments at 6 weeks may have been attributable to the skeletal immaturity of the experimental animals so that the ligaments avulsed from the bone. These investigators found that rabbit medial collateral ligaments allowed to heal spontaneously continued to be abnormal even after 40 weeks of healing. This they demonstrated in terms of deficient collagen content, cross-linking, and organization. Additionally, much of the collagen present was type III, rather than type I, collagen. Mechanically, the scar continued to be the weakest point even after 40 weeks.

Effects of Joint Motion

The effect of appropriate joint exercise on the healing of injured ligaments has been shown by several investigators to result ultimately in stronger repairs, although some protective immobilization may confer greater strength in the early stages of healing.[17,35,36,43] Exogenous administration of interstitial cell–stimulating hormone or testosterone has been shown to improve the strength of ligamentous repair whereas thyroid-stimulating hormone, thyroxine, adrenocorticotropic hormone, and growth hormone may impair it.[41] Electromagnetic stimulation has been used to effect healing of repaired rabbit medial collateral ligament by Frank et al with initially favorable results.[14] Beneficial effects of acute local cooling of injured ligaments were in one study attributed to the decreased edema and inflammatory reaction in the ligaments themselves, although the overlying soft tissues became more swollen.[11]

Effects of Reconstruction and Repair

Considerable clinical evidence has been accumulated which documents the long-term effects of ligamentous instability on joints. These are described elsewhere in this volume in regional sections. At this point it is unclear whether surgical repair of ligaments either acutely or late can alter these sequelae. Reconstruction of anterior cruciate ligament, in particular, by various autogenous and even allogeneic tissues has been shown histologically to result in a fibroblastic response which may represent conversion of the graft into a ligamentous structure. Although the use of vascularized synovial pedicles may improve procedures, the long-term outcome of ligament reconstruction is uncertain. However, joint instability consistently leads to long-term degenerative changes in the joint itself.[19,28,34,38,39]

REFERENCES

1. Akeson, W.H., Amiel, D., and LaViolette, D. The connective tissue response to immobility: A study of the chondroitin-4 and -6 sulfate and dermatan sulfate changes in periarticular connective tissue of control and immobilized knees of dogs. Clin Orthop 51:183–196 1967.

2. Akeson, W.H., Woo, S.L.Y., Amiel, D., Coutts, R.D., and Daniel, D. The connective tissue response to immobility: Biochemical changes in periarticular connective tissue of the immobilized rabbit knee. Clin Orthop 93:356–361, 1973.

3. Alm, A., and Stromberg, B. Vascular anatomy of the patellar and cruciate ligaments. A microangiographic and histologic investigation in the dog. Acta Chir Scand 445:25–35, 1974.

4. Amiel, D., Ing, D., Akeson, W.H., Harwood, F.L., Frank, C.B. Stress deprivation effect on metabolic turnover of the medial collateral ligament collagen. A comparison between nine and 12-week immobilization. Clin Orthop 172:265–270, 1983.

5. Amiel, D., Frank, C., Harwood, F.L., Fornek, J., and Akeson, W.H. Tendons and ligaments—A morphological and biochemical comparison. J Orthop Res 1:257, 1984.

6. Amiel, D., Woo, S.L.Y., Harwood, F.L., Akeson, W.H. The effect of immobilization on collagen turnover in connective tissue: A biochemical-biomechanical correlation. Acta Orthop Scand 53:325–332, 1983.

7. Arnoczky, S.P., Rubin, R.M., and Marshall, J.C. Microvasculature of the cruciate ligaments and its response to injury. An experimental study in dogs. J Bone Joint Surg 61-A:22;–1228, 1979.

8. Clayton, M.L., Miles, J.S., and Abdulla, M. Experimental investigations of ligamentous healing. Clin Orthop. 61:146–153, 1968.

9. Cooper, R.R., and Misol, S. Tendon and ligament insertion. A light and electron microscopic study. J Bone Joint Surg 52A:1, 1970.

10. *Dorland's Illustrated Medical Dictionary,* 25th ed. Philadelphia, Saunders, 1974.

11. Farry, P.J., Prentice, N.G., Hunter, A.C., and Wakelin, C.A. Ice treatment of injured ligaments: An experimental model. New Zealand Med 91:12–14, 1980.

12. Fitton-Jackson, S. The morphogenesis of collagen, in Gould, B.S. (ed): *Treatise on Collagen,* vol 2, *Biology of Collagen,* part B. London, Academic Press, 1968.

13. Frank, C.B., Amiel, D., Woo, S.L.Y., Akeson, W.H. Normal ligament properties and ligament healing. Clin Orthop 196:15–23, 1985.

14. Frank, C., Schacher, N., Dittrich, D., Shrive, N., Dehaas, W., and Edwards, G. Electromagnetic stimulation of ligament healing in rabbits. Clin Orthop 17E:263–271, 1983.

15. Frank, C., Woo, S.L.Y., Amiel, D., Harwood, F., Gomez, M., and Akeson, W. Medial collateral ligament healing. A multidisciplinary assessment in rabbits. Am J Sports Med 11:379–389, 1983.

16. Goldberg, V.M., Burstein, A, and Dawson, M. The influence of experimental immune synovitis on the failure mode and strength of

the rabbit anterior cruciate ligament. J Bone Joint Surg 64-A:900–905, 1982.

17. Goldstein, W.M., and Barmada, R. Early mobilization of rabbit medial collateral ligament repairs: Biomechanic and histologic study. Arch Phys Med Rehabil 65:239–242, 1984.

18. Jack, E.A. Experimental rupture of the medial collateral ligament of the knee. J Bone Joint Surg 32-B:396, 1950.

19. Jokl, P., Kaplan, N., Stovell, P., and Keggi, K. Non-operative treatment of severe injuries to the medial and anterior cruciate ligaments of the knee. J Bone Joint Surg 67-A:741–744, 1984.

20. Kennedy, J.C., Hawkins, R.J., Willis, R.B., and Danylchuk, K.D. Tension studies of human knee ligaments. Yield point, ultimate failure, and disruption of the cruciate and tibial collateral ligaments. J Bone Joint Surg 58-A:350–355, 1976.

21. Klein, L., Player, J.S., Heiple, K.G., Bahniuk, E., and Goldberg, V.M. Isotopic evidence for resorption of soft tissues and bone in immobilized dogs. J Bone Joint Surg 64-A:225–230, 1982.

22. Laros, G.S., Tipton, C.M., and Cooper, R.R. Influence of physical activity on ligament insertions in the knees of dogs. J Bone Joint Surg 53-A:275–285, 1971.

23. Leeson, T.S., and Leeson, C.R. *Histology*. Philadelphia, Saunders, 1970.

24. Mathews, M.B. Biophysical aspects of acid muco-polysaccharides relevant to connective tissue structure and function, in Wagner, B.M., and Smith, D.E. (eds): *The Connective Tissue*. Baltimore, Williams and Wilkins, 1967.

25. Miltner, L.J., Hu, C.H., and Fang, H.C. Experimental joint sprain. Arch Surg 35:234, 1934.

26. Minns, R.J., Soden, P.D., and Jackson, D.S. The role of the fibrous components and ground substance in the mechanical properties of biological tissues. A preliminary investigation. J Biomech 6:153–165, 1973.

27. Noyes, F.R. Functional properties of knee ligaments and alterations induced by immobilization. A correlative biomechanical and histological study in primates. Clin Orthop 123:210–139, 1977.

28. Noyes, F.R., Butler, D.L., Grood, E.S., Zernickle, R.F., and Hefzy, M.S. Biomechanical analysis of human ligament grafts used in knee-ligament repairs and reconstructions. J Bone Joint Surg 66-A:344–352, 1984.

29. Noyes, F.R., DeLucas, J.L., and Toruik, P.J. Biomechanics of anterior cruciate ligament failure: An analysis of strain-rate sensitivity and mechanisms of failure in primates. J Bone Joint Surg 56-A:236–253, 1974.

30. Noyes, F.R., and Grood, E.S. The strength of the anterior cruciate ligament in humans and rhesus monkeys. Age-related and species-related changes. J Bone Joint Surg 58-A:1074–1082, 1976.

31. Noyes, F.R., Grood, E.S., Nussbaum, N.S., and Cooper, S.M. Effect of intra-articular corticosteroids on ligament properties. Clin Orthop 123:197–207, 1977.

32. Noyes, F.R., Nussbaum, N.S., Torvik, P.J., and Cooper, S. Biochemical and ultrastructural changes in ligaments and tendons after local corticosteroid injections. Proceedings of the orthopedic research society, 1975 Annual Meeting. J Bone Joint Surg 57A:876, 1975.

33. Noyes, F.R., Torvik, P.J., Hyde, W.B., and DeLucas, J.L. Biomechanics of ligament failure, II. An analysis of immobilization, exercise, and reconditioning effects in primates. J Bone Joint Surg 56-A:1406–1417, 1974.

34. Odensten, M., Lysholm, J., and Gillguist, J. Suture of fresh ruptures of the anterior cruciate ligament. Acta Orthop Scand 55:270–272, 1984.

35. O'Donoghue, D.H., Frank, G.R., Jeter, G.L., Johnson, W., Zelders, J.W., and Kenyon, R. Repair and reconstruction of the anterior cruciate ligament in dogs. J Bone Joint Surg 53-A:710–718, 1971.

36. O'Donoghue, D.H., Rockwood, C.A., Jr., Frank, G.R., Jack, S.C., and Kenyon, R. Repair of the anterior cruciate ligament in dogs. J Bone Joint Surg 48-A:503–518, 1966.

37. Oxlund, H. The influence of a local injection of cortisol on the mechanical properties of tendons and ligaments and the indirect effect on skin. Acta Orthop Scand 51:231–238, 1980.

38. Shino, K., Kawasaki, T., Hirose, H., Gotoh, I., Inove, M., and Ono, K. Replacement of the anterior cruciate ligament by an allogenic tendon graft. An experimental study in the dog. J Bone Joint Surg 66-B:672–681 1984.

39. Tegner, Y., Lysholm, J., Gillquist, J., and Oberg, B. Two-year follow-up of conservative treatment of knee ligament injuries. Acta Orthop Scand 55:176–180, 1984.

40. Tipton, C.M., James, S.L., Mergner, W., and Tcheng, T. Influence of exercise on strength of medial collateral ligaments of dogs. Am J Physiol 218:894–901, 1970.

41. Tipton, C.M., Matthes, R.D., Maynard, J.A., and Carey, R.A. The influence of physical activity on ligaments and tendons. Med Sci Sports 7:165–175, 1975.

42. Vailas, A.C., Tipton, C.M., Laughlin, H.L., Tcheng, T.K., and Matthes, R.D. Physical activity and hypophysectomy on the aerobic capacity of ligaments and tendons. J App Physiol 44:542–546, 1978.

43. Vailas, A.C., Tipton, C.M., Matthes, R.D., and Gart, M. Physical activity and its influence on the repair process of medial collateral ligaments. Connect Tissue Res 9:25–31, 1981.

44. Viidik, A. Biomechanics and functional adaptation of tendons and joint ligaments, in Evans, E.G. (ed): *Studies on the Anatomy and Function of Bones and Joints*. Berlin, Springer, 1966, pp 17–39.

45. Viidik, A. Elasticity and tensile strength of the anterior cruciate ligament in rabbits as influenced by training. Acta Physiol Scand 74:372–380, 1968.

46. Viidik, A. Functional properties of collagenous tissues. Int Rev Connect Tissue Res 6:127–215, 1973.

47. Whiteside, L.A., and Sweeney, R.E., Jr. Nutrient pathways of the cruciate ligaments. J Bone Joint Surg 62-A:1176–1180, 1980.

48. Zuckerman, J., and Stull, G.A. Ligamentous separation force in rats as influenced by training, detraining, and cage restriction. Med Sci Sports 5:44–49, 1973.

CHAPTER 7

Bone: Structure and Function

Roger Dee and Mark Sanders

THE DEVELOPMENT OF BONE

At the primary centers of ossification and the region of the growth plate bone formation occurs by the process known as *endochondral ossification.* Cartilage cells replicate, producing longitudinal growth. A sequence of chondrocyte calcification and then of chondrocyte death precedes vascular ingrowth leading to the production of osteoid.

Intramembranous ossification is the mechanism whereby clusters of mesenchymal cells differentiate into osteoblasts,

which secrete the organic matrix of bone. Since there is no cartilaginous phase or cell division in this mechanism, as the osteoblasts become surrounded by matrix and convert into osteocytes it is necessary for a new population of osteoblasts to be formed from osteogenic cells in the mesenchyme. Growth occurs by a process of appositional bone formation. In this type of ossification, spicules of bone are formed with the bone-forming cells closely applied to their surface. Intramembranous ossification occurs in some flat bones such as the skull. It is also periosteal appositional bone growth in long bones which accounts for the increase in diameter of these bones (Fig. 7-1). Increase in length occurs by endochondral ossification at the growing physis. In the early embryo a thin bony collar of periosteally derived intramembranous bone is first produced and may precipitate nutritional changes in the cartilaginous model, particularly oxygen deprivation to the cartilage cells, which in turn triggers the ingrowth of blood vessels and the formation of the primary ossification centers[69](Figs. 7-2, 7-3, and 7-4).

Bone formed by these two methods is qualitatively identical. Throughout the body, however, there are considerable variations in the design of individual bones associated with particular structural requirements. Dense, compact cortical bone is seen characteristically in the diaphysis of long bones, and spongy cancellous bone with its internal network of fine

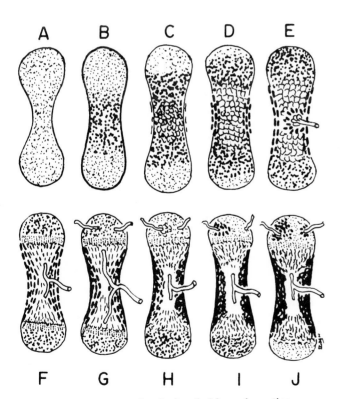

Figure 7-1 Schematic of endochondral bone formation. **A.** Mesenchymal anlage. **B.** Central chondrification. **C.** Central cartilage hypertrophy. **D.** Formation of primary bone collar. **E.** Vascular interruption to form the primary ossification center. **F.** Development of contiguous endochondral (at the bone ends) and membranous (periosteal, diaphyseal) ossification; well-developed physeal cytoarchitecture. **G.** Cartilage canal formation within the epiphysis. **H.** Diaphyseal remodeling and cavitation; formation of epiphyseal preossification center. **I.** Formation of secondary ossification center. **J.** Formation of accessory epiphyseal ossification centers (e.g., greater trochanter). *(From Ogden, J.A.: Skeletal Injury in the Child. Philadelphia, Lea & Febiger, 1982. Reproduced with permission.)*

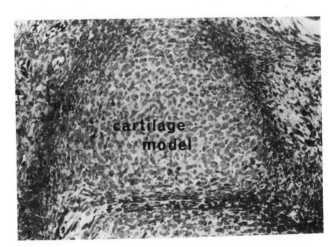

Figure 7-2 Cartilage model of the metatarsal bone from a chick embryo incubated for 10 days. Epon section toluidine blue stain, ×200. Note the central region of young hyaline cartilage surrounded by the primitive perichondrium (Pch). *(From Warshawsky, H., in Cruess, R.L., ed: The Musculoskeletal System. New York, Churchill Livingstone, 1982. Reproduced with permission.)*

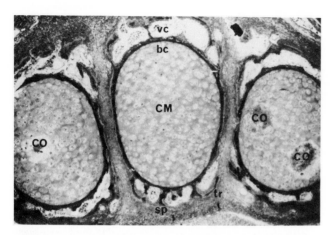

Figure 7-3 Eroded regions within the cartilage model (CM) represent the primitive center of ossification (CO). These contain blood vessels and connective tissue cells. Also seen are bone collars (bc), spicules (sp), trabeculae (tr), and large vascular channels (vc). Thirteen-day chick embryo metatarsal. Epon section toluidine blue stain, ×75. *(From Warshawsky, H., in Cruess, R.L., ed: The Musculoskeletal System. New York, Churchill Livingstone, 1982. Reprinted with permission.)*

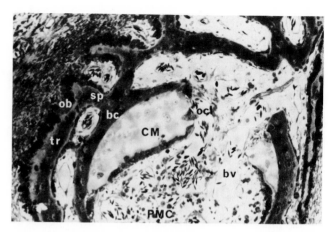

Figure 7-4 The primitive marrow cavity (PMC) is filled with blood vessels (bv), connective tissue, and hematopoietic marrow elements. What is left of the cartilage model (CM) is being eroded by osteoclasts (Oc1) and mononuclear cells. Spicules (sp) and trabeculae (tr) project from the original bony collar (bc). They are surrounded by osteoblasts (ob). Thirteen-day-old embryo metatarsal. Epon section toluidine stain, ×200. *(From Warshawsky, H., in Cruess, R.L., ed: The Musculoskeletal System. New York, Churchill Livingstone, 1982. Reproduced with permission.)*

trabeculae enclosing marrow spaces is characteristically present in the metaphysis of a long bone and in bones of the tarsus and carpus.

The first bone to appear during embryonic development resembles that produced in fracture callus and is described as *woven bone.* In this type of bone the collagen fibers have no recognizable pattern of arrangement and run in a haphazard fashion in numerous directions. It is unevenly mineralized and characterized by a higher content of proteoglycans than mature lamellar bone. The lacunae which contain the osteocytes in woven bone also tend to be more irregularly shaped than those in mature bones. Embryonic woven bone is replaced during growth by mature bone, which has a much more orderly structure.

Compact Cortical Bone

The majority of mature bone is compact cortical bone, which is responsible for much of the mechanical strength of long bones. Replacement of woven bone by cortical bone occurs by means of vascular channels which invade the embryonic bone from its periosteal and endosteal surfaces. During growth, periosteal blood vessels become enclosed on the surface of the developing long bone. This occurs with the development first of a ripplelike elevation which becomes a longitudinal trenchlike channel on the periosteal surface. This closes over to form a longitudinally running tunnel within which the periosteal vessel is then entrapped for part of its course. At the point at which it runs at right angles to the axis of the shaft to enter this tunnel, the vessel traverses a channel termed a *Volkmann's canal.*

In the walls of the tunnels around the invading blood vessels, resorption cavities ("cutting cones") lined by osteo-

clasts remove the woven bone. Closely adjacent osteoblasts meanwhile deposit new bone in an organized lamellar form (Fig. 7-5). The layers of collagen bundles are parallel to each other in one lamella but change direction in the adjacent lamella in an alternating fashion. This lamellar arrangement of collagen fibers has a birefringent pattern when viewed in cross section with polarized light (Figs. 7-6 and 7-7). The resorption cavity lined with osteogenic cells and surrounded by circular plates of bone is called an *osteon,* or a *haversian system.* The mechanical strength of cortical bone is due to the compact packing of osteons. Separating the osteons in mature bone are irregular fragments of interstitial bone representing remnants of the earlier bone replaced by the osteon. Each osteon is separated from adjacent osteons and from interstitial bone by cement lines which can be identified on histological sections. The remodeling brought about by osteoclastic resorption of bone and the simultaneous deposition of new matrix by osteoblasts and its mineralization continues during adult life and is controlled by numerous factors including changes in the mechanical environment and the endocrine status of the skeleton.

Trabecular Bone

Trabecular bone is found in the metaphyses of long bones and in areas of the axial skeleton, such as vertebral bodies and pelvis. It has very few haversian systems. In trabeculae the lamellar bone is laid down in the form of bony plates connected together by transverse supporting struts of bone (Fig. 7-8). The plates vary in shape, depending upon the structural requirements of the particular site. During growth the metaphyseal bony trabeculae consist of bone surrounding a calcified cartilage core. During longitudinal growth some woven

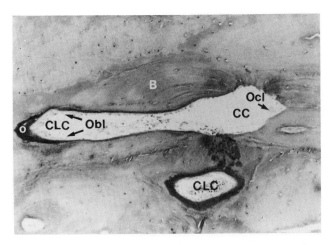

Figure 7-5 Events in cortical bone remodeling, shown in this longitudinal section of an osteon. Bone (B) is being reabsorbed by osteoclasts (Ocl), eroding a cutting cone (CC). The canal is being progressively filled by the deposition of osteoid (o) laid down by osteoblasts (Obl), forming a closing cone (CLC), which also appears circular in transverse section in the lower part of the slide. Undecalcified, Goldner stain; 5-μm section of human cortical bone $\times 100$. *(From Marie, P.J., in Cruess, R.L., ed: The Musculoskeletal System. New York, Churchill Livingstone, 1982.)*

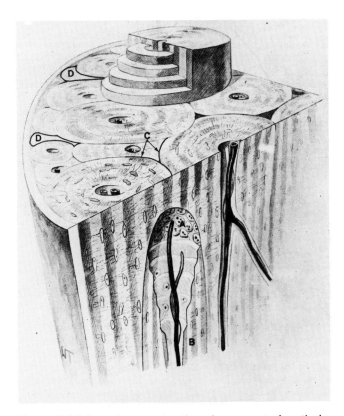

Figure 7-6 Schematic reconstruction of a segment of cortical bone. **A.** The cutting cone where osteoclasts are actively creating a tunnel along which new bone is laid. **B.** Creation of a new osteon. **C.** Cement lines **D.** Interstitial lamellae. *(From Bullough, P.G., in Wren, R., Goodfellow, J., and Bullough, P.: Scientific Foundations of Orthopaedics and Traumatology. Philadelphia, Saunders, 1980. Reproduced with permission.)*

bone may also be present adjacent to the epiphyseal plate, but at maturation the woven bone has been entirely replaced by lamellar bone; also, the cartilage core is no longer present. Trabecular bone, like cortical bone, continually undergoes remodeling at the endosteal bone surfaces (Fig. 7-9). It has a larger relative proportion of bone surface available for remodeling than dense cortical bone.

THE CELLS OF BONE

All osteogenic stem cells originate in the mesoderm, which is in itself a product of embryonic mesenchyme. The precursor cells have been differentiated by Friedenstein[16] into *determined precursor cells* that will form bone without inducer substances and into other called *inducible osteogenic precursor cells,* which will not. Determined cells will form bone when transplanted heterotopically.

The Osteoblast

Bone surfaces are lined with a cellular envelope of osteoprogenitor cells[42] (Fig. 7-10). There are three varieties of cellular envelopes: periosteal, endosteal, and haversian (cutting cones). These cells can be stimulated to form *osteoblasts,* which are the cells that produce the bone matrix (prebone). An osteoblast will lay down three times its own volume of matrix over a 3- or 4-day period before becoming an osteocyte, which may be thought of as an imprisoned osteoblast surrounded by its matrix.[65] Osteoblasts contain intracellular structures consistent with their important role in the synthesis of collagen, mucopolysaccharides, and glycoprotein. Thus, golgi apparatus, an abundance of mitochondria, and endoplasmic reticulum are present. Their cytoplasm is rich in alkaline phosphatase activity.[25] Elevation of the alkaline phos-

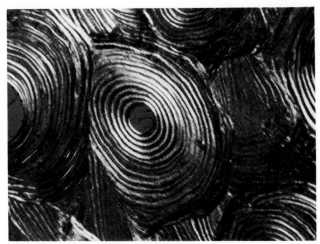

Figure 7-7 Lamellar bone viewed with polarized light. The collagen-rich bundles are arranged in concentric rings approximately 7-μm thick about the haversian canal. Straight, rather than circular, bundles are interstitial lamellae ($\times 350$). *(From Sokoloff, L., and Bland, J.H., eds: The Musculoskeletal System. Baltimore, Williams & Wilkins, 1975.)*

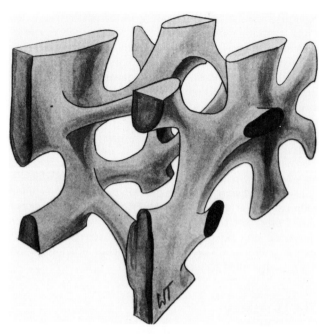

Figure 7-8 Reconstruction of cancellous bone to show three-dimensional appearance of a thin section. *(From Bullough, P.G., in Owen, R., Goodfellow, J., and Bullough, P., eds: Scientific Foundations of Orthopaedics and Traumatology. Philadelphia, Saunders, Co., 1982.)*

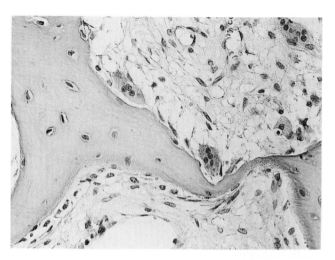

Figure 7-9 An osteoclast in Howship's lacuna absorbing bone on the surface of a trabecula. The patient has secondary hyperparathyroidism, and the adjacent marrow is fibrous (osteitis fibrosa) H&E, ×350. *(From Sokoloff, L., and Bland, J.H., eds: The Musculoskeletal System, Baltimore, Williams & Wilkins, 1975.)*

phatase level in the blood (above 21 to 100 international King Armstrong units per liter) is indicative of osteoblastic activity. In Paget's disease a fall in the blood level of alkaline phosphatase upon treatment with calcitonin measures the therapeutic response. If measurement of 5-nucleotidase or gamma-glutamyl transferase shows these two enzymes to be normal, the raised blood alkaline phosphatase level is probably due to osteoblastic activity rather than to liver alkaline phosphatase.[13] The level is often raised in bone-forming metastases.

The osteoblast's subcellular organelles are involved in the transduction of signals from physical forces and chemical factors to the biological response expressed by the genome.[52] The osteoblast contains adenylate cyclase and protein kinase systems, and since the osteoblast is now considered to be a target cell for parathyroid hormone (PTH), it is considered that these systems probably represent a mode of action of that hormone.[32] The interaction between PTH and its receptors on the osteoblast plasma membrane promotes the activity of membrane-located adenylate cyclase and the entry of calcium into the cell. Cyclic AMP is cyclic adenosine 3′,5′ monophosphate and is formed from ATP by adenylate cyclase. The rise in cellular cyclic AMP and in calcium levels then triggers a cascade of metabolic events that culminate in purposive cell behavior.[17] Prostaglandins of the E series similarly influence osteoblastic function by specifically binding to osteoblastlike cells and stimulating cyclic AMP formation.[12] The acidic peptide *calmodulin*, with four calcium-binding domains, has been shown to be present in a wide variety of different cells in mammals. It is a heat- and acid-stable protein with a molecular weight of about 17,000 daltons and may

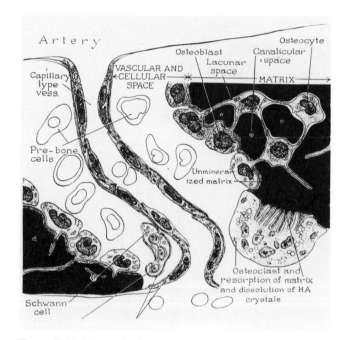

Figure 7-10 Schematic drawing representing the concept of a physiological unit of bone tissue. The bone cells consisting of osteoblasts and osteoclasts line the bone and communicate via tight junctions and the canaliculi with cytoplasmic processes of osteocytes deep in the bone. This cellular membrane separates the bone fluid compartment from the extracellular fluid compartment. A continuous basement membrane covers the endothelial cells of blood sinusoids and capillaries, which are an integral part of cancellous and compact bone. The extracellular fluid space extends from the basement membrane of the blood capillaries to the cellular membrane. *(From Dotty, S.B., Robinson, R.A., and Schofield, B., in Auerbach, G.D., ed: Handbook of Physiology, sec 7, vol 7. Baltimore, Waverly Press, 1976. Reproduced with permission.)*

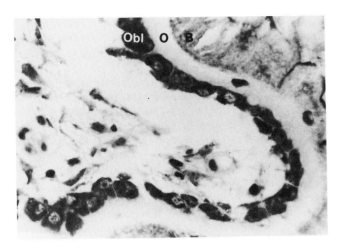

Figure 7-11 Osteoblasts (Obl) actively synthesizing osteoid (O) along a trabecular bone (B) surface. Undecalcified toluidine blue stain, 5-μm thick section of iliac crest bone biopsy, ×500. *(From Marie, P.G., in Cruess, R., ed: The Musculoskeletal System. New York: Churchill Livingstone, 1982. Reproduced with permission.)*

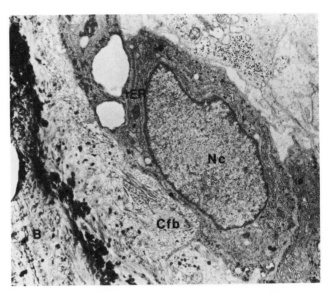

Figure 7-12 Electron micrograph of an osteoblast. There is a well-developed rough endoplasmic reticulum (rER) close to the nucleus (Nc); along the bone (B) surface are disposed several collagen fibers (Cfb). Decalcified bone, ×7200. *(From Marie, P.G., in Cruess, R., ed: The Musculoskeletal System. New York: Churchill Livingstone, 1982. Reproduced with permission.)*

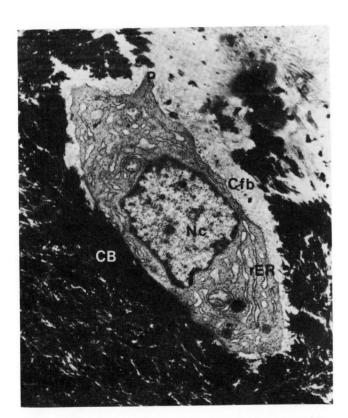

Figure 7-13 Electron micrograph of a young osteocyte within its lacuna. It is surrounded by collagen fibers (Cfb). It possesses a large nucleus (Nc) and has well-developed rough endoplasmic reticulum (rER). A process from the osteocyte (P) extends into the calcified bone (CB). Undecalcified bone, ×6600. *(From Marie, P.G., in Cruess, R., ed: The Musculoskeletal System. New York, Churchill Livingstone, 1982. Reproduced with permission.)*

regulate numerous enzyme functions in the osteoblast including phosphodiesterase (PDE) activity, adenylate cyclase, and some membrane kinase.[5,17] Calmodulin has a structural resemblance to troponin.

Osteoblasts tend to be columnar in shape with the nucleus at the end farthest from the bone surface (Figs. 7-11 and 7-12). They may be spindle-shaped when inactive. On routine decalcified hematoxylin and eosin (H&E) preparations, they appear as large blue cells with nuclei indistinct from the cytoplasm. The cells have many fine cytoplasmic projections that penetrate the osteoid and calcified matrix and communicate with the osteocytes through tight gap junctions.[40] The matrix channels through which these processes traverse are known as *canaliculi*. Osteoblasts probably play a role in the physiological transfer of calcium and phosphorus and in the mineralization of osteoid.

Osteocytes

The osteocytes are by far the majority of cells of the mature skeleton. Like the osteoblasts, these cells also have a full complement of intracellular organelles, indicating their ability to participate in bone function. They have well-developed endoplasmic reticulum (Fig. 7-13) and posses golgi apparatus and mitochondria. Although they are usually within the bone matrix, some remain as surface osteocytes. They lie within lacunae in the matrix and both the cells and their lacunae are larger in new woven bone compared to those in mature bones where the lacunae have a more flattened appearance.

The surface osteocytes and osteoblasts connect to one another by cell processes (Figs. 7-13 and 7-14) and are termed *bone lining cells*. It is believed that they function as a physio-

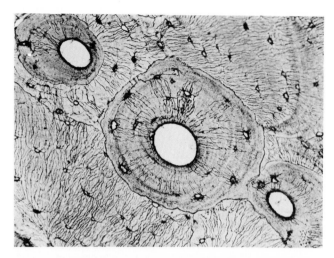

Figure 7-14 Nutritional pathways through bone. The cement line is seen encircling the osteon with its large central canal and circumferentially arranged lamellae. The fine filaments extending radially from the lacunae are canaliculi. Bodian, ×250. *(From Sokoloff, L., and Bland, J.H., eds: The Musculoskeletal System. Baltimore, Williams & Wilkins, 1975. Reproduced with permission.)*

logical membrane separating the fluid which bathes the inorganic nonliving portion of bone from the extracellular fluid compartment.[42] These cells are concerned with the control of extracellular concentrations of calcium and phosphorus. They are target cells for the action of such hormones as PTH and calcitonin, which thus exercise their metabolic functions.

The Osteoclasts

The *osteoclast* is a fully differentiated bone cell that functions to absorb both bone mineral and matrix. Stained with H&E, osteoclasts appear as large cells containing as many as a dozen uniform nuclei with one or two nucleoli. Their cytoplasm exhibits basal staining which becomes acidophilic as the cell ages. Osteoclasts are seen on the bone surface within small erosions known as *Howship's lacunae* (Figs. 7-9 and 7-10). They always occur adjacent to the vascular channels, forming cutting cones, and their action is probably coupled with that of osteoblasts during the remodeling process (Fig. 7-5). Recently, a coupling factor linking the actions of these two types of cell in human bone has been postulated.[14] The concept of "coupling" of osteoclastic resorption and osteoblastic formation in bone remodeling units is of considerable importance in analysis of bone metabolism in the aging adult skeleton.[49]

The osteoclast possesses a ruffled (brush) border apparatus that is active in resorbing bone in contact with it (Figs. 7-10 and 7-15). The cell forms a seal upon the surface of the bone and develops a local acid pH which promotes dissolution of the mineral. Crystalloids are then dislodged in the region of the brush border and pass into the cell by extracellular clefts that are continued intracellularly in tubular fashion into the vesicles of the nearby cytoplasm. Crystalloids are thereby taken into the osteoclasts, where they lose all structural identity and pass out into the bloodstream as calcium ions. The loss of mineral exposes the collagen fibers of the matrix to the action of lysosomal proteases, particularly ca-

thepsin B and collagenolytic cathepsin.[70] The ruffled border disappears and intracellular changes occur when the osteoclast leaves the bone's surface, suggesting a quiescent state.[28]

Dispute over the origin of osteoclasts seems to have been resolved by recent work by Burger and co-workers,[6] who explained earlier failures to demonstrate production of osteoclasts from the suspected cell of origin, the phagocytic monocyte. At one time it was postulated that there might be different pools of monocytes, only some of which give rise to the osteoclasts. Burger has shown that no osteoclast will develop from blood monocytes or tissue macrophages since these populations all contain only mature, nondividing latestate mononuclear phagocytes. It seems from Burger's work that it is the proliferating *immature* mononuclear phagocyte which is the precursor of the osteoclast.

Bone remodeling is the process by which bone is continuously removed and replaced. Some 10 percent of the skeleton is replaced annually in young adults. Remodeling occurs at the cellular envelopes at haversian, endosteal, and periosteal bone surfaces. The resorption cavity (cutting cone) is developed by osteoclasts and is the mechanism whereby the remodeling cycle is initiated.[39] Bone remodeling is influenced locally by prostaglandins of the E series, coupling factor, osteoclast-simulating factors; also by endocrine effects, particularly thyroxine, growth hormone, insulin, glucocorticoids, and androgens. Mechanical factors play an important role in overall direction of the remodeling process.

BONE MATRIX

The tunnel made by an advancing osteoclast cutting cone is progressively obliterated by the coupled deposition of matrix

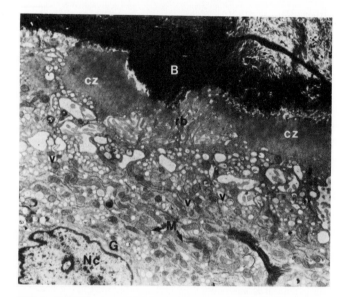

Figure 7-15 Electron micrograph of an osteoclast, showing one nucleus (Nc), a large number of mitochondria (M), golgi apparatus (G), and numerous vacuoles (V). The ruffled border (rb) is surrounded by a clear zone (cz) and applied to the bone matrix (B). Undecalcified bone, ×5400. *(From Marie, P.G., in Cruess, R.L. ed: The Musculoskeletal System. New York, Churchill Livingstone, 1982.)*

by active osteoblasts. Approximately two-thirds of adult bone is inorganic material and only one-third organic. Only a small percentage makes up the bone cell mass, and there is approximately 10 percent water. Of the organic matrix approximately 90 percent is collagen and only 1 percent mucopolysaccharides.

Collagen

The collagen of bone is the genetically distinct type I collagen. This is the most common collagen found in the body and is present in skin and tendon as well as in bone.

Collagen imparts to bone a great deal of its mechanical strength, particularly in tension. The biosynthesis of collagen is described in Chap. 2.

Within the collagen fiber the individual collagen molecules (each molecule consisting of a triple helix of alpha chains) are specifically aligned in a quarter stagger arrangement. This means that although the collagen molecules are the same length and the gap size between molecules is constant since the fibril has a three-dimensional arrangement and the layering of the molecules one upon the other is staggered, the intermolecular gaps are not in alignment. The regularity of the stagger overlap gives the typical banded pattern seen with electron microscopy. The dark zones correspond to low molecular density (intermolecular gaps or holes regions) and the light zones to overlap regions of greater molecular density. The exact three-dimensional organization of the staggered molecule is not known but a pentafibril macromolecular model has been proposed.

The osteoblast is the cell responsible for the synthesis of bone collagen.[26] The hole zones are thought to be important with regard to mineral fluxes within bone. During calcification early mineral is deposited in the hole zones of the bone collagen.[19,21]

Noncollagenous Proteins

These usually constitute just under 20 percent of osteoid but progressively decrease with maturity of bone and its degree of calcification so that a figure as low as 6 percent may be reached.[66]

A phosphorylated glycoprotein with a molecular weight in the region of 62,000 daltons has been identified in fetal and growing bone. A smaller molecule (molecular weight 32,000 daltons), which is also a phosphorylated gylcoprotein, is found associated with new bone matrix formation in the region of the calcified cartilage framework of endochondral ossification and also in the region of newly formed bone ossicles during intramembranous ossification. This smaller molecule is called *osteonectin*. Based on immunologic criteria, this material has been found to be bone-specific with a strong affinity for apatite and is an excellent marker for osteogenesis. It facilitates the binding of free calcium ions to type I collagen fibers, regardless of collagen tissue source.[61]

Although osteonectin has a strong affinity for collagen, it has been noted that it is not as strong a collagen binder as fibronectin, which can totally block the ability of osteonectin to bind calcium ions to collagen. Fibronectin is a large glyco-

protein of 220,000 molecular weight which has two disulfide-linked subunits containing different binding sites for collagen, heparin, and cell surfaces. It occurs on many different types of cells and affects cell shape. There is considerably more osteonectin than fibronectin in developing bone.[62]

Bone matrix also contains phosphoproteins. These have molecular weights in the region of 24,000 daltons and contain hydroxyproline. They may have importance in calcium binding.[23,61] The first bone-specific noncollagenous protein completely characterized was *osteocalcin*.[30,45] Two-thirds of this material is firmly attached to the bone apatite phase and resists extraction.[61] This material is one of the gamma-carboxyglutamic-acid–containing proteins (GLA proteins). These proteins are vitamin K–dependent, and osteocalcin is sometimes known as bone gamma-carboxyglutamic-acid–containing protein (BGP). The protein only seems to accumulate after the peak of mineralization in bone.[44] Treating bones with vitamin K antagonists depletes the bone of this protein but does not affect either the proline content or the mechanical strength of the bone.[4]

Proteoglycans

Mineralized bone contains a small proteoglycan that is chemically and immunologically distinct from other tissue proteoglycan.[61] The molecular weight is 120,000 daltons, and the molecule contains 25 percent protein. Proteoglycans are thought to retard the deposition of hydroxyapatite crystals so that modifications in the proteoglycans may be necessary to facilitate mineralization in those tissues that are actively calcifying.[10] The hydrodynamic size of the molecule seems important, and experimental results show that proteoglycan aggregate is more effective than monomer (and monomer is more effective than the component glycosaminoglycan chain) in inhibiting hydroxyapatite growth during epiphyseal growth plate calcification. Buckwalter has shown that proteoglycans are altered in structure and size in calcifying cartilage.[5]

Lipids

Lipids account for a relatively small proportion of the organic matrix of bone (7 to 14 percent).[4] Lipids are present in the membranes of extracellular matrix vesicles and are also distributed throughout cell membranes, as intracellular structures and in extracellular deposits. Acidic phospholipids appear to be involved in the calcification process by forming complexes with calcium phosphate. Calcifiable proteolipids have been shown to peak in concentration as the epiphyseal cartilage begins to calcify.[4]

FACTORS INVOLVED IN THE MINERALIZATION OF BONE

Organization of Collagen

Under polarized light the lamellar structure of collagen appears as successive white and dark layers. This lamellar birefringence is absent when the collagen fibers are not oriented in this regular way, such as in woven bone. Since it is the collagen fiber that ultimately becomes mineralized, the first step in the integrated sequence of events leading to mature bone is initiated by the specific way in which the collagen fiber is laid down by the osteoblasts. Tetracycline is a useful marker of bone mineralization, and fluorescent study of undecalcified sections clearly shows the mineralization front.

Role of Mitochondria

The regulation of calcification of bone matrix has not yet been fully elucidated. It seems that by using ATP generated by oxidative phosphorylation, the mitochondria in cells of a calcifying matrix can accumulate calcium and phosphate. In the growth plate, the chondrocytic mitochondria become increasingly loaded with calcium and phosphate prior to calcification.[4] In the hypertrophic cells of the growth plate, the mitochondria lose their calcium, and mineral then appears in organelles in the extracellular matrix (except when the animal is rachitic).

Role of Matrix Vesicles

Extracellular matrix vesicles are often present and associated with the process of mineralization. They are present in endochondral ossification when it occurs in immature or woven bone with a large amount of osteoid, but they seem unnecessary and may be absent when mineralization occurs in lamellar bone where many mineral crystals are already present. Matrix vesicles have been seen to be formed by the budding of chondrocytes.[7] These vesicles are rich in phosphatases, and acid phospholipids are present in their membranes.

Role of Osteoinductive Matrix Proteins

In view of the affinity of fibronectin for collagen, it is thought that fibronectin may play a role in attachment and recruitment of osteoprogenitor cells by chemotaxis as a necessary first step to osteoinduction. It has recently become possible to dissociate the osteoinductive components of matrix from collagen residues by means of differential matrix breakdown and extraction. It has been shown that the collagenous matrix alone will not induce bone formation without the replacement of the osteoinductive components of matrix. However, it has been shown that substituting for bone collagen residues with tendon residues will not induce bone formation despite the addition of the noncollagenous osteoinductive portion of the matrix.[56] This, despite the fact that tendon is type I collagen as is the collagen of bone matrix. It would seem that there is something specific about the function of the bone collagen molecule in inducing the production of mineralization. The role of osteonectin and osteocalcin has already been referred to. The process is presumably held in balance by a series of inhibitors such as the proteoglycan molecules in the aggregated state.[56]

A *bone morphogenetic protein* fraction can be extracted from demineralized bovine bone matrix and will induce dif-

ferentiation of determined osteoprogenitor mesenchymal cells when implanted in the thigh muscles of mice.[41] The molecular weight of these fractions seem to be between 500 and 10,000 daltons.[62] How these substances work has not yet been determined, but a clue may be found in the discovery of factors resembling fibronectin that are chemotactic for osteoblasts in extracts of demineralized bone, e.g., *bone chemotactic factor* (BCF).[59]

A calcium-binding protein termed *chondrocalcin* with a strong affinity for hydroxyapatite has been identified in growth plate cartilage. This substance is present in intracellular vacuoles of chondrocytes in the proliferation, maturation, and upper hypertrophic zones of the epiphysis. It is not seen in the lower hypertrophic chondrocytes but appears there in the extracellular matrix to which it presumably has been transported. There is no observable morphological relationship between the geographical location of matrix vesicles and the major sites of calcification where chondrocalcin is concentrated.[46] Chondrocytes have the ability to induce calcification in the matrix, and endochondral ossification has been produced by transplanting a culture of growth plate chondrocytes from one animal into a dorsal ectopic site in a host animal.[71] The production of chondrocalcin is a specific property of the epiphyseal chondrocytes, and articular chondrocytes do not induce the same response. Osteoblasts seem to originate from separate mesenchymal progenitor cells rather than from differentiating chondrocytes in endochondral ossification.[71]

Mechanism of Bone Mineralization

There has been some dispute as to the exact nature of bone mineral. It has been shown to consist mainly of calcium and inorganic phosphorus. It contains a significant amount of carbonate and has the x-ray structural characteristics of poorly crystallized hydroxyapatite.[47,48] There is still lack of agreement about the details of its molecular structure or chemical composition. There is agreement, however, that the bone crystals are of very small size, offering a large surface area for chemical interactions consistent with the role of bone as the body's large reservoir of ionic reserves of calcium and magnesium (about two-thirds of the body's magnesium is in the skeleton). Of importance is the fact that progressive changes occur in the x-ray diffraction patterns of bone mineral as a function of the age of the tissue, the animal species, or the age of the mineral itself.[19,21]

During endochondral ossification in the growth plate, there is evidence to suggest that the process of mineralization is heterogeneous. It can be initiated by differing trigger mechanisms in various parts of the tissue but with the same underlying physicochemical process of mineral nucleation.

Cartilaginous matrix consists of type II collagen, whereas bone matrix contains type I collagen, and the mechanism of this change occurring during endochondral ossification has been studied using amino histochemical staining.[72] These studies have shown that mesenchymal cells (presumably invading osteoblasts) lay down type I collagen on the surface on the eroded cartilage. However, eventually type I collagen appears together with type II collagen within the territorial matrix of the hypertrophic chondrocytes, indicating that as they degenerate, the chondrocytes switch over to initiating synthesis of type I collagen, which seems to be a necessary precursor for the formation of osteoid.

According to Glimcher[19] the solid phase particles of calcium phosphate seen within the matrix vesicles or the mitochondria cannot themselves play a direct physical role in the calcification of relatively remote components, for example, the collagen fiber. In different geographical sites during different modes of calcification, matrix vesicles are not present. The theory that matrix vesicles may initiate nucleation, which then spreads to the hole zones of the collagen fiber by secondary nucleation, also does not seem to stand up since in most instances the spaces *between* the collagen fibers are *not* first filled up with a solid mineral phase of calcium phosphate before mineralization of the collagen fiber begins. According to Glimcher the striking feature of early mineralization is the deposition of the initial crystals within the collagen fiber in the hole zone region at a time when there is generally little or no mineral between the collagen fibril. This author and coworkers have suggested a unifying hypothesis that crystals are initially formed de novo within collagen fibrils from a solution phase of calcium phosphate and that these crystals do not form spontaneously in the extracellular fluid in the intervening space between the fibrils.[19,27,54] This hypothesis supposes that collagen fibrils in their configuration within bone act as a heterogeneous nucleation catalyst and are themselves responsible for de novo formation of initial calcium phosphate solid-phase particles in the hole zones of the fibrils.[20] This hypothesis is supported by the work referred to on the specific nature of the osteoinductive properties of bone collagen matrix residues.[56] Collagen fibrils in bone are potent nucleation catalysts probably because they contain specific nucleation sites where calcification can be initiated. Glimcher has concluded, therefore, that calcification of mitochondria matrix vesicles, collagen, and other spatially distinct components are independent physicochemical events. An arrangement of specific organic macromolecules in each of these regions provides the correct circumstances to form a solid calcium phosphate phase of bone mineral from calcium phosphate solutions.[19,54] These molecular changes may be modulated not only by facilitatory factors but also by enzyme inhibitor systems. The affinity of tetracycline for sites of mineralization of osteoid is well known, and it has now been demonstrated that this antibiotic can inhibit the breakdown of connective tissue mediated by excessive collagenolytic activity because of its ability to inhibit tissue collagenase activity.[24] Glimcher has recently suggested that phosphoproteins synthesized by bone osteoblasts link the mineral phase of bone to the organic matrix. He suggests that specific binding occurs between the phosphoproteins and particular sites in the collagen fibers which may be near hole zone regions.[19] The particular phosphoproteins involved link the mineral and organic phase by phosphomonoester bonds of phosphoserine and phosphothreonine. The serine and threonine concentration seems to be highest in the earlier stage of mineralization but falls with increased mineralization. This suggests that the mechanism described is responsible for the nucleation of the first mineral particles but that further mineralization occurs by secondary nucleation.

BONE MARROW

Marrow occupies the medullary cavity and the space between the trabeculae of cancellous bone.

Red marrow is hematopoietic and is the only marrow type found in the neonate. In adults, the presence of red marrow in the diaphyses of the appendicular skeleton is always pathological. It is normally restricted to the axial skeleton and the epiphyses of long bones. It is the principal source of both erythrocytic and granulocytic cells and is also a source of osteoprogenitor cells. Hematopoietic stem cells colonize the marrow during development and are derived from blood in the fetal liver.[66]

Yellow marrow has its characteristic color because of the large quantity of fat it contains. Yellow marrow is the norm in most areas of bone in the adult skeleton. It may revert to its hematopoietic function, however, and become red in certain pathological states, for example, Paget's disease.[13]

THE BLOOD SUPPLY OF BONE

The nutrient artery enters a long bone by traversing the cortex of the diaphysis obliquely. This artery supplies not only the medullary cavity but the diaphyseal cortex by vessels which penetrate the cortex from within. The direction of blood flow, therefore, is centrifugal. This always seems to be so where the muscles are only loosely attached to the external surface of the cortex, although in regions such as the linea aspera, additional vessels may supply a small piece of cortex from its external surface.[52] This supply from attachments of major septa, such as to the linea aspera, is by periosteal arteries. In addition to these vessels metaphyseal arteries enter and anastomose with terminal branches of the nutrient artery; this anastomotic circulation becomes significant following trauma. The centrifugal flow of blood in bone is confirmed by the appearance of the oozing cortex of the long bone after the periosteum has been stripped at surgery (Fig. 7-16).

The venous drainage of bone (the efferent system) consists of capillary efflux into medullary sinuses, which form veins traversing the cortex to reach the periosteum. Thus the full thickness of the cortex is drained to the periosteal surface. Unlike the arterial supply the venous drainage is similar even at the fascial attachments.[52]

Rhinelander has carried out valuable work to show the effect of various surgical insults on the blood supply of bone. He has disproved the long-standing belief that a circlage wire loop could seriously damage the blood supply of the long bone but has demonstrated that an encircling band of greater width, such as a Parham-Martin band or a plate, applied to bone can affect the afferent outflow of both arterial and venous blood in that situation. Similarly, he has shown how the clover leaf nail, both by its large surface area in contact with the endosteal bone surface and by its elasticity causing it to maintain such contact over a long period, can seriously affect the blood supply of a long bone. From purely vascular considerations a fluted nail is less harmful. His review article[52] contains important fundamental knowledge of the effect of other surgical insults including that from acrylic cement. The ex-

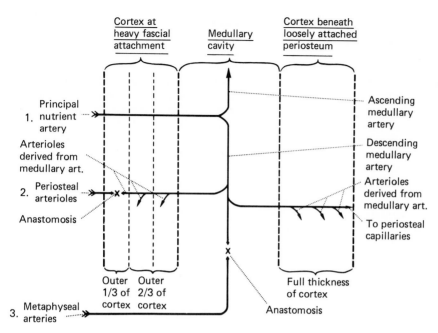

Figure 7-16 Diagram showing the distribution of the afferent vascular system of a mature long bone. Components (1), (2), and (3) are its sources of blood. Blood flow is centrifugal from medulla to periosteum (direction indicated by arrow.) *(From Rhinelander, F.W., in Bourne, G.H., ed: The Biochemistry and Physiology of Bone, 2d ed, vol 2. New York, Academic Press, 1972.)*

tensive cortical necrosis achieved with this material may be due in part to its effect in preventing reestablishment of a medullary blood supply after its destruction by diaphyseal reaming. With the advent of porous ingrowth materials such fundamental knowledge is critical, and this article should be read in full.

Altered hemodynamics of the bone may occur in several disease states. Pathological increases in bone blood flow occur in the active phase of Paget's disease. The early phases of reflex sympathetic dystrophy also cause bone hyperemia. Plethysmographic studies demonstrate a 30 percent increase in blood flow to an affected limb.[29] Immobilization of uninjured rabbit limbs, while causing regional osteopenia, did not produce changes in regional blood flow rates.[70]

Bone marrow pressure is dependent on arterial perfusion and resistance within the venous system. Normal bone marrow pressure is 20 mmHg. Sustained increases over 30 mmHg are likely etiologic factors in idiopathic osteonecrosis of bone.[15]

Living bone receives blood flow at the rate of 10 ml/g of tissue per minute. This accounts for approximately 11 percent of the cardiac output. Control of bone hemodynamics is mediated by neural, humeral, and local mechanisms. A 25 percent increase in bone blood flow has been shown to occur following sympathectomy or neurectomy.[57] Unmyelinated autonomic nerve fibers are seen around bone marrow vessels, and norepinephrine and adrenaline have been shown to produce vasoconstriction and vasodilation, respectively, in bone and bone marrow. Local metabolic modulation of bone hemodynamics has also been demonstrated. Hypercapnia, acidosis, and acid metabolites cause local vasodilation and increased blood flow.[57]

BONE METABOLISM

Calcium

Bone is the reservoir for 99 percent of the body's calcium; 1 percent of the calcium in bone may be considered as a readily exchangeable reservoir. Access to the rest of the bone calcium is only by some combination of cellular (e.g., osteoclast), paracrine (e.g., osteoclast stimulating factor), or endocrine (e.g., PTH) factors (Table 7-1, Fig. 7-17).

Control of extracellular calcium concentration is important. The excitability of the muscle cell membrane is proportional to the ratio,

$$\frac{(HCO_3^-)\,(HPO_4^-)}{(Ca^{++}Mg^{++})\,(H^+)}$$

According to the formula, a fall in the level of the calcium in the extracellular fluid can promote tetany. This is the basis of the well-known Chvostek's sign, when tapping the masseter muscle often induces spasm in that muscle. There may be associated carpopedal spasm. The treatment of hypocalcemia is an appropriate infusion of calcium. (See Chap. 20, Sect. A.)

Excessive administration of vitamin D preparations together with oral calcium supplements can result in hypercalcemia which in excess of 40 mg/dl can be rapidly fatal. The treatment of life-threatening hypercalcemia is urgent rehydration and the administration of furosemide. The symptoms of hypercalcemia may vary from mental depression and lethargy to psychosis. The effect on the muscles is to induce hypotonia and weakness, and there may be cardiac arrhythmias. Alterations may be seen on the EEG as well as the ECG.[53] The differential diagnosis includes malignancy with bone involvement, primary hyperparathyroidism, vitamin D intoxication,

TABLE 7-1 Some Agents Affecting Bone Metabolism and Their Actions at Different Target Sites

Agent	Gut	Kidney	Bone
PTH	Increases Ca^{2+} absorption via effect on $1,25(OH)_2D_3$ production.	Increases renal reabsorption of $Ca.^{2+}$	Acts on osteoblasts (via cyclic AMP and $Ca.^{2+}$ Second messengers).
		Inhibits active reabsorption of phosphate: phosphaturia (via cyclic AMP). Stimulates $1,25(OH)_2D_3$ production by renal 1α hydroxylase.	Indirect stimulation of osteoclasts.
$1,25(OH)_2D_3$	Promotes binding and absorption of Ca^{2+} from lumen.	Inhibits activity of renal 1α hydroxylase.	$\downarrow$ Bone matrix synthesis.
		Promotes $24,25(OH)_2D_3$ pathway.	$\uparrow$ Osteocalcin synthesis. $\uparrow Ca^{2+}$ in ECF* (active transport across bone cells).
Calcitonin		Increases excretion of sodium and phosphate.	Induces quiescence in osteoclasts. Phosphate enters BF† and bone cells; probably Ca^{2+} also.

*ECF: extracellular fluid.
†BF: bone fluid.

and sarcoidosis. There are also rare inherited forms of hypercalcemia.

Plasma calcium exists in three forms: 48 percent of it is present in the free ionized form; 46 percent is ionized but bound to serum proteins, mainly albumin; and the remainder is complexed with citrate and phosphates.[37] It will be seen from the equation described above that even in the presence of normal serum calcium, an alkaline pH, such as one induced by hyperventilation, may cause the physiological effects of hypocalcemia. Other causes include surgically produced hypoparathyroidism, pseudohypoparathyroidism, malabsorption syndromes, and vitamin D deficiencies.

Calcium absorption from the gut is by means of active transport in the brush border of certain lining epithelial cells. This process is regulated by 1,25-dihydroxy vitamin D_3 $[1,25(OH)_2D_3]$. At the luminal surface of the mucosal cell, the absorption of calcium *into* the cell is mediated by a $1,25(OH)_2D_3$-dependent calcium carrier in the brush border. Calcium transport *from* the mucosal cell into the blood is enhanced by $1,25(OH)_2D_3$, but the necessary calcium transporting ATPase may also be enhanced by stimulation of alpha-adrenergic receptors (e.g., by epinephrine).[31]

The rate of production of $1,25(OH)_2D_3$ at the kidney is increased when the plasma calcium level is decreased, and it is reduced when the plasma calcium is elevated (Fig. 7-18). Calcium absorption is thus adjusted to body needs. Calcium is also possibly secreted into the gut, by different cells from that which reabsorb it, by means of a calmodulin-dependent calcium transporting ATPase.[31] Some calcium is absorbed by passive diffusion and by certain substances that form insoluble compounds with calcium, for example, oxylates. Phosphates may therefore have some effect on decreasing absorp-

tion of alimentary calcium. Severe dietary calcium deficiency or intestinal malabsorption of calcium produces defective skeletal mineralization (osteomalacia). Calcium ingestion varies greatly and is often subnormal in the elderly.

Reabsorption of almost all filtered calcium is accomplished by the kidney. Sixty percent of the reabsorption occurs in the proximal tubule. The remainder takes place in the distal tubule and is regulated by parathyroid hormone.

Phosphate

Plasma levels of phosphate vary from 2.4 to 4.4 mg/dl. Most of this is in a diffusable form, only 12 percent being bound to protein. Apart from its role in key cellular enzyme systems and molecular interactions, phosphate is a component of bone mineral. It is not surprising, therefore, that of the total body phosphorus of 500 to 800 g, some 85 to 90 percent is found in the skeleton.

The movement of calcium and phosphate ions is often linked (Fig. 7-18). Phosphate is the normal accompanying anion in the calcium transport system during absorption from the gut, but an independent phosphate absorption system that shows vitamin D dependence has been postulated. The absorption of phosphate from the gut seems to be linearly proportionate to dietary intake.[17]

Only 10 percent of the phosphate passing through the glomerulus is excreted in the urine, the rest being reabsorbed. There are two mechanisms for reabsorption. Active reabsorption in the proximal tubule of the nephron is by active transport, a process which when inhibited by PTH, is responsible for the phosphaturic action of that hormone. A sec-

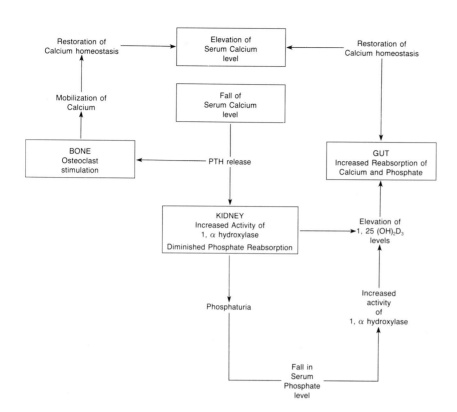

Figure 7-17 Feedback mechanisms affecting kidney, bone, and gut that maintain calcium homeostasis.

ond mechanism seems to be independent of parathyroid gland functions so that as the serum level of inorganic phosphate rises, renal tubular reabsorption of phosphate diminishes; this can be shown to occur in isolated tubular segments. It is not simply dependent upon variations in the amount of phosphate filtered at the glomerulus.

A feedback mechanism exists between the level of plasma phosphate and the activity of the renal 1α-hydroxylase enzyme responsible for converting $25\text{-}OH\text{-}D_3$ to the more active form $1,25(OH)_2D_3$ (Figs. 7-18). Production of the active metabolite is reduced by the inhibition of this enzyme by high plasma phosphate levels. Plasma phosphate levels seem to have no effect upon parathyroid gland production of PTH.

A decrease in blood calcium level is caused by hyperphosphatemia (such as that which may occur with the low filtration rates of chronic renal disease) related to diminished production of calcitriol. The low calcium stimulates increased parathyroid activity, which will increase the renal clearance of phosphate as well as blood calcium levels to restore homeostasis (Fig. 7-18). If the kidney cannot respond with increased phosphate loads, since PTH is also mobilizing phosphate from the bone, phosphate levels will remain high. Eventually, however, the low levels of $1,25(OH)_2D_3$ will affect the ability to maintain adequate calcium balance. There may be undiminished stimulation of the parathyroids and renal osteodystrophy results. Inadequate levels of $1,25(OH)_2D_3$ lead to osteomalacia; the secondary hyperparathyroidism may cause changes of osteitis fibrosa cystica.

In renal tubular diseases, there may similarly be low levels of $1,25(OH)_2D_3$, associated however with abnormally high levels of phosphate excretion by the kidney.[34]

Parathyroid hormone

The stimulus for the release of stored PTH from the production site—the chief cells in the parathyroid glands—is a diminution in the level of ionized calcium in the extracellular fluid (Fig. 7-18). When serum calcium levels are elevated, secretion is inhibited. According to Rosenblatt [53] the relationship of calcium to parathyroid hormone is linear within a narrow physiological range, but below 8 mg/dl, hormone secretion decreases dramatically. The hormone mobilizes calcium from bone by action upon cells lining the bone surfaces and also mobilizes phosphate from bone. At the kidney it has a phosphaturic action and also influences vitamin D metabolism.

There is data to suggest that cyclic AMP and, perhaps, ionic calcium (Ca^{2+}) function as second intracellular messengers in response to parathormone.[18,32] This certainly seems to be true in bone, where the osteoblast is the target cell for PTH. In bone, PTH interacts with receptors on the osteoblast cell membrane, promoting the activity of adenylate cyclase located on the membrane and the entry of calcium into the cell. The changes in levels of calcium and cyclic AMP inside the cell produce the desired cellular result. At the kidney, cyclic AMP can be detected in the urine after exposure to PTH, and such a finding can be used clinically as an indicator of hormone activity.

At the kidney the phosphaturic effect of PTH occurs rapidly. The half-life of the polypeptide hormone is less than 20 min, and it is quickly metabolized by liver Kupffer cells.[17]

Parathyroid hormone provides an appropriate physiological response to low ionic calcium by stimulating the production of $1,25(OH)_2D_3$ by 1α-hydroxylase in the kidney. The

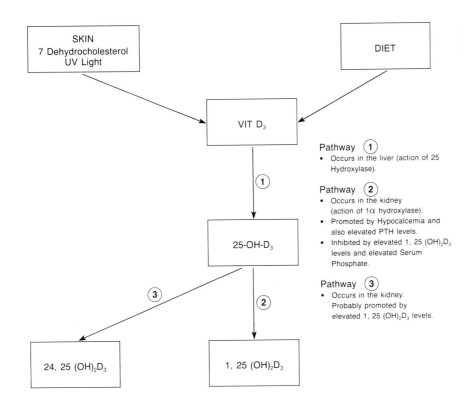

Figure 7-18 The metabolic pathways for vitamin D_3 and factors that affect them. Vitamin D_3 is the naturally occurring animal form, but synthetically produced D_2 is the usual supplement in the diet. Vitamin D_2 produces metabolic analogues similar to the D_3 compounds shown in the figure.

hormone acts directly on bone to increase bone resorption and mobilize calcium, which contributes to restoration of appropriate blood levels (Fig. 7-18).

Since the resorption of bone is associated with osteoclastic stimulation and yet the osteoblast is the *primary* target cell of this hormone, it is now evident that both in bone morphogenesis and, in response to hormonal stimulation, many of the functions of the osteoclasts seem to be mediated via the osteoblast[9] (Table 7-1).

There is evidence that hormones such as PTH, $1,25(OH)_2D_3$, and PGE_2 (one of the prostaglandin E series) stimulate osteoclasts indirectly following a primary hormonal interaction with osteoblasts.[8,9] In addition to inducing changes in the osteoblasts on the bone surface, which change into a spindlelike shape, PTH inhibits bone collagen synthesis by altering the activity of procollagen messenger RNA.[49]

Vitamin D

The naturally occurring animal form of vitamin D is termed D_3 and has minor chemical differences from the synthetic form (D_2). The precursor 7-dihydrocholesterol is stored in the skin and may be converted to cholecalciferol (vitamin D_3) by the effect of ultraviolet irradiation in sunlight.

At the liver, vitamin D_3 is converted to 25-hydroxycholecalciferol ($25\text{-}OH\text{-}D_3$). Like all vitamin D derivatives, this metabolite is transported bound in the plasma to a specific globulin (vitamin D–binding protein). Within the mitochondria of cells of the proximal renal tubules, $25\text{-}OH\text{-}D_3$ is converted by the action of the enzyme renal 1α hydroxylase

to 1,25-dihydroxycholecalciferol $[1,25(OH)_2D_3]$ (Fig. 7–17). The activity of renal 1α hydroxylase in the production of $1,25(OH)_2D_3$ is inhibited both when the plasma phosphate level is high and when the level of PTH is low. This provides a mechanism for controlling extracellular fluid calcium levels. Further specific hydroxylation in the kidney of $25\text{-}OH\text{-}D_3$ also produces another metabolite, 24,25-dihydroxycholecalciferol $[24,25(OH)_2D_3]$, this pathway being facilitated by elevated $1,25(OH)_2D_3$ levels (Fig. 7-18).

It follows from this description of the production of active metabolites that vitamin D is more appropriately thought of as a hormone and one with critical roles within the body whose depletion or absence induces severe bone disease. The action of the active metabolite, $1,25(OH)_2D_3$, in regulating calcium absorption from the gut has been described, but it also has important actions directly upon the bone. It can have similar reactions to PTH on bone matrix synthesis, which it may diminish in vitro by as much as 50 percent.[67] It also increases the synthesis and serum concentration of osteocalcin (Table 7-1).

It has been suggested that the role of vitamin D in inhibiting bone collagen synthesis (studied in tissue culture) is a mechanism useful when calcium and phosphate are in short supply.

Recent work has shown that $1,25(OH)_2D_3$ inhibits the proliferation of first-generation mesenchymal cells in the bone induction promoted by intramuscular implants of demineralized bone graft. There is a delay in mesenchymal tissue proliferation and the beginning of chondrogenesis. However, at a later stage in the induction of bone, when capillary sprouts are prominent, the hormone stimulates the differentiation of the cells associated with the vascular ingrowth. These cells differentiate into osteoblasts with an increase in alkaline phosphatase levels which can be measured.[67] The evidence suggests also that a receptor for $1,25(OH)_2D_3$ is present in osteoblasts. Its action may be similar upon osteoblasts that line bone surfaces as is its action upon gut mucosal cells, where it modulates calcium transport across the cells.

It has been observed that serum levels of $1,25(OH)_2D_3$ do not increase in the summer months. There are, however, seasonal trends for the incidence of such conditions as osteomalacia and certain fractures, which tend to increase in the winter months, and for renal nephrolithiasis, which seems to increase in the summer months. The data would seem to suggest that metabolites of vitamin D other than $1,25(OH)_2D_3$ may have an important physiological role.[11] The metabolite $24,25(OH)_2D_3$ was thought to represent a shunting of hormone that might act as a storage mechanism when high levels of calcitriol were not required. However, it is now believed that this metabolite has a role of its own since it seems to be necessary together with $1,25(OH)_2D_3$ for adequate healing in experimental rickets and also has a potent influence on chondrogenesis and mineralization during endochondral bone development and in fracture repair.[43]

Calcitonin

Calcitonin is a polypeptide hormone synthesized and secreted by parafollicular cells derived from the ultimobranchial body. These cells are identified in humans as clear cells (C cells) primarily in the thyroid gland. In fishes, where calcitonin is probably more important metabolically, the ultimobranchial body is distinct from the thyroid. The exact role of the hormone is uncertain (Table 7-1), but it is secreted when the thyroid gland is perfused with solutions containing high calcium concentration, and it seems to have a half-life of only about 10 min.[17] Calcitonin seems to induce quiescence in osteoclasts and consequently lowers serum calcium. Thyroidectomy does not affect plasma calcium levels if the parathyroid glands are preserved.

Osteoclasts have membrane receptors for calcitonin, and the hormone causes loss of ruffled borders on these cells associated with a rise in intracellular cyclic AMP levels. Prostaglandin PGI_2 has a similar effect, increasing intracellular levels of cyclic AMP in osteoclasts and inducing cytoplasmic quiesence. Prostaglandin PGE_2, PTH, and $1,25(OH)_2D_3$ can reactivate quiescent osteoclasts and stimulate osteoblasts in vivo but not affect those cells directly in vitro, suggesting that they act indirectly by means of a primary interaction with osteoblasts.[9]

Other Hormones

Mineral homeostasis is normally maintained primarily by the mechanisms described, and these mechanisms function smoothly during growth and normal bone remodeling. The changes that occur in metabolic and endocrine bone disease are described in Chap. 20, Sect. A.

Although changes in levels of other hormones do not cause such dramatic skeletal manifestations, nevertheless gross changes will lead to bone disease. With thyroid hormone excess, for example, there is a generalized increase in bone turnover with a balance tipped toward bone reabsorption and the development of osteoporosis.

Patients chronically treated with glucocorticoid demonstrate a decrease in bone formation associated with inhibition of collagen synthesis. Increase in bone reabsorption is also observed and is thought to be due in part to increased PTH activity.[18] Certainly an increase in the blood level of parathyroid hormone and alkaline phosphatase coupled with an increase in calcium excretion was observed after the administration of prednisone in human subjects.[18] There is an increase in urinary cyclic AMP levels as a response to the raised PTH. It seems that at the gut, glucocorticoids stimulate active calcium secretion by mucosal cells, resulting in a decrease of net calcium absorption in that portion of the gut concerned with active transport of calcium. However, there is some increase in the passive diffusion of calcium in the duodenum mediated by glucocorticoid, which seemed to cancel out the effect on active transport.

The mechanism by which postmenopausal bone loss is associated with diminished estrogen levels is presently unknown, and estrogens do not seem to have a direct effect on bone cells or matrix synthesis but may moderate the action of other hormones such as PTH.[36]

Insulin seems to participate in the regulation of bone growth,[66] and, in particular, it is necessary for the anabolic effect of growth hormone.

Growth hormone increases calcium excretion in urine but also increases intestinal absorption of calcium, with a resulting positive calcium balance.[17] Normal thyroid hormone levels are also necessary for normal maturation and growth. Some of the effects of growth hormone on epiphyseal cartilage are mediated by the somatomedins. The latter are a group of five separate peptides released in the liver by the effect of growth hormone.[17]

REFERENCES

1. Ane, W.P., Roufosse, A.H., Glimcher, M.J., and Griffin, R.C. Solid-state phosphorus-31 nuclear magnetic resonance studies of synthetic solid phases of calcium phosphate: Potential models of bone mineral. Biochemistry 23:6110, 1984.
2. Baxter, L.A., and DeLuca, A.H. Stimulation of 25 hydroxy vitamin D3 one alpha hydroxylase by phosphate depletion. J Biol Chem 251:315–318, 1976.
3. Bonar, N.C., Lees, S., and Mook, H.A. Neutron diffraction studies of collagen in fully mineralised bone. J Mol Biol 181:265–270, 1985.
4. Boskey, A.L. Current concepts of the physiology and biochemistry of calcification. Clin Orthop 157:225–257, 1981.
5. Buckwalter, J.A. Proteoglycan structure in calcifying cartilage. Clin Orthop 172:207–232, 1983.
6. Burger, E.H., Vandermeer, J.W.M., Vandergabel, J.S., Giribnan, J.C., Thesingh, C.W., and Van Furth, R. Origin of osteoclasts from immature mononuclear phagocytes in Silbermann, M., and Slavkin, H.C. (eds): *Current Advances in Skeletogenesis.* Excerpta Medica. Amsterdam, Elsevier, 1982, pp. 87–92.
7. Cecil, R.N.A., and Anderson, H.C. Freeze fracture studies of matrix vesicle calcification in epiphyseal growth plate. Metab Bone Dis. 1:89, 1978.

8. Chambers, T.J., and Dunne, C.J. Osteoclast activities determined by intracellular AMP levels, in Silbermann, M., and Slavkin, H.C. (eds.): *Current Advances in Skeletogenesis.* Excerpta Medica. Amsterdam, Elsevier, 1982, pp. 154–157.

9. Chambers, T.J. and Dunne, C.J. Prostacyclin inhibits the cytoplasmic activity of isolated osteoclasts, in Silbermann, M., and Slavkin, H.C. (ed): *Current Advances in Skeletogenesis.* Excerpta Medica. Amsterdam, Elsevier, 1982, pp. 149–153.

10. Chen, C.C., Boskey, A.L., and Rosenberg, L.C. The inhibitory effect of cartilage proteoglycans on hydroxyapatite growth. Calcif Tissue Int 36:285–290, 1984.

11. Clayton, J., Clayton, J., Guilland-Cumming, D.F., Johnson, S.K., Challa, A., Russell, R.G.G., and Kanis, J.A. Seasonal trends in vitamin D metabolism in Silbermann, M., and Slavkin, H.C. (eds): *Current Advances in Skeletogenesis.* Excerpta Medica. Elsevier, Amsterdam, 1982, pp. 224–229.

12. Dezik, A.M., Hard, D., Migasaki, K.T., Brown, M., Weinfeld, N., and Housmann, E. Prostaglandin E2 binding and cyclic AMP production in isolated bone cells. Calcif Tissue Int 34:57, 1983.

13. Duthie, R., and Bentley, G. *Mercer's Orthopaedic Surgery,* 8th ed. Baltimore, University Park Press, 1983, p. 30.

14. Farley, J.R., Howard, G.A., Drivdahl, R.H., and Baylink, D.J. Characterisation of a putative coupling factor from human bone, in Silbermann, M., and Slavkin, H.C. (eds): *Current Advances in Skeletogenesis.* Excerpta Medica. Amsterdam, Elsevier, 1982, pp. 112–116.

15. Ficat, R.P. Idiopathic bone necrosis of the femoral head. J Bone Joint Surg 67B: 3–10, 1985.

16. Friedenstein, A.J. Determined and indetermined osteogenic precursor cells, in *Hard Tissue, Growth Repair and Mineralisation,* vol. 11. Ciba Foundation Symposium. Excerpta Medica. Amsterdam, Elsevier, 1973, pp. 1169–1185.

17. Ganong, W.P. *Review of Medical Physiology,* 11th ed. Lange Medical Publications, Los Altos, Calif. 1983.

18. Gennari, C., Imbimbo, B., Montagnani, M., Bernini, M., Nardi, P., and Avioli, L.V. Effects of prednisone and deflazacort on mineral metabolism and parathyroid hormone activity in humans. Calcif Tissue Int 36:245–252, 1984.

19. Glimcher, M.J. Recent studies of the mineral phase in bone and its possible linkage to the organic matrix by protein-bound phosphate bonds. Philos Trans R Soc Lond B304:479–508, 1984.

20. Glimcher, M.J. The role of collagen and phosphoproteins in the calcification of bone and other collagenous tissues, in Rubin R.P., Weis, G.B., and Putney, J.W. (eds): *Calcium in Biological Systems.* Plenum Pub. Co., 1985, pp. 607–615.

21. Glimcher, M.J., and Krane, S.N. The organization and structure of bone and the mechanism of calcification, in Ramchandran, G.N., and Gould, B.S. (eds): *Treatise on Collagen,* vol. 2. London, Academic Press, 1968, pp. 67–251.

22. Glimcher, M.J., Shapiro, F., Ellis, R., and Eyre, D.R. Changes in tissue morphology and collagen composition during the repair of cortical bone in the adult chicken. J Bone Joint Surg 62A:964–973, 1980.

23. Glorieux, F.H. Mineral, in Cruess, R.L. (ed): *The Musculoskeletal System.* New York, Churchill Livingstone, 1982, p. 103.

24. Golub, L.N., Ramamurthy, N., McNamara, T.F., Gomes, B., Wolff, M., Casino, A., Kapoor, A., Zambow, J., Ciancio, M., Schneir, M., and Perry, H. Tetracycline inhibits tissue collagenase activity. J Periodont Res 19:651–655, 1984.

25. Gomori, C. Microtechnical demonstration of phosphatase in tissue sections. Proc Soc Exp Biol 42:23, 1939.

26. Grant, M.G., and Prockop, D.J. The biosynthesis of collagen. N Eng J Med 286:194–199, 242–249, 291–300, 1972.

27. Grynpas, M.D., Bonar, L.C., and Glimcher, M.J. Failure to detect an amorphous calcium-phosphate solid phase in bone mineral. A radial distribution function study. Calcif Tissue Int 36:291–301, 1984.

28. Halthrop, M.E., Racz, L.C., and Simmons, H.A. The effects of parathyroid hormones, colchicine and calcitonin on the ultrastructure and activity of osteoclasts. J Cell Biol 60:346, 1974.

29. Hartley, J. Reflex hyperemic deossification (Sudeck's atrophy) J Mt Sinai Hosp 22:268, 1955.

30. Hauscher, P.V., Lin, J.B., and Gallop, P.N. Proc Nat Acad Sci USA 73:1447, 1976.

31. Hyun, C.S., Cragoe, J.E., Jr., and Field, M. Adrenergic receptor mediated regulation of internal calcium transport. Am J Physiol 249:117–123, 1985.

32. Kohler, G., Schen, U., and Peck, W.A. Adriamycin inhibits PTH-mediated but not PGE2-mediated stimulation of cyclic AMP formation in isolated bone cells. Calcif Tissue Int 36:279–284, 1984.

33. Kowarski, S., and Schacter, D. Effects of vitamin D on phosphate transport and incorporation in the mucosal constituents of rat intestinal mucosa. J Biol Chem 244:211–217, 1969.

34. Krane, S.M., and Near, R.M. Connective tissue, in Smith, L.H., and Thier, S.O. (eds): *Pathophysiology: The Biological Principles of Disease.* Philadelphia, Saunders, 1985.

35. Lane, J. Current concepts review. Osteoporosis. J Bone Joint Surg 65A:274–278, 1983.

36. Langeland, N. The in vitro effect of oestradiol on collagen metabolism in metaphyseal rat bone. Acta Orthop Scand 48:226–272, 1977.

37. Lingarde, F. Potentiometric determination of serum ionised calcium in the normal human population. Clin Chem Acta 40:477–484, 1972.

38. Manezel, J., Posner, A.S., and Harper, R.A. Age change in the crystallinity of rat bone apatite. Isr J Med Sci 1:251, 1965.

39. Marie, P.G. Bone: structure organization and healing, in Cruess, R.L. (ed): *The Musculoskeletal System.* New York, Churchill Livingstone, 1982, p. 143.

40. Matthes, J.L., Kennedy, J.W., III, and Collins, E.J. An ultrastructural study of calcium and phosphate deposition in hard tissues. *Hard Tissue Growth, Repair and Mineralisation.* Ciba Found Symp 11:187–211, 1973.

41. Mitzutani, H., and Urist, M.R. The nature of bone morphogenetic protein (BMP). Factors derived from bovine bone matrix gelatin. Clin Orthop 171:213–223, 1982.

42. Norimatsu, H., Vanderwiel, C.J., and Talmage, R.V. Morphological support of a role for cells lining bone surfaces in maintenance of plasma calcium concentration. Clin Orthop 138:254–262, 1979.

43. Norman, A.W., and Edelstein, S. Overview of vitamin D sessions, in Silbermann, M., and Slavkin, H. C. (eds): *Current Advances in Skeletogenesis.* Excerpta Medica. Amsterdam, Elsevier, 1982, pp. 230–232.

44. Price, P.A., Lothringer, J.W., Baukol, S.A., and Reddi, A.H. Developmental appearance of the vitamin K-dependent protein of bone during calcification. J Biol Chem 256:3781, 1981.

45. Price, P.A., Otsuka, A.S., Poser, J.W., Kristaponis, J., and Raman, N. Characterization of a -carboxyglutamic acid-containing protein from bone. Proc Natl Acad Sci USA 73:1447, 1976.

46. Poole, A. R., Pridoux, I., Reiner, A., Choi, H., and Rosenberg, L. C. Association of extracellular protein (chondrocalcin) with the calcification of cartilage in endochondral bone formation. J Cell Biol 98:54–65, 1984.

47. Posner, A.S. Crystal chemistry of bone mineral. Physiol Rev 49:760–792, 1969.

48. Posner, A.S., and Betts, F. Bone mineral, in Owen, R., Goodfellow, J., and Bullough, P. (eds): *Scientific Foundation of Orthopaedics and Traumatology.* Philadelphia, Saunders, 1980, pp. 42–49.

49. Raisz, L.G., and Kream, B.E. Regulation of bone formation. New Engl J Med 309:29–35, 1983.

50. Ray, R.D., Aouad, R., and Kawabata, M. Experimental study of peripheral circulation in bone growth. Clin Orthop 52:221-232, 1967.

51. Reddi, A.H. Local and systemic mechanisms regulating bone formation and remodeling an overview, in Silbermann, M., and Slav-

kin, H.C. (eds): *Current Advances in Skeletogenesis.* Excerpta Medica. Amsterdam, Elsevier, 1982.

52. Rhinelander, F.W. The blood supply of the limb bones, in Owen, R., Goodfellow, J., and Bullough, P. (eds): *Scientific Foundations of Orthopaedics and Traumatology.* Philadelphia, Saunders, 1980, pp. 126–154.

53. Rosenblatt, M. Hormonal regulation of calcium metabolism, in Smith, L.H., and Thier, S.O. (eds): *Pathophysiology: The Biological Principles of Disease.* Philadelphia, Saunders, 1985.

54. Roufosse, A.H., Ane, W.P., Roberts, J.E., Glimcher, M.J., and Griffin, R.C. Investigations of the mineral phase of bone by solid state phosphorus-31 magic angle sample spinning nuclear magnetic resonance. Biochemistry 23:6115, 1984.

55. Roufousse, A. H., Landis, W. J., Sabine, W. K., and Glimcher, M.J. Identification of bushite in newly deposited bone mineral from embryonic chicks. J Ultrastruct 68:235, 1979.

56. Sampath, T.K., DeSimone, D.P., and Reddi, A.H. The role of extracellular matrix in local bone induction, in Silbermann, M., and Slavkin, H.C. (eds): *Current Advances in Skeletogenesis.* Excerpta Medica. Amsterdam, Elsevier, 1982, pp. 66–73.

57. Shim,S.S. Physiology of blood circulation of bone. J Bone Joint Surg, 50A:812–824, 1968.

58. Smith, J.W. Molecular patterns in native collagen. Nature 219:157, 1968.

59. Somerman, M., Hewitt, A.T., Varne, H.H., Varner Schiffmann, E., Reddi, H.H., and Termine, J.D. The role of chemotaxis in bone induction, in Silbermann, M., and Slavkin, H.C. (eds): *Current Advances in Skeletogenesis.* Amsterdam, Elsevier, 1982, pp. 56–57.

60. Strawich, E., and Glimcher, M.J. Differences in the extent and heterogeneity of lysyl hydroxylation in embryonic chick cranial and long bone collagens. J Biol Chem 258:555–562, 1983.

61. Termine, J.D. Phenotypic protein of calf lamellar bone, in Silbermann, M., and Slavkin, H.C. (eds): *Current Advances in Skeletogenesis.* Excerpta Medica. Amsterdam, Elsevier, 1982, pp. 3–7.

62. Termine, J.D. Chemical characterization of fetal bone matrix, in Silbermann, M., and Slavkin, H.C. (eds): *Current Advances in Skeletogenesis.* Exerpta Medica, Amsterdam, Elsevier, pp 349–352, 1982.

63. Thielemann, F.W., Alexa, M., Herr, G., and Schmidt, K. Matrix induced intramembranous osteogenesis, in Silbermann, M., and Slavkin, H.C. (eds): *Current Advances in Skeletogenesis.*Excerpta Medica. Elsevier, Amsterdam, 1982, pp. 56–57.

64. Uhthoff, H.K., Sekaly, G., and Jaworski, Z.F.G. Effects of long term nontraumatic immobilisation on metaphysical spongiosa of adult and old beagle dogs. Clin Orthop 192:278–283, 1985.

65. VanderRest, M. Collagen structure and biosynthesis, in Cruess, R. L. (ed): *The Musculoskeletal System.* New York, Churchill Livingstone, 1982, p. 67.

66. Vaughan, J. *The Physiology of Bone,* 2nd ed. Oxford, Clarendon Press, 1975.

67. Vukicevoc, S., et al. One alpha dihydroxy vitamin D_3 stimulates alkaline phosphatase activity and inhibits soft tissue proliferation in implants of bone matrix. Clin Orthop 196:285–291, 1985.

68. Walser, M. Ion association and interaction between calcium, magnesium, inorganic phosphate, citrate and protein in normal human plasma. J Clin Invest 40:723–730, 1961.

69. Warshawsky, H. Embryology in development of the skeletal system, in Cruess, R.L. (ed): *The Musculoskeletal System.* New York, Churchill Livingstone, 1982, p. 37.

70. Woessner, J.F., Jr., and Howell, D.S. The enzymatic degradation of connective matrices, in Owen, R., Goodfellow, J., and Bullough, P. (eds): *Scientific Foundations of Orthopaedics and Traumatology.* Philadelphia, Saunders, 1980, pp. 232–241.

71. Wright, G. C., Miller, F., and Sokoloff, L. Induction of bone by xenografts of rabbit growth plate chondroyctes in the nude mouse. Calcif Tissue Int 37:250–256, 1985.

72. Yasui, N., Ono, K., Konomi, H., and Nagai, Y. Transitions in collagen types during endochondral ossification in human growth cartilage. Clin Orthop 183:215–218, 1984.

CHAPTER 8

Bone Healing

Roger Dee

STAGES OF HEALING

Hematoma

When a long bone fractures, the associated soft tissue injury disrupts the bone blood supply and devascularizes the bone ends. There is usually periosteal rupture and associated muscle damage on one side of the bone, but the soft tissue may be intact on the other side, forming a hinge useful in reducing fractures by closed manipulation. Histologically empty lacunae are seen lying within dead bone ends where cell death has occurred. The fracture hematoma is soon colonized by inflammatory cells, including macrophages and polymorphonuclear leukocytes but also by mast cells capable of secreting heparin. Typical changes during the inflammatory phase include vasodilatation, exudation of plasma, and the migration of the leukocytes.[23]

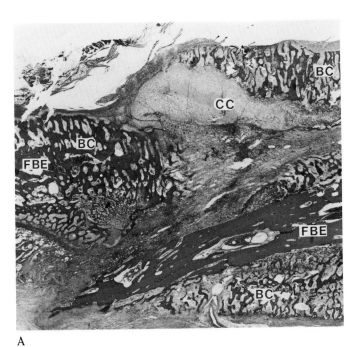
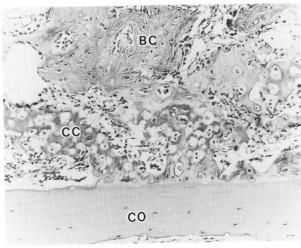

A

B

Figure 8-1 Bone formation in early external callus. **A.** Fracture in a child aged 2 years showing proliferative bone and cartilage formation. H & E, × 9.6. **B.** Same fracture as in *A.* BC, bony callus; CC, chondroid callus; CO, cortex; FBE, fracture bone ends; H & E, × 193. *(Courtesy of Dr. L. Sokoloff.)*

Callus Formation

The fracture hematoma is next invaded by a mantle of capillaries and cells including fibroblasts that are capable of laying down collagen. There is rapid replacement of the fracture hematoma by granulation tissue. Organization of the hematoma may be termed the *reparative phase* of fracture healing and leads to the formation of soft callus. Osteoprogenitor cells proliferate in the endosteum, also in the cambial layer of the periosteum and surrounding soft tissues. This produces osteoblasts, which proceed to lay down woven bone. Cartilage is produced at the most peripheral portion of the callus which is later converted to bone by a process of endochondral ossification. According to Lane and co-workers[11] types I, II, and III collagen may be seen during the stage of early soft callus production. The appearance of chondral material, however, is accompanied by predominantly type II collagen production associated with territorial matrix of the condrocytes. During the period of woven bone formation, type I collagen once again predominates. (These are similar to the changes in collagen types seen in mineralization of epiphyseal cartilage.)

The periosteal blastema of cells, with actively dividing cells in the vanguard, originates near the fracture. It approaches a similar growth of callus from the adjacent fragment of bone and will form bridging callus if other soft tissues are not interposed or if the gap is not too large. In a fracture that has not been treated by rigid fixation and where there is therefore some movement at the fracture site during healing, the external callus formation may be considerable and may cause a noticeable swelling in the region of the fracture (Fig. 8-1).

REGIONAL DIFFERENCES IN BONE HEALING

Glimscher and co-workers[9] have observed variations in bone repair in different regions of the bone. They used a liquid nitrogen probe to create an area of dead compact cortical bone. They noted that initially almost all differentiating cells became osteoclasts and began reabsorbing the dead cortical bone. Later, osteoblasts appeared on the scene, and the characteristic coupled cutting cone type of activity of both kinds of cells was observed. It took about 3 years, however, for the majority of the dead bone to be resorbed and replaced by new living bone. They obtained a different response to a liquid nitrogen lesion in cancellous bone,[9] where osteoprogenitor cells proliferate and then differentiate mainly into osteoblasts. They also observed that osteoprogenitor cells did not differentiate into bone cells in the living bone at the sites where they proliferate but that they differentiated only after they had invaded the dead bone. In cancellous bone there is, therefore, initially an increase in the mass of bone with trabecular thickening. Cutting cones with osteoclasts remove the dead trabecular bone eventually, but this process is very slow and may take several decades.[6]

McKibbin points out that in cancellous bone, since the cells are never very far away from blood vessels, bone apposition or replacement can take place on the surface of the trabeculae by creeping substitution, and cutting cones may not be required.[13] This type of bone obeys Wolff's law only sluggishly if at all.[9] In compact subchondral bone, resorption seems to take place at the expense of new bone formation, so that collapse and fracture in the region of the bone articular cartilage junction is common.

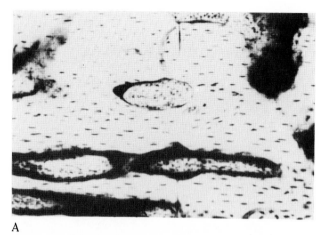

A

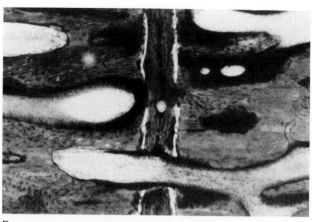

B

Figure 8-2 A. Histology of the cortex of the sheep tibia beneath a rigid plate, 12 weeks after operation. Primary fracture healing is seen in spite of full weight bearing. No specific resorption of the compressed surfaces is visible. **B.** Histology of the opposite side of the same tibia shown in *A.* The gap between the fragments is first filled by lamellar bone ("transverse osteon"), which in turn will be remodeled later in an axial direction. Fluorescent label given 3 weeks after the operation is found in such a transverse osteon. This animal was sacrificed at 12 weeks. *(From Perren, S.M., et al, Acta Orthop Scand (suppl) 125, 1969. Reproduced with permission.)*

FACTORS AFFECTING FRACTURE HEALING

Effect of Mechanical Environment: Osteonal Healing

When a fracture is rigidly immobilized, for example, by rigid compression plates, minimal external callus is produced and the fracture may heal by a mechanism resembling normal bone remodeling (Figs. 8-2*A* and 8-3). It is possible for a remodeling cutting cone to traverse the fracture and for the space to become filled with a new osteon that traverses the fracture (Fig. 8-2*B*). It appears that this process is extremely slow, as would seem to be confirmed by Glimcher's work, and most of the revascularization occurs from vessels lying in the medullary canal.[13]

Woo et al[22] believe it is unlikely that direct osteonal union occurs without some initial callus being formed, even with the most rigid compression plate. They point out that the micromotion between bone ends immobilized by even the most rigid plate will generate stresses which exceed the ultimate strain (failure point) of osteons of haversian bone crossing the fracture line under these circumstances, because of the small size of the gap (Fig. 8-4). Since the ultimate strain of callus is about twice that of bone, much more micromotion is permissible without rupture of the tenuous union during the early stage of union if callus is the first material laid down.[22]

It seems likely then that direct osteonal union across the bone ends does not occur under clinical conditions, even with the most rigid plate, without a preliminary phase of medullary callus. Also, osteons cannot cross gaps in fibrous tissue so that if there is any appreciable gap between the bone ends after plating, preliminary replacement by medullary callus certainly must occur (Fig. 8-2).[13] Leaving a gap between the bone ends invites failure when using a plate. McKibbin[13] points out that if a fracture has been plated with a rigid plate and with any appreciable gap between the bone ends, then it is unlikely that that fracture will be healed by an external bone graft. He also points out that remodeling by primary union is a very slow way of achieving union, and so the implant is necessary for a long period of time.

It seems certain that alterations of the electrical properties of bone and injury potentials affect osteogenesis. An appropriate mechanical stimulus to a molecule such as collagen or a proteoglycan, which has a fixed charge, may influence its activity with regard to the formation of nucleation sites for mineralization.[19] Bassett[1] has termed such molecules "electrets" and has suggested that mechanical changes may influence the bone cells in such a way as to modify their behavior. The factors which may influence the release of such inductive proteins, such as bone morphogenic protein or osteonectin, await elucidation.

The remodeling of newly deposited woven bone during fracture healing is obviously affected by the mechanical forces imposed upon the fracture. The primary callus is relatively uninfluenced by mechanical factors until it becomes external bridging callus.[13] When bridging has occurred, inductive mechanisms come into play that speed up or delay the mineralization of chondroosteoid. They may influence the outcome and even contribute to nonunion. Fractures treated with intramedullary rods show more periosteal callus than fractures treated with rigid compression plates.[16] The bone porosity is increased in fractures treated either with a compression plate or with a rigid intramedullary rod, when compared with a loosely fitted intramedullary rod.[16] On the other hand, the presence of a loose intramedullary rod delays union by damaging the formation of endosteal callus. Indeed, biomechanical maturation is delayed in all fractures treated with intramedullary rods compared with compression plates, although once union is achieved, the biomechanical quality of the union is similar with either plate or nail.[16] Primary bone healing occurring during rigid fixation produces an area of bone beneath the plate which, because it is protected from

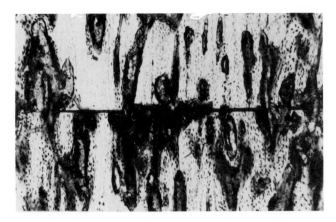

Figure 8-3 Histology of a transverse tibial osteotomy in a sheep 8 weeks after fixation with two DCP gauge plates. At this time the osteotomy is only partially remodeled. The gap at this particular site of the osteotomy measures about 20 μm. *(From Perren, S.M., et al, Acta Orthop Scand (suppl) 125, 1969. Reproduced with permission.)*

stress, can subsequently produce fatigue fracture.[21] This effect is diminished in experimental animals by using less rigid plates—a procedure that produces bone with better mineralization and mechanical properties. Microradiography shows this bone to have undergone less endosteal resorption than with rigid plates.[20] Some authors have designed their fracture treatment around the precept that some motion at the fracture site must be perpetuated for early rapid healing, and this is the basis for the search for less rigid internal fixation devices and also for the functional bracing of fractures.[17]

Medullary callus has been shown to be independent of mechanical influences.[13] This probably explains why if there is a 50 percent transverse displacement in a diaphyseal fracture, union is often vigorous since the osteogenic endosteal

blastema from the medullary cavity will unite with the periosteal blastema of the opposite fragment.[13] It would seem that once the stage of bridging callus is reached, successful differentiation into bone is influenced considerably by mechanical factors.[13]

Woo and his co-workers[23] have considered the theoretical requirements for fixation plates to maximize the environmental conditions necessary for fracture union using various materials and designs. They have concluded that during the early stage of fracture management, the plate must be stiff enough in bending and torsional directions to prevent bone angulation or implant failure. They caution against using more flexible materials without great consideration because of these reasons. They point out that in the late phases of callus or bone remodeling, the plate must be stiff enough under axial loading to ensure that the underlying bone shares a higher proportion of the physiological stresses needed to facilitate its normal remodeling and avoid osteoporosis (Fig. 8-5). Their preliminary results have shown a tubular cross-sectional plate composed of titanium alloy has suitable properties in this regard.

Blood Supply and Fracture Healing

There is good correlation between the increased blood supply seen during fracture healing and the mineralization at the fracture site. The blood supply to the whole bone increases in addition to the regional increase in flow at the fracture site. This was demonstrated by Paradis and Kelly[16] in dog tibias. They also demonstrated that the blood flow at the fracture site reached its maximum on the tenth day and then progressively decreased. It may be 2 months, however, before blood flow to a fracture approaches normal levels.

In a review, Brighton[3] has drawn attention to the paradox between the increased local blood flow which can be measured with radioisotopes and the finding of diminished oxygen

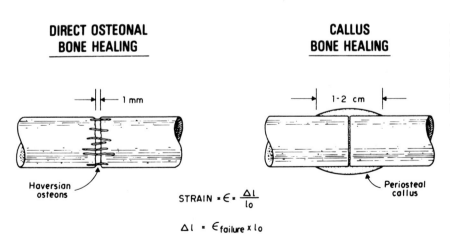

Figure 8-4 Diagram showing that the maximum permitted motion of 1 to 2 mm occurring at a fracture site healing by callus is many orders of magnitude higher than that permissible for successful direct osteonal healing to occur (5 μm). *(From Woo, S.L.Y., et al, J Orthop Res 1:431–449, 1984. Reproduced with permission.)*

tension in fracture hematoma and in newly formed fracture cartilage. It seems that despite a rich capillary bed into the fracture callus, hypoxia does exist at the cellular level. During mineralization of osteoid in fracture callus, this cellular hypoxia may be a trigger for chondrocyte mitochondria to release accumulated calcium into the matrix by exocytosis in the same way that this process occurs in the hypertrophic zone at the growth plate.[3] A cartilaginous phase is, however, not essential for the mineralization of osteoid in all modes of bone repair (see below).

The blood supply to a fracture is changed dramatically by surgical intervention. It has been shown by Rand and coworkers,[16] that higher values exist for whole bone and fracture site blood flows when the fracture is fixed with an intermedullary rod than when a similar fracture is fixed with a rigid compression plate and that the high levels persist for a longer period with the rod. These changes presumably reflect alteration in the pattern of interosseous flow to accommodate the new circulatory dynamics caused by the fixation device, as well as the fracture. When the normal centrifugal blood supply is interfered with by a large intermedullary rod, the periosteal supply becomes more important. Whether the plate is placed subperiosteally or extraperiosteally, there were similar effects on bone blood flow and the rate of fracture union was the same.

It has been shown that marginal bone necrosis and bone resorption at the bone ends does not occur under a compression plate, as had been previously believed[12] (Figs. 8-1 and 8-2). If a medullary device is inserted, the periosteal blood supply must be meticulously preserved so that it may nourish the bone until the endosteal circulation has recovered from the surgical insult. When a plate is applied, the intramedullary blood supply becomes the major source of blood to the bone.

Factors Contributing to Impair Union

A whole host of systemic factors have been said to impede fracture healing, and these have been enumerated by Brighton.[3] These factors include steroids, indomethacin and estrogens, anemia, vitamin A and D excess, and also vitamin D deficiency associated with malabsorption. Similarly, factors which may promote fracture healing include vitamins A and D, calcitonin, thyroid derivatives, insulin, and growth hormone[3] (although there are also some negative reports concerning the effect of calcitonin and growth hormone). The rate of callus production in some experimental animals has also been thought to be accelerated by hyperbaric oxygen.[14] Denervation has been shown to have some effect upon the rate of cellular mitosis in the periosteum following amputation.[5] Increased healing of fibular fractures in sciatically denervated rats has been reported.[6]

A distinction has been drawn between fractures caused by high-energy absorption of bone before failure and those lesser injuries where there will probably be less extensive associated soft tissue damage. It has been suggested that with severe soft tissue injury, there may be conflicting priorities to heal bone or soft tissues and consequently the activation of structural genes may cause differentiation at an early stage in

fracture healing to produce fibroblasts rather than osteogenic cells.[10] A similar suggestion attributed to Pritchard is quoted by McKibbin.[13] This author differentiated between the repair process initiated from the outer fibrous layer of the periosteum and that which emanated from the cambial layer. He considered it possible for the fibrous tissue to invade the fracture gap under certain circumstances and impair the ingrowth of the osteogenic blastema.

Failure to develop an adequate anastomotic blood supply to the fracture area is a probability in high-velocity injuries and may be responsible for the so-called atrophic nonunion where all cellular activity seems to be suppressed. No callus is produced, the bone ends are sclerotic, and the medullary cavities are closed over at the fracture site. There may be a fully developed pseudarthrosis with a "joint cavity" after a period of time. Such radiological changes indicate cessation of reparative biological activity, support a diagnosis of nonunion, and differentiate from the condition of delayed union. This latter condition exists when union has not occurred within the expected time frame but there are as yet no clinical or radiological changes to indicate that it cannot. In hypertrophic nonunion there may be abundant proliferative radio-

PRE-UNION

LOADS ON PLATE: BENDING AND TWISTING

POST-UNION

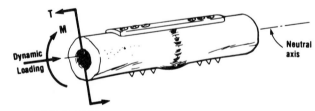

LOADS ON PLATE: TENSION OR COMPRESSION

Figure 8-5 Diagram demonstrating the changes in the loading conditions on the internal fixation plates between the pre- and postunion stages of a long bone fracture. Under identical dynamic in vivo loads, the plate is subjected to bending and torsional loads in the early healing phase because of the discontinuity of bone. However, as healing progresses, the neutral axis of the plate-bone structure shifts toward the bone and the plate is subjected to tensile or compressive loads. *(From Woo, S.L.Y., et al, J Orthop Res 1:431–449, 1984. Reproduced with permission.)*

paque callus, but none of it bridges the fracture, which is still visible as a lucent line. Presumably, here differentiation has been to cartilage and fibrous tissue, but not to bone. Such a response with proliferative external callus but no bridging bony callus is less common than atrophic nonunion. It may also, if untreated, produce a fully developed pseudarthrosis. The role of "inadequate immobilization" in producing nonunion is unclear but certainly it would appear to affect the differentiation of pluripotential cells during the phase of bridging callus.

Other factors which may contribute to nonunion include infection and ischemia or similar unfavorable factors affecting tissue nutrition. In an established nonunion, the capacity to form bone is not lost and endochondral ossification has been shown to continue with the typical arrangement of hypertrophic cartilage cells in columns in the tissue separating the bone ends. A barrier seems to be established between the bone ends with proliferation of cartilage cells similar to the situation existing in a growth plate. Surgical intervention is usually necessary at this stage to alter the physical environment in favor of union. This can be done by altering the mechanical condition of the fracture with some kind of fixation device (either internal or external) or, alternatively, by introducing autogenous bone graft together with whatever osteoinductive proteins it may contain. The operative procedure itself will dramatically affect the blood supply to the fracture, which will contribute in a major way to the outcome of the surgery.[2] The use of electrical stimulation is described elsewhere.

Intraarticular fractures, in the past, achieved a reputation for nonunion, and there has been speculation that synovial fluid interposes itself between the fragments. However, with modern methods of early, accurate open reduction of these fragments and internal fixation, they have been found to heal, as does most cancellous bone, with a lower rate of nonunion than diaphyseal fractures.

With regard to pathological fractures, there has been controversy in the past concerning their rate of union. This is important when making a decision whether to insert methyl methacrylate cement together with a fixation device into a pathological fracture. In many cases this technique will give enough structural support for the limited life span of the terminal patient. In individual cases, depending on the prognosis and the loads expected on the bone, bony union can be achieved and may be a preferable solution. In such cases cement may be omitted; however, the problem is that irradiation and chemotherapy in themselves may significantly delay union in pathological fractures.[7] The long bone pathological fractures that heal most predictably are those in patients who have been internally fixed and irradiated with less than 3000 rad. In patients with nonlung tumors who survived longer than 6 months, 74 percent of such fractures united. Internal fixation improved the rate of fracture union by 23 percent compared with cast and immobilization.[7]

REFERENCES

1. Bassett, C.A.L., and Becker, R.O. Generation of electric potentials by bone in response to mechanical stress. Science 137:1063–1064, 1962.
2. Bohr, H. Bone formation in case of delayed fracture union and pseudarthrosis. Calcif Tissue Res 4(suppl):117:119, 1970.
3. Brighton, C. The biology of fracture repair. Instruct Course Lect 33:60–82, 1984.
4. Brookes, M. *The Blood Supply of Bone.* New York, Appleton-Century-Crofts, 1971, p 270.
5. Bunch, W.H., Deck, J.D., and Roma, J. The effect of denervation on bony overgrowth after below knee amputation in the rat. Clin Orthop 122:333–339, 1977.
6. Frymoyer, J.N., and Pope, M.H. Fracture healing in the sciatically denervated rat. J Trauma 17:355–361, 1977.
7. Gainor, B.J., and Buchert, P. Fracture healing in metastatic bone disease. Clin Orthop 178:297–302, 1983.
8. Glimcher, M.J., Shapiro, F., Ellis, R.D., and Ayre, D.R. Changes in tissue morphology and collagen composition during the repair of cortical bone in the adult chicken. J Bone Joint Surg 62A:964–972, 1980.
9. Glimcher, M.J. The nature of the mineral component of bone and mechanism of calcification. Instruct Course Lect 36:49–69, 1987.
10. Hulth, D. Fracture healing, a concept of competing healing fractures. Acta Orthop Scand 51:5–8, 1980.
11. Lane, J.M., et al.: A temporal study of collagen, proteoglycans, lipids and mineral constituents in a model of endochondral osseous repair. Metab Bone Dis Relat Dis 1:319, 1979.
12. Mayer, G., and Wolf, E. Animal experiments to examine the histology of fracture healing in osteosynthesis with external fixation and compression. Arch Orthop Trauma Surg 101:111–120, 1983.
13. McKibbin, B. The biology of fracture healing in long bones. J Bone Joint Surg 60B:150–162, 1978.
14. Ninikoski, J., et al.: Effect of hyperbaric oxygen on fracture healing in the rat. A biochemical study. Calcif Tissue Res 4(suppl):115–116, 1970.
15. Paradis, G.R., and Kelly, P.J. Blood flow and mineral deposition in canine tibial fractures. J Bone Joint Surg 57A:220–226, 1975.
16. Rand, J.A., An, K.N., Chao, E.Y.S., and Kelly, P.J. A comparison of the effect of open intramedullary nailing and compression plate fixation on fracture site blood flow and fracture union. J Bone Joint Surg 63A:427–442, 1981.
17. Sarmiento, A., et al.: Principles of fracture healing. Instr Course Lect 33:84, 1984.
18. Schenk, R., and Willenegger, H. Morphological findings in primary fracture healing. Symp Biol Hung 7:75, 1967.
19. Tornberg, D.N., and Bassett, C.A.L. Activation of the resting periosteum. Clin Orthop 129:305–312, 1977.
20. Torino, A.J., Davidson, C.L., Klopper, P.J., and Linclau, L.A. Protection from stress in bone and its effects. Experiments with stainless steel and plastic plates in dogs. J Bone Joint Surg 58B:107–113, 1976.
21. Uhthoff, H.K., and Dubuc, F.L. Bone structure in the dog under rigid internal fixation. Clin Orthop 81:165–171, 1971.
22. Woo, S.L.Y., et al.: Rigid internal fixation plates: Historical perspectives and new concepts. J Orthop Res 1:431–449, 1984.
23. Wray, J.B. Acute changes in femoral arterial blood flow after closed tibial fractures in dogs. J Bone Joint Surg 46A:1261–1268, 1964.

CHAPTER 9

Bone Grafting and Transplantation

Gary E. Friedlaender

Bone grafts are frequently used to repair or replace skeletal deficits associated with a wide variety of bony disorders spanning congenital, traumatic, degenerative, and neoplastic causes. Specific applications include the filling of cystic defects, repairing nonunions, supplementing arthrodeses, and providing segmental replacements.[15]

In one form or another, bone grafts have been used for centuries, as documented by numerous biblical, ecclesiastical, and ancient medical records of varying credibility.[2] The modern science associated with bone grafts began in the nineteenth century with contributions by Ollier[27] and Macewen[24] and practical applications were further developed in the early twentieth century by Albee,[1] Lexer,[23] and Phemister,[29] to name only a few.

BONE GRAFT APPROACHES

Today, the armamentarium of bone graft approaches is extensive. Cortical and cancellous autograft can be transplanted alone or as composites with soft tissues, and the procedures may be effected with or without an intact or reestablished blood supply. Similarly, a variety of allogeneic and even xenogeneic preparations treated and preserved by a wide spectrum of approaches are available. Indeed, the choice of appropriate bone graft material is now as complex as the diversity of disorders for which these transplants are employed. Nonetheless, autografts remain the standard by which all other approaches must be measured and for which our knowledge, while incomplete, is most comprehensive.

Autografts

Autografts are tissues removed from one place in the body and returned to another site in that *same individual* (whether animal or human). By definition, these tissues are histocompatible, and transfer of disease from donor to recipient is not an issue. Consequently, the biological potential of autogenous tissues is considered to represent the maximum achievable.

Much of the physiological control over bone graft incorporation remains unknown or a matter of speculation, but the histological sequence of events has been well described and serves as a basis for discussing rational clinical applications of these tissues.[5,7,19]

Bone graft incorporation is an interactive process between the graft and the host bed, with contributions from each source that can either enhance or detract from the process. In general, grafts must be invaded by blood vessels. The blood vessels emanate from the recipient site and carry with them multipotential cells that differentiate into populations specialized in bone formation or resorption. The graft itself serves as a passive scaffold or template for this influx of activity (osteoconduction) and may also provide active signals to the host response capable of influencing, if not regulating, the process (osteoinduction).[37] The goal of incorporation is replacement of preexisting bone graft with host-bed-derived osteogenic activity; this new bone eventually enters into the normal homeostatic routine of remodeling, a process that responds to physiological stresses, be they mechanical or biological.

Nonvascularized Grafts

The histological pattern observed with nonvascularized bone graft incorporation—that is, a graft transferred without an intact blood supply or without immediate reestablishment of blood flow by vascular reanastomosis—begins with hematoma formation (similar to fracture repair) followed by a gradual transformation to a fibrovascular response. The graft itself undergoes substantial cell necrosis, except for those cells within approximately 0.1 to 0.3 mm of the surface, which can survive by diffusion.[20] The necrosis causes an inflammatory response within the contiguous fibrovascular stroma, the tissue that is also responsible for ingrowth of new blood vessels into the bony architecture.

Up to this point, cortical and cancellous grafts behave in a similar fashion, but significant differences can be identified both qualitatively and quantitatively in the now-ongoing repair processes. Cancellous grafts are rapidly revascularized by virtue of their porous structure. Osteoblastic activity then follows with the deposition of osteoid on surfaces of necrotic trabeculae, and mineralization proceeds to engulf the osteogenic cell population. This new bone activity causes cancellous grafts to initially appear increased in radiographic density. Osteoclastic activity begins later in this sequence, and eventually the preexisting necrotic graft is resorbed and replaced as remodeling ensues. The incorporation process of cancellous bone is relatively rapid and relatively complete compared to cortical grafts.

Cortical bone revascularizes more slowly, with an initial ingrowth of blood vessels occurring peripherally and through preexisting haversian canals. Revascularization is aided and, in part, is dependent upon a vigorous osteoclastic response, and this response causes increased porosity (decreased radiographic density) and reduced mechanical strength during the early stages of cortical graft incorporation. Resorption is followed by osteoblastic activity, resulting in "creeping substitution" of the original cortex, along with an increased mechanical strength, and this phase of repair is followed by an ongoing remodeling mode. Cortical bone graft incorporation is slower and less complete than that seen with cancellous tissue, but the end result is substantial and is both biologically and biomechanically effective.

Vascularized Grafts

Revascularized grafts—those tissues transferred along with their vascular pedicle which are reanastomosed at their site of implantation and those grafts transferred limited distances such that their usual blood supply remains intact—do not undergo the incorporation process described for nonvascularized grafts. Instead, they unite to the recipient-site skeleton by a process analogous to fracture repair.[38] Theoretically, these grafts remain in a remodeling mode and do not sustain the initial cell necrosis, matrix resorption, and transient loss of mechanical strength characteristic of nonvascularized tissues.

Allografts

Allografts are tissues transferred between members of the *same species* (human to human, rabbit to rabbit, etc.). Unlike autografts, they do not require sacrifice of a normal structure when recovered from cadavers or when removed incidentally from a living donor in the course of an unrelated operative procedure. Furthermore, the potential morbidity associated with a second operative site required to obtain autograft is avoided, and the limits in size, shape, and quantity of autogenous tissues is circumvented by allogeneic sources. On the other hand, allografts raise issues relevant to their biological potential: possible transfer of disease from donor to recipient and immune responses to clearly foreign tissues.

At the present time, allografts cannot be transferred with an intact blood supply because of the consequences of immunologic rejection on vascular endothelium. Instead, allogeneic bone is usually subjected to some form of long-term preservation, especially freezing or lyophilization. In any case, cell viability within the graft is lost. This cellular activity is not prerequisite to biological efficacy of bone grafts, but the few cells that remain viable in fresh autografts undoubtedly contribute to the biological momentum observed during the initial stages of bone graft incorporation. Allografts, therefore, incorporate more slowly and, perhaps, less completely but are otherwise qualitatively similar to autografts. Various preservation techniques can, however, influence subsequent allograft repair.[5,7,19,21] For example, demineralization of allogeneic bone appears to enhance the osteoblastic response but reduces the initial strength of the graft. Lyophilization and high-dose irradiation contribute to long-term storage but also sacrifice mechanical characteristics.[15,28]

Xenografts

Xenografts are tissues transferred *between species* (cow to human, etc.), and although they are used clinically in some countries, past experience in the United States has been unsatisfactory. Lack of reliable bone incorporation, in particular, has detracted from the clinical application of these tissues. Efforts to combine xenografts with autogenous marrow are being explored and may stimulate renewed interest and reconsideration of the role of xenogeneic bone grafts in the future.[33]

IMMUNOLOGIC CONSIDERATIONS

Foreign tissues evoke immune responses, the nature and scope of which are influenced by a variety of factors. The degree of genetic disparity between donor and recipient, the route of immunization as well as dose and time of exposure to antigen, and the general immunocompetence of the recipient—all influence the expression of transplantation immunity. In addition, immune responses are manifest by both cellular and humoral components that are interrelated, often apparently reciprocal in intensity and, in the case of bone, rarely of straightforward significance. Immunologic rejection is usually defined as an adverse influence on biological function resulting from a specific immune response. It is difficult to quantitate bone graft biology or function in vivo and noninvasively. In contrast, renal, hepatic, and cardiac function can be monitored easily. Therefore, most approaches to assessing bone graft immunology and its significance have relied upon animal models.[10,12]

Investigational approaches to transplantation immunobiology require choices between animal models, potential graft-related antigens, and various assays of immunity. Each of these separate issues is further complicated by many variables that must be kept in perspective when trying to ascribe significance to the results of these studies. These issues must be added to a baseline of problems when assessing biological function of the grafts. Different animals, for example, have their own immunologic idiosyncrasies that may infringe upon their relevance to human transplantation. The induction of tolerance is much easier to achieve in mice than in humans. Reagents for manipulating immune responses and quantitating results also vary among different species, as does our understanding of immunogenetics and the availability of well-defined inbred strains. The choice of appropriate assays of immunity are another source of variation among different investigational approaches. In vivo methods such as skin graft rejection patterns may not provide results analogous to in vitro quantitation of lymphokine production, mixed lymphocyte reactivity, or cytotoxicity. The dose of reagents, dilution of sera, numbers of cells or specific fractionation of cell populations, and assay conditions including timing and temperature may all influence results.

Antigens

Of particular interest is the choice of appropriate antigen(s) to represent "bone graft" in immunologic assays. Bone includes mineral, matrix, collagen, and a heterogeneous cell population. Of these various components, only the mineral phase has been excluded as a potential immunogen. Matrix, collagen, and cell-surface antigens have all been implicated as sources of immunogenicity and, therefore, sensitization associated with bone grafts. Each have been explored to varying degrees in both animals and humans.

Although little is known about the production of anticollagen antibodies following bone graft transplantation, there is no question that collagen is immunogenic.[36] In allogeneic systems and, indeed, xenogeneic models, collagen is a weak antigen but cannot be excluded as a significant factor in sensitizing recipients to bone. Matrix components have only recently been purified to the point where they can be evaluated as immunogens with confidence. Results to date suggest that hyaluronic acid and the sugar side chains of the large proteoglycan aggregate molecules (chondroitin-4-sulfate and chondroitin-6-sulfate) lack detectable immunogenicity. On the other hand, xenogeneic and probably allogeneic proteoglycan subunits and link protein do evoke immune responses in laboratory animals.[13,30,31]

Undoubtedly the most potent source of sensitization from bone grafts is associated with cells and their surface transplantation antigens, expressions of the major histocompatibility complex (HLA-A in man, H-2 in mice, RLA-A in rabbits, etc.). Despite the heterogeneity of cell types in bone (e.g., osteogenic, chondrogenic, fibrous, hematopoietic, fatty, neural, etc.), all bone cells share common transplantation antigens, and these antigens have routinely been used to evaluate the immunogenicity of bone.

Animal Studies

Numerous approaches have been used to define bone allograft antigenicity in animals over the past 30 years. The earliest studies were based upon histological examination of cellular infiltrates associated with various implants and from which immunogenicity was inferred.[3,8,9] In fact, histology alone cannot be used to differentiate a nonspecific inflammatory reaction from a specific immune response. Other early approaches included observation of skin graft rejection patterns and both histological and morphological evaluation of lymph nodes draining the site of bone graft transplantation.[4,6,9] Virtually all these studies suggested that fresh allografts were strongly immunogenic, that deep-freezing prior to implantation significantly reduced the intensity of response, and that lyophilization decreased immunogenicity to negligible levels.

More recently a variety of sophisticated and objective in vitro assays of humoral and cell-mediated immunity have been applied in animal models.[10,12,16] Qualitative as well as quantitative differences have been observed between various laboratory animals, but the majority of studies support the earlier conclusions previously cited.

Human Studies

The evaluation of bone graft immunogenicity in humans has been relatively limited; however, available information paral-

lels that obtained in animals.[11] Human recipients of fresh bone allografts usually develop humoral antibodies following allogeneic bone graft transplantation.[22] The response seen after implantation of massive frozen allograft appears to be reduced modestly in both frequency and intensity and even more so if the bone has been freeze-dried.[17,32]

Significance of Allograft Antigenicity

Even though the occurrence of sensitization following osteochondral allograft transplantation has been substantiated in animal models and humans, the significance of these responses remains unclear. It has not been possible to correlate the nature of histological repair in animals with either the presence or intensity of immune responses, and there is virtually no clinical material available with which to address these questions in humans. There is, nonetheless, reason to believe that sensitization to any tissue will, to some degree, influence biological behavior, and, most probably, the more intense reactions observed with fresh allografts are associated with the most adverse effects on biological function. This contention is extrapolated from experience with solid organ transplantation, but confirmation will require some sophisticated and extensive human studies.

BONE BANKING

The goals of bone banking are to provide adequate quantities of biologically useful tissues at times dictated by clinical circumstance and without concern for transferring disease from donor to recipient. Guidelines and standards have been developed by the American Association of Tissue Banks that address these requirements.[14,34]

Donor Criteria

Bone grafts can be recovered from living donors "incidentally" in the course of operative procedures necessitating the removal of bone (e.g., femoral heads during joint replacement) or from cadaveric sources. In either event, appropriate authorization of the individual or next of kin is required, and the history of the potential donor is carefully reviewed. The basic principle in screening donors is to avoid the use of bone as a vector for transmission of a potentially serious illness to the recipient and to avoid the use of bone whose biological or physical properties may be compromised or may be viewed as unpredictable. Contraindications to tissue donation include evidence of sepsis or infection of the bone to be recovered; malignancies, particularly those with a propensity to metastasize to the skeleton; viral diseases, including hepatitis, rabies, Creutzfeldt-Jakob disease (and other slow-virus disorders), and acquired immunodeficiency syndrome (AIDS); venereal diseases; the presence of toxic substances in toxic amounts; systemic collagen disorders; and diseases of unknown etiology.

Tissue Recovery and Preservation

Bone may be recovered in a sterile fashion using an operating room environment and customary technique, or tissues may be removed under clean conditions that require secondary sterilization. High-dose irradiation and chemicals (e.g. ethylene oxide or concentrated acids) have been used widely to render tissues free from pathogens, but these may, in turn, influence the mechanical properties of bone.

Once removed, tissues may be preserved for later application by a wide variety of approaches including deep-freezing, lyophilization, or combinations of chemical extraction and chemosterilization. Again, manipulation of the graft may cause changes in its biological or biomechanical properties,[28] but the importance of these changes will vary with intended clinical applications. For example, lyophilization causes gross structural cracks that render bone less capable of withstanding loads. Such tissue may not be suitable for segmental replacements, unless methods of internal fixation compensate for this weakness; however, loss of mechanical strength will be of no significance when such tissue is used to fill cystic defects. The author's preferred method of tissue acquisition and long-term preservation is sterile recovery and frozen storage at -70°C to -80°C.

Unlike bone, cartilage preservation requires retention of cell viability. For this purpose, the articular surface is exposed to either glycerol or dimethyl sulfoxide (DMSO) prior to freezing. This results in viability of approximately 40 percent of chondrocytes and appears to be compatible with matrix homeostasis.[35]

Record keeping should document the donor's medical history as well as results of laboratory tests including those for hepatitis and venereal diseases. Records also provide an opportunity to identify donor-recipient combinations in the event of adverse reactions that may be related to the bone graft.

CLINICAL APPLICATIONS

The choice of appropriate graft material should be based upon knowledge of the biological and biomechanical advantages and disadvantages of specific types of bone as well as a clear understanding of the clinical circumstances and goals of the reparative procedure. As such, there may be more than one satisfactory solution for specific problems, but there are also relative inadequacies inherent to some alternatives.

Autografts (Nonvascularized)

In general, the biological potential of autografts is maximal, if not superior, when compared to all other bone graft preparations.[5,7,19] Autografts must be highly considered for all circumstances requiring bone graft and especially where failure of biological potential has occurred (e.g., such as fracture nonunion) or where rapid incorporation, especially across large surfaces, is crucial to success (e.g., arthrodeses of major

joints). Decisions regarding the choice of cortical or cancellous bone reflect the specific need for the graft material. It may have to act as a structural element characteristic of cortex (struts, wafers, blocks, plates, etc.), or it may be used in filling cystic defects or in some other intrinsically stable circumstances.

Autografts (Revascularized)

Revascularized autografts do not depend upon the host bed for their success, and their potential applications reflect this uniqueness.[38] Vascularized grafts are not as dependent upon recipient site contributions as nonvascularized grafts. They can function, therefore, in locations compromised by irradiation-induced changes (characterized by fibrosis and obliteration of small blood vessels) or even by infection. Host contributions to graft repair can also be compromised by systemic factors, such as chemotherapy. Adriamycin and methotrexate, for example, are toxic to both osteoblastic and osteoclastic cells, in addition to their adverse influence on neoplastic tissues.[18] For example, these grafts can be used in circumstances that may involve infection, generally a contraindication to the use of nonvascularized autografts or allografts. They also function in a superior fashion, compared to alternatives, when the host bed has been compromised by irradiation, when there has been loss of adequate soft tissue coverage (e.g., trauma, after tumor resection) or when the patient is more generally (systemically) impaired (e.g., chemotherapy). Vascularized bone autografts also offer the opportunity to bridge substantial distances of segmental loss with a tissue that rapidly unites at each osteosynthesis site and remains viable rather than undergoing necrosis followed by creeping substitution.

Potential disadvantages to this approach include its technically demanding and time-consuming nature and the limitations imposed by available donor sites, currently confined to the fibula, rib, or iliac crest. The shape and quantity of vascularized autograft is also obviously limited as is the scope of mechanical properties, e.g., the fibula alone may be structurally inadequate to compensate properly for femoral or tibial bone stock.

Allografts

Allografts avoid the need for a donor site (postoperative discomfort, sacrifice of normal structures, etc.) and are available in virtually unlimited supply and any anatomic shape. At the present time, only nonvascularized allografts are feasible, but these can be preserved for elective reconstructive approaches, making them particularly well-suited for trauma and limb-sparing tumor resections. Available clinical information suggests that 70 to 80 percent of massive frozen osteochondral allografts are associated with successful resolution of the problem for which they are employed.[26] Unsuccessful circumstances usually involve infection, failure to unite at the osteosynthesis site, or graft fracture.[25] The use of systemic chemotherapy also appears to have an adverse effect on bone graft repair.[18] Animal studies suggest that the biological capacity of allografts, especially those which have been deep-frozen, is qualitatively similar to autografts but temporally prolonged in terms of repair.[7,21]

Allografts should be highly considered where massive segmental loss is incurred, provided that adequate soft tissue coverage and an aseptic environment can be anticipated. Allografts have also been used for filling cystic defects, in joint arthrodeses, and in fracture repair, and clinical observations support their efficacy in these circumstances as well.[15]

In summary, the future will undoubtedly provide opportunities to use fresh vascularized allografts, but their applications and logistics will remain complex and limited. Other forms of providing reliable osteogenic potential, either by treatment of allogeneic or xenogeneic bone or by using extracts of skeletal tissues, will emerge and decrease reliance upon autografts. In addition, methods to enhance the body's own osteogenic activity, either by systemic drugs or electric signals, will continue to be pursued. It is important to understand the biological aspects of bone graft repair, including the contributions of the graft and of the recipient site. Only then can one appreciate the biomechanical consequences of graft incorporation and use this knowledge to make an appropriate choice of graft material and of surgical application and method. Further, one can then also recognize and utilize responsible ways to bank allografts for later clinical applications. The surgeon must clearly understand the goals of the operative procedure in which bone graft will play a role and match these circumstances (including changes anticipated over time) with the graft material appropriate for such intended use.

REFERENCES

1. Albee, F.H. *Bone-Graft Surgery.* Philadelphia, Saunders, 1915.
2. Bick, E.M. *Source of Orthopaedics.* New York, Hafner, 1968.
3. Bonfiglio, M., Jeter, W.S., and Smith, C.L. The immune concept: Its relation to bone transplantation. *Ann NY Acad Sci* 59:417–432, 1955.
4. Brooks, D.B., Heiple, K.G., Herndon, C.H., and Powell, A.E. Immunological factors in homogeneous bone transplantation, IV: The effect of various methods of preparation and irradiation on antigenicity. J Bone Joint Surg 45A:1617–1626, 1963.
5. Burchardt, H. The biology of bone graft repair. Clin Orthop 174:28–42, 1983.
6. Burwell, R.G. Studies in the transplantation of bone, V: The capacity of fresh and treated homografts of bone to evoke transplantation immunity. J Bone Joint Surg 45B:386–401, 1963.
7. Burwell, R.G. The fate of bone grafts, in Apley, A.G. (ed): *Recent Advances in Orthopaedics.* Baltimore, Williams and Wilkins, 1963, pp. 115–207.
8. Burwell, R.G., and Gowland, G. Studies in the transplantation of bone, III: The immune response of lymph nodes draining components of fresh homogeneous bone treated by different methods. J Bone Joint Surg 44B:131–148, 1963.
9. Chalmers, J. Transplantation immunity in bone homografting. J Bone Joint Surg 41B:160–179, 1959.
10. Elves, M.W. Newer knowledge of the immunology of bone and cartilage. Clin Orthop 120:232–259, 1976.
11. Friedlaender, G.E. Immune responses to preserved bone allografts in humans, in Friedlaender, G.E., Mankin, H.J., and Sell, K.W. (eds): *Osteochondral Allografts: Biology, Banking and Clinical Applications.* Boston, Little, Brown, 1983, pp. 159–164.
12. Friedlaender, G.E. Immune responses to osteochondral allografts. Current knowledge and future directions. Clin Orthop 174:589–568, 1983.
13. Friedlaender, G.E., Ladenbauer-Bellis, I., and Chrisman, O.D. Cartilage matrix components as antigenic agents in an osteoarticular model. Trans Orthop Res Soc 5:170, 1980.
14. Friedlaender, G.E., and Mankin, H.J. Bone banking: Current methods and suggested guidelines. Instruct Course Lect 30:36–55,1981.
15. Friedlaender, G.E., Mankin, H.J., and Sell, K.W. *Osteochondral Allografts: Biology, Banking, and Clinical Applications.* Boston, Little, Brown, 1983.
16. Friedlaender, G.E., Strong, D.M., and Sell, K.W. Studies on the antigenicity of bone, I. Freeze-dried and deep-frozen bone allografts in rabbits. J Bone Joint Surg 58A:854–858, 1976.
17. Friedlaender, G.E., Strong, D.M., and Sell, K.W. Studies on the antigenicity of bone, II. Donor-specific anti-HLA antibodies in human recipients of freeze-dried bone allografts. J Bone Joint Surg 66A:107–112, 1984.
18. Fridlaender, G.E., Tross, R.B., Doganis, A.C., Kirkwood, J.M., and Baron, R. Effects of chemotherapeutic agents on bone, I: Short-term methotrexate and doxorubicin (Adriamycin) treatment in a rat model. J Bone Joint Surg 66A:602–607, 1984.
19. Heiple, K.G., Chase, S.W., and Herndon, C.H. A comparative study of the healing process following different types of bone transplantation. J Bone Joint Surg 45A: 1593–1616, 1963.
20. Heslop, B.F., Zeiss, I.M., and Nisbet, M.W. Studies on transference of bone, I: A comparison of autologous and homologous bone implants with reference to osteocyte survival, osteogenesis and host reaction. Br J Exp Pathol 41:269–287, 1960.
21. Kreuz, F.P., Hyatt, G.W., Turner, T.C., and Bassett, A.L. The preservation and clinical use of freeze-dried bone. J Bone Joint Surg 33A:863–872, 1951.
22. Langer, F., Gross, A.E., West, M., and Urovitz, E.P. The immunogenicity of allograft knee joint transplants. Clin Orthop 132:155–162, 1978.
23. Lexer, E. Joint transplantation and arthroplasty. Surg Gynecol Obstet 40:782, 1925.
24. Macewen, W. Observations concerning transplantation of bone. Illustrated by a case of inter-human osseous transplantation, whereby over two-thirds of the shaft of a humerus was restored. Proc R Soc Lond 32:232, 1881.
25. Mankin, H.J. Complications of allograft surgery, in Friedlaender, G.E., Mankin, H.J., and Sell, K.W. (eds): *Osteochondral Allografts: Biology, Banking and Clinical Applications.* Boston, Little, Brown, 1983, pp. 259–274.
26. Mankin, H.J., Doppelt, S.H., Sullivan, T.R., and Tomford, W.W. Osteoarticular and intercalary allograft transplantation in the management of malignant tumors of bone. Cancer 50:613–630, 1982.
27. Ollier, L. *Traite Experimental et Clinique de la Regeneration des Os.* Paris, Victor Masson et Fils, 1867.
28. Pelker, R.R., Friedlaender, G.E., and Markham, T.C. Biomechanical properties of bone allografts. Clin Orthop 174:54–57, 1983.
29. Phemister, D.B. The fate of transplanted bone and regenerative power of its various constituents. Surg Gynecol Obstet 19:39–33, 1914.
30. Poole, A.R., Reiner, A., Choi, H., and Rosenberg, L.C. Immunological studies of proteoglycan subunit from bovine and human cartilages. Trans Orthop Res Soc 4:55, 1979.
31. Poole, A.R., Reiner, A., Tang, L.H., and Rosenberg, L.C. Immunologic studies of link protein from bovine nasal cartilage. Trans Orthop Res Soc 4:56, 1979.
32. Rodrigo, J.J., Fuller, T.C., and Mankin, H.J. Cytotoxic HLA anti-

bodies in patients with bone and cartilage allografts. Trans Orthop Res Soc 1:131, 1976.

33. Salama, R. Xenogeneic bone grafting in humans. Clin Orthop 174:113–121, 1983.
34. Tomford, W.W., and Friedlaender, G.E. 1983 bone banking procedures. Clin Orthop 174:15–21, 1983.
35. Tomford, W.W., and Mankin, H.J. Investigational approaches to articular cartilage preservation. Clin Orthop 174:22–27, 1983.

36. Trentham, D.E., Townes, A.S., Kang, A.H., David, J.R. Humoral and cellular sensitivity to collagen: Type II collagen-induced arthritis in rats. J Clin Invest 61:89–96, 1978.
37. Urist, M.R., Silverman, B.G., Buring, K., Dubue, F.L., and Rosenberg, J.M. The bone induction principle. Clin Orthop 53:243, 1967.
38. Weiland, A.J., Moore, J.R., and Daniel, R.K. Vascularized bone autografts: Experience with 41 cases. Clin Orthop 174:87–95, 1983.

CHAPTER 10

Response of Bone to Mechanical Stimulation

Clinton T. Rubin

Wolff's Law

A change in the primary form and function of bone or even its function alone, results in definite changes in the internal architecture according to self ordered mathematical rules, as well as secondary changes in the external form of the bone, following the same rules.

Julius Wolff (1892)[102]

BONE REMODELING AND ADAPTATION

Bone possesses the intrinsic capability to identify changes in its functional environment and to subsequently stimulate an "appropriate" adaptive response. In fact, the skeleton's capacity to successfully withstand external loading is only achieved and maintained because the adaptive remodeling of bone tissue is so responsive to the functional mechanical demands made upon it. This morphology can be assumed to be the "optimal compromise" between the skeleton's structural needs (i.e., mass, strength, and form) and the metabolic advantages inherent in tissue efficiency and economy. Changes in either the positive or negative osteoregulatory parameters will quickly alter the morphology, and therefore the structural capacity, of the bone.

The concept that the course and balance of bone remodeling can be affected by mechanical function is one of the oldest in modern medicine, and is widely referred to as Wolff's law (see Roesler[71] for a review). However, the nature of this structure-function relationship is undetermined, and the causal link between function and adaptive remodeling usually receives attention only in the context of structural inadequacy (e.g., implant surgery, fracture fixation).

It has been proposed that bone remodeling, both locally and throughout the skeleton, is continually influenced by the level and distribution of the functional strains within the bone.[76] Throughout adult life, mechanically related stimuli are the primary agents responsible for the positive balance of bone remodeling, and thus the maintenance of the skeleton's structural competence (Fig. 10-1).

This hypothesis is consistent with a significant body of literature reporting the response of bone to changes in its functional environment. These studies have considered the response of bone to whole body exercise,[55,60,80,104–106] differential exercise on one of the two sides of body,[46,95] changes in gravitational force,[81,82,84,94,98] mechanical changes adjacent to fracture plates of varied stiffness,[59,87,89,95] femoral components of different design,[5,26,63] strain reorganization following selective osteotomy,[16,17,20,33,49,50] artificially applied loading,[23,24,25,41,43,52,61] and immobilization.[42,45,84,92] A distinct pattern of response between bone remodeling and mechanical circumstances exists; increase in the level of activity consistently leads to an increase in bone mass, and reduction in activity leads to a decrease.

Even in paralyzed appendages, however, bone does not disappear completely, and the balance of remodeling finds a new "stable" level.[38,48,54] This may represent the genetically determined "baseline" level, normal bone mass being developed from this baseline equilibrium by the osteogenic effect of functional load bearing.

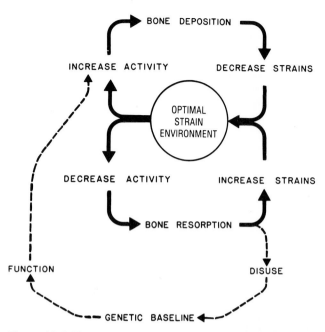

Figure 10-1 The skeleton regulates its mass to maintain an "optimal strain environment" predetermined genetically for each specific location on the bone. As activity increases at skeletal strains beyond the optimal level, osteogenesis is stimulated, which in turn ultimately reduces the functional strain. Decreased activity stimulates resorption. Complete disuse, however, causes bone mass to decrease only as far as the genetic baseline, not to disappear completely. *(From Rubin, C.T., Calcif Tissue Int vol. 36, 1984. Reproduced with permission.)*

Although this lower baseline level exists, no upper limit has ever been established. An increase in functional activity in exercised swine resulted in a 17 percent increase in cortical thickness of the femur over a 1-year experimental period.[104–106] Interestingly, changes in the geometric (i.e., architectural) properties of the bone were achieved without changing the mechanical properties of the bone tissue. In professional tennis players, Jones et al[46] compared the humeral mass of the racquet arm to the side which simply throws the ball into the air. They observed a 35 percent increase in men, and a 28 percent increase in women, in the cortical thickness of the more active humerus. In skeletally immature pigs, following ulna osteotomy, a 50 percent increase in cross-sectional area of the "overloaded" radius occurred within 3 months.[33]

Although this evidence clearly demonstrates a distinct structural adaptive response to function, there is no evidence that an additional increase in activity could not have increased bone mass even further. However, the functional level of bone mass will only be maintained as a result of a continuing "positive" stimulus arising from the appropriate strain environment engendered within the bone.

The sensitivity of the adaptive remodeling process, which protects the skeleton from structural damage, is not without disadvantages and can produce deleterious results. Immobilization and bed rest can cause negatively balanced bone remodeling affecting either the whole skeleton or a part

of it. Healthy adult males restricted to complete bed rest for up to 36 weeks showed a total body calcium loss during the entire bed rest period averaging 4.2 percent. Using photon absorption densitometry, bone mineral content measurements of the calcaneus demonstrated a mean decrease of 34 percent, and in one case as much as 45 percent was lost.[29] The weight-bearing bones contributed the major portion of the mineral resorbed during bed rest; removal of the "functional environment" resulted in unacceptable loss of bone mass. However, recovery of the bone mineral content began upon reambulation, and the rate of remineralization was similar to that measured during the initial loss.

Encasing the right forelimb of young dogs in plaster resulted in a 30 to 50 percent loss of bone at 32 weeks, but, interestingly, the loss of bone mass stabilized at this level.[92] The conclusion was that the cause of bone loss was mechanical in nature. Sequential studies[93,45] have monitored the effect of immobilization on skeletally mature dogs. In the metacarpal, disuse caused approximately 33 percent loss of bone mass. This bone loss was reversed on remobilization, demonstrating the sensitivity of the adaptive mechanism, even in the mature adult animal.

The shift from earth's gravitational pull to a weightless environment reduces the magnitude of functional loading, resulting in loss of bone mass. This occurs particularly in the axial and appendicular skeleton directly committed to weight bearing. In growing animals, periosteal growth is inhibited and appositional increase in bone girth ceases. Normal longitudinal growth, however, continues.[97] During a flight of only 19 days, there is a startling 47 percent reduction in periosteal bone formation on the tibia of growing rats.[58] The effect of weightlessness on the human differs according to specific location and function of the bone. The adaptive response in negligible in the mandible (whose principal loading is derived from bite forces), small in the upper extremities (where the main component of the loading regime is probably reproduced), and most marked in the lower limbs (where gravity-related loading from ground contact is essentially eliminated).[69,81,88,94] The extent of the bone loss during extended periods of weightlessness is speculative, and is naturally subject to individual variation and previous levels of activity. Nevertheless, a loss of 9.5 percent of total body calcium per month,[88] and perhaps up to 10 times that for the calcaneus,[69] represents a structurally significant reduction in skeletal mass. In fact, the rate of total body calcium loss may be up to three times that which occurs during bed rest.[32] Obviously, these problems of structurally inadequate bone mass must be overcome to ensure a successful long-term space flight and return to normal gravity.

The remodeling adjacent to orthopaedic implants is not always desirable. Although a bone plate must be strong and tough enough to immobilize and support a fracture, it may also be so stiff as to deprive the bone of a functional strain environment. This strain protection, or "shielding," may stimulate a resorptive remodeling response in the bone adjacent to the trauma, creating the potential for a second fracture following removal of the plate.[67]

The attachment of bone plates alters the stress distribution about the bone cortex[16,17] and is directly related to the bone remodeling that follows fixation.[91] The degree of osteoporosis is influenced by the stiffness of the plate material; the stiffer the bone plate, the greater the stress shielding afforded to the underlying bone, and the greater the bone loss.[89] The remodeling changes only the structural architecture (e.g., distribution of bone mass, geometry, etc.), but the basic material (bone mineral and matrix) appears not to change.[103] Composite and resorbable implants are being developed. However, until these new developments are optimized in terms of mechanical integrity and biocompatability, conventional implants should be used and only after careful consideration of the extremely adaptive nature of bone. When a fracture has healed, the implant can be removed. In the case of prosthetic replacement, the implant must coexist permanently with the bone and its adaptive changes.

Following total hip arthroplasty, radiographic evidence of resorption in the calcar femorale has been reported as early as 13 months.[12] Appearance of a radiolucent line of more than 2 mm in diameter is interpreted as indicating a loose prosthesis. Signs of early radiolucency may occur in as many as 24 percent of cases within a 4 to 7-year period. Radiolucency has been documented in 30 percent of cases at 10 years [79] and as high as 70 percent at 15 years.[11]

Although the exact sequence of events is unclear, progressive lucency adjacent to a prosthesis is related to micromovement and shifting of the cement mantle, which often precede the failure of the component.[2,5,6,7,8,63,68]

Osteoporosis is one of the major public health problems in medicine today. In the United States alone, 1.3 million fractures annually can be attributed to this condition in the over-45 age group, accumulating over $3.8 billion in medical costs. The ever-increasing elderly population can only exacerbate this problem.

Although the etiology of osteoporosis in not well understood, it has been proposed that this condition consists of at least two components: the approximately 0.3 percent annual bone loss identified in all persons beyond the age of 40 and the superimposed accelerated loss of bone tissue, estimated as high as 2 percent per year, which follows the menopause.[40] The cumulative bone loss creates a staggering effect; in the 30 to 40 years which follow the menopause, the average woman can expect to lose one-quarter of her cortical bone and more than one-half of her trabecular bone.[28] One of every two women who have undergone such bone loss suffers some fracture due to structurally inadequate bone mass.[22]

Recent clinical surveys demonstrate that what was once considered to be an inevitable age-related decline in bone mass may be slowed and even reversed by a regimen of exercise. Physical activity in elderly women (normal bone loss: -1.1 percent per year) can be more effective in increasing bone mass (+0.8 percent/per year) than calcium or vitamin D supplementation (+0.5 percent/per year).[83] Despite their success, the exercise regimes employed in this and other studies on the aged[1] were chosen with little regard to the specific factors of the mechanical environment likely to maximize the exercise regime's osteogenic potency.

Exercise for the elderly must be prescribed with caution. It is potentially dangerous since it may cause the fracture that it was intended to prevent. Therefore, in order to minimize the duration of the exercise regime while maximizing its osteogenic potential, it would be of great benefit to first isolate those specific parameters of the mechanical regime which are identified as "osteogenic" by the skeleton, and thus stimulate an "appropriate" adaptive response.

EXPERIMENTAL BASIS FOR WOLFF'S LAW

The peak functional strains developed on the surface of bone can be measured with strain gauges in a variety of vertebrates. During vigorous activity the highest strains generated are remarkably similar, resulting in "identical" safety factors to yield and ultimate failure (Table 10-1).

Although the range of peak functional strain levels is remarkably narrow, the strain distributions engendered during customary activity are maintained at each location with even greater precision. In the limb bones, the ratio of the principal strains on opposing cortices, the orientation of the principal strains on each cortex, and the distribution of strains across the cortex are kept constant throughout the stance phase, thus indicating that the mode of loading remains constant throughout the limb's contact with the ground, and is maintained through the animal's complete range of speed, regardless of change of gait.[74]

This restricted manner of loading creates a unique structural requirement for functional activity. Through functional adaptation, it should produce a structure optimally designed for this functional demand, ultimately allowing considerable economy in the skeleton's final morphology.

Structurally, the smallest level of strain is engendered if loads are applied axially. Therefore, it has been assumed that the objective of bone morphology is to resist, reduce, or inhibit strains caused by functional load bearing. However, some bones (horse metacarpus) are loaded predominantly in axial compression,[10] whereas in others (radius, tibia, femur, humerus, ulna) bending accounts for up to 90 percent of the total strains engendered.[74] Some features of bone architecture (e.g., curvatures) do not appear to counteract external bending moments but in some cases actually accentuate the total bending moment developed.

Strain gauge measurement from the metacarpus, radius, and tibia in dogs, sheep, turkeys, and horses also demonstrates that the orientation of the elliptical cross section in these bones is directed not to inhibit bending but to provide the minimal resistance to the direction in which bending normally occurs during locomotor loading[78] (Fig. 10-2). While the orientation of the elliptical cross section may increase the magnitude of strains generated during normal loading, it certainly coordinates their direction.

Reduction of strain would appear not to be the primary objective of adaptations within the skeleton. Indeed, both curvature and cross-sectional shape combine to create the high strains engendered by bending, rather than conspiring to lower strain levels. Provided that functional strains do not induce an unacceptable degree of fatigue damage (and bone does enjoy a twofold safety factor to yield point), these strains do not, by themselves, constitute a danger to the bone structure. Indeed, functional strains may be beneficial by increasing the perfusion of the tissue or maintaining a beneficial "flux" of strain-generated electric charge.

Table 10-1 Peak Functional Strains (Pϵc in Microstrain) Measured from Bone Bonded Strain Gauges in a Range of Animals during the Customary Activity which Generated the Highest Strain Magnitude

Bone	Activity	Pϵc	Yld.*	Ult.*
Horse radius	Trotting	−2800	2.4	5.6
Horse tibia	Galloping	−3200	2.1	4.9
Horse metacarpus	Accelerating	−3000	2.3	5.2
Dog radius	Trotting	−2400	2.8	6.5
Dog tibia	Galloping	−2100	3.2	7.4
Goose humerus	Flying	−2800	2.4	5.6
Cockerel ulna	Flapping	−2100	3.2	7.4
Sheep femur	Trotting	−2200	3.1	7.1
Sheep humerus	Trotting	−2200	3.1	7.1
Sheep radius	Galloping	−2300	3.0	6.8
Sheep tibia	Trotting	−2100	3.2	7.4
Pig radius	Trotting	−2400	2.8	6.5
Fish hypural	Swimming	−3000	2.3	5.2
Macaca mandible	Biting	−2200	3.1	7.1
Turkey tibia	Running	−2350	2.9	6.6

*The safety factors to yield (Yld), and ultimate (Ult) failure were calculated using values of 6800 and 15,700 microstrain for yield and ultimate tensile strain, respectively, The primary role of these bones is load bearing rather than protection or display. It appears that, regardless of location or origin of loading, the maximum peak strains induced during functional activity are remarkably similar.
Source: Rubin, C.T., Calcif Tissue Int 36:S11–S18, 1984. Reproduced with permission.

Behavioral mechanisms can also regulate skeletal loads and the strain magnitude levels that they engender. Peak strains achieved are directly dependent upon the mode of gait. During walking, the peak strains within the radius and tibia of both horse and dog increase with increasing speed and then jump incrementally (up to 59 percent) when the animals change to a trot.[74] When the change is from a trot to a canter, the peak strain in the limb bones (and the peak force on the ground) is reduced substantially (a decrease of up to 42 percent; Fig. 10-3). Only at the highest speeds (fast gallop) are the same levels of peak strain attained as those engendered during the trot. This regulation of limb loading also limits the stress developed in tendons, ligaments, and muscles. Although the primary benefit from such an arrangement may be a minimization of metabolic energy expenditure, gait change can be seen as a behavioral adaptation by which increased performance can be attained (in terms of speed) without placing additional requirements on either the material or the structural properties of the load-bearing elements involved. The decreased limb loading, which occurs at this gait transition, permits increased speed without progressive erosion of the bone's safety factors to failure.

Although the gross architecture of skeletons is certainly different in different locations, at the levels of small volumes of bone tissue the diverse range of loading activities all resolve into strain. The small range of peak functional strains which has been measured over a wide range of animals during a variety of activities would suggest that a strain-sensitive cellular population exists within each of these bones that has a universal mechanism and objective for structural adaptation. Perhaps this cellular population is responsible for adjusting bone mass and architecture to achieve and maintain

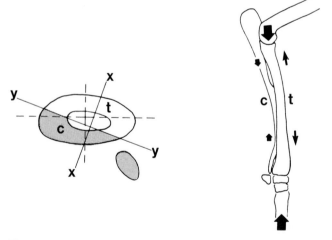

Figure 10-2 A diagram of a sheep radius and ulna, showing the elliptical cross section (left), and the bone's slight craniocaudal curvature. Axial loading through the joint surfaces (large black arrows) generates bending strains and places the cranial surface in tension (t) and the caudal surface in compression (c). Tension in the extensor muscle group (concave side), which is most active during weight bearing, contributes to the bending rather than opposing it. The transverse section of the radius and ulna show the principal axis of the midshaft; the greatest resistance to bending is about the x-x axis, the least in the y-y direction. This elliptical cross section appears to have a strong influence on the distribution of strains about the cortex during locomotion. It would appear that bone curvature is developed not to inhibit bending but to accentuate it, while cross-sectional morphology does not resist loads but orients them.

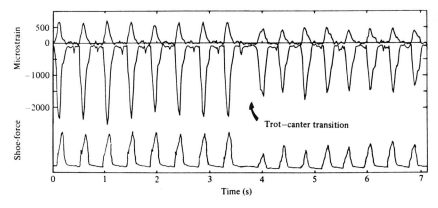

Figure 10-3 Tensile strains (*upper trace*) and compressive strains (*middle trace*) at caudal surface of horse's radius during transition from trot to canter at a constant speed on a treadmill. Lowest trace is from load-sensitive shoe attached to same forefoot when gait change was repeated 1 year after completion of strain gauge experiments. Peak compressive strain decreases 42 percent at the transition. A similar decrease in peak force is recorded from the shoe. Change in gait allows an increase in speed without progressive increase in strain. (*From Rubin, C.T., and Lanyon, L.E., J Exp Biol 101:187–211, 1982. Reproduced with permission.*)

an "optimal strain environment" for each specific location within the skeleton.

Primarily, the search for the stimuli behind Wolff's law has depended upon osteotomy or tenotomy experimentation to first alter the mechanical environment of a specific skeletal element and, therefore, engender an adaptive skeletal change. A major disadvantage of this sort of experimentation is that since it is the animal which applies the loads to the bone under study, the investigator has little or no control in selecting which parameters are to be evaluated.

Such disadvantages were minimized by Hert et al using the externally applied loading technique.[41] They concluded that since the adaptive response is inherent to the bone itself, it requires no central nervous system supply.[42] In addition, they found positive remodeling to be influenced only by intermittent loading; static loads were ignored as an adaptive remodeling stimulus.[43] In subsequent studies by other investigators, loading the sheep metacarpus demonstrated a correlation between the amount of stress engendered and the quantity of new bone formed,[23] as well as a difference in the bone's response between bending and compressive loads.[25] Intermittent load regimes externally applied to the sheep radius demonstrated strain rate to be an effective osteogenic determinant,[62] and strain distribution was shown to be of prime importance in the osteoregulatory processes of a "balanced" skeleton.[50]

The functionally isolated bird ulna has also been used as a model. Functional isolation of the left ulna diaphysis was achieved by removing the bone's articular extremities, covering the transversely cut ends of the shaft with stainless steel caps, which were then penetrated by Steinman pins. The unloaded, isolated bones, showed little change in bone mineral content (BMC) for 2 weeks. Then a steady decline ensued which, by 6 weeks, appeared to stabilize at 88 percent plus or minus 2 percent of the original BMC value (Fig. 10-4). This bone loss monitored by photon absorption densitometry was accomplished by endosteal resorption and incomplete Haversian remodeling, accompanied by some subperiosteal new bone formation. The disuse osteopenia which developed in this model (Fig. 10-5A) closely resembled the changes reported in the human metacarpus in senile/postmenopausal osteopenia.[28]

Surprisingly, in bones which were loaded for only four load reversals per day (cycles/day) at a rate of 0.5 Hz, the BMC

did not decline but remained essentially unchanged over the 6-week experimental period (6-week value = 103 plus or minus 4 percent). Few remodeling changes of any kind were apparent, and, in fact, it was difficult to distinguish these isolated ulnae from their contralateral pairs which had received no surgical intervention (Fig. 10-5B).

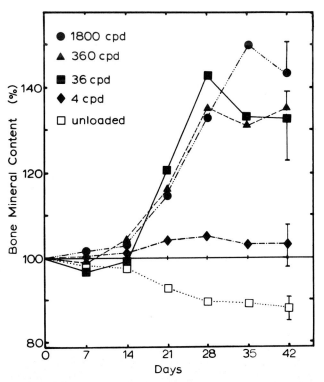

Figure 10-4 Percentage change in bone mineral content at the midshaft of the rooster ulna preparation over a 6-week experimental period in bones subjected to zero, 4, 36, or 1800 consecutive loading reversals (cycles) per day of an indentical mechanical regimen. The vertical lines for 6-week values indicate standard deviations. The transverse scans were made using an I^{125} source. It would appear from this data that the maximum osteogenic response is triggered by a very few cycles of load. (*From Rubin, C.T., and Lanyon, L.E., J Bone Joint Surg vol. 66A 1984. Reproduced with permission.*)

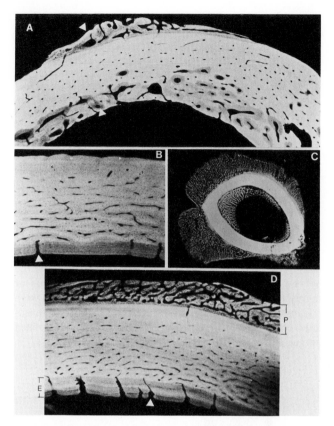

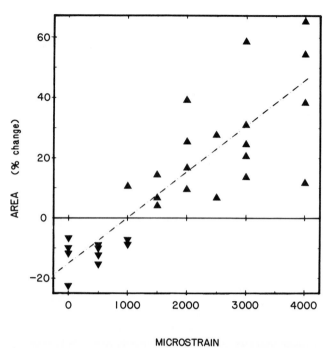

Figure 10-5 Transverse microradiographs of the rooster ulna midshaft following specific applied loading conditions. **A.** Following 6 weeks of complete disuse, partially infilled haversian systems and cortex thinning primarily by endosteal resorption occurs. Some subperiosteal new bone formation is also evident. **B.** Following loading at only four reversals (cycles) per day, remodeling is inhibited, making the experimental ulnae from this series difficult to distinguish from their untouched contralateral pairs. The arrow shows a Volkmann's canal traversing the normal band of less well mineralized bone of the endosteal surface that had been completely removed in the nonloaded ulnae (*A*) **C.** At 24 days, 36 load reversals/day stimulated calcification of osteoid fronds and an explosive hyperplastic reaction. **D.** This bone remodeled by 6 weeks to a more consolidated formation deposited in the entire thickness of the periosteal band (P). Note that there is no remodeling within the preexisting cortex and that the endosteal area looks quite similar to that seen in *B*. *(From Rubin, C.T., and Lanyon, L.E., J Bone Joint Surg vol. 66A, 1984. Reproduced with permission.)*

The BMC in ulnas subjected to 36 cycles/day showed a rapid increase between 2 and 3 weeks following the onset of loading. Values peaked around 28 days and stabilized by 6 weeks at 133 plus or minus 11 percent above normal. This increase in new bone formation was accounted for by periosteal and endosteal circumferential lamellae and primary osteon formation. Sections from birds killed throughout the experimental period showed that remodeling occurred in two phases. In the first phase, fronds of osteoid tissue developed vertically from the bone surface. The peak of BMC coincided with the mineralization of these fronds (Fig. 10-5*C*). By the end of the experimental period, nearly all of these vertical

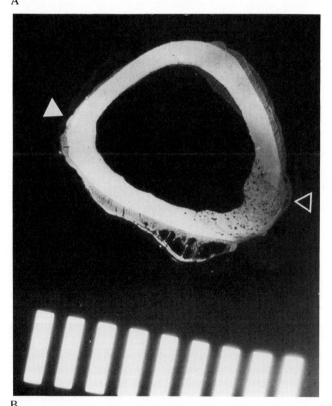

Figure 10-6 A. Percentage change in bone area of an isolated bird ulna preparation after 8 weeks of 100 load reversals per day. Comparison is with intact contralateral control. Inverted triangles below baseline represent bone loss relative to the intact side. *(From Rubin, C.T., and Lanyon, L.E., Calcif Tissue Int 37:411–417, 1985. Reproduced with permission.)* **B.** The new bone formed on the ulna preparation is not necessarily at the points of the cortex subjected to the highest strains. (Solid arrow indicates peak compressive strain; open arrow indicates peak tensile strength.)

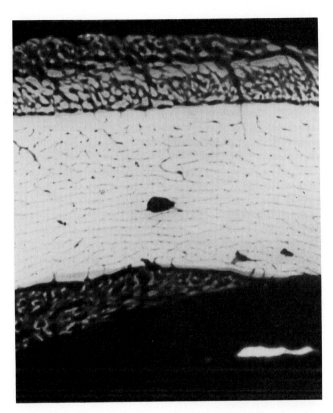

Figure 10-6 (Cont.) C. New bone, both endosteal and periosteal, forms in the absence of remodeling within the cortex. Hence this is an adaptive, rather than a reparative, response.

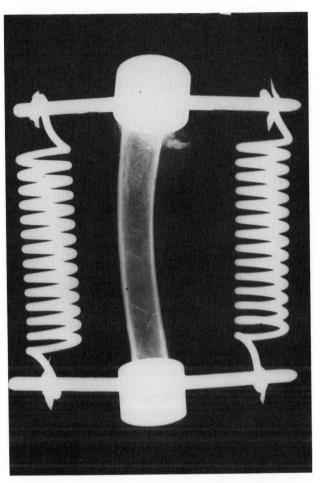

Figure 10-7 A radiograph of the turkey ulna preparation, following 8 weeks of static loading with springs. This plate was taken postmortem and shows the 110 mm portion of the bone's diaphysis, with caps and transfixing pins in place. The percutaneous pins are shown joined by the loading springs, which are situated outside the wing. *(From Lanyon, L.E., and Rubin, C.T., J Biomech vol. 17, 1984. Reproduced with permission.)*

fronds had been remodeled away. However, the portions nearest to the periosteal surface become incorporated within the bone's original cortex (Fig. 10-5*D*).

Interestingly, the increase in BMC in bones subjected to 360 or 1800 strain cycles/day followed the same pattern as those subjected to only 36. Neither the character nor the amount of new bone formation showed any substantial difference between ulnas subjected to more than 36 cycles/day (136 plus or minus 3 percent and 143 plus or minus 6 percent, respectively).

These results are a dramatic illustration of the sensitivity of the remodeling response of bone to a short exposure of an "osteogenic" stimulus. An osteogenic response had been triggered and maximized by only 72 s of load bearing. A fiftyfold increase in the number of strain cycles above 36/day caused no increase in the amount of new bone formed. Remarkably, only 4 cycles/day of this strain regime, requiring only 8 s of load bearing, were necessary to prevent disuse osteoporosis from occurring. It would appear that it is the nature and not

the duration of the functional stimulus that is most potent in determining skeletal morphology.

NATURE OF THE ADAPTIVE RESPONSE

Subsequent studies demonstrate a distinct "dose-response" curve for an adaptive stimulus (Fig. 10-6). Strains well within the physiological range, but applied at numbers of loading cycles not sufficient to engender microdamage and thus evoke a reparative response, generate a substantial adaptive response.[76] It would appear that simply the change from a "normal" strain distribution can be perceived by the bone as a stimulus for adaptation.

While 100 cycles/day of an intermittent load regime engendering 2000 microstrain produced an increase in bone area of up to 40 percent, microradiographs of ulnae exposed to a static mechanical environment of a similar magnitude, engendered by springs attached to the pins (Fig. 10-7) showed

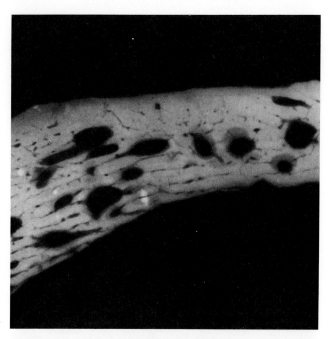

Figure 10-8 Microradiograph of a section of a turkey ulna following 8 weeks of a constant *static* load regime. Whereas a *dynamic* load regime engendering the same strain magnitude (2000 microstrain) was sufficient to stimulate a 24 percent increase in bone mass (see Fig. 10-7), the bones subjected exclusively to a static load regime suffered negatively balanced remodeling resulting in a 13 percent loss of bone mass, a net change of 37 percent from the dynamically loaded preparation. Static load regimes are "ignored" as an osteogenic stimulus, and bone morphology is attained only as the result of the dynamic strain environment.

no evidence of surface new bone formation. In fact, the remodeling response was identical to that in bones subjected only to disuse, involving cortical thinning and intracortical porosis (Fig. 10-8).

This data suggest that static strains have little or no influence on the maintenance of a "balanced" remodeling process.[52] If the static load environment is essentially ignored as an osteoregulatory stimulus, the functional influence on bone architecture could only be derived from the dynamic loading environment.

Laboratory data then suggest that adaptive bone remodeling (alterations in bone mass, tissue turnover, and internal replacement) in a "balanced" system is sensitive to alterations in the magnitude, distribution, and rate of strain generated within the bone tissue. An "appropriate" loading regime is one which is dynamic in nature but needs to be applied for only a very short period of time for it to provide an effective stimulus to maintain a remodeling "balance." The potency of the stimulus appears to be dependent on the magnitude of the strain engendered. Strain levels that are acceptable in one location induce adaptive remodeling in others, suggesting that each region of each bone is *genetically programmed* to accept a particular amount and pattern of intermittent strain as normal. Deviation from this optimal strain environment will stimulate changes in the bone's remodeling balance, resulting in adaptive increases or decreases in its mass.

The control of functional adaptation using this hypothesis requires a population of cells that are directly or indirectly sensitive to mechanical strain and achieve and maintain this predetermined strain environment for each specific location of the skeleton. The remarkably few numbers of cycles necessary to induce adaptive remodeling suggest a specific cellular response triggered within a receptive cellular population rather than an indirect effect such as increased perfusion or a reparative process generated by tissue damage. The remodeling response generated by so few strain reversals is in sharp contrast to the large numbers of cycles necessary to cause fatigue damage,[17,19] even when the latter are applied at the highest functional strain levels we have recorded.[73,74] The adaptive mechanism appears to be a dose-response mechanism; the higher the strains, the more potent the stimulus, but the strains must be perceived by the bone as dynamic in nature, and static loads are ignored. This suggests that the bone mass in a balanced skeletal system is most influenced by a strain situation engendered by short periods of particularly osteogenic activity (e.g., vigorous, diverse activity), rather than by the strain situation experienced during the predominant activity (e.g., walking) or by fatigue damage.

By determining the effects of various aspects of a bone's functional regime on adaptive remodeling, we have begun to define the criteria in human subjects for a minimum effective mechanical regime which is capable of maintaining a state of balanced remodeling.

ACKNOWLEDGMENT   This work has been funded by grants from the MRC (U.K.), NASA Grant #NAG 9-25, Electro-Biology Inc., and NIH Grant #AM36080-01.

REFERENCES

1. Acoia, J.F., Cohn, S.H., Ostuni, J.A., Cane, R., and Ellis, K. Prevention of involutional bone loss by physical exercise. Calcif Tissue Res 24(suppl):2, 1977.
2. Amstutz, H.C. Complications of total hip replacement: Part I. Skeletal fixation and loosening of total hip replacements. Instr Course Lect 23:201–209, 1974.
3. Amstutz, H.C., Ma, S.M., Jinnah, R.H., and Mai, L. Revision of aseptic loose total hip arthroplasties. Clin Orthop 170:21–23, 1982.
4. Andersson, G.B.J., Freeman, M.A.R., and Swanson, S.A.V. Loosening of the cemented acetabular cup in total hip replacement. J Bone Joint Surg 54B(4):590–599, 1972.
5. Andriacchi, T.P., Galante, J.O., Belytschko, T.B., and Hampton, S. A stress analysis of the femoral stem in THR. J Bone Joint Surg 58A:618–624, 1976.
6. Baggott, D.G., and Lanyon, L.E. An independent postmortem calibration of electrical resistance strain gauges bonded to bone surfaces in vivo. J Biomech 10:615–622, 1977.
7. Bechtol, C.O. Failure of femoral implant components in total hip replacement operations. Orthop Rev 4:23–29, 1975.
8. Beckenbaugh, R.D., and Ilstrup, D.M. Total hip arthroplasty. J Bone Joint Surg 60A:306–313, 1978.
9. Bergstrom, B., Lidgren, L., and Lindberg, L. Radiographic abnormalities caused by postoperative infection following total hip arthroplasty. Clin Orthop 99:95–102, 1974.
10. Biewener, A.A., Thomason, J., Goodship, A., and Lanyon, L.E. The stresses in the horse forelimb: A comparison of two experimen-

tal techniques. J Biomech 16:577–589, 1984.

11. Blacker, F., and Charnley, J. Changes in the upper femur after low friction arthroplasty. Clin Orthop 137:15–23, 1978.

12. Bocco, F., Langan, P., and Charnley, J. Changes in the calcar femoris in relation to cement technology in total hip replacement. Clin Orthop 128:287–295, 1977.

13. Burr, D.B., Martin, R.B., and Lefever, S. The prevention of disuse osteoporosis in sedentary rabbits. Trans Orthop Res Soc 9:146, 1984.

14. Caler, W.E., Carter, D.R., and Harris, W.H. Technical note: Technique for implementing an in vivo bone strain gage system. J Biomech 1981.

15. Carlsson, A.S., and Gentz, C.F. Mechanical loosening of the femoral head prosthesis in the Charnley total hip arthroplasty. Clin Orthop 147:262–270, 1980.

16. Carter, D.R., Harris, W.H., Vasu, R., and Caler, W.E. The mechanical and biological response of cortical bone to in vivo strain histories, in Cowin, S. (ed): *Mechanical Properties of Bone.* ASME Publ AMD 45:81–92, 1981.

17. Carter, D.R., Vasu, R., Spengler, D.M., and Dueland, R.T. Stress fields in the unplated and plated canine femur calculated from in vivo strain measurements. J Biomech 14:63–70, 1981.

18. Carter, D.R., and Vasu, R. Plate and bone stresses for single and double-plated femoral fractures. J Biomech 14:55–62, 1981.

19. Chamay, A. Mechanical and morphological aspects of experimental overload and fatigue in bone. J Biomech 3:262–270, 1970.

20. Chamay, A., and Tschantz, P. Mechanical influence in bone remodelling: Experimental research on Wolff's law. J Biomech 5:173–180, 1972.

21. Charnley, J., and Cupic, Z. The nine and ten year results of the low-friction arthroplasty of the hip. Clin Orthop 95:9–25, 1973.

22. Christiansen, C., Rodbro, P., and Drewson, B. Acta Med Scand 200:293–295, 1976.

23. Churches, A.E., Howlett, C.R., Waldron, K.J., and Ward, G.W. The response of living bone to controlled time varying loading: Method and preliminary results. J Biomech 12:35–45, 1979.

24. Churches, A.E., Howlett, C.R., and Ward, G.W. Bone reaction to surgical drilling and pinning. J Biomech 13:203–209, 1980.

25. Churches. A.E., and Howlett, C.R. The response of mature cortical bone to controlled time varying loading, in Cowin, S.C. (ed): *Mechanical Properties of Bone.* ASME, AMD 45:81–92, 1981.

26. Crowninshield, R.D., Brand, R.A., and Johnston, R.C. et al. Analysis of femoral component stem design in total hip arthroplasty. J Bone Joint Surg 62A:68–78, 1980.

27. Crowninshield, R.D., Brand, R.A., and Johnston, R.C. et al. The effect of femoral stem cross-sectional geometry on cement stresses in total hip reconstruction. Clin Orthop 146:71–77, 1981.

28. Dequeker, J. Bone and aging. Ann Rheum Dis 34:100–113, 1975.

29. Donaldson, C.L., Hulley, S.B., Vogel, J.M., Hattner, R.S., Bayers, J.H., and McMillan, D.E. Effect of prolonged bed rest on bone mineral. Metabolism 19:1071–1084, 1970.

30. Eftekhar, N.S. Complications of total hip replacement: Part III. Mechanical failure in low-friction arthroplasty. Instr Course Lect 23:230–242, 1974.

31. Galante, J. Total hip replacement. Orthop Clin North Am 2:139–255, 1971.

32. Goode, A. Man in space. Nature 283:525–526, 1980.

33. Goodship, A.E., Lanyon, L.E., and MacFie, H. Functional adaptation of bone to increased stress. J Bone Joint Surg 61A:539–546, 1979.

34. Gould, S.J. Darwinism and the expansion of evolutionary theory. Science 206:380–387, 1982.

35-36. Green, T.A., McNeice, G.M., and Amstutz, H.C. Modes of failure of cemented stem-type femoral components. A radiographic analysis of loosening. Clin Orthop 141:17–27, 1979.

37. Griffith, M.J., Seidenstein, M.K., Williams, D., and Charnley, J.

Eight year results of Charnley arthroplasties with special reference to the behavior of cement. Clin Orthop 137:24–36, 1978.

38. Harris, W.H. Revision surgery for failed nonseptic total hip arthroplasty. The femoral side. Clin Orthop 170:8–20, 1982.

39. Heaney, R.P. Radiocalcium metabolism in disuse osteoporosis in man. Am J Med 33:188, 1962.

40. Heaney, R.P. Paradox of irreversibility of age related bone loss, in Menczel, J., Robin, G.C., Makin, M., and Strenberg, R. (eds): *Osteoporosis.* New York, Wiley, 1981, pp 15–20.

41. Hert, J., Liskova, M., and Landgrot, B. Influence of the long-term continuous bending on the bone. An experimental study on the tibia of the rabbit. Folia Morphol 17:389–399, 1969.

42. Hert, J., Skelenska, A., and Liskova, M. Reaction of bone to mechanical stimuli: Part 5. Effect of intermittent stress on the rabbit tibia after resection of the peripheral nerves. Folia Morphol 19:378–387, 1971.

43. Hert, J., Liskova, M., and Landa, J.L. Reaction of bone to mechanical stimuli: Part 1. Continuous and intermittent loading of tibia in rabbit. Folia Morphol 19:290–317, 1971.

44. Horsman, A., Nordin, B.E., Aaron, J., and Marshall, D.H. Cortical and trabecular osteoporosis and their relation to fracture in the elderly, in Deluca, H.F., Frost, H.M, Jee, W.S.S., Johnston, C.C., and Parfitt, A.M. (eds): *Osteoporosis, Recent Advances in Pathogenesis and Treatment.* Baltimore, University Park Press, 1980.

45. Jaworski, Z.F.G., Liskova-Kiar, M., and Uhthoff, H.K. Effect of long term immobilization on the pattern of bone loss in older dogs. J Bone Joint Surg 62B:104–110, 1980.

46. Jones, H.H., Priest, J.D., Hayes, W.C., Tichenor, C.C., and Nagel, D.A. Humeral hypertrophy in response to exercise. J Bone Joint Surg 59A:204–208, 1977.

46. Jones, H.H., Priest, J.D., Hayes, W.C.,Tichenor, C.C., and Nagel, D.A. Humeral hypertrophy in response to exercise. J Bone Joint Surg 59A:204–208, 1977.

47. Lanyon L.E. Measurement of bone strain in vivo. Acta Orthop Belg 42:98–108, 1976.

48. Lanyon, L.E. The influence of function on the development or bone curvature. J Zool Lond 192:457–466, 1980.

49. Lanyon, L.E. The measurement and significance of bone strain in vivo, in Cowin, S. (ed): *Mechanical Properties of Bone.* ASME Publ AMD 45:93–106 (1981).

50. Lanyon, L.E., Goodship, A.E., Pye, C., and McFie, H. Mechanically adaptive bone remodelling. A quantitative study on functional adaptation in the radius following ulna osteotomy in sheep. J Biomech 15:141–154, 1982.

51. Lanyon, L.W., and Rubin, C.T. Static vs. dynamic loads as an influence on bone remodelling. J Biomech 17:897–906, 1984.

52. Liskova, M., and Hert, J. Reaction of bone to mechanical stimuli: Part I. Periosteal and endosteal reaction of the tibial diaphysis in rabbits to intermittent loading. Folia Morphol 19:301–317, 1971.

53. Marmor, L. Femoral loosening in total hip replacement. Clin Orthop 121:116–119, 1976.

54. Marotti, B., and Marotti, F. Topographic quantitative study of bone tissue formation and reconstruction in inert bones, in Fleisch, H., Blackwood, H.J., and Owen, M. (eds): *Proc Third Europ Symp Calcif Tissues,* Berlin, Springer, 1965.

55. Miller, E.M., Schneider, H.J., Bronson, J.C., and McLain, D. A new consideration in athletic injuries: The classical ballet dancer. Clin Orthop 111:181–189, 1975.

56. Mirra, J.M., Marder, R.A., and Amstutz, H.C. The pathology of failed total joint arthroplasty. Clin Orthop 170:175–183, 1982.

57. Moreland, J.R., Gruen, T.A., Mai, L., and Amstutz, H.C. Aseptic loosening of total hip replacement. Incidence and significance. *The Hip: Proceedings of the 8th Open Scientific Meeting of the Hip Society.* St. Louis, Mosby, 1980, pp 281–291.

58. Morey, E.R., and Baylink, D.J. Inhibition of bone formation during space flight. Science 201:1138–1141, 1978.

59. Moyen, B.M.L., Lahey, P.J., Weinberg, E.H., and Harris W.H. Effects on intact femora of dogs of the application and removal of metal plates. J Bone Joint Surg 60A:940–947, 1978.
60. Nilsson, B.E., Anderson, S.M., Hardrup, T.V., and Westlin, N.E. Bone mineral content in ballet dancers and weight lifters. *Proceedings of the 4th International Conference on Bone Measurement.* University of Toronto, 1978, pp 81–86.
61. O'Connor, J.A., Goodship, A.G., Rubin, C.T., and Lanyon, L.E. The effect of externally applied loads on bone remodelling in the radius of the sheep, in Stokes, I.A.F. (ed): *Mechanical Factors and the Skeleton.* London, John Libbey, 1981.
62. O'Connor, J.A., Lanyon, L.E., and McFie, H. The influence of strain rate on adaptive bone remodelling. J Biomech 15:767–781, 1982.
63. Oh, I., and Harris, W.H. Proximal strain distribution in the loaded femur. J Bone Joint Surg 60A:75–85, 1978.
64. Patterson, F.P., and Brown, C.S. Complications of total hip replacement arthroplasty. Orthop Clin North Am 4:503–512, 1973.
65. Pellicci, P.M., Salvati, E.A., and Robinson, H.J. Mechanical failures in total hip replacement requiring reoperation. J Bone Joint Surg 61A:28–36, 1979.
66. Pellicci, P.M., Wilson, P.D., Jr., Sledge, C.B., Salvati, E.A., Ranawat, C.S., and Poss, R. Results of revision total hip replacement. *The Hip: Proceedings of the 9th Open Scientific Meeting of the Hip Society.* St. Louis, Mosby, 1981, pp 57–68.
67. Perren, S.M. Physical and biological aspects of fracture healing with special reference to internal fixation. Clin Orthop 138:175–196, 1979.
68. Radin, E.L., Rubin, C.T., Thrasher, E.L., Lanyon, L.E., Crugnola, A.M., Schiller, A.S., Paul, I.L., and Rose, R.M. Femoral component loosening after total hip replacement: An in vivo animal study. J Bone Joint Surg 64A:1188–1200, 1982.
69. Rambaut, P.C., Smith, M.C., Mack, P.B., and Vogel, J.M. Skeletal response, in Johnston, R.S., and Dietlein, L.F. (eds): *Biomedical Results of Apollo.* NASA publication, 1975.
70. Reckling, F.W., Asher, M.A., and Dillon, W.L. A longitudinal study of the radiolucent line at the bone-cement interface following total joint-replacement procedures. J Bone Joint Surg 59A:355–358, 1977.
71. Roesler, H. Some historical remarks on the theory of cancellous bone structure (Wolff's law), in Cowin, S. (ed): *Mechanical Properties of Bone.* ASME Publ AMD 45:27–42, 1981.
72. Rubin, C.T., DeLaura, R.A., and Lanyon, L.E. A mathematical model bone bonded strain gauges. (1987) (in preparation)
73. Rubin, C.T., Harris, J., Jones, B., Ernst, H., and Lanyon, L.E. Stress fractures: The remodelling response to excessive repetitive loading. Trans Orthop Res Soc 9:303, 1984.
74. Rubin, C.T., and Lanyon, L.E. Limb mechanics as a function of speed and gait: A study of functional strains in the radius and tibia of horse and dog. J Exp Biol 101:187–211, 1982.
75. Rubin, C.T., and Lanyon, L.E. Dynamic strain similarity in vertebrates: An alternative to allometric limb bone scaling. J Theor Biol 107:321–327, 1984.
76. Rubin, C.T., and Lanyon, L.E. Regulation of bone formation by applied dynamic loads. J Bone Joint Surg 66A:397–402, 1984.
77. Rubin, C.T., and Lanyon, L.E. Regulation of bone mass by mechanical strain magnitude. Calcif Tissue Int 37:411–417, 1985.
78. Rubin, C.T. Skeletal strain and the functional significance of bone architecture. Calcif Tissue Int 36:S11–S18, 1984.
79. Salvati, E.A., Wilson, P.D., Jr., Jolley, M.N., Vakili, F., Aglietti, P., and Brown, G.C. A ten-year follow-up study of our first one hundred consecutive Charnley total hip replacements. J Bone Joint Surg 63A:753–767, 1981.
80. Saville, P.D., and Whyte, M.P. Muscle and bone hypertrophy: Positive effect of running exercise in the rat. Clin Orthop 65:81–88, 1969.
81. Simmons, D.J., Russell, J.E., Winter, F., Baron, R., Vignery, A., Thuc, V.T., Rosenberg, G.D., and Walker, W. Space flight and the non-weight bearing bones of the rat skeleton. (Cosmos 1129.) Trans Orthop Res Soc 4:65, 1981.
82. Smith, M.C., Rambaut, P.C., Vogel, J.M., and Whittle, M.W. Bone mineral measurement—Experiment M078, in Johnston, R.S., and Dietlein, L.F. (eds): *Biomedical Results from Skylab.* NASA publication, 1977.
83. Smith, E.L., Reddan, W., and Smith, P.E. Physical activity and calcium modalities for bone mineral increase in aged women. Med Sci Sports Exerc 13:60–64, 1981.
84. Spengler, D.M., Morey, E., Carter, D., Turner, R., and Baylink, D. Effect of space flight on bone strength. Physiologist s:75–76, 1979.
85. Stauffer, R.N. Ten year follow-up study of total hip replacement with particular reference to roentgenographic loosening of the components. J Bone Joint Surg 64A:983–990, 1982.
86. Sutherland, C.J., Wilde, A.H., Borden, L.S., and Marks, K.E. A ten year follow-up of one hundred consecutive Muller curved-stem total hip-replacement arthroplasties. J Bone Joint Surg 64A:970–982, 1982.
87. Szivek, J.A., Cameron, H.U., Weatherly, G.C., and Pilliar, R.M. A study of bone remodelling using biologically attached composite on-lay plates. Trans Orthop Res Soc 6:61, 1981.
88. Tilton, F.E., Degioanni, J.C., and Schneider, V.A. Long term follow-up of skylab bone demineralization. Aviat Space Environ Med 51:1209–1213, 1980.
89. Tonino, A.J., Davidson, C.L., Klopper, P.J., and Linclau, L.A. Protection from stress in bone and its effects. J Bone Joint Surg 58B:107–112, 1976.
90. Tschantz, P., and Rutishauser, E. La Surharge Mechanique de L'Os Vivant. Ann Anat Pathol 12:223–248, 1967.
91. Uhthoff, H.K., and Dubuc, F.L. Bone structural changes in the dog under rigid internal fixation. Clin Orthop 81:165–170, 1978.
92. Uhthoff, H.K., and Jaworski, Z.F.G. Bone loss in response to long term immobilization. J Bone Joint Surg 60B:420–429, 1978.
93. Uhthoff, H.K., Jaworski, Z.F.G., and Liskova-Kiar M. Age specific activities of bone envelopes in experimental disuse osteoporosis and its reversal. Trans Orthop Res Soc 4:125, 1979.
94. Vogel, J.M. Bone mineral changes in the Apollo astronauts, in Mazess, R.B. (ed): *Int Conf Bone Mineral Measurement.* U.S. DHEW, NIH, 1973, pp 352–360.
95. Watson, R.C. Bone growth and physical activity in young males, in Mazess, R.B. (ed): *Int Conf Bone Mineral Measurement.* U.S. DHEW, NIH, 1973, pp 380–386.
96. Weber, B.C. Total hip replacement: Problem of implant-loosening, Chapchal, G. (ed): *Symposium on Arthroplasty of the Hip*, Stuttgart, Thieme, 1973, pp 11–21.
97. Whedon, G.D. Hearing before the Subcommittee on Aerospace Technology and National Needs of the Committee on Space Sciences, 94th Cong, 2 Sess, 1976.
98. Whedon, G.D., Lutwak, L., Rambaut, P., Whittle, M., Leach, C., Reid, J., and Smith, M. Effect of weightlessness on mineral metabolic studies on Skylab orbital space flight. Calcif Tissue Res 21(suppl):423–430, 1977.
99. Willert, H.G. Tissue reactions around joint implants and bone cement, in Chapcal, G. (ed): *Symposium on Arthroplasty of the Hip.* Thieme, 1973, pp 11–21.
100. Wilson, J.N., and Scales, J.T. Loosening of total hip replacements with cement fixation. Clin Orthop 72:145–157, 1970.
101. Wolf, J.W., White, A.A., Panjabi, M.M., and Southwick, W.O. Comparison of cyclic loading versus constant compression in the treatment of long bone fractures in rabbits. J Bone Joint Surg 63A:805–810, 1981.
102. Wolff, J. Das Gesetz der Transformation der Knochen. Verlag Von August Hirshwald, 1892. As translated by R.A. Brand, 1987, per-

sonal communication.

103. Woo, S.L.-Y., Akeson, W.H., Coutts, R.D., Rutherford, L., Doty, D., Jemmott, G.F., and Amiel, D. A comparison of cortical bone atrophy secondary to fixation with plates with large differences in bending stiffness. J Bone Joint Surg 58A:190–195, 1976.

104. Woo, S.L.-Y., Gomez, M.A., Amiel, D., Cobb, N.G., Hayes, W.C., and Akeson, W.H. The effect of short and long term exercise training on cortical bone hypertrophy. Orthop Res Soc 6:63, 1981.

105. Woo, S.L-Y, Kuei, S.C., Amiel, D., Gomez, M.A., Hayes, W.C., White, F.C., and Akeson, W.H. The effect of prolonged physical training on the properties of long bone: A study of Wolff's law. J Bone Joint Surg 63A:780–787, 1981.

106. Woo, S.L-Y. The relationships of changes in stress levels on long bone remodelling, in Cowin, S. (ed): *Mechanical Properties of Bone*. AMD ASME publ. 45:107–130, 1981.

107. Wroblewski, B.M. Revision surgery in total hip arthroplasty: Surgical techniques and results. Clin Orthop 170:56–61, 1982.

CHAPTER 11

Response of Bone to Electrical Stimulation

Joseph A. Spadaro

Descriptions of the application of electric currents to healing fractures first appeared in the British literature during the early nineteenth century as part of the general popularity of "electrotherapy."[73,80]

More recently, observations of the electromechanical properties of bone by Yasuda and Fukada in the 1950s,[47,91] and by Bassett, Becker et al in the 1960s[8] did much to stimulate further research. Bone, in both fresh and dry states, produces small electric potentials on its surface when placed under an appropriate mechanical stress. It was suggested that bone remodeling as an adaptive response to mechanical stress was mediated by means of these electric potentials which subsequently trigger osteoblastic and osteoclastic activity.[15,91] This hypothesis, which remains unproven, influenced researchers to apply exogenous electric current to bone in vivo in order to stimulate bone formation.[10,30,92] This led to further definition of effective parameters[44,45] and to electrical treatment of nonunited fractures in humans in 1971.[46,63]

CLINICAL APPLICATIONS

In 1974, Bassett, Pilla, and co-workers suggested the possibility of applying an electrical stimulus to bone tissue using pulsed magnetic fields without the necessity of implanting electrodes.[11] More recently, the application of electric currents through the skin with surface electrodes, originally studied by Cziesynski,[30,31] has been improved and explored as a potential clinical tool.[26]

While the biological effects of electrical and magnetic stimuli have been demonstrated under laboratory conditions, there remains some controversy over their efficacy in human fracture healing and bone augmentation.[6,13,37,40,68] Well-controlled clinical trials have been lacking, generally, despite active commercial development.

Several clinical devices have evolved for electrically stimulating bone formation and fracture healing. They illustrate the basic concepts and mechanisms which are the subject of this discussion (Fig. 11-1). They have been used in the treatment of nonunions, pseudarthroses, and failed fusions; for the enhancement of fresh fracture healing[12,51] and bone grafting,[9,71] and in the treatment of avascular necrosis[86] and loosened prostheses.[61] Their clinical results are described in Chap. 18, Sect. A.

The invasive devices (Fig. 11-1*A* and *B*) typically employ a cathode (negative electrode) placed into the fracture site. Direct currents and pulsing or alternating currents have been used. Noninvasive devices (Fig. 11-1*C* and *E*) rely on currents induced or transmitted without surgery. Hybrid devices are also in use (Fig. 11-1*D*).[60]

Most case reports with any method demonstrate a 75 to 90 percent rate of nonunion healing and an approximately 50 percent rate for congenital pseudarthrosis. For a more detailed discussion of the clinical methodology and results with each method, a number of recent reviews are available.[2,5,20,49,82,88] The subject of clinical application is further discussed in Chap. 18, Sect. A.

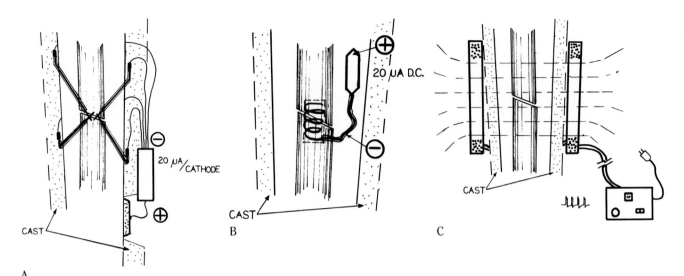

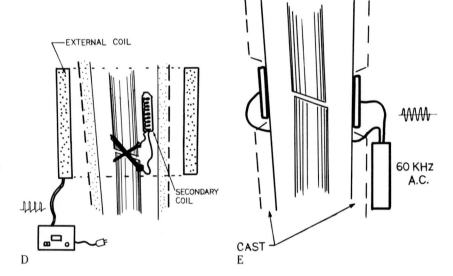

Figure 11-1 Several forms of electrical stimulation in clinical use predominantly for nonunited fractures and pseudo-arthroses: **A.** Percutaneous cathode, direct-current method (Brighton, C.T.)[26] **B.** Totally implanted direct-current cathode method (Patterson, D.)[2] **C.** Pulsed magnetic field induced-current method (Bassett, C.)[2] **D.** Magnetically driven induced electrode current method (Kraus, W.)[60] **E.** Skin-coupled alternating-current method (Brighton, C.T.)[26] Note that methods *A, B,* and *D* rely on an electrode proximate to the target site. Methods *C* and *E* are surgically noninvasive. *(From Spadaro, J., in Frumer, L. ed: Product Liability. New York, Mathew Bender, 1985. Reproduced with permission.)*

STIMULATION METHODS

The term *electrical stimulation* encompasses many different techniques for providing some sort of electric current in tissue. It is uncertain whether they have a common underlying mechanism of stimulation or whether any are related to the natural physiological processes which trigger bone formation. Four types can be distinguished, based on the electrical conditions produced in the target tissue.

1. Proximate Electrodes

These are implanted or inserted into, or immediately adjacent to, the target or fracture site, producing nonuniform electric currents in nearby tissue, as well as electrochemical (faradic) reactions and products. This form of stimulation has been successful in inducing osteogenesis in animal experiments and has been used extensively in human fracture healing. (Fig. 11-1*A* and *B*).

2. Distant Electrodes

These electrodes are implanted into or placed on the skin several centimeters from the target area where they produce electric currents which tend to be spatially more uniform. Electrochemical (faradic) reactions can and do occur, but they are usually too far from the target tissue to be of direct influence. Any extraneous effects due to the presence of the electrodes or to the trauma of their insertion are also fairly well excluded from influencing osteogenesis (Fig. 11-1*E*).

3. Time-Varying Magnetic Fields

Pulsing or sinusoidal external magnetic fields induce time-varying electric currents (and electric fields) in tissue without electrode reactions. The fields are applied with various types of coils usually placed over the target area (see Fig. 11-1*C*). The induced currents are circular in nature in planes perpendicular to the magnetic field lines (parallel to the coil faces) and pervade the entire region under the coil.[69] Their magnitude and pathways are determined by the local conductivities and geometry within the complex tissue layers as well as by the strength and rate of change of the applied magnetic field.[67,70] Near the bone, for example, current tends to run parallel to the surface. At the cellular level, tissue and membrane boundaries and their electrical characteristics play an important role in the way in which such currents form.

4. Electric Fields

Constant and time-varying electric fields are applied externally using capacitor plates without electrical contact to the body. A voltage applied to the plates results in an electric field which induces relaxation currents within the nearby tissue, generally perpendicular to the plane of the plates. Electrode reactions are not involved. This method has been used experimentally, but the high voltages required may limit its usefulness clinically.[69]

STIMULUS CHARACTERISTICS

The electric current resulting from any of the above methods can be characterized by the total current, current density (charge flow per unit area), or voltage gradient at the target site. These are not independent parameters and are related by the impedance and geometry of the tissues and the nature and location of the electrical source. Although total currents from 0.01 to 1000 μA have been used to stimulate bone formation, results are best when tissue current densities are in the range of 0.01 to 1 μA/mm,[2] corresponding to a voltage gradient of 0.1 to 10 mV/cm in tissue fluid.[18,82]

When electrodes are used, the applied electric potential and electrode material largely determine the electrochemical reactions that occur on the electrode surface.[81,83] Total electric charge delivered to the tissue is also important.[23] Cathodic negative electrode potentials in excess of 1.2 V (measured against a calomel reference electrode) can cause tissue necrosis due to the formation of toxic reaction products.[19,81] Below this level, proximate cathode electrodes carrying direct currents have been most successful as bone-stimulating electrodes. Anodic (positive) electrodes promote corrosion and have not been as successful, although there have been some exceptions[30,44,62]

To stimulate tissue with sufficient electric current density using distant electrodes or electric or magnetic fields, alternating or pulsed waveforms of various frequencies and shapes have been employed. This is partly due to the improvement in coupling efficiency between tissue and electrode or between tissue and electromagnetic fields.[69] Specificity of waveforms and frequencies has been claimed and has some theoretical basis, but remains an area of active research.[12,42,48,52,65,75,]

BIOLOGICAL RESPONSES
In Vivo Response of Bone

A large number of connective tissue responses to electrical stimuli have been observed in animals and in humans, of

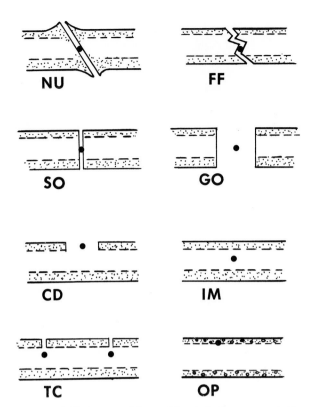

Figure 11-2 Various models used to study the response of bone to electrical stimuli in vivo. NU, nonunion or pseudoarthroses; FF, fresh fracture model; SO, simple osteotomy; GO, gap osteotomy; CD, cortical defect model; IM, intramedullary implant model; TC, transcortical implant model; OP, osteoporosis model. The dots mark the target site in each case. *(From Spadaro, J.A., J Bioelec 1:99–129, 1982. Reproduced with permission.)*

which stimulation of bone formation is perhaps the most prevalent.[18,80,82] A number of experimental models have been used to demonstrate this (Fig. 11-2). They usually involve an attempt at augmentation of normal reparative processes in bone, making evaluation complicated.[18,82] Endochondral and/or intramembranous bone, appropriate to the target site, is formed and may undergo subsequent remodeling. Electrically stimulated bone is generally indistinguishable from that formed by trauma or mechanical stimulation and may often be confused with it.[45,83,85] In some animals fresh fractures, osteotomies, or cortical defects have shown an early enhancement (2 to 3 weeks) of bone, osteoid, or mechanical strength which may not be evident at a later time.[12,50,71]

The most successful osteogenic response model, uncomplicated by repair, has been the IM model with proximate electrodes, defined initially by Friedenberg et al in rabbits.[45] New bone formation in the medullary canal is easily visualized and quantifiable. Figure 11-3 shows a similar osteogenic response for three successful cathode materials using this model.[83] Bone formed by the trauma of electrode insertion is short-lived, whereas that induced by continuous electric current persists for at least 3 weeks.[24,43]

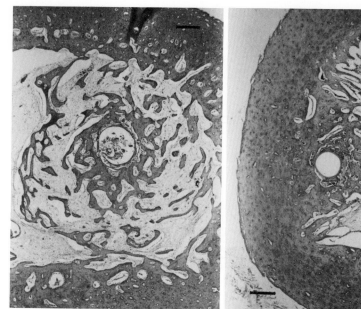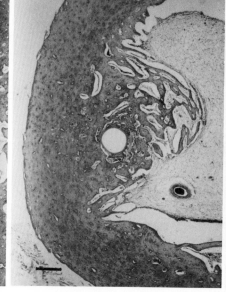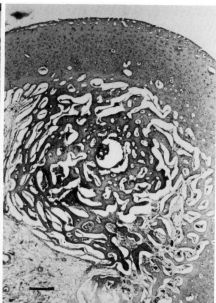

Figure 11-3 Photomicrographs of rabbit femora, 3 weeks after implantation of various cathodes, using the IM model in Fig. 11-2. **A.** Platinum (0.02 μA/mm^2; **B.** Silver (0.2 μA/mm^2); **C.** Stainless steel 316L (0.2 μA/mm^2). The cancellous new bone formation near the electrode space is clearly evident and tends to incorporate with the endosteal bone. H&E, stained cross section; bars = 0.5 mm. *(B and C reprinted with permission from Spadaro, J.A., in J Biomed Mater Res 16, 1982.)*

Bone and Bone Cell Responses in Vitro

Bone cells (osteocytes, osteoblasts, or osteoblastlike sarcoma cells), chick embryo fibroblasts as well as limb rudiments, and embryonic bone fragments have been exposed in culture to electrodes or induced electric currents. Because of the more precise control possible in such systems, biochemical responses can be more directly studied. Electrical stimuli have been found in various studies to increase DNA synthesis, increase tissue and cell proliferation, cause changes in cyclic AMP accumulation, increase collagen synthesis, increase mineralization, interfere with PTH activation, increase prostaglandin synthesis, or cause specific changes in genetic transcription.[22,89] Interest in pulsed magnetic and electric fields has led to increased experimental output in recent years. A comprehensive, critical review of this complex in vitro work has not yet emerged, but the majority of reports indicate that many mesenchymal cells of embryonic and adult origin are sensitive to several types of electrical stimuli.[89]

In Vivo Responses of Cartilage

Attempts to stimulate articular cartilage repair or epiphyseal cartilage growth in animals have not been as successful as for bone. Pulsed magnetic fields do not seem to promote epiphyseal growth in length in young animals,[78,84] and mixed results have been seen with electrode implants[1,3,58] and with externally applied 60-kHz currents.[27] Becker and others reported electrical stimulation of epiphyseal bone regeneration in rats.[16]

Cartilage Response in Vitro

Cartilage explants and cartilage cells have been subjected to electrode stimulation and induced currents in vitro with more positive results. Costochondral junction growth was increased in response to induced electric currents, electric fields, and proximate electrode implantation.[54,74,90] Cartilage cells in culture have shown changes in glycosaminoglycan (GAG) synthesis and in DNA synthesis in response to several types of stimuli.[27,72,77]

MODES OF ACTION

Direct Interactions of Electric Currents and Fields with Cells

Induced electric currents and fields can interact directly with connective tissue cells in several different ways. There is evidence that strong pulsed currents (1 to 50 V/cm) as well as the weaker, clinically applicable type (< 1mV/cm) can modify transmembrane potentials.[59,87] The electric field may displace membrane-bound ions and influence ionic fluxes within the cell.[36,38] Calcium ion flux changes across the plasma membrane, and calcium release from intracellular stores have been implicated experimentally and theoretically.[7,28,32,33,56,59] Electrochemical relaxation processes at cell membranes have been suggested to explain waveform specificity with pulsed magnetic field stimuli,[75] and biophysical calculations of membrane-binding affinity and reaction rate show that induced currents affect ligand-receptor interactions and transport kinetics.[29,53]

Recently, Liboff et al have proposed that "ionic cyclotron resonance" can couple exogenous fields to Ca^{2+} and other ions in or near cell membrane channels.[65a] In this mechanism, a weak low-frequency magnetic field (10–100 Hz, <1 gauss) combined with a weak constant magnetic field (<1 gauss) selectively affects the transport of specific ionic species. The method is potentially a very powerful clinical tool. Experimental confirmation has been found so far in human lymphocytes and marine diatoms in vitro.[65b,70a]

Indirect Interaction Mechanisms

Osteogenesis can be indirectly stimulated by faradic electrochemical reactions near an electrode. At a direct-current cathodic electrode, the electrochemical reduction of molecular oxygen can produce a slight decrease in local oxygen concentration (PO_2) as well as a change in pH and so modify osteoblast or chondrocyte activity.[19,21,81] In vivo experiments have confirmed a PO_2 decrease near a cathode[4,76] but have failed to confirm a change in pH at reasonable current levels and have also shown oxygen decrease at stainless *anodes*.[76] Equally likely is the possibility that the products of oxygen reactions such as the free radicals O_2, OH, and hydrogen peroxide can trigger membrane- or enzyme-mediated cellular activity.[34,81,82] Such electrochemical reactions may account for the relative differences in bone formation at different electrode materials and can be considered the most likely mechanism for the osteogenic response to implanted (proximate) electrodes.[21,83] However, as frequency increases or as pulse rise times decrease, the contribution of faradic reaction products decreases in favor of the more direct forms of cell stimulation noted previously.[23]

On a more speculative basis, the possibility of electroosmosis[39] or electromechanical responses (electric fields inducing mechanical stresses that stimulate osteogenesis) have also been considered as alternate forms of indirect stimulation by electricity.[57]

Cellular Response Mechanisms

Cellular activity can be modulated by membrane interaction with peptide hormones, mechanical forces, and exogenous electric forces. In bone cells, it has been shown that peptide hormones, such as parathyroid hormone (PTH), bind to membrane receptors, change calcium fluxes, and trigger release of adenyl cyclase and phosphodiesterase intracellularly. These in turn cause cyclic AMP accumulation and, ultimately, DNA synthesis and protein production. Mechanical forces, on the other hand, seem to modulate bone cell activity by prostaglandin E_2 (PGE_2) synthesis followed by cyclic AMP accumulation.[79] Electric fields and currents seem to be able to activate adenyl cyclase as well as PGE_2, but the latter is not required for activation of the cyclic AMP second messenger system.[17,35,55,56] In general, capacitively induced, strongpulsed electric fields as well as weak, magnetically induced pulsed currents and weak sinusoidal currents seem to share this characteristic. Cartilage cells also respond to mechanical

and electrical stimuli, but may not use the PGE_2 pathway for either stimulus.[17,64] Increased calcium flux into cells and intracellular calcium accumulation is nevertheless thought to be a common trigger in bone and cartilage cells.

In addition, induced electric currents can interfere with the response to PTH by bone cells.[25,66] This prevents PTH-induced bone resorption and is another possible mechanism leading to net bone formation.

Nonelectromagnetic Stimuli

In animal experiments and clinical applications, the use of electrical stimuli can also be accompanied by other potent stimuli of bone formation. An electrode can provide a mechanical stimulus arising from muscle activity and locomotion, as well as surgical trauma, producing an osteogenic response.[24,85] In patients treated with pulsed magnetic fields to stimulate fracture healing, significant immobilization is often required by the constraints of the apparatus, which itself promotes early bone union. Reactivity to implant materials can result in a hypertrophic osteogenic response, possibly confused with an electrically stimulated process.[24,83] In electromagnetic systems, resistive heating can produce a slight temperature increase in the cell culture or target tissue, contributing yet another stimulus to cellular activation.[41,74]

In conclusion, the weight of evidence now suggests that exogenous electrical stimuli can promote bone formation in vitro and in vivo. Electrochemical reactions and products may be the primary trigger for cells in the vicinity of an electrode carrying direct or very low frequency current. In other cases, calcium channel modulation followed by AMP accumulation seems to be one of the most likely cellular response mechanisms.

Future research will seek a more precise understanding of the underlying biophysical and biochemical mechanisms and a comprehensive evaluation of waveform specificity for various cellular responses. Clinically, an unambiguous determination of efficacy in musculoskeletal applications is being pursued. New applications such as peripheral and central nervous system repair, enhancement of chemotherapy, and soft tissue healing are being evaluated. There may also be genetic and developmental applications. However, we should also be alert for undesirable or unexpected responses.[13,14,37]

REFERENCES

1. Abraham, E. The long term effect of electrical stimulation on longitudinal growth. Orthop Res Soc 10:200, 1985.
2. Bassett, C., Brighton, C., Patterson, D. Ununited fractures, in Frankel, V. (ed): Instruct Course Lect 31:88–113, 1982.
3. Baker, B., Becker, R.O., and Spadaro, J. A study of electrochemical enhancement of articular cartilage repair. Clin Orthop 102:251–267, 1974.
4. Baranowski, T., Black, J., and Brighton, C. Microenvironmental changes assoicated with electrical stimulation of osteogenesis by direct current. Trans Bioelect Repair Growth Soc 2:47, 1985.
5. Barker, A., and Lunt, M. The effects of pulsed magnetic fields of

the type used in the stimulation of bone fracture healing. Clin Phys Physiol Meas 4:1–27, 1983.

6. Barker, A., Dixon, R., Sharrard, W., and Sutcliff, M. Pulsed magnetic field therapy for nonunion; interim results of a double-blind trial. Lancet, 5:994–996, May 1984.

7. Bassett, C.A.L. Biomedizinische und biophysikalische Wirkung pulsierender elecktromagnetisher Felder. Orthopade 13:64–67, 1984.

8. Bassett, C.A.L., and Becker, R.O. Generation of electric potentials in bone in response to mechanical stress. Science 137:1063–1064, 1962.

9. Bassett, C.A.L., and Hess, K. Synergistic effects of pulsed electromagnetic fields and fresh canine cancellous bone grafts. Trans Orthop Res Soc 9:49, 1984.

10. Bassett, C.A.L., Pawluk, R.J., and Becker, R.O. Effects of electric currents on bone in vivo. Nature 204:652–654, 1964.

11. Bassett, C.A.L., Pawluk, R., and Pillar, A.A. Augmentation of bone repair by inductively coupled electromagnetic fields. Science 184:575–577, 1974.

12. Bassett, C.A.L., Valdes, M., and Hernandez, E. Modification of fracture repair with selected pulsing electromagnetic fields. J Bone Joint Surg 64A:888–895, 1982.

13. Becker, R.O. The significance of electrically stimulated osteogenesis; more questions than answers. Clin Orthop 141:266–274, 1979.

14. Becker, R.O. Electrostimulation and undetected malignant tumors. Clin Orthop 161:336–339, 1981.

15. Becker, R.O., Bachman, C.H., and Friedman, H. The direct current control system: A link between environment and organism. NY J Med 62:1169–1962, 1962.

16. Becker, R.O., and Spadaro, J. Electrical stimulation of partial limb regeneration in mammals. Bull NY Acad Med 48:627–641, 1972.

17. Binderman, I., Shimshoni, Z., and Somjen, D. Biochemical pathways involved in the translation of physical stimulus into biological message. Calcif Tissue Int 36:S82–S85, 1984.

18. Black, J. Tissue response to exogenous electromagnetic signals. Orthop Clin North Am 15:15–31, 1984.

19. Black, J., and Brighton, C.T. Mechanisms of stimulation of osteogenesis by direct current, in Brighton, C.T., Brighton, C.T., Black, J., and Pollack, S.R. (eds): *Electrical Properties of Bone and Cartilage.* New York, Grune and Stratton, 1979, p 215.

20. Brighton, C.T. The treatment of nonunions with electricity; current concepts review. J Bone Joint Surg 63-A:847–851, 1982.

21. Brighton, C.T., Adler, S., Black, J., Itada, N., and Friedenberg, Z. Cathodic oxygen consumption and electrically induced osteogenesis. Clin Orthop Rel Res 107:277–282, 1975.

22. Brighton, C.T., Black, J., and Pollack, S. (eds): *Electrical Properties of Bone and Cartilage: Experimental Effects and Clinical Applications.* New York, Grune and Stratton, 1979.

23. Brighton, C.T., Friedenberg, Z., and Black, J. Electrically induced osteogenesis: Relationship between charge, current density, and amount of bone formed. Clin Orthop 161:122–132, 1981.

24. Brighton, C.T., and Hunt, R. Initial ultrastructural changes occurring in the vicinity of active and dummy cathodes in the rabbit medullary canal, in Brighton C.T., Black, J., and Pollack, S.R. (eds): *Electrical Properties of Bone and Cartilage.* New York, Grune and Stratton, 1979.

25. Brighton, C.T., and McClusky, W. The early response of bone cells in culture to a capacitively coupled electric field. Trans Bioelectr Repair Growth Soc 3:10, 1983.

26. Brighton, C.T., and Pollack, S.R. Treatment of nonunion of the tibia with a capacitively coupled electric field. J Trauma 24:153–155, 1984.

27. Brighton, C.T., Unger, A., and Stambough, J. In vitro growth of bovine articular cartilage chondrocytes in various capacitively coupled electric fields. J Orthop Res 2:15–22, 1984.

28. Chiabrera, A., Caratozzolo, F., Gianetti, G., Grattarola, M., and Parodi, A. Modulation of Ca^{++} influx due to electromagnetic exposure. Trans Bioelect Growth Repair Soc 4:31, 1984.

29. Chiabrera, A., and Rodan, G. The effect of electromagnetic fields on receptor-ligand interaction. J Bioelectr 3:509–521, 1984.

30. Cieszynski, T. Studies on regeneration of ossal tissue; treatment of bone fractures in experimental animals with electrical energy. Arch Immunol Ther Exp 11:191–208, 1963.

31. Cieszynski, T. Electric factors in bone regeneration. Report on studies in vitro and in vitro. Symp Biol Hungary 7:269–273, 1967.

32. Colacicco, G., and Pilla, A.A. Electromagnetic modulation of biological processes: Influence of culture media and significance of methodology in the Ca-uptake by embryonal chick tibia in vitro. Calcif Tissue Int 36:167–174, 1984.

33. Cullen, J., and Spadaro, J. Axonal regeneration in the spinal cord: A role for applied electricity. J Bioelectr 2:57–75, 1983.

34. Darolles, J., Sechaud, P., Dahhan, P., and Buvet, R. Oxygen reduction and peroxide production at cathodes used for tissue growth stimulation. Trans Bioelectr Repair Growth Soc 2:78, 1982.

35. Davidovitch, Z., Shanfield, J., Montgomery, P., et al. Biochemical mediators of the effects of mechanical forces and electric currents on mineralized tissues. Calcif Tissue Int 36:S86–S97, 1984.

36. Delport, P. Cheng, N., Mullier, J., Sansen, W., and DeLoecker, W. Metabolic effects of pulsed elecromagnetic fields on rat skin. Trans Biolectr Repair Growth Soc 4:44, 1984.

37. Editorial. Electromagnetism and bone. Lancet 11:815–816, April 1981.

38. Eisenberg, S., Grodzinsky, A., and Fechner, P. Changes in membrane permeability and interactions between connective tissue macromolecules induced by an applied electric current. Trans Bioelectr Repair Growth Soc 2:36, 1982.

39. Elwood, W., and Smith, S.D. Electroosmosis in compact bone in vitro. J Bioelectr 3:409–425, 1984.

40. Enzler, M., Blumlein, H., Gerber, H., Jacobs, R., and Perren, S. Experimentelle Untersuchungen uber die Wirksamkeit elektrischer und electromagnetischer Stimulation bei Heilungsvorgangen am knochen. Helv Chir Acta 49:663–666, 1982.

41. Fitton-Jackson, S., Marsland, T., and Boutle, A. Biological effects of electromagnetic fields and temperature: A comparison. Trans Bioelectr Repair Growth Soc 3:38, 1983.

42. Fitton-Jackson, S., Marsland, T., Farndale R., and Boutle, A.: Physical factors involved in biological responses to pulsed magnetic fields. Trans Bioelectr Repair Growth Soc 2:31, 1982.

43. Friedenberg, Z., Brighton, C.T., Black, J., and Esterhai, J. Quantitative analysis of progressive bone formation in response to constant direct current stimulation. Trans Orthop Res Soc 3: 198, 1978. See also: Esterhai, J.L., Friedenberg, Z.B., Brighton, C.T., and Black, J. Temporal course of bone formation in response to constant direct current stimulation. J Orthop Res 3:136–139, 1985.

44. Friedenberg, Z., and Kohanim, M. Effect of direct current on bone. Surg Gynecol Obstet 127:97–102, 1968.

45. Friedenberg, Z., Zemsky, L., Pollis, R., and Brighton, C. The response of non-traumatized bone to direct current. J Bone Joint Surg 54-A:1023–1030, 1974.

46. Friedenberg, Z., Harlow, M., and Brighton, C.T. Healing of nonunion of the medial malleolus by means of direct current. J Trauma 11:883–885, 1971.

47. Fukada, E., and Yasuda, I. On the piezoelectric effect in bone. J Physiol Soc Japan 12:1158–1162, 1957.

48. Hassler, C.R., Rybicki, E., Diegle, R., and Clark, L. Studies of enhanced bone healing via electrical stimuli. Clin Orthop 124:9–19, 1977.

49. Haupt, H.A. Electrical stimulation of osteogenesis. South Med J 77:56–64, 1984.

50. Hellewell, A., and Beljan, J. The effect of a constant direct current on the repair of an external osseous defect. Clin Orthop 142:219–

222, 1979.

51. Hinsenkamp, M., Burny, F., Donkerwolcke, M., and Coussarert, E. Electromagnetic stimulation of fresh fractures treated with Hoffmann external fixation. Orthopedics 7:411–416, 1984.

52. Hozack, W., and Brighton, C.T. Capacitively coupled electrical stimulation and fracture healing: The effect of varying the signal parameters. Trans Orthop Res Soc 9:182, 1984.

53. Hsieh, S., and Seto, Y. A two dimensional model for ELF electric fields interaction with biochemical systems. J Bioelectr 3: 469–482, 1984.

54. Iannacone, W., Pollack, S., Brighton, C.T., and Pienkowski, D. Pulsing electromagnetic field stimulation of in vitro epiphyseal plate growth. Trans Bioelectr Repair Growth Soc 3:39, 1883.

55. Johnson, D., and Rodan, G. The effect of pulsating electromagnetic field on prostaglandin synthesis in osteoblast-like cells. Trans Bioelectr Repair Growth Soc 2:7, 1982.

56. Jones, D. B. The effect of pulsed magnetic fields on cyclic AMP metabolism in organ cultures of chick embryo tibia. J Bioelectr 3:427–450, 1984.

57. Kavesh, N., Frank, E., and Grodzinsky, A. Electromechanical transduction mechanisms in cartilage: Implications for mechanical and electrical stimulation. Trans Bioelectr Repair Growth Soc 4:9, 1984.

58. Klems, H. Tierexperimentelle Studie zur Stimulation des Extremitatenwachstums durch elektrischen Gleichstrom. Z Orthop 119:315–319, 1981.

59. Korenstein, R., Somjen, D., Fischler, H., and Binderman, I. Capacitive pulsed electric stimulation of bone cells. Induction of c-AMP changes and DNA synthesis. Biochem Biophys Acta 803:302–307, 1984.

60. Kraus, W. Magnetfeldtherapie und magnetisch induzierte Elektrostimulation in der Orthopadie. Orthopade 13:78–92, 1984.

61. Kraus, W., Lechner, F., Ascherl, R., and Blumel, G. On the treatment of loosening of endoprosthesis by means of pulsing electromagnetic fields. Trans Bioelectr Repair Growth Soc 2:15, 1982.

62. Lagey, Cl., Roelofs, J., Lentferink, R. Experimental study of bone remodeling influenced by DC currents. Trans Bioelectr Repair Growth Soc 2:66, 1982.

63. Lavine, L.S., Lustrin, I., Shamos, M., Rinaldi, R., and Liboff, A. Electric enhancement of bone healing. Science 175:118–1121, 1972.

64. Lee, R., Rich, J., Kelley, K., Weiman, D., and Mathews, M. A comparison of in vitro cellular responses to mechanical and electrical stimulation. Am Surg 48:567–574, 1982.

65. Liboff, A., Williams, T., Strong, D., and Wistar, R. Time varying magnetic fields: Effect on DNA synthesis. Science 223:818–819, 1984. See also J Bioelectr 6:1–12, 1987.

65a. Liboff, A.R. Geomagnetic cyclotron resonance in living cells. J Biol Phys 13:99–102, 1985.

65b. Liboff, A.R., Rozek, R., Sherman, M., McLeod, B.R., and Smith, S.D. Ca^{+2}-45 cyclotron resonance in human lymphocytes. J Bioelectr 6:13–22, 1987.

66. Luben, R., Cain, C., Chi-Yun, M., Rosen, D., and Adey, W. Effects of electromagnetic stimuli on bone and bone cells in vitro: Inhibition of responses to PTH by low energy, low frequency fields. Proc Nat Acad Sci USA 79:4180–4184, 1982.

67. Lunt, M.J. Magnetic and electric fields produced during pulsed electromagnetic field therapy for nonunion of the tibia. Med Biol Eng Comput 20:501–511, 1982.

68. Marino, A. Electrical stimulation in orthopedics: Past, present and future. J Bioelectr 3:235–244, 1984.

69. Martin, R.B. Comparison of capacitive and inductive bone stimulation devices—Analysis of sinusoidal electromagnetic fields. Ann Biomed Eng 7:387–409, 1979.

70. McLeod, B., and Parker, R. Electromagnetic fields, biological systems and their connection in electromagnetic biostimulation.

Reconstr Surg Traumatol 19:19–31, 1985.

70a. McLeod, B.R., Smith, S.D., Cooksey, K.E., and Liboff, A.R. Ion cyclotron resonance frequencies enhance Ca-dependent motility in diatoms. J Bioelectr 6:1–12, 1987.

71. Miller, G., Burchhardt, H., Enneking, W., and Tylkowski, C. Electromagnetic stimulation of canine bone grafts. J Bone Joint Surg 66-A:693–696, 1984.

72. Norton, L.A. Pulsed electromagnetic field effects on chondroblast culture. Reconstr Surg Traumatol 19:70–86, 1985.

73. Peltier, L.F. A brief historical note on the use of electricity in the treatment of fractures. Clin Orthop 161:4–7, 1981.

74. Pienkowski, D., Pollack, S., Iannacone, W., and Brighton, C.T. Thermal effects during electromagnetic field stimulation of in vitro epiphyseal plate growth. Trans Bioelectr Growth Repair Soc 4:47, 1984.

75. Pilla, A.A. The rate modulation of cell and tissue function via electrochemical information transfer, in Becker, R.O. (ed): *Mechanisms of Growth Control.* Springfield, Ill., CC Thomas, 1981, pp 211–236.

76. Renooij, W., Janssen, L., Akkermans, L., Lagey, C., and Wittebol, P. Electrode oxygen consumption and its effects on tissue oxygen tension. Clin Orthop 173:239–244, 1983.

77. Rodan, G., Bourret, L., and Norton, L.A. DNA synthesis in cartilage cells is stimulated by oscillating electric fields. Science 199:690–691, 1978.

78. Smith, R.L., and Nagel, D. Effects of pulsing electromagnetic fields on bone growth and articular cartilage. Clin Orthop Rel Res 181:277–282, 1983.

79. Somjen, D., Binderman, I., Berger, E., and Harell, A. Bone remodeling induced by physical stress is prostaglandin E2 mediated. Biochim Biophys Acta 627:91–100, 1980.

80. Spadaro, J.A. Electrically stimulated bone growth in animals and man: Review of the literature. Clin Orthop 122:325–332, 1977.

81. Spadaro, J.A., and Becker, R.O. Function of implanted electrodes in electrode induced bone growth. Med Biol Eng Comput 17:769–775, 1979.

82. Spadaro, J. Bioelectric stimulation of bone formation: Methods, models and mechanisms. J Bioelectr 1:99–128, 1982.

83. Spadaro, J. Electrically enhanced osteogenesis at various metal cathodes. J Biomed Mater Res 16:861–873, 1982.

84. Spadaro, J., and Webster, D. A study of skeletal growth in young mice treated with pulsed magnetic fields. Trans Bioelectr Growth Repair Soc 4:21, 1984.

85. Spadaro, J., Mino, D., Chase, S., Werner, F., and Murray, D. Mechanical factors in electrode-induced osteogenesis. J Orthoped Res 4(1):37–44, 1986.

86. Steinberg, M., Brighton, C., Steinberg, D., Tooze, S., and Hayken, G. Treatment of avascular necrosis of the femoral head by a combination of bone grafting, decompression and electrical stimulation. Clin Orthop 186:137–153, 1984.

87. Strope, E., Findl, E., Conti, J., and Acuff, V. Pulsed electric fields and the transmembrane potential. J Bioelectr 3:329–346, 1984.

88. Symposium on electrically induced osteogenesis. Orthop Clin N Am 15:1–87, 1984. Current reviews of clinical applications by major contributors.

89. *Transactions of the Bioelectric Repair and Growth Society,* vols. 2–7, 1982–1987. For numerous examples of these responses the reader is directed to these concise reports.

90. Treharne, R., Brighton, C., Korostoff, E., and Pollack, S. An in vitro study of electrical osteogenesis using direct and pulsating currents. Clin Orthop 145:300–306, 1979.

91. Yasuda, I. Fundamental aspects of fracture treatment. J Kyoto Med Soc 4:395–406, 1953; reprinted in: Clin Orthop 124:5–8, 1977.

92. Yasuda, I., Noguchi, K., Sata, T. Dynamic callus and electric callus. J Bone Joint Surg 37-A:1292–1293, 1955.

CHAPTER 12

The Growth Plate: Structure and Function

Donald P. Speer

STRUCTURE OF THE PHYSIS

The growth plate, most commonly designated as the *epiphyseal plate,* or *epiphyseal growth plate,* is probably best considered as morphogenetically separate from the epiphysis. Certainly no growth plate is truly flat, or platelike. The most consistent current term for the growth plate is *physis. (Physis will be used generically to refer to the entire growth apparatus between the epiphysis and metaphysis of a growing bone.)* Thus, the cartilaginous growth zones that support endochondral ossification in the mandibular condyles or the proximal end of the metacarpals where a secondary ossification center is not present are not physes in this strict sense, in spite of their contribution to increased size of these bones. They do, however, exhibit the familiar columnar orientation of chondrocytes and the same sequence of cellular and matrix changes as long bone physes. A similar argument can be made for the circular (spherical) growth zone that is characteristic of the secondary ossification centers.

Most of the structural, physiological, and biochemical information on growth plates is derived from studies of higher mammals. These studies and less frequent observations on human specimens span several generations of admirable work which has been reviewed and/or advanced recently by numerous clinical and basic scientists.[5,6,13,18,40,41,48,87,93,99] Comparative aspects of physeal anatomy have also been evaluated.[14,68,69,97] Conclusions from animal data must be applied to humans with care. In general, the principles of structure and function of the growth plate apparatus among mammals, and vertebrates as a class, show biological variation about a central theme of mechanisms of bone growth.

The physis is a true synchondrosis, a cartilaginous junction between the epiphyseal and metaphyseal portion of a bone.[126] Although commonly illustrated as a component of a long bone, a physis is present in association with apophyseal centers (traction epiphyses) of flat or cuboidal bones such as the ilium or calcaneus. Each physis is unique to the species and bone from which it came with respect to the pattern of central and peripheral contours of the plate.[110] Largely as a consequence of the geometry of these contours in association with the tensile restraints of highly oriented collagen fiber systems, the physis is able to withstand potentially damaging forces in childhood while serving as the primary organ of axial and diametric growth of the bone.[54,70,88,102,105,106,107]

Even though the general principles of design and function are applicable to any physis, the geometric uniqueness of growth plates in each bone and species demands flexibility in application of these principles in a specific instance. This is extremely critical in a clinical setting, for example, where a surgical approach or physical diagnosis depends upon an accurate assessment of the specific physeal anatomy. It is equally critical in experimental design and in interpretation of biomechanical data with respect to growth plate studies. The growth plate is a constantly changing structure, and it is essential to develop a cinematic and three-dimensional conceptualization of the physes within their resident bones. The structural and biochemical features of the plate differ as a function of age, growth rate, loading history, and pathological conditions and also show variation within the substance of the physis.

Central and Peripheral Contours of the Growth Plate

Each growth plate shows a precise system of contours that are unique to both physis and species, much like a fingerprint.[70,110] Examination of the opposing bony surfaces of epiphysis and metaphysis reveals the complex topography (Fig. 12-1).

A systematic nomenclature of the major topographical features of each specific growth plate is now being developed. Definition of these features is extremely useful in the precise localization of posttraumatic crossunions across the plate and in the biomechanical analysis of the growth plate and its injuries.[4,10,102,105,110] The convention of using the contours of the *metaphyseal* side to name the contours was adopted. Thus, a named mammillary process, ridge, or peripheral process on the metaphysis corresponds to a mating depression, groove, or facet on the epiphyseal bone.[110] The transverse diameter of most epiphyses is greater at the physeal junction than the diameter of the metaphysis, creating an overlapping lappet formation.[70] As bone formation progresses laterally in the secondary ossification center, the epiphyseal bone may curve about the circumference of the metaphysis creating a circumferential process-and-facet relationship that affords further stabilization of the physis.

The peripheral margin of a growth plate is not in a constant transverse plane. Although capsular ligament attachments are generally to the epiphysis, the line of attachment may pass proximal or distal to the physeal line at various points on the circumference of the bone.[56] When the capital femoral epiphysis and greater trochanteric apophysis are removed from the metaphysis (Fig. 12-1), the complex pattern of grooves, depressions, ridges, and mammillary processes can be seen. In other bones, peripheral facets and processes may be present as well.[104] In addition, the overall or average contour of the epiphyseal bone surface is concave, whereas that of the metaphysis is convex, resulting in the periphery of the growth plate being located more toward the diaphysis than the central portion of the plate.

The surface of the epiphysis is a precise mold of the metaphysis and the two fit together like pieces of a jigsaw puzzle, separated from one another in life by the thickness of the growth cartilage. Clinical radiographs belie the complex three-dimensional structures of the physis due to superimposition of interdigitating bone images (Fig. 12-2). This radiographic averaging or voluming effect is a source of error in all imaging techniques to some degree. It is apparent that more sophisticated measurement and imaging techniques are essential to accurately map normal or pathological foci in the intact growing bone.[10] Three-dimensional reconstruction from computed tomography or magnetic resonance imaging

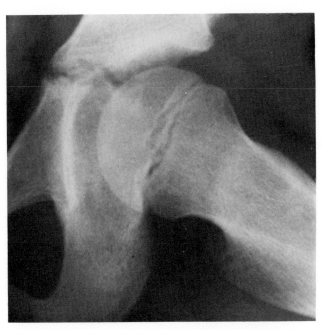

Figure 12-2 Lateral radiograph of normal proximal femur of a 9-year-old male. The x-ray beam was oriented perpendicular to the average plane of the proximal femoral physis. The images of the bony contours of opposed epiphyseal and metaphyseal surfaces are superimposed on the two-dimensional radiograph.

may offer a more complete and accurate standard in the future.

The interdigitating contours defining the topography of the physis have important biomechanical consequences (Fig. 12-3). Shear strain through the growth cartilage is prevented or minimized by the interlocking structures acting as stress concentration points.[14,102,106] Crack failure of the epiphyseal and/or metaphyseal bone begins experimentally at these points of stress concentration, and this can be histologically demonstrated (Fig. 12-3A). Radiological confirmation is provided in clinical cases of growth plate injuries where the mechanism of injury can be reconstructed.[54,70,88,105,106,107] Circumstances that result in increased physeal thickness such as rickets, hypothyroidism, growth hormone excess, or the condition of the bones of young or fast-growing children, may unlock the interdigitating structure of the plate and render the physis more susceptible to shear strain in response to loading (Fig. 12-3*B*). The thicker physes present in young or fast-growing children more commonly show Salter-Harris type I injuries, whereas older children who have thinner or partially closed physes show greater frequency of types II to IV after similar mechanisms of injury.

The pattern of major topographical features of the metaphyseal surface of the long bones is constant in all age groups studied from 4 to 17 years. These contours increase in amplitude with age. In addition, increasing complexity and numbers of minor topographical features of low amplitude are also observed as the child gets older. Radiographs may not show the epiphyseal concavity in the younger child who has not yet sufficiently ossified the secondary ossification center (Fig. 12-2).

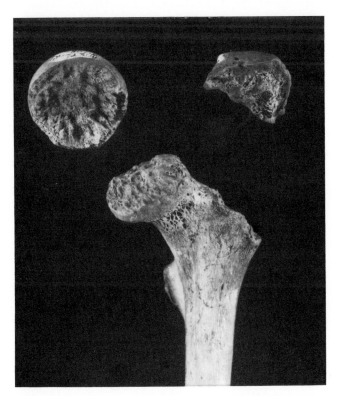

Figure 12-1 Proximal femur from a 14-year-old skeletally normal child. Separation of epiphysis and apophysis from metaphysis reveals central contours of the opposing bone surfaces. Note the undulating course of the peripheral margin which in life would correspond to the perichondral groove. *(Courtesy of the University of Arizona, Department of Anthropology.)*

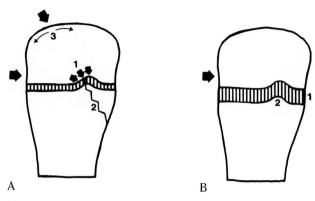

Figure 12-3 Biomechanical consequences of contours of the growth plate. **A.** Any irregularity can concentrate stresses (1) which may result in crack failure and propagation (2). Loads applied obliquely to the plane of the growth plate result in failure of the metaphyseal (2) and/or epiphyseal (3) bone more frequently than pure transverse shear forces. **B.** Increased thickness of the growth plate (1) may unlock the interdigitating bony contours (2) and increase susceptibility to separation through the growth plate.

Zones and Matrix Compartments of the Physis

The chondrocytes of the physis are organized into columns which are axially oriented with respect to the long axis of the bone and perpendicular to the plane of the growth plate[6,18,23,47,70,90] (Fig. 12-4). The growth cartilage is bounded on its epiphyseal side by an end plate of epiphyseal cartilage or epiphyseal bone, depending upon age, joint, species, and stage of development of the secondary ossification center.[3,6,119] This epiphyseal bone plate is continuous with the subchondral bone supporting the articular cartilage, emphasizing that the morphogenesis of the secondary ossification center functionally resembles a spherical growth plate. The deep zone of reserve cells of the physis may be homologous with the deep layer of the articular cartilage which has been shown in growing animals to have two zones of cell division.[60] One zone contributes chondrocytes to the enlarging articular surface and the other to the deeper zone of chondrocytes that are replaced in endochondral bone formation at the subchondral bone plate of the secondary ossification center. Cells of the physeal reserve zone undergo division, but with a low mitotic index. Their precise fate is uncertain, but it is possible that some of these cells contribute to development of the epiphyseal bone plate as well as to the growth plate.[48] The epiphyseal bone plate is initially cartilaginous, at a later stage it is calcified cartilage (chondroidal bone II),[3] and ultimately it is lamellar bone.

The physis is divided classically into several transverse and peripheral zones (Table 12-1) and to an increasing degree into distinct matrix zones as well. Although there is little substantive disagreement regarding these divisions, there is considerable confusion resulting from inconsistent use of a plethora of terms defining the regions. The convention of defining three major transverse zones based upon descriptive cellular growth phenomena has the advantage of simplicity and descriptive accuracy. These three major zones are: (1) zone of reserve cells, (2) zone of proliferation, and (3) zone of

hypertrophy[6] (Fig. 12-4). The zone of the epiphyseal bone (or cartilage) plate and the zone of ossification are not of the physis as such but are functionally and physically related. Furthermore, their appearance distinguishes the presumptive from the definitive growth plate.[119]

Each of the primary zones is subdivided in a variety of ways which reflect identification of metabolic, secretory, or synthetic activity of the cells or matrix of the area[5,7,18,23,70,90,119] (Table 12-1). The metaphyseal level of vascular invasion and spongiosae and early deposition of osteoid are often referred to, respectively, as zones of transformation and zones of remodeling. The noncalcified portion of the zone of hypertrophy is similarly referred to as the zone of maturation.[70] These terms reflect dynamic activity of the cells or matrix rather than a specific anatomical structure or appearance.

Matrix Compartments

The matrix compartments of the growth plate are commonly differentiated by histochemical criteria. Recent work suggests that these matrix compartments might be better defined on the basis of their collagen fiber content and organization.[18,102] A useful distinction is made between the territorial matrix, which is immediately surrounding the chondrocytes, and the interterritorial matrix, which is further removed from the cell and confined to the longitudinal cartilage bars between the cell columns. The classical and practical distinction between territorial and interterritorial matrix was refined as a result of recent improvements in fixation of proteoglycans, permitting demonstration of a noncollagenous, proteoglycan-rich peri-

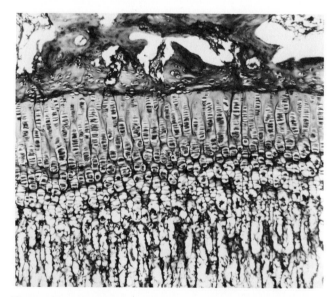

Figure 12-4 Histological section of definitive growth cartilage from the central portion of the proximal femoral physis of an 18-week-old pig. Shown in its anatomical setting between epiphyseal bone plate (top) and metaphyseal bone (bottom). The successive tissues or zones shown include epiphyseal bone, calcified cartilage (chondroid bone II), zone of resting cells, zone of proliferating cells, zone of hypertrophic cell with calcification and degeneration, and spongiosa. H&E, X100.

TABLE 12-1 Stratification of the Growing Bone End Including the Growth Plate and Juxtaposed Epiphyseal and Metaphyseal Structures (In Sequential Order from Epiphysis to Metaphysis)

Epiphyseal bone plate	Present in older age group. Not present in all bones or all species. Evolves as cartilage, then as calcified cartilage (chondroid bone II), and finally as bone in definitive growth plate.
Zone of reserve cells	Also called *zone of round cells* and, sometimes, *germinative zone,* but these are not accurate terms.
Zone of proliferation	True germinative zone with cell division, palisading or columnation. Subzones based upon the metabolic, secretory, and synthetic activity of the cells.
Zone of hypertrophy	Enlargement of cells chiefly in long axis of bone. Diametric hypertrophy at expense of matrix of cartilage bars.
Maturation	Subzone based chiefly on changes in metabolic, secretory, and synthetic activity of the cells.
Calcification	Appearance of Ca-PO$_4$ species in interterritorial matrix.
Degeneration (senescence)	Progressive loss of structural integrity.
Zone of ossification (metaphyseal)	Metaphysis begins at the level of the last intact transverse septum.
Vascular invasion Primary spongiosa Secondary spongiosa	

cellular matrix immediately surrounding the cell membrane. This pericellular matrix, which is not considered a part of the territorial matrix, is penetrated by cell processes that reach the territorial matrix. There are differences in properties of the proteoglycans of the pericellular and territorial matrices that may be due to variation in aggregation and/or the species and distribution of glycosaminoglycans.[1,21,22,95] The territorial matrix surrounds pericellular matrix and is characterized by a dense population of collagen fibers. These fibers are aligned parallel to the cell columns in the region abutting the interterritorial matrix but are randomly oriented where adjacent territorial matrices intermesh to form the transverse septae. The territorial matrix and its derivative

transverse septae do not undergo calcification. The transverse septum is the first structural component of the matrix to be destroyed by invasion of metaphyseal capillaries.[6,40]

The interterritorial matrix extends from the zone of reserve cells to the spongiosa. Collagen fibers within the interterritorial matrix are less densely packed than those of the territorial matrix, but they form larger fiber bundles and show a greater degree of orientation (anisotropy). They are oriented longitudinally, presumably as a result of local mechanical influences of hypertrophy of the chondrocytes, producing axial tension and transverse compression of the interterritorial matrix. It is the interterritorial matrix that supports the important process of calcification in the growth plate and then persists as a cartilaginous scaffold upon which osteoid is laid down following vascular invasion from the metaphysis.

Growth cartilage shares many biochemical and biophysical features with other hyaline cartilages but demonstrates a major distinctive difference in the degree of anisotropy of its cellular and fibrillar components acting in concert with matrix proteoglycan. Proteoglycans associated with collagen fibers are generally oriented perpendicular to those fibers. Thus, orientation of the collagen fibers of the territorial and interterritorial matrices confers a precise orientation to the proteoglycans of the matrix. It is the specific and high order of orientation of these components that in part distinguishes the growth plate from other hyaline cartilages and enables the growth plate to serve as the organ of growth for bones and to withstand the considerable stresses of normal function.[2,18,35,36,38,53,65,66,76,102,117,118]

Cartilages as a class of tissue are structural composites with proteoglycans and cells acting as hydrophilic-hydrostatic components and collagen fiber systems that provide tensile restraints within the tissue.[2,15,33,35] Cells, by proliferation and hypertrophy, and proteoglycans, by binding large domains of water, provide tissue pressures that are literally the force that both produces growth and gives resilience and shape to the tissues. Collagen fibers, on the other hand, maintain the structural integrity of the tissue and serve to restrain and guide the matrix and cells.[36,87,117] The interaction of collagen fibers and proteoglycans is enhanced by the linkage of the two to localize and stabilize the proteoglycans in the matrix. Disaggregation of proteoglycans or disruption of the collagen fiber systems results in loss of resilience of cartilages, in general, and impaired growth of cartilage, in particular. Changes in the state of proteoglycan aggregation or localization may affect normal morphogenetic mechanisms as well as calcification.[25,61,62,82,83] Glycosaminoglycans have been implicated both as inhibitors and mediators of calcification of cartilage because of their ability to combine with calcium.[95,120] Many earlier studies and conclusions are subject to reinterpretation as a result of the observations that methods of tissue fixation may remove, displace, or alter proteoglycans.[21,22,95]

Cellular Compartments (Zones)

Zone of Reserve Cells

Typical of this zone are small rounded cells surrounded by a relatively large amount of matrix. This zone is not metabolically inert as its name implies. These cells are actively synthesizing proteoglycans, collagen, and noncollagenous proteins as well as giving rise in some instances to matrix vesicles.[6,22,43] Cell mitoses are not prominent in this area of cells. The cells contain glycogen, lipid bodies, and vacuoles, indicating a storage function, but they are generally poor in their content of enzymes and minerals to support calcification or anaerobic metabolism. The collagen content of the matrix of this zone is high[123] and is organized into fiber systems that are in both axial and transverse orientation.[102]

Zone of Proliferating Cells

The distinguishing cellular characteristic of this zone is flattening of the chondrocyte with its long axis parallel to the plate. This flattening is already evident in the initial histogenesis of the growth plate before development of the secondary ossification center.[38,87] It is in this zone that cell division occurs in a predominantly transverse plane providing a morphogenetic mechanism that produces columnar alignment of chondrocytes of the growth plate.[18,87] The first "flattened" cell to appear in embryonic limb cartilage is the true germinal cell of the growth plate, and such a cell and its successors may have a finite number of programmed cell divisions that determine the ultimate number of cells available for axial growth.[6,48]

The highest oxygen tension of the growth plate is found in this zone. Aerobic metabolic activity supports storage of glycogen in the cells, production of adenosine triphosphate by the mitochondria anticipating calcium uptake by the mitochondria, and very active synthesis of glycosaminoglycans, collagen, and other noncollagenous proteins.[6] The concentration of collagen is lower than in the resting zone,[123] but its birefringence is more intense, indicating larger fiber systems, denser packing of aligned fibers, and/or loss of matrix components that interfere with birefringence.[102] The orientation of collagen fibers is longitudinal in the interterritorial matrix and increasingly random in closer proximity to the chondrocyte. Matrix vesicles are produced and are localized in the territorial matrix.[6,18,43] An increasingly heterogeneous population of proteoglycans is distributed through the pericellular matrix and the territorial and interterritorial matrices.[21,22,95] The zone has been further subdivided to demonstrate and measure gradients of metabolic, synthetic, and enzymatic activity.[6]

Zone of Hypertrophic Cells

The chief characteristics of the zone of hypertrophy are increase in the length of the cell columns as a result of the hypertrophy, accretion and release of calcium by mitochondria, calcification of the interterritorial matrix, and progressive degeneration of the chondrocyte. Since the cells of this zone are no longer dividing but are assuming their functional roles, they are in this sense undergoing maturation.

The cells of the hypertrophic zone progressively and forcefully increase their volume, chiefly expanding along the longitudinal axis of the bone and by this mechanism contributing to the growth of bone in length. Hypertrophy is the most important mechanism to growth in length, and it occurs even in experimentally produced absence of cell division.[117] The

forces generated by the distal femoral physis, representing effects of both proliferation and hypertrophy, range from 30 to 40 newtons.[74]

Oxygen tension is progressively reduced in this zone and the glycogen stored in the zone of resting and proliferating cells is used in an increasingly anaerobic metabolism. Mitochondria which begin to store calcium in the zone of proliferation continue to do so at a faster rate and at the expense of ATP production in the zone of maturation of hypertrophic cells. The mitochondria gradually lose their stored calcium as the cells assume a more anaerobic metabolism in the zone of degeneration.[6] As calcium is lost from the mitochondria, there is a temporally associated appearance of calcium in the matrix vesicles located in the adjacent interterritorial matrix of the axially oriented cartilage bars. These initial deposits are amorphous calcium phosphate complexes that eventually form calcium hydroxyapatite as the predominant species of crystal. Apart from matrix vesicles, mineral deposition occurs in association with specific foci on collagen fibers in the interterritorial matrix. Alkaline phosphatase, which is associated with mineralization, is abundant in this zone as are enzymes supporting anaerobic metabolism. Calcium, phosphorus, and alkaline phosphatase are present in the matrix vesicles, and recent evidence points to increased content of specific proteoglycans in the region of these matrix vesicle mineral deposits.[6,42,43,64,91,95]

The zone of hypertrophy has the lowest concentration of collagen and of glycosaminoglycans of any region of the plate.[6,122] The magnitude of loss of proteoglycans and changes in their distribution may be overemphasized in published studies due to artifactual loss and diffusion of these substances in fixation or preparation.[18,21,22,95] Recent work shows a fairly homogeneous distribution of proteoglycans. Probably differences in the state of aggregation or fixation of proteoglycans accounts for many of the reported differences in staining properties and ultrastructural appearances. The axial collagen fiber system in the interterritorial matrix shows its smallest transverse diameter at this level, in part because of compression by the hypertrophied chondrocytes of the cell columns but also because of enzymatic degradation of the matrix[6,20,27,115](Fig. 12-4).

The metaphyseal border of the growth plate is defined by the last intact transverse septum separating the dead or dying chondrocyte from the invading metaphyseal capillaries. Between the cells the cartilage columns themselves are more resistant to degradation than the transverse septae, and this cartilage persists as a substrate for the deposition of osteoid in the formation of the primary spongiosa. The ultimate fate of the chondrocyte is death and displacement by invading capillaries. This process of degeneration of the cell in the zone of hypertrophy is biologically a form of physiological senescence. That is, it is a programmed set of events for this cell.

PERICHONDRAL COMPLEX

The *perichondral complex* is the region at and adjacent to the periphery of the physis and metaphysis. It is characterized by a group of structures that serve critical roles in axial and diametric growth, remodeling, and stability of the physis in the growing ends of bones.

The specific components of this (Fig. 12-5) complex include the perichondral ossification groove[79] or, simply, zone of Ranvier;[70] the perichondral bone ring of LaCroix,[50] which is a subdivision of the zone of Ranvier; the perichondrium; the marginal germinative zone or juxtaepiphyseal apparatus;[37,85,94] and three major longitudinal, circumferential, and transverse collagen fiber systems.[102]

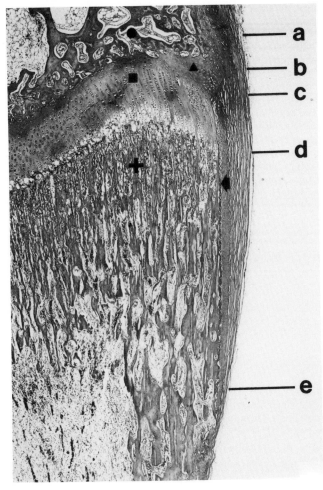

Figure 12-5 Longitudinal coronal plane section of the distal end of the third metacarpal of an 8-week-old New Zealand white rabbit. One of the mammillary processes is shown contouring the plane of the growth plate (square). Epiphyseal bone of the secondary ossification center is at the top (circle) and metaphyseal bone at the bottom (cross). The marginal germinative zone (triangle) is part of the perichondral groove which extends between the transverse planes defined by *b* and *e*. This cellular area contains the perichondral bone ring (arrow). A fibrous perichondrium inserts into the epiphysis and is thickened throughout the longitudinal extent of the perichondral groove before continuing as the substantially thinner periosteum. Lowercase letters define approximate planes of transverse sections shown in Fig. 12-6. H&E, ×32. *(From Speer, D.P., J Bone Joint Surg 64A:399–407, 1982. Reproduced with permission.)*

The perichondral groove anatomically defines the peripheral line of the growth plate. In addition to describing the groove, Ranvier[79] noted that the cells of the groove produced fibers (subsequently identified as collagen) and a ring of bone which became better known as the perichondral bone ring of LaCroix.[50] This ring extends from the physeal plane for a variable distance over the metaphysis to define a segment of bone called the *metaphyseal pedestal* (socle metaphysaire).[37,71]

The ring delimits the portion of the metaphysis that has not yet begun remodeling or funnelization. Furthermore, the ring is of variable length, in general in inverse proportion to the degree of funnelization characteristic of a particular bone. Thus in the distal metacarpal (Fig. 12-5), which undergoes modest remodeling, the ring is elongated and prominent, whereas in the proximal femur, which undergoes extensive remodeling, it is extremely short, and is usually fibrous rather than bony.[102] A similar variability is noted with respect to the location of the epiphyseal border of the perichondral ring, depending upon the specific physis and also upon the age. In the infant the perichondral ring spans the entire growth plate,[6,70] whereas in older age groups it may at least extend over the zone of hypertrophic cells.

At the epiphyseal border, a cellular zone conjoins the perichondrium and perichondral ring, and the growth cartilage and the epiphyseal cartilage (or bone). The articular cartilage is also included in some bone ends such as the proximal femur. This region is appropriately named the *marginal germinative zone* (Figs. 12-5 and 12-6)[37] because it contributes chondroblasts for diametric growth of the physis, osteoblasts for axial proliferation of the bone ring, and fibroblasts for both axial and circumferential growth of the perichondrium.[37,51,52,85,86,94,100] On the epiphyseal side of the marginal germinative zone (Fig. 12-6B) are cells which largely contribute to formation of epiphyseal bone and perichondrium; they are relatively small and randomly distributed with abundant intercellular matrix. On the metaphyseal side of the marginal germinative zone (Fig. 12-6C) are cells which are not only larger than those on the epiphyseal side but which show columnation much like the growth plate but in a radial direction, reflecting the role of this portion of the zone in diametric growth of the physis.[102] Within its circumference, the position of the perichondral ring limits diametric proliferation and hypertrophy of chondrocytes. Importantly, the ring restricts such proliferation and hypertrophy of growth plate chondrocytes to the longitudinal axis of the bone (Fig. 12-5). By these mechanisms, a major role of the perichondral ring is in the control of morphogenesis.

At its diaphyseal limit the perichondral ring begins to undergo osteoclastic resorption from the endosteal side (Figs. 12-5e and 12-6E).[93,102] Toward the diaphysis beyond the border of the perichondral ring and groove tissue, subperiosteal osteoclasis also contributes to the process of funnelization of the bone. The medullary bone at this level contains cartilage core remnants surrounded by bone, which is an identifying characteristic of the metaphyseal region.

The perichondrium superficial to the perichondral groove is typically thicker than the periosteum of the same bone (Fig. 12-5). Most of this increased thickness can be attributed to an abundance of circumferential fiber groups.

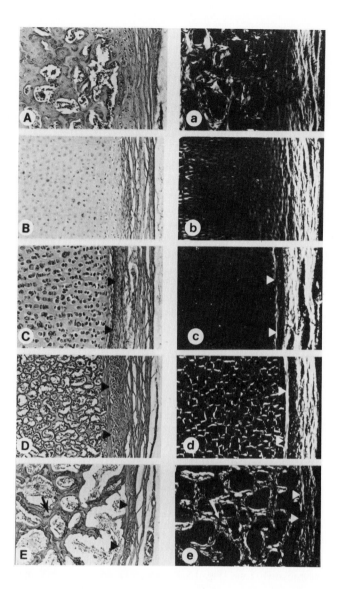

Figure 12-6 Transverse sections of third metacarpal of 8-week-old New Zealand white rabbit, corresponding to the planes shown in Fig. 12-5. Uppercase letters on the left are under bright field, and the lowercase letters on the right are polarized light views of serial sections of the same histological specimen. **Aa.** Epiphyseal bone and cartilage with perichondrium containing circumferential and longitudinal collagen fiber groups. **Bb.** Epiphyseal cartilage from the epiphyseal side of the marginal germinative zone portion of the perichondral groove. There are radially oriented collagen fibers in the cartilage interdigitating with those of the perichondrium, which contains both circumferential and longitudinal collagen fiber groups. The cartilage cells are smaller and closer together near the perichondrium. **Cc.** Metaphyseal side of the marginal germinative zone, at junction with growth plate and beginning of the perichondral bone ring (arrowheads). Both chondrocytes and adjacent collagen fibers are oriented radially. The perichondrium has longitudinal fibers, and both the ring and the perichondrium show circumferentially oriented collagen fiber groups. The perichondral groove is cellular with negligible collagen fiber content. **Dd.** Primary spongiosa is present. The perichondral ring (arrow), perichondral groove cells, and perichondrium are similar to that seen at *Cc.* Circumferential collagen fiber groups in the osteoid of the primary spongiosa are laid down on calcified cartilage. **Ee.** Metaphyseal bone with retained cartilage cores is seen. The perichondral bone ring (arrow) is undergoing osteoclastic resorption from the endosteal side. Minimal circumferential collagen fibers are found in the periosteum compared to the more distal sections. *(From Speer, D.P., J Bone Joint Surg 64A:399–403, 1982. Reproduced with permission.)*

These are seen between the longitudinal fiber groups of the perichondrium and are more prominent in deeper than superficial regions of the perichondrium (Fig. 12-6). The perichondral groove region is significantly and specifically characterized by its content of circumferential fiber systems.[102] A basis for the production of these circumferential fibers is discussed below.

COLLAGEN FIBER ARCHITECTURE

In contrast to the classical separation of histological regions of the physis and adjacent perichondral structures, a consideration of the three-dimensional architecture of the collagen fiber framework of the bone and physis provides an integrated picture of the continuous whole structure.[18,50,51,79,102] This conceptualization based upon the orientation and interconnections of collagen fiber systems permits a synthesis of many structural biomechanical and morphogenetic principles of the growing bone.

The collagen of growth cartilage is predominantly type II, but there are small and often transient quantities of other types.[26,36,84,113,124,125] Type II collagen is more heavily glycosylated and contains different species of cross-links than type I collagen of skin and bone, probably accounting for its greater resilience.[34,125]

Although several corroborating techniques are required to fully assess collagen fiber systems, polarized light microscopy is an excellent method for study and illustration of the collagen fiber systems in bone and cartilage[18,101,102,103,108] (Figs. 12-6, 12-7, and 12-8). When either stained or unstained histological sections are used, collagen fibers are easily demonstrated by their typical birefringence. Orientation is inferred from the relationship of observed planes of maximal and minimal intensity of birefringence to the known planes of polarizing optics in the microscope (Fig. 12-7) and is confirmed using serial cross sections of the same specimen (Fig. 12-6). This information can then be used to reconstruct the collagen fiber architecture in three dimensions (Fig. 12-9).

Six major collagen fiber systems have been identified in the physis and adjacent perichondral region. Each major fiber system shows a group of aligned collagen fibers with precise

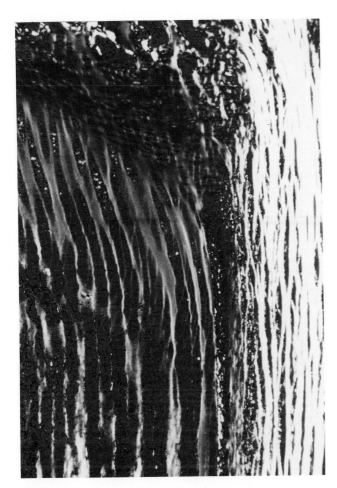

Figure 12-7 Longitudinal coronal plane section of the distal end of third metacarpal of an 8-week-old New Zealand white rabbit showing the perichondral ossification groove and adjacent structures under polarized light. *(From Speer, D.P., J Bone Joint Surg 64A:399–407, 1982. Reproduced with permission.)*

spatial orientation extending over a wide area of tissue and generally traversing or bordering a classical histological zone of the bone. Two of these fiber systems are longitudinal, three are circumferential, and one is radial or transverse (Fig. 12-8). The longitudinally oriented transphyseal fiber groups arise from the epiphyseal bone plate, traverse the growth plate within the territorial matrix of the cartilage bars, and persist in cartilage cores of the metaphysis where they achieve attachment to the spongiosa (Figs. 12-8 and 12-9). Collagen fibers in the primary spongiosa are deposited chiefly circumferentially within the columnar tubes of calcified cartilage that remain after vascular invasion exposes the chondrocyte lacunae (Figs. 12-6 and 12-9).

The perichondrium-periosteum is a tube also consisting of longitudinally oriented collagen fiber groups that extend from the level of the diaphysis and achieve insertion into the epiphysis (Figs. 12-5 through 12-8). The epiphyseal insertion of these longitudinal fibers may be into epiphyseal cartilage, epiphyseal or subchondral bone, and/or articular cartilage, depending upon the age and specific bone. As noted above, the perichondrium is rendered substantially thicker by the presence of a system of circumferential fibers which are more numerous in the deeper layers of the perichondrium.

The collagen fiber system of the perichondral ring is intensely birefringent and almost exclusively circumferentially oriented (Fig. 12-9). The ring is analogous to the hoops about a barrel encircling the periphery of the growth plate and adjacent metaphysis. There are a few longitudinal collagen fibers in the cellular perichondral groove tissue over the ring.

Transverse collagen fibers are located in the epiphyseal cartilage and zone of resting cells (Figs. 12-8 and 12-9). These radially oriented fibers form a cap over the growth plate centrally and pass through and over the epiphyseal border of the marginal germinative zone to interdigitate with the perichondrium peripherally.

In experimental Salter-Harris type I injuries to the growth plate produced by transverse shear loading, the growth plate separates through the zone of hypertrophy and specifically

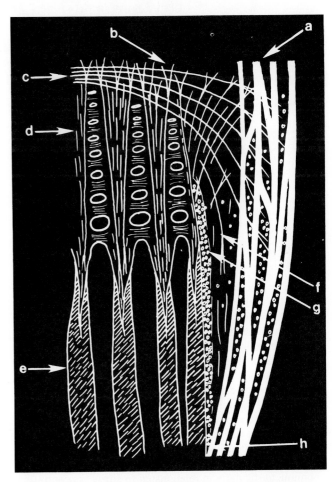

Figure 12-8 Drawing of the perichondral complex shown in Fig. 12-7 showing only the collagen fibers as revealed by their birefringence. **a.** Perichondral fibers. **b.** Transphyseal fibers originating in the epiphyseal bone plate. **c.** Radial or transverse fibers in bone plate and zone of resting cells. **d.** Transphyseal fibers in interterritorial matrix. **e.** Metaphyseal bone collagen fibers. **f.** Perichondral groove with almost no fibers in cellular area. **g.** Perichondral bone ring. *(From Speer, D.P., J Bone Joint Surg 64A:399–403, 1982. Reproduced with permission.)*

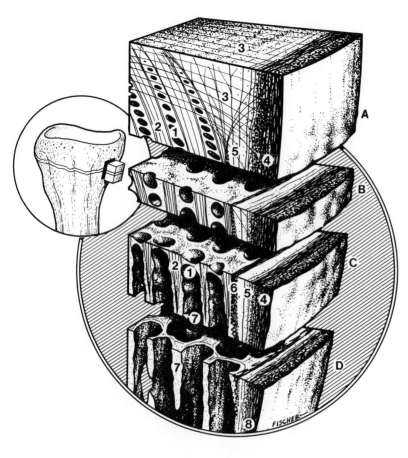

Figure 12-9 Reconstruction of the three-dimensional architecture of the major collagen fiber systems of the growth plate, perichondral ossification groove, perichondral bone ring, and adjacent structures of the growing bone. The reconstruction is based upon analysis of serial transverse and longitudinal histological sections by both bright field and polarized light microscopic techniques. **A.** Epiphyseal bone plate, zones of reserve and proliferating cells, and epiphyseal end of perichondral groove with early ring. **B.** Zone of hypertrophy and thickest portion of perichondrium. **C.** Beginning of metaphysis shown at the last intact transverse septum. **D.** Metaphyseal bone with retained cartilage cores. (1) Chondrocyte columns. (2) Longitudinal transphyseal collagen fibers in the interterritorial matrix. (3) Radial (transverse) collagen fibers in the epiphyseal bone plate and cartilage and zone of resting cells. These form a fibrous "cap" over the epiphyseal side of the physis. (4) Longitudinal perichondral collagen fibers continuous with those of the periosteum toward the diaphysis. In deeper layers of perichondrium, increasing numbers of circumferential collagen fibers are found over the region of the perichondral groove. (5) Perichondral groove. This cellular region has few collagen fibers and those present are almost entirely longitudinally oriented. (6) Circumferential collagen fibers of the perichondral bone ring. (7) Circumferential collagen fibers of the osteoid in primary spongiosa. (8) Longitudinal fibers of the perichondrium continue in the periosteum beyond the diaphyseal border of the perichondral groove.

through its junction with the zone of calcification (Fig. 12-10). This region of the plate is the most deficient in collagen fibers and collagen content[102,123] and is probably more brittle (higher modulus of elasticity) as a result of calcification. For both these reasons, this portion of the zone of hypertrophic cells tolerates displacement (strain) poorly. Although the specific direction and loading characteristics of applied force influences the type of disruption of the growth plate in animal experiments, the initial disruption is uniformly within the substance of the physis with subsequent disruption of the perichondrium. Furthermore, the zone of hypertrophy is consistently separated in some degree, but propagation of the plane of failure into other zones of the plate and/or bone is common, particularly in relationship to stress concentrating topographical features of the physis and adjacent bone (Fig. 12-3).[102,105,107]

In experimental Salter-Harris type I shear injury, the plane of failure peripherally is also defined by the collagenous architecture. The separation line passes over the epiphyseal end of the perichondral ring and disrupts the perichondrium along the course of the interdigitating radially oriented fibers (Figs. 12-8 and 12-10 (arrow)).

BLOOD SUPPLY OF THE PHYSIS

The pattern of blood supply to the physis differs with the age and stage of development as well as with the specific bone and species of animal.[8,12,24,49,68,69,119] Interest in the blood supply to specific growth plates accompanies contemporary efforts to achieve transplantation of physes using microvascular surgical techniques.[67,72,116] The most complete morphological assessment with substantial pathophysiological correlations of physeal blood supply is of the proximal femoral physis.[9,12]

There are two sources of blood supply to the definitive physis. These are the epiphyseal arteries and the perichondral arteries. Metaphyseal and nutrient vessels are critical in support of endochondral bone formation but do not supply the physis itself once the epiphyseal bone plate is formed. Communication between epiphyseal and metaphyseal vessels across the zone of the growth plate does occur, however, prior to development of the secondary ossification center (stage of presumptive growth plate) and during the process of physiological closure of the growth plate.[17,20,28,68,69,119] It is also recognized that calcification of

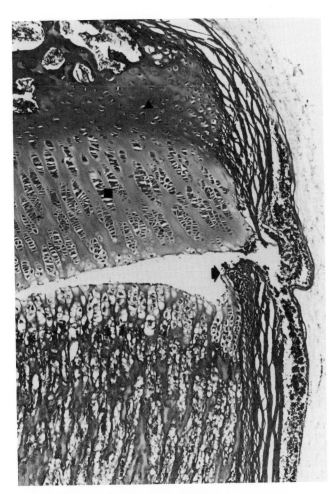

Figure 12-10 Photomicrograph of Salter type I growth plate injury produced experimentally in the distal metacarpal of a 10-week-old New Zealand white rabbit. A transverse shear force was applied at 2.5 cm/s until separation occurred. The plane of separation passes through the zone of hypertrophy at the junction with the zone of calcification, over the epiphyseal border of the perichondral bone ring, and through the perichondrium in the plane of interdigitation with the radially oriented collagen fiber system.

the growth cartilage fails to occur if the metaphyseal blood supply is ablated, indicating that diffusion from the metaphyseal side occurs and is physiologically important.[119] Cartilage canals transmit vessels from the epiphyseal and perichondral systems but may not provide blood supply in a physiological sense along their entire course through regions of the chondroepiphysis including, at various early stages, the growth cartilage itself. A major secondary role of cartilage canals is to provide stem cells for osteogenesis and interstitial cartilage growth.[57]

Epiphyseal arteries provide the major source of blood supply to the central portion of the physis. Usually, several arteries enter the epiphysis and give branches which supply the secondary ossification center, subchondral bone, and physis as end arterial systems. Those vessels which supply the physis penetrate the epiphyseal bone plate, and the zone of reserve cells then arborize to terminate as capillary com-

plexes supplying the zone of proliferating cells directly. Although epiphyseal vessels are multiple to most epiphyses, each vessel may supply only a limited volume of the epiphysis or corresponding area of the growth plate and so are functional end arteries. This is reflected clinically in the segmental necrosis of the capital femoral epiphysis and physis occurring in such conditions as Legg-Perthes disease and congenital hip disease. Subsequent changes in the physeal inclination angle, epiphyseal shape, and femoral neck length have been directly related to partial vascular involvement of the physis.[9,11,12,13]

The peripheral portion of the physis is supplied by several perichondral arteries which enter in the region of the perichondral groove. Although these perichondral vessels surround the physis with an extensive network of vessels, they rarely communicate with the epiphyseal vessels. They may, however, at an early age serve as a route of infection to the epiphysis via the epiphyseal arteries.[70] The blood supply to the portion of the physis responsible for diametric growth is therefore relatively independent from the portion supporting axial growth of the bone. Damage to the perichondral vessels can produce a peripheral growth arrest or retardation.[70]

The metaphyseal arteries penetrate the metaphyseal cortex to supply the peripheral region of the metaphysis. Branches of the nutrient artery supply the central portion of the metaphysis subjacent to the growth plate. Each of these vessel systems supply capillary loops which penetrate the last transverse septae of the chondrocyte columns of the physis and support initial deposition of osteoid on the calcified cartilage.

It was shown in an avian model that the capillary loops of the metaphysis form venous sinusoids, which are characterized by endothelial gaps and absence of a basement membrane, whereas the epiphyseal vessels terminate at the zone of cell proliferation as capillary-venule plexuses in which the endothelium is continuous.[41] Most likely, this is the case in humans as well. The arrangement may, in part, reflect the predominance of synthesis and cell division of the epiphyseal side versus degradation and resorption on the metaphyseal side of the physis, but controversy remains regarding the afferent or efferent roles of specific vessels.[16] Most information concerning the circulation to the growing end of bone is morphological and concerns the arterial vessels. Much less is known of the venous drainage from these areas, and there is very little data on flow, uptake, or other physiological parameters to correlate with the excellent morphological information.

MORPHOGENETIC CONTROL MECHANISMS DURING GROWTH

The fact that embryonic bone will continue to grow in both length and diameter while maintaining its characteristic gross morphology[38,87,111,116] reflects a high level of morphogenetic control intrinsic to the bone itself. Many of these control mechanisms are based upon the dynamic interaction of the cells and matrix components.[36,39,51,52,81,109,117,118] Modulation of these intrinsic morphogenetic control mechanisms to enhance or arrest growth may be produced by extrinsic factors such as pressure,[122] absence of loading,[63] excessive loading,[98] or altered blood supply.[45] Extrinsic control may in part be mediated by hormonal receptors demonstrated in the growth cartilage.[13,44,46,55,59,75,112] When the chondrocytes of the growth plate proliferate and, especially, hypertrophy, tension is produced in the perichondrium-periosteum since the perichondrium is firmly inserted into the epiphysis. This tension is thought to provide a specific stimulus for axial progression of subperiosteal osteogenesis, necessarily in the perichondral bone ring, resulting in increased length of the shaft of the bone by an intramembranous mechanism. This same tension also results in a proportional increase in axial loading of the growth cartilage chondrocyte columns and serves as negative feedback inhibiting proliferation and/or hypertrophy by these cells. Conversely, release of this periosteal-perichondral tension will accelerate proliferation and/or hypertrophy. The latter effects are seen after circumcision of the periosteum, which was once used clinically in attempts to lengthen short extremities and may be a mechanism of accelerated growth of long bones in children after diaphyseal fractures. These effects are examples of and possible mechanisms for the *Hueter-Volkman law of bone growth* which states that axial pressure slows and axial tension accelerates the growth contribution of the physis.

Diametric or transverse growth of the physis occurs by both interstitial and appositional mechanisms.[37,38,51,63,70,77,78,85,89,99,100,102] The proliferation and hypertrophy of cells from the marginal germinative region of the physis progresses centrifugally providing progenitor cells for the formation of additional longitudinal cell columns and coincidentally increasing the diameter of the growth plate. As they grow in a transverse direction, the chondrocytes are radially aligned as are the collagen fibers, giving the appearance of a radially oriented growth plate located just beyond the epiphyseal border of the perichondral bone ring (Fig. 12-6).

The circumferential collagen fiber system of the perichondral ring becomes an effective restraint to diametric expansion of the hypertrophying chondrocytes of the longitudinal cell columns. These cells are guided in a longitudinal axis with resulting growth in length of the bone. On the epiphyseal side of the ring, however, there is less restraint and diametric expansion occurs until restrained by further extension of the ring. Experimental defects of the perichondral ring result in cartilaginous outgrowths having the appearance of clinical osteochondromata, suggesting a possible basis for this disease and supporting the proposed morphogenetic role of the ring.[85]

The cells of the zone of proliferation are flat with their long axes parallel to the plane of the growth plate and, therefore, perpendicular to the long axis of the bone. When these cells divide, their plane of cleavage is also parallel to the plane of the growth plate, and cell division alone contributes to the columnar stacking of the resulting daughter cells. The appearance of the flattened chondrocyte is a key morphogenetic event in the embryological development of a bone as well, for it is among the first events leading to the columnar architecture of the growth plate. Matrix secretion signals the beginning of chondrification in embryonic limb, and this occurs first in the cell condensation that will eventually become the primary center of ossification.

The cellular change of flattening of the chondrocytes occurs as the volume of the matrix increases in the face of peripheral restraint by the primitive perichondrium. Flattening of successive layers of chondrocytes between the hypertrophic cells and the rounder cells located toward and ultimately within the epiphysis may be a predominantly mechanical effect. It is also postulated that the transversely oriented layer of collagen fibers aligned with these flattened cells influences successive populations of rounded cells to flatten by assuming an orientation parallel with the long axis of the collagen fibers.[87]

Although the interaction of collagen fibers and cells has been emphasized, the noncollagenous matrix components, particularly the proteoglycans, also influence the described morphogenetic mechanisms. Proteoglycans produce and maintain the swelling or turgor of cartilages, and in this way place collagen fibers under constant physiological tension. The glycosaminoglycans are also able to bind cations, and when stabilized as proteoglycans in collagen fiber matrices, the matrix is analogous to an ion exchange column which may serve to modify and maintain the local ionic environment. Both ionic strength and species may affect the conformation of proteoglycan chains and thus may also affect diffusion within the matrix as well as cell membrane and mineralization phenomena. The distribution of several anion and cation species in normal growth cartilage and of calcium and phosphorus in rachitic growth cartilage was reported.[31,80,94] Their roles other than in calcification remain to be studied.

Calcification of cartilage in the growth plate is of direct morphogenetic importance. Calcification of the interterritorial matrix about the hypertrophying chondrocyte may preclude further axial elongation of the matrix and arrest hypertrophy. It is also postulated that diffusion of nutrients to the chondrocyte is retarded by calcification of the matrix. Uncalcified cartilage is resistant to both degradation and invasion by blood vessels, and failure of calcification arrests endochondral bone formation, as illustrated by the increased height of the growth plate in rickets.

Even though the principle of mutual morphogenetic influences of cells and collagen fibers is well demonstrated, knowledge of the complex interplay between mechanical, chemical, and cell kinetic factors is limited. Studies of morphogenetic mechanisms of bone, and of the growth apparatus in particular, may offer many avenues to both understand them biologically and, potentially, control them therapeutically.

REFERENCES

1. Axelsson, I., Berman, I., and Pita, J. C. Proteoglycans from rabbit articular and growth plate cartilage. Ultracentrifugation, gel chromatography, and electron microscopy. J Biol Chem 258:8915–8921, 1983.
2. Bayliss, M. T. Proteoglycans: Structure and molecular organization of cartilage, in Hukins D. W. L. (ed): *Connective Tissue Matrix.* Deerfield Beach, Fla., Verlag-Chimie, 1984.
3. Beresford, W. A. *Chondroid Bone: Secondary Cartilage and Metaphysis.* Baltimore, Urban and Schwarzenberg, 1981.
4. Birch, J. G., Herring, J. A., and Wenger, D. R. Surgical anatomy of selected physes. J Pediatr Orthop 4:224–231, 1984.
5. Brighton, C. T. Structure and function of the growth plate. Clin Orthop 136:22–32, 1978.
6. Brighton, C. T. The growth plate. Orthop Clin North Am 15:571–595, 1984.

7. Brighton, C. T., Sugioka, Y., and Hunt, R. M. Quantitative zonal analysis of cytoplasmic structures of growth-plate chondrocytes in vivo and in vitro. J Bone Joint Surg 64A:1336–1349, 1982.

8. Brookes, M. *The Blood Supply of Bone.* London, Butterworth, 1971.

9. Buckholz, R. W., and Ogden, J. A. Patterns of ischemic necrosis of the proximal femur in non-operatively treated congenital hip disease, in *The Hip,* vol 6. St. Louis, Mosby, 1978.

10. Carlson, W. O., and Wenger, D. R. A mapping method to prepare for surgical excision of a partial physeal arrest. J Pediatr Orthop 4:232–238, 1984.

11. Catterall, A. *Legg-Calve-Perthes Disease.* New York, Churchill Livingstone, New York, 1982.

12. Chung, S. M. The arterial supply of the developing proximal end of the human femur. J Bone Joint Surg 58A:961–971, 1976.

13. Cruess, R. L. Binding sites in fetal and growth plate cartilage. J Orthop Res 3:109–120, 1983.

14. Curry, J. *The Mechanical Adaptation of Bones.* New Jersey, Princeton University Press, 1984.

15. Dorrington, K. L. The theory of viscoelasticity in biomaterials, in Vincent, J. F. V., and Currey, J. D. (eds): *The Mechanical Properties of Biological Materials.* New York, Cambridge University Press, 1980, pp. 289–317.

16. Draenert, K., and Draenert, Y. The role of the vessels in the growth plate: Morphological examination. Scan Electron Microsc Part 1:339–344, 1985.

17. Dronch, V. M., and Bunch, W. H. Pattern of closure of the proximal femoral and tibial epiphyses in man. J Pediatr Orthop 3:498–501, 1983.

18. Eggli, P. S., Herrmann, W., Hunziker, E. B., and Schenk, R. K. Matrix compartments in the growth plate of the proximal tibia of rats. Anat Rec 211:246–257, 1985.

19. Ehrlich, M.G., Armstrong, A., and Mankin, H. J. Isolation and partial purification and characterization of the growth plate neutral proteoglycanase. Trans Orthop Res Soc 6:109, 1981.

20. Ehrlich, M. G., Mankin, H. J., and Treadwell, B. V. Biochemical and physiological events during closure of the stapled distal femoral epiphyseal plate in rats. J Bone Joint Surg 54A:309–322, 1972.

21. Farnum, C. E., and Wilsman, N. J. Pericellular matrix of growth plate chondrocytes: A study using postfixation with osmium-ferrocyanide. J Histochem Cytochem 31:765–775, 1983.

22. Farnum, C. E., and Wilsman, N. J. Lectin-binding histochemistry of non-decalcified growth plate cartilage: A postembedment method for light microscopy of epon-embedded tissue. J Histochem Cytochem 32:593–607, 1984.

23. Fawcett, D. W. *A Textbook of Histology,* 11th ed. Philadelphia, Saunders, 1986.

24. Firth, E. C., and Poulos, P. W. Blood vessels in the developing growth plate of the equine distal radius and metacarpus. Res Vet Sci 33:159–166, 1982.

25. Goetinck, P. F. Mutations affecting limb cartilage, in Hall, B. K. (ed): *Cartilage,* vol 3. New York, Academic Press, 1983, pp. 172–191.

26. Grant, W. T., Sussman, M. D., and Balian, G. A disulfide-bonded short chain collagen synthesized by degenerative and calcifying zones of bone growth plate cartilage. J Biol Chem 260:3798–3803, 1985.

27. Gross, J. An essay on biological degradation of collagen, in Hay, E. D. (ed): *Cell Biology of Extracellular Matrix.* New York, Plenum Press, pp. 217–258.

28. Haines, R. W. The histology of epiphyseal union in mammals. J Anat 120:1–25, 1975.

29. Hall, B. K. *Developmental and Cellular Skeletal Biology.* New York, Academic Press, 1978.

30. Hall, B. K. (ed). *Cartilage,* vol 1: *Structure, Function, and Biochemistry;* vol 2: *Development, Differentiation and Growth;* vol 3: *Biomedical Aspects.* New York, Academic Press, 1983.

31. Hargest, T. E., Gay, C. V., Schraer, H., and Wasserman, A. J. Vertical distribution of elements in cells and matrix of epiphyseal growth plate cartilage determined by quantitative electron probe analysis. J Histochem Cytochem 33:275–286, 1985.

32. Harkness, E. M., and Trotter, W. D. Growth of transplants of rat humerus following circumferential division of the periosteum. J Anat 126:275–289, 1978.

33. Harris, B. The mechanical behavior of composite materials, in Vincent, J. F. V., and Currey, J. D. (eds): *The Mechanical Properties of Biological Materials: Symposia of the Society for Experimental Biology,* XXXIV. New York, Cambridge University Press, 1980, pp. 37–74.

34. Harris, E. D., Jr., and Krane, S. M. Collagenases. Specific involvement of collagenase in normal physiology and pathology. N Engl J Med 291:652, 1974.

35. Hascall, V. C., and Hascall, G. K. Proteoglycans, in Hay, E. D. (ed): *Cell Biology of Extracellular Matrix.* New York, Plenum Press, 1981, pp. 39–64.

36. Hay, E. D. Collagen and embryonic development, in Hay, E. D. (ed): *Cell Biology of Extracellular Matrix.* New York, Plenum Press, 1981, pp. 379–410.

37. Hert, J. Growth of the epiphyseal plate in circumference. Acta Anat 82: 420–436, 1972.

38. Hinchliffe, J. R., and Johnson, D. R. Growth of cartilage, in Hall, B. K. (ed): *Cartilage,* vol 1. New York, Academic Press, 1983, 255–295.

39. Houghton, G. R., and Dekel, S. The periosteal control of long bone growth. Acta Orthop Scand 50:635–637, 1979.

40. Howlett, C. R. The fine structure of the proximal growth plate and metaphysis of the avian tibia: Endochondral osteogenesis. J Anat 130:745–768, 1980.

41. Howlett, C. R., Dickson, M., and Sheridan, A. K. The fine structure of the proximal growth plate of the avian tibia: Vascular supply. J Anat 139:115–132, 1984.

42. Hsu, H. H. T., Munoz, P. A., Barr, J., Oppliger, I., Morris, D. C., Vaananen, H. K., Tarkenton, N., and Anderson, H. C. Purification and partial characterization of alkaline phosphatase of matrix vesicles from fetal bovine epiphyseal cartilage. J Biol Chem 260:1926–1831, 1985.

43. Iannotti, J. P., Brighton, C. T., Stambough, J. L., and Storey, B. T. Calcium flux and endogenous calcium content in isolated mammalian growth-plate chondrocytes: Hyaline-cartilage chondrocytes, and hepatocytes. J Bone Joint Surg 67A:113–120, 1985.

44. Isaksson, O. G. P., Eden, S., and Jansson, J. O. Mode of action of pituitary growth hormone on target cells. Am Rev Physiol 47:483–499, 1985.

45. Janes, J. M., and Musgrove, J. E. Effect of arteriovenous fistula on growth of bone. Proc Mayo Clin 24:405–408, 1949.

46. Kan, K. W., Cruess, R. L., Posner, B. I., Guyda, H. J., and Solomon, S. Hormone receptors in the epiphyseal cartilage. J Endocrinol 103:125–131, 1984.

47. Kelly, D. E., Wood, R. L., and Enders, A. C. *Microscopic Anatomy.* Baltimore, Williams and Wilkins, 1984.

48. Kember, N. F. Cell kinetics and cartilage, in Hall, B. K. (ed): *Cartilage,* vol 1. New York, Academic Press, 1983.

49. Kuettner, K. E., and Pauli, B. U. Vascularity of cartilage, in Hall, B. K. (ed): *Cartilage,* vol 1. New York, Academic Press, 1983, pp. 281–312.

50. LaCroix, P. *The Organization of Bone.* London, Churchill Livingstone, 1951.

51. Langenskiold, A. Normal and pathological bone growth in the light of development of cartilagenous foci in chondrodysplasia. Acta Chir Scand 95:367–386, 1947.

52. Langenskiold, A., and Edgren, W. The growth mechanism of the epiphyseal cartilage in the light of experimental observations. Acta Orthop Scand 19:19–24, 1949.

53. Lash, J. W., and Vasan, N. S. Glycosaminoglycans of cartilage, in Hall, B. K. (ed): *Cartilage,* vol 1. New York, Academic Press, 1983, pp. 215–251.

54. Lee, K. E., Pelker, R. R., Rudicel, S. A., Ogden, J. A., and Panjabi, M. M. Histologic patterns of capital femoral growth plate fracture in the rabbit: The effect of shear direction. J Pediatr Orthop 5:32–39, 1985.

55. Liakakos, D., Vlachos, P., Doulas, N. L., Litsios, B., and Alexiou, D. Effect of ascorbic acid (vitamin C) on the epiphyseal plate of young guinea pigs receiving prednisone. Dev Pharmacol Ther 2:69–79, 1981.

56. Lockhart, R. D., Hamilton, G. F., and Fyfe, F. W. *Anatomy of the Human Body.* Philadelphia, Lippincott, 1959, pp. 31, 92.

57. Lutfi, A. M. Mode of growth, fate, and functions of cartilage canals. J Anat 106:135–145, 1970.

58. Lutfi, A. M. The role of cartilage in long bone growth: A reappraisal. J Anat 117:413–417, 1974.

59. Madsen, K., Makower, A. M., Fribert, U., Eden, S., and Isaksson, O. Effect of human growth hormone on proteoglycan synthesis in cultured rat chondrocytes. Acta Endocrinol 108:338–342, 1985.

60. Mankin, H. J. Localization of tritiated cytidine in articular cartilage of immature and adult rabbits after intra-articular injection. Lab Invest 12:543–548, 1963.

61. Maynard, J. A., Ippolito, E. G., Ponseti, I. V., and Mickelson, M. R. Histochemistry and ultrastructure of the growth plate in metaphyseal dysostosis: Further observations on the structure of the cartilage matrix. J Pediatr Orthop 1:161–169, 1981.

62. Maynard, J. A., Ippolito, E. G., Ponseti, I. V., and Mickelson, M. R. Histochemistry and ultrastructure of the growth plate in achondroplasia. J Bone Joint Surg 63A:969–979, 1981.

63. Meikle, M. C. The influences of function in chondrogenesis of the epiphyseal cartilage of a growing long bone. Anat Rec 182:387–400, 1975.

64. Morris, D. C., Vaananen, H. K., and Anderson, H. C. Matrix vesicle calcification in rat epiphyseal growth plate cartilage prepared anhydrously for electron microscopy. Metab Bone Dis Relat Res 5:131–137, 1983.

65. Mourao, P. A. S., Rozenfield, S., Laredo, J., and Dietrich, C. P. The distribution of chondroitin sulfates in articular and growth cartilages of human bones. Biochem Biophys Acta 428:19–26, 1976.

66. Mourao, P. A. S., and Dietrich, C. P. Chondroitin sulfates of the epiphyseal cartilages of different mammals. Comp Biochem Physiol 62B:115–117, 1979.

67. Nettelbald, H., Randolph, M. A., and Weiland, A. J. Free microvascular eipiphyseal-plate transplantation. An experimental study in dogs. J Bone Joint Surg 66A:1421–1430, 1984.

68. Ogden, J. The development and growth of the musculoskeletal system, in Albright, J. A., and Brand, R. A. (eds): *The Scientific Basis of Orthopedics.* Appleton-Century-Crofts, New York, 1979.

69. Ogden, J. Chondro-osseous development and growth, in Urist, M. R. (ed): *Fundamental and Clinical Bone Physiology.* Philadelphia, Lippincott, 1980.

70. Ogden, J. A. Injury to the growth mechanisms of the immature skeleton. Skeletal Radiol 6:237–253, 1981.

71. Oligo, N., Laval-Jeantet, M., and Juster, M. Le socle metaphysaire de l'os normal en croissance et ses rapports avec la variole perichondral. Compt. rend. Assoc Anat 136:745–755, 1967.

72. Olin, A., Creasman, C., and Shapiro, F. Free physeal transplantation in the rabbit. An experimental approach to focal lesions. J Bone Joint Surg 66A:7–20, 1984.

73. Pease, C. N. Local stimulation of growth of long bones. J Bone Joint Surg 34A:1–24, 1952.

74. Peruchon, E., Bonnel, F., Baldet, P., and Rabischong, P. Evaluation and control of growth activity of epiphyseal plate. Med Biol Eng Comput 18:396–400, 1980.

75. Plachot, J. J., Du Bois, M. B., Halpern, S., Cournot-Witmer, G., Garabedian, M., and Balsan, S. In vitro action of 1,25–dihydroxycholecalciferol and 24,25-dihydroxycholecalciferol on matrix organization and mineral distribution in rabbit growth plate. Metab Bone Dis Relat Res 4:135–142, 1982.

76. Poole, B.P. Glycosaminoglycans in morphogenesis, in Hag, E. D. (ed): *Cell Biology of Extracellular Matrix.* New York, Plenum Press, 1981, 259–294.

77. Pratt, C. W. M. Observations on osteogenesis in the femur of the foetal rat. J Anat Lond 91:533–544, 1957.

78. Pratt, C. W. M. The significance of the perichondral zone in a developing long bone of the rat. J Anat 93:110–122, 1959.

79. Ranvier, L. A. Traite technique d'histologie, 2d ed. Sary, Paris, 1889, pp. 249–268, 359–365.

80. Ream, L. J., and Pendergrass, P. B. Scanning electron microscopy of the femoral epiphyseal plate and metaphysis of the rat after short-term fluoride ingestion. J Submicrosc Cytol 14:73–80. 1982.

81. Redd, E. H., Miller, S. C., and Jee, W. S. Changes in endochondral bone elongation rates during pregnancy and lactation in rats. Calcif Tissue Int 36:97–701, 1984.

82. Reinholt, F. P., Engfeldt, B., Heinegard, D., and Hjerpe, A. Proteoglycans and glycosaminoglycans of epiphyseal cartilage in florid and healing low phosphate, vitamin D deficiency rickets. Coll Relat Res 5:55–64, 1985.

83. Reinholt, F. P., Hjerpe, A., Jansson, K., and Engfeldt, B. Stereological studies on matrix vesicle distribution in the epiphyseal growth plate during healing of low phosphate vitamin D deficiency rickets. Virchows Arch [Cell Pathol] 44:257–266, 1983.

84. Ricard-Blum, S., Tiollier, J., Garrone, R., and Herbage, D. Further biochemical and physicochemical characterization of minor disulfide-bonded (type IX) collagen, extracted from foetal calf cartilage. J Cell Biochem 27:147–158, 1985.

85. Rigal, W. M. The use of tritiated thymidine in studies of chondrogenesis, in Lacroix, P., and Budy, A. (eds): *Radioisotopes and Bone.* Philadelphia, F.A. Davis, 1962, p. 197.

86. Rigal, W. M. Experimental metaphyseal exostoses. The role of perichondrial ring of the growth cartilage (juxtaepiphyseal apparatus or ossification groove of Ranvier), in Gaillard, L., van der Hoof, A., and Steendijk, J. R., (eds): *Fourth European Symposium on Calcified Tissues,* abridged proceedings. Amsterdam, Excerpta Medica, 1966, p. 91.

87. Rooney, P., Archer, C., and Wolpert, L. Morphogenesis of cartilaginous long bone rudiments, in Trelstad, R. L. (ed): *The Role of Extracellular Matrix in Development.* New York, Alan R. Liss, 1984, pp. 305–322.

88. Rudicel, S., Pelker, R. R., Lee, K. E., Ogden, J. A., and Panjabi, M. M. Shear fractures through the capital femoral physis of the skeletally immature rabbit. J Pediatr Orthop 5:27–31, 1985.

89. Sakakida, K., and Yamashita, B. An experimental study on the proliferation of epiphyseal cartilage cells after partial resection of epiphyseal plate. Arch Jap Chir 45:201–221, 1976.

90. Schenk, R. K. Basic histomorphology and physiology of skeletal growth, in Weber, B. G., Brunner, C. H., and Freuler, F. (eds): *Treatment of Fractures in Children and Adolescents.* New York, Springer-Verlag, 1980, pp. 3–19.

91. Schenk, R. K., Hunziker, E. B., and Herrmann, W. Structural properties of cells related to tissue mineralization, in Nancollas, G. H. (ed): *Biological Mineralization and Demineralization.* Dahlem Konferenzen. New York, Springer-Verlag, 1982, pp. 143–160.

92. Sebek, J., Skalova, J., and Hert, J. Reaction of bone to mechanical stimuli. Local differences in structure and strength of periosteum. Folia Morphol 20:29–37, 1972.

93. Shapiro, F., Holtrop, M. E., and Glimcher, M. J. Organization and cellular biology of the perichondral ossification groove of Ranvier. J Bone Joint Surg 59A:703–723, 1977.

94. Shapiro, I. M., and Boyde, A. Microdissection—Elemental analysis of the mineralizing growth cartilage of the normal and rachitic chick. Metab Bone Dis Relat Res 5:317–326, 1984.

95. Shepard, N., and Mitchell, N. Ultrastructural modifications of

proteoglycans coincident with mineralization in local regions of rat growth plate. J Bone Joint Surg 67A:455–464,1985.

96. Shinozuka, M., Tsurui, A., Naganuma, T., Moss, M., and Moss-Salentijn, L. A stochastic-mechanical model of longitudinal long bone growth. J Theor Biol 108:413–436, 1984.

97. Simmons, D. J. Comparative physiology of bone, in Bourne, G. H. (ed): *Biochemistry and Physiology of Bone,* vol IV. New York, Academic Press, 1971, pp. 445–516.

98. Simon, M. R., and Holmes, K. R. The effects of simulated increases in body weight on the developing rat tibia: A histologic study. Acta Anat (Basel) 122:105–109, 1985.

99. Sissons, H. A. The growth of bone, in Bourne, G. H. (ed): *Biochemistry and Physiology of Bone,* vol III. New York, Academic Press, 1971, pp. 145–180.

100. Solomon, L. Diametric growth of the epiphyseal plate. J Bone Joint Surg 58B:170–177, 1966.

101. Speer, D. P. The pathogenesis of amputation stump overgrowth. Clin Orthop 159:294–307, 1981.

102. Speer, D. P. The collagenous architecture of epiphyseal growth cartilage and perichondrial ossification groove. J Bone Joint Surg 64A:399–407, 1982.

103. Speer, D. P. The collagenous architecture of antler velvet, in Brown, R. D. (ed): *Antler Development in Cervidae.* Proc Int Symp on Development of Antler in Cervidae. Kingsville, Texas, Caesar Kleberg Wildlife Research Institute, 1983, pp 273–278.

104. Speer, D. P. Peripheral and central contours of the distal tibial physis. Trans Orthop Res Soc 10:198, 1985.

105. Speer, D. P. and Braun, J. K. Effect of varying force vectors on injuries to the growth plate. Trans Orthop Res Soc 7:57, 1982.

106. Speer, D. P. and Braun, J. K. The biomechanical basis of growth plate injuries. Phys Sports Med 13:72–78, 1985.

107. Speer, D. P., Braun, J. K., and Reinecke, C. Effect of loading rate on growth plate injuries. Trans Orthop Res Soc 9:1871, 1984.

108. Speer, D. P., and Dahners, L. The collagenous architecture of articular cartilage: Correlation of scanning electron microscopy and polarized light microscopy observations. Clin Orthop 139:267–275, 1979.

109. Speer, D. P., Kischer, C. W. Developing antler as a model system of fibrillogenesis, in Bailey, G. W. (ed): *Proceedings of the 40th Annual Meeting Electron Microscopy Association of America.* Washington, D.C., 1982, pp. 298–299.

110. Speer, D. P., and Pitt, M. J. Peripheral and central contours of the growth plate. Trans Orthop Res Soc 7:53, 1982.

111. Strangeways, T. S. P., and Fell, H. B. Experimental studies on the differentiation of embryonic tissues growing in vivo and in vitro. Proc R Soc Lond [Biol] 99:340–364, 1926.

112. Suda, S., Takahashi, N., Shinki, T., Horiuchi, N., Yamaguchi, A., Yoshiki, S., Enomoto, S., and Suda, T. 1 alpha, 25-Dihydroxyvitamin D3 receptors and their action in embryonic chick chondrocytes. Calcif Tissue Int 37:82–90, 1985.

113. Sussman, M. D., Ogle, R. C., and Balian, G. Biosynthesis and processing of collagens in different cartilagenous tissues. J Orthop Res 2:134–142, 1984.

114. Tachdjian, M. O. *Pediatric Orthopedics.* Philadelphia, Saunders, 1972, pp. 41–44.

115. Tebor, G. B., Ehrlich, M. G., Armstrong, A., and Mankin, H. J. A comparative study of neutral proteoglycanase activity by growth plate zone. Trans Orthop Res Soc 7:54, 1982.

116. Teot, L., Bosse, J. P., Gilbert, A., and Tremblay, G. R. Pedicle graft epiphysis transplantation. Clin Orthop 180:206–218, 1983.

117. Thorogood, P. Morphogenesis of cartilage, in Hall, B. K. (ed): *Cartilage,* vol 1. New York, Academic Press, pp. 255–295, 1983.

118. Toole, B. P. Glycosaminoglycans in morphogenesis, in Hay, E. D. (ed): *Cell Biology of Extracellular Matrix.* New York, Plenum Press, 1981, pp. 259–294.

119. Trueta, J. *Studies of the Development and Decay of the Human Frame.* Philadelphia, Saunders, 1968.

120. Urist, M. R., Speer, D. P., Ibsen, K. J., and Strates, B. S. Calcium binding by chondroitin sulfate. Calcif Tissue Res 2:253–261, 1968.

121. Vaananen, K., and Korhonen, L. K. Histochemistry of epiphyseal plate. Cell Mol Biol 23:105–111, 1978.

122. Van Kampen, G. P. J. Veldhuijzen, J. P., Kuijer, R., van de Stadt R. J., and Schipper, C. A. Cartilage response to mechanical force in high-density chondrocyte cultures. Arthritis Rheum 28:419–424, 1985.

123. Vaughan, J. *The Physiology of Bone.* Oxford, Clarendon Press, 1975.

124. von der Mark, K., and von der Mark, H. The role of three genetically distinct collagen types in endochondral ossification and calcification of cartilage. J Bone Joint Surg 59B:458–464, 1977.

125. Weiss, J. B. Collagens and collagenolytic enzymes, in Hukins, D. W. L. (ed): *Connective Tissue Matrix.* Deerfield Beach, Fla., Verlag-Chemie, pp. 17–53, 1984.

126. Williams, P. L., and Warwick, R. (eds): *Gray's Anatomy.* Philadelphia, Saunders, 1980.

CHAPTER 13

Muscle: Structure and Function

Marie A. Badalamente and Roger Dee

STRUCTURE OF SKELETAL MUSCLE

The muscle cell is termed a *myofiber.* It contains contractile elements called *myofibrils,* which extend throughout its length. Myofibrils consist of contractile proteins,[19,31,68] regulatory proteins,[6,14,15] and scaffold, or backbone, proteins.[22,52,54,56] The most abundant of these are the contractile proteins *actin* and *myosin.* Actin, termed *thin filament,* is a globular protein made of a single polypeptide chain which can bind to the other contractile protein, myosin, termed the *thick filament.* Actin may also bind one molecule each of nucleotide adenosine di- or triphosphate (ADP or ATP) and divalent cation (Ca^{2+} or Mg^{2+}). Myosin is composed of two large polypeptide chains (Fig. 13-1) called *heavy chains* and four small *light chains.* The heavy chains are folded into an alpha-helical configuration through their length, with one end folded into the light chains forming a globular head. These myosin globular heads also possess ATPase activity.

The major regulatory proteins are *troponin*[16] and *tropo-myosin.*[6] Troponin is the only calcium-receptive protein of a myofibril.[65] It is located on the thin (actin) filaments and is bound to tropomyosin. A number of studies have further clarified that the troponin molecule consists of three components—troponins C,[26] I,[58] and T.[16] Troponin C can bind calcium at four molecule sites[39] or, in addition, magnesium[42] at two sites. Troponin I inhibits actin-myosin interaction in the presence of ATP,[55] and troponin T is tropomyosin-binding.[16] Tropomyosin is an alpha-helical coiled molecule composed of an alpha[67] and a beta chain.[59] Tropomyosin binds to actin and troponin T (Fig. 13-1).

The minor regulatory proteins may be associated with actin or myosin filaments. They are a small part of the total muscle protein and are mainly concerned with regulation of filamentous structure. The following are minor regulatory proteins capable of binding to myosin: M protein,[46] C protein,[53] F protein,[53] and I protein.[55] The actinins, alpha,[14] beta,[44] gamma,[40] Eu,[41] and filamin,[27] are minor regulatory proteins that regulate the physical state of actin.

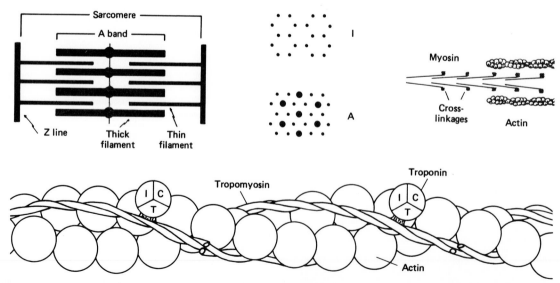

Figure 13-1 *Top left,* the arrangements of thin (actin) and thick (myosin) filaments in skeletal muscle. *Middle, I* represents a cross section of the I band; *A* represents a cross section through the lateral portion of the A band. *Top right,* the interlinking structure of myosin and actin. *Bottom,* the arrangement of actin, tropomyosin, and the three subunits of troponin. *(From Ganong, W.F., ed: Review of Medical Physiology. Los Altos, Lange Medical, 1983. Reproduced with permission.)*

The elasticity of the myofibril has been shown to be due to very thin filaments of scaffold protein, called *connectin,* which links neighboring Z lines.[45] The remaining scaffold proteins are Z protein, which constitutes the lattice structure of Z lines,[57] and *desmin* (skeletin), which links neighboring Z lines.[22,23]

The Ultrastructure of the Myofiber[13,31,36,61]

Mature myofibers are somewhat cylindrical and when sectioned transversely appear rounded or polygonal. In transverse section at high magnifications, the central myosin (thick) filament possesses six cross-bridges on each pitch of the helical chain binding to six actin (thin) filaments in the region of the A band (Fig. 13-1). Thin and thick filaments are arranged in parallel order and show a regular repeat pattern between adjacent Z lines. The tissue limited by two Z lines, is called a *sarcomere,* and there is a median, dense A band and two lateral I bands as well. Additionally, the A band possesses a dense center, the M line, which is limited on both sides by the lighter H zone. The myofibrillar protein localization in these banding patterns is summarized in Table 13-1. The ultrastructural arrangement of these banding patterns is depicted in longitudinal orientation in Fig. 13-2.

TABLE 13-1 Myofibrillar Protein Localization in Muscle Bands

Proteins	Localization
Myosin	A band
Actin	I band
Troponin (C, I, T)	I band
Tropomyosin	I band
M protein	M line
C, F, I proteins	A band
Alpha actinin, Eu actinin, and filamin	Z line
B actinin	Free end of actin filaments
Gamma actinin	I band (?)
Connectin	A band, I band, Z line
Z protein	Z line
Desmin	Periphery of Z line

Source: Modified from Obinata, T., et al, Muscle Nerve, 4:456, 1981.

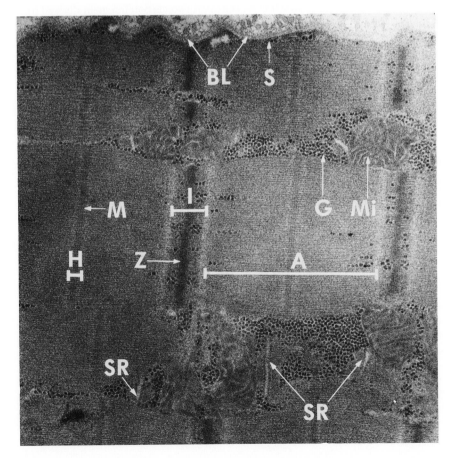

Figure 13-2 Electron micrograph of human peroneus brevis in longitudinal orientation. The sarcolemma (*S*) and basal lamina (*BL*) limit the myofiber. Mitochondria (*Mi*), glycogen (*G*) deposits, and cisterns of sarcoplasmic reticulum (*SR*) are shown between myofibrils. The A, I, Z, H, and M bands are labeled. ×30,000.

Myofibers vary in length, depending on the length of a muscle, and in diameter from 10 to 100 μm. Each myofiber is limited by a cell membrane, called the *sarcolemma,* and by a basal lamina. Each myofiber contains many nuclei located at the periphery of the fiber just under the sarcolemma. Satellite cells, possessing a large nucleus and scanty cytoplasm, are often confused with myofiber nuclei as they are located at the fiber periphery and are enclosed by the fiber's basal lamina. Unlike mature myofibers, satellite cells retain the ability to undergo myogenesis. They therefore function in muscle regeneration.

The sarcolemma of the myofiber invaginates to extend to the interior in the form of narrow transverse T tubules. These occur at the junction of the A and I bands. The T tubule is bordered on each side by a terminal cistern of agranular sarcoplasmic reticulum. These structures make up the membrane *triad.* There are two triads per sarcomere. The sarcoplasmic reticulum is the intracellular longitudinal membrane system which regulates calcium concentration.

Other subcellular organelles in myofibers include numerous mitochondria, which may form small collections at the periphery of the cell near nuclear poles or lie in between myofibrils. Glycogen is also present in the form of beta particles and may be widely distributed between myofibrils according to fiber type. Lipid droplets are seen; their content varies according to fiber type. The Golgi complex is located near nuclear poles. Membrane-bound lysosomes are occasionally observed in normal myofibers.

Muscle-Tendon Junction

The muscle-tendon junction is a specialized region at the ends of the myofiber where force is transmitted from the intracellular filaments across the sarcolemma and basal lamina to extracellular collagen fibers.[69,70] The main structural feature is a folding of the interface between muscle and tendon, increasing its area and consequently producing a decrease in stress. The parallelism of the interface causes the junction to be loaded in shear more than in tension.[69,70] The molecular architecture of the extracellular matrix of the muscle-tendon interface is not, at present, entirely delineated. Recent studies have reported the presence of a protein termed *laminin.*[69,70] Type IV collagen and heparan sulfate proteoglycan are macromolecules which connect actin filaments of the terminal sarcomere to tendon collagen fibrils.

Motor End Plate

Motor nerve endings lie in a depression of the myofiber surface, forming the neuromuscular junction. The myofiber membrane and basal lamina at this site are highly folded into the typical synaptic cleft. Acetylcholine receptor protein is localized in the myofiber membrane at the neuromuscular junction. Acetylcholinesterase activity is associated with the basal lamina. The sarcoplasm of the myofiber at this site is characterized by numerous filaments, microtubules, ribosomes, clusters of mitochondria, and nuclei.

PHYSIOLOGY OF STRIATED MUSCLE CONTRACTION[20,50,68]

The hydrolysis of ATP releases energy for muscle contraction according to the following reaction:

$$ATP + H_2O \xrightarrow{ATPase} ADP + P_i + H^+ \ (+energy\ for\ contraction)$$

where P_i is inorganic phosphate. The ADP formed by this reaction cannot be further utilized to release energy useful for the contractile system. It leaves the myofibrils by diffusion and must be rephosphorylated back to ATP by one of the following pathways:

1. *Phosphocreatine Rephosphorylation.* Phosphocreatine has a high-energy phosphate bond which can be used to rephosphorylate ADP back to ATP by means of the enzyme creatine phosphokinase. This energy store is, however, very rapidly depleted.
2. *Anaerobic Rephosphorylation.* This makes use of the glycolytic pathway but yields only two molecules of ATP per glucose molecule metabolized, which is much less than is formed in the aerobic process. A by-product of this anaerobic reaction is lactic acid, which may accumulate in muscle. Lactic acid is eventually metabolized in the liver. This mechanism is commonly utilized by the fast glycolytic (type IIB, or white) fibers.
3. *Aerobic Rephosphorylation.* This reaction makes use of the oxidative phosphorylation of acetyl coenzyme A, which is an activated two-carbon fragment derived from glucose or glycogen. This process takes place within mitochondria. The reaction produces a high yield (36 molecules) of ATP per molecule of glucose metabolized. This is the mechanism favored by both fast oxidative and slow oxidative fibers, type IIA and type I fibers, respectively.
4. *Transphosphorylation.* Muscle contains the enzyme myoadenylate kinase, which catalyzes the reversible reaction of two ADP molecules to form one molecule of ATP and one molecule of adenosine monophosphate.

Assuming the availability of ATP from the preceding reactions, the following chain of events effects skeletal muscle contraction. As an efferent nerve impulse reaches the neuromuscular junction, acetylcholine is released from the axon terminal and depolarizes the sarcolemma and its invaginations—the T tubules. Acetylcholinesterase antagonizes the action of acetylcholine. The T-tubule system channels this impulse to the sarcoplasmic reticulum at the triads. Calcium bound in the reticulum, at $10^{-9}\ M$ in the resting state, flows out into the sarcoplasm and binds to troponin C. This weakens the binding of troponin I to actin, permitting tropomyosin to move laterally and expose actin binding sites.[20] ATPase located on the globular heads of the myosin chains splits ATP to ADP. The energy set free by the splitting of these bonds induces myosin chains to join actin sites which were activated by calcium (Fig. 13-3). Each myosin globular head is attracted by a succession of actin sites, resulting in a sliding of thin filaments into spaces between the thick filaments.

The results of contraction cause the H band to narrow, or

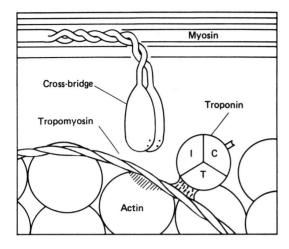

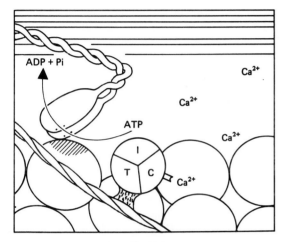

Figure 13-3 Initiation of muscle contraction by calcium (Ca^{2+}). The cross-bridges (heads of myosin molecules) attach to binding sites on actin (*striped areas*) and swivel when tropomyosin is displaced laterally by binding of Ca^{2+} to troponin C. *(From Ganong, W.F., ed: Review of Medical Physiology. Los Altos, Lange Medical, 1983. Reproduced with permission.)*

to be obliterated in maximum contraction. The length of the I bands and sarcomeres is also reduced, with the entire myofiber being shortened.

Relaxation is brought about by the active transport of calcium back into the sarcoplasmic reticulum, thus forcing calcium to dissociate from troponin and the tropomyosin chain to assume its resting configuration.

Muscle Fiber Types (See Table 13-2)

Not all myofibers are identical in contractile behavior. Characteristic myofiber types may be identified on the basis of whether their energy supply is largely oxidative, eliciting a slow, type I, contractile response, or glycolytic, demonstrating fast, type II, contractile behavior. The division is by no means so simple, however, as intermediate fibers designated type IIA (fast oxidative/glycolytic) and type IIB (fast glyco-

lytic) exist. Fiber typing based on these energy mechanisms involves histochemical methods of testing for enzymatic activity such as succinic dehydrogenase activity, which is oxidative and occurs largely in mitochondria. Phosphorylase activity may also be utilized in this typing method as an indication of glycogen breakdown (glycolytic).

By far the most common classification of myofiber typing is based on the use of histochemical staining procedures for myosin ATPase activity.[18] It is important to understand that qualitative differences in the myosin ATPase structure, not the myosin content, control the ATPase activity and thus the speed of contraction.[19] Fast glycolytic fibers (type IIB) have a high content of fast-acting myosin ATPase, as do fast oxidative/glycolytic fibers (type IIA), enabling them to respond rapidly. By contrast, type I fibers have relatively slow acting myosin ATPase. Depending on whether the histochemical procedure uses acid or alkaline incubations, the staining result differs. For example, at pH 9.4, type I slow-twitch fibers appear light pink, reflecting low ATPase activity. At the same pH, type II fast-twitch fibers appear dark brown, indicative of high ATPase activity. Tables 13-2 and 13-3 summarize myofiber type discrimination based on various histochemical staining procedures and their energy characteristics.

A third type II fiber, designated type IIC, may also be distinguished by use of these various histochemical staining methods. However, the type IIC fiber is an undifferentiated precursor of types IIA and IIB.[8]

Ultrastructural differences between myofiber types have been demonstrated in experimental animal muscle,[17] but not in humans. For example, slow fibers have been shown by electron microscopy to possess a wider Z line and smaller amounts of T-tubule system and terminal cisterns of sarcoplasmic reticulum than fast fibers. There is also a greater volume of mitochondria in slow-twitch fibers.

Fiber type composition differs in various muscles. For example, the human soleus is 75 percent to 90 percent type I and the triceps only about 20 percent to 40 percent type I.[1,63,64] After remaining constant for seven decades, there is a relative decrease in the number of type IIB fibers thereafter.[35]

Muscle Metabolism During Exercise

Skeletal muscle can increase its rate of utilization of ATP by several hundredfold in the transition from rest to heavy exercise. ATP generation via the anaerobic and aerobic phosphorylation pathways differs between muscles. A work rate sustained by anaerobic metabolism in one muscle may result in rapid fatigue. However, the same work rate may be supported without fatigue in another muscle by the aerobic process.[28] The difference in energy metabolism between muscles may reflect myofiber type and level of training.[64]

In humans, type I fibers have the highest capacity for aerobic metabolism, while type IIA fibers vary in their metabolic capacity by combining aerobic and anaerobic pathways. These two fiber types do not become fatigued rapidly and are usually recruited during endurance work of light or moderate intensity.

In contrast, type IIB fibers have a low aerobic capacity

TABLE 13-2 Skeletal Muscle Fiber Typing

Fiber type	ATPase			Succinic dehydrogenase	Phosphorylase
	pH 9.4	4.3	4.6		
Type I (slow oxidative)	Low	High	High	High	Low
Type IIA (fast oxidative/glycolytic)	High	Low	Low	Moderate	High
Type IIB (fast glycolytic)	High	Low	High	Low	High

Source: Brooke, M.H., and Kaiser, K.K., Arch Neurol 23:369, 1970.

and derive their supply of ATP by anaerobic (glycolytic) mechanisms. They are recruited during work of short burst intensity, which results in the rapid accumulation of lactate and the development of fatigue. Therefore, periods of contraction of type IIB fibers must be separated by periods of recovery in order for lactate to be removed via the blood.[29]

Effects of Physical Training on Muscle

When contractile activity is increased, as during endurance exercise, all myofiber types can respond by increasing their rates of synthesis of mitochondria,[7] concomitant with increases in the levels of mitochondrial enzymes necessary for the aerobic pathway. This pathway is further facilitated during endurance exercise by an increase in muscle capillaries and an increase in the levels of muscle myogloblin, both of which contribute more oxygen to the aerobic mechanism. Of all the fiber types, the IIB fibers when subjected to endurance training demonstrate the smallest increase in the number of mitochondria.

Endurance exercise also induces an increase in a muscle's capacity to metabolize glycogen and fat.[30] Fat may be utilized only through the aerobic metabolism. It is interesting to note that glycolysis is inhibited by fatty acid oxidation.[60] Therefore, the greater the percentage of energy derived from fatty acids, the longer it will be before glycogen stores are depleted and the individual has to stop exercising. Athletes derive a greater percentage of their energy from fatty acids than untrained individuals do.[28]

Muscle mass, as measured by cross-sectional area of myofibers, increases during weight training, and this is accompanied by increased synthesis of contractile protein. But these changes in the muscle do not seem to be able to account for the increase in the force of voluntary muscle contraction which accompanies training. For example, increases in muscle cross-sectional area are negligible in the early phases of training, but increases in voluntary force are substantial.[47] Even with longer periods of training, up to 14 weeks, the increase in cross-sectional area accounts for only 25 percent of the gains in maximal voluntary contraction.[32] McDonagh and his co-workers found that training produces a 20 percent increase in the force of maximal voluntary isometric contraction in human elbow flexor muscles, but the forces produced by electrically evoked twitch and tetany, which are directly proportional to muscle cross-sectional area, show no increase. Thus they postulate that the increase in muscle forces associated with training must be related to factors other than the force-generating capacity of the myofibers themselves. This concurs with the finding that training produces an increase in the maximal integrated electromyogram (EMG) in the femoral muscles concomitant with an increase in the force of maximal voluntary contraction. The EMG activity increased by 38 percent and the muscle force 20 percent in 12 weeks.[38] It seems likely that in the untrained individual recruitment is not maximal for all motor units in a muscle (see Control in the Spinal Cord, below). Training brings more motor units into play and also increases muscle force by alterations "in a spacial and temporal pattern which is optimal for maximal force development by the whole muscle."[47]

TABLE 13-3 Energy Characteristics of Muscle Fiber Types

Fiber type	Contraction velocity	Myoglobin content	Principal mode of energy production
Type 1 (slow oxidative)	Slow	High (red)	Aerobic (oxidative phosphorylation)
Type IIA (fast oxidative/glycolytic)	Fast	High (red)	Oxidative glycolysis
Type IIB (fast glycolytic)	Fast	Low (white)	Anaerobic glycolysis

Source: Modified from Kidd, G.L., in Owen, R., Goodfellow, J., and Bullough, P., eds: *Scientific Foundations of Orthopaedics and Traumatology.* Philadelphia, Saunders, 1980, p 166.

MUSCLE HEALING

Injury and Repair in Muscle

Muscle strains are commonly seen. Athletes are especially susceptible in such areas as the groin, hamstring, and calf muscles. Strains are thought to be acute partial tears in the musculotendinous unit.

Both animal and human studies indicate that the distal myotendinous junction is the common location of failure in response to increasing stretch.[4,5] Microscopically, the muscle tear at this location reveals mild hemorrhage, an inflammatory response, myofiber separation, and disruption along the distal myotendinous junction.[48] If the injury is not sufficient to tear the myotendinous junction, the result may be only a minimal inflammatory response with mild myofiber disruption.

Myofiburs have a limited ability to regenerate following injury. Usually, scar formation prevents myofiber bridging of any significant gaps.[2] In ischemic contracture of the forearm muscles, there is no significant regeneration after muscle necrosis. By contrast, following some types of damage, such as transient ischemia or toxin damage, muscle may completely recover.[9] Determination of change in the ultrastructural appearance of the muscle (e.g., mitochondrial and sarcoplasmic reticulum dilatation) is the best way to assess the effects of ischemia in muscle. More than 3 h of tourniquet-induced ischemia causes irreversible changes in the myofibrils. Atrophic denervation changes are also seen, but, in fact, the associated peripheral nerve may show no change.[71] It should be noted that inflating a pneumatic tourniquet substantially above systolic pressure has the capacity to mechanically deform and damage peripheral nerve locally.[37]

The nuclei of mature myofibers do not divide and regenerate. However, a varying proportion of satellite cells, which may account for one-third of all muscle nuclei, are found in the newborn (these cells constitute less than 5 percent in the mature adult).[1] After injury, satellite cells recapitulate the normal embryonic development of skeletal muscle (see Chap. 1). Myotube formation occurs maximally at 10 days post injury in newborn muscles, and at 3 weeks there is an increased number of fully mature myofibers.[34,43] When young adult muscles are tenotomized at the Achilles tendon, they show some indication during healing of a change in fiber type characteristics from type I slow-twitch fibers to type II fast-twitch fibers.[66] Immobilization significantly impairs the ability of muscle to recover from injury.[51] Active joint and muscle movement seem to provide the ideal tissue environment for rapid regeneration of muscles in the injured limb.[3,10,11] Muscles severed at their midpoint and resutured lose considerable function.[21] Fibroblasts lay down collagen fibrils at right angles to the axis of a surgical incision in muscle whether the line of incision is parallel to the direction of existing muscle fibers or perpendicular to it.[62]

REGULATION OF MUSCLE FORCE

Control in the Spinal Cord

The nerve supply to myofibers is by fibers originating from alpha motoneurons in the anterior horn of the spinal cord.

The summation of all facilitatory and inhibitory influences upon its cell membrane determines whether an individual alpha motoneuron will fire. An alpha motoneuron provides a single axon which supplies numerous neuromuscular junctions on adjacent myofibers. The number of myofibers supplied per motoneuron is known as the *innervation ratio*. It varies from a relatively high number (2000) for muscles like the gastrocnemius to a small value (10) for rectus muscles of the eye. The combination of the motoneuron plus myofibers it supplies is known as a *motor unit*. Probably at no time do all the motor units in one individual skeletal muscle contract simultaneously.[33] During increasing demand, however, an increasing number of motor units are recruited to increase the force and strength of muscular contraction. This process is known as *recruitment*. It follows that this level of control is determined by the number of alpha motoneurons that reach threshold at a particular moment.

Central Mechanisms

Central control over the alpha motoneurons is achieved by means of descending axons in the principal efferent tracts of the spinal cord (cortico- and vestibulospinal). These enable a programmed pattern of movement to occur. At the spinal level, afferent fibers with their endings in the muscle spindles exert facilitatory influences monosynaptically on alpha motoneurons. They are responsible for the well-known stretch reflex so useful in clinical practice.

Peripheral Mechanisms

Other important influences impinging upon motoneurons are the afferent fibers from joint and muscle receptors, as well as those from skin, tendon, and fascia.

Joint Afferent Fibers

It is believed that mechanoreceptors in the capsule and ligaments exert powerful reflex influences upon control of posture. These exert both facilitatory and inhibitory influences. Their reflex effects are polysynaptic, thus affecting the tone in muscles innervated by alpha motoneurons at several spinal cord levels. Wyke has classified joint receptors histologically.[72] Halata and co-workers have described afferent endings in primate joint capsules by ultrastructural methods.[25] Type I receptors are the spray endings of Ruffini. They are slowly adapting and signal static joint position. Type II receptors, which are corpuscular (resembling Vater-Pacinian corpuscles), are rapidly adapting and signal briefly during changes in joint position. These joint receptors, which are histologically distinct, can be shown to exert powerful influences on the reflex control of muscles controlling the joints which contain them (proprioception). A type III receptor, which is primarily inhibitory to alpha motoneurons in the neuraxis, is a high-threshold receptor present in ligaments; it seems to be similar structurally to the Golgi tendon organ. The type IV receptor is the pain-receptor system and responds to nociceptive stimulation primarily by strongly stimulating, in reflex fashion, flexor motoneurons polysynaptically at several levels in the neuraxis. Since joint receptors are afferents which communicate to the higher centers of the brain, it is thought that they may also play a role in perception of joint position (kinesthesia).

Muscle Spindles

Until recently, it was thought that the afferent input from muscle spindles was not represented in the cortex. Thus, muscle sense was thought to be limited to joint receptors. However, it is now known that muscle spindles indeed contribute to joint-position sense and that their afferent discharge is represented in the cortex. Figure 13-4 shows the structure of the muscle spindle. The spindle consists of 8 to 10 myofibers called *intrafusal fibers* which run within a capsule in parallel with normal myofibers (sometimes called *extrafusal fibers)*. In the equatorial region of each intrafusal fiber is a large aggregation of nuclei. One may differentiate, primarily according to appearance of the nuclei, two kinds of fibers, the so-called nuclear-bag and nuclear-chain fibers. The primary afferent ending consists of annulospiral terminals form large alpha afferent axons (with a diameter of 12 to 20 μm) which supply the central parts of both bag and chain fibers. Somewhat smaller beta afferent axons (4 to 12 μm) form the secondary, flower-spray endings, which supply the less central regions of the fibers, primarily the chain fibers. The two types of endings respond differently. The primary endings are sensitive mainly to the rate of change of stretch, so their frequency of discharge is maximal while the stretch is

applied but subsides to a resting level while the stretch is maintained (dynamic response). The secondary endings, on the other hand, are relatively unaffected by the rate of stretch but are sensitive to a particular steady level of tension (static response) (see Fig. 13-4).

The intrafusal fibers are separately innervated from gamma motoneurons in the spinal cord, ensuring a sophisticated servomechanism.[24] The gamma fibers control the contraction of the intrafusal fibers and thereby adjust the level of sensitivity of the muscle spindle and its afferent rate of discharge during muscle stretch. The gamma motoneurons themselves are influenced by polysynaptic peripheral reflex and also central control mechanisms. The balance of these is normally inhibitory. When gamma motoneurons are released from central control (which may occur, for example, in spinal cord transection), there are changes in the level at which the muscle spindle is set. This accounts for the spasticity which then develops. Changes in the higher centers are known to exert influence upon the alpha and gamma motoneurons, particularly the reticular formation and the cerebellum. This explains the various changes in muscle tone which accompany brain damage.

There is more than one kind of termination from fusimotor axons. They vary from a structure which closely resembles a motor end plate to another kind of termination described as a trail ending, in which the axon seems to be distributed on the fiber through diffuse branching. To further complicate the matter, intrafusal myofibers may each be innervated by several motor axons. There may be more than one type of gamma motoneuron, each responding differently to dynamic and static parameters.

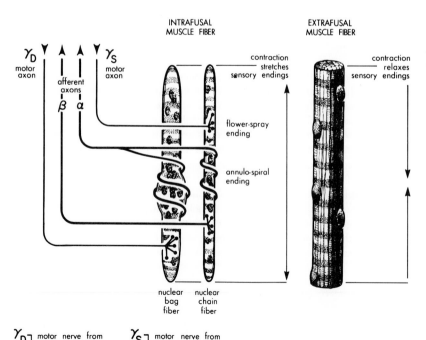

Figure 13-4 The mammalian muscle spindle consists of intrafusal and extrafusal fibers. Contraction responses of both fibers are schematically represented.

Control at the Neuromuscular Junction

Interference with muscle contraction at the neuromuscular junction is well known to anesthesiologists. Paralysis may be produced by blockade at the neuromuscular junction in two ways. The first is by competitive block, in which the drug administered competes for acetylecholine receptors on the postsynaptic membrane (e.g., d-tubocurarine). The second mechanism is by depolarization block, which occurs if cholinesterase is inhibited by anticholinesterase drugs such as neostigmine.

Control at the Level of Muscle Fiber

When motor units are recruited, the motor goal is achieved by increasing the firing rate of motoneurons.[49] Although in the laboratory repetitive stimulation of a myofiber within its relative refractory period (but not within its even shorter absolute refractory period) produces tetanic contraction, this probably rarely occurs in vivo. It should be emphasized that depolarization, both at the neuromuscular junction and at the myofibril membrane, is an all-or-none phenomenon.

Pathological contractions of muscle fibers can occur if there are gross changes in the environment. Changes in the pH or in the level of critical ions (particularly magnesium and calcium) affect the myofiber. Tetany is caused by levels of calcium in the extracellular fluid which are sufficiently low to cause membrane depolarization. Rigor occurs when muscles are depleted of ATP and phosphocreatine, for example, post mortem. This is accompanied by fixed bonding of actin and myosin.[20]

Biomechanics of the Single Fiber

The *resting length* of a muscle is the length at which it develops maximum tension. This concept follows from the properties of muscle fibers. The active tension developed in a muscle when contracting can be increased by increasing the intial fiber length up to the value of the resting length (Fig. 13-5). The tension then falls off, however, if the muscle is stretched beyond resting length when the contraction occurs. Although the active tension developed beyond resting length falls off as a proportion of the total tension developed, passive tension progressively rises. This is particularly important in muscles which cross two joints, for example, the hamstrings.[12]

Muscles can still exert tension even while they are elongating. The velocity of muscle contractions varies inversely in relation to its load. This occurs until the velocity equals zero at isometric tension. Beyond that point elongation of the muscle occurs in spite of the muscle contraction (eccentric contraction).

Other important considerations in estimating the action of a muscle include its ability to generate useful moments around a joint. The moment generated around a joint is perpendicular to the line of muscle action. In many muscles the body is engineered so that the maximum moment is generated when the joint is flexed to 90° (e.g., brachialis). The importance of the various fascial straps at the foot and ankle in improving the mechanical advantage of some calf and shin muscles can be similarly explained.

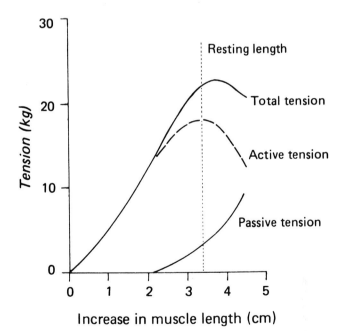

Figure 13-5 Length-tension diagram for human triceps muscle. Note that beyond the muscle's resting length, no further active tension is developed. There is a continuing increase in passive tension, however. The total tension curve is the tension developed when the muscle contracts isometrically in response to a maximal stimulus. *(From Ganong, W.F., ed: Review of Medical Physiology. Los Altos, Lange Medical, 1983. Reproduced with permission.)*

REFERENCES

1. Aard, E., Graham, T. and Wahren, J. Muscle fiber characteristics in healthy men and patients and with juvenile diabetes. Diabetes 28(1): 93–99, 1979.
2. Allbrook, D.B. Muscle breakdown and repair, in Owen, R., Goodfellow, J., and Bullough, P.W.B. (eds): *Scientific Foundations of Orthopedics and Traumatology.* Philadelphia, Saunders, 1980, p. 307.
3. Allbrook, D.B., Baker, N. de C., Kirkaldy-Willis, W.H. Muscle regeneration in experimental animals and man. J Bone Joint Surg 48B: 153–169, 1966.
4. Almekinders, L.C., Garrett, W.E., and Seaber, A.V. Histopathology of muscle tears in stretching injuries. Trans 30th Orthop Res Soc, 9:306, 1984.
5. Almekinders, L.C., Garrett, W.E., and Seaber, A.V. Pathophysiologic response to muscle tears in stretching injuries. Trans 30th Orthop Res Soc 9:307, 1984.
6. Bailey, K. Tropomyosin: A new asymmetric protein component of the muscle fibril. Biochem J 43:271–279, 1948.
7. Boothe, F.W., and Holloszy, J.O. Cytochrome turnover in rat skeletal muscles. J Biol Chem 252:416–419, 1977.
8. Brooke, M.H., and Kaiser, K.K. Muscle fiber types: How many and what type? Arch Neurol 23:369–379, 1970.
9. Carlson, B.N. The regeneration of skeletal muscle. A review. Am J Anat 137:119–144, 1973.

10. Chierici, G., and Miller, A.J. Experimental study of muscle reattachment following surgical detachment. J Oral Maxillofac Surg 42:485–490, 1984.

11. Cooper, R.R. Alterations during immobilization and regeneration of skeletal muscle in rats. J Bone Joint Surg 54:919–925, 1972.

12. Crawford, G.N.C., and James, N.T. The design of muscles, in Owen, R., Goodfellow, J., and Bullough, P. (eds): *Scientific Foundations of Orthopedics and Traumatology.* Philadelphia, Saunders, 1980, pp. 67–74.

13. Dubowitz, V., Brooke, M.H., and Neville, H.E. *Muscle Biopsy: A Modern Approach.* Philadelphia, Saunders, 1973.

14. Ebashi, S., and Ebashi, F. Alpha-actinin, a new structural protein from skeletal muscle. I. Preparation and action on actomyosin-ATP interaction. J Biochem (Tokyo) 58:7–12, 1965.

15. Ebashi, S., Endo, M., and Ohtsuki, I. Control of muscle contraction. Q Rev Biophys 2:351–384, 1969.

16. Ebashi, S. Separation of troponin into its three components. J Biochem (Tokyo) 58:7–12, 1965.

17. Eisenberg, B.R., and Kuda, A.M. Discrimination between fiber populations in mammalian skeletal muscle by using ultrastructural parameters. J Ultrastruct Res 54:76–88, 1976.

18. Engel, W.K. Essentiality of histo- and cytochemical studies of skeletal muscle in investigation of neuromuscular disease. Neurology (Minneapolis) 12:778–794, 1962.

19. Furukawa, T., Sugita, H., and Toyokura, Y. Comparative studies on myofibrillar proteins in different types of skeletal muscle fibers. Exp Neurol 37:515–521, 1972.

20. Ganong, W.F. *Review of Medical Physiology.* Los Altos, Calif., Lange Publications, 1983, p. 49.

21. Garrett, W.E., Boxwick, J.M., Davenport, W.C., and Seaber, A.V. Contractile and functional properties of partially and totally surgically transected muscle. Trans Orthop Res Soc 8:280, 1983.

22. Granger, B.L., and Lazarides, E. Synemin: A new high molecular weight protein associated with desmin and vimentin filaments in muscle. Cell 22:727–738, 1980.

23. Granger, B.L., and Lazariudes, E. The existence of an insoluble disc scaffold in chicken skeletal muscle. Cell 15:1253–1268, 1978.

24. Granit, R. *Muscle Afferents and Motor Control.* New York, Wiley, 1966.

25. Halata, Z., Badalamente, M.A., Dee, R., and Propper, M. Ultrastructure of sensory nerve endings in monkey (*Macaca fascicularis*) knee joint capsule. J Orthop Res 2:169–176, 1984.

26. Hartshorne, D.J., and Mueller, H. Fractionation of troponin into two distinct proteins. Biochem Biophys Res Commun 31:647–653, 1968.

27. Hartwig, J.H., and Stossel, T.T. Isolation and properties of actin myosin and a new actin-binding protein in rabbit alveolar macrophage. J Biol Chem 250:5696–5705, 1975.

28. Holloszy, J.O., Winder, W.W., Fitts, R.H., Rennie, M.J., Hickson, R.C., and Connie, R.K. Regulatory mechanisms in metabolism during exercise, in Landry, F., and Orgin, W.A.R. (eds): *International Symposium on Biochemistry of Exercise.* Miami, Symposia Specialists, 1978, pp. 61–74.

29. Holloszy, J.O. Muscle metabolism during exercise. Arch Phys Med Rehabil 63:231–234, 1982.

30. Holloszy, J.O., and Boothe, F.W. Biochemical adaptations to endurance exercise in muscle. Ann Rev Physiol 38:273–291, 1976.

31. Huxley, H.E. Electron microscope studies on the structure of natural and synthetic protein filaments from striated muscle. J Mol Biol 7:281–308, 1963.

32. Ikai, M., and Fukunaga, T. A study of training effect on strength per unit cross-sectional area of muscle by means of ultrasonic measurement. Int Z Angew Physiol 28:173–180, 1970.

33. Ikai, M., and Steinhouse, A.H. Some factors modifying the expression of human strength. J Appl Physiol 16:157–163, 1961.

34. Jarvinen, M., Aho, A.J., Lehto, M., and Toivonen, H. Age dependent repair of muscle rupture. Acta Orthop Scand 54:64–74, 1983.

35. Jerusalem, F., Engel, A.G. and Peterson, H.A. Human muscle fiber fine structure: morphometric data on controls. Neurology (Minneapolis) 25:127–134, 1975.

36. Johannessen, J.V. *Electron Microsopy in Human Medicine,* vol 4. New York, McGraw-Hill, 1981, pp 257–310.

37. Klenerman, L. Tourniquet paralysis. J Bone Joint Surg 65B:374–375, 1983.

38. Komi, P.V., Vitasalo, J.T., Raurama, R., and Vihko, V. Effecting isometric strength training on mechanical, electrical and metabolic aspects of muscle function. Eur J Appl Physiol 40:45–55, 1978.

39. Kretsinger, R.H., and Barry, C.D. The predicted structure of the calcium-bonding component of troponin. Biochem Biophys Acta 405:40–52, 1975.

40. Kuroda, M., and Maruyama, K. Gamma-actinin, a new regulatory protein from rabbit skeletal muscle. I. Purification and characterization. J Biochem (Tokyo) 80:315–322, 1976.

41. Kuroda, M., Tanaka, T., and Masaki, T. Eu-actinin, a new structural protein of the Z-line of striated muscles. J Biochem (Tokyo) 89:279–310, 1981.

42. Leavis, P.C., Rosenfeld, S.S., Gergely, J., Grabarik, Z., and Drabikowski, W. Proteolytic fragments of troponin C. Localization of high and low affinity calcium binding sites and interactions with troponin I and troponin T. J Biol Chem 253:5452–5495, 1978.

43. Lipton, B.H., and Schultz, E. Developmental fate of skeletal muscle satellite cells. Science 205:1292–1294, 1979.

44. Maruyama, K. A new protein factor hindering network formation of actin in solution. Biochem Biophys Acta 94:208–225, 1965.

45. Maruyama, K. Elastic structure of connectin muscle, in Ebashi, S., Maruyama, K., and Endo, M. (eds): *Muscle Contraction, Its Regulatory Mechanisms.* Tokyo, Japan Science Society Press, 1980 pp. 485-496.

46. Masaki, T., and Takaiti, O. Purification of M-protein. J Biochem (Tokyo) 71:355–357, 1972.

47. McDonagh, M.J.N., Haynard, C.M., and Davies, C.D.N. Isometric training in human elbow flexor muscles. The effect on voluntary and electrically evoked forces. J Bone Joint Surg 65B:355–358, 1983.

48. Miller, W.A., Rupture of the musculotendinous juncture of the medial head of the gastrocnemius muscle. Am J Sports Med 5:191–193, 1977.

49. Milner-Brown, H.S., Stein, R.B., and Yemor, R. The orderly recruitment of human motor units during voluntary isometric contractions. J Physiol 230:359–370, 1973.

50. Morel, J.E., and Pinset-Harstrom, I. Ultrastructure of the contractile system of striated skeletal muscle and the processes of muscular contraction. I. Ultrastructure of the myofibril and source of energy. Biomedicine 22:88–96, 1975.

51. Nystrom, B., and Holmlund, D. Experimental evaluation of immobilization in operative and non-operative treatment of Achilles tendon rupture. Acta Chir Scand 149:669–673, 1983.

52. Obinata, T., Maruyama, K., Sugita, H., Kohama, K., and Ebashi, S. Dynamic aspects of structural proteins in vertebrate skeletal muscle. Muscle Nerve 4:456–488, 1981.

53. Offer, G., Moos, C., and Starr, R. A new protein of the thick filaments of vertebrate skeletal myofibrils. Extraction, purification and characterization. J Mol Biol 74:653–676, 1973.

54. Ohashi, K., and Maruyama, K. A new structural protein located on the Z-line of chicken skeletal muscle. J Biochem (Tokyo) 85:1103–1105, 1979.

55. Ohashi, K., Kimura, S., Deguchi, K., and Maruyama, K. I-protein, a new regulatory protein from vertebrate skeletal muscle. I. purification and characterization. J Biochem (Tokyo) 81: 233–236, 1977.

56. Ohashi, K., Murakami, F., Honda, S., and Eguchi, G. Connectin and elastic protein of muscle. Characterization and function. J Biochem (Tokyo) 82:317–337, 1977.

57. Ohashi, K., and Maruyama, K. A new structural protein located on the Z-line of chicken muscle, in Ebashi, S., and Maruyama, K. (eds): *Muscle Contraction, Its Regulatory Mechanisms.* Tokyo,

Japan Society Press, 1980, pp 497–505.

58. Perry, S.V. Structure and interactions of myosin. Prog Biophys Mol Biol 17:325–381, 1967.

59. Phillips, G.N., Lattman, E.E., Cummins, P., Lee, K.Y., and Cohen, C. Crystal structure and molecular interactions of tropomyosin. Nature 278:413–417, 1979.

60. Rennie, M.J., and Holloszy, J.O., Inhibition of glucose uptake and glycogenolysis by availability of oleate in well oxygenated perfused skeletal muscle. Biochem J 168:161–170, 1977.

61. Rhodin, J.A.G. *Histology, a Text and Atlas.* New York, Oxford University Press, 1974, pp 221–234.

62. Rizk, N.N. SEM of the structural reconstruction of the abdominal wall after experimental paramedian incision. J Surg Res 35:354–364, 1983.

63. Saltin, B., Henriksson, J., Nygaard, E., and Anderson, P. Fiber types and metabolic potentials of skeletal muscles in sedentary man and endurance runner. Ann NY Acad Sci 301–329, 1977.

64. Saltin, B., Houston, M., Nygaard, E., Graham, T., and Wahren, J. Muscle fiber characteristics in healthy men and patients with juvenile diabetes. Diabetes 28(1):93–99, 1979.

65. Schaub, M.C., and Perry, S.V. The relaxing protein system of striated muscle. Presolution of the troponin complex into inhibitory and calcium-sensitizing factors and their relationship to tropomyosin. Biochem J 115:993–1004, 1969.

66. Sjostrom, M., and Nystrom, B. Achilles tendon injury. Virchows Arch [Pathol Anat] 399:177–189, 1983.

67. Sodek, J., Hodges, R.S., and Smillie, L.B. Amino acid sequence of rabbit skeletal muscle-tropomyosin and COOH-terminal half. J Biol Chem 253:1129–1136, 1978.

68. Szent-Gyorgyi, A. *Chemistry of Muscular Contraction,* 2d ed. New York, Academic Press, 1951.

69. Trotter, J.A., Corbett, K.A., and Avner, B.T. Structure and function of the murine muscle-tendon junction. Anat Rec 201:293–302, 1981.

70. Trotter, J.A., Ebehard, S., and Samora, A. Structural connections of the muscle tendon junction. Cell Motil 3:431–438, 1983.

71. Tountas, C.P., and Bergman, R.A. Tourniquet ischemia. Ultrastructural and histochemical observations of ischemic human muscle and of monkey muscle and nerve. J Hand Surg 2:31–37, 1977.

72. Wyke, B.D. The neurology of joints. Ann R Coll Surg Engl 41:25, 1967.

CHAPTER 14

Nerve: Structure and Function

Roger Dee

The structure of individual peripheral nerve depends upon its makeup of individual fibers and varies from nerve to nerve. The principal categories of nerve fibers, each of which differs with regard to fiber diameter, electrical properties, and function, are shown in Table 14-1.

The unmyelinated fibers, the myelinated fibers, and the Schwann cells are surrounded by individual sheaths of *endoneurium,* which contributes to the elasticity of nerve.[9] The individual fibers are furthermore grouped into bundles, termed *fascicles,* within the peripheral nerve. Each fascicle

TABLE 14-1 Classification of Nerve Fibers

Fiber type	Fiber diameter, μm	Nerve fiber function
A	α 12–20	Motor; propriception
	β 5–12	Touch; pressure
	δ 2–5	Pain; temperature; touch
B	<3	Preganglionic autonomic
C (unmyelinated)	<1.3	Dorsal root sensory Postganglionic sympathetic

Note: C fibers are most sensitive to local anesthetic and least susceptible to hypoxia and pressure. A fibers are most sensitive to pressure but least sensitive to local anesthetic.
Source: Modified from Ganong, W.F., ed: *Review of Medical Physiology.* Los Altos, Lange Medical, 1983. Reproduced with permission.

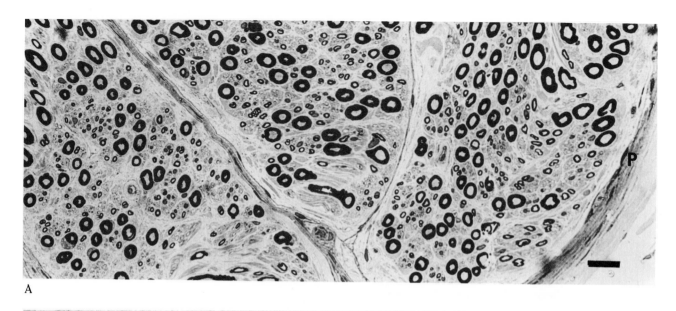

A

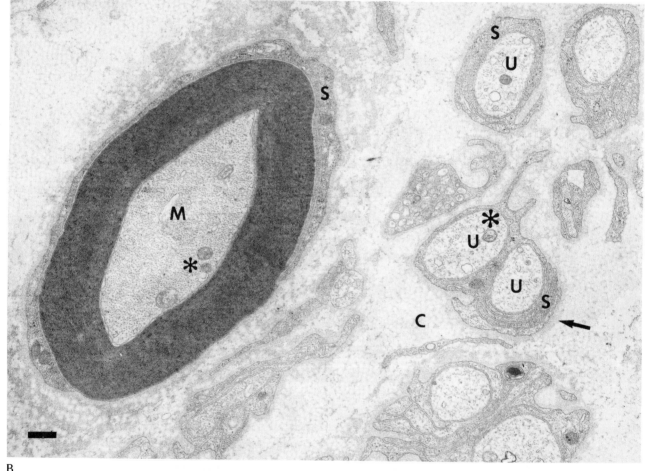

B

Figure 14-1 A. Light micrograph of a 1-μm-thick epoxy cross section through a portion of a human sural nerve. This bundle of fascicles is surrounded by perineurium (P). Within each fascicle, many myelinated axons are seen. The myelin sheaths appear as black circles in this preparation. Unmyelinated axons cannot be seen at this magnification. (Bar = 10 μm.) **B.** An electron micrograph of one small region of the same nerve. Note the presence of a myelinated axon (M) and several unmyelinated axons (three of which are labeled U). Each axon is surrounded by satellite cells (S), and each satellite cell is enveloped in a basal lamina (*arrow*). Between the cells are many collagen fibrils cut in cross section (C). Within the axons can be seen a variety of organelles, including mitochondria (*). The "speckling" of the axoplasm reflects the presence of neurofilaments and microtubules, which cannot be easily resolved at this magnification. (Bar = 0.5 μm.) *(Courtesy of Dr. J. Halperin.)*

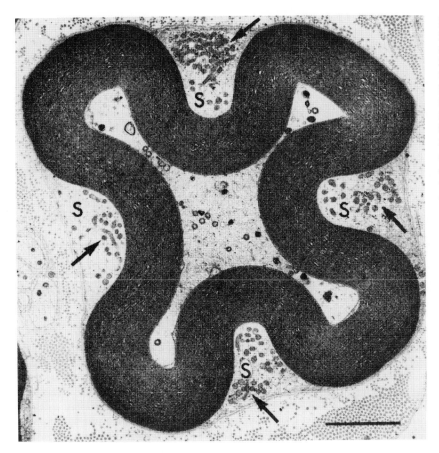

Figure 14-2 Transverse section through the paranodal region of a large myelinated nerve fiber (12 μm). The myelin is folded into ridges and grooves. The contained axon, which conforms to the myelin's inner contour, is compressed and fluted. The grooves on the external surface of the myelin sheath are filled with Schwann cell cytoplasm (S) containing many mitochondria (*arrows*). Bar = 2 μm. *(From Landon, D.N., in Swash, M., and Kennerd, C., eds: Scientific Basis of Clinical Neurology. New York, Churchill Livingstone, 1985. Reproduced with permission.)*

has its own sheath termed the *perineurium* (Fig. 14-1). The *epineurium* is connective tissue that invests the peripheral nerve as a loose sheath *(epineurial sheath)* and also binds the fascicles together *(interfascicular epineurium)*. Within the interfascicular epineurium runs the vascular supply of the nerve and its lymphatic drainage.

Peripheral nerves provide a means of transmitting information between the central nervous system and peripheral sensors and effectors. Each individual nerve fiber is the axon of a single neuron (nerve cell body), which in the case of a motor fiber is an anterior horn cell and in the case of a sensory fiber is the cell body located in the dorsal root ganglion.

THE NEURON

The nucleus of the cell plus its soma (called the *perikaryon*) are together termed the *cell body*.[2] Cytoplasmic extensions consist of a half dozen or so *dendrites* that extend out from the cell body, arborize extensively, and provide a receptor membrane zone for the neuron to receive modulating influences from other cells. The efferent cytoplasmic extension process is the *axon*, which is usually singular for each neuron. Axons arising from sensory neurons of the dorsal root ganglion branch, one portion passing distally to the sensory receptor, the other passing centrally up the dorsal root. The soma gives evidence of synthetic capability; the presence of

rough endoplasmic reticulum and associated ribosomes gives a floccular appearance termed *Nissl substance* (Fig. 14-2).[6] The slightly thickened area of the cell body from which the axon originates is termed the *axon hillock*.

The metabolic activity of the neuron relates primarily to three processes. The first is the maintenance of the ionic gradients necessary to conduct impulses. The second is synthesizing neurotransmitters and transporting them to their sites of action. The third is providing energy for these transport systems, since the mechanism of nerve transmission is not passive but requires energy for amplification during the transmission of the impulse down the nerve fiber.

The Axon

The neural membrane of the axon is continuous with the cell membrane of the cell body and is termed the *axolemma*. This membrane consists of two layers of phospholipids and possesses a series of ion-specific channels within it which can be open or closed to permit bioelectric conduction. Its surface also has receptor proteins involved in the permeability changes.[6] Microtubules which provide a cytoskeleton are seen both within dendrites and axons. Neurofilaments are strandlike structures which also contribute to the cytoskeleton. Both these elements may have a role in axon transport.

Throughout its course the axon is surrounded by satellite cells. Larger-diameter axons have *Schwann cells* sur-

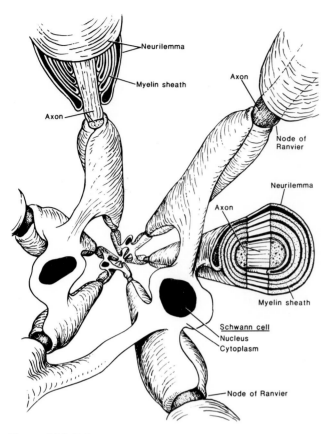

Figure 14-3 Relationship of Schwann cells to axons. *(From Tortora, G.J., and Agnostakos, N.P.: Principles of Anatomy and Physiology, 4th ed. New York, Harper & Row, 1984. Reproduced with permission.)*

rounding them (Fig. 14-3). The cell membrane of the Schwann cell rolls itself around the axon in a spiral fashion (Fig. 14-4) and produces myelin. It seems that the axon's attainment of a certain critical diameter is a major stimulus for myelinization. The myelin sheath develops longitudinal grooves, giving it a crenated or fluted appearance in transverse section as well as being increased in diameter on either side of the node of Ranvier. The axon also develops a fluted transverse section in the paranodal area (Fig. 14-2). It appears that Schwann cells also have a nutritional function, providing the axon with metabolic support. This is important since Schwann cells are the nerve elements most vulnerable to ischemia.[9]

In the central nervous system, the oligodendroglial cell produces myelin in a fashion similar to that of the Schwann cells in the peripheral nervous system. *Remak cells* are those satellite cells which surround smaller-diameter axons. They are biologically identical to Schwann cells, but they do not myelinate the very fine axons with which they are associated.

In both the central and peripheral nervous systems, myelin-free intervals termed the *nodes of Ranvier* leave areas of the axon membrane of myelinated fibers unprotected from the insulating properties of myelin and therefore available for ionic exchange in the process of saltatory conduction, which

transmits the nerve impulse. The interval between each node of Ranvier, i.e., the unmyelinated segment, is termed the *internode* and is typically about 200 to 2000 mμ long. In general the larger the diameter of the axon, the longer the internode. The thicker the myelin sheath, the faster the conduction. In addition, these fibers with thick myelin sheaths and large diameters are less susceptible to local anesthetic but more susceptible to hypoxia and pressure effects (see Table 14-1).

Large axons convey very precisely modulated information. They are heavily myelinated and conduct impulses at high speed (50 to 60 m/s). These include those axons that sense joint position and muscle stretch as well as motor axons. These are all functions requiring frequent and precise readjustments. The smaller unmyelinated axons (called C fibers) are far more numerous (Table 14-1). They slowly conduct impulses (1 to 2 m/s) which do not require rapid modulation, e.g., vasoconstrictor fiber.

Intracellular Transport Mechanisms

The specific mechanisms of intracellular transport are highly specialized, associated with the neuron's peculiar configuration. Synthesis in the cell body is a long way from where the resulting products are required; this is particularly true of substances required for neurotransmission and in the case of axon growth or repair. The axons are involved in the transport of material between the cell bodies and the periphery. Transportation occurs both centrifugally and centripetally along the length of the axon via this complex transport system. There is both a rapid transport system (several hundred millimeters per day) and a slower transportation system, the latter associated with the structural axonal skeleton (about 1 mm/day). Transmission from the cell body is known as *anterograde transport.*

A more homogeneous system is responsible for *retrograde transport* of materials toward the cell body, and this occurs typically at a rate approaching that of fast anterograde transport. This process is probably used to return material not needed at the axon terminal and the metabolic debris of the axon; it also samples substances brought into the axon terminal from its environment by endocytosis.

Nerve Injury

The specialized configuration of neurons and their processes render these cells very susceptible to injuries.

Since axons lack the ability to synthesize the substances essential for their survival, transecting them renders their distal portions lifeless. A severed distal portion typically remains functional and intact several days following the injury, but thereafter the effects of the injury slowly propagate down the axon at the rate of slow transport as the distal portion gradually expends its unreplenishable metabolic stores. The stump remains electrically excitable until the axon gradually undergoes wallerian degeneration. Usually the proximal end

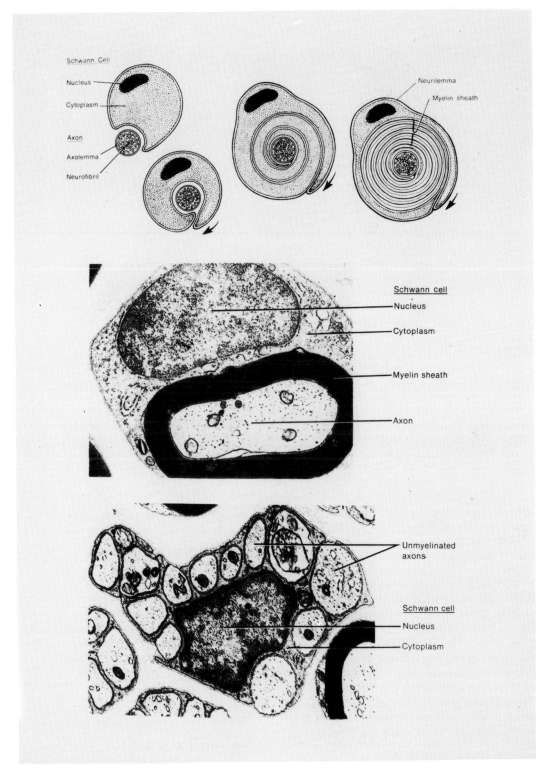

Figure 14-4 Myelinization of the axon. *Top,* the Schwann cell rolls around the axon in a spiral manner, forming the sheath. *Middle,* the relation of the Schwann cell nucleus to the myelinated nerve fiber. *Bottom,* one Schwann cell related to several unmyelinated axons. *(From Tortora, G.J., and Agnostakos, N.P.: Principles of Anatomy and Physiology, 4th ed. New York, Harper & Row, 1984. Reproduced with permission.)*

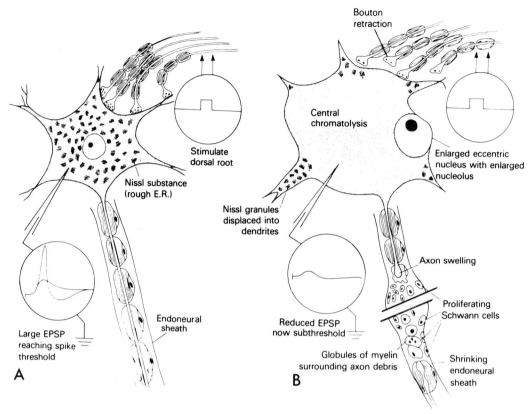

Figure 14-5 The proximal changes seen following axonal division in mammalian spinal motoneurons. **A.** Normal motoneuron. **B.** Appearance after ventral root transection. *(From Selzer, M.E., in Sumner, A.J., ed: The Physiology of Peripheral Nerve Disease. Philadelphia, Saunders, 1980. Reproduced with permission.)*

undergoes some retrograde degeneration, and if the site of the injury is near the cell body, the cell itself may be lethally injured. During wallerian degeneration the axon swells and a beaded appearance precedes fragmentation. Globules of the disorganized myelin sheath are ingested by macrophages and satellite cells.[8] The retrograde reaction involves breakup and dispersion of Nissl substance (chromatolysis) and changes in the intracellular organelles of the cell body (Fig. 14-5).

Axonotmesis is the term used to describe disruption of the axon (e.g., by severe crush) causing its distal degeneration but preserving the endoneurium. A usually transient loss of the function of a nerve fiber associated with preservation of the intact axon is termed *neuropraxia*. The term *neurotmesis* describes disruption not only of the axon but also of the associated Schwann cells and connective tissue structure.[7] The details of these changes and nerve repair are described in Chap. 40, Sect. A.

Myofibers are very dependent on interactions with their innervating motor neuron for maintaining their usual function. After damage to the motor axon, myofibrils atrophy and become more sensitive to acetylcholine. The fibers become prone to spontaneous fibrillations, which is attributable to this hypersensitivity to acetylcholine, and this phenomenon appears typically 7 to 14 days following the injury. In general, the longer it takes for the regenerating axon to reach the denervated myofiber, the less the likelihood of obtaining a useful functional result. For a detailed review of the biochemistry of nerve regeneration, the reader is referred to Selzer's stimulating review.[8]

REFERENCES

1. Aguamo, A.J., and Bray, G.M. Cell interactions studied in the peripheral nerves of experimental animals, in Dyck, P.J., Thomas P.K., Lambert, E.H., and Bunge, R. (eds): *Peripheral Neuropathy,* 2d ed, chap 16. Philadelphia, Saunders, 1984, pp 360–377.

2. Ganong, W.F. *Review of Medical Physiology.* Los Altos, Lange, 1983.

3. Ochoa, J., Fowler, T.J., and Gilliatt, R.W. Anatomical changes in peripheral nerves compressed by a pneumatic tourniquet. J Anat 113:433, 1972.

4. Ochs, S. Basic properties of axoplasmic transport, in Dyck, P.J., Thomas, P.K., Lambert, E.H., and Bunge, R. (eds): *Peripheral Neuropathy,* 2d ed, chap 21. Philadelphia, Saunders, 1984, pp 453–476.

5. Olum, F. and Posner, J.B. Neurobiologic essentials in pathophysiology. in Smith, L.H., and Thier, S.O. (eds): *Pathophysiology* Philadelphia, Saunders, 1985, pp 1009–1036.

6. Plum, P., and Posner, J.B. Neurobiologic essentials, in Smith, L.H., and Thier, S.O. (eds): *Pathophysiology.* Philadelphia, Saunders, 1985, pp 1009–1036.

7. Seddon, H. *Surgical Disorders of Peripheral Nerves,* 2d ed, chap 2.

New York, Churchill Livingstone, 1975, pp 9–31.
8. Selzer, M.E. Regeneration of peripheral nerve, in Sumner, A.J. (ed): *The Physiology of Peripheral Nerve Disease.* Philadelphia, Saunders, 1980, pp 358–431.
9. Terzis, J.K. Nerve structure organization and healing, in Cruess,

R.L. (ed): *The Musculoskeletal System.* New York, Churchill Livingstone, 1982, pp 357–382.
10. Wujeck, J.R., Lasek, R.J. Correlation of axonal regeneration and slow component B in two branches of a single axon. J Neurosci 3:243–251, 1983.

<hr>

CHAPTER 15

Electrodiagnostic Tests

John Halperin

Neurophysiological testing is now used routinely in the assessment of clinical disorders of the peripheral nervous system. Although technical advances have made the task of the electromyographer much simpler, it is important to remember that even with sophisticated instrumentation, obtaining useful data still requires detailed knowledge of the anatomy of the peripheral nervous system, as well as of the potential technical pitfalls inherent in these techniques. A carefully planned study can localize a lesion to a specific nerve root, a small region of a nerve plexus, or a segment of a peripheral nerve. A poorly performed one inflicts considerable discomfort and expense on the patient but provides no useful information.

NERVE CONDUCTION STUDIES

Tests of nerve conduction are performed by applying electric impulses to peripheral nerves while electronically recording their responses. Such studies can be used to assess selectively the function of motor or sensory nerves at virtually any point along their course.

Pathological processes may affect peripheral nerves in one of two ways—either the axon itself or the myelin sheath surrounding it may be damaged.[2] Axonal damage affects nerve conduction in an all or none fashion—an injured axon either conducts essentially normally or, if the damage is severe enough, it stops conducting completely.[3] Transection of a nerve or avulsion of a root obviously interrupts all conduction through the point of injury. Lesser insults to axons may be electrophysiologically inapparent.

Myelin sheath damage results in a graded slowing of conduction.[3] Conduction is slowed in proportion to the length of nerve demyelinated until ultimately conduction stops. Compressive lesions of nerves tend to produce demyelination of the largest fibers at the site of compression, thereby slowing

nerve conduction locally.[10] Consequently, nerve conduction studies are often useful in localizing entrapments or pressure palsies of individual nerves.

The nerve is stimulated by means of a pair of electrodes applied to the skin surface. The stimulus is generally a square wave pulse of up to 500 V in amplitude and from 0.1 to 1 ms in duration. Stimulation is gradually increased in intensity, causing more and more axons to be depolarized. As additional axons depolarize, the amplitude of the recorded response gradually increases. When the stimulus intensity is such that all axons are being depolarized, the response amplitude plateaus; a further increase in stimulus strength has no additional effect on the recorded response. For all nerve conduction studies, the stimulus intensity must be adjusted so as to elicit this maximal response consistently.

The response to the stimulus is usually recorded with surface electrodes, which may be placed over the nerve itself (Fig. 15-1) or over a muscle (Fig. 15-2) it innervates. Recording from a muscle offers the advantage of considerable intrinsic electrical amplification. When recorded from the skin surface, a nerve potential is typically 5 to 10 μV in amplitude, while a muscle potential is usually 1000 times larger. On the other hand, recording from a muscle provides no information about the function of sensory axons.

The stimulus and response are recorded electronically. Response amplitude and latency (the time between the onset of the stimulus and that of the response) are measured. It is important to remember that the response recorded from the skin represents the summated activity of a large number of axons. Its amplitude is proportional to the number of functional axons present in the nerve. Loss of axons causes a corresponding decrease in the response amplitude. Therefore, the response amplitude can be used as a measure of the total number of functioning axons present in the nerve. In contrast, the conduction velocity calculated from such a summated response reflects only the function of the fastest-conducting fibers (since latencies are measured to the onset of the sum-

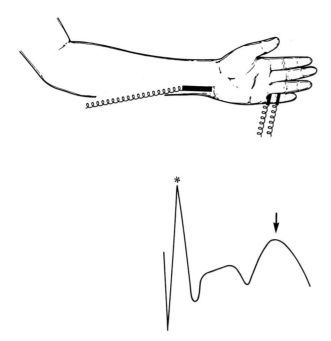

Figure 15-1 Technique for recording the ulnar nerve sensory potential. Electrodes around the small finger stimulate the digital nerves.

The compound nerve action potential (CNAP) is shown in the lower diagram as recorded from a surface electrode at the wrist. In this case the time from the stimulus artifact (*) to the first upward deflection of the CNAP (arrow) is 2.5 ms. Since the distance between stimulating and recording electrodes was 13.5 cm the conduction velocity (CV) was calculated as 54 m/s. The amplitude of the CNAP is 24 μV.

mated response, the most clearly identifiable point). Since a nerve contains many different axons conducting at differing velocities, conclusions concerning slower-conducting fibers are limited. In fact, if most of a nerve is destroyed but a small number of rapidly conducting fibers remain, the calculated conduction velocity may be normal! Fortunately (for the electromyographer) most traumatic or compressive neuropathies affect the largest fibers.

Once the latencies are measured, a conduction velocity can be readily calculated. If the response is recorded directly from a nerve (Fig. 15-1), the conduction velocity can be determined by measuring the distance between the site of stimulation and the site of recording and dividing this by the response latency. If the response is recorded from a muscle (Fig. 15-2), the calculation is slightly more complex. The measured latency in this case includes delays resulting from the slower conduction of impulses in the small, unmyelinated terminal branches of the motor axons, and in addition, from neuromuscular transmission, which involves the release of acetylcholine and its diffusion from the nerve terminal to the muscle end plate. These two phenomena typically increase the latency by about 1 ms. Because of this additional delay, the terminal latency (the time between distal stimulation of a

motor nerve and the recorded muscle activation) cannot be used to calculate a meaningful conduction velocity. On the other hand, the amount of the delay introduced by these factors is fairly consistent, so the terminal latency can be compared with an empirically determined range of normal values and described as normal or abnormal, without converting it to a conduction velocity.

To determine a conduction velocity in a motor nerve, it is necessary to stimulate the nerve at at least two sites while recording the compound muscle action potential (CMAP) from an innervated muscle (Fig. 15–2). By subtracting the terminal latency from the latency obtained with more proximal stimulation, it is possible to determine the time for conduction of impulses between the two stimulation sites. Once the distance between the two sites is measured, the conduction velocity of this segment of nerve can be calculated. This process can be repeated by stimulating at additional, more proximal sites, providing information on conduction in different segments of the nerve. For example, when the examiner is trying to demonstrate an abnormality of ulnar nerve function, the signal is recorded from the hand intrinsic muscles, and the nerve is stimulated first at the wrist, then below the ulnar groove, and finally above the ulnar groove. By calculating

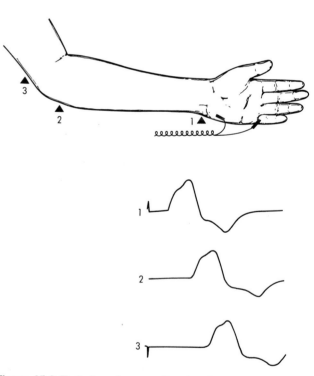

Figure 15-2 Technique for recording the ulnar nerve motor potential. Small disk electrodes overlying the abductor digiti minimi muscle are used to record the response as the ulnar nerve is stimulated at the wrist (trace 1), below the elbow (trace 2), and above the elbow (trace 3). Latencies of each wave (measured to the onset of each response) are 3.2 ms, 6.8 ms, and 8.8 ms. The distance between the above elbow stimulation site and the below elbow site is 12 cm, so the conduction velocity (CV) across the elbow is 60 m/s. The response amplitude is 10 mV.

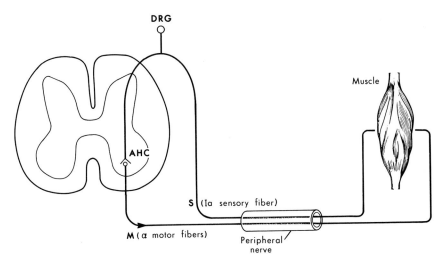

Figure 15-3 Motor axons (m) arise from anterior horn cells (AHC) and join sensory fibers (S) to make up the peripheral nerve. Sensory fibers arise from cell bodies in the dorsal root ganglia (DRG). Central processes of some of these fibers project directly into the anterior horns, providing the anatomic basis for the monosynaptic reflex (tendon jerk).

H reflex: A low-amplitude stimulus of the peripheral nerve will selectively depolarize the large rapidly conducting Ia sensory axons involved in this reflex. The monosynaptic reflex stimulation of the AHC produces the H reflex response.

F response: A supramaximal stimulus at the same location will depolarize all axons of the peripheral nerve. In particular it will result in an antidromic volley ascending the motor axons back to the AHC, some of which will produce a recurrent volley returning orthodromically in the same motor axons—the F response.

conduction velocities in each of these segments, the examiner can demonstrate focal slowing.

F Response and H Reflex

In the case of many commonly occurring injuries of peripheral nerves, it is technically simple to stimulate the nerve in question on one side of the suspected lesion and record from the other. However, in the case of nerve roots and other very proximal lesions (such as disorders of the intrapelvic nerves or the lumbosacral plexus), this is technically difficult. In recent years several techniques have become available to aid in the assessment of these disorders.

One of these techniques involves the study of what are referred to as *late responses,* a term encompassing two different tests, one called the *F response* and the second, the *H reflex.*[7,8,12] Both entail stimulation of a peripheral nerve and recording over a peripherally located muscle while the applied impulse travels toward the spinal cord on the stimulated nerve and then returns (Fig. 15-3). As might be expected, this round trip to the spinal cord and back takes considerably longer than the response to direct stimulation. In the arm, typically the direct muscle response (*M response*) occurs about 3 ms after stimulation, while the F response occurs about 25 to 30 ms later. This impulse traverses the entire course of the nerve being studied and therefore provides valuable information about the proximal segments.

The two tests differ in several important ways. The H reflex is the electrical equivalent of a deep tendon reflex and is performed by stimulating a mixed peripheral nerve (typically the tibial nerve, which innervates the gastrocnemius-

soleus) with a relatively weak, submaximal stimulus (Figs. 15-3 and 15-4). Sensory fibers are more easily depolarized than motor axons, and the most easily depolarized ones are the large myelinated fibers that convey information about

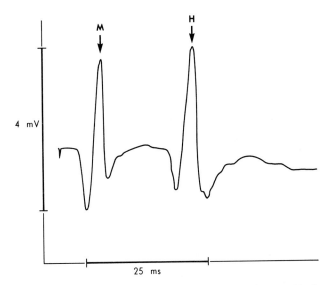

Figure 15-4 Illustration of the H reflex. A single low-amplitude stimulus was applied to the tibial nerve in the popliteal fossa, while the response was recorded from the soleus muscle. Note that there is a double response. The first is the direct motor (M) response and occurs approximately 4.5 ms following the stimulus. The second slightly larger response (H), begins 29 ms after the stimulus and is the H reflex response. Both the M and H are about 4 mV in amplitude.

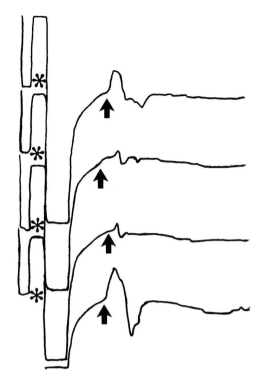

Figure 15-5 The F response. For each of these four tracings, a single stimulus was applied to the ulnar nerve at the wrist while the response was recorded from the abductor digiti minimi muscle, exactly as depicted in Figure 15-2; however, a longer time period is recorded following each stimulus, and the amplification is increased. As a result, the initial direct response appears as a narrow early wave that is off scale (*).

The F responses are represented by a later second wave (arrow) which varies in shape as well as latency. The amplitude of the largest trace (bottom) is about 0.4 mV.

muscle stretch—the same ones that are tested when the Achilles tendon is tapped with a reflex hammer. Therefore, following a relatively weak stimulus these sensory fibers are selectively depolarized, producing a volley of impulses that ascends to the spinal cord, where it passes through the same monosynaptic reflex arc that is involved in the tendon reflex. This results in the depolarization of the anterior horn cells, causing a secondary volley of impulses in the motor axons, with a resultant muscle contraction. This is called the *H reflex* and is characterized by having a highly consistent latency and by being elicited by a stimulus so small that it does not cause significant direct muscle contraction. This is a very useful technique that allows measurement of conduction in the proximal portions of sensory and motor fibers. Unfortunately, in normal subjects it can only be easily elicited in the tibial nerve.

The F response (Figs. 15-3 and 15-5), which is readily elicited from a much larger number of nerves, occurs when the stimulus amplitude is increased to supramaximal inten-

sity. When this is done, the motor axons themselves are directly depolarized. Like all axons, these conduct impulses equally well in both directions. This results in two volleys of impulses. One goes in the "normal" orthodromic direction, directly to the muscle, where it produces a typical M response. The other volley ascends "backward" (antidromically) in the motor axon to the spinal cord, where the anterior horn cell which gives rise to the stimulated axon is directly depolarized. This depolarization propagates slowly through the cell body and its appendages. Initially during this phase, the axon itself is refractory to further depolarization. However, after a brief period it once again becomes excitable, and if the adjacent portion of the cell body is still depolarized, a recurrent discharge ensues, propagating back down the same axon. (After any particular antidromic volley, this occurs in a small proportion of the anterior horn cells, typically about 5 to 10 percent.) This recurrent discharge propagates back to the periphery, producing a small muscle contraction, the F response. This entire "round trip" occurs in a single motor neuron.

Although F responses can be elicited from far more nerves than the H reflex can, there are technical factors limiting their applicability. In particular, they can only be easily measured in muscles in which the late response occurs after the initial M response (direct contraction) is over, i.e., only those muscles located far enough away from the spinal cord that the round trip takes over about 15 to 20 ms. Their other shortcoming is that they only study the function of motor axons, providing no information about sensory fibers.

Somatosensory Evoked Potentials (SEPs)

In order to study the function of the proximal portions of nerves which do not contain many motor axons, or nerves in which no muscle is sufficiently far away from the spinal cord to permit observation of late responses, in recent years researchers have focused increasing interest on the use of the somatosensory evoked response.[4,5,6,7,8,11] This technique differs from routine conduction studies in several important ways. A small electric stimulus is applied to a nerve repeatedly (typically approximately 5 stimuli per second, a total of 1000 to 2000 times), and the response is recorded from the brain and spinal cord. By computer averaging, all randomly occurring noise (and background EEG activity) is eliminated from the signal, and the very small amplitude responses (about 1 μV) can easily be discerned. The low-intensity stimulus selectively affects the large myelinated sensory axons, sending an afferent volley to the spinal cord. Recording electrodes are placed over the spinal cord and over the appropriate part of the cerebral cortex. By measuring the time of arrival of the volley of impulses at the spinal cord and at successively higher levels of the neuraxis, the examiner can detect abnormalities of peripheral nerves, roots, the spinal cord, or the brain. When the site of stimulation is carefully selected, individual peripheral nerves or roots can be studied.

This technique has proved particularly useful in studying disorders of the brachial plexus and of multiple sensory nerve roots.[6,7,8,13] In brachial plexus injuries the evoked response to peripheral nerve stimulation is recorded at the parietal sensory cortex and also at Erb's point (or if intraoperative, directly from the suspect roots). Information such as the identification of irreparable high proximal avulsion of nerve roots from the spinal cord thus can be obtained.

Sensory nerve roots which may be compressed by an osteophyte or herniated nucleus pulposus or avulsed as a result of trauma are virtually impossible to study by other electrophysiological techniques, except in those few nerves where the H reflex is elicitable. Since the cells of origin of sensory fibers lie outside the spinal canal in the dorsal root ganglia, when sensory roots are damaged the ganglion cell and the peripheral axon typically survive in continuity. Because of this, the peripherally recorded sensory potentials remain completely normal, even when the root is severely damaged. By recording the SEP, continuity through the root zone can sometimes be assessed.

SEPs have also been used to assess spinal cord integrity during spinal instrumentation, in an effort to detect motor dysfunction early enough to remedy it. The posterior tibial nerve is stimulated while the scalp SEP is monitored for surgically induced changes. While this appears to be of some utility,[11] it does not provide a foolproof method of monitoring, since the signal being recorded is carried in the posterior columns of the spinal cord (where it is relatively immune to compromise of the anterior spinal artery) while motor control is located far more anteriorly in the cord, in the descending corticospinal tracts.

SEPs may also be of some use in the diagnosis of radiculopathies (such as occur in lumbar disc disease), particularly those with prominent sensory signs and symptoms.[7,8] Attempts have been made to use dermatomal stimulation, using surface disc electrodes applied to the skin in the dermatome being studied. While some authors have reported excellent results,[5] it must be remembered that there is tremendous overlap in innervation between adjacent dermatomes, so it is not surprising that other authors[1] have met with much less success.

Electromyography

Nerve conduction studies are complemented by the findings of the needle electromyography exam.[9] Potentials can be recorded from individual motor units if a patient is asked to activate a muscle following the insertion of an intramuscular needle electrode. In normal muscle, each motor unit (which consists of all the myofibers controlled by a single anterior horn cell) fires fairly synchronously. Since the different myofibers of the motor unit are typically scattered over a small area, their potentials all reach the needle electrode at about the same time, resulting in a single, brief, smoothly summated motor unit potential. This potential typically has one or two subcomponents.

When muscle is affected by a myopathy, individual myofibers become quite small, producing much smaller amplitude myofiber potentials. These small potentials do not summate smoothly into a single large monophasic motor unit potential but rather form a small-amplitude, often somewhat polyphasic (consisting of many subcomponents), waveform. Because the myofibers of each motor unit are no farther apart

than normal, the duration of this small-amplitude polyphasic potential is typically about the same as that of a normal monophasic potential. In contrast, when a muscle is denervated and reinnervated, each motor unit comes to contain many more myofibers than normal. Since many more myofibers contribute to each summated response, the resulting motor unit potentials are increased in amplitude and have many phases. Since the myofibers are spread out over a larger area than in a normal motor unit, the overall duration of the potential is typically prolonged.

In addition to looking at the shape of voluntary potentials, the examiner can examine the extent to which the patient is able to control the muscles' activity. A normal muscle is electrically silent at rest. About 1 to 2 weeks following damage to its nerve, a denervated muscle becomes "irritable"—it starts to depolarize spontaneously, giving rise to small brief electric discharges called *fibrillations*. These fibrillation potentials (and a similar, related spontaneous discharge with a slightly different shape, referred to as a *positive sharp wave*) are the hallmark of acute denervation. Unfortunately, similar potentials may occur in other situations, particularly in inflammatory myopathies (in which low-amplitude polyphasics may also be seen).

Other peculiar spontaneous discharges can be seen in certain disease states. One unique abnormality—called *myotonia*—occurs in myotonic dystrophy and myotonia congenita. This abnormal spontaneous discharge consists of a long train of impulses, occurring at high frequency, waxing and waning in amplitude. A somewhat similar, sustained high-frequency discharge may be seen in denervated muscle and in certain other settings.

Another aspect of muscle function studied by electromyographer is the manner in which motor units are *recruited*. Normally when a muscle is relaxed, it is electrically silent. When minimal effort is exerted, a single motor unit begins to fire. To maintain constant force, this unit fires at a constant rate. To increase the strength of contraction, initially the firing rate of that unit is increased. As more force is needed, a second unit is recruited to help and fires together with the first unit. As additional force is required, additional motor units join in, one at a time, until finally all those available are involved. By examining the *recruitment pattern,* the examiner can determine how much effort the subject is exerting and whether the units being used are normal or abnormal. Characteristic abnormalities are seen in myopathies, denervation, hysteria, and other disease states.

Most such examinations are done seeking evidence of denervation. As should be evident from the above discussion, denervation is not manifest by a single, pathognomonic finding but rather is characterized by an evolving constellation of abnormalities which follow a typical evolution in time. During the first 1 or 2 weeks following an injury to a nerve, the only abnormality seen on EMG is that the patient cannot activate the muscle. (Unfortunately this observation is not very specific and is indistinguishable from the appearance of the EMG when the patient is not exerting any effort.) Interestingly, during much of this time the distal nerve stump is electrically excitable; however, if nerve conduction can be tested through the area of injury, impairment of conduction through this region should be demonstrable.

TABLE 15-1 Median Nerve

1. Site:	Ligament of Struthers.
Cause:	Rare; due to supracondylar bony spur with ligament to humeral medial epicondyle. Affects median nerve, proximal to branch to pronator teres and proximal to origin of anterior interosseous nerve.
Nerve conductions:	
Motor (APB):	Normal velocity in forearm and hand but loss of CMAP amplitude.
Sensory (digit II):	Decreased median CNAP amplitude.
F responses (APB):	Prolonged.
EMG:	Denervation in APB, FPL, pronator teres, FCR, FDP.
2. Site:	Pronator teres.
Cause:	Caused by trauma or repeated pronation. Lesion of median nerve, distal to branch to pronator teres, proximal to origin of anterior interosseous nerve.
Nerve conductions:	
Motor (APB):	Slowed velocity in forearm and hand with loss of CMAP amplitude.
Sensory (digit II):	Decreased median CNAP amplitude.
F responses (APB):	Prolonged.
EMG:	Denervation in FPL, APB, FDP (median). Generally spares pronator teres.
3. Site:	Anterior interosseous nerve.
Cause:	Local trauma, fibrous band attached to FDS. Isolated lesion of proximal anterior interosseous nerve.
Nerve conductions:	
Motor (APB)	Normal CV and CMAP amplitude in forearm and hand. Prolonged conduction to pronator quadratus.
Sensory (digit II):	Normal median CNAP amplitude and CV.
F responses (APB):	Normal.
EMG:	Denervation in FPL, FDP (median), pronator quadratus.
4. Site:	Carpal tunnel.
Cause:	Local trauma or ligamentous thickening; affects median nerve after origin of palmar cutaneous branch.
Nerve conductions:	
Motor (APB):	Normal CV in forearm; prolonged terminal latency; decreased CMAP amplitude.
Sensory (digit II):	Decreased median CNAP amplitude and CV.
Mixed:	Disproportionate slowing in palm-to-wrist segment.
F responses (APB):	Prolonged.
EMG:	Denervation in APB; sparing of FPL, FDP, pronator teres, pronator quadratus.

Abbreviations: APB, abductor pollicis brevis; FPL, flexor pollicis longus; FCR, flexor carpi radialis; FDP, flexor digitorum profundus; FDS, flexor digitorum superficialis; CMAP, compound muscle action potential; CNAP, compound nerve action potential; CV, conduction velocity.

The earliest EMG evidence of denervation occurs about 1 to 2 weeks following the injury, corresponding to the time it takes the distal nerve stump to degenerate. Because the individual myofibers have lost contact with the nerves that formerly controlled them, the myofibers start to depolarize spontaneously, producing fibrillations. As time goes by, if portions of the injured nerve regenerate, reinnervation occurs. In this situation, single regenerated axons control many more myofibers than normally, producing large-amplitude polyphasic potentials.

Difficulties in interpreting electromyograms arise from the potentially confusing overlap between some of the findings in denervation and those in myopathies and also from a failure to find electrical evidence of muscle dysfunction when it is clinically suspected. The latter arises because even the most thorough EMG examination is merely a sampling procedure. In the course of the examination, the needle electrode is used to explore different areas of each muscle. Even the most stoic patient will only permit a certain amount of sampling. If a muscle is only partially denervated (particularly if the denervation has been evolving over a long period of time), and if the denervated motor units happen to be in an area that is not sampled, minor lesions may be missed. Despite these difficul-

ties, in most, but not all, cases it is possible to diagnose denervation with EMG.

After the characteristic changes of denervation in a symptomatic muscle are identified, the procedure is then used to identify the site of the lesion more precisely. This entails determining if similar electrical abnormalities are present in other muscles which share a common peripheral nerve, portion of the plexus, or root with the symptomatic muscle. By carefully sampling different muscles, the examiner can accurately localize lesions (Tables 15-1 to 15-6). One particularly useful technique to assess nerve root function is to study the electrical activity in the paraspinal muscles. Since these are innervated segmentally by fibers arising very early in the nerves' course, abnormal activity at a single level is strong confirmatory evidence of a radiculopathy. Absence of abnormal activity in these muscles suggests that the lesion is more peripheral than the root.

By combining these different techniques—nerve conductions, late responses, and a careful analysis of EMG abnormalities—and interpreting them in the light of a detailed knowledge of the neuroanatomy involved, the examiner can usually identify the location of peripheral nerve damage accurately.

TABLE 15-2 Ulnar Nerve

1. Site:	Ulnar groove.	3. Site:	Guyon's canal.
Cause:	Injury to elbow (chronic or acute); "Tardy ulnar palsy." Affects nerve proximal to ulnar contribution to FDP and usually proximal to supply to FCU.	Cause:	Injuries to wrist or palm. Affects ulnar nerve distal to origin of dorsal cutaneous branch. Usually proximal to branches to hypothenar muscles.
Nerve conductions:		Nerve conductions:	
Motor (ADM):	Slowed CV around the elbow (by > 10 m/s); loss of CMAP amplitude in same segment.	Motor (ADM):	Prolonged terminal latency; loss of CMAP amplitude; normal forearm CV.
Sensory (digit V):	Decreased CNAP amplitude; +/– slowing; dorsal cutaneous branch affected.	Sensory (digit V):	Decreased CNAP amplitude and slowed CV. Spares dorsal cutaneous branch.
F responses (ADM):	Prolonged.	F responses (ADM):	Prolonged.
EMG:	Denervation in hypothenar muscles, FDI, FDP (ulnar half), and FCU.	EMG:	Denervation in hypothenar muscles and FDI; spares FCU, FDP (ulnar).
2. Site:	Cubital tunnel.		
Cause:	Repeated elbow flexion?		
Nerve conductions:		4. Site:	Palmar branch.
Motor (ADM):	Slowed CV in cubital tunnel segment, with loss of CMAP amplitude in same segment.	Nerve conductions:	
		Motor (ADM):	Normal. Relative prolongation of terminal latency measured to FDI.
Sensory (digit V):	Decreased CNAP amplitude; +/– slowing. Dorsal cutaneous branch affected.	Sensory (digit V):	Normal, as is dorsal cutaneous branch.
F responses (ADM).	Prolonged.	F responses (ADM):	Normal. Prolonged if measured to FDI.
EMG:	Denervation in hypothenar muscles, FDI, FDP (ulnar half), sparing FCU.	EMG:	Denervation of FDI, sparing FCU, FDP (ulnar) hypothenar muscles.

ADM, abductor digiti minimi; FDP, flexor digitorum profundus; FCU, flexor carpi ulnaris; FDI, first dorsal interosseous; CV, conduction velocity; CMAP, compound muscle action potential; CNAP, compound nerve action potential.

TABLE 15-3 Radial Nerve

Site:	Radial groove.
Cause:	"Saturday night palsy"; humeral fractures. Injury to radial nerve distal to supply to triceps and anconeus; proximal to supply to forearm extensors and usually to brachioradialis.
Nerve conductions:	
Motor (EIP):	Slowed conduction, upper arm to elbow segment; loss of CMAP amplitude.
Sensory (digit I):	Low amplitude; +/– slowing.
F responses (EIP):	Prolonged.
EMG:	Denervation in brachioradialis, forearm extensors; spares triceps, anconeus.

EIP, extensor indicis proprius; CMAP, compound motor action potential.

TABLE 15-4 Brachial Plexus

Site:	Thoracic outlet (rare).
Cause:	Cervical rib, fibrous band. Affects lower trunk of brachial plexus.
Nerve conductions:	
Motor:	Normal velocities in median and ulnar; loss of CMAP amplitude in median (APB); +/– loss of CMAP amplitude in ulnar (ADM).
Sensory:	Low-amplitude ulnar CNAP. Usually normal median.
F responses:	+/– prolonged median and ulnar.
EMG:	Denervation of APB, opponens, +/– ADM, FDI.

APB, abductor pollicis brevis; ADM, abductor digiti minimi; FDI, first dorsal interosseous; CMAP, compound muscle action potential; CNAP, compound nerve action potential.

TABLE 15-5   Lower Extremity

Tibial nerve		Peroneal nerve	
Site:	Tarsal tunnel.	Site:	Fibular head.
Cause:	Local trauma (old fracture).	Cause:	Local injury, crossing legs, stretch.
a. Medial plantar nerve			Damages common peroneal or its branches (superior and deep).
Nerve conductions:			
Motor (AHB):	Prolonged terminal latency. Normal conduction in leg. Normal conduction to ADQ.	Nerve conductions:	
Sensory (digit I):	Slowed conduction; decreased CNAP amplitude; normal to digit V.	Motor (EDB):	Focal slowing and loss of CMAP amplitude around fibular head.
F responses (AHB):	Prolonged.	Sensory:	Normal or slowed with decreased CNAP amplitude.
EMG:	Denervation in AHB.	(superficial peroneus)	Sural normal.
b. Lateral plantar nerve		F responses (EDB):	Prolonged.
Nerve conductions:		EMG:	Denervation in EDB, tibialis anterior, peronei.
Motor (ADQ):	Prolonged terminal latency. Normal conduction in leg. Normal conduction to AHB.		
Sensory (digit V):	Slowed conduction; decreased CNAP amplitude; normal to digit I.		
F responses (ADQ):	Prolonged.		
EMG:	Denervation in ADQ.		

EDB, extensor digitorum brevis; CMAP, compound muscle action potential; CNAP, compound nerve action potential; ADQ, abductor digiti quinti; AHB, abductor hallucis brevis.

TABLE 15-6   Radiculopathies

EMG finding	Denervation in appropriate segmental paraspinal muscles (early) and limb muscles (later).		
	Root	**Nerve**	**Recorded from**
H reflex	S1	tibial	soleus
F response	If motor root affected, often abnormal in appropriate segmentally innervated muscles; eg:		
	C6	radial	brachioradialis
	C7	radial	extensor indicis proprius
	C8-T1	median	abductor pollicis brevis
		ulnar	abductor digiti minimi
	L3-L4	femoral	vastus medialis
	L5-S1	peroneal	extensor digitorum brevis
	S1	tibial	abductor digiti quinti
SEP finding	If sensory root affected, often abnormal in appropriate segment; e.g.:		
	Root	**Nerve**	**Stimulation at**
	C5	musculocutaneous	nerve
	C6	median	digit I
	C7	median	digits II or III
	C8	ulnar	digit V
	L3	lateral femoral cutaneous	nerve
	L4	saphenous	nerve
	L5	superficial peroneal	nerve
	S1	sural	nerve

Additional information concerning electrodiagnostic testing including single-fiber electromyography is provided in Chap. 30.

REFERENCES

1. Aminoff, M.J., Goodin, D.S., Parry, G.J., Barbaro, N.M., Weinstein, P.R., and Rosenblum, M.L. Electrophysiologic evaluation of lumbosacral radiculopathies. Neurology 35:1514–1518, 1985.

2. Asbury, A.K., and Johnson, P.C. *Pathology of Peripheral Nerve.* Philadelphia, Saunders, 1978.

3. Buchthal, F., Rosenfalck, A., and Behse, F. Sensory potentials of normal and diseased nerves, chap 43, in Dyck, P.J., and Lambert, E.H. (eds): *Peripheral Neuropathy,* 2d ed., vol 1. Philadelphia, Saunders, 1984, pp 981–1015.

4. Cracco, J.B., and Cracco, R.Q. Somatosensory evoked potentials, chap 12 in Goodgold, J., and Eberstein, A. (eds): *Electrodiagnosis of Neuromuscular Diseases,* 3d ed. Baltimore, Williams & Wilkins, 1983, pp 282–304.

5. Dvonch, V., et al. Dermatomal somatosensory evoked potentials: Their use in lumbar radiculopathy. Spine 9:291–293, 1984.

6. Eisen A. Use of lumbar, cervical and scalp-recorded SEP's for diagnosing peripheral nerve lesions, in *Course B: Special Topics in EMG.* American Association of Electromyography and Electrodiagnosis, 1982.

7. Eisen, A., and Hoirch, M. The electrodiagnostic evaluation of spinal root lesions. Spine 8:98–106, 1983.

8. Haldeman, S. The electrodiagnostic evaluation of nerve root function. Spine 9:42–48, 1984.

9. Kimura, J. Electromyography, chaps 12 and 13, in Kimura, J. (ed): *Electrodiagnosis in Diseases of Nerve and Muscle.* Philadelphia, F. A. Davis, 1983, pp 235–282.

10. Ochoa, J., Fowler, T.J., and Gilliatt, R.W. Anatomical changes in peripheral nerves compressed by a pneumatic tourniquet. J Anat 113:433, 1972.

11. Spielholz, N.I., et al. Somatosensory evoked potentials during decompression and stabilization of the spine. Spine 4:500–505, 1979.

12. Shahani, B.T., and Young, R.R. The blink, H, and tonic vibration reflexes, in Goodgold, J., and Eberstein, A. (eds): *Electrodiagnosis of Neuromuscular Diseases,* 3d ed. Williams & Wilkins, Baltimore. pp 263–274, 1983

13. Yiannikas, C. Short latency somatosensory evoked potentials, Chap 7, in Chiappa, K. (ed): *Evoked Potentials in Clinical Medicine.* New York, Raven Press, 1983, pp 271–286.

CHAPTER 16

Properties of Musculoskeletal Tissues and Biomaterials

James Pugh and Roger Dee

SECTION A

Properties of Musculoskeletal Tissues

THE RESPONSE OF MATERIALS TO LOAD

Force Deformation Curves

The application of a force to a material results in finite *deformation* (Fig. 16-1). Deformation is expressed as length in both the International System of Units (SI) and the English systems. The slope of the elastic region of the force deformation curve is the *stiffness* of a material. The *compliance* of a material is the inverse of the stiffness.

Units Relating to Stress and Strain

When a material is loaded in axial tension or compression, the resulting stress is measured by dividing the applied force by the cross-sectional area of the material perpendicular to the applied force. In the SI system, this results in units of newtons per meter squared, which are called pascals (Pa). A newton (N) is that force required to accelerate a mass of 1 kg at a rate of 1 m/s. More commonly, the unit of stress is expressed as newtons per millimeter squared, or megapascals (MPa). In the English system, the corresponding units are pounds per square inch (lb/in.^{2}). Strain, however, is the deformation normalized by the original length of the material. This has the units of length per length in both systems and is therefore dimensionless. Strain is commonly expressed as millimeters per millimeter.

Stress-Strain Curve

The stress-strain curve is useful in comparing the mechanical response of two samples of different geometry, because these curves are normalized to eliminate the effects of sample dimensions. The slope of the elastic portion of the stress-strain curve is *Young's modulus.* Young's modulus necessarily must have the units of stress since strain is dimensionless. Thus in SI the units are gigapascals (GPa) and in English, pounds per square inch.

A material also changes shape in a direction perpendicular to the direction of the applied force. The modulus controlling this deformation is termed *Poisson's ratio* and is the negative ratio of the strain in the direction perpendicular to the direction of the applied force to the strain in the direction of the applied force. Poisson's ratio is usually 0.3 for most materials.

Stress can be either *compressive, tensile,* or *shear.* The shear modulus is computed by division of the shear stress by the angular change in shape of the material specified by radians. Thus the shear modulus has the same units as Young's modulus.

The *rigidity* of a structure is a function of both the material of which the structure is fabricated and the configuration of the specific design. Rigidity is specified as the product of Young's modulus and a quantity called the *area moment of inertia.* The latter is computed by taking an element of area and multiplying it by the square of the distance of that element from the center of rotation of the cross section. This rotation center is also called the *neutral axis,* since about it there exist zero compressive and tensile stresses. The area moment of inertia is specified in the SI system as meters to the fourth power. Another term in use is the *section modulus.* This is not really a modulus at all but the cross section of the material divided by the maximum distance away from the neutral axis and still inside the material. The section modulus has units of meters cubed.

The plastic properties of a material are *yield strength, ultimate strength,* and *fracture strength.* The yield strength is that stress at which the material takes on a permanent deformation as contrasted to an elastic deformation, which is completely recovered upon removal of the load (Figs. 16-1, 16-2). The ultimate strength is the maximum stress sustained by the material, which paradoxically may or may not be the same as the fracture strength, or stress at which the material breaks into at least two pieces. All the strengths are specified in terms of megapascals and pounds per square inch in SI and English units, respectively.

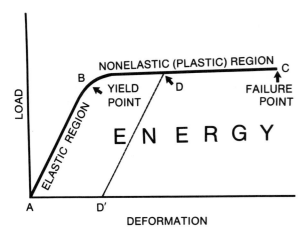

Figure 16-1 Load versus deformation for a ductile material showing the elastic region, the yield point, the plastic region, and the failure point. *A–B* is the elastic region. *B–C* is the plastic region. If the specimen is loaded to point *D* and unloaded, it springs back to point *D'* leaving an amount of permanent deformation *A–D'*. The area under this curve has the units of energy and is termed the *toughness. (From Frankel, V.H., and Nordin, M.: Basic Biomechanics of the Skeletal System. Philadelphia, Lea and Febiger, 1980. Reproduced with permission.)*

Another parameter of significance is the *ductility, or deformability,* of a material. This is the stretch or strain to failure and is the sum total of the amount of elastic stretch and plastic stretch. Ductility is expressed in corresponding units of strain, or as a percentage of the original length, or as actual amount of stretch in meters or inches. A structure which is *brittle* exhibits little deformation before fracture.

The energy or work required to fracture a specimen is given by taking the area under the stress-strain curve. This is termed the *toughness.* The units of toughness are joules per cubic meter or pounds-feet per cubic inch. The actual work required to fracture a specimen must be computed by multiplication of the toughness by the volume of the specimen in cubic meters or cubic inches. The toughest materials have an optimum combination of high yield strength, high fracture strength, and high deformability.

Materials are said to be *purely elastic* if their mechanical response is independent of time or duration of loading. If the mechanical properties of a material change with rate of loading, the material is said to be *viscoelastic.* This means that the material has part elastic (Hookean) and part fluid (Newtonian) properties. Notice that at a high rate of loading, all the mechanical properties are enhanced. The stiffness, yield strength, fracture strength, deformability, and toughness all increase with increase in loading rate. This rate sensitivity of the mechanical properties of materials is especially the case with dynamic loading.

STATICS

Statics is that aspect of mechanics dealing with systems in force and moment equilibrium. The two criteria for static equilibrium are the following: (1) The sum of the forces in any and all directions must equal zero, and (2) the sum of the moments about any and every point must be zero. The first criterion ensures that there are no net forces on the system and that the system is not linearly accelerating. The second criterion ensures that there are no net moments and that the system is not angularly accelerating. Examples of static systems include passive weight bearing, as well as activities occurring over protracted periods of time, such as very slow leg raising, and similar exercises. Even when there is motion, implying nonzero net force and net moment and therefore net linear and angular accelerations, each increment of time can be broken down into quasistatic increments for individual analysis and final summation into the observed action.

The usefulness of static analysis, such as the freebody technique, lies in its potential for predicting the nominal forces, and hence the stresses, on and in the components involved in a structure.[10,13]

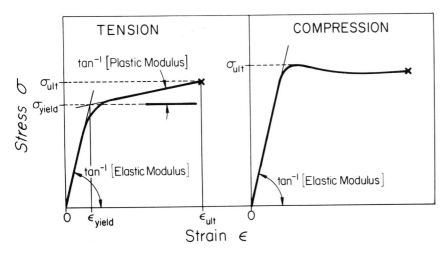

Figure 16-2 Stress-versus-strain curves for human cortical bone specimens tested in tension (*left*) and in compression (*right*). Note that in tension there is a plastic modulus defined as the slope of the curve in the plastic region. *(From Carter, D.R. and Spengler, D.M., Clin Orthop 135:192, 1978. Reproduced with permission.)*

DYNAMICS

Dynamics differs from statics in that there *are* net forces and moments. Dynamics is the study of systems not in static equilibrium. There are net linear accelerations and net angular accelerations.

Dynamics also encompasses systems in which forces are rapidly applied. In contrast to the analysis of static systems, in which loads are applied over periods of approximately 10 min, in the analysis of dynamic systems loads are applied over periods of approximately 1 s or less. Thus, any activity involving rapidly applied loads is a problem in dynamics.

Fatigue situations also fall in the realm of dynamics. Fatigue failures are produced by repeated applications of a load that would not fracture the specimen were it to be applied only once.

BIOMECHANICAL PROPERTIES OF HARD AND SOFT TISSUES

General Tissue Properties

Table 16-1 shows the relative mechanical properties of various tissues. Tendon, ligament, and muscle are relatively weak but exhibit considerable enhancement of properties at dynamic rates of loading. The relative strengths of these tissues shown in Table 16-1 are inversely proportional to their relative efficiency as shock absorbers. Such data are helpful in the analysis of mechanical function and dysfunction.

Bone

Bone is a composite whose mechanical properties are determined by the contributions of collagen fibers and hydroxyapatite crystals and the elusive bond between them.[28] Microstructurally, mature bone is a composite with tissue arranged in an organized pattern and separated by relatively weak interfaces. The pattern of microstructural organization is found to vary with species and age.

Work on isolated haversian systems (slices of single osteons) by Ascenzi and co-workers has shown that a high correlation exists between mechanical properties of a single system and the mechanical properties of the overall compact bone.[1] Black's work addressed the statistical variability of orientation of osteons in diaphyseal bone.[2] When Ascenzi's and Black's work are taken together, an even higher correlation exists between the properties of the component haversian systems and the overall piece of bone. The directional variability of the mechanical properties of bone is also effectively explained by this model. Such variation of properties with direction is termed *anisotropy.*

Since cancellous bone is composed of plates of lamellae bone with cross struts, Wright and co-workers have taken the approach of modeling this structure as a continuum of lamellar bone with a variability of porosity.[29] They found a correlation between mechanical properties and porosity.

Because bone shows viscoelastic behavior, a whole family of stress-strain curves may be produced under different loading conditions (Fig. 16-2).[22] Panjabi and White observed that bone absorbs 67 percent more energy and has 33 percent more torque and torsional deformation and also 5 percent more stiffness when deformed at a high testing rate compared with a low testing rate. Since the energy absorbed is released at failure, the degree of comminution seen in fractures incurred by high-velocity injury is explained by these facts.

Burstein and associates believe that the mechanical properties of cortical bone are consistent with an elastic—perfectly plastic model for the *mineral* phase of bone tissue in which the mineral contributes the major portion of the tension yield strength (Fig. 16-3).[5] The slope, or stiffness, of the plastic region of the stress-strain curve is then a function only of the collagenous matrix, which itself plays a surprisingly minor role in the tension yield strength of bone. These authors suggest that bone mineral behaves in this way because

TABLE 16-1 Tissue Properties

Tissue	Young's modulus, GPa (lb/in^2)	Tensile strength, MPa (lb/in^2)	Compressive strength, MPa (lb/in^2)
Cortical bone			
Femur	17.2 (2.5×10^6)	121 (17,500)	167 (24,200)
Tibia	18.1 (2.6×10^6)	140 (20,300)	159 (23,000)
Fibula	18.6 (2.7×10^6)	146 (21,100)	123 (17,800)
Cancellous bone			
Vertebrae	0.09 (0.013×10^6)	1.2 (174)	1.9 (276)
Distal femur	1.7 (0.25×10^6)	2.0 (290)	3.0 (435)
Tendon	—	53 (7,690)	—
Collagen	0.1 (0.015×10^6)	3000 (43,500)	—
Articular cartilage	0.01 (0.0015×10^6)	3.4 (493)	

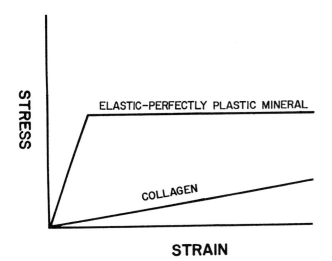

Figure 16-3 Hypothetical curve illustrating elastic–perfectly plastic behavior of the *mineral* phase of cortical bone in tension. The lower curve represents the elastic behavior of collagen. (Compare with Fig. 16-2.) *(From Burstein, A.H., J Bone Joint Surg 57A:956, 1975. Reproduced with permission.)*

multiple cracks occur in the bone when critical stress is reached. These cracks then propagate for a limited distance during plastic deformation, the process continuing until a sufficient amount of strain energy has been put into the material and catastrophic failure then occurs. They point out, however, that for such a model to work the mineral phase has to exhibit this elastic–perfectly plastic behavior only when it is in conjunction with the collagen.

Burstein also showed a decrease in the mechanical properties of cortical bone with decreases in mineral content.[7] This may also explain the decrease in mechanical properties with increasing age, documented by Currey.[11] Sedlin, in an exhaustive study of the effects of various variables on the mechanical properties of bone, examined the effects of fixation, freezing, age, test conditions, and a host of other variables.[24] He found bone to be strongest in compression and weakest in tension.

Burstein has also shown that the mechanical properties of bone seem to vary even between different parts of the lower limb. Their data suggest that femoral tissue undergoes a progressive but slow degradation in mechanical properties with age, with an increase in the slope of the plastic portion of its stress-strain curve. Tibial tissue, on the other hand, does not show this characteristic, and this change may reflect different levels of bone turnover in tibia and femur.[6] On the other hand, both bones show a decrease in ultimate strain in tension of 5 to 7 percent per decade, with associated diminution in the amount of energy absorbed during tensile stress with increasing age. This suggests that ultimate strain is dependent upon some property of bone tissue which decreases in an age-dependent manner.[7]

Compact cortical bone has a porosity of only 5 to 30 percent, whereas the porosity of trabecular bone may range from 30 percent to more than 90 percent.[9] Carter and Hayes believe that the compressive strength of bone is approximately proportional to the apparent density squared, and that this relation is valid for the entire range of bone density in the skeleton from compact bone to trabecular bone.[9] Trabecular bone fails by buckling and bending of the trabeculae and the cross struts that support them. The trabecular bone is surrounded by a shell of compact bone, and this together with the presence of bone marrow enhances the compressive strength of the material. However, the presence of marrow increases the strength modulus and energy absorption of specimens only at a high rate of strain. In specimens without marrow the strength of the material follows the proportionality of the density previously described.[9] Other studies suggest that the cortical shell only provides a modest structural role and, at least in the vertebral body, the role of the central trabeculae is most important in uniaxial compressive loading where there may be a reduction in strength of only 10 percent when the cortex is removed.[14] Because of the relation between vertebral compressive strength and central trabecular density, the authors hope that quantitative computed tomography may be a useful predictor of the risk of vertebral fracture.

A brittle material such as bone fails in tension in a transverse manner. Ductile materials such as metals fail in the plane of maximum shear to produce an oblique fracture. Compression invariably produces oblique shear failures in both ductile and brittle materials.

The application of a torsional force to a cylinder of material builds up significant shear stresses. Torsional forces can be applied to the tibia by a pivoting action on the foot. The shear stresses in a bone under torsional loading are maximal at the periphery of the bone. Bones have a high resistance to bending and torsion largely because the bony material is located where the stresses are highest, at the outer circumference of the shaft.

A bone under torsional loading tends to fail along a plane 45° to the length of the bone (Fig. 16-4). The fracture line tends to spiral around the shaft, which leads to the classification of this as a spiral fracture. The side opposite the spiral shows a component parallel to the long axis of the bone, because the fracture itself must have continuity. An analysis resolving the resulting forces and stresses on the 45° plane reveals that this is invariably a tension plane. The plane parallel to the bone axis is a shear plane. Burstein asserts that torsional fractures begin on this shear plane.[8]

Bone is weakest in tension and shear; strongest in compression. Given a particular loading condition, the fracture occurs in a tension or shear region and on a tension or shear plane. Knowing the orientation of the fracture surface often leads to a deeper understanding of the internal stresses in the bone prior to fracture, and to the possible loading condition leading to that fracture.

The tendency exhibited by bone for enhancement of mechanical properties by rate of loading explains why they can sustain forces higher than their breaking strengths as long as these loads are of short duration. If such loads are sustained, however, a large volume of bone will be loaded in excess of its static breaking strength. When the duration of loading is long enough to create a fracture, there may be so much energy stored in the bone that the fracture is comminuted.

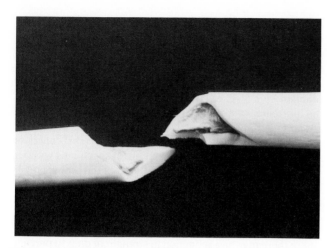

Figure 16-4 Torsional or spiral fracture produced by a twisting of the bone. Note the spiral and the axial components of the fracture.

Fatigue Fractures in Bone

Fatigue failure is failure under cyclic loading. Often this occurs within the apparent elastic limit of a material. The fracture typically begins at a stress concentration such as the junction of the hip nail and the plate, and the crack progresses along a microscopic amount with the application of each cycle of loading.

Fatigue failure is a common mode of failure of components of the human body, since the musculoskeletal system is subjected to many types of cyclic loads of varying magnitude. Morris and Blickenstaff have documented numerous sites of fatigue fractures.[17] Fatigue fractures may occur with osteopenia and in people who lead sedentary lives for a time and then engage in strenuous physical activity. Also, abnormal stresses can be produced in bone by an athlete, especially if there are special circumstances, e.g., imperfect technique or equipment or environmental factors. Possibly the bone cannot remodel in time to be able to repair fatigue damage, and failure occurs. Common sites are the second metatarsal, the lower fibula, and the tibial shaft.

Fatigue fracture data in the laboratory are generally plotted as stress versus cycles to failure, or force applied versus cycles to failure. The higher the force, the shorter the life expectancy (or cycles to fatigue failure).

Some materials exhibit what is known as an *endurance limit*. This is a load below which the material can be expected to withstand an unlimited number of cycles without failure.

Bone tested in the laboratory ex vivo shows no endurance limit. Failure always occurs after a sufficient number of cycles.

Ligament and Tendon

Polymeric materials, of which collagenous materials constitute a subgroup, can be generally characterized by their de-

gree of viscoelasticity or degree of rate dependence of their mechanical properties. As a rule, materials with a higher fluid content, higher polymer fraction, and lower stiffness exhibit a greater rate dependence of mechanical properties. This is especially germane for ligaments and tendons.

It is appropriate in this regard to refer to the work of Noyes, DeLucas, and Torvik, who showed that ligaments exhibit less of a strain-rate hardening (enhancement of properties) than bone.[21] Theoretically, one would expect the opposite. In fact, Noyes's experiments showed that at moderate strain rates, ligament-bone preparations fail at the bony insertion. At rates 100 times higher, the ligaments predominantly fail. This implies a higher strain-rate dependence of the mechanical properties of bone relative to that of ligaments. The bone, at the attachment, becomes stronger relative to the ligaments at the higher strain rates.

In bone, the collagen is already organized in a direction roughly parallel to the direction of tension loading. In the relaxed ligament, the collagen fibers are slightly crimped (see Chap. 6). On application of a load, the collagen fibers tend to align. An interpretation of Noyes's experiments is that the collagen of the ligaments does not align as well at high strain rates as at low rates. This fact compromises its mechanical properties and its resistance to failure at the highest strain rates.

Data typical of that obtained by Noyes and co-workers is shown in Fig. 16-5. The fracture strength, toughness, and ductility are all enhanced by a 100-fold increase in rate of loading. Tendon shows a similar behavior.

Another phenomenon exhibited by the softer polymeric materials such as tendon and ligament is *viscoelastic creep*. This is a tendency for the material under load to show an increasing deformation which is time-dependent. Upon application of the initial load, there is some immediate lengthening, followed by a gradual elongation with time. When the load is removed, there is an immediate snapback, followed by a time-dependent recovery of the lengthening produced by the load.

Stress relaxation is another manifestation of the time dependence of the properties of viscoelastic materials (Fig. 16-6). It is similar to creep and also occurs by time-dependent deformation after stretching a material to a fixed deformation. The stress gradually drops off with time, since the material is elongating with time. Stress relaxation is sometimes disadvantageous, e.g., with synthetic polymeric ligaments. Prestretching a synthetic ligament prior to insertion seems to control this stress relaxation to some degree by aligning the polymeric chains in the direction of applied load.

Articular Cartilage

Typical viscoelastic behavior of articular cartilage is shown in Fig. 16-6. Cartilage does show a time-dependent deformation, which is thought by Torzilli to be due to escape of the aqueous component from the cartilage matrix.[26] This is thought by Mow to be essential to the lubrication process, insofar as

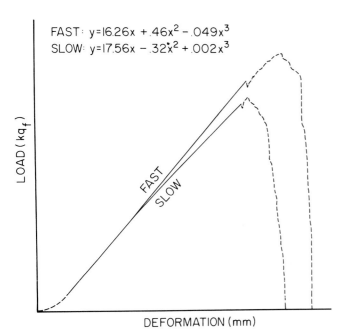

$$\text{FAST}: \quad y = 16.26x + .46x^2 - .049x^3$$
$$\text{SLOW}: \quad y = 17.56x - .32x^2 + .002x^3$$

Figure 16-5 Typical ligament data for 17 knees tested at fast and slow rates of load deformation. The knees had been dissected to allow loading of the anterior cruciate ligament in a physiological direction. Note the difference in properties with a 100-fold difference in loading rate. *(From Noyes, F.R., DeLucas, J.L., and Torvik, P.J., J Bone Joint Surg 56A:241, 1974. Reproduced with permission.)*

such a mechanism is capable of providing an almost constant supply of lubricant to the opposing surfaces in a joint.[18]

The materials of which joints are composed all increase in stiffness as the distance from the cartilage surface increases. The cartilage itself increases in stiffness in proximity to the compact underlying bone called the subchondral plate. The stiffness in the subchondral region is then relatively constant, but higher than in the deepest region of the articular cartilage. Finally, the compact cortical bone has the highest stiffness of any of the joint materials.

With increasing load the actual contact area of cartilage on cartilage is increased. This increasing congruity is an example of a variable surface bearing with functional advantages provided by the stiffness of the material. Increasing the load further causes subsequent bone deformation up to and through the point of failure. The cartilage-bone assembly thus provides an important shock-absorbing function around the joint.

In certain disease states, the effects of this shock absorption are diminished. In osteoarthritis, the Young's modulus of the cartilage is reduced from the normal value and the bone in the subchondral region is stiffer. Changes in these values alter the functioning of the joint.

SECTION B

Properties of Orthopaedic Materials

Over the years, several materials have been accepted for manufacture of components of total joint replacements. These are shown in Tables 16-2 and 16-3 along with their mechanical properties.[2,10,19,28,33,38,40]

Generally, orthopaedic materials can be classified into three groups: metals, ceramics, and polymers. Metals consist of metallically bonded atoms and are characterized by opac-

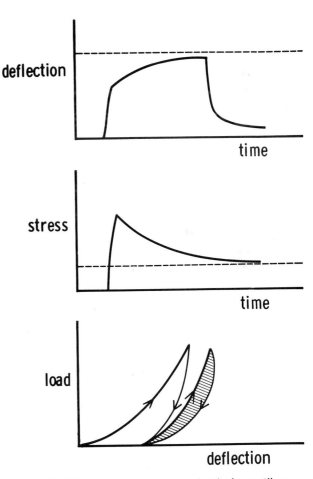

Figure 16-6 Viscoelastic functioning of articular cartilage showing (*top to bottom*) creep, stress relaxation, and hysteresis during cyclic loading. The phenomenon of hysteresis is the absorption of energy when subjected to temporary loading. Repetitive loading may diminish the hysteresis, diminishing shock absorption ability of the material (bottom graph). *(From Walker, P.S., in Resnick, D., and Niwayama, G. eds: Diagnosis of Bone and Joint Disorders with Emphasis on Articular Abnormalities. Philadelphia, Saunders, 1981.)*

TABLE 16-2 **Properties of Orthopaedic Materials**

Material	Tensile strength, MPa (lb/in^2)	Ductility %	Young's Modulus, GPa (lb/in^2)	Fatigue Strength, MPa (lb/in^2)
316L stainless steel, annealed	650 (94,000)	45	211 (30 × 10)	280 (41,000)
316 stainless steel, cold-worked	1000 (145,000)	9	230 (33 × 10)	300 (43,500)
Wrought Co-Cr	1540 (223,000)	9	240 (35 × 10)	490 (71,000)
Cast Co-Cr	690 (100,000)	—	240 (35 × 10)	300 (43,500)
MP 35N	1670 (242,000)	13	240 (35 × 10)	—
Ti-6Al-4V	1000 (145,000)	12	120 (17 × 10)	617 (89,500)
Ceramic (Al$_2$O$_3$)	270 (40,000)	0	350 (50 × 10)	—

ity, strength, ductility, electrical conductivity, and rigidity. Ceramics are aggregates of ionically bonded metal and non-metal atoms having the characteristics of opacity, strength, brittleness, electrical resistance, and rigidity. Polymers are aggregates of covalently bonded atoms arranged into long chains having the properties of radiolucency, weakness, ductility, electrical resistance, and compliance. Composites offer the mixing of the best properties of metals, ceramics, and polymers into a configuration more supportive of an intended function than a single-component device.

TYPE 316L STAINLESS STEEL

Of the metals available for implantation, Type 316L stainless steel has shown a notable susceptibility for crevice corrosion that has limited its current applications to those devices such as bone plates that are intended for removal after serving their function.[17,20,32] Type 316L stainless steel is not considered a superalloy (Table 16-3) since its yield strength is less than 1000 MPa in most configurations.

Despite a generally very high resistance to corrosion, stainless steels are notably subject to crevice, pitting, intergranular, and stress corrosion. All these processes can severely degrade the mechanical properties of the alloy.

Type 316L stainless steel has the following chemical composition: 17 to 20 percent chromium, 1 to 14 percent nickel, 2 to 4 percent molybdenum, 0.08 percent carbon maxi-

mum, 2 percent manganese maximum, 0.75 percent silicon maximum, and the balance iron.

The advantages of the use of Type 316L stainless steel are economy and ease of fabrication. The material is quite ductile and can be worked easily without cracking. In addition, it easily takes a high polish of the type required on femoral heads. In the annealed condition, the material is quite ductile but of lowest strength. In the cold-worked condition, an amount of ductility is sacrificed to increase the yield strength.

COBALT ALLOYS

Cast Cobalt-Chromium

The specifications for cast cobalt-chromium alloy call for 27 to 30 percent chromium, 5 to 7 percent molybdenum, 0.35 percent carbon maximum, and the balance cobalt. Cobalt alloys have a notable advantage over stainless steels in their increased resistance to corrosion, particularly crevice corrosion. This alloy is not regarded as a superalloy, since its yield strength is less than 1000 MPa.

The mechanical properties of this alloy are improved by subjecting the final products to a combination of high temperature and high pressure. This technique is known as hot isostatic pressing (HIP) and results in implants with a clean, void-free microstructure and increased resistance to breakage, notably by fatigue mechanisms.

TABLE 16-3 **Compromise in Fatigue Strengths of Superalloys**

Alloy	Condition	Fatigue strength, MPa (lb/in^2)
Co-Cr	Solution treated	250 (36,000)
Co-Cr	Sintered (porous coated)	175 (25,000)
Ti-Al-V	Solution treated	617 (89,000)
Ti-Al-V	Sinter annealed	377 (55,000)
Ti-Al-V	ST and notched	230 (33,000)
Ti-Al-V	Sintered (porous coated)	138 (20,000)

Wrought Cobalt-Chromium

Wrought cobalt-chromium alloy has a composition of 19 percent to 21 percent chromium, 14 percent to 16 percent tungsten, 9 percent to 11 percent nickel, 0.05 percent to 0.15 percent carbon, and the balance cobalt. Like stainless steel, this alloy can be cold-worked without cracking. It also offers superior resistance to crevice corrosion.

TITANIUM AND ITS ALLOYS

Titanium and titanium-based alloys offer superior biocompatibility and corrosion resistance when compared with either stainless steel or cobalt-based alloys. It can be worked to increase its yield strength.

The alloy specifications for titanium-aluminum-vanadium (Ti-6Al-4V) are as follows: 5.5 percent to 6.5 percent aluminum, 3.5 percent to 4.5 percent vanadium, 0.25 percent iron maximum, 0.05 percent nitrogen maximum, 0.08 percent iron maximum, 0.0125 percent hydrogen maximum, 0.1 percent other impurities maximum, and the balance titanium.

Titanium and its alloys offer a modulus of elasticity roughly one third that of the stainless steels and cobalt-based alloys. This lower modulus offers the potential for reduced stress shielding of the surrounding bone, since the metal carries a smaller fraction of the load due to its reduced modulus.

SUPERALLOYS

Only wrought cobalt-chromium, MP35N, and Ti-6Al-4V are considered to be superalloys, in view of their tensile strength (Table 16-2) and resistance to corrosion. It is for this reason that most metallic components of total joint replacements are now fabricated of one of these three alloys.

Unfortunately, when porous coatings are applied to these superalloys, the mechanical properties, most notably the fatigue strength, are compromised, as shown in Table 16-3.[33] It is arguably worth the compromise in mechanical properties to increase the propensity for direct biological locking. Plasma coatings, on the other hand, if carefully applied, offer the opportunity to increase surface roughness conducive to bone ingrowth without significant compromise in mechanical properties since the base metal is heated for only a very short length of time.[27]

CORROSION

With the introduction of the superalloys listed in Table 16-3, the problems of metallic corrosion in the body disappeared. Nevertheless, the superalloys have a finite dissolution rate. There is increasing concern about the formation of ill-characterized metalloproteins and the role these complexes play in mutagenesis and carcinogenesis.

Of all the alloys listed in Table 16-2, Type 316L stainless steel suffers the greatest rate of corrosion in the body. It is notably susceptible to crevice corrosion, which is an electrochemical cell set up between regions of a device that are oxygen-deficient relative to those areas exposed to a higher oxygen potential.[5,9] The oxygen-deficient region is anodic relative to the higher-oxygen cathodic region. The anode undergoes an oxidation reaction of the type productive of metallic ions. The cathode undergoes a reduction reaction of the form productive of the formation of hydroxyl ions. The presence of an active infection can accelerate the process by changing oxygen concentrations and the local pH. Typical crevices are scratches on the surface of an implant, the interface between bone and an implant, the cement-metal interface, and any other sharp interface likely to be depleted of oxygen relative to another oxygenated area.

Documented cases of galvanic corrosion have occurred with the use of dissimilar metals in the human body.[37,42] Such a cell is set up when two devices fabricated of different metals are in electrical contact. They must actually be touching for this to occur. The more active metal corrodes, i.e., stainless steel when touching a cobalt-chromium alloy. For this reason, cobalt-chromium wires and screws must be used with implants of this alloy.

Galvanic effects do not seem to be of significance in combinations of cobalt-chromium and Ti-6Al-4V alloy.[42] The wear properties of titanium-based material against polyethylene are not as good as those of cobalt-chromium against polyethylene. However, the mechanical properties and biocompatibility of titanium-based alloy are superior. Therefore, titanium-based implants often have a cobalt-chromium component where they articulate with polyethylene. Such is the case with titanium alloy total hip prostheses. The stem is Ti-6Al-4V and the head is cobalt-chromium. Galvanic corrosion does not occur due to the specific electrochemical characteristics of the two alloys.

The third basic type of corrosion is produced by differences in ion concentration and is likely to occur as a result of prior crevice corrosion.[9] Where a crevice is liberating ions into surrounding tissue, a concentration gradient of ionic material builds up. Eventually, the areas away from the highest concentration of ions will become anodic and corrode. A metallic device in a concentration gradient of its own ions invariably corrodes in the region relatively depleted of ions. Again, perturbations in local pH and oxygen affect this type of corrosion.

CERAMICS

The only ceramic of significant use in orthopaedics is aluminum oxide (Al_2O_3). Since this is a compound, the proportions of aluminum and oxygen are fixed 2:3 by the stoichiometry. Aluminum oxide is highly biocompatible and very strong.

The chief disadvantage of aluminum oxide is its extreme brittleness (Table 16-2). When overloaded, the material tends to fragment. This does not preclude its application as thin coatings on metallic substrates. Ceramic does offer a notable biocompatibility advantage over metallic components.[3,14,16]

Ceramic-on-ceramic bearing surfaces have a low coeffi-

TABLE 16-4 Properties of Solid Polymeric Materials

Material	Modulus, GPa (lb/in²)	Tensile strength, MPa (lb/in²)	Ductility, %	Fatigue strength, MPa (lb/in²)
Polyethylene	0.15 (21,800)	30 (4,350)	800	9 (1,300)
Polymethylmethacrylate	3 (435,000)	70 (10,150)	5	22 (3,190)
Polysulfone	2.3 (334,000)	65 (9,430)	75	4 (500)
Silicone rubber	0.01 (1,450)	5 (730)	600	—

cient of friction. However, they do exhibit wear in excess of what one would predict based solely on friction.

POLYMERS

Table 16-4 lists the mechanical properties of the major polymeric materials that have significant applications in orthopaedics.[2,19,29,38,40] A comparison of the fatigue strengths with those of the metals in Table 16-2 shows the major drawback to the use of polymers in the body—they do not stand up readily to cyclic loads.

Polyethylene

Polyethylene falls into the classification of a polyvinyl, with the basic structure

$$-(-CH_2-CH_2-)_n$$

It is generally used as the polymeric component articulating with a polished metallic counterface.

The density of commercially available polyethylene varies from 0.92 g/cm^3 to 0.98 g/cm^3. The former is termed a *low-density polyethylene* and the latter a *high-density polyethylene.* Because of the way a long-chain molecule packs itself into a given volume, the higher-molecular-weight polymer actually has a lower density than the lower-molecular-weight materials.

Ultrahigh-molecular-weight polyethylene has evolved as a material of choice in most total joint prostheses. High molecular weight is necessary for wear resistance. When the molecular weight of polyethylene is compromised, as with deficient manufacturing procedures, or when an abrasive foreign body such as fragmented polymethylmethacrylate bone cement becomes lodged in the joint, significant wear (three-body wears) occurs.

Clinical and experimental data have confirmed that the major mode of shape change in polyethylene components is through *cold flow.*[35] The cold flow (i.e., creep rate) of the polyethylene is effectively controlled by metallic backings to give a rigid encapsulation to the relatively lower modulus plastic.[1,10,17] The coefficient of friction of metal on polyethylene is 0.01 as opposed to 0.1 for metal-on-metal bearings.

Polysulfone

Polysulfone has the structure

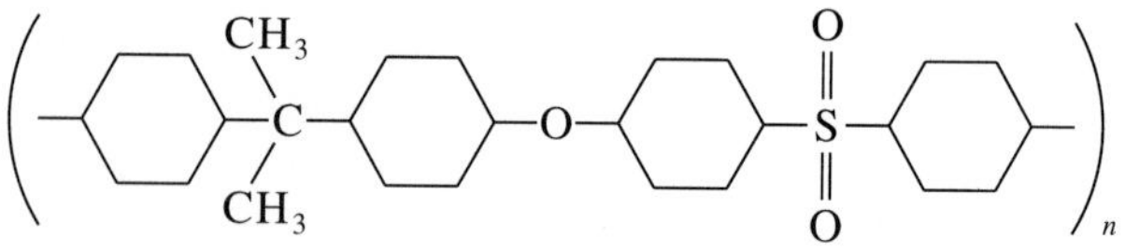

As a biomaterial, it is currently used in a porous configuration as a coating for metallic substrates such as total hip prostheses. It is thought that porous polymers, because of their low moduli of elasticity, reduce the deleterious effects of stress shielding.

Silicone Rubber

Silicones are also known as *polysiloxanes* and are characterized by a backbone consisting of silicon and oxygen atoms. They have the following structure:

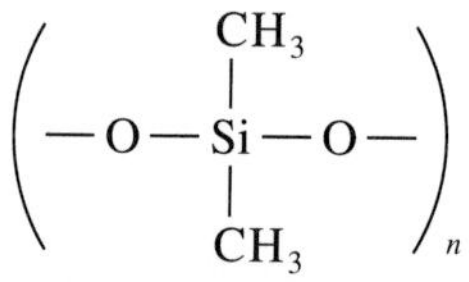

The silicone rubbers are highly resilient materials. They are used as finger joint prostheses and wrist spacers, and for smaller bone replacements. They have a tendency to degrade in situ.[19,32,34]

Polymethylmethacrylate (PMMA)

PMMA is in the class termed *vinylidene* and has the structure

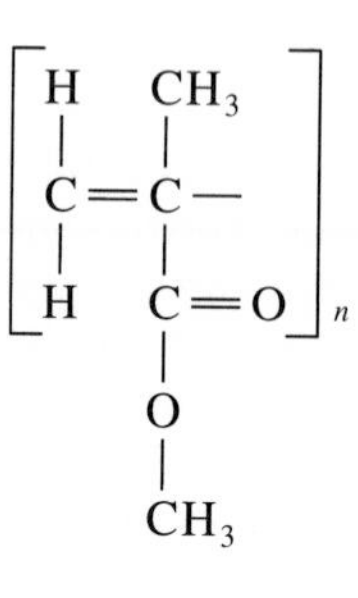

As acrylic bone cement, it comes as a two-part system. The liquid is methylmethacrylate monomer with a polymerization inhibitor such as hydroquinone. The powder is a mixture of beads of PMMA and polystyrene (which has a structure similar to that of polyethylene except that a benzene ring replaces one of the hydrogen atoms), flakes of both polymers, and barium sulfate added for radiopacity.

PMMA is a brittle material with a compromised fatigue strength. It has no inherent bonding capacity to bone or any other material. As such, it is used as a grout rather than as a glue. Bonding occurs by interdigitation. Thus, a roughened surface must be used in conjunction with PMMA bone cement.

Two major disadvantages of PMMA are obvious from the data in Table 16-4. It possesses low ductility relative to other polymers and metals, and low fatigue strength compared with that of metals. Thus, in the interface of a metallic device with acrylic bone cement fatigue failure of the acrylic is likely before any gross damage occurs to the metallic component. Efforts to increase its resistance to fatigue have resulted in improvements in its performance. These include vacuum mixing,[24] centrifugation prior to insertion, and pneumatic syringes and pressurization techniques.[4,6,30,31] Precoats of cement on the prosthesis and alloying the cement with another material have also shown beneficial effects.[18] Nevertheless, in total joints fixed with acrylic, the first evidence of failure is fatigue fracture of the acrylic. This is usually accompanied by resorption of bone around the acrylic mantle.

LOOSENING OF CEMENTED IMPLANTS

Newer techniques of handling acrylic cement in the operating room have reduced the incidence of short-term failure due to areas of inadequate thickness of the cement mantle or lamination, the inadvertent production of voids due to mixing with air and blood, and imperfect penetration of the cement into the interstices of bone. Despite these advances, however, and more meticulous preparation of the bone, long-term studies reveal a high incidence of radiolucent lines progressing to clinical loosening, an incidence which appears to increase with time after surgery.[18] Acetabular loosening occurring late has been a significant problem in the young patient undergoing arthroplasty. In this category of patients, one in four patients may require revision within a decade due to acetabular loosening. The incidence of femoral component lucency may be up to 70 percent in some series.[21] Using PMMA at revision surgery has also revealed the inadequacies of this method of fixation. Even when competent revision surgery is performed for what is considered a technically inadequate first operation exhibiting an inadequate cement technique, the failure rate is unacceptable.[8,22]

In some cases the cause of the loosening can be related to a technically unacceptable operation such as the insertion of a femoral component in varus or the acetabular component too lateral or too superior. The cement mantle will similarly fail if the joint design is unsatisfactory and generates unacceptable stresses. Examples are the earlier use of fully constrained cemented hinge joints, now a thing of the past

except under the most exceptional circumstances, and the use of high-friction metal-metal bearings.[43,44,45] There is still disagreement on whether loosening is primarily a mechanically initiated event or whether biological factors are responsible. Most authors believe that aseptic loosening is mechanically initiated but that the progress of loosening is then influenced by biological events.[23] The membrane present at the cement-bone interface in the loose implant has the histological and histochemical characteristics of synovial-like lining. Macrophages predominate, and this tissue has the capacity to generate prostaglandin E_2 and collagenase, which may then produce the progressive bone lysis.[15] It has also been suggested that the macrophages may become activated in response to wear particles and that clinical loosening is then primarily due to wear debris concentrating at the interface.[34]

The cement-bone interface may also fail because of significant stress shielding of the surrounding bone, which stimulates its resorption. The resulting loss of support for the cement produces fatigue failure in the mantle associated with subsidence and the development of hoop stresses. A different method of failure associated with fatigue of the cancellous bone a distance away from the cement-bone interface has also been documented.[36] This type of failure is particularly likely if there are significant amounts of cancellous bone remaining after preparation to receive cement.

Failure at the implant-cement interface may also be an initiating factor causing subsequent failure at the cement-bone interface. Once the implant-cement interface degrades, significant stresses are placed upon the cement mantle and failure is then likely. Recently implants have become available precoated with PMMA to reduce the likelihood of this mode of failure. Their introduction has also brought into consideration design modifications of implants and instruments which may be necessary to overcome any problems.

Metal backings applied to polyethylene components have contributed to a reduction in the incidence of loosening for reasons already given.[1,11,17,26]

UNCEMENTED PROSTHESES

There is a new generation of prostheses with special surfaces to allow biological locking of the prosthesis into the bony substrate. The introduction of porous surfaces may overcome some of the problems associated with the use of PMMA. The first generation of porous implants showed bony ingrowth only over about 20 percent of the available porous surface. Current designs have restricted the area of porous surface available to strategic areas. These take into account the mode of load transmission and the possibility that the implant will have to be removed.[13] Any pore size in the range of 50 to 500 μm is essentially equivalent with regard to ingrowth rate and bone-implant interface strength.[13] Direct bone apposition to the implant with an approximately 100-nm-thick glycoprotein monolayer is observed at the interface.[23] Ingrowth seems to occur whether the implant is situated adjacent to cancellous or cortical bone.[13] It is important that the implant be sufficiently stabilized at the time of surgery to eliminate or minimize micromotion at the interface, so a press fit is preferred.

The design of the component is of great importance in this situation where stress shielding may be much more important than with cemented implants. The ultimate success of these implants depends on the pattern of bone remodeling. Additional concerns are metal toxicity relating to the release of cobalt and chromium ions in chrome-cobalt alloy implants and the metal corrosion which seems to be a concern with fiber metal-coated titanium implants.[23]

Porous Sintered Coatings

Porous sintered coatings consist of fine titanium or cobalt chrome beads that have been sintered (a high-temperature diffusion bonding process) to produce a layer of metal into which bone grows and locks the prosthesis firmly in place. A wide variety of bead sizes and other parameters are associated with these prostheses, but there is general agreement that the pore size optimum for bone ingrowth lies in the range of 50 to 500 μm.[13]

Plasma Spray Coatings

These prostheses have a surface of a specific roughness applied by a plasma (a stream of ionized particles at a very high temperature, usually produced by ionizing argon with an electric arc under high vacuum).[27] This surface differs from the porous coatings in that it consists of only a specific roughness rather than a true porous coating. Such a roughened surface is believed to offer fixation mechanically comparable to that of the porous coatings. Plasma coating requires expertise in its application, as do sintered porous coatings, and is extremely unforgiving of uncontrolled variables such as temperature, time, and cooling rates to room temperature from the plasma or sintering temperature. Metals, ceramics, and polymers can be plasma-sprayed.

Low-Modulus Coatings

Low-modulus coatings include porous polyethylene and porous polysulfone.[12] The low-modulus coatings may be plasma sprayed, or they can be bonded by adhesives or mechanical interlock. Low-modulus coatings offer a mechanical buffer zone between the high-modulus metal and the high-but-lower-modulus bone and in theory could promote supportive bone growth. These coatings, however, are often mechanically insufficient to support fixation.

Screw Threads

Some acetabular prosthetic components are designed with screw-thread fixation. These devices function well, but such designs may not be suitable for long-term fixation.

Press Fit

These prostheses often resemble the conventional cemented prostheses, but the intent is to accurately machine the bony bed and to simply press the prosthesis in place. Fixation relies primarily on generating an appropriate mechanical environment for the remaining bone to functionally adapt to the press-fit prosthesis. Usually such prostheses have macroscopic surface structure to assist with this.

Combinations

The technology has been developed to the point that it is possible to combine porous and screw configurations in a single component, perhaps offering the advantages of both systems. Press-fit and plasma or porous configurations can also be combined. This may lead to improved longevity of such devices.

REFERENCES

Section A: Properties of Musculoskeletal Tissues

1. Ascenzi, A., and Bonucci, E. Mechanical similarities between alternate osteons and cross-ply laminates. J Biomech 9:65-71, 1976.
2. Black, J., Mattson, R., and Korostoff, E. Haversian osteons: Size, distribution, internal structure, and orientation. J Biomed Mater Res 8:299-319, 1974.
3. Bu Park, Joon. *Biomaterials, an Introduction.* New York, Plenum Press, 1979.
4. Burstein, A.H., and Frankel, V.H. A standard test for laboratory animal bone. J Biomech 4:155-158, 1971.
5. Burstein, A.H., Currey, J.D., Frankel, V.H., and Reilly, D.T. The ultimate properties of bone tissue: The effects of yielding. J Biomech 5:35-44, 1972.
6. Burstein, A.H., Zika, J.M., Heiple, K.G., and Klein, L. Contribution of collagen and mineral to the elastic-plastic properties of bone. J Bone Joint Surg 57A:956-960, 1975.
7. Burstein, A.H., Reilly, D.T., and Martens, M. Aging of bone tissue: Mechanical properties. J Bone Joint Surg 58A:82–86, 1976.
8. Burstein, A.H., Reilly, D.T., and Frankel, V.H. Failure characteristics of bone and bone tissue, in Kennedi, R.M. (ed): *Perspectives in Biomedical Engineering.* Baltimore, University Park Press, 1973, pp 131–134.
9. Carter, D.R., and Hayes, W.C. The compressive behavior of bone as a two phase porous structure. J Bone Jt Surg 59A:954–961, 1977.
10. Crandall, S.H., and Dahl, N.O. *An Introduction to the Mechanics of Solids.* New York, McGraw-Hill, 1959.
11. Currey, J.D. The mechanical properties of bone. Clin Orthop 73:210-231, 1970.
12. Eisenberg, S.R., and Grodzinsky, A.J. Swelling of articular cartilage and other connective tissues: electromechanochemical forces. J Orthop Res 3:148–159, 1985.
13. Frankel, V.H., and Nordin, M. *Basic Biomechanics of the Skeletal System.* Philadelphia, Lea & Febiger, 1980.
14. McBroom, R.J., Hayes, W.C., Edwards, W.T., Goldberg, R.P., and White, A.A. Prediction of vertebral body compressive fracture using quantitative computed tomography. J Bone Joint Surg 67A1206–1213, 1983.

15. McCutchen, C.W. Joint lubrication. Bull Hosp Jt Dis Orthop Inst 43:118–129, 1983.

16. McCutchen, C.W. A note on weeping lubrication, in Kennedi, R.M. (ed): *Perspectives in Biomedical Engineering.* Baltimore, University Park Press, 1974, pp 109–110.

17. Morris, J.M., and Blickenstaff, L.D. *Fatigue Fractures—A Clinical Study.* Springfield, Illinois, Charles C Thomas, 1967.

18. Mow, V.C., Holmes, M.H., and Lai, W.M. Fluid transport and mechanical properties of articular cartilage: A review. J Biomech 17:377–394, 1984.

19. Muir, I.H.M. The chemistry of the ground substance of joint cartilage, in Sokoloff, L. (ed): *The Joints and Synovial Fluid,* vol 2. New York, Academic Press, 1980, pp 27–94.

20. Muir, I.H.M. A molecular approach to the understanding of osteoarthrosis. Ann Rheum Dis 36:199–208, 1977.

21. Noyes, F.R., DeLucas, J.L., and Torvik, P.J. Biomechanics of anterior cruciate ligament failure: An analysis of strain-rate sensitivity and mechanisms of failure in primates. J Bone Joint Surg 56A:236–253, 1974.

22. Panjabi, M.M., and White, A.A. Mechanical properties of bone as a function of rate of deformation. J Bone Joint Surg 55A:322–330, 1973.

23. Reilly, D.T., and Burstein, A.H. The mechanical properties of cortical bone. J Bone Joint Surg. 56A:1001, 1974.

24. Sedlin, E. A rheological model for cortical bone. A study of the physical properties of human femoral samples. Acta Orthop Scand 36 (Suppl 83), 1965.

25. Sokoloff, L. Elasticity of articular cartilage: Effects of ions and viscous solutions. Science 141:1055–1057, 1963.

26. Torzilli, P.A., Rose, D.E., and Dethemers, D.A. Equilibrium water partition in articular cartilage. Biorheology 19:519–537, 1982.

27. Voloshin, A., and Wosk, J. An in vivo study of low back pain and shock absorption in the human locomotor system. J Biomech 15:21–27, 1982.

28. Wright, T.M., and Carter, D.R. Macroscopic directionality in bone, in Ducheyne, P., and Hastings, G.W. (eds): *Functional Behavior of Orthopaedic Biomaterials,* vol 1: *Fundamentals.* Boca Raton, Florida, CRC Press, 1984, pp 38–49.

29. Wright, T.M., and Hayes, W.C. Tensile testing of bone over a wide range of strain rates: Effects of strain rate, microstructure, and density. Med Biol Eng 14:671–680, 1976.

Section B: Properties of Orthopaedic Materials

1. Baxtel, D.L. Effect of metal backing on stresses in polyethylene acetabular components. Hip 229–239, 1983.

2. Bement, A.I. (ed): *Biomaterials.* Seattle, University of Washington Press, 1971.

3. Blencke, B.A., Bromer, H., and Deutscher, K.K. Compatibility and long-term stability of glass-ceramic implants. J Biomed Mater Res 12:307–316, 1978.

4. Bourne, R.B., Oh, I., and Harris, W.H. Femoral cement pressurization during total hip arthroplasty: The role of different femoral stems with reference to stem size and shape. Clin Orthop 183:12–16, 1984.

5. Brown, S.A., and Simpson, J.P. Crevice and fretting corrosion of stainless steel plates and screws. J Biomed Mater Res 15:867–878, 1981.

6. Burke, D.W., Gates, E.I., and Harris, W.H. Centrifugation as a method of improving tensile and fatigue properties of acrylic bone cement. J Bone Joint Surg 66A:1265–1273, 1984.

7. Cahoon, J.R., Jr., and Holte, R.N. Corrosion fatigue of surgical stainless steel in synthetic physiological solution. J Biomed Mater Res 15:137–146, 1981.

8. Callaghan, J.J., Salvati, E.A., Pellicci, M.D., Wilson, P.D., Jr., and Ranawat, C.S. Results of revision for mechanical failure after cemented total hip replacement (1979–1982). J Bone Joint Surg 67A:1074–1085, 1985.

9. Cohen, J., and Wulff, J. Clinical failure caused by corrosion of a Vitallium plate: Case report, new testing methods for crevice corrosion, and new techniques for fashioning cobalt chromium alloys to be used in surgical implants. J Bone Joint Surg 54A:617–628, 1972.

10. Cook, S.D., Georgette, F.S., Skinner, H.B., and Haddad, R.J. Fatigue properties of carbon-and porous-coated Ti-6Al-4V alloy. J Biomed Mater Res 18:467–512, 1984.

11. Crowninshield, R.D. Analytical support for acetabular component metal backings. Hip 207–215, 1983

12. Ducheyne, P., and Hastings, G.W. (eds) *Functional Behavior of Orthopaedic Biomaterials,* vols I and II. Baca Raton, Florida, CRC Press, 1984.

13. Engh, C.A., and Bobyn, J.D. *Biological Fixation in Total Hip Arthroplasty.* Thorofare, New Jersey, Slack Incorporated Publishers, 1985.

14. Gibbons, D.F. Biocompatibility of Macor glass ceramic. J Biomed Mater Res 14:177–180, 1980.

15. Goldring, S.R., Schiller, A.L., Roelke, M., Rourke, C.M., O'Neill, D.A., and Harris, W.H. The synovial-like membrane at the bone cement interface in loose total hip replacements and its proposed role in bone lysis. J Bone Joint Surg 65A:575–583, 1983.

16. Harms, J., and Mausle, E. Tissue reaction to ceramic implant material. J Biomed Mater Res 13:67–88, 1979.

17. Harris, W.H. Advances in total hip arthroplasty: The metal-backed acetabular component. Clin Orthop Rel Res 183:4–11, 1984.

18. Harris, W.H. Quoted in Lewis, J.L., and Gallante, J.O.: Workshop on the Bone-Joint Interface. J Orthop Res 3:380–386, 1985.

19. Hertzberg, R.W., and Manson, J.A. *Fatigue of Engineering Plastics.* New York, Academic Press, 1980.

20. Hierholzer, S., Hierholzer, G., Sauer, K.H., and Paterson, R.S. Increased corrosion of stainless steel implants in infected plated fractures Arch Orthop Trauma Surg 102:198–200, 1984.

21. Kaufer, H., et al. Symposium lower extremities joint reconstruction in very young patients. Contemp Orthop 12:79–108, 1986.

22. Kavanaugh, B.F., et al. Revision total hip arthroplasty. J Bone Joint Surg 67A:517–526, 1985.

23. Lewis, J.L., and Galante, J.O. Workshop on bone-joint implant interface. J Orthop Res 3:380–386, 1985.

24. Lidgren, L., Drar, H., and Miller, J. Strength of polymethylmethacrylate increased by vacuum mixing. Acta Orthop Scand 55:536–541, 1984.

25. Lim, W.T., Landrum, K., and Weinberger, B. Silicone lymphadenitis secondary to implant degeneration. J Foot Surg 22:243–246, 1983.

26. Mattingly, D.A., Hopson, C.N., Kahn, A., and Giannestras, N.J. Aseptic loosening in metal-backed acetabular components for total hip replacement: A minimum five-year follow-up. J Bone Joint Surg 67A:387–391, 1985.

27. Mayer, C.A. Thermal spray coating—A money-saving technology. Weld Design Fabrication 66–79, February 1982.

28. Mears, D.C. *Materials in Orthopaedic Surgery,* vol 1. Baltimore, Williams & Wilkins, 1972, 64–112.

29. Neville, H.L.L.K. *Handbook of Biomedical Plastics.* Pasadena, California, Pasadena Technology Press, 1971.

30. Oh, I., Merckx, D.B., and Harris, W.H. Acetabular cement compactor: An experimental study of pressurization of cement in the acetabulum in total hip arthroplasty. Clin Orthop 177:289–293, 1983.

31. Panjabi, M.M., Goel, V.K., Drinker, H., Wong, J., Kamire, G., and Walter, S.D. Effect of pressurization on methylmethacrylate-bone interdigitation: An in vitro study of canine femora. J Biomech 16:473–480, 1983.

32. Pazzaglia, U.E., Minoia, C., Ceciliani, L., and Riccardi, C. Metal determination in organic fluids of patients with stainless steel hip arthroplasty. Acta Orthop Scand 54:574–579, 1983.

33. Pilliar, R.M. Powder metal-made orthopaedic implants with porous surface for fixation by tissue ingrowth. Clin Orthop 176:42–51, 1983.

34. Roberts, V. In Lewis, J.L., and Galante, J.O.: Workshop on Bone Joint Implant Interface. J Orthop Res 3:380–386, 1985.

35. Rose, R.M., Nusbaum, H.J., Schneider, H., Ries, M., Paul, I., Crugnola, A., Simon, S.R., and Radin, E.L. On the true wear of ultra high molecular weight polyethylene in the total hip prosthesis. J Bone Joint Surg 62A:537–549, 1980.

36. Rose, R.M., Martin, R.B., Orr, R.B., and Radin, E.L. Architectural changes in the proximal femur following prosthetic insertion: Preliminary observations on an animal model. J Biomech 17:241–249, 1984.

37. Rose, R.M., Schiller, A.L., and Radin, E.L. Corrosion-accelerated mechanical failure of a Vitallium nail-plate. J Bone Joint Surg 54A:854–862, 1972.

38. Rudin, A. *The Elements of Polymer Science and Engineering.* New York, Academic Press, 1982.

39. Sollitto, R.J., and Shonkweiler, W. Silicone shard formation: A product of implant arthroplasty. J Foot Surg 23:362–365, 1984.

40. Swanson, S.A.V., and Freeman, M.A.R. *The Scientific Basis of Total Joint Replacement.* New York, Wiley, 1977.

41. Telaranta, T., Solonen, K.A., Tallroth, K., and Nickels, J. Bone cysts containing silicone particles in bones adjacent to a carpal silastic implant. Skel Radiol 10:247–249, 1983.

42. Thompson, N.G., Buchanan, R.A., and Lemons, J.E. In vitro corrosion of Ti-6Al-4V and type stainless steel when galvanically coupled with carbon. J Biomed Mater Res 13:35–44, 1979.

43. Walker, P.S., Salvati, E., and Hotzler, R.K. The wear on removed McKee-Farrar total hip prostheses. J Bone Joint Surg 56A:92–100, 1974.

44. Weightman, B.O., Paul, I.L., Rose, R.M., Simon, S.R., and Radin, E.L. A comparative study of total hip replacement prostheses. J Biomech 6:299–311, 1973.

45. Wilson, P.D., Jr., Amstutz, H.C., Czerniecki, A., Salvai, E.A., and Mendes, D.G. Total hip replacement with fixation by acrylic cement: A preliminary study of 100 consecutive McKee-Farrar prosthetic replacements. J Bone Joint Surg 54A:207–236, 1972.

46. Woodman, J.L., Black, J., and Jimenez, S. Isolation of serum organometallic corrosion products from 316L stainless steel and Haynes Stellite 21 in vitro and in vivo. *Transactions of Seventh Annual Meeting of the Society for Biomaterials,* May 1981, p 18.

PART II

General Considerations in Trauma

CHAPTER 17

The Patient with Multiple Injuries: Treatment and Complications

Richard Hindes and Lonnie Frei

EARLY MANAGEMENT OF MULTIPLE INJURIES

Trauma is the leading cause of death in patients under the age of 40 in the United States. Proper treatment of the multiply injured patient is dependent upon the smooth functioning of a designated trauma team. This begins in the field with paramedics or emergency medical technicians trained to stabilize and transport the patient. Advance notification by radio to the

hospital by the transport team provides time to gather physicians and ancillary personnel who in some circumstances may not ordinarily be present in the emergency room. The team approach is stressed since the patient with multiple-system injuries cannot be managed by a single physician. However, this team must have a designated leader who is responsible for resuscitation and decision making in the early period after injury (Fig. 17-1).[1] This person is the general surgeon in most instances. The contribution of the orthopaedic

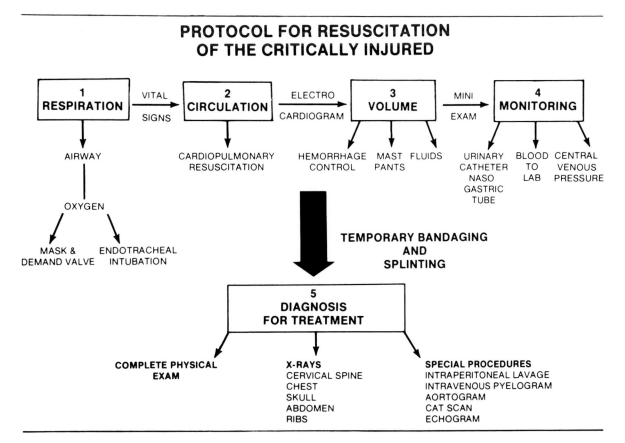

Figure 17-1 Protocol for the initial management of the critically injured patient. Team approach with a physician, nurse, and respiratory therapist assigned to respiration (1) and circulation (2), and a physician and nurse assigned to volume replacement (3) and monitoring (4). Trauma team leader supervises efforts and direction of resuscitation methods. *(From Wilder, R.J., Prog Crit Care Med 1:1, 1984. Reproduced with permission.)*

surgeon in the early decision-making period is vital to avoid possible complications from improperly treated bony injuries. This is especially true in head-injured patients, in whom a poor prognosis is occasionally incorrect.

Airway

The establishment and maintenance of an adequate airway is the first priority in a multiply injured patient. Mechanical blocks including blood, vomitus, and dentures must be removed. Once the oropharynx has been cleared, the physician must decide which type of device, if any, is best suited for maintenance of the airway.

Increasing the angle of the jaw will open the airway in an alert conscious patient. An oropharyngeal airway may be used if spontaneous breathing is present and there is no upper airway obstruction. If the upper airway is partially blocked, a nasopharyngeal airway can be utilized. The decision to perform intubation is a difficult one and must be taken seriously. Attempts to intubate an awake patient can result in severe complications. Endotracheal intubation should be performed in the unconscious patient if adequate respiratory function is not present, or if positive pressure is needed. Patients with severe facial trauma may require tracheostomy, as oro- or nasopharyngeal intubation may prove too difficult. Evaluation of chest injuries is also mandatory, as pneumo- or hemothorax requires placement of a chest tube.

Circulation

Once an adequate airway has been established, attention is then turned toward the identification and control of hemorrhage, and restoration of circulating-fluid volume. Bleeding may be present in the thorax or abdomen (intraperitoneal or retroperitoneal) or from the extremities. Intrathoracic hemorrhage can be identified by examination of the chest x-ray film and by thoracentesis. Abdominal bleeding is best diagnosed by peritoneal lavage.[1,42,47] CT scan unfortunately uses precious time, but may be invaluable for intracapsular injury to spleen or liver. Extremity bleeding is controlled by pressure dressings and judicious use of the tourniquet. The use of hemostats and clamps should be avoided, as this can cause permanent damage to vessels which could otherwise ultimately be repaired.

Use of the pneumatic antishock garment applied at the scene of the accident has gained popularity in recent years and increases peripheral resistance in the lower extremities.[39,48] However, there are several drawbacks associated with the use of this device. These include decreased venous return from overcompression of the inferior vena cava, which in turn prevents emptying of the peripheral veins.[34] In addition, the inflated garment can make examination of the lower extremities difficult. Removal of the trousers must be done slowly and only after adequate fluid replacement has been performed.

In the emergency room, two large-bore catheters should be inserted in the peripheral veins and blood samples sent for typing and cross matching, a complete blood cell count, and measurement of electrolyte levels, amylase levels, prothrombin time (PT), and partial thromboplastin time (PTT).

Fluid resuscitation should begin with Ringer's lactate until whole blood becomes available. Ringer's lactated solution is preferable to isotonic saline because large infusions of saline have been associated with acidosis secondary to high chloride load.[53] Colloid solutions containing albumin have not been found to be more effective than crystalloid in the treatment of hemorrhagic shock.[43]

Normal blood volume is approximately 5 liters in the adult. During resuscitation it is important to keep in mind that some injuries are associated with marked blood loss which may not be readily apparent. For example, femoral fractures may result in a loss of 1000 to 2000 ml of blood into the thigh, and pelvic fractures may result in considerably more blood loss and near exsanguination.

Careful monitoring of the patient's hemodynamic state must be instituted. This can be done through placement of a central venous pressure (CVP) line. However, some authors feel that CVP is inaccurate and misleading, and placement of a Swan-Ganz catheter has been suggested as a routine procedure.[58]

Monitoring of the urinary output is done through placement of a Foley catheter. An output of 1 ml/kg per hour is desirable.[53] However, in the presence of a pelvic fracture, a retrograde urethrogram must be obtained to rule out urethral injury prior to catheterization. Attempted catheterization in the face of urethral injury could result in more damage. In males, rectal examination may show elevation of the prostate, which is associated with urethral injury. If urethral injury is present, a suprapubic catheter should be inserted. Frank hematuria is an indication for performance of a cystogram examination, and if this is negative, an intravenous pyelogram is obtained.[64] A protocol for the initial resuscitation of the multiply traumatized patient is outlined in Fig. 17-1.

Physical Examination

When the patient's ventilatory and circulatory status is stabilized, attention is then turned toward evaluation of specific injuries. The history of the type of trauma is important, and details of the injury should be obtained from the ambulance team. Information such as whether the patient was wearing a seat or lap belt can be quite helpful in the evaluation of blunt trauma.

The patient's level of consciousness as well as motor and sensory function to the extremities is determined. The scalp should be checked for lacerations or contusions, and cerebral spinal fluid leakage from the nose and ears should be looked for. If intracranial trauma is suspected, arrangements should be made to obtain a CT scan of the head without delay.

If the patient is unconscious, a cervical spine injury should be assumed and the head splinted until an adequate portable-cross-table lateral x-ray film of the cervical spine is obtained. In addition, skull, chest, abdominal, and pelvic x-ray examinations should be performed in the unconscious patient.

Evaluation of the abdomen is done by physical examination with specific reference to tenderness, guarding, bowel sounds, and the presence of free fluid in the abdomen. Peritoneal lavage is mandatory in the unconscious patient. Once life-threatening injury has been managed or excluded, attention can then be turned toward evaluation of specific orthopaedic injuries.

The orthopaedic examination of a multiply injured patient begins with the spine. Palpation of the spinous processes may elicit pain, and there may be malalignment or increased space between the spinous processes, both of which are associated with a spinal injury. A neurological examination should be performed as the patient's level of consciousness permits. Specific findings such as sustained priapism are indicative of spinal cord injury and are present even in the unconscious patient.

Compression of the iliac crest elicits pain in patients with pelvic fractures. In addition, scrotal ecchymosis is associated with these injuries. Patients with a pelvic fracture should be assumed to have a concomitant injury to the genitourinary tract, and evaluation is performed as outlined above.

A brief physical examination of the extremities discloses any obvious deformity, crepitus, swelling, or ecchymosis. A careful neurovascular examination of all extremities must be performed, and the amount of information obtained depends upon the patient's level of consciousness. In the unconscious patient, an attempt should be made to observe spontaneous motion. An x-ray examination should be performed on all areas of suspected injury.

Frank dislocations of joints should be reduced as early as possible. Fractures are splinted until the patient is stabilized, when definitive treatment consisting of cast immobilization, traction, or surgical stabilization is performed.

Open fractures present more of a challenge to the orthopaedic surgeon. Sterile dressings are applied to the open wound. After blood for cultures has been taken, intravenous antibiotics are begun. Cephalosporins, for staphylococcal coverage, are usually the drugs of choice.[15] Some authors advocate administration of an aminoglycoside in addition to a cephalosporin. Studies by Gustilo have shown a definite substantial decrease in the incidence of infection with the use of prophylactic antibiotics.[30] Antibiotics are usually continued for 4 to 5 days, although this varies from institution to institution. Open fractures are debrided in the operating room as soon as the patient's condition allows. Use of the jet lavage is recommended.

Definitive Management of Fractures

The decision on how to best manage multiple fractures is a difficult one and is dependent largely on the personal experience of the surgeon and the equipment available. Ill-conceived surgical procedures attempted in the middle of the night without adequate equipment or personnel can end in disaster. This is particularly the case if adequate fluid replacement has not been achieved and the patient's condition remains unstable. However, an increasing number of authors recommend the immediate rigid stabilization of multiple fractures to allow mobilization of a polytraumatized patient. Mobilization to the sitting position is associated with a reduced incidence of pulmonary complications and decreased mor-

bidity and is advantageous to the patient's psychological welfare. The use of external fixators and also the internal fixation of open fractures has been reported with good results.[2,13] Open intraarticular fractures are also best treated with immediate rigid internal fixation. This allows early mobilization of the joints. It is important to stress that primary wound closure is not necessarily performed along with internal fixation of open fractures. Management of the wound is handled on an individual basis. The recent tendency toward operative stabilization of fractures is because many physicians believe that the multiply injured patient is in optimum condition for surgery at the time of admission to the hospital and that as much skeletal stabilization as possible should be performed immediately, as opportunity for a second attempt might not be available for some time.[38]

NUTRITIONAL SUPPORT IN PATIENTS WITH MULTIPLE INJURIES

Adjusting Basal Requirements

One of the most detrimental effects of the altered metabolism in stress is the breakdown of native protein to provide amino acids for the creation of new proteins and to provide carbon skeletons for gluconeogenesis. The protein which is lost may be from muscle or from any of the circulating proteins in the body, e.g., immunoglobulins, coagulation factors, or carrier proteins. This manifests clinically as decreases in serum levels of total protein, albumin, and transferrin. Such decreases may predispose the body to the development of further complications such as sepsis or organ failure. When dietary intake is normal, the mobilization of body stores can be arrested or stopped. However, in the setting of trauma, patients are frequently unable to ingest adequate amounts. This may be the result of gastrointestinal tract dysfunction or altered mental status. Nutritional support must then be provided. This may be by parenteral or enteral routes, using various formulations.

A generally accepted figure for the basal energy requirement (BER) of an adult is 25 to 30 kcal/kg per day. It is possible to use the Harris-Benedict equations to calculate these *basal* requirements.[31]

For males: BER = 66.5 + 13.8(wt) + 5(hgt) − 6.8(age)
For females: BER = 66.5 + 9.6(wt) + 1.8(hgt) − 4.6(age)

Body weight (wt) refers to ideal body weight in kilograms, height (hgt) is in centimeters, and age is in years.[9] BER in kilocalories is then multiplied by a factor which takes into account the amount of injury and associated stress response. In patients with multiple trauma, it may be doubled.[9] An accepted range of basal requirements for nitrogen is 0.8 to 1.0 g of protein per kilogram of lean body weight per day.[14] In the multiple-trauma patient, calculations may be made on the basis of 1.5 to 3.0 g of nitrogen per kilogram, or alternatively 1 g of nitrogen per 150 kcal.[9]

Whenever the gastrointestinal tract is functional, it is the preferred route to use in providing nutritional support. The head-injured patient with an altered mental status and the ventilator-dependent patient are good examples of the type of patient in whom enteral support can be used. Many different formulations of the enteral diets are available, varying in caloric content, osmolarity, viscosity, lactose level, protein source, and cost. Additionally, special formulations are available to meet the special needs imposed by cardiac, hepatic, and renal failure, as well as the needs imposed by severe stress. The feedings are administered through nasogastric feeding tubes or through surgically placed gastrostomy or enterostomy tubes. The major complications are aspiration, especially important in the patient with impaired mental status, and gastrointestinal motility problems such as diarrhea, cramping, and distension.[54]

The alternative to enteral feeding is parenteral nutrition, which may be provided by peripheral veins or by central venous cannulation. The formulation of the fluids which are administered can vary greatly. The standard glucose-containing intravenous fluids which are routinely used in the hospitalized patient (usually 5% glucose solutions) are a form of nutritional support but provide only 17 kcal/100 ml. To meet the caloric needs of the normal 70 kg man would require more than 10 liters of fluid! When these standard intravenous formulations are the only parenteral support provided, caloric needs are not usually met. The increased requirements in the stress situation further decrease the effectiveness of standard intravenous fluids in meeting the body's needs. It has been shown that glucose in hypocaloric amounts has a protein-sparing effect, decreasing both the breakdown of endogenous protein and the negative nitrogen balance without completely stopping either.[10,19] Infusion of amino acid solutions without dextrose also exerts a protein-sparing effect by providing substrate for gluconeogenesis and protein metabolism, but again is ineffective in completely blocking protein catabolism and negative nitrogen balance.[1,7] The development of parenteral hyperalimentation has overcome the limitations imposed by hypocaloric solutions and has made possible the nutritional support of patients whose basic or increased nutritional needs cannot be met by standard means.

Hyperalimentation solutions are hypertonic, hyperosmolar mixtures of glucose and amino acids, also containing electrolytes, minerals, and vitamins. Total parenteral nutrition (TPN) is the most calorically dense solution and must be given through the central veins only. It usually provides 1 kcal/ml and 40 g of protein per liter of solution. Peripheral parenteral nutrition (PPN) is less calorically dense, less hypertonic, and less hyperosmolar and hence can be tolerated by peripheral veins. Because of its lower caloric content, however, larger volumes must be used to meet nutritional needs; more preferably, it is given in combination with lipid solutions which have higher caloric content. The cost of hyperalimentation is much higher than that of enteral alimentation, and this may be one consideration in its use. The complications associated with hyperalimentation are multiple; hyperosmolar states, glucose intolerance from the large glucose loads delivered, hepatic dysfunction, and sepsis. Just as with the enteral diets, there are special hyperalimentation formulations for hepatic and renal failure.[16,65]

One important aspect of the successful management of trauma patients is a consideration of normal metabolism and the alterations introduced by trauma. The application of prin-

ciples of metabolic support then follows and becomes a vital part of the overall management plan.

COMPLICATIONS OF MULTIPLE INJURIES

Adult Respiratory Distress Syndrome

Adult respiratory distress syndrome (ARDS) is a convenient term for a disease process which results from a heterogeneous group of causes (Table 17-1).[5] ARDS is the most commonly accepted name from a long list of synonyms which includes "shock lung," "Da Nang lung," "wet lung," and "white lung syndrome." A significant counterpoint to the heterogeneity of the names and the causes is the homogeneous picture that the syndrome produces: hypoxemia, decreased pulmonary compliance, and a noncardiogenic pulmonary edema that manifests radiologically as a diffuse "whiteout" of the lungs. The diffuse causes have no known common denominator. Additionally, ARDS does not develop each time one or more of the causes occurs. Once it does develop, the course of the disease is variable and quite unpredictable. The purpose of this section is to provide a basis for understanding the disease, and managing it when it develops.

Diagnosis

ARDS should be suspected when, in the setting of one or more of the causes listed in Table 17-1, the patient develops hypoxemia (defined as a $PO_2 < 60$ on room air, $PO_2 < 60$ with supplemental oxygen fraction $FiO_2 > 0.6$), tachypnea (respiratory rate > 30), and a radiological picture of diffuse interstitial infiltrates (see Table 17-2).[4] The radiological findings may lag behind the development of the syndrome by 12 to 24h. Cardiac failure should be ruled out as a cause of the derangements. Chronic obstructive pulmonary disease (COPD) may confuse the picture since some of the characteristics of COPD are common also to ARDS (e.g., hypoxemia, tachypnea), but ARDS should be suspected when the normally compensated COPD patient acutely deteriorates in the setting of one of the known causes of the syndrome. Further support for the diagnosis comes from data obtained from some of the adjunctive measures used in the treatment of ARDS. When central hemodynamics are monitored, the pulmonary edema is found to be of a noncardiogenic basis as verified by wedge pressures < 18. The shunt fraction (the ratio of that part of the circulation which flows past lung units, not participating in gas exchange, to total pulmonary blood flow) is usually in excess of 15 percent. Pulmonary compliance (dV/dP, or the change in lung volume with pressure change) is reduced, often to the range of 20 to 30 ml/cmH_2O. Vital capacity and functional residual capacity (FRC) both decrease. The ratio of dead space ventilation to total ventilation (V_D / V_t) is also increased.

Pathophysiology of ARDS

Injury to the alveolar capillary membrane is central to the development of ARDS. Known to produce this injury are both

TABLE 17-1 Disorders with Etiologic Significance in Adult Respiratory Distress Syndrome

Blood-borne or Vascular Source of Injury

*Trauma
*Sepsis
Fat embolism
Pancreatitis
Shock
Multiple transfusions
  Microemboli
  Leukoagglutinin reaction
Disseminated intravascular coagulation
Surface burns
Miliary tuberculosis
Drug overdoses
  Heroin, methadone,
  ethchlorvynol, acetylsalicyclic acid,
  propoxyphene
Drug idiosyncratic reaction
Thrombotic thrombocytopenic purpura
Leukemia
Venous air embolism
Head injury
Paraquat
Cardiopulmonary bypass/hemodialysis

Inhalation of Airway Source

*Aspiration of gastric contents
*Diffuse infectious pneumonia
  Viral, mycoplasma,
  Legionnaires', pneumocystis
*Near-drowning
Irritant gas inhalation
  NO_2, Cl_2, SO_2, NH_3
Smoke inhalation
O_2 toxicity

Direct or Physical Source

Lung contusion
Radiation
High altitude
Hanging
Reexpansion

*Common cause of ARDS.
Source: Hudson, L.D., Clin Chest Med 3(1):196, 1982. Reprinted with permission.

humoral and cellular factors, including neutrophils and their toxic products; circulating metabolites such as leukotrienes, thromboxane, and prostaglandins; and the direct injury caused by bacterial toxins. The lung epithelium may be injured primarily, as in aspiration, allowing extravasation of fluids and cells into the alveolar space. The damage to the capillary membrane causes a capillary leak, with movement of fluid into the interstitium. Platelets and leukocytes aggregate at the site of injury, and fibrin thrombi may be deposited in small vessels. With progression of the disease, hyaline

membranes form and there is capillary congestion. Lung epithelium may undergo necrosis. This is followed by a proliferation of the pulmonary epithelium in an attempt to resurface the denuded alveolus. Interstitial fibrosis occurs, causing a thickening of the alveolar-capillary membrane and a decrease in capillarity. In progressive ARDS, the final pathological presentation is one of total or near total obliteration of normal pulmonary architecture. This is associated with diffusion abnormalities and the clinical picture of pure respiratory failure.[52,60]

The pathological picture helps explain the alterations in physiology which occur. The interstitial and alveolar edema prevent alveoli from participating in gas exchange, thus causing hypoxemia. Fibrotic capillary membranes cause diffusion abnormalities, adding to the hypoxemia. A major contributor to the hypoxemia is the aggregation, inactivation, or loss of surfactant. This leads to alveolar collapse, or atelectasis, and increased intrapulmonary shunting, both of which are causes of hypoxemia. Loss of surfactant also makes the lung more difficult to expand, or noncompliant. The loss of these alveoli to respiration causes a decrease in the FRC.

Treatment of ARDS

The treatment of ARDS is directed at the major life-threatening symptom, namely, hypoxemia. This usually involves intubation of the patient and the administration of supplemental oxygen. However, there are limits to the amount of O_2 which can be used. A quick review of the etiology of ARDS reveals that oxygen toxicity is also one of the causes of this syn-

TABLE 17-2 Criteria for Diagnosing Adult Respiratory Distress Syndrome

Clinical setting
  Catastrophic event
    Pulmonary
    Nonpulmonary, e.g., shock
  Exclusions
    Chronic pulmonary disease
    Left heart abnormalities
  Respiratory distress (judged clinically)
    Tachypnea > 20, usually greater
    Labored breathing
X-ray film: Diffuse pulmonary infiltrates
  Interstitial (initially)
  Alveolar (later)
Physiological
  $PO_2 < 50$ with $FiO_2 > 0.6$
  Overall compliance < 50 ml/cm—usually 20 to 30 ml/cm
  Increased shunt fraction Q_s/Q_t and deadspace
  ventilation $\dot{V}_D/\dot{V}_t$
Pathological
  Heavy lungs, usually > 1000 g
  Congestive atelectasis
  Hyaline membranes
  Fibrosis

Source: Petty, T.C., Clin Chest Med, 3:3, 1982. Reprinted with permission.

drome. Oxygen concentrations in excess of 50 percent are considered toxic; hence this becomes a limiting factor in the usefulness of oxygen as a treatment modality.

To supplement the oxygen and to directly treat some of the underlying pathological changes it is necessary to add positive end-expiratory pressure (PEEP) to the ventilator circuit. PEEP works by distending the alveoli which have collapsed because of the underlying disease process. With reexpansion of collapsed alveoli, gas exchange can again occur and hypoxia can be lessened. This process of reexpansion is called *recruitment* and is associated with a decrease in the shunt fraction, an increase in pulmonary compliance, and better oxygenation. The amount of PEEP which is used varies from patient to patient and also depends on the particular end point which is being treated. Thus one may treat to an adequate level of oxygenation ($P_{O_2} = 60$–65) on nontoxic levels of oxygen,[26] to the best compliance,[62] to a certain level of shunt ($Q_s/Q_t < 15\%$),[23,37] or to optimal O_2 delivery to the tissues. This is a controversial area, and much has been written in support of each method, with no proven advantage of one over another. It is usually true, however, that more PEEP must be used to achieve the desired end point as the severity of the ARDS increases. Once the end point is reached and the ARDS shows signs of resolving (as manifested by clearing of the chest film, increasing compliance, and improved oxygenation), the PEEP is removed in a stepwise fashion, or weaned, to the point that the patient no longer needs the ventilatory support.[56,66]

Since PEEP has been shown to be effective in the treatment of ARDS, some investigators have advocated the use of "prophylactic PEEP," that is, administering PEEP to patients who have risk factors for the development of ARDS. There has been little data to support this practice.[50] The ineffectiveness of prophylactic PEEP only serves to emphasize that there is, as yet, no good way to predict who will develop the syndrome.

The next component in the treatment of ARDS is fluid management. Since interstitial and alveolar edema are major defects caused by ARDS, the overzealous or injudicious use of fluids may worsen the clinical picture by causing an increase in the edema. Patients with ARDS should be maintained in a relatively balanced fluid state, while allowing enough volume to ensure sufficient cardiac output. Maintaining a balanced fluid status may be difficult if high levels of PEEP are employed, and hemodynamic monitoring may be necessary to aid in fluid management.

The final component in the management of ARDS is the treatment of the underlying cause of the problem. Thus, if sepsis has caused the syndrome, antibiotics, drainage of an abscess, or debridement of dead or devitalized tissue is indicated. If the underlying cause persists, the syndrome will persist and may progress to an irreversible state. It must be emphasized at this point that progression may occur even when the underlying cause has been or is being treated.

Outcome of Treatment

As mentioned briefly above, ARDS may follow several paths, and the outcome is not always predictable. The first and most favorable outcome is the complete recovery of the patient with no residual pulmonary dysfunction. The chest film re-verts to normal and studies of lung function are normal. A second outcome is recovery, but with residual pulmonary dysfunction, usually in the form of diffusion defects. Some of these patients may require supplemental oxygen therapy in order to lead a functional existence. The final outcome is the development of a progressive deterioration which results in pure respiratory failure as manifested by progressive hypoxemia, subsequent hypercarbia, and finally the inability to provide respiratory support. In the end stage this is fatal. The mortality associated with ARDS approaches 50 percent in some published series.[17] Because of our ability to support and maintain patients with ARDS, we now see less than 50 percent mortality directly attributable to ARDS; more often ARDS presents as a part of the complex of multisystem organ failure, or in conjunction with sepsis which is now the more common cause of mortality.

Fat Embolism Syndrome

The fat embolism syndrome (FES) is one of the less clearly understood complications of multiple trauma. Zenker is credited with the first demonstration (in 1862) of fat droplets in the pulmonary circulation. In 1873 Von Bergmann was the first physician to detail the clinical presentation of this syndrome.

Gossling and Pelligrini have defined FES as "a complex alteration of homeostasis which occurs as an infrequent complication of fracture of the pelvis and long bones, and manifests clinically as acute respiratory insufficiency."[28] The significance of FES lies in the fact that a mortality approaching 15 percent has been identified in the overt syndrome. However, it should be noted that FES may not be solely the result of trauma. It has been linked with other conditions including diabetes and other metabolic disorders as well as in the postoperative periods of total hip and total knee replacement surgery.[33,38,55]

Incidence

FES has been reported to occur in 0 to 55 percent of multiply injured patients.[46] In order to determine the incidence,[46] it is essential to differentiate the subclinical entity from the clinically apparent syndrome of respiratory distress, cerebral changes, fever, and tachycardia.

Subclinical FES is felt by many authors to occur in a majority of all multiply injured patients. Gossling has stated that nearly all patients with long-bone fractures can be shown to have histological evidence of fat droplets in the lungs. McCarthy studied 50 patients with long-bone fractures and found that only 26 percent of them maintained a $P_{O_2} >80$ mmHg,[27] 46 percent had decreased platelet counts, and 50 percent had hyperfibrinogenemia. However, even in the face of these laboratory abnormalities, none of the 50 patients showed any clinical signs of respiratory distress.

In another prospective study by Riseborough, 63 percent of 118 patients with long-bone fractures developed a notable decrease in P_{O_2}.[41] In addition, a significant number of these 63 patients had a reduction in hemoglobin levels and platelet counts. Only 2 of the 63 patients developed clinically evident FES.

In a more recent study by Chan, 80 fracture patients were studied prospectively.[53] Of the patients with a single fracture, 64 percent had a decrease in P_{O_2}, 33 percent had tachycardia (>100/min), 55 percent had an increase in temperature, and 36 percent had hemoglobin levels of less than 10 g/100ml; 8.8 percent of these patients developed overt FES. The corresponding percentages in patients with multiple fractures were higher.

Clinical FES Gossling has noted that clinically apparent FES is noted in 0.5 to 2 percent of patients with single long-bone fractures, and in 5 to 10 percent of patients with multiple fractures.[28]

Pathophysiology

Most of the controversy about FES concerns its pathophysiology. The exact source and fate of the fat globules seen in the lungs are unknown. However, clinical and experimental studies performed during the past 10 years have shed much light on this subject.

There have been two major theories concerning the source of the fat in this syndrome: the *marrow globular theory,* and the *biochemical fat embolization theory.* These have been well-organized and well-presented by Ooh and Mital.[46]

Proponents of the marrow globular theory feel that trauma from a long-bone fracture results in the release of marrow fat, which is then filtered and trapped by the lung. This theory has been substantiated by experimental studies in dogs.[36,51] Proponents of the biochemical theory feel that an alteration in lipid stability within the blood results in the spontaneous production of free fat globules, which are filtered by the lung. It is plausible that both these mechanisms may play a role in the production of free fat globules in the blood. Once trapped in the lung, fat is metabolized to free fatty acids, which have been shown to be toxic to the lung parenchyma.[3,49]

In addition, it seems clear that concurrent alterations in platelet function (increased aggregation) and release of catecholamines also occur, and the clotting mechanism appears to be activated as well.[41,53] The biochemical abnormalities just outlined lead to decreased lung and cardiopulmonary function, which in turn produce the observed clinical manifestations.

Clinical and Laboratory Findings

FES usually presents as respiratory distress occurring between 24 and 72 h after injury. Typically, a patient initially shows an increased heart rate, tachypnea, and fever as high as 103° F. This is followed by an alteration in mental status which may range from slight agitation and disorientation to coma.

Petechiae appear in 50 to 60 percent of patients and are most typically found in the axillae, conjunctivae, and anterior chest wall (Fig. 17-2). There is usually a delay of approximately 24 h between the onset of FES and the petechiae. Retinal lesions also occur in approximately 50 percent of patients.

The most consistent laboratory finding is a decrease in the arterial P_{O_2} that coincides with the onset of symptoms.

However, as discussed earlier, arterial hypoxemia may be present without any other laboratory or clinical findings and as such represents subclinical FES.

Chest roentgenographic changes occur in approximately one-third of patients. These consist of small fluffy exudates which may progress to extensive infiltrates. Electrocardiographic changes are nonspecific and usually consist of ST-segment changes indicative of ischemia.

There may be a fall of 3 to 5 g in the hemoglobin level and a decrease in the number of circulating platelets. Lipuria has been noted in 50 percent of patients, but its significance is not yet understood.

Gurd reported on a test to determine the presence and concentration of fat droplets in the blood and stated that this may be diagnostic for FES.[29] However, other studies[44] have failed to confirm this finding, and fat droplets of similar size and concentrations were identified in normal controls.

Treatment

The cornerstone of management of FES centers around early diagnosis and respiratory support. Hypoxemia must be corrected by treatment with oxygen. Further ventilatory support including intubation and PEEP may be required in order to keep arterial P_{O_2} greater than 70 mmHg. Hemodynamic abnormalities must be corrected by adequate fluid and blood replacement, and the fractured extremity should be properly immobilized.

Several types of chemical and drug regimens have been evaluated for the treatment of FES. Heparin has been suggested because of its ability to increase serum lipase levels and therefore decrease serum fat levels, and also because of its antiplatelet activity.[20] However, the efficacy of heparin therapy has not been determined by adequate prospective studies, and there have been reports of negative effects.[24]

Corticosteroids have been advocated for both the treatment and the prevention of FES. Two prospective randomized studies have shown a statistically significant decrease in the incidence of FES in steroid-treated patients with long-bone fractures.[55,61] In addition, in patients who developed the syndrome, oxygen concentration remained at high levels in the steroid-treated group. The efficacy of steroid treatment is felt to be secondary to a decreased inflammatory response in the lungs.

Low-molecular-weight dextran has also been advocated in the treatment of FES because of its anticoagulant effect. However, as with heparin, there have been no controlled studies to support its use, and the risk of bleeding in fracture patients must be considered. Awareness of this complication and early diagnosis combined with proper ventilatory support will in most cases lead to a satisfactory outcome.

Multiple System Organ Failure

Tilney in 1973 described a syndrome of sequential multiple system organ failure (MSOF) developing in patients who survived the initial insult of ruptured aortic aneurysm.[63]

The name of the syndrome implies the involvement of more than one organ system, but which systems are involved

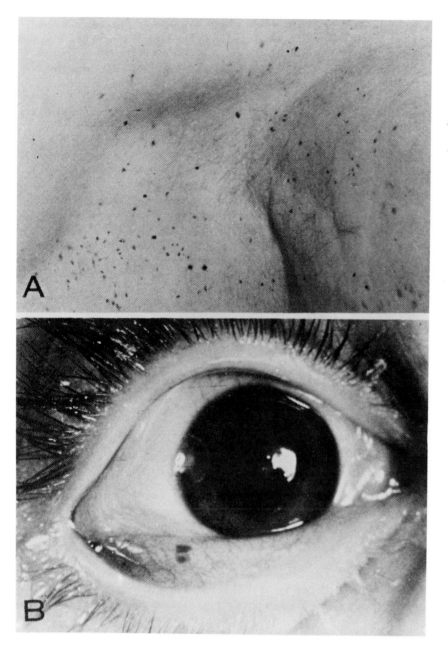

Figure 17-2 Petechial hemorrhages associated with (**A**) fat embolism over the lateral chest wall and axilla and (**B**) in the conjunctiva of the lower lid. Two days previously the patient had sustained fractures of both femora in an automobile accident. *(From Salter, R.B.: Textbook of Disorders and Injuries of the Musculoskeletal System. Baltimore, Williams & Wilkins, 1970. Reproduced with permission.)*

and how many systems must fail to be included in the MSOF syndrome are controversial matters. However, there is universal agreement on the inclusion of the pulmonary, renal, hepatic, and gastrointestinal systems. The coagulation and cardiovascular systems are also included by the majority of authors.[5,21,22,40,45] Manship defines MSOF as the failure of three or more of six designated organ systems,[40] but most authors define MSOF as the failure of two systems.

The patients who ultimately develop MSOF are a heterogeneous group and include trauma patients as well as elective surgical patients. However, common factors that may predispose them to the development of MSOF have been identified. As with the list of organ systems involved, there is uncertain predictability of associated risk factors, but invasive infection, periods of shock, and multiple blood transfusions are those which occur most commonly.[1] In addition, other risk factors may include "severe trauma" (Eiseman includes chest and head injuries and long-bone fractures in this category)[18] and Manship's "pre-insult limitations," which include COPD, diabetes, heart disease, and chronic renal failure.

Of those factors which seem to predispose patients to the development of the syndrome, sepsis appears to play a major role. Sepsis was present in over 50 percent of the patients in each of the series reviewed. Eiseman noted that in approximately 70 percent of his patients with MSOF, the onset correlated with the development of infection.[18] Faist described two patterns of development of the syndrome, single-phase multiple organ failure, and two-phase multiple organ failure, which developed with a lag phase that frequently involved sepsis, usually pneumonia.[21] The primary sites of infection are the lungs and the abdominal cavity. The organisms most commonly isolated in MSOF patients are *Pseudomonas aeruginosa, Escherichia coli,* and *Staphylococcus aureus.*

Perhaps in keeping with the primary sites of infection, the organ systems that most commonly fail are the pulmonary and renal systems. Norton found the combination of these two systems failing in almost three-quarters of the nonsurvivors in his series.[40] Additionally, as the number of involved systems increases, so does the mortality, ranging from 60 percent with two-organ failure to 100 percent with four-organ failure.[22]

The treatment of MSOF is perhaps the most difficult problem. Fry discusses alterations in ATP metabolism because of deficient delivery or utilization of oxygen and substrate as possible cellular mechanisms underlying the etiology of MSOF.[22] Pulmonary support with positive pressure ventilation and PEEP, and cardiac support with the use of volume assistance, inotropes, and vasoactive agents, are in part directed to these problems. Much work has been done looking at the metabolic profiles of the MSOF patients, and nutritional therapy has been directed at correcting some of the problems noted, including the provision of branched-chain amino acid formulations, proper nutritional "fuel mixes," and adequate amounts of nutritional support.[32] Antibiotics are the mainstay of treatment. However, if improperly chosen, antibiotics may predispose patients to the development of resistant organisms or allow the emergence of organisms which are usually nonpathogenic but which can become so in the immunocompromised host (which many of the MSOF patients are). The use of antibiotics may also cause damage to other organ systems, such as the well-known nephrotoxicity of the aminoglycosides.

Perhaps the most important part of the therapy of MSOF is prevention.[6] Analysis of the factors which predispose to the development of the syndrome make up the guidelines for preventive therapy. Since sepsis is on the top of the list, control of infection through the judicious use of antibiotics and prompt drainage of septic foci is important. The recognition of respiratory insufficiency with intubation and ventilatory support must occur early, and support should be continued until the patient demonstrates no further need for support. Shock should be treated vigorously to prevent damage to the kidneys, the brain, and the heart. Nutritional support should be instituted early and in adequate amounts to prevent the late sequelae of malnutrition. In cases of massive transfusions, filters should be used when administering the blood. Renal blood flow and urine output should be maintained, and dialysis should be used early to preserve function and prevent volume overload and tissue toxicity.

REFERENCES

1. Ahmad, W., and Polk, H.C., Jr. Blunt abdominal trauma: A prospective study with selected peritoneal lavage. Arch Surg 111:489, 1976.
2. Anderson, J.T., and Gustilo, R.D. Immediate internal fixation in open fractures. Orthop Clin North Am 11:569–578, 1980.
3. Baker, P.L., Pazzeo, J.A., and Peltier, L.F. Free fatty acids, catecholamines, and arterial hypoxemia in patients with fat embolism. J Trauma 11:1026–1030, 1971.
4. Balk, R., and Bone, R.C. The adult respiratory distress syndrome. Med Clin North Am 67:685–700, 1983.
5. Baue, A.E. Multiple, progressive, or sequential systems failure, a syndrome of the 1970's. Arch Surg 110:779–781, 1975.
6. Baue, A.E., and Chaudry, I.H. Prevention of multiple systems failure. Surg Clin North Am 60:1167–1178, 1980.
7. Blackburn, G.L., Flatt, J.P., and Clowes, G.H.A., Jr., et al. Peripheral intravenous feeding with isotonic amino acid solutions. Am J Surg 125:447–454, 1973.
8. Blackburn, G.L., Flatt, J.P., and Clowes, G.H.A., Jr., et al. Protein sparing therapy during periods of starvation with sepsis or trauma. Ann Surg 177:588–594, 1973.
9. Braun, R.M., and Schorr, R. Surgical nutrition in the patient with multiple injuries. J Bone Joint Surg 65A:123–127, 1983.
10. Cahill, G.F. Starvation in man. N Engl J Med 282:668, 1970.
11. Canizaro, P.C., Prager, M.D., and Shires, G.T. The infusion of Ringer's lactate solution during shock. Am J Surg 122:494–501, 1971.
12. Chan, K.M., Tham, K.T., Chiu, H.S., Chow, Y.N., and Leung, P.C. Post-traumatic fat embolism: Clinical and subclinical manifestations. J Trauma 24:45–49, 1984.
13. Chapmann, N.W. The use of immediate internal fixation in open fractures. Orthop Clin North Am 11:579–591, 1980.
14. Committee on Dietary Allowances, Committee on Interpretation of the Recommended Dietary Allowances: *Recommended Dietary Allowances,* 8th ed. National Academy of Sciences, Washington, DC, 1974.
15. Dabezies, E.J., and D'Ambrosia, R.D. Treatment of the multiply injured patient: Plans for treatment and problems of major trauma, in Murray, J.A. (ed): *American Academy of Orthopaedic Surgeons, Instructional Course Lectures,* vol 33. St. Louis, Mosby, 1984.
16. Daly, J.M., and Long, J.M., III. Intravenous hyperalimentation: Technique and potential complications. Surg Clin North Am 61:583–592, 1981.
17. Demling, R.H. The pathogenesis of respiratory failure after trauma and sepsis. Surg Clin North Am 60:1373–1390, 1981.
18. Eiseman, B., Beart, R., and Norton, L. Multiple organ failure. Surg Gynecol Obstet 144:323–326, 1977.
19. Elwyn, D.H., Gump, F.E., and Iles, M., et al. Protein and energy sparing of glucose added in hypocaloric amounts to peripheral infusions of amino acids. Metabolism 27:325–331 1978.
20. Evarts, C.M., and Mayer, P.J. The fat embolism syndrome, in Rockwood, C.A., and Green, D.P. (eds): *Fractures in Adults,* 2d ed. Philadelphia, Lippincott, 1984.
21. Faist, E., Baue, A.E., Dittmer, H., and Heberer, G. Multiple organ failure in polytrauma patients. J Trauma 23:775–787, 1983.
22. Fry, D.E., Perlstein, L., Fulton, R.L., and Polk, H.C., Jr. Multiple system organ failure: The role of uncontrolled infection. Arch Surg 115:136–140, 1980.
23. Gallagher, T.J., Civetta, J.M., and Kirby, R.R. Terminology update: Optimal PEEP. Crit Care Med 6:323–326, 1978.
24. Gardner, A.M., and Harrison, M.H. Report of the treatment of experimental fat embolism with heparin. J Bone Joint Surg [Br] 39:538–541, 1957.
25. Gil, K.M., Askanazi, J., and Hyman, A.I. Substrate utilization in the acutely ill: Implications for nutritional support, in *Critical Care: State of the Art,* vol 5. Society of Critical Care Medicine, 1984.
26. Gong, H., Jr. Positive-pressure ventilation in the adult respiratory distress syndrome. Clin Chest Med 3:69–88, 1982.
27. Gossling, H.R., Ellson, L.H., and Degraff, A.C. Fat embolism. The role of respiratory failure and its treatment. J Bone Joint Surg [AM] 56:1327–1337, 1974.
28. Gossling, H.R., and Pellegrini, V.D. Fat embolism syndrome: A re-

view of the pathophysiology and physiological basis of treatment. Clin Orthop 165:68–82, 1982.

29. Gurd, A.R. Fat embolism: An aid to diagnosis. J Bone Joint Surg [Br] 52:732–737, 1970.

30. Gustillo, R.D., and Anderson, J.T. Prevention of infection in treatment of 1,025 open fractures of long bones. J Bone Joint Surg [Am] 58:453–458, 1976.

31. Harris, J.A., and Benedict, F.G. *A Biometric Study of Basal Metabolism in Man.* Washington, DC, Carnegie Institute of Washington, no. 279, 1919.

32. Hassett, J., Cerra, F., Siegel, J., Moyer, E., Caruana, J., Yu, L., Peters, D., Border, J., and McMenamy, R. Multiple systems organ failure: Mechanisms and therapy. Surg Annual 14:25–72, 1982.

33. Herndon, J.H., Bechtol, C.O., and Crickenberger, D.P. Fat embolism during total hip replacement: A prospective study. J Bone Joint Surg [Am] 56:1350–1362, 1974.

34. Holcroft, J.W. Venous return and pneumatic anti-shock garment in hypovolemic baboons. J Trauma 24:928, 1984.

35. Hudson, L.D. Causes of the adult respiratory distress syndrome—Clinical recognition. Clin Chest Med 3:195–212, 1982.

36. Kerstell, J. Pathogenesis of post-traumatic fat embolism. Am J Surg 121:712–715, 1971.

37. Kirby, R.R., Downs, J.B., and Civetta, J.M., et al. High level positive end-expiratory pressure (PEEP) in acute respiratory insufficiency. Chest 67:156–163, 1975.

38. Lachiewicz, P.F., and Ranawat, C.S. Fat embolism syndrome following bilateral total knee replacement with total condylar prosthesis: Report of two cases. Clin Orthop 160:106–108, 1981.

39. Lee, H.R., Blank, W.S., Massion, W.H., and Wilder, R.J. Venous return in hemorrhagic shock after application of military anti-shock trousers. Am J Emer Med 6:288, 1983.

40. Manship, L., McMillan, R.D., and Brown, J.J. The influence of sepsis and multisystem organ failure on mortality in the surgical intensive care unit. Am Surg 50:94–101, 1984.

41. McCarthy, B. Mammen, E., Leblanc, L.P., and Wilson, R.F. Subclinical fat embolism: A prospective study of 50 patients with extremity fractures. J Trauma 13:9–16, 1973.

42. Moore, J.B., Moore, E.E., and Markovchick, V.D. Diagnostic peritoneal lavage for abdominal trauma: Superiority of the open technique at the infraumbilical ring. J Trauma 21:570–572, 1981.

43. Moss, G.S., Lowe, R.J., and Jilek, J. Colloid or crystalloid in the resuscitation of hemorrhagic shock: A controlled clinical trial. Surgery 89:434–438, 1981.

44. Nolte, W.J., Olofsson, T., Schersten, T., and Lewis, D.H. Evaluation of the Gerr Test for fat embolism. J Bone Joint Surg [Br] 56:417–420, 1974.

45. Norton, L.W. Does drainage of intraabdominal pus reverse multiple organ failure? Am J Surg 149:347–350, 1985.

46. Ooh, W.H., and Mital, M.A. Fat embolism: Current concepts of pathogenesis, diagnosis, and treatment. Orthop Clin North Am 9:769–779, 1978.

47. Pachter, H.L., and Hofstetter, S. Open and percutaneous paracentesis and lavage for abdominal trauma: A randomized prospective study. Arch Surg 116:318–319, 1981.

48. Pelligra, R., and Sandberg, E.D. Control of intractable abdominal bleeding by external counter pressure. JAMA, 241:708, 1979.

49. Peltier, L.F. Fat embolism: III. The toxic properties of neutral fat and free fatty acids. Surgery 40:665, 1956.

50. Pepe, P.E., Hudson, L.D., and Carrico, C.J. Early application of positive end-expiratory pressure in patients at risk for the adult respiratory-distress syndrome. N Engl J Med 311:281–286, 1984.

51. Raffer, R.K., Montemurno, R., Scudese, V., and Sherr, S. Experimental production and recovery of pulmonary fat embolism in dogs: Origin of the fat. Surg Forum 22:446–448, 1971.

52. Rinaldo, J.E., and Rogers, R.M. Adult respiratory distress syndrome. N Engl J Med 306:900–909, 1982.

53. Riseborough, S., and Herndon, J.H. Alterations in pulmonary function, coagulation, and fat metabolism in patients with fractures of the lower limbs. Clin Orthop 115:248–267, 1976.

54. Rombeau, J.L., and Barot, L.R. Enteral nutritional therapy. Surg Clin North Am 61:605–620, 1981.

55. Schonfeld, S.A., Ploysongsang, Y., Oilisco, R., Chrissman, J.D., Miller, E., Hammerschmidt, D.E., and Jacob, H.S. Fat embolism: Prophylaxis with corticosteroids: A prospective study in high-risk patients. Ann Intern Med 99:438–443, 1983.

56. Shapiro, B.A., Cane, R.D., and Harrison, R.A., Positive end-expiratory pressure in acute lung injury. Chest 83:558–563, 1983.

57. Shires, G.T. Principles and management of hemorrhagic shock, in Shires, G.T. (ed): *Principles of Trauma Care,* 3d ed. New York, McGraw-Hill, 1985.

58. Smith, T.K., Day, L.J., Hansen, S.T., and Johnson, R.M. Management of the multiply injured patient, in Murray, D.G. (ed): *American Academy of Orthopaedic Surgeons, Instructional Course Lectures,* vol 30. St. Louis, Mosby, 1981.

59. Spengler, D.M., Costenbader, M., and Bailey, R. Fat embolism syndrome following total hip arthroplasty. Clin Orthop 121:105–107, 1976.

60. Stevens, J.H., and Raffin, R.A. Adult respiratory distress syndrome. I. Aetiology and mechanisms. Postgrad Med J 60:505–513, 1984.

61. Stoltenberg, J.J., and Gustilo, R.B. The use of methyl-prednisolone and hypertonic glucose in the prophylaxis of fat embolism syndrome. Clin Orthop 143:211–221.

62. Suter, P.M., Fairley, H.B., and Isenberg, M.D. Optimum end-expiratory airway pressure in patients with acute pulmonary failure. N Engl J Med 292:281–289, 1975.

63. Filney, N.L., Bailey, G.L., and Morgan, A.P. Sequential system failure after rupture of abdominal aortic aneurysms: An unsolved problem in postoperative care. Ann Surg 178:117–122, 1973.

64. Walt, A.J. Initial assessment and management of the injured patient, in Walt, A.J. (ed): *Early Care of the Injured Patient.* Philadelphia, Saunders, 1982.

65. Watters, J.M., and Freeman, J.B. Parenteral nutrition by peripheral vein. Surg Clin North Am 61:593–604, 1981.

66. Weisman, I.M., Rinaldo, J.E., and Rogers, R.M. Positive end-expiratory pressure in adult respiratory failure. N Engl J Med 307:1381–1384, 1982.

CHAPTER 18

General Principles of Management of Fractures and Dislocations

Kenneth Zaslav, Robert Moriarty, Bruce Meinhard, Paul Levin, Stuart Polisner, and Roger Dee

SECTION A

Fractures and Dislocations in Adults

Kenneth Zaslav, Robert Moriarty, Bruce Meinhard, Paul Levin, and Roger Dee

DEFINITIONS

A *fracture* may be defined as a discontinuity in the structure of bone.

Fractures occur when an injuring force exceeds the mechanical strength of the involved bone. These forces may be applied directly or indirectly.[141] Direct injuries can be caused not only by such things as a car bumper or a hammer but also by an unrestrained passenger in a car striking the doors or dashboard. Bullets may also inflict direct injury to the bone. Indirect fractures may result from violent muscular contractions. Falls on an outstretched hand or bending and twisting of the leg on a fixed foot can also cause indirect fractures at a distance from the point of application of the force. Biomechanically, failure of the bone leading to a fracture results from tension, compression, and/or shear forces acting on the bone.[86]

Open Fractures

An *open fracture* communicates externally through a break in the overlying soft tissue integument (skin or mucous membrane). In distinction to a closed fracture, an open fracture is more often complicated by severe soft tissue injury,[86,134] infection,[86,249] delayed union,[342] and nonunion.[86,220]

Open fractures have been classified by Gustilo et al into three types (Table 18-1).[133,135] A type I open fracture represents an injury in which a spike of bone from within has pierced the skin and immediately retracted back into the affected extremity. They are low-energy injuries and consequently have a simple fracture pattern. Type II open fractures have larger skin wounds with moderate soft tissue injuries. The wounds are not grossly contaminated with dirt or other substance, and true soft tissue loss is minimal. Type III open fractures are severe open injuries with significant soft tissue injury as well as contamination. They have been further subdivided into three types, and the subdivisions have prognostic significance (Table 18-1).

TABLE 18-1 Classification of Open Fractures

Type	Classification
I	Open fracture with clean laceration <1 cm long
II	Open fracture with clean laceration >1 cm long without extensive soft tissue injury, flaps, or avulsions
III	Open fractures with extensive damage to soft tissue including muscle, skin, and neurovascular structures
IIIa	Adequate soft tissue coverage of fracture despite extensive soft tissue damage
IIIb	Extensive soft tissue injury with periosteal stripping, bone exposure, and/or massive contamination
IIIc	Open fractures associated with arterial injury requiring repair

Source: Modified Gustilo classification. From Meinhard, B., and Moriarty, R.V., Infect Surg, August 1985, p. 621. Reprinted with permission.

Comminution

Comminuted fractures are fractures in which more than one fracture line is present. Two frequently seen comminuted patterns are segmental fractures, in which a middle segment of bone is separated by fracture lines, and the butterfly fragment, in which a triangular portion of bone is separated from the major oblique or spiral fracture. Comminuted fractures reflect a high energy injury and have significant soft tissue damage. These injuries tend to have greater delays in healing when compared with simple linear fractures.[9]

Regional Definitions of Fracture

Fractures are described using regional terms such as intra-, juxta-, or extraarticular; metaphyseal or diaphyseal. Diaphyseal fractures are further described as located in the proximal, middle, or distal third.

Definitions Related to Deformity

Fractures are also characterized by their displacement, angulation, and rotation. By convention, the position of the distal fragment is described in respect to its relation to the proximal fragment. Displacement can be anterior, posterior, medial, or lateral and is measured as a percentage of the diameter of the fractured bone. Angulation, which is measured in degrees, is properly described by the location of the apex of the fracture. Rotation is primarily a clinical diagnosis but is detectable on an x-ray film when adjacent joints are seen in different projections, or the diameters of the fracture surfaces are different.

Stress Fractures

Devas defines *stress fracture* as "a fracture occurring in the normal bones of healthy people doing every day activities without injuries."[88] The sites of these fractures vary with age and activity. They are often seen in healthy athletes and armed forces recruits, and occur more frequently than previously suspected. A prospective study of a population subjected to strenuous physical training showed the incidence of stress fractures to be 31 percent.[221] Pain usually begins after activity. Symptoms recur earlier in subsequent outings and may eventually curb the activity. Radiological confirmation is most often delayed. If a fracture pattern does materialize, it is most commonly of an oblique type.[88] The bone scan may be of great diagnostic value when the x-ray films are normal. Milgrom et al noted that 68 percent of the femoral stress fractures in military recruits are either minimally symptomatic or totally asymptomatic. In a group of similar patients with tibial stress fractures, only 8 percent were found to be asymptomatic. If diagnosed early and treated conservatively, with simple rest, most of these fractures heal.[221]

Pathologic Fracture

A fracture through preexisting diseased bone is a *pathologic fracture.* The fracture occurs with trivial injury or spontaneously. These fractures may be found in both benign and ma-

lignant primary bone neoplasms as well as in metastatic lesions. Pathologic fracture may also occur in bones afflicted with generalized disease processes such as osteoporosis and osteomalacia.

DIAGNOSIS OF FRACTURE

Clinical Presentation

Pain and tenderness over a localized area are the most reliable presumptive evidence of fracture. Swelling is usually present. Loss of function or deformity may also accompany a fracture. However, nondisplaced or impacted fractures may not exhibit these signs, and one may be deceived by their absence. Definitive evidence of fracture is present if there is abnormal mobility within a bone.

Radiological Diagnosis

The clinical suspicion of a fracture must always be confirmed by x-ray examination. Although the type of x-ray view that is needed may vary according to anatomical location, one should adhere to the following two general principles: (1) Routinely obtain at least two radiographic views at right angles to one another; and (2) include the entire bone, as well as the joints above and below the fracture.

DISLOCATIONS

A *dislocation* is a capsular, ligamentous, or osseous disruption of a joint resulting in a complete loss of contact of the two articulating surfaces. A *subluxation* is a partial loss of congruity in which articular surfaces maintain contact without their normal anatomical relations.

Clinical Presentation

The clinical features of dislocation include pain, loss of normal contour of the overlying soft tissues, and loss of the relations of bony prominences. Gross limitation of both active and passive motion are usually present.[141] The position or attitude of the extremity upon presentation is at times diagnostic of the direction of the dislocation. For example, the classic position of the leg following a posterior dislocation of the hip is adduction, flexion, and internal rotation.

A complete neurological examination should always accompany evaluation of a dislocation as the incidence of associated nerve injury is well-described.[141]

Radiological Diagnosis

Once again, obtaining two x-ray views is mandatory. One of the most commonly missed musculoskeletal injuries is the posterior dislocation of the shoulder, which may appear normal on the anteroposterior (AP) film. Adequate lateral x-rays in the scapular plane or transaxillary lateral views clearly show this dislocation.

FRACTURE REDUCTION

Anatomical Criteria

The anatomical parameters necessary to obtain a good result vary depending on the bone involved, the type of deformity, the region of the bone involved, and the age of the patient. Significant degrees of shortening, rotation, or angulation are less acceptable than displacement. However, persisting displacement of such magnitude that there is little or no bone-on-bone contact is suboptimum. Shortening is more acceptable in the upper limb, for example, in the humerus, than in the bones of the lower limb. The type of joint above and below the fracture also determine what deformity is functionally tolerable. Hinged joints can compensate well for AP bowing, as in the forearm, whereas ball-and-socket joints can compensate for malrotation, as in proximal humeral shaft fractures.[6] Large degrees of rotation are not well-tolerated even by ball-and-socket joints.

Connolly considers rotation "the forgotten third dimension of treatment." Frequently overlooked when reading two-dimensional x-ray films, malrotation is a more common reason for malunion than simple varus or valgus angulation in the frontal plane.[73]

Mayfield studied 75 femoral shaft fractures treated with traction. Rotational malunion was present in 34 of the 75 fractures. He found that patients with significant rotation, or patients with shortening of greater than 2 cm, exhibited a gluteus medius limp. When both existed, the limp was worse. He believed that rotation decreases the efficiency of the gluteus medius by shifting the greater trochanter to a more posterior position. Shortening causes a similar decrease in its function by causing laxity in the iliotibial tract and its attached muscles.[211]

Intraarticular Fracture

Most authors agree that precise anatomical realignment is necessary after an intraarticular fracture to avoid future traumatic arthritis.[2,7,62,169,224,283] If displaced, even small bone fragments may obstruct smooth motion of a joint. Acceptance of less than anatomical reduction in joints can also lead to joint instability, as bony disruption near ligament attachments may cause an alteration in ligament length.[224]

CLOSED REDUCTION

Analgesia and Anesthesia

One of the major obstructions to obtaining an adequate reduction is muscle spasm. This is increased greatly by pain. Anesthesia can be achieved in the emergency room with local hematoma infiltration. This is especially the case in upper extremity fractures. Fractures can also be manipulated with the use of intravenous narcotics that have predictable actions and can be easily reversed pharmacologically. At times, general anesthesia may be required to overcome strong muscle forces.

Manipulation

Sir John Charnley in his classic monograph has discussed the use of the intact soft tissue hinge to aid in the manipulation of fractures.[66] An appropriately molded cast provides three-point fixation and maintains these intact tissues in a stretched position preserving the reduction (Fig. 18-1). A sound knowledge of muscle attachments is required if manipulative reduction is to succeed.

The distal fragment of a fracture is more easily controlled than the proximal fragment, which adopts the position dictated by the muscles attached to it. During manipulative reduction one normally aligns the distal fragment with the position of the proximal fragment.

Skeletal Traction

Skeletal traction involves the use of transfixion pins and these apply traction force directly to the skeleton. Many surgeons seem to prefer threaded Steinmann pins to Kirschner wires

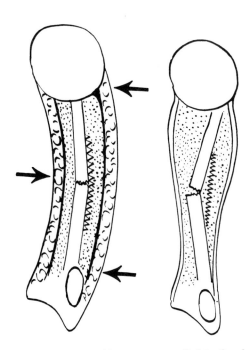

Figure 18-1 Illustration of how a cast applied to the shape of an injured extremity may allow loss of reduction. However, application of a cast with three-point fixation helps achieve and maintain reduction of a fracture by placing the intact soft tissue hinge under tension. *(From Charnley, J.: The Closed Treatment of Common Fractures. Edinburgh, Churchill Livingstone, 1968. Reproduced with permission.)*

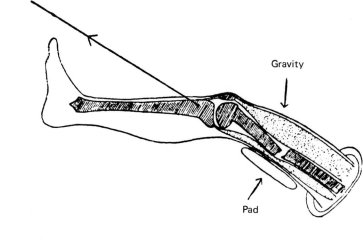

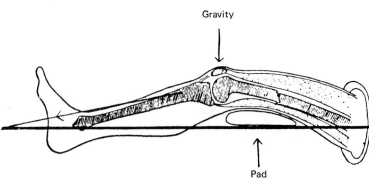

Figure 18-2 Despite longitudinal traction applied to a midshaft femur fracture, the effect of gravity may produce a posterior sag at the fracture site; the sag may be reduced by application of a pad posterior to the fracture site, and by flexing the knee with traction in the axis of the tibia. Note that the limb is cradled by a Thomas splint. *(From Charnley, J.: The Closed Treatment of Common Fractures. Edinburgh, Churchill Livingstone, 1968. Reproduced with permission.)*

for this purpose. The larger size and grasp of the Steinmann pin allows better purchase on the bone. This improved purchase decreases motion at the bone-pin interface and helps prevent pin tract problems.

Traction is a method of restoring alignment to a fracture through gradual neutralization of muscular forces. In fixed traction systems, the limb rests on a splint and the end of the traction cord is tied to the distal end of the splint. Countertraction is then achieved proximally by the other end of the splint, which may "dig in" and ulcerate the skin at the root of the limb unless the whole fixed system is then pulled away from the patient with a second traction application. In sliding traction, which is the system more commonly in use, the traction cord is run over a pulley at the base of the bed and the patient's body weight is the counterweight. Such a system can be used with or without a supporting splint which cradles the limb (Fig. 18-2). Simple longitudinal or vectored traction, through the axis of the bone, realigns fracture fragments within the soft tissue envelope (Fig. 18-3).[198]

Traction alone may be unable to overcome some cases of interlocking of fragments. Also interposition of soft tissue may block reduction. Furthermore, excessive swelling around the fracture site due to bleeding may increase the hydrostatic pressure so that the soft tissue does not allow elongation during traction.[66]

It is important that one does not overdistract the fragments. Overdistraction may result in delayed fracture healing and leg length discrepancies.

In fractures of the femur, posterior bowing due to gravitational forces persists after length has been regained. Increasing the traction weight may result in overdistraction and still not correct the posterior angulation. Lewis suggests that a traction sling be placed beneath the apex of the femoral fracture and weight then be applied to reverse the posterior angulation.[198] However, Charnley used a modification of the Thomas splint with a pad to achieve the same result (Fig. 18-2).

Skin Traction

Skin traction is a technique in which adhesive strapping is secured to the involved extremity for the purpose of applying a traction weight. It is imperative that the strapping encompass a large area of skin such that the force of traction is distributed evenly. Traction by this technique is limited to 10 percent of body weight with a maximum of 5 to 7 lb. It is used primarily on small children, adults awaiting hip surgery, and postoperative or postinjury care in which a small amount of weight is indicated for muscle relaxation.

Maintenance of Reduction

Once reduction is achieved, it must be maintained. In closed treatment this may be provided by casts, splints, or continuous skeletal traction.

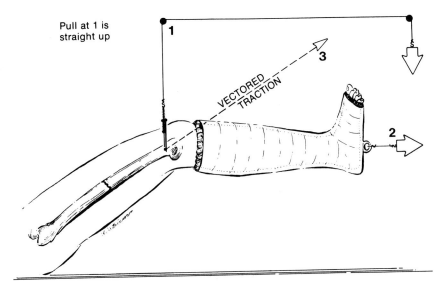

Pull at 1 is straight up

VECTORED TRACTION

Figure 18-3 Vectored traction. The resultant of vector force 1 and vector force 2 is vector force 3, which produces a traction force through the longitudinal axis of the fractured femur. *(From Lewis, R.: Handbook of Traction, Casting, and Splinting Techniques. Philadelphia, Lippincott, 1977. Reproduced with permission.)*

Use of Traction to Maintain Reduction

Skeletal traction and balanced suspension may be utilized to maintain reduction. The main disadvantages of traction include prolonged bed rest and the attendant systemic complications: deep venous thrombosis, pulmonary embolism, pneumonia, and muscle atrophy. In addition, nerve palsy due to traction or compression, pressure sores on the skin, and pin tract infection may complicate this form of treatment.

Fractures may be treated by skeletal traction until callus formation has stabilized the bone. Displaced pelvic fractures and femur fractures are the skeletal injuries most frequently treated by this technique. Some investigators advocate traction treatment for comminuted tibial plateau and plafond fractures as well as comminuted diaphyseal fractures. When treating these intraarticular fractures by traction, one attempts to achieve articular congruency by ligamentotaxis acting on the major displaced articular fragments. If this is successful, an early range-of-motion program may be instituted. On occasion intraarticular fractures with comminuted metaphyseal and diaphyseal extension may be treated by minimal internal fixation to restore articular congruency and then continuous skeletal traction. Again early range-of-motion programs may be begun.

Traction may be discontinued when early fracture consolidation is demonstrated radiographically. Shortening will no longer be a significant problem, but malalignment due to angulation may still develop. Supplemental casting, cast bracing, or splinting must be instituted at this time and must be continued until complete bony union has been achieved.

Use of Cast to Maintain Reduction

Despite the advent of newer materials over the past 5 to 10 years, plaster of Paris is still the most popular cast material. The plaster is applied over a layer of cotton wadding. This padding should be placed in smooth overlapping layers so as to avoid wrinkles, which can cause irritation to the skin.

Areas with superficial neurological structures (i.e., peroneal and ulnar nerves) as well as bony areas with increased prominence, such as the heel, should be padded with an extra layer for protection. The use of stockinette is optional. However, several studies have shown that its use provides greater patient comfort.[189,331] Plaster setting is an exothermic reaction by which plaster of Paris ($CaSo_4 \cdot \frac{1}{2}H_2O$) is converted to gypsum ($CaSo_4 \cdot 2H_2O$). The amount of heat imparted to the patient's skin is related to the cast thickness, water temperature, and humidity. LaValette et al measured peak skin temperatures during plaster setting in relation to the temperature of the dip water. They noted that when the temperature of the dip water is greater than 24°C there is a risk of skin burn.

One should use an even motion during cast application to equally distribute the plaster in all areas. For maximum strength of the cast, joint motion must be avoided during drying. A cast which is molded to the shape of the limb, although cosmetically pleasing, may not always maintain the best reduction. Charnley's concept of three-point fixation involves the application of three points of force to the drying plaster as a means of placing the intact soft tissue hinge under tension. This adds stability to the fracture and helps prevent loss of reduction (Fig. 17-2).

Complications of Casting *Decubitus Ulcers* Ulceration beneath a cast or splint may be related to the initial soft tissue trauma, folds in the cast padding or casting material, or a combination of both. Any complaints of localized pressure, pain, or burning must be investigated either by removing the cast or by cutting an appropriate window.

Neurovascular Compromise Casts may also greatly increase intracompartmental pressures in a swollen extremity and be of etiologic significance in the development of a compartment syndrome. The key to diagnosis and treatment of this condition is a high degree of suspicion and early intervention. The management of this complication is further discussed later in this chapter.

Joint Stiffness Effective immobilization often necessitates immobilization of the joint both above and below the injured bone. Joint stiffness is a potential complication. It rarely occurs in children but is a common problem with adults, especially if the fracture has an intraarticular extension.[264] Functional bracing, and hinged casts or orthoses, may prevent these problems. These forms of treatment will be discussed later in this chapter.

Cast Wedging

Cast wedging is of great value in correcting angulation of certain fractures, especially in the tibial shaft.[43,55,141,326] Several authors have recommended opening wedges,[43,55,326] while others prefer the closing wedge technique.[66] A theoretical analysis of cast wedging by Schulak et al supports a combined opening-closing wedging technique, in which the opening wedge is performed at the level where the long axis of the two major fragments intersect and not at the fracture site. This best corrects both angulation and translation.[300] Other authors agree that this provides the best fulcrum for adjustment of reduction with the least risk of pressure injury to the skin.[15] Extreme care is necessary when wedging a cast immediately after a tibia fracture. The increased tension placed on the swollen traumatized skin may precipitate a skin breakdown.

Windows

For the care of small wounds and surgical incisions, windows may be cut in casts. When this technique is used, the window must be replaced and secured with an Ace wrap. This avoids herniation of edematous tissue, and necrosis of skin edges through the window.

Fiberglass

New, improved materials have made fiberglass casting products easier to apply. The lighter weight of fiberglass is especially helpful in long leg casts for the elderly or weakened patient. However, fiberglass casting materials are more difficult to apply and less forgiving. Small folds of casting materials in the layers closest to the skin are extremely uncomfortable and can lead to pressure sores. As a result the indication for the use of these materials in acute injuries is limited. When crossing joints during application it is advisable to use the narrower-width rolls to prevent creasing. Although fiberglass is water-resistant, it is important to warn patients that the skin and padding beneath the cast will not dry without exposure to the air. Therefore, frequent immersion is not advisable, or skin maceration will result.

Use of Splints to Maintain Reduction

When severe soft tissue swelling is present or can be anticipated with a comminuted fracture pattern, the use of splinting techniques is required and circumferential plaster casts must be avoided. Some injuries may be definitively treated with splints. Several types of basic splints are commercially available or can be fabricated. The Sugar tong splint, which is constructed from layers of plaster slab, effectively immobilizes and maintains reduction of wrist, forearm, and humeral shaft fractures and may be converted to a complete cast when appropriate. Nondisplaced ankle fractures and fractures of the bones of the feet may be comfortably and safely immobilized with either plaster U splints and foot plates, or commercially available splints.

Closed Functional Bracing of Fractures

Appley was one of the first to advocate early functional treatment with cast bracing instead of rigid immobilization after closed reduction of certain fractures.[18] The principles of functional cast bracing have expanded the indications of closed treatment. Sarmiento has provided experimental and clinical evidence supporting the use of fracture bracing for the closed treatment of select fractures of the upper and lower extremity. Proponents of this technique emphasize that prolonged immobilization is nonphysiological and predisposes to fracture disease. In contrast to rigid internal fixation, which leads to primary osseous union, closed treatment relies on motion at the fracture site to stimulate callus formation. At times, mild shortening and displacement occur but within acceptable functional parameters.[292,293]

Sarmiento reported on 2000 appendicular fractures treated with cast bracing, with a rate of nonunion less than 1 percent.[293] Others confirm the value of this technique when used in tibial,[55,84] femoral,[226,227] and humeral fractures[23] (Fig. 18-4). These data have shown functional bracing to be an effective method to achieve union while allowing early restoration of function.

Contraindications Functional bracing is not indicated for all fractures. Sarmiento includes the following as contraindications:[293]

1. Diabetes with peripheral neuropathy
2. Uncooperative patients
3. Fractures of the proximal half of the femur, which tend to angulate into varus
4. Isolated fractures of the radius with distal radioulnar joint disruption, which may yield late deformity and a painful radioulnar joint due to late arthritis
5. Fractures of both bones of the forearm which cannot be reduced
6. Monteggia's fractures
7. Intraarticular fractures, since joint congruity must be reestablished
8. Fractures in spastic patients, which commonly undergo angular deformity because of uncontrollable muscle forces

It is important to note that this treatment protocol cannot correct shortening. However, Sarmiento has shown that shortening will not increase beyond that which occurred at the time of the initial injury.[292] His follow-up of tibial fractures treated with fracture bracing suggests that some diaphyseal shortening will not affect extremity function.

Fracture bracing has also become an important adjunctive treatment of fractures that have undergone internal fixation when absolutely rigid fixation has not been achieved. For example, a fracture brace may help prevent angular or rota-

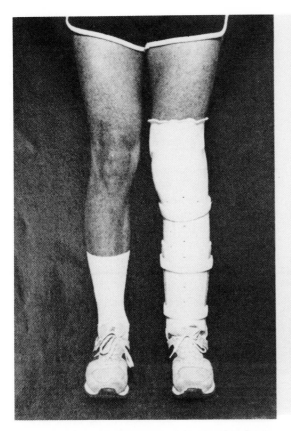 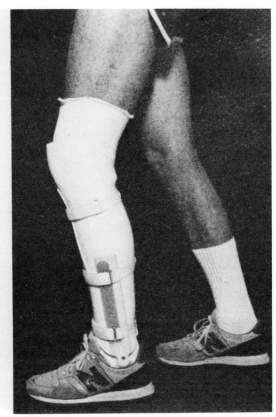

Figure 18-4 Prefabricated tibial functional fracture bracing as popularized by Sarmiento. *(From Tarr, R.T., et al, Orthop Rev 12:25, 1984. Reproduced with permission.)*

tional deformity from occurring when weight bearing occurs on a tibial fracture that has been internally fixed with a flexible intramedullary rod.

Pins and Plaster

Cast immobilization is unable to maintain the length of an injured extremity in the presence of inherently unstable fracture patterns. In the past a popular technique used for unstable diaphyseal fractures was the application of transfixing Steinmann's pins proximal and distal to the fracture, with incorporation of these pins into the plaster cast. While this technique did help maintain length, it was associated with numerous complications including infection and nonunion. Other forms of internal or external skeletal fixation are now preferred for the treatment of long bone fractures.

Some authors still prefer the pins-and-plaster techniques for maintaining length in comminuted distal radius fractures. This preference is due to a high incidence of reflex sympathetic dystrophy when external fixators have been utilized.[129]

External Fixation

This technique is usually utilized in maintaining reduction after an open procedure and is described in a later section. It should be noted, however, that external fixation is also occasionally used to control unstable closed reduction.

OPEN REDUCTION

Indications

No single treatment is right for any specific fracture in all individuals. It is important to take into consideration the general health, vocation, expectations, and needs of each patient. In addition, not all surgeons are equally adept at all forms of treatment. Ill-judged surgical treatment is the worst of all possible options, exposing the patient to the risk of infection and nonunion without gaining any of the potential benefits.[6,141,173]

The only absolute indications for operative reduction and stabilization in closed fractures is the inability to obtain or maintain an acceptable reduction by closed methods.

Internal Fixation

The goal of internal fixation is to achieve a circumstance in which external splinting of the fractured extremity is superfluous, and full, active, pain-free mobilization of the surrounding joints and muscles is possible. This is accomplished by the use of techniques that obtain anatomical reduction and neutralize external forces about the fracture site.

Over the past decade, members of the Association for the Study of Internal Fixation (Arbeitsgemeinshaft für Osteosyntesefragen) of Switzerland have worked to compile scientific and clinical data supporting theories behind internal fixation. Their work has shown that excellent functional results can be obtained with both-bone fractures of the forearm,[14] intraarticular joint fractures,[8,278] and multiply injured patients.[47] In addition, when the procedures are carefully performed by surgeons adhering to their method, the overall infection rate has been 0.5 to 1.5 percent with closed fractures and 7 percent with open fractures.[7,8] With tibial fractures alone, Allgower reported a series of 4400 tibia fractures treated with open reduction and internal fixation. Although 10 percent of these fractures were open, the overall infection rate was only 1.7 percent.[8]

Techniques of Internal Fixation

Lag Screw Technique The lag screw technique is the most important method to provide static interfragmental compression. This well-described technique allows the screw threads to gain purchase on the far cortex but not engage the near cortex.[233] As the screw is tightened, the fracture surfaces are compressed together. The lag screw should be utilized whenever the fracture pattern permits its use.

Compression Plates Static compression across the fracture site can also be achieved by the use of plates. Plate osteosynthesis has been especially effective in forearm fractures.[233,235] In oblique fractures of the lower extremity, compression should not be applied without lag screws because of the high levels of axial compressive forces.[233] The dynamic compression plate (DCP) is the mainstay of this method. The oblong-shaped screw holes allow compression to be placed across a fracture site without the need to prestress the plate. Screws may also be inserted at various angles through these plates. When the eccentric drill guide is used to insert screws through the screw hole closest to the fracture, this places the screw 1 mm from the neutral position. As it is tightened, it engages the spherical-shaped hole and pushes the plate, and therefore the attached bone, 1 mm toward the fracture. This yields 50 to 80 kilopounds of axial compression.[6,253] A second screw may be placed in the eccentric position in the closest screw hole on the same or opposite side of the fracture. The remaining screws are placed in the neutral position.

Standard AO plates may also be used to achieve compression across the fracture site of an eccentrically loaded long bone. According to the tension band principle, if the plate can be applied to the tension side of the fractured bone, the tensile forces will be converted to compressive forces.[253] The technique of tension band wiring of fractures of the patella and olecranon also produces a similar compression across the fracture site.[233]

Intramedullary Nailing First used by Hey Groves during World War I, medullary rods have been used to internally fix selected long bone fractures, especially diaphyseal fractures of the femur and tibia. In contrast to interfragmental compression, this technique does not achieve rigid fixation. The intramedullary rod acts as an internal splint. It provides a method of maintaining accurate reduction and alignment while allowing prompt mobilization of the patient and the adjacent muscles and joints.[233]

Modern radiographic techniques have permitted the routine use of closed intramedullary nailing techniques. This method is attractive in that surgical dissection in the vicinity of the fracture is not necessary. While displaced fractures disrupt the medullary and endosteal blood supply, the periosteal blood supply remains largely intact and provides continued vascularity to bone.[83] Studies have shown that medullary reaming further damages the endosteal vessels. Experiments with rabbits have demonstrated that endosteal vessel fragments are often seen in subperiosteal vessels following tibial reaming. These fragments may actually add further stimulus to osteogenesis,[298] and may explain the healing of delayed unions after intramedullary nailing. In addition, it has been shown that endosteal blood supply reconstitutes after intramuscular rodding.[268]

Because dissection at the fracture site is avoided, the incidence of infection is dramatically decreased and the rate of union is markedly increased (when compared with other techniques of internal fixation).[83,139,268] Winquist and Hansen have reported a 1 percent infection rate with closed intramedullary nailing as opposed to a 3 to 8 percent incidence of infection with open nailing.[341] The reported rate of union of 99 percent with closed nailing is equally impressive.

When the technique was first introduced, the indications for intramedullary nailing were limited to noncomminuted fractures at the isthmus. Shortening and rotational and angular malalignment were common sequelae when standard intramedullary nails were used in the event of comminuted, proximal, or distal fracture patterns.

Most recently, interlocking nail devices have been used to control these difficult fractures (Fig. 18-5).[1,42,131,165,166] These devices have effectively expanded the indication of intramedullary nailing to include long spiral and oblique fractures, comminuted fractures, and proximal or distal one-third fractures.[131] In the event of a noncomminuted proximal or distal fracture, a closed nailing can be performed with an interlocking screw placed into the smaller bone fragment. This dynamic interlocking technique allows for rotational stability as well as impaction at the fracture site as the patient ambulates. Comminuted fracture patterns can be treated with both proximal and distal interlocking (static mode) to maintain both appropriate length and rotational stability.

Flexible Intramedullary Rods Flexible intramedullary rods were first introduced by Ender to treat intertrochanteric and subtrochanteric fractures.[102] However, more recently, others have shown their effectiveness in fractures of the humerus, tibia, and femoral shaft.[147,210,218,243] Flexible rods do not require reaming; therefore, minimal damage occurs to the endosteal blood supply. This is an attractive technique especially in closed tibial fractures with severe soft tissue injuries. In these cases, reaming of the acutely injured tibia may result in a compartment syndrome or devitalize the bone enough to lead to an infection. The stability achieved is not as great as with interlocking nails, and postoperative casting is often necessary. Comminuted and proximal or distal fractures are also susceptible to rotational and angular malunion. However, as these implants do not share load, no stress shielding occurs, and therefore no weight-bearing restriction is necessary following their removal.[243,244]

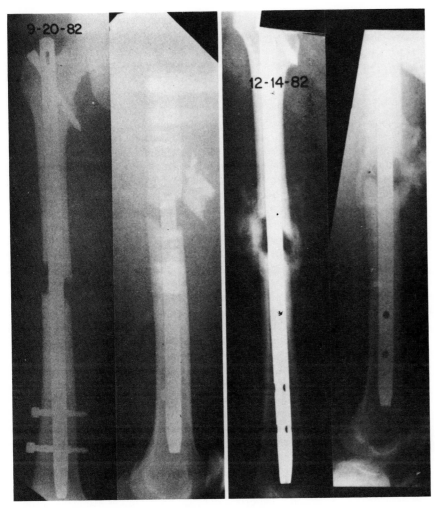

Figure 18-5 A Grosse-Kempf interlocking nail was used initially in a static mode for internal fixation of an unstable, comminuted midshaft fracture of the femur. (Film dated 9/20/82.) The distal screws were removed 12 weeks later, and the remaining films (dated 12/14/82) demonstrate early healing of the fracture. *(From Johnson, K.D., J Bone Joint Surg 66A:1231, 1984. Reproduced with permission.)*

Complications of Internal Fixation

The application of internal fixation changes a previously closed fracture to an open one. Thus, infection is always a potential complication. Most wound infections following the internal fixation of closed injuries are superficial.[58,186] Deep wound infections are less frequent but potentially disastrous complications of orthopaedic surgery.[186,263]

Fortunately, the incidence of wound sepsis in the operative management of closed fractures is less than 2 percent.[58,186] Precise surgical technique, prophylactic broad-spectrum antibiotics, and closed suction drainage all contribute to a lower wound sepsis rate.[58]

In addition to the immediate threat of sepsis, deep infection involving the fracture site may lead to acute and chronic osteomyelitis or to an infected nonunion. Infected nonunions are perhaps the most difficult conditions to treat in orthopaedics.[58] Their treatment will be discussed later in this chapter.

Complications of internal fixation may arise directly from failure of the implanted appliance. Although material defects may play causative roles, more often poor operative technique, delayed union or nonunion of the fracture, and excessive, premature weight bearing are the factors that are responsible for bending, breaking, loosening, or even migration

of internal fixation devices.[1,119,141,303] Bone of increased porosity is the end result of stress shielding by a rigid plate or a tight, load bearing intramedullary rod (but is less likely with a flexible rod). The risk of refracture may persist for months or years following the removal of such an implant. This is further discussed in Chap. 8.

External Fixation

Indications

External fixation of fractures has become a versatile method of treating a variety of osseous injuries. The most frequent indication is for Gustilo-Anderson type II and type III open tibia fractures (Table 18-I). It is also used for type III open femur fractures, as well as other open injuries about the appendicular and axial skeleton.[35,311,325]

External fixation has also proved to be a rapid, safe, and reliable technique to stabilize unstable pelvic fractures and fracture dislocations. In the hemodynamically unstable multiply injured patient, this form of fixation has been demonstrated as a lifesaving technique to obtain hemostasis in the pelvic region.[216]

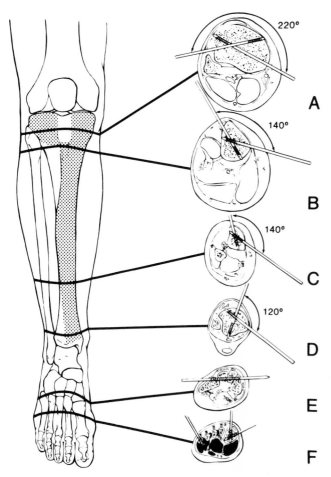

Figure 18-6 The safe corridor for insertion of external fixation pins in the lower leg. At level *A,* proximal to the tibial tubercle, pins can be inserted within an arc of 220°. This arc reduces as one moves distally. At *C,* the anterior tibial vessels and deep peroneal nerve become vulnerable as they cross the lateral tibial cortex. At levels *E* and *F,* pins may be placed in the tarsal or metatarsal bones to splint the ankle joint. The dotted area indicates the subcutaneous regions of the tibia where pin insertion is safe. *(From Behrens, F., and Searls, K., J Bone Joint Surg 68B:247, 1986. Reproduced with permission.)*

Additional indications for external fixation include treatment of closed fractures on extremities with other significant soft tissue injuries such as burns and deglovings.[282,318] It has also proved useful in the reduction of displaced intraarticular fractures of the distal radius by permitting controlled application of a traction force and reduction by ligamentotaxis.[214,311] External fixation may be used to neutralize the deforming forces across a bone which has been treated by minimal internal fixation.[233,311] Finally, its efficacy in compression arthrodesis, leg-lengthening procedures, and stabilization of infected nonunions has been well-demonstrated.[3,149,311]

Techniques of External Fixation

Regardless of indication, several important factors must be universally considered when applying external fixators. Be-

hrens has divided these factors into three major groups: anatomical, clinical, and mechanical.[35] The most important anatomical consideration is the window of safe pin application. This window must be analyzed separately for each extremity to avoid damage to neurovascular structures. The tibia is the most common site of fixator application. Its window describes a 220° arc anteriorly at the proximal one-third. However, it decreases in width from 140° below the tibial tubercle to a 120° arc in the distal one-third (Fig. 18-6).

Mechanical considerations include adequate rigidity of components and an analysis of the deforming forces that may be active on the involved extremity. These forces must each be considered and counteracted by the geometric configuration of the external fixator in order to provide adequate stability.[35,310]

Six configurations are commonly used today: unilateral, bilateral, quadrilateral, triangular, half circular, and circular (Fig. 18-7). For lower limb and pelvic stabilization, 5- or 6-mm pins provide maximal support. However, pin diameter should not exceed 20 percent of the diameter of the bone or the pin tract may diminish the structural integrity of the bone. Pins should be threaded, and they should be inserted with a hand drill after predrilling with power to avoid producing bony necrosis and subsequent pin loosening.[35,167,214,310]

The use of unilateral frames is preferable when the bone and fracture pattern permit. The virtues of this technique include increased mobility for the patient because of the lighter-weight frames, improved access to soft tissues for wound management, and greater safety with the use of half pins. As half pins only penetrate skin, soft tissue on one side of the bone, and both cortices, the risk of neurovascular impalement, and joint stiffness due to muscle tethering, is greatly reduced.[35,214]

It is important to neutralize all forces acting on the bone when applying unilateral frames to weight-bearing bones such as the tibia. In the tibia, sagittal forces are three to four times greater than those acting along the frontal plane. Therefore, one should place the frame in the sagittal plane whenever possible. If this is contraindicated because of wound location, one should consider adding a second half frame to obviate the need for a sagittally placed frame. The most common combinations would be anteromedial and medial half frames. Half pins should not be placed midlaterally in the tibia because of the risk of neurovascular injury and muscle impalement (Fig. 18-6).[35]

Greater degrees of comminution, as well as lesser degrees of inherent fracture stability, demand more complex configurations which may require application of the external fixator above and/or below adjacent joints. Bilateral and quadrilateral frames afford excellent compression across an unstable fracture.[214] If significant bone loss has occurred, bone graft must be utilized to fill in gaps which will most likely not be bridged by local bone healing alone. As the graft incorporates and stability increases, supplementary fixation may be removed to lighten the patient's load.

Complications of External Fixation

The most common problem that occurs with the use of external fixation devices is pin tract infection. Reports on the inci-

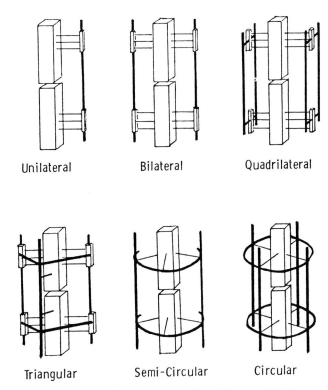

Unilateral   Bilateral   Quadrilateral

Triangular   Semi-Circular   Circular

Figure 18-7 The various configurations of external fixators. *(From Sisk, T., Clin Orthop 180:11, 1983. Reproduced with permission.)*

dence vary from 10 to 100 percent depending on how one defines infection.[129] Colonization of the pin tract most probably occurs in 100 percent of cases. However, the incidence of true cellulitis or dermal infection is considerably less. The incidence of chronic osteomyelitis was found in one series to have occurred in 4 percent of 129 cases.[192] Careful pin insertion technique and meticulous pin care is essential. Several studies have shown that the use of threaded pins surrounded by bulky dressings to decrease motion of the skin-pin interface, along with compulsive antiseptic pin care three times daily, aids in avoiding this complication.[129,130] In addition, reduction of skin-pin tension by adequate skin release around the pin minimizes soft tissue necrosis and resultant infection. Once the pins are removed, most of the superficial infections appear to resolve with continued wound care.

Neurovascular damage is a potential risk when inserting pins without respect to the anatomical topography. In the upper extremity, the most commonly injured nerves are the radial nerve at the distal one-half of the upper arm and at the proximal one-half of the forearm. The dorsal sensory radial nerve at the wrist may also be injured when Colles' fractures are treated by external fixation. In the lower extremity, the most common injuries involve the anterior tibial artery and the deep peroneal nerve at the junction of the distal quarter of the leg.[310] The use of half pins and a thorough knowledge of anatomical "safe windows" decrease the incidence of these dreaded complications.

Ankle stiffness is commonly seen when transfixion pins are used to stabilize tibia fractures and less commonly when half pins are used. Failure to dorsiflex the ankle before pin insertion, and failure to encourage active joint motion above and below the fixator, may lead to stiffness and plantar flexion deformity. Commercially available or custom-made dorsiflexion splints may be attached to the fixator by elastic bands. This allows the patient to actively exercise the ankle and yet maintain a neutral position when resting.

Delayed union is commonly associated with the use of external fixation. In the absence of rigid fixation, bony healing relies upon macromotion at the fracture site, and impaction forces to allow cyclic loading, which helps stimulate callus formation. To avoid this complication, adequate autologous bone graft should be used to fill all gaps and early fixator removal should be a prime goal.[129] It is important to bear in mind that, in most cases, the external fixation device is best used to allow treatment of soft tissue injury. Many centers are now investigating the use of various fixator designs and stiffness characteristics which will allow enough stability for treating the soft tissues as well as enough flexibility to permit complete bony union while the fixator is in place.

REHABILITATION AND THE ROLE OF CONTINUOUS PASSIVE MOTION

Adams stated that "reduction is often unnecessary, immobilization is often unnecessary; whereas rehabilitation is always essential."[2] This statement should remain in the back of every orthopaedist's mind who approaches the treatment of fractures. Although fracture union is important, it is not our only goal. Functional rehabilitation of the extremity is achieved through the judicious and timely use of passive motion, active exercise, and functional use of the extremity.

A cooperative team relationship between the orthopaedic and rehabilitation departments is essential. Physical therapy should be instituted at the earliest appropriate time in the care of the fracture. However, the patient must be reminded that this is only one segment of his or her rehabilitation program. It is essential that the patients be motivated to perform their exercises for any protocol to be successful.

Animal studies have shown that joint immobilization is detrimental to joint architecture and function.[286,322] Irreversible degenerative changes develop in articular cartilage within 4 weeks in rats and 10 weeks in rabbits. Additional changes include contracture of the capsule and periarticular structures, encroachment on the joint by connective tissue, and eventual obliteration of the joint.

Salter has demonstrated that these changes can be prevented by early, continuous passive motion.[284,286,288,289] In addition, this treatment has proved to be well-tolerated by the patient, and it may have some effect on decreasing postoperative pain.[287] This may be partially due to a reduced clearance time of any hemarthrosis.[240]

Continuous passive motion has also been quite effective in regaining early joint motion in tibial plateau and other intraarticular fractures of hinged joints.

CONSIDERATIONS IN SPECIAL FRACTURES

Open Fractures

Successful management of open fractures is dependent upon adequate debridement,[134] judicious antibiotic usage,[133,249] rigid fracture stabilization,[107,173] and timely wound coverage.[334] The contaminated open fracture must be converted to a healthy, noninfected stable environment that is conducive to both bony and soft tissue healing.[140]

In the emergency room, the open fracture wound should be cultured for both aerobic and anaerobic organisms, and a Gram stain should also be performed in order to allow early identification of contaminating organisms.[78,134,163] The wound should then be promptly covered with a sterile dressing to avoid further contamination. Excessive probing, scrubbing, or soaking of the wound should be avoided. The fracture should be temporarily splinted, but vigorous attempts at reduction, especially prior to debridement of the wound, is not recommended.[163]

Admission cultures demonstrate wound contamination in most cases.[249] In those wounds that subsequently become infected, the organisms that are cultured are often grown in the initial wound cultures.[36,249] *Staphylococcus epidermidis,* and *Corynebacterium* species are often isolated.[236] However, gram-negative and polymicrobial infections are becoming more frequent.[133,236] Gas gangrene and tetanus, although uncommon, are still considerable threats with this type of injury.[236]

Since open fractures are contaminated,[249] the use of antibiotics should be considered as a therapeutic rather than a prophylactic treatment in the management of these injuries.[249] A broad-spectrum cephalosporin is the initial drug of choice[133,249] and should be administered parenterally in the emergency room once the Gram stain and cultures of the open wound have been obtained. The addition of an aminoglycoside and penicillin are indicated with severely injured or grossly contaminated open fractures.[133] Optimal antibiotic delivery is dependent upon thorough surgical debridement and rigid fracture stabilization so as to provide a stable and viable soft tissue bed.[220] Antibiotics are administered for 48 to 72 h. Therapy is then reassessed when culture and sensitivity reports become available from the postdebridement cultures.

Debridement

Surgical debridement is the mainstay of open fracture management.[133,134,236] Adequate debridement mandates the removal of all foreign matter and necrotic tissue about the wound. Soft tissue viability is often difficult to assess in high-energy type III injuries, and necrosis may progress over several days.[134] The patient should therefore be returned to the operating room if necessary within 24 to 48 h, and every 1 to 3 days thereafter until all nonviable soft tissue of bone can be identified and removed.[133]

Stabilization: Use of Internal Fixation

Prompt stabilization of open fractures enhances initial soft tissue survival, as well as the delivery of host defense fac-

tors.[220] Fracture stabilization may be achieved by a variety of treatment modalities ranging from cast immobilization to internal[55] or external[140] fixation or through a combination of both methods. The higher-grade open injuries demand greater stability to achieve successful soft tissue healing. The selection of a particular method of stabilization depends on the type of open fracture, the extent of associated injuries, and the surgeon's familiarity with each technique.[173]

Some still regard as controversial the use of plates, screws, and intramedullary devices for the primary fixation of open fractures.[69,133,135] Historically, a higher rate of infection was associated with the internal fixation of open fractures.[65,135] Further soft tissue and periosteal stripping as well as the introduction of hardware into a contaminated, open wound are the reported disadvantages.[65,237] Recently, however, excellent results with infection rates comparable to those of external stabilization methods have been reported.[36,129] These improved results are associated with improved patient selection, sound wound management, good surgical technique, and an experienced surgical team.[129] The technique used to stabilize open fractures must be determined based on the bone injured, the location within the bone (whether intraarticular or extraarticular), and the severity of the soft tissue injury.

Closure of Open Fractures

Primary wound closure should be avoided even in type I injuries, in which a small, clean, low-energy type wound is present.[133] Delayed primary closure is considered to be the procedure of choice in most open fractures, and it is generally performed within 5 to 7 days after the initial debridement, when wound viability can be most accurately assessed.[69,133,237] Split-thickness skin grafting is a technique which allows prompt, reliable wound coverage. It may be used to provide coverage of portions of wounds that could not be treated by delayed primary closure, or to cover local muscle flaps. Type III open fractures with extensive soft tissue loss often require local muscle and myocutaneous flaps for wound coverage.[99,116] Free microvascular flaps are employed when local flaps are precluded.[334] However, these free flaps have significant complications and failure rates of 21.5 percent for purely soft tissue flaps and 14.3 percent for bone composites.[343]

Bone grafting is often required in the treatment of open fractures, particularly where severe comminution or bone loss is present.[65,133] Delayed autogenous cancellous bone grafting is usually preferred.[133] Devitalized cortical bone grafts should not be used because of their predilection for infection, sequestrum, and resorption.[56,64,104] Larger bone defects may be bridged with a free, vascularized fibular or iliac crest transfer. A noninfected, viable soft tissue envelope is mandatory for the successful incorporation of bone grafts.[58]

Penetrating Injuries

Penetrating injuries can be inflicted by a variety of agents ranging from low- or high-energy projectiles to objects such

TABLE 18-2 Comparison of Kinetic Energy Calculated for Commonly Used Bullets

Weapon type	Projectile mass, grain	Muzzle velocity, f/s	Kinetic energy*, ft/lb
.22 caliber rifle	49	1180	124
.38 caliber pistol	158	800	263
.45 caliber pistol	230	850	370
12-gauge shotgun	656	1315	2519
M-16 (AR 15) rifle	55	3250	1290

$*KE = \dfrac{MV^2}{2}$

as bullets, knives, glass, splinters, or nails.[308] The common denominator is the focal area of skin laceration relative to the depth of the underlying tract. The differentiating feature is the extent of the tissue injury that surrounds the penetrating tract.[308]

The diagnosis and management of nonprojectile penetrating injuries are generally straightforward. The location and severity of the injury dictate the extent of surgical intervention. Local debridement, exploration, antibiotic prophylaxis, and neurovascular repair when indicated are the essentials of treatment.[308]

The vast majority of civilian projectile injuries are gunshot wounds.[150,204] They are classified either as low- or high-velocity injuries. Firearms with muzzle velocities greater than 2500 ft/s are considered high-velocity weapons.[37] Most civilian firearms have muzzle velocities less than 1000 ft/s (Table 18-2).[97]

Tissue destruction is related to the projectile's kinetic energy that is carried to the target and dissipated upon impact.[158] A close-range shotgun blast, although low-velocity by definition, exceeds many high-velocity injuries in tissue damage.[305] A more precise classification would divide these wounds into low- and high-energy injuries.[305]

High-energy missile injuries include most military gunshot and shrapnel wounds. Characteristically, these wounds are severe with tissue damage occurring at a distance from the obvious wounding tract.[150] A cavitation effect occurs, largely due to a momentary formation of a cavity along the high-energy missile tract as tissue particles are accelerated radially.[96,344] This effect is also said to be responsible for creating a momentary negative suction pressure which pulls bacteria and other foreign material into the wound.[96,323]

Shotgun injuries are distinctly different from single-bullet wounds.[87,204,305] Depending on the distance the target is from the weapon, these injuries vary from mild, superficial pellet wounds to lethal close-range blast injuries.[204] Although they are low-velocity, close-range shotgun blasts impart high-energy injuries because of the large combined mass of the pellets and filler wadding.[305] A direct blast injury secondary to the rapidly expanding gases of combustion also contributes to the severe tissue damage at close range.[305] Devastating segmental bone and soft tissue loss is not uncommon.[204] Cavitation usually does not occur in shotgun injuries.[305]

The successful management of high-energy gunshot wounds is derived from the military experience.[50] The essentials of treatment include radical and serial debridements, fasciotomy, delayed closure, and appropriate antibiotic and tetanus prophylaxis.[71] Bony stabilization is performed in conjunction with this aggressive soft tissue management. Only accessible bullets and pellets need to be removed.[245] In shotgun injuries an effort should be made to remove all wadding material from the wound in order to prevent a severe local inflammatory reaction.[245]

In contrast to military injuries, most civilian gunshot wounds arise from small-caliber, low-velocity weapons that produce a low-energy type of wound.[50,150] In these injuries the damage is confined primarily to the immediate projectile pathway.[150] Tissue cavitation, blast injury, and extensive soft tissue involvement are not typically encountered.[122,150]

Most low-energy gunshot wounds involving the extremities can be managed safely, and with a low complication rate, utilizing the principles of limited wound-margin excision, irrigation, antibiotic and tetanus prophylaxis, and delayed primary closure. Formal surgical debridement or exploration is appropriate in the presence of neurovascular injury, gross contamination, or uncertainty regarding the type of weapon.[50]

The decision to remove a bullet should be based upon a consideration of the hazards of its remaining in its present position compared with the hazards of its attempted removal.[193] Most retained bullets are subsequently encapsulated in scar tissue and seldom present future problems.[261]

Bullets in the hands and feet should be removed if possible, as these often become painful at a later time. Similarly, intraarticular and periarticular bullets should be removed, as lead can induce an arthropathy,[261] and as systemic lead toxicities have been reported following these injuries.[34]

Pathologic Fractures

Pathologic fractures can be secondary to systemic metabolic diseases, infection, primary neoplastic lesions, or metastatic disease. The most common group consists of those related to postmenopausal osteoporosis such as Colles' fractures, humeral neck fractures, and hip fractures. Of patients with metastatic disease, 15 to 20 percent develop detectable skeletal metastases.[164] Of this population, 10 to 15 percent who have radiographic evidence of skeletal metastasis develop pathologic fractures.[307] Of all pathologic fractures through skeletal metastasis, 40 percent occur in the femur. Of metastatic lesions to bone, 20 percent present in the upper extremity; the largest percentage of these are found in the humerus.[168] Tumors which commonly metastasize to the bone include breast (50 percent), lung (12 percent), kidney, prostate, gut and thyroid.

Surgical Indications in Pathologic Fractures

As the number of pathologic lesions detected early has increased, the diagnosis of impending pathologic fracture has gained increased importance. Studies have shown that 85 percent of lesions which were internally fixed before a fracture occurred and then irradiated showed restitution of bony architecture and bony healing.[33,109] In contrast, pathologic fractures which were fixed and then postoperatively irradiated showed a nonunion rate as high as 65 percent in some studies.[35,45] Additionally, it has been demonstrated that when tumor bone is irradiated, the first local response is hyperemia followed by bone softening, which may greatly increase the risk of fracture.[144]

Lesions encompassing 50 percent of cortical circumference have been shown to have a 50 percent risk of fracture.[109] As a result most authors agree that there are definite indications for internal fixation as a prophylactic measure. Recent data suggests that prophylactic internal fixation of the femur should be performed for lesions which are greater than 2.5 cm in diameter and show cortical destruction over 50 percent or greater of the circumference of the bone. It may also be considered for somewhat smaller lesions with persisting pain after adequate radiation therapy.[33,109,144]

The goals of surgery must be carefully considered when contemplating orthopaedic fixation of a pathologic fracture. These goals should primarily be aimed at relief of pain, restoration of function, and facilitation of nursing care.

In the series of Habermann and co-workers, 80 to 90 percent of patients with pathologic fractures that were internally fixed had good to excellent pain relief.[136]

The goal with a terminally ill cancer patient can involve restoring to ambulation a patient with a pathologic femur fracture or enabling patients with a pathologic fracture of the upper extremity to feed and dress themselves. Several series have reported that 80 to 90 percent of patients who walked

prior to the occurrence of a pathologic fracture were able to walk for the remainder of their life after their fractures were internally fixed.[136,144] In addition, even for patients who would not be able to ambulate, internal fixation of lower extremity fractures facilitates nursing care and allows the patient to turn, or to move from bed to chair.

Prognosis in Pathologic Fractures

Because of advances in modern oncology, including improved chemotherapy protocols, radiotherapy, and early detection screening programs, patients with metastatic lesions are now living longer than they have in the past. Breast cancer patients who sustain pathologic fractures have the best prognosis for prolonged survival, with the 1-year survival rate approaching 75 percent. Fractures secondary to breast cancer, prostate cancer, multiple myeloma, and lymphomas unite far more frequently than those in patients with malignant tumors of lung, kidney, or gastrointestinal tract. Although pathologic fractures have slower healing rates than fractures of normal bone, patients whose postoperative survival is greater than 3 months have been shown in several studies to have a union rate of up to 89 percent.[136,144,183]

Cement Fixation in Pathologic Fractures

The use of polymethylmethacrylate is strongly recommended to supplement fixation of pathologic fractures with insufficient bone stock. This addition has been shown to dramatically improve the symptomatic results. These patients are observed to have a noticeable decrease in pain with the use of cemented, as opposed to noncemented, fixation devices.[11,33,92,111,164,183] When cement is used with good cortical contact, the fracture ends may unite through endochondral bone formation, and the rate of union appears to be based solely on the survivability of the patients.[101,144,234]

Cement is an important adjunct in providing mechanical integrity, as cortical destruction secondary to tumor invasion often extends for some distance proximal and distal to the fracture. This is most commonly a problem in the trochanteric and subcapital fracture of the femur. Bone grafting these defects has been shown to be ineffective if performed within 9 months following irradiation.[143] In addition, cement may provide enhanced rotatory stability of devices such as intramedullary nails. Cement has not been shown to have any adverse effects on radiotherapy.[234] In patients whose survivability is low, i.e., less than 6 months to 1 year expected survival, the use of cement is almost always advisable.

COMPLICATIONS ASSOCIATED WITH FRACTURES

Complications associated with fractures may arise from the initial injury or from its subsequent management. Complications may be confined to the site of injury or may have systemic manifestations. Systemic complications include shock, adult respiratory distress syndrome, thromboembolic disease, fat emboli, and hypercalcemia.

Local sequelae include delayed union, malunion, nonunion, avascular necrosis, Sudeck's type of atrophy, posttraumatic arthritis, and heterotopic ossification. In addition, complications associated with vascular, nerve, and other soft tissue injuries may occur.

Soft Tissue Injury

Since successful fracture healing is dependent on a viable soft tissue envelope, careful attention to the soft tissue injury is important.[86,100,259,324] Local soft tissue destruction following blunt trauma involves vascular and lymphatic destruction as well as increased local vasodilatation and increased capillary permeability.[194,291] The ensuing edema, hemorrhage, and increased tissue pressure lead to local tissue hypoxia.[291] If the initial injury or the subsequent swelling is severe, dermal and epidermal nutrition may become impaired, with resultant skin blistering, skin necrosis, and impaired wound healing.[304] Fracture blisters, although innocuous in appearance, represent the end product of altered skin nutrition with epidermal necrosis.[54,304] Skin and soft tissue necrosis may change a relatively simple fracture into a limb-threatening injury.[60,148]

The injured skin and soft tissue are particularly vulnerable to pressure necrosis from an overlying cast, occlusive bandage, or poorly applied traction device. This is especially true in the region of the lower extremity where this skin is often less than 3 mm thick and devoid of underlying muscle and subcutaneous fat.[304]

Immobilization of the affected area to prevent further injury, elevation to promote venous and lymphatic drainage, and ice compresses applied to the injury to decrease local vasodilatation are the essentials of soft tissue treatment.[262] Although some investigators question their value,[304] compressive, bulky dressings seem to limit soft tissue swelling.

Preoperatively, the overlying skin must be carefully assessed for viability. The presence of massive edema, fracture blisters, or a history of a severe crush injury is often indicative of compromised soft tissue vascularity. In such cases, surgical intervention should be postponed since incisions through an already compromised skin and soft tissue bed may be the insult leading to its subsequent necrosis.[304]

Muscle injury accompanying fracture varies from severe trauma associated with high-energy types of injuries[133] to local contusions, stretches, and tears. In the latter types of injuries, muscle healing occurs via fibrosis and/or muscle regeneration and is usually uneventful.[108] Myositis ossificans, an unpredictable sequelae of muscle injury, occurs infrequently.[202,342]

Vascular Injury

Significant vascular injury is an infrequent complication of bone and joint injury,[306] but its prevalence is greater than is clinically appreciated.[125,319] Accurate diagnosis requires a high index of suspicion, knowledge of the common sites of vascular injury,[306] and aggressive use of arteriography.[122,319]

Approximately 75 percent of all major vascular injuries occur in the extremities,[44,254] with concurrent orthopaedic trauma in 10 to 40 percent of cases.[63] The overall incidence of arterial injury with associated long bone fracture is 0.3 to 3.0 percent.[63,306] However, certain orthopaedic injuries may have concurrent vascular injury in up to one-third of cases.[178,266]

Blunt trauma accounts for the majority of vascular injuries encountered in civilian orthopaedic practice.[342] In contrast to penetrating injuries, in which vascular disruption is either apparent or suspected, the closed injury is less likely to arouse clinical suspicion.[259,265] The diagnosis is often delayed or missed, especially in the unconscious polytrauma victim when attention is directed to the more obvious and life-threatening injuries.[259]

Intimal tears with associated thrombosis occur in most cases.[124,217] Vessel laceration, transection, kinking, and compression are less frequent.[44,72,75] Clinically significant arterial spasm as a result of injury is rare.[72,75,290] Concomitant soft tissue injury, venous trauma, and disruption of collateral circulation occur commonly with blunt injuries.[138,265]

Vascular insufficiencies secondary to orthopaedic trauma may be classified as acute, delayed, or remote.[90,257,259] Delayed insufficiency may result from an enlarging thrombus, an expanding hematoma, compartment swelling, or occlusive dressings. Remote insufficiency from arteriovenous fistulas and vascular aneurysm have been reported but are rare.[63,257]

Vascular injury may accompany any fracture or dislocation.[181] Vessels in fixed apposition to bone are more prone to injury. Particularly at risk are the subclavian artery beneath the distal clavicle, the brachial artery along the shaft and supracondylar regions of the humerus, the superficial femoral artery in the adductor canal, and the popliteal artery as it spans the popliteal fossa.[181,327]

The diagnosis of arterial injury is suspected by history or by the presence of pulsatile bleeding, an expanding hematoma, or findings of peripheral ischemia.[181,306] The earliest signs of vascular insufficiency are often subtle and include hypesthesia and a small relative difference in limb temperatures in the affected limb.[259,306] The absence of a palpable pulse is the most reliable indicator of arterial injury,[217,265] although pulses may be found initially in up to 20 percent of limbs sustaining a major vascular injury.[63,217,319] Capillary refill is an unreliable sign.[259]

The presentation of vascular injury may be delayed; thus, an initial careful examination with frequent follow-up is recommended.[257] Doppler flow meters are very accurate indicators of peripheral flow in suspected cases.[297] Arteriography should be performed expeditiously in all suspected cases of arterial injury.[213,342] However, in cases of obvious limb ischemia, corrective intervention should not be delayed by time-consuming trips to the angiography suite. Intraoperative arteriography may be appropriate in these cases.[265]

When combined orthopaedic and vascular trauma occur, opinions differ regarding the proper sequence of treatment.[124,217,259,265,306,319,342] Close cooperation between the orthopaedist and vascular surgeon is necessary.[124,217] Often a temporary Gore-Tex (polytetrafluoroethylene) bypass graft should be placed initially. This is followed by definitive bony stabilization and then definitive vascular repair.[259,265] Fracture stabilization may be obtained by an external fixator, or by internal fixation when indicated.[265,269,312,319,342] Fasciotomies should be performed routinely at the initial operative procedure. Muscle swelling increases for several hours, with the restoration of circulation following vascular repair.[217,259,319,342] The period of time from injury to vascular repair should be kept to a minimum. The advocated safe time lag of 6 h[223] is an arbitrary interval and is dependent on several factors including the location and extent of the injury and the presence or absence of collateral circulation.[259,265,302]

An extensive time lag,[223] massive soft tissue injury,[312,319] or infection[124,319] all contribute to a poor result in the management of these injuries.[265]

Nerve Injuries

The majority of peripheral nerve injuries are the result of deep lacerations and penetrating wounds.[258,302] The overall incidence of nerve injury complicating orthopaedic trauma is relatively low.[301] However, certain skeletal injuries may be associated with nerve injury in as much as 30 percent of cases.[40]

Direct contusion and stretch injuries account for most orthopaedically related nerve injuries.[179,301] Lacerations of nerves by bone fragments are rare.[24,301] Nerve injury may also occur as a late complication of skeletal trauma through scar tissue,[201] fracture callus,[301] and heterotopic bone formation.[154,180]

Glenohumeral dislocations and humeral shaft fractures account for most of the nonpenetrating nerve injuries in the upper extremity.[40,179,301] Nerve injury occurs in as many as one-third of patients sustaining shoulder dislocations.[40,179,301] The axillary nerve is most frequently involved, with brachial plexus and musculocutaneous nerve injuries occurring less frequently.

Fractures of the humerus, especially spiral midshaft fractures, are associated with radial nerve injury in 5 to 15 percent of cases.[120,179,301] A small percentage of these nerve injuries reportedly occur during and after reduction of the fracture.[179] Thus, in most radial nerve injuries associated with humeral fractures, conservative expectant management with a cockup-type wrist splint and dynamic finger extension is indicated.[179,301]

Any fracture or dislocation of the elbow may damage a contiguous nerve.[200] Ulnar nerve injury may accompany elbow dislocations.[270] The radial nerve, specifically the posterior interosseous branch, is occasionally injured with a fracture or dislocation of the radial head.[201,313] Median nerve injury is uncommon at the elbow[150] but may be associated with supracondylar fractures of the humerus.[260]

Forearm fractures rarely produce injury to the nerves of the forearm.[14] Transient median nerve lesions may be occasionally noted with distal radius[77,197] and carpal fractures and dislocations.[302] Injuries to the hook of the hamate, or pisiform bones of the wrist, may infrequently injure the ulnar nerve in Guyon's canal.[157,302]

Fracture dislocations of the pelvis, especially in conjunction with sacroiliac disruption, produce a wide variety of neural injuries in approximately 1 to 10 percent of cases.[248] Nerve injuries may include lumbosacral root avulsion,[25] obturator palsy,[86] or sciatic nerve involvement.[127] Since pelvic fractures are often encountered in the setting of major trauma, nerve injuries are often initially overlooked.[248] As in the upper extremity, treatment is expectant, but recovery is seldom complete although overall functional results may be good.[248]

Posterior dislocations and fracture dislocations of the femoral head are associated with sciatic nerve injury in 10 to 15 percent of cases.[105,301] The peroneal division of the sciatic nerve is especially vulnerable.[301] Early recognition and treatment of these nerve compromises is important. Functional recovery is expected in 60 to 70 percent of cases in 3 to 30 months.[161,301]

In the leg, the common peroneal nerve is quite vulnerable to injury as it passes the fibular head.[270] Most often the nerve is injured by extrinsic pressure applied at this point from an occlusive bandage, venous stocking, cast, or traction bar.[46] Posterior dislocation of the knee, or any severe knee adduction injury, may be associated with a traction injury to this nerve.[295,301] Proximal fibular fractures and dislocations may cause a peroneal nerve injury. Fractures of the femoral shaft, tibial diaphysis, ankle, and foot are infrequent causes of nerve injury.[22]

Compartment Syndromes

A *compartment syndrome* is defined as a progressive condition in which increased tissue pressure within a confined limb compartment exceeds capillary pressure and ultimately compromises the circulation to the muscle.[207,229,336] Unrecognized, this condition may lead to the devastating complication of Volkmann's ischemic contracture.[96] Compartment syndromes may arise from any condition which increases intracompartmental pressure. These include localized extrinsic pressure, restrictive dressings, or the tight closure of a fascial defect.[207] Elevated pressure may also be secondary to increased volume of compartmental contents from hemorrhage, muscle swelling, or muscular hypertrophy. Trauma, ischemia, exercise, burns, drugs, surgery, venous obstruction, and nephrotic syndromes may be inciting causes.[206]

Increased tissue pressure is the key to the pathogenesis of compartment syndromes (Fig. 18-8).[207] Elevated local tissue pressure decreases the local arteriovenous gradient. Local blood flow and oxygenation is diminished, thereby compromising tissue function and viability. The pressure necessary to impede the microcirculation is usually less than arterial blood pressure so that the larger arterial vessels that pass through the affected compartment remain patent, and the distal blood flow is intact.[207] As a result, distal pulses are almost invariably present in the face of a compartment syndrome.

The tolerance of local tissue to increased pressure is variable. This tolerance is dependent upon the magnitude and the duration of pressure, and the metabolic needs of that tissue. Traumatized tissue may require a greater blood flow than that of resting uninjured muscle.[206,207]

The compartments most often affected in the upper extremity include the dorsal and volar compartments of the forearm, and the intrinsic compartments of the hand. In the lower extremity, typical locations include the anterior, lateral,

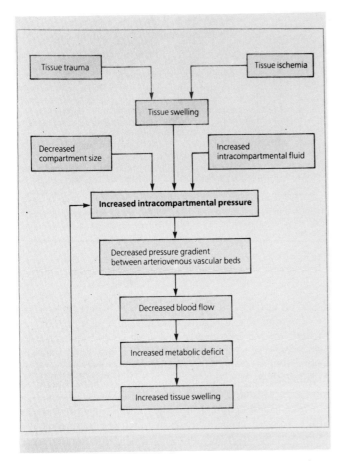

Figure 18-8 The vicious cycle of hemodynamic changes that occurs in the development of a compartment syndrome. *(From Rorabeck, C.H., and Armstrong, R.D., J Musculoskel Med 2(9):54, 1985. Reproduced with permission.)*

superficial posterior, and deep posterior compartments of the leg.[142,186] Crush injuries, and fractures of the forearm, supracondylar humerus, and tibial shaft are particularly susceptible to the syndrome.[229]

Diagnosis

The diagnosis of this condition begins with the identification of patients at risk. Since the compartment syndrome is usually progressive, frequent repeated examination is indicated in questionable cases.[207]

Pain out of proportion to the injury and not controlled with the usual mild analgesics can be the earliest symptom of an impending compartment syndrome.[207] The most reliable physical findings include a swollen, palpably tense compartment and a sensory deficit. Paresthesia is the first sign of nerve ischemia, with anesthesia being a relatively late sign. The nerve affected is indicative of the compartment involved. Pain with passive muscle stretch is a common and usually reliable finding. Motor weakness and paralysis are late signs.

The diagnosis is often difficult, particularly in the unresponsive or neurologically impaired patient. An important adjunct is the direct measurement of intracompartmental tissue pressure by the Whitesides' needle manometer[335] or slit catheter[229] techniques (Fig. 18-9). Normal tissue pressure is around 0 mmHg.[274] Ischemia may begin when compartment pressures rise to within 30 to 40 mmHg of diastolic blood pressure.[274]

Treatment

The treatment of choice for compartment syndrome is early decompression.[274,336] Initially, all casts and dressings must be split to skin level or removed completely.[274] This in itself is capable of reducing compartmental pressures by as much as 85 percent.[121] The persistence of the typical symptoms and signs of a compartment syndrome with intracompartmental tissue pressure greater than 30 mmHg mandates immediate and complete fasciotomy of involved compartments.[208,229,274,336] The two-incision technique is preferred (Fig. 18-10). Delayed primary closure of the open wounds is performed after the swelling diminishes.[274]

Infection

Infection and osteomyelitis are well-recognized complications of open fractures[133,135] and after the open treatment of closed fractures.[57,250]

The development of infection in a closed fracture managed nonsurgically is rare, with only a small number of cases having been reported.[4,60,80,98] In these cases, infection followed soon after the fracture. Although clinical evidence of infection was usually present, the diagnosis was often delayed.[80,98]

Delayed Union and Nonunion

Union of a fracture has been achieved when a pain-free, functional status has returned. Clinically, there is no mobility at the fracture site. No pain is present either from firm palpation at the fracture site or from application of a deforming stress. Radiographically visible callus is noted bridging the fracture site and there is diminution or dissolution of the fracture line.

Delayed union exists when a fracture has failed to unite within an expected time frame. If a radiographic progression of healing is noted, then most probably the fracture will eventually achieve complete union. If serial x-ray views demonstrate no progression of the healing process (increasing callus or diminution of the fracture line), then one can predict that the delayed union will lead to a nonunion.

Primary bone healing is not guaranteed by anatomical reduction. However, inadequate reduction without bony opposition or with persisting interposed soft tissues contributes to delayed union or nonunion. Inadequate immobilization also has deleterious effects but more so in some bones such as the tibia than in others like the clavicle.

Severe open fractures are more prone to develop nonunions, and this is probably secondary to soft tissue stripping and poor local vascularity.

Injuries most commonly associated with delayed union or nonunion include open fractures, segmental or highly

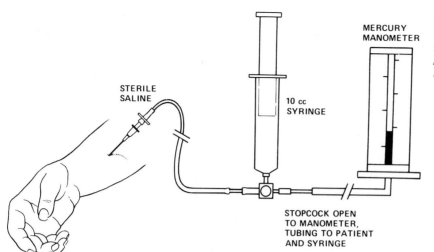

Figure 18-9 Whitesides' technique of intracompartmental pressure measurement. *(From Halpern, A.A., and Nagel, D.A., J Hand Surg 4:258, 1979. Reproduced with permission.)*

comminuted fractures, and fractures iatrogenically devitalized at the time of open reduction. An increased likelihood of nonunion in fractures associated with multiple injuries has also been reported. No single factor in and of itself, however, causes nonunion of a fracture. It is usually a combination of these factors which adversely affect the fracture healing process and culminate in nonunion.[49]

Nonunion can be recognized radiologically as well as clinically. In atrophic nonunion the bone ends are avascular and produce little or no callus; the medullary cavities are closed off by caps of sclerotic bone. In the hypertrophic variety of nonunion, exuberant callus is visible on x-ray but the fracture line remains clearly visible on serial films and may even widen. The hypertrophic nonunion has good biologic healing potential and will probably benefit from more rigid immobilization. Atrophic nonunion will probably require a bone graft to bridge the avascular region.

Established nonunion of either variety may progress to form a synovial pseudarthrosis in which the bone ends are covered by fibrocartilage and separated at the fracture by a

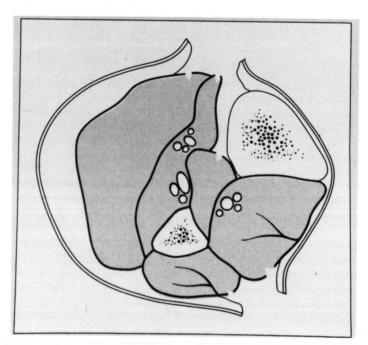

Figure 18-10 Section through the proximal calf indicating the five compartments decompressed by double-incision fasciotomy. The lateral and anterior compartments are approached via a lateral incision which carefully preserves the superficial peroneal nerve. The superficial and deep posterior compartments and the centrally situated compartment of the tibialis posterior muscle are approached through a medial incision. At least 7 cm of intact skin should be maintained between incisions, and compartments should be decompressed along their entire length. *(From Rorabeck, C.H., and Armstrong, R.D., J Musculoskel Med 2(9):54, 1985. Reproduced with permission.)*

false joint with a pseudocapsule.[330] This condition may be suspected in a long established nonunion if the bone scan shows increased uptake at the bone ends with a photopenic (cold spot) area of uptake in between. The MRI scan may also be useful in diagnosis of this condition.

The most important factor in the prevention of a nonunion is effective, primary treatment of the fracture. Some authors believe that 90 percent of nonunions are preventable by following basic tenets of fracture care, which include preservation of blood supply, proper fracture reduction, and adequate immobilization.[17] Careful handling of soft tissues, with adequate irrigation and debridement of open wounds, prevents many of the problems associated with open injuries. In addition, certain fractures should be recognized for their potential to develop a nonunion and followed closely. Severely comminuted fractures in which open reduction and internal fixation are performed should be bone-grafted. Open fractures treated with external fixation must be closely followed for evidence of delayed union and grafted early if necessary.

Treatment of Established Nonunion

Bone Grafts Bone graft surgery plays an important role in treatment of nonunions. It is estimated that nearly 200,000 bone grafts are performed each year.[151] Cortical bone graft does not in itself have the ability to form new bone, but its resorption can induce new bone formation.[130] Cancellous bone has osteoinductive properties and is preferable as graft material. In the Phemister technique, corticocancellous strips of autogenous bone are interleaved around the nonunion site without freshening the bone ends. The graft becomes vascularized proximal and distal to the fracture and forms bridging bone.

A different technique is necessary for a synovial pseudarthrosis. Bone grafting without resection of a pseudarthrosis has been shown to be associated with a high rate of failure.[130,151] Studies by several authors have shown that the best results with these ununited fractures are achieved with debridement of the pseudarthrosis, provision of osteogenic potential with bone graft, and rigid immobilization with internal fixation.[220,329,330,348] Aseptic nonunion without synovial pseudarthrosis has been shown to respond well to closed intramedullary rodding. This technique, which is particularly useful in the femur and the tibia, is not accompanied by any open surgery in the region of the nonunion so that the periosteal blood circulation is left intact and bone graft augmentation to the fracture site is provided by the reamings, which accumulate at the fracture site during the intramedullary procedure.[63,165,185,341]

Operative Intervention for Infected Nonunion Operative intervention is also essential for treating infected nonunions. Adequate, serial debridement of necrotic and infected soft tissue and bone must be performed. Provision of stability, soft tissue coverage, and osteogenic potential has been shown to achieve success rates of 86 percent.[177,199,329,348] Additional studies have shown that if rigid internal fixation is achieved, union can occur in the face of persistent infection, which subsides once bony union is complete and the metal is removed.[63,276,330,339] The use of open bone grafting with stability

provided by external fixation devices has been shown to be equally effective.[130,149] This technique is of greatest value when multiple soft tissue procedures must be performed in order to gain adequate bony coverage. The use of vascularized bone grafting techniques in these situations is similar to their use in the treatment of osteomyelitis, described in Chap. 22.

Electric Stimulation Currently, three types of electric stimulation are approved for use in the United States. These include the totally implanted system using direct current first developed by Dwyer and Wickham of Australia,[94,95] the semiinvasive system developed by Brighton and his colleagues at the University of Pennsylvania,[51] and the noninvasive system of pulsed electromagnetic fields (PEMF) developed by Bassett.[26-32]

Implanting both the electrode and the power source involves an extensive open procedure and these methods are no longer used by the authors. In the semiinvasive method the electrodes are inserted percutaneously to the site of the nonunion but are then attached to an external power source. Patients are placed in a long leg cast and with this method they do not bear the weight for at least 12 weeks. Contraindications include: (1) bone loss greater than one-half the bone diameter, (2) synovial pseudarthrosis, (3) infection, (4) a patient unable to comply with the treatment.[51]

The PEMF patient is treated without electrodes, the field generated between externally applied coils producing the necessary effect at the nonunion. These patients must also be non–weight bearing in a long leg cast for the first portion of the 3-month period but are allowed protected weight bearing once the "coil" effect is seen on x-rays to have produced changes indicating bridging callus. Contraindications to PEMF include: (1) bone loss greater in length than one-half the diameter of the bone, (2) fragment separation greater than 1 cm, (3) synovial pseudarthrosis, (4) a patient unable to cooperate with 10 h of required daily treatment.[52]

No complications are reported with the use of pulsed electromagnetic field (PEMF). The semi-invasive method is, however, associated with several complications, including pin tract infection, cathode or anode displacement, and wire breakage.[51,52]

Brighton reported a 73 percent rate in 418 patients with nonunion treated with the semi-invasive method.[51] Heppenstall reported 85 percent success treating tibial nonunion with this method.[152] Bassett's own multicenter evaluation of PEMF revealed an 81 percent success rate in 220 patients treated at Columbia Presbyterian Hospital, and 76 percent in 625 patients treated in other American centers.[30] The success rate for this method outside the United States was 79 percent in 233 patients.[29]

Conflicting reports on the effects of combining electromagnetic stimulation with bone grafts have recently been published.[30,222]

The bulk of the evidence described has earned electric stimulation a place in the therapeutic armamentarium when treating nonunion. However, several studies suggest that the technique cannot substitute for proper fracture management. Optimism about its efficacy should not lead to overextending its indications.[255,348] At our institution we have found that the most common reason for failure of electric stimulation remains improper patient selection. Recent attempts to utilize electric stimulation for the treatment of acute fractures has led to equivocal results at this time.[70,155]

SECTION B

Fractures and Dislocations in Children

Stuart Polisner and Roger Dee

Fractures and fracture dislocations are more common in children than ligament disruptions and uncomplicated dislocation. The skeletal tissues are more likely to fail. This tendency gradually reverses through the period of adolescence and no longer applies at physeal closure.

Children's bone has increased porosity and wider haversian canals than adult bone, and consequently has different biomechanical properties. Also, in children the periosteum is thicker and more elastic and may prevent completion of a tension fracture or limit displacement of bone in a complete fracture.[23,24] It provides a strong soft tissue hinge which helps maintain reduction. Occasionally a fragment of bone can become buttonholed through this strong periosteum, and this then impedes reduction. Juvenile periosteum creates ample callus.[23]

CLASSIFICATION

Certain unique modes of failure result after trauma in children (Fig. 18-11). Increased metaphyseal porosity permits the buckle typical of the *torus* fracture which occurs as a result of compressive load. The localized outward buckling of the cortex may require several x-ray views for adequate visualization. Another pattern of childrens' fractures is the *greenstick* type, in which there is an incomplete fracture on the tension side of the bone, but the cortex and periosteum may remain intact on the compression side. Yet another pattern is *plastic deformation,* which occurs when the elastic limit is exceeded and an irreversible deformation occurs. This takes the form of a gentle bowing of the bone rather than a localized angulation. In the case of the forearm, the diagnosis may be missed since one bone may be bowed and the other not so affected. This contrasts with the characteristic angular deformation usually seen with fractures of both bones of the forearm. None of these fracture types occur in adult bone.[17,18,23,24]

TREATMENT

Angulated greenstick fractures may be reduced by appropriate manipulation. A slight manipulative overcorrection stretching the intact periosteum is used by some surgeons who consider that otherwise there is a tendency to underreduce these fractures. The authors' preference is to reduce to a neutral position and then prevent subsequent recurrence of the deformity with the use of a well molded cast. In the case of displaced or overriding fractures, it is necessary to have a very cooperative and relaxed patient. Regional blocks or local anesthesia with general analgesia is adequate in a calm patient. Usually, however, general anesthesia is required; this is also true for dislocations in children when an atraumatic reduction is essential.

The usual techniques of manipulative reduction are used. These include, when necessary, the application of longitudinal traction to disimpact fragments. Sometimes an exaggeration of the deformity to hitch the ends of a fracture is helpful before correcting the angulation and achieving reduction (Fig. 18-12). Rarely an open reduction may be required in long bone fractures if good alignment is not achieved. This may be the case when a fragment is buttonholed through the periosteum or when there is plastic deformation. In the latter case, osteotomy and internal fixation in the corrected position may be required. This is occasionally the case in forearm bone fractures in the older child. Use of the external fixator has been described, particularly in fractures of the lower limb, and the device is useful when there is associated skin loss or burns.

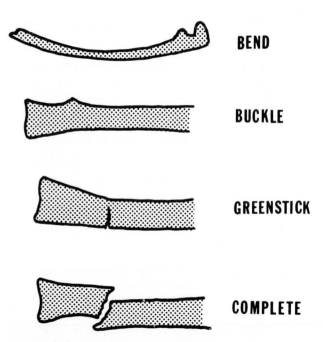

Figure 18-11 Patterns of injury in children's bones. From above downward they are plastic deformation, torus-type compression injury (buckling), greenstick fracture, and complete fracture. *(From Rang, M.: Children's Fractures, 2nd ed. Philadelphia, Lippincott, 1983. Reproduced with permission.)*

As in adult fractures, cast wedging is an effective way of correcting minor degrees in malalignment.[4] Plastic wedges are commercially available in various sizes.[3] During the initial period of any cast immobilization, the neurovascular status of the extremity should be checked at regular intervals and immediately following any report of increasing discomfort. Unstable fractures should have serial x-ray examinations on a weekly basis for at least 3 weeks in the case of physeal injuries and for at least 6 weeks in diaphyseal fractures. Immobilization is continued until union is secure enough for ordinary gentle daily activities. A rule of thumb is that physeal healing requires approximately half the healing time required for the adjacent diaphysis to heal.[3] In general, for secure healing of physeal fractures, toddlers require 3 weeks, children 4 weeks, and adolescents 5 weeks of immobilization. These times may be approximately doubled for diaphyseal fractures, but the final determination is made by visualizing adequate bone callus on the x-ray film.

The use of crutches in young children may be hazardous due to limited strength and coordination. In adolescents also, tripping and falling is common. If crutches are required, three-point-touchdown partial weight bearing is safer and easier to perform than attempting non–weight bearing. Walkers and walkerettes are preferable, particularly in younger children.

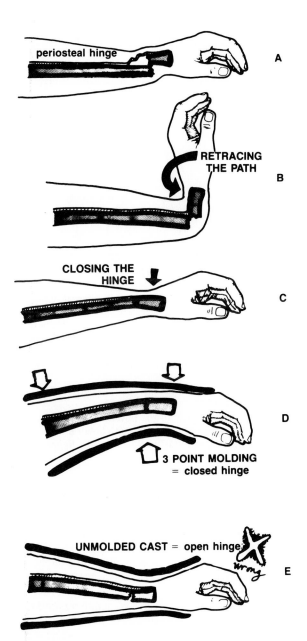

Figure 18-12 Use of intact soft tissue hinge to obtain and maintain reduction. **A.** The periosteum is usually intact on one side of a fracture, and it may prevent reduction when simple traction alone is attempted. **B** and **C.** Achieving reduction by retracing the path of the fracture, followed by closing the periosteal hinge. **D.** The cast should be applied with three-point molding in order to keep the periosteal hinge in tension and the fracture reduced. **E.** Failure to properly mold the cast allows the periosteal hinge to open, and loss of reduction may then occur. *(From Rang, M.: Children's Fractures, 2nd ed. Philadelphia, Lippincott, 1983. Reproduced with permission.)*

FACTORS AFFECTING FRACTURE HEALING IN CHILDREN

1. *Age.* The younger the child, the more rapid the healing[1,20,24] and the more complete the bony remodeling.[27] Furthermore, the younger the child, the greater the capacity to correct deformities (e.g., malunions) through growth.[27]

2. *Nutrition.* Although malnutrition may retard healing, enhanced nutrition has not been proved to be an accelerator of healing.[3] A routine, well-rounded diet is adequate to allow normal healing. In children, calcium stores in the body are generally adequate to heal even multiple fractures. Supplemental calcium may promote hypercalciuria and the formation of kidney stones. Vitamin supplements in recommended daily doses are an innocuous adjunct if dietary deficiencies are suspected.

3. *Mechanism of Injury.* The rate of healing is generally inversely proportional to the violence of the injury (e.g., the greater the violence, the slower the rate of healing).[4]

4. *Type of Fracture.* Oblique and spiral fractures with relatively large areas of bone contact achieve functional union more quickly than transverse fractures. Separation of fracture fragments slows healing, although children fill in bony gaps faster than adults. With multiple or segmental fractures, healing tends to be slower in at least one fracture site.

5. *Adjacent Injury.* The less the local soft tissue damage and damage to blood supply of bone and periosteum, the more rapid the healing.

6. *Location of Fracture.* The closer the fracture is to a growth center, the more rapid the healing, the less abundant the callus, and the greater the remodeling potential. Conversely, the middiaphysis is the slowest-healing portion of the bone.[13]

7. *Head Injury.* With associated severe head injury, especially if there is associated spasticity or convulsions,

healing is rapid and callus abundant. Thus, realignment of the fracture without delay by closed or open means is essential to avoid malunion.

FRACTURE REMODELING IN CHILDREN

Children form rapid and abundant callus during closed fracture healing.[28] Callus formation is most impressive in the diaphysis of the bone. In subcutaneous loci (e.g., clavicular, tibial, metacarpal, and phalangeal shafts) where there is little soft tissue covering the exuberant fracture callus, the patient and parents should be forewarned of the visibility, and palpability, of the impending callus formation. This callus is often mistaken for a tumor or a malunion. Preparing the family reduces unwarranted fears.

The younger the child, the more rapidly and completely the callus dissipates during the remodeling process. The majority of this remodeling occurs within the first 2 years after fracture healing. In prepubertal children, the callus generally disappears completely. In adolescents the callus matures, smooths, and shrinks, leaving some permanent bony enlargement at the fracture site.[28] Remodeling is controlled by factors that determine the final shape and size of bones during growth. The following are important aspects of the remodeling process:

1. *Bone Length.* Physeal stimulation causes a long bone to overgrow in length within the first 2 years after fracture.[9,27] This is probably due to the hyperemia of healing, which stimulates the adjacent growth plates.[7] In general, 0.5 to 1 cm of overgrowth can be expected,[5,9,19,26] although 2 cm of gain in length is common and there have been sporadic reported cases of 3 cm or more of overgrowth.[8,24] Overriding of 1.5 cm can be compensated for in the femur; overgrowth is most for fractures in the proximal one-third, indicating that location is important.[10]

2. *Angulation.* In prepubertal children deformity of up to 30° may correct spontaneously in the sagittal plane (which is in the same plane as the movement of the adjacent joint), and up to 20° of correction may be achieved in the coronal plane.[10]

3. *Rotation.* Although rotational correction does occasionally occur, it is generally minimal. Rotational correction is not to be expected with fracture remodeling in children.[14,27]

4. *Translocation.* Partial side-to-side displacement or complete (bayonet) translocation corrects extremely well in growing children, especially in those that are prepubertal. This deformity generally remodels within 1 to 2 years after fracture, leaving no residual cosmetic or functional disability.

PHYSEAL INJURIES

Classification

Several anatomical classifications of physeal injury have been suggested. Such classifications are valuable in relating the

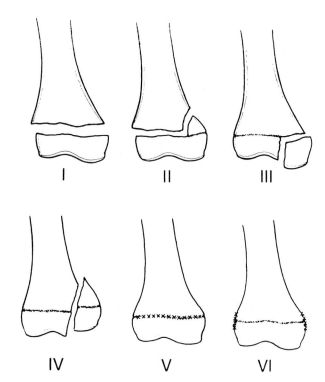

Figure 18-13 Salter's classification of physeal injuries with Rang's type VI added.
Salter I: The fracture extends through the physis only.
Salter II: The fracture extends through the physis and part of the metaphysis.
Salter III: The fracture extends through the physis and the epiphysis.
Salter IV: The fracture extends through the metaphysis, physis, and epiphysis.
Salter V: Crush injury to the physis.
Rang VI: Fracture through the perichondral ring.
(From Denton, J.R., Orthop Rev 12:130, 1983. Reproduced with permission.)

anatomy of the fracture to the specific nature of the injury and also some guide to prognosis.

The most commonly quoted classification is that of Salter and Harris.[22] They described five types of injury (Fig. 18-13).

Type I is a fracture in which a complete separation of the epiphysis from the metaphysis has occurred.

Type II is a fracture in which the fracture separation extends into the metaphysis and a triangular metaphyseal bony fragment remains attached to the epiphysis. The x-ray appearance of this fragment of varying size is termed the *Thurston-Holland sign.*

Type III is a fracture through the epiphysis from the articular surface.

Type IV is a vertical fracture through the epiphysis, the physis, and the metaphysis.

Type V is radiologically normal, a compression-type injury being inferred by delay or cessation of subsequent growth.

Rang suggests a sixth type (Fig. 18-13) when localized physeal injury to the perichondral rim (zone of Ranvier) occurs.[17]

While the classification has been of great value, Ogden has suggested that it requires amplification to include additional important patterns of injury. The salient features of Ogden's categorization are summarized in the legend to Fig. 18-14.

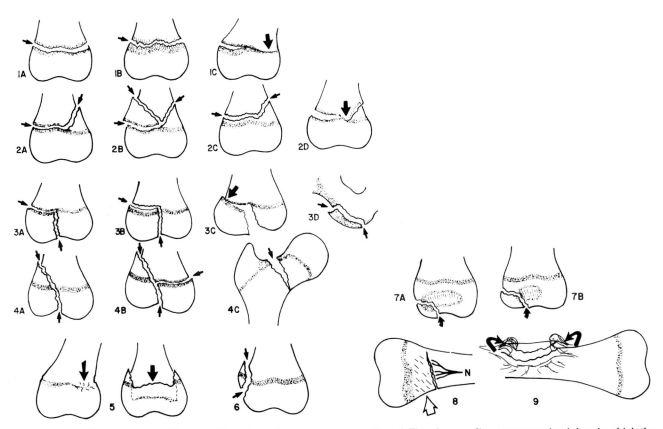

Figure 18-14 The revised classification of injuries in the region of the growth plate proposed by Ogden.

Type 1. This is a fracture through the hypertrophic zone and the zone of provisional calcification. In type 1B the fracture extends more deeply into the degenerating myeloproliferative diseases. In type 1C there is associated local damage to the germinal layer of the physis.

Type 2. This injury shows a large metaphyseal fragment (2A). The presence of this fragment is called the Thurston Holland sign. The periosteum is intact on the compression side. In type 2B there is a free metaphyseal fragment. In type 2C there is a smaller piece of metaphysis than in type 2A. In type 2D associated localized damage to the physis has occurred.

Type 3. This has a transverse fracture line through the physis at the same level as in type 1A. In type 3B this transverse fracture is through the primary spongiosa. In type 3C there is localized damage to the physis, and in type 3D a nonarticular epiphysis is avulsed from the metaphysis.

Type 4. This shows a vertical failure through all layers plus the secondary center of ossification when present. In type 4B there is in addition a transverse fracture causing an accompanying type 3 injury. In type 4C, commonly seen in the neck of the femur, there is a fracture through nonarticular cartilage, an injury which extends from the conjoint physis into the metaphysis.

Type 5. This shows a direct compression injury in which the radiographic appearance is normal but there may be disruption of the germinal layer. Other etiologies have been proposed to explain the consequent growth retardation (see text). It is possible for the metaphysis to be driven through the growth plate into the epiphysis.

Type 6. In this type there is involvement of the peripheral margin of the growth plate in the region of the zone of Ranvier. A localized contusion or slicing laceration may cause this lesion, which can produce a peripheral osseous bridge.

Type 7. This injury is a completely intraepiphyseal injury involving the secondary center of ossification. Type 7B is similar but extends entirely through cartilage and is consequently difficult to diagnose on x-ray films.

Type 8. This is a specialized type of injury in which there is interference with the metaphyseal growth and remodeling region associated with vascular damage. Epiphyseolysis may follow as a result of the temporary metaphyseal ischemia.

Type 9. In type 9 injury there is damage to the diaphyseal growth mechanisms that control appositional membraneous new bone formation. Direct trauma to the periosteum is the cause.

(From Ogden, J.A., J Pediatr Orthop 2:371, 1982. Reproduced with permission.)

Prognostic Considerations in Physeal Injuries

Injuries in this region may be complicated by subsequent growth abnormalities or joint incongruity. Growth may be temporarily or permanently retarded. Alternatively a bony bar may form across a localized area of physeal damage either centrally or peripherally, causing the development of an angular growth deformity. If the bar is central, cupping of the metaphysis occurs with relative shortening of the bone.[15]

The Salter-Harris type IV injury is likely to lead to formation of a bony bar if displaced and unreduced. A similar potential, however, exists for type III fractures.[8,15,22] Although Blount believed that open reduction was rarely required in physeal injuries,[8] several modern authors believe that open reduction and anatomical reduction are essential for success in most type III and type IV injuries that are displaced.[3,8] Kling and co-workers believe that particularly in the distal tibial physis, type III fractures should be treated identically to type IV fractures with regard to the need for absolutely accurate reduction.[8] These authors believe that any residual gap, even the 2 mm often cited as acceptable, is in fact too much to accept and may lead to subsequent growth abnormalities. These authors also point out that in the region of the ankle, displacement in type II fractures may also be unacceptable and open reduction may be necessary. If reduction of a physeal fracture is delayed beyond 5 to 7 days, some authors recommend that it be permitted to heal since operative intervention at that stage may interfere with early union between the cartilaginous portions of the physis and consequently encourage nonunion.[3]

Even if one accepts the position of a type III fracture which is undisplaced, there is always the tendency for subsequent displacement during closed cast treatment, so repeated observation is necessary, particularly over the critical first week after the injury. If 2 mm is too much displacement, there is certainly little margin for error and any displacement of an undisplaced injury indicates the need for open reduction, particularly in the region of the ankle joint.

One of the problems is accurate assessment of the nature of the injury, and for this purpose standard radiographs are inadequate. For a fracture to be accepted as undisplaced or in a satisfactory position after closed reduction, not only must the physeal gap be closed but also there must be restoration of any malrotation of the fragment.[8] Computed tomography has been recommended as a useful adjunct in assessing these fractures.[29] Hypocycloidal tomography performed at 0.25- to 0.5-cm intervals with a growth plate perpendicular to the plane of the film is a valuable technique for the early detection of a bony bar. Because of the configuration of the physis false-positive and false-negative findings may be attained with standard tomography when looking for a bony bar.[15]

The development of growth abnormalities can occur following all five types of Salter-Harris injury. Peterson has questioned whether in fact the type V injury ever occurs, pointing out that many factors can be responsible for the growth arrest following injury in the region of the physis. He believes that alterations in local blood flow associated with immobilization are of particular importance. He also points out that bony bars may occur following many types of physeal injury, e.g., electrical burns, frostbite, metabolic abnormality (vitamin A intoxication), infection, tumors, or irradiation, fol-

lowing the insertion of metal crossing the physis. Injury is particularly important when internal fixation is required following open reduction. If there is a metaphyseal fragment, it can be fixed without using pins crossing the physis.

Transepiphyseal fixation can also be used. In the case of an unstable type I or type II fracture, as Bright points out, transphyseal pins are unfortunately inevitable, but they should be smooth, not threaded pins. They should be removed as soon as possible.[3,8] Removal of the metaphyseal fragment to permit visualization of the physis and its accurate reduction has been recommended.[3,8]

Other important facts concerning bony bars have been summarized by Peterson. He points out that although the distal radius is the most frequent injured physis, it is an uncommon site of a bony bar. The proximal tibia and distal femur account for only 3 percent of all physeal injuries but are responsible for the majority of bars. He suggests that the contour of the physis and its rate of growth or its size may be of significance and points out that at the knee the physes are large in area, irregular in contour, and account for most of the growth of their respective bones.[15]

The age of the patient and the proximity to skeletal maturity are important. Most type III fractures occur near skeletal maturity, and according to Peterson they therefore infrequently produce bony bars with much clinical deformity.[15] In a younger patient, with more growth remaining, the deformity may be considerable and require such measures as corrective osteotomy, leg lengthening, or contralateral epiphyseodesis for its control.

The treatment of leg length inequality is dealt with elsewhere in this volume. With regard to the excision of bony bars, the technique varies depending on whether the bar is peripheral or central. A central bar may be approached through an opening in the metaphysis. A transepiphyseal approach is not used because it means transgressing the joint. Accurate localization using the techniques described is first necessary. The bar is best removed with a motorized burr (techniques have been well-described by Peterson[15]).

Rehabilitation

A young child is usually his or her own best therapist![3,17] However, range-of-motion exercises to the surrounding joints, followed by a stretching program, and a progressive resistive strengthening program are useful in rapidly restoring normal function in the older child. With fractures that are prone to growth disturbance, degenerative joint changes, or avascular necrosis, reexamination with repeat x-ray films are indicated at 6-month intervals for approximately 2 years after injury.[3] Some surgeons recommend that physeal injuries be followed until skeletal maturity.

REFERENCES

Section A: Fractures and Dislocations in Adults

1. Acker, J.H., Murphy, C., and D'Ambrosia, R. Treatment of fractures of the femur with Grosse-Kempf rod. Orthopedics 8:1393–1401, 1985.

2. Adams, J.C. *Outline of Fractures,* 6th ed. Baltimore, Williams & Wilkins, 1972.

3. Ahmadi, B., Akbarnia, B.A., Ghobadi, F., Ganjavian, M.S., and Nasseri, D. Experience with 141 tibial leg lengthenings in poliomyelitis; comparison of 3 different methods. Clin Orthop 145:150–153, 1979.

4. Abrahams, M.A., and Tytlkowski, M.S. Brucella osteomyelitis of a closed femur fracture. Clin Orthop 195:194–196, 1985.

5. Ahl, T., Anderson, G., Herberts, P., and Kalen, R. Treatment of non-united fractures. Acta Orthop Scand 55:585–588, 1984.

6. Albright, J.A., Johnson, T.R., and Sahn, S. Principles of internal fixation, in Ghista, R. (ed): *Orthopaedic Mechanics Procedures and Devices.* New York, Academic Press, 1978, p 130.

7. Allgower, M. Cinderella of surgery: Fractures. Surg Clin North Am 58:1071–1093, 1978.

8. Allgower, M., and Spiegel, P.G. Internal fixation of fractures: Evolution of concepts. Clin Orthop 138:26–29, 1979.

9. Allum, R.L., and Mowbray, M.A.S. A retrospective review of the healing of fractures of shaft of tibia with special reference to the mechanism of injury. Injury 11:304–308, 1980.

10. Alms, M. Fracture mechanics. J Bone Joint Surg [Br] 43:162–166, 1961.

11. Altman, M. Intramedullary nailing for pathological impending and actual fractures of long bones. Bull Hosp Jt Dis Orthop Inst 13:239–239, 1952.

12. American Academy of Orthopaedic Surgery, sec 11: Metals used in orthopaedic surgery, in *Orthopaedic Knowledge Update I Home Study Syllabus.* AAOS, Chicago, 1984, pp 89–90.

13. Anderson, L. Use of plates in patients with multiple injuries. Orthop Clin North Am 1:151–167, 1970.

14. Anderson, L.D. Fractures of the shafts of the radius and ulna, in Rockwood, C.A., and Green, D.P. (eds): *Fractures.* Philadelphia, Lippincott, 1975.

15. Anderson, L.D., Hutchins, W.C., Wright, P.E. and Duney, J.M. Fractures of tibia and fibula treated by casts and transfixing pins. Clin Orthop 105:179–191, 1974.

16. Anderson, L.D., Sisk, T.D., Tooms, R.E. and Parks, W.C. Compression-plate fixation of acute diaphyseal fractures of radius and ulna. J Bone Joint Surg [Am] 57:287–297, 1975.

17. Anderson, R., and Burgess, E. Delayed union and nonunion. J Bone Joint Surg 25:427–1445, 1943.

18. Appley, G. *Appley's System of Orthopedics and Fractures,* 7th ed. Boston, Butterworth Scientific, 1982, pp 337–338.

19. Arzimanoglou, A., and Skiadaressis, G. A study of internal fixation by screws of oblique fractures on long bones. J Bone Joint Surg [Am] 34:219–223, 1952.

20. Auxhausen, G. Histologische untersuchen uber knochen Transplantation am Menschen. Disc Chir 91:388–393, 1907.

21. Bacorn, R.W., and Kurtzke, J.F. Colles' fracture: A study of two thousand cases from the New York State workmen's compensation board. J Bone Joint Surg [Am] 35:643–658, 1953.

22. Baker, B.I., and Rankin, E.A. Complications of treatment of fractures of the femoral shaft, in Epps, C. (ed): *Complications in Orthopaedics.* Philadelphia, Lippincott, 1978, pp 451–469.

23. Balfour, G.W., Mooney, V., and Ashby, M.E. Diaphyseal fractures of the humerus treated with a ready-made fracture brace. J Bone Joint Surg [Am] 64:11–13, 1982.

24. Banskota, A., and Volz, R.G. Traumatic laceration of the radial nerve following supracondylar fracture of the elbow: A case report. Clin Orthop 184:150–152, 1984.

25. Barnett, H.G., and Connolly, E.S. Lumbosacral nerve root avulsion report of a case and review of the literature. J Trauma 15:532–535, 1975.

26. Bassett, C.A., and Becker, P.O. Generation of electrical potential by bone in response to mechanical stress. Science 137:1063–1065, 1962.

27. Bassett, C.A., Becker, P.O., and Pawluk, R.J. Effects of electric currents on bone in vivo. Nature 204:652–684, 1964.

28. Bassett, C.A.L., Mitchell, S.N., and Gaston, S.R. Treatment of ununited tibial diaphyseal fractures with pulsing electromagnetic fields. J Bone Joint Surg [Am] 63:511–522, 1981.

29. Bassett, C.A.L., Mitchell, S.N., and Gaston, S.R. Pulsing electromagnetic field treatment of ununited fractures and failed arthrodeses. JAMA 247:623–628, 1982.

30. Bassett, C.A.L., Mitchell, S.N., and Schink, M.M. Treatment of therapeutically resistant non-unions with bone grafts and pulsing electromagnetic fields. J Bone Joint Surg [Am] 64:1214–1230, 1982.

31. Bassett, C.A.L., Pawluk, R.J., and Becker, R.L. Effects of electric currents on bone in vivo. Nature 204:652–684, 1964.

32. Bassett, C.A.L., Pawluk, R.J., and Pilla, A.A. Augmentation of bone repair by inductively coupled electromagnetic fields. Science 184:575–577, 1974.

33. Beals, R.K., Lawton, G.D., and Snell, W.E. Prophylactic internal fixation of the femur in metastatic breast cancer. Cancer 28:1350–1354, 1971.

34. Beazley, W.C., and Rosenthal, R.E. Lead intoxication 18 months after a gunshot wound. Clin Orthop 190:199–203, 1984.

35. Behrens, F. Basic concepts of external fixation and application in open tibial fractures. Instr Course Lect 33:124–130, 1984.

36. Benson, D.R., Riggins, R.S., Lawrence, R.M., Hoeprich, P., Huston, A., Harrison, J. Treatment of open fractures: A prospective study. J Trauma 23:25–30, 1983.

37. Beyer, J.C. *Wound Ballistics.* Washington, DC, Office of the Surgeon General, Department of the Army, 1962.

38. Black, F., Duckworth, N., and Hunter, N. *Atlas of Plaster Cast Techniques,* 2d ed. Chicago, Year Book, 1974.

39. Blake, D.D. Radiation treatment of metastatic bone disease. Clin Orthop 73:89–100, 1970.

40. Blom, S., and Dahlback, L.O. Nerve injuries in dislocations of the shoulder and fractures of the neck of the humerus. A clinical and electromyographic study. Acta Chir Scand 136:461, 1970.

41. Blount, W.P. *Fractures in Children.* Huntington, NY, Kreger (Williams & Wilkins), 1977.

42. Blyznak, N., Thompson, A., and Meinhard, B.M. Experience with interlocking intramedullary fixation devices, 1984. Personal communication.

43. Bohler, L. *The Treatment of Fractures,* 5th ed. New York, Grune and Stratton, 1958.

44. Bole, P.V., Purdy, R.T., Munda, R.T., et al. Civilian arterial injuries. Ann Surg 183:1, 1975.

45. Bonarigo, B.C., and Rubin, P. Nonunion of pathological fracture after radiation therapy. Radiology, 88:889–891, 1967.

46. Bora, F.W., Jr., and Osterman, A.L. Compression neuropathy. Clin Orthop 163:20–32, 1982.

47. Border, J., Chenier, R., McMenamy, R., LaDuca, J., Seibel, R., Birkhahn, R., and Yu, L. Multiple systems organ failure. Surg Clin North Am 56:1147–1167, 1976.

48. Bradshear, M.R., Jr., and Raney, R.B. Fracture principles and fracture healing, in *Handbook of Orthopedic Surgery,* 9th ed. St. Louis, Mosby, 1978.

49. Brashear, H.R. Diagnosis and prevention of nonunion. J Bone Joint Surg [Am] 47:174–178, 1965.

50. Brettler, D., Sedlin, E.D., and Mendes, D.G. Conservative treatment of low velocity gunshot wounds. Clin Orthop 140:26–30, 1979.

51. Brighton, C.T. The semi-invasive method of treating nonunion with direct current. Orthop Clin North Am 15:33–45, 1984.

52. Brighton, C.T., Black, J., Friedenberg, Z.B., Esterhai, J., Day, L., and Connelly, J.F. Multicenter study and treatment of non-union with constant direct current. J Bone Joint Surg [Am] 63:2–11, 1981.

53. Bromage, P. Local anesthetic procedures for the hand and arm. Surg Clin North Am 44:919–922, 1964.

54. Brostom, L., and Sidlin, P. Histological changes in recent chronic ligament ruptures. Acta Chir Scand 132:248, 1936.

55. Brown, P.W., and Urban, J.G. Early weight-bearing treatment of open fractures of the tibia: An end-result study of sixty-three cases. J Bone Joint Surg [Am] 51:59–74, 1969.

56. Burchardt, H., Busbee, G.A., and Enneking, W.F. Repair of experimental autologous grafts of cortical bone. J Bone Joint Surg [Am] 57:814–818, 1975.

57. Burnett, J.W., Gustilo, R.B., Williams, D.N., and Kind, A. Prophylactic antibiotics in hip fractures: A double blind, prospective study. J Bone Joint Surg [Am] 62:457–461, 1980.

58. Burri, C. *Posttraumatic Osteomyelitis.* Berne, Betne, Hans, Huber, 1975.

59. Canale, S.T., and Kelly, F.B., Jr. Fractures of the neck of the talus: Long-term evaluation of 71 cases. J Bone Joint Surg [Am] 60:143–156, 1978.

60. Canale, S.T., Puhl, J., Watson, F.M., and et al. Acute osteomyelitis following closed fractures: Report of 3 cases. J Bone Joint Surg [Am] 57:415–418, 1975.

61. Cass, C.A. Some experiences with a battery stimulator in fractures with well established non-union. J Bone Joint Surg [Br] 57:251, 1970.

62. Cedell, C.A. Supination outward rotation injuries of the ankle: A clinical and roentgenological study with special reference to operative treatment. Acta Orthop Scand 110(suppl):3–148, 1967.

63. Chapman, M.W. Closed intramedullary bone-grafting and nailing of segmental defects of the femur: A report of three cases. J Bone Joint Surg [Am] 62:1004–1008, 1980.

64. Chapman, M.W. The use of immediate internal fixation in open fractures. Orthop Clin North Am 11:579–690, 1980.

65. Chapman, M.W., and Mahoney, M. The role of early internal fixation in the management of open fractures. Clin Orthop 138:120–130, 1979.

66. Charnley, J. *The Closed Treatment of Common Fractures,* 3d ed. Edinburgh, Churchill Livingstone, 1968.

67. Ciesynski, T. Stimulation and depression of bone regeneration by electric polarization in humans. Calcif Tissue Res 4:134.

68. Ciesynski, T. Studies on regeneration of ossil tissue, II: Treatment of bone fractures in experimental animals with electrical energy. Arch Immunol Ther Exp 11:191, 1963.

69. Clancey, G.J., and Hansen, S.T., Jr. Open fractures of the tibia: A review of 102 cases. J Bone Joint Surg [Am] 60:118–122, 1978.

70. Cochran, G.V.B., Johnson, M.W., Kadaba, M.P., Vosburgh, F., Ferguson-Pell, M.W., and Palmieri, V.R. Piezoelectric internal fixation devices. A new approach to electrical augmentation of osteogenesis. J Orthop Res 3:50–13, 1985.

71. Cohen, S.M., and Shubenberg, C.A.R. Treatment of war wounds of the limb. Lancet 239:351–356, 1940.

72. Collins, H.A., and Jacobs, J.K. Acute arterial injuries due to blunt trauma. J Bone Joint Surg [Am] 43:193–197, 1961.

73. Connolly, J.F. Torsional fractures and the third dimension of fracture management. South Med J 73:884–891, 1980.

74. Connolly, J.F. Selection, evaluation, and indications for electrical stimulation of ununited fractures. Clin Orthop 161:39–53, 1981.

75. Connolly, J.F., Whittaker, D., and Williams, E. Femoral and tibial fractures combined with injuries to the femoral or popliteal artery: A review of the literature and analysis of fourteen cases. J Bone Joint Surg [Am] 53:56–67, 1971.

76. Connolly, W.B. Cold therapy: An improved method. Med J Aust 2:424–425, 1972.

77. Cooney, W.P., Dobyns, J.H., and Linscheid, R.L. Complications of colles fractures. J Bone Joint Surg [Am] 62:613–619, 1980.

78. Cooney, W.P., III, Fitzgerald, R.H., Jr., Dobyns, J.H., and Washington, J.A. Quantitative wound cultures in upper extremity trauma. J Trauma 22:112–117, 1982.

79. Cotton, F.J. Elbow dislocation and ulnar artery injury. J Bone Joint Surg 11:348, 1929.

80. Cozen, L.N. Four unusual cases of osteomyelitis in adults, in Proceedings of the Western Orthopaedic Association. J Bone Joint Surg [Am] 39:454, 1957.

81. Cruess, R.L. Healing of bone tendon and ligament, in Rockwood, C.A., and Green, D.P. (eds): *Fractures,* vol. 1, 2d ed. Philadelphia, Lippincott, 1984.

82. Danis, R. Theorie et pratique de l'osteosynthesis. Paris, Libraire del Acadamie Med, 1941. Reprinted in Clin Orthop 138:23, 1974.

83. Danckwardt-Lilliestrom, G., et al. Intracortical circulation after intramedullary reaming with reduction of pressure in the medullary cavity: A microangiographic study on the rabbit tibia. J Bone Joint Surg [Am] 52:1390–1394, 1970.

84. Dehne, E. Nonoperative treatment of fractures of the tibia by immediate weight bearing. J Trauma 1:514–535, 1961.

85. Dehne, E. The spinal adaptation syndrome. Clin Orthop 5:211–220, 1955.

86. Dehne, E., Deffer, P.A., and Hall, R.M. The natural history of the fractured tibia. Surg Clin North Am 41:1495, 1961.

87. Deitch, E.A., and Grimes, W.R. Experience with 112 shotgun wounds of the extremities. J Trauma 24:600–603, 1984.

88. Devas, M. *Stress Fractures.* New York, Churchill Livingstone, 1975.

89. Dorph, M.H. The cast syndrome. N Engl J Med 243:445, 1950.

90. Doporto, J.M., and Rafique, M. Vascular insufficiency complicating trauma to the lower limb. J Bone Joint Surg [Br] 51:680–685, 1969.

91. Doty, D.B., Trieman, R.L., Rothschild, P.D., et al. Prevention of gangrene due to fractures. Surg Gynecol Obstet 125:284–, 1967.

92. Douglass, H.O., Jr., Shukla, S.K., and Mindell, E. Treatment of pathological fractures of long bones excluding those due to breast cancer. J Bone Joint Surg [Am] 58:1055–1061, 1976.

93. Dowden, J.W. The principle of early active movement in treating fractures of the upper extremity. Clin Orthop 146:4–8, 1980.

94. Dwyer, A.F., The use of electrical current in spinal fusion. Orthop Clin N Am 6:265–273, 1975.

95. Dwyer, A.F., and Wickham, G.G. Direct current stimulation in spinal fusion. Med J Aust 1:73–75, 1974.

96. Dziemian, A.J., and Herget, C.M. Milit Surg 106:204, 1950.

97. Dziemian, A.J., Mendelson, J.A., and Lindsey, E.D. Comparison of the wounding characteristics of some commonly encountered bullets. J Trauma 1:341–353, 1961.

98. Ebong, W.W. Acute osteomyelitis three years after a closed fracture in an adult with sickle cell anemia: A case report. J Bone Joint Surg [Am] 62:1196–1197, 1980.

99. Edwards, C.C. Staged reconstruction of complex open tibial fractures suing Hoffmann external fixation: Clinical decisions and dilemmas. Clin Orthop 178:130–161, 1983.

100. Edwards, P. Fractures of the shaft of the tibia: 492 consecutive cases in adults. Acta Orthop Scand 76(suppl):39, 1965.

101. Eftekhar, N.J., and Thurston, C.W. Effect of irradiation or acrylic cement with special reference to fixation of pathologic fracture. J Biomech 8:53, 1975.

102. Ender, H.G. Treatment of peritrochanteric and subtrochanteric fractures of femur with ender pins. Hip 1978, 187–206.

103. Enneking, W.F., and Howowitz, M. The intraarticular effects of immobilization on the human knee. J Bone Joint Surg [Am] 54:973–985, 1972.

104. Enneking, W.F., Burchardt, H., Puhl, J.J., and Piotrowski, G. Physical and biological aspects of repair in dog cortical bone transplants. J Bone Joint Surg [Am] 57:237–252, 1975.

105. Epstein, H.C. *Traumatic Dislocations of the Hip.* Baltimore, Williams & Wilkins, 1980.

106. Esterhai, J.L., Jr., Brighton, C.T., Heppenstall, R.B., Alavi, A., and

Mandell, G.A. Technetium and gallium scintigraphic evaluation of patients with long bone fracture nonunion. Clin Orthop 15:125–130, 1974.

107. Etter, C., Burri, C., Claes, H.L., Kinzl, L., and Raible, M. Treatment by external fixation of open fractures associated with severe soft tissue damage of the leg: Biomechanical principles and clinical experience. Clin Orthop 173:80–88, 1983.

108. Jackson, D.W., and Feagin, J.A. Quadriceps contusions in young athletes: Relation of severity of injury to treatment and prognosis. J Bone Joint Surg [Am] 55:95–105, 1973.

109. Fidler, M. Prophylactic internal fixation of secondary neoplastic deposits in long bones. Br Med J 1:341–344, 1973.

110. Fischer, D.A. External fixation in adult fracture management: Current indications, techniques, and successes. Adv Orthop Surg :240–243, 1984.

111. Foster, R.J., Dixon, G., Bach, A., Appleyard, R., and Green, T. Internal fixation of fractures and non-unions of the humeral shaft: Indications and results in a multi-center study. J Bone Joint Surg [Am] 67:857–864, 1985.

112. Friedenberg, Z.B., and Brighton, C.T. Bioelectric potentials in bone. J Bone Joint Surg 48:915–923, 1966.

113. Friedenberg, Z.B., and Brighton, C.T. Electrical fracture healing. Ann NY Acad Sci 238:564, 1964.

114. Friedenberg, Z.B., Dwyer, R.H., and Brighton, C.T. Electrosteograms of long bones of immature rabbits. J Dent Res 50:635, 1971.

115. Friedenberg, Z.B., Harlow, M.C., and Brighton, C.T. Healing of non-union of the medial malleolus by means of direct current: A case report. Trauma 11:883–885, 1971.

116. Friedrich, B., and Klaue, P. Mechanical stability and post-traumatic osteitis: An experimental evaluation of the relation between infection of bone and internal fixation. Injury 9:23–29, 1977.

117. Garrat, A.C. Electrophysiology and electrotherapeutics in electrically stimulated bone growth: A review of literature. Clin Orthop 122:325–332, 1977.

118. Gates, D.J., Alms, M., and Cruz, M.M. Hinged cast and roller traction for fractured femur: A system of treatment for the third world. J Bone Joint Surg [Br] 67:750–756, 1985.

119. Galante, J., and Rostoker, W. Corrosion-related failure in metallic implants: An experimental study. Clin Orthop 86:237–244, 1972.

120. Garcia, A., and Maec, B.N. Radial nerve injuries in fractures of the shaft of the humerus. Am J Surg 99:665, 1960.

121. Garfin, S.R., Mubarak, S.J., Evans, K.L., and Akevon, W. Quantification of intracompartmental pressure and volume under plaster casts. J Bone Joint Surg [Am] 63:449–453, 1981.

122. Gaspar, M.R., Treiman, R.L., Payne, J.M., and et al. Special problems in vascular trauma. Surg Clin North Am 48:1355, 1968.

123. Ger, R. The management of open fractures of the tibia with skin loss. J Trauma 10:112–121, 1970.

124. Gill, S.S., Eggleston, F.C., Singh, C.M., Abraham, K.A., Kumar, S., and Lobo, L.H. Arterial injuries of the extremities. J Trauma 16:766–772, 1976.

125. Goldman, B.S., Firor, W.B., and Key, J.A. The recognition and management of peripheral arterial injuries. Can Med Assoc J 92:1154, 1965.

126. Goldthwait, J.R. The backgrounds and foreground of orthopaedics. J Bone Joint Surg 14:279, 1933.

127. Goodell, C.L. Neurological deficits associated with pelvic fracture. J Neurosurg 24:837, 1966.

128. Granberry, W.M., and Janes, J.M. The effect of electric current on the epiphyseal cartilage. Proc Conf Mayo Clin 38:87, 1963.

129. Green, S.A. Complications of external skeletal fixation. Clin Orthop 180:109–116, 1983.

130. Green, S.A., and Dlabar, T.A. The open bone graft for septic nonunion. Clin Orthop 180:117–124, 1983.

131. Kempf, I., Grosse, A., and Beck, G. Closed locked intramedullary nailing: Its application to comminuted fractures of the femur. J Bone Joint Surg [Am] 67:709–719, 1985.

132. Gundry, S.R., Burney, R.E., Mackenzie, J.R., Wilton, G., Whitehouse, W., Wu, S.C., and Kirsh, M. Assessment of mediastinal widening associated with traumatic rupture of the aorta. J Trauma 23:293–299, 1983.

133. Gustilo, R.B. *The Management of Open Fractures.* As presented at the Eli Lily Symposium on Infections in Orthopedics, San Francisco, 1985.

134. Gustilo, R.B., and Meindoza, R.M. Results of treatment of 1400 open fractures, in Gustilo, R.B. (ed): *Management of Open Fractures and Their Complications.* Philadelphia, Saunders, 1982.

135. Gustilo, R.B., Simpson, L., Nixon, R., and Ruiz, A. Analysis of 511 open fractures. Clin Orthop 66:148–154, 1969.

136. Habermann, E.T., Sachs, R., Stern, R., Hirsh, D., and Anderson, W. The pathology and treatment of metastatic disease of the femur. Clin Orthop 169:70–82, 1982.

137. Hambury, H.J., Watson, J., Silyer, A., and Ashley, D.J.B. Effective micro ampular electric currents on bone in vivo and its measurement using strontium 85 update. Nature 231:190, 1971.

138. Hammerberg, K.W., Berkson, M.H., Skeinkop, M.B., et al. Care of fractures and other trauma with vascular injury. Orthop Rev 10:83–88, 1981.

139. Hansen, S.T., Jr., and Winquist, R.A. Technical considerations in intramedullary nailing. Instr Course Lect 27:90–108, 1978.

140. Hardaker, W.T., Jr., Ward, W.T., and Goldner, J.L. External fixation in the management of severe musculoskeletal trauma. Orthopedics 4:437–444, 1981.

141. Harkess, J.W., Ramsey, W.C., and Ahmadi, B. Principles of fractures and dislocations, in Rockwood, C.A., and Green, D.P. (eds): *Fractures in Adults.* Philadelphia, Lippincott, 1984, pp 1–135.

142. Harper, M.C. Fractures of the femur treated by open and closed intramedullary nailing using fluted rod. J Bone Joint Surg [Am] 67:699–708, 1985.

143. Harrington, K.D. The management of acetabular insufficiency secondary to metastatic malignant disease. J Bone Joint Surg [Am] 63:653–663, 1981.

144. Harrington, K.D., Sim, F.H., Enis, J.E., Johnston, J.O., Dick, H., and Gristina, A.G. Methyl methacrylate as an adjunct in internal fixation of pathological fractures: Experience with 375 cases. J Bone Joint Surg [Am] 58:1047–1055, 1976.

145. Harrington, K.D. New trends in the management of lower extremity metastases. Clin Orthop 169:53–61, 1982.

146. Harris, W.H., Thrasher, E.L., Moyen, B.J., Cobben, R.H., Davis, L.A., McKenzie, T.A., and Sywinski, J.K. Stimulation of fracture healing by direct current: An experimental study in dogs. Trans Orthop Res Soc 1:106, 1976.

147. Hasenhutti, K. The treatment of unstable fractures of the tibia and fibula with flexible medullary wires: A review of 235 fractures. J Bone Joint Surg [Am] 63:921–931, 1981.

148. Hawkins, L.G. Fractures of the neck of the talus. J Bone Joint Surg [Am] 52:991–1002, 1970.

149. Hedley, A.K., and Bernstein, M.L. External fixation as a secondary procedure. Clin Orthop 173:209–215, 1983.

150. Hennessy, M.J., Banks, H.H., Leach, R.B., and Quigley, T.B. Extremity gunshot wound and gunshot fracture in civilian practice. Clin Orthop 114:296–302, 1976.

151. Heppenstall, R.B. The present role of bone graft surgery in treating nonunion. Orthop Clin North Am 15:113–123, 1984.

152. Heppenstall, R.B. Constant-direct current treatment for established nonunion of the tibia. Clin Orthop 178:179–184, 1983.

153. HeyGroves, E.W. Methods of transplantation of bone in repair of defects caused by injury or disease. Br J Surg 5:185–242, 1918. Cited in Harkess, J.W., Ramsey, W.C., and Ahmadi, B. Principles of fractures and dislocations, in Rockwood, C.A., and Green, D.P.

(eds): *Fractures in Adults.* Philadelphia, Lippincott, 1984.

154. Hirasawa, Y., Oda, R., and Nakatani, K. Sciatic nerve paralysis in posterior dislocation of the hip: A case report. Clin Orthop 126:172–175, 1977.

155. Hinsenkamp, M., Burny, F., Donkerwolcke, M., and Coussaert, E. Electromagnetic stimulation of fresh fractures treated with Hoffman external fixation. Orthopedics 7:411–416, 1984.

156. Hojer, J., Gillquist, J., and Liljedahl, S.O. Combined fractures of the femoral and tibial shafts in the same limb. Injury 8:206–212, 1977.

157. Howard, F.M. Ulnar-nerve palsy in wrist fractures. J Bone Joint Surg [Am] 43:1197–1201, 1961.

158. Howland, W.S., Jr., and Ritchey, S.J. Gunshot fractures in civilian practice: An evaluation of the results of limited surgical treatment. J Bone Joint Surg [Am] 53:47–55, 1971.

159. Hudson, O.C. Multiple fractures. J Bone Joint Surg 22:354–360, 1940.

160. Hughes, J.L. External skeletal fixation: Part V. Wagner apparatus as portable traction device for the femur. Instr Course Lect 13:158–167, 1984.

161. Hunter, G.A. Posterior dislocation and fracture-dislocation of the hip: A review of fifty-seven patients. J Bone Joint Surg [Br] 51:38–44, 1969.

162. Itay, S., and Haggai, T. Thermal osteonecrosis complicating Steinmann pin insertion in plastic surgery: Case report. Plast Reconstr Surg 72:557–561, 1983.

163. Iversen, L.D., and Clawson, D.K., *Manual of Acute Orthopaedic Therapeutics,* 2d ed. Boston, Little, Brown, 1982.

164. Jaffe, H.L., and Campbell, C.J. Palliation of metastatic bone disease, in Hickey, J. (ed): *Palliative Care of the Cancer Patient.* Boston, Little, Brown, 1967.

165. Johnson, K.D. Indications, instrumentation, and experience with locked tibial nails. Orthopedics 8:1377–1383, 1985.

166. Johnson, K.D., Johnston, D.W.C., and Parker, B. Comminuted femoral-shaft fractures: Treatment by roller traction, cerclage wires and an intramedullary nail, or an interlocking intramedullary nail. J Bone Joint Surg [Am] 66:1222–1235, 1984.

167. Johnson, W. Comparison of multiplane fixation devices. Clin Orthop 180:34–43, 1983.

168. Johnston, A.D. Pathology of metastatic tumors in bone. Clin Orthop 73:8–32, 1970.

169. Jones, R. An orthopaedic view of treatment of fractures. Clin Orthop 75:4–16, 1971.

170. Jorgensen, T.E. The effect of electric current on the healing time of crural fractures. Acta Orthop Scand 43:421–437, 1972.

171. Kaplan, S.S. Burns following application of plaster splint dressings: Report of two cases. J Bone Joint Surg [Am] 63:670–672, 1981.

172. Karlstrom, G., and Olerud, S. Ipsilateral fracture of femur and tibia. J Bone Joint Surg [Am] 59:240–243, 1977.

173. Karlstrom, G., and Olerud, S. Fractures of tibial shaft: A critical evaluation of treatment alternatives. Clin Orthop 105:82–115, 1974.

174. Kasman, R.A., and Chao, E.Y.S. Fatigue performance of external fixator pins. J Orthop Res 2:377–387, 1984.

175. Kaufer, H. Non-operative ambulatory treatment for fracture of the shaft of the femur. Clin Orthop 87:192–199, 1972.

176. Keon-Cohen, B.T. Fractures at the elbow. J Bone Joint Surg [Am] 48:1623–1639, 1966.

177. Kelly, P.J. Infected non-union of femur and tibia. Orthop Clin North Am 15:481–490, 1984.

178. Kennedy, J.C. Complete dislocation of the knee joint. J Bone Joint Surg 45:889–904, 1963.

179. Kettelkamp, D.B., and Alexander, H. Clinical review of radial nerve injury. J Trauma 7:424–432, 1967.

180. Kleiman, S.G., Stevens, J., Kolb, L., and Pankowich, A. Late sciatic nerve palsy following posterior fracture-dislocation of the hip. A case report. J Bone Joint Surg [Am] 53:781–782, 1971.

181. Klingensmith, W., Olis, P., and Martinez, H. Fracture with associated blood vessel injury. Am J Surg 110:849–852, 1965.

182. Knight, R.A., and Purvis, G.D. Fractures of both bones of the forearm in adults. J Bone Joint Surg [Am] 31:755–764, 1949.

183. Koskinin, E.V.S., and Nieman, R.A. Surgical treatment of metastatic pathological fracture of major long bones. Acta Orthop Scand 44:539–549, 1973.

184. Kuntscher, G. Die Markinagelong von konchebrucher. Arch Kluscher 200:443, 1940.

185. Kuntscher, G. *Practice of Intramedullary Nailing.* Springfield, IL, Thomas, 1967, pp 85–96.

186. Kyle, R.F., Gustilo, R.B., and Premer, R.F. Analysis of six hundred and twenty-two intertrochanteric hip fractures: A retrospective and prospective study. J Bone Joint Surg [Am] 61:216–221, 1979.

187. Laduca, J.N., Bone, L.L., Seibel, R.W., and Border, J.R. Primary open reduction and internal fixation of open fractures. J Trauma 20:580–586, 1980.

188. LaFollette, B.F. Rehabilitation of fractures. Instr Course Lect 24:405, 1985.

189. LaValette, R., Pope, M.H., and Dickstein, H. Setting temperatures of plaster casts: The influence of technical variables. J Bone Joint Surg [Am] 64:907–911, 1982.

190. Laros, G.S., and Spiegel, P.G. Rigid internal fixation of fractures: Editorial comments. Clin Orthop 138:2–22, 1979.

191. Lavine, L.S., Lustrin, I., Shamos, N.H., Rinaldi, R.I., and Lieboff, L.R. Electric enhancement of bone healing. Science 175:1118–1120, 1972.

192. Lawyer, J.R., and Lubbers, L.M. Use of Hoffman apparatus in the treatment of unstable tibial fractures. J Bone Joint Surg [Am] 62:1264–1272, 1980.

193. Ledgerwood, A.M. The wandering bullet. Surg Clin North Am 57:97–109, 1977.

194. Leffert, R.D. Anterior submuscular transposition of the ulnar nerves by the Learmonth technique. J Hand Surg 7:147–155, 1982.

195. Levy, M. Peroneal nerve palsy due to superior dislocation of the head of the fibula and shortening of the tibia. Acta Orthop Scand 46:1020–1025, 1975.

196. Lewis, D.H., and Lim, R.C., Jr. Studies on the circulatory pathophysiology of trauma: I. Effect of acute soft tissue injury on nutritional and nonnutritional shunt flow through the hindleg of the dog. Acta Orthop Scand 41:17–36, 1970.

197. Lewis, M.H. Median nerve decompression after Colles's fracture. J Bone Joint Surg [Br] 60:195–196, 1978.

198. Lewis, R. *Handbook of Traction, Casting and Splinting Techniques.* Philadelphia, Lippincott, 1977.

199. Lifeso, R.M., and Al-Saati, F. The treatment of infected and uninfected non-union. J Bone Joint Surg [Br] 66:573–579, 1984.

200. Linscheid, R.L., and Wheeler, D.K. Elbow dislocations. JAMA 194:1171–1176, 1965.

201. Lichter, R.L., and Jacobsen, T. Tardy palsy of the posterior interosseous nerve with a Monteggia fracture. J Bone Joint Surg [Am] 57:124–125, 1975.

202. Loomis, L.K. Reduction and after treatment of posterior dislocation of the elbow. Am J Surg 63:56–60, 1944.

203. Lottes, J.L. Intramedullary fixation of fractures of the shaft of the tibia. South Med J 45:407–414, 1952.

204. Luce, E.A., and Griffen, W.O. Shotgun injuries of the upper extremity. J Trauma 18:487–492, 1978.

205. Luck, J.V. Plaster of paris. An experimental and clinical analysis. JAMA 124:23–29, 1944.

206. Martz, C.D. Studies on stress and strain in treatment of fractures. J Bone Joint Surg [Am] 46:409–11, 1964.

207. Matsen, F.A., III. Compartment syndrome: A unified concept.

Clin Orthop 113:8–14, 1975.

208. Matsen, F.A., III. Compartment syndromes definitions, theory and pathogenesis. Instr Course Lect 32:88–92, 1983.

209. Matsen, F.A., III. Effect of local cooling on postfracture swelling: A controlled study. Clin Orthop 109:201–206, 1975.

210. Mayer, L., Werbie, T., Schwab, J.P., and Johnson, R.P. The use of Ender nails in fracture of the tibial shaft. J Bone Joint Surg [Am] 67:446–455, 1985.

211. Mayfield, G. Rotational malunion of femoral shaft fractures and its functional significance. J Bone Joint Surg [Am] 56:1309, 1974.

212. Mays, J., and Neufeld, A.J. Skeletal traction methods. Clin Orthop 102:144–151, 1974.

213. McDonald, E.J., Goodman, P.C., and Winestock, D.P. The clinical indications for arteriography in trauma to the extremity: A review of 114 cases. Radiology 116:45–46, 1975.

214. Mears, D. External Skeletal Fixation. Baltimore, Williams & Wilkins, 1985.

215. Mears, D.C., and Rothwell, G.P. The structure and properties of materials, in Mears, D.C. (ed): Materials and Orthopaedic Surgery. Baltimore, Williams & Wilkins, 1979, p 404.

216. Mears, D.C., and Rubash, H.E. External skeletal fixation: Part IV. External and internal fixation of pelvic ring. Instr Course Lect 33:144–157, 1984.

217. Meek, A.C., and Robbs, J.V. Vascular injury with associated bone and joint trauma. Br J Surg 71:341–344, 1984.

218. Merianos, P., Cambouridis, P., and Smyrnis, P. The treatment of 143 tibial shaft fractures by Ender's nailing and early weight-bearing. J Bone Joint Surg [Br] 67:576–580, 1985.

219. Merriam, W.F., and Mifsud, R.P. Internal fixation in patients with multiple injuries. Injury 15:78–86, 1983.

220. Meyer, S., et al. The treatment of infected nonunion of fractures of long bones: Study of sixty-four cases with a five to twenty-one-year follow-up. J Bone Joint Surg [Am] 57:836–841, 1975.

221. Milgrom, C., Giladi, M., Stein, M., Kashtan, H., Margulies, J.Y., Chisin, R., Steinberg, R., and Aharonson, Z. Stress fractures in military recruits: A prospective study showing an unusually high incidence. J Bone Joint Surg [Br] 67:732–735, 1985.

222. Miller, G.J., Burchardt, H., Enneking, W.F., and Tylkowski, C.M. Electromagnetic stimulation of canine bone grafts. J Bone Joint Surg [Am] 66:693–698, 1984.

223. Miller, H.H., and Welch, C.S. Quantitative studies on time factors in arterial injuries. Ann Surg 130–428, 1949.

224. Miller, J. Characteristics and management of joint fracture. Instr Course Lect 28:94–102, 1979.

225. Monroe, J.K. The history of plaster of Paris in the treatment of fractures. Br J Surg 23:257, 1935.

226. Montgomery, S.P., and Mooney, V. Femur fractures: Treatment with roller traction and early ambulation. Clin Orthop 156:196–200, 1981.

227. Mooney, V., Nickel, V.L., Harvey, J.P., and Snelson, R. Cast-brace treatment for fractures of the distal part of the femur: A prospective controlled study of one hundred and fifty patients. J Bone Joint Surg [Am] 52:1563–1578, 1970.

228. Moore, J.R. The closed fracture of the long bones. J Bone Joint Surg [Am] 42:869–874, 1960.

229. Mubarak, S.J. Compartment syndrome. A practical approach to diagnosis. Instr Course Lect 32:92–101, 1983.

230. Mubarak, S.J., and Hargens, A.R. Diagnosis and management of compartment syndromes, in AAOS Symposium on Trauma to the Leg and its Sequelae. St. Louis, Mosby, 1981.

231. Mubarak, S.J., Hargens, A.R., Lee, Y.F., Lundblad, A.F., Castle, G.S.P., and Rorabeck, O.H. Slit catheter: A new technique for measuring intra-compartmental pressures. Orthop Trans 5:324, 1981.

232. Muller, J., Schenk, R., and Willnegger, H. Experimentelle Untersuchungen über die entstehung Reaktiver pseudarthorsen am

Hunderadius. Helv Chir Acta 35:301, 1968.

233. Muller, M.E., Allgower, M., Schneider, R., and Willnegger, N. Manual of Internal Fixation Techniques Recommended by the A-O group, 2d ed. New York, Springer-Verlag, 1979.

234. Murray, J.A., Bruels, M.C., and Lindberg, R.D. Irradiation of polymethylmethacrylate: In vitro gamma radiation effect. J Bone Joint Surg [Am] 56:311–312, 1974.

235. Naiman, P.T., Schein, A.J., and Siffert, R.S. Use of ASIF compression plates in selected shaft fractures of the upper extremity: A preliminary report. Clin Orthop 71:208–216, 1970.

236. Nelson, J.P. Musculoskeletal infection. Surg Clin 60:213–222, 1980.

237. Nelson, J.P., Ferris, D.U., and Ivins, J. The cast syndrome. Postgrad Med 42:457–461, 1967.

238. Netz, P., Erikson, K., and Stromberg, L. Non-linear properties of diaphyseal bone: An experimental study on dogs. Acta Orthop Scand 50:139–144, 1979.

239. Neufeld, A.J., Mays, J.D., and Naden, C.J. A dynamic method for treating femoral shaft fractures. Orthop Rev 1:19–21, 1972.

240. O'Driscoll, S.W., Kumar, A., and Salter, R.B. The effect of continuous passive motion on the clearance of a hemarthrosis from a synovial joint: An experimental investigation in the rabbit. Clin Orthop 176:305–311, 1983.

241. Olerud, C. Orthopedic traction device: An analysis of forces. Injury 15:341–346, 1984.

242. Pankovich, A. Manual of Flexible Nailing Techniques. OEC (Orthopedic Equipment Co.) Publication, 1983.

243. Pankovich, A.M., Tarabishy, I.E., and Yelda, S. Flexible intramedullary nailing of tibial-shaft fractures. Clin Orthop 160:185–195, 1981.

244. Pankovich, A.M. Adjunctive fixation in flexible intramedullary nailing of femoral fractures: A study of twenty-six cases. Clin Orthop 157:301–309, 1981.

245. Paradies, L.H., and Gregory, C.F. The early treatment of close-range shotgun wounds to the extremities. J Bone Joint Surg [Am] 48:425–435, 1966.

246. Paterson, D. Electrical stimulation: An implantable system. Orthop Clin North Am 15:47–59, 1984.

247. Paterson, D., Lewis, G.N., and Cass, C.A. Clinical experience in Australia with implanted bone growth stimulator from 1976 to 1978. Orthop Trans 3:288, 1979.

248. Patterson, F.P., and Morton, K.S. Neurological complications of fractures and dislocations of the pelvis. J Trauma 12:1013–1023, 1972.

249. Patzakis, M.J., Wilkins, J., and Moore, T.M. Use of antibiotics in open tibial fractures. Clin Orthop 178:31–35, 1983.

250. Pavel, A., Smith, R.L., Ballard, A., and Larsen, I.J. Prophylactic antibiotics in clean orthopaedic surgery. J Bone Joint Surg [Am] 56:777–782, 1974.

251. Perren, S.M. Physical and biological aspects of fracture healing with special reference to internal fixation. Clin Orthop 138:175–196, 1979.

252. Perren, S.M., Huggler, A., Russenberger, M., Allgower, M., Mathys, R., Willeneger, H., and Müller, M.E. The reaction of cortical bone to compression. Acta Orthop Scand 125(suppl):19–29, 1969.

253. Perren, S.M., and Cardy, J. Russenberger development of compression plate techniques for internal fixation of fractures. Prog Surg 12:152–179, 1973.

254. Perry, M.O., Thal, E.R., and Shires, G.T. Management of arterial injuries. Ann Surg 173:403–408, 1971.

255. Pess, G.M., Waugh, T.R., and Melone, C.P., Jr. Treatment of nonunions with electrical stimulation: A review paper. Orthop Rev 14:17–27, 1985.

256. Phemister, D.B. The rate of transplanted bone and regenerative power of its various constituents. Surg Gynecol Obstet 19:303, 1914.

257. Porter, M.F. Delayed arterial occlusion in limb injuries: Report of three cases. J Bone Joint Surg [Br] 50:138–140, 1968.

258. Posch, J.L., and Dela Cruz-Saddul, F. Nerve repair in trauma surgery: A ten-year study of 231 peripheral injuries. Orthop Rev 9:35–45, 1980.

259. Pradhan, D.J., Juanteguy, J.M., Wilder, R.J., and Michaelson, E. Arterial injuries of the extremities associated with fractures. Arch Surg 105:582–585, 1972.

260. Prietto, C.A. Supracondylar fractures of the humerus: A comparative study of Dunlop's traction versus percutaneous pinning. J Bone Joint Surg [Am] 61:425–428, 1979.

261. Primm, D.D., Jr. Lead arthropathy—progressive destruction of a joint by a retained bullet: Case report. J Bone Joint Surg [Am] 66A:292–293, 1984.

262. Quigley, T.B. Management of the ankle injuries sustained in sports. JAMA 169:1431–1436, 1959.

263. Quinn, T.P., and Slager, R.F. Delayed deep wound sepsis five years after hip nailing: A case report. Clin Orthop 158:117–119, 1981.

264. Rang, M. *Children's Fractures.* Philadelphia, Lippincott, 1974.

265. Ransom, K.J., Swatney, C.H., Soderstrom, C.A., and Cowle, R.A. Management of arterial injuries in blunt trauma of the extremity. Surg Gynecol Obstet 153:241–246, 1981.

266. Reckling, F.W., and Peltier, L.F. Acute knee dislocations and their complications. J Trauma 9:181–191, 1969.

267. Reid, R.L., and Gamon, R.S., Jr. The cast syndrome. Clin Orthop 79:85–88, 1971.

268. Rhinelander, F. Intramedullary nailing of long-bone fractures—Current concepts: Effects of medullary nailing on the normal blood supply of diaphyseal cortex. Instr Course Lect 22:161–187, 1973.

269. Rich, N.M., Matz, C.W., Hutten, J.E., Jr., Baugh, H., Jr., and Hughes, C.W. Internal versus external fixation of fractures with concomitant vascular injuries in Vietnam. J Trauma 11:463–473, 1971.

270. Roberts, P.H. Dislocation of the elbow. Br J Surg 56:806–815, 1969.

271. Rockwood, C.A., Jr. Dislocations about the shoulder, in Rockwood, C.A., and Green, D.P. (eds): *Fractures,* 2d ed. Philadelphia, Lippincott, 1984, pp 742–948.

272. Rogers, J.F., Bennett, J.B., and Tullos, H.S. Management of concomitant ipsilateral fractures of the humerus and forearm. J Bone Joint Surg [Am] 66:552–556, 1984.

273. Romano, R.L., Burgess, E.M., and Rubenstein, C.P. Percutaneous electrical stimulation for clinical tibial fracture repair. Clin Orthop 114:290–294, 1976.

274. Rorabeck, C. Management of compartment syndromes. Instr Course Lect 32:192–212, 1983.

275. Rorabeck, C.H., and Macnab, I. Anterior tibial-compartment syndrome complicating fractures of the shaft of the tibia. J Bone Joint Surg [Am] 58:549–550, 1976.

276. Rosen, H. Operative treatment of nonunion of long bone fractures. JCE Orthop 7:13–39, 1979.

277. Rowe, C.R. Management of fractures in elderly patients is different. J Bone Joint Surg [Am] 47:1043–1059, 1965.

278. Ruedi, T.P., and Allgower, M. Fractures of the lower end of the tibia into the ankle joint. Injury 1:92–99, 1969.

279. Ruedi, T.P., and Luscher, J.N. Results after internal fixation of comminuted fractures of the femoral shaft with dc plates. Clin Orthop 138:74–76, 1979.

280. Ruedi, T., Webb, J.K., and Allgower, M. Experience with the dynamic compression plate (DCP) in 418 recent fractures of the tibial shaft. Injury 7:252–257, 1976.

281. Rush, L. *Atlas of Rush Pin Techniques: A System of Fracture Treatment.* Meridian, MS, Berivan, 1955.

282. Saffle, J.R., Schnelby, A., Hoffman, A., and Warden, G. The management of fractures in thermally injured patients. J Trauma 23:902–910, 1983.

283. Salter, R.B. Healing of intraarticular fractures with continuous passive motion. Instr Course Lect 37:102–117, 1979.

284. Salter, R.B., Bell, R.S., and Keeley, F.W. The protective effect of continuous passive motion on living articular cartilage in acute septic arthritis: An experimental investigation in the rabbit. Clin Orthop 159:223–247, 1981.

285. Salter, R.B., Simmonds, D.F., Malcolm, B.W., Rumble, E.J., Macmichael, D., and Clements, N.D. The biologic effect of continuous passive motion full-thickness defects in articular cartilage. J Bone Joint Surg [Am] 62:1232–1250, 1980.

286. Salter, R.B., and Field, P. The effect of continuous compression on living articular cartilage: An experimental investigation. J Bone Joint Surg [Am] 42:31–48, 1960.

287. Salter, R.B., et al. Clinical application of basic research on continuous passive motion for disorders and injuries of synovial joints: A preliminary report of a feasibility study. J Orthop Res 1:74–91, 1986.

288. Salter, W. Address to the British academy on continuous passive motion. J Bone Joint Surg 64:251–254, 1982.

289. Salter, W. Proceedings of university lecture on review of 10 years experience of continuous passive motion. J Bone Joint Surg [Br] 64:640, 1952.

290. Samson, R., and Pasternak, B.M. Traumatic arterial spasm—Rarity or nonentity. J Trauma 20:607–609, 1980.

291. Sandegard, J. Vasodilatation in extremity trauma. Immediate hemodynamic changes in the dog hindleg. Acta Chir Scand 447(suppl):1–32, 1974.

292. Sarmiento, A., Latta, L., Zilioli, A., and Sinclair, W. The role of soft tissues in the stabilization of tibial fractures. Clin Orthop 105:116–129, 1974.

293. Sarmiento, A., and Latta, C.S. *The Closed Treatment of Fractures.* New York, Springer-Verlag, 1981.

294. Schatzker, J.A. *Primer on the AO/ASIF Method of Internal Fixation.* Berlin, Springer-Verlag, 1974.

295. Schatzker, J., McBroom, R., and Bruce, D. The tibial plateau fracture: The Toronto experience 1968–1975. Clin Orthop 138:94–104, 1979.

296. Schaubel, H.J. Local use of ice after orthopaedic procedures. Am J Surg 72:711–714, 1946.

297. Scheur, J. Tissue-viability assessment with the Doppler ultrasonic flowmeter in acute injuries of extremities J Bone Joint Surg [Am] 55:157–161, 1973.

298. Schneider, M. Closed intramedullary nailing of fractures of the femoral shaft: Historical, physiologic, and biomechanical aspects. Instr Course Lect 27:88–108, 1978.

299. Schonholtz, G.J., and Jahnke, E.J., Jr. Occult injury of the thoracic aorta associated with orthopaedic trauma. J Bone Joint Surg [Am] 46:1421–1430, 1964.

300. Schulak, D.J., Duyar, A., Schlicke, L.M., and Gradisar, I.A. A theoretical analysis of cast wedging with practical applications. Clin Orthop 130:239–246, 1978.

301. Seddon, H.J. *Surgical Disorders of the Peripheral Nerves.* Baltimore, Williams & Wilkins, 1975.

302. Seddon, H.J. *Peripheral Nerve Injuries.* Medical research council special report, series no. 282. HM stationary, office, London, 1954.

303. Seitz, W.H., Jr., Berardis, J.M., Giannaris, T., and Schreiber, G. Perforation of the rectum by a Smith-Petersen nail: Case reports. J Trauma 22:339–340, 1982.

304. Shelton, M.L., and Anderson, R.L. Complications of fractures and dislocations of the ankle, in Epps, C.H. (ed): *Complications in Orthopaedic Surgery.* Philadelphia, Lippincott, 1978, p 535.

305. Shepard, G.H. High energy, low-velocity close range shotgun wounds. J Trauma 20:1065–1067, 1980.

306. Sher, M.H. Principles in the management of arterial injuries associated with fracture/dislocations. Ann Surg 182:630–634, 1975.
307. Sherry, H.S., Levy, R.N., and Siffert, R.S. Metastatic disease of bone in orthopedic surgery. Clin Orthop 169:44–52, 1982.
308. Shires, G.T. Infections following penetrating injuries, in Shires, G.T. (ed): *Care of the Trauma Patient,* 2d ed. New York, McGraw-Hill, 1979.
309. Schulak, D.J., Duyar, A., Schlicke, L.H., and Gradisar, I.A. A theoretical analysis of cast wedging with practical applications. Clin Orthop 130:239–246, 1978.
310. Sisk, T.D. External fixation: Historic review, advantages, disadvantages, complications, and indications. Clin Orthop 180:15–22, 1983.
311. Sisk, T.D. General Principles and techniques of external skeletal fixation. Clin Orthop 180:96–100, 1983.
312. Snyder, W.H. Vascular injuries near the knee. An updated series and overview of the problem. Surgery 91:502, 1982.
313. Spar, I. A neurological complication following Monteggia fracture. Clin Orthop 122:207–209, 1977.
314. Spencer, F.C., and Imparato, A.M. Peripheral arterial disease, in Schwartz, S., et al (eds): *Principles of Surgery.* New York, McGraw-Hill, 1974.
315. Spiegel, P.G., and Mast, J.W. Internal and external fixation of fractures in children. Orthop Clin North Am 11:405–421, 1980.
316. Spiegel, P.G., and Vanderschildren, J.L. Minimal internal and external fixation in the treatment of open tibial fractures. Clin Orthop 178:96–102, 1983.
317. St. Pierre, R.K., Holmes, H.E., and Fleming, L.L. Cast-bracing of femoral fractures: Experience at Emory University Hospitals. Orthopedics 5:739–745, 1982.
318. Stern, H., et al. The Wagner external fixator: Its use in devascularizing injuries of upper and lower extremities. Instr Course Lect 33:35–42, 1984.
319. Sturm, J.T., Bodily, K.C., Rothenberger, D.A., and Perry, J.F., Jr. Arterial injuries of the extremities following blunt trauma. J Trauma 20:933–936, 1980.
320. Suzuki, Y. Bone proliferation induced by electrical stimulation and tibial fracture, case report: Kyoto Second Red Cross Hospital, Kyoto, 1975, in Spadaro, J.A.: Electrically stimulated bone growth—a review of the literature. Clin Orthop 122:325–367, 1977.
321. Swearinger, R.L., and Dehne, E. A study of pathologic muscle function following injury to a joint. J Bone Joint Surg [Am] 46:1364, 1964.
322. Thaxter, T.H., Mann, R.A., and Anderson, C.E. Degeneration of immobilized knee joints in rats: Histological and autoradiographic study. J Bone Joint Surg [Am] 47:567–585, 1965.
323. Thoresby, F.P., and Darlow, H.M. The mechanisms of primary infection of bullet wounds. Br J Surg 54:359, 1967.
324. Tonnesen, P.A., Heerfordt, J., and Pers, J. 150 open fractures of the tibial shaft: The relation between necrosis of the skin and delayed union. Acta Orthop Scand 46:823–835, 1975.
325. Vidal, J. External fixation: Yesterday, today, and tomorrow. Clin Orthop 180:7–14, 1983.
326. Watson-Jones, R. *Fractures and Joint Injuries,* 4th ed. Baltimore, Williams & Wilkins, 1955.
327. Weaver, F.A., Rosenthal, R.E., Waterhouse, G., and Adkins, R.B. Combined skeletal and vascular injuries of the lower extremities. Am Surg 50:189–197, 1984.
328. Webb, J.K. The orthopedic management and rehabilitation of patients with multiple skeletal injuries. Orthop Clin North Am 9:569–579, 1978.
329. Weber, B.G., and Brunner, C. The treatment of nonunions without electrical stimulation. Clin Orthop 161:24–32, 1981.
330. Weber, B.G., and Cech, O. *Pseudoarthrosis.* New York, Grune and Stratton, 1976.
331. Wehbe, A. Plaster uses and misuses. Clin Orthop 167:242–249, 1982.
332. Weiland, A.J., and Daniel, R.K. Microvascular anastomoses for bone grafts in the treatment of massive defects in bone. J Bone Joint Surg [Am] 61:98–104, 1979.
333. Weiland, A.J., Kleinert, H.E., Kutz, J.E., and Daniel, R.K. Free vascularized bone grafts in surgery of the upper extremity. J Hand Surg 4:129–144, 1979.
334. Weiland, A.J., Moore, J.R., and Hotchkiss, R.N. Soft tissue procedures for reconstruction of tibial shaft fractures. Clin Orthop 178:42–53, 1983.
335. Whitesides, T.E., Jr., Haney, T.C., Harada, H., Holmes, H., and Morimoto, K. A simple method for tissue pressure determination. Arch Surg 110:1311–1313, 1975.
336. Whitesides, T.E., Jr., Harada, H., and Morimoto, K. Compartment syndromes and the role of fasciotomy, its parameters and technique. Instr Course Lect 26:179–198, 1977.
337. Whittaker, R.P., Heppenstall, R.B., Menkowitz, E., and Montique, F. Comparison of open vs. closed rodding of femurs utilizing a Sampson rod. J Trauma 22:461–468, 1982.
338. Wilhelm, K., Feidmeier, C.H., and Hower, G. Die behandlung von mavikulare, fracturen und navikulare, pseudarthrosen mit elektrichen und magnetischen potentialen, Munich Med WSCR 116:2191, 1974.
339. Willenegger, H., Meyer, S., and Weiland, A.J. The treatment of infected non-union of fractures of long bones: Study of sixty-four cases with a five to twenty-one-year follow-up. J Bone Joint Surg [Am] 57:836–841, 1975.
340. Winquist, R.A., and Hansen, S.T., Jr. Comminuted fractures of the femoral shaft treated by intramedullary nailing. Orthop Clin North Am 11:633–643, 1980.
341. Winquist, R.A., Hansen, S.T., Jr., and Clawson, D.K. Closed intramedullary nailing of femur fractures: A report of five hundred and twenty cases. J Bone Joint Surg [Am] 66:529–539, 1984.
342. Wolma, F.J., Larrieu, A.J., and Alsop, G.C. Arterial injuries of the legs associated with fractures and dislocations. Am J Surg 140:806–809, 1980.
343. Wood, M.B., Cooney, W.P., and Irons, G.B. Lower extremity salvage and reconstruction by free-tissue transfer: An analysis of results. Clin Orthop 201:151–161, 1985.
344. Woodruff, L.E. NY Med J 67:593, 1898.
345. Wray, J.B. Fractures and the pathogenesis of nonunion. J Bone Joint Surg [Am] 47:168–173, 1965.
346. Yasuda, I. Fundamental aspects of fracture treatment. Clin Orthop 124:5–8, 1977.
347. Yasuda, I.N., Jr. Dynamic callus and electrical callus. J Bone Joint Surg [Am] 37:1293–1294, 1955.
348. Zaslav, K.R., and Meinhard, D.M. Management of resistant pseudarthrosis of long bone after failure to achieve union with electromagnetic stimulation. Clin Orthop, 1988.
349. Zimmerman, K.W., and Klasen, H.J. Mechanical failure of intramedullary nails after fracture union. J Bone Joint Surg [Br] 65:274–275, 1983.

Section B: Fractures and Dislocations in Children

1. Blount, W.P. *Fractures in Children.* Baltimore, Williams & Wilkins, 1955.
2. Bowen, A. Plastic bowing of the clavicle in children. A report of two cases. J Bone Joint Surg 65A:403–405, 1983.
3. Bright, R.W. Physeal injuries, in Rockwood, C.A., Jr., Wilkins, K.E., and King, R.E. (eds): *Fractures in Children,* vol III. Philadelphia, Lippincott, 1984.
4. Charnley, J. *The Closed Treatment of Common Fractures,* 3d ed. Edinburgh, Churchill Livingstone, 1974.

5. Denton, J. Trauma to the growing skeleton. Orthop Rev 12:129–133, 1983.

6. Godfrey, J.D. Trauma in children. J Bone Joint Surg 46A:422–446, 1964.

7. Karrholm, J., Hansson, L.I., and Svennson, K. Prediction of growth pattern after ankle fractures in children. J Pediatr Orthop 3:319–325, 1983.

8. Kling, T.F., Bright, R.W., and Hensinger, R.N. Distal tibial physeal fractures in children that may require open reduction. J Bone Joint Surg 66A:647–657, 1984.

9. Langenskiold, A. Consideration of growth factors in the treatment of fractures of long bones in children, in Chapchal, G. (ed): *Fractures in Children.* New York, Thieme-Stratton, 1981, p 16.

10. Malkawi, H., Shannak, A., and Hadidi, S. Remodeling after femoral shaft fractures in children treated by modified Blount's method. J Paediatr Orthop 6:421–429, 1986.

11. Neer, C.S., II, and Horwitz, B.S. Fractures of the proximal humeral epiphyseal plate. Clin Orthop 41:24–31, 1965.

12. Ogden, J.A. Skeletal growth mechanism injury patterns. J Pediatr Orthop 2:371–377, 1982.

13. Ogden, J. *Skeletal Injury in the Child.* Philadelphia, Lea & Febiger, 1982.

14. Ogden, J. The uniqueness of growing bone, in Rockwood, C.A., Jr., Wilkins, K.E., and King, R.E. (eds): *Fractures in Children.* Philadelphia, Lippincott, 1984, pp 1–86.

15. Peterson, H.A. Partial growth arrest and its treatment. J Paediatr Orthop 4:264–268, 1984.

16. Peterson, H.A., and Burkhart, S.S. Compression injury of the epiphyseal growth plate: Fact or fiction. J Paediatr Orthop 1:377–384, 1981.

17. Rang, M. *Children's Fractures,* 2d ed. Philadelphia, Lippincott, 1983.

18. Reed, M.H. Fractures and dislocations of the extremities in children. J Trauma 17:351–354, 1977.

19. Reynolds, D.A. Growth changes in fractured long-bones: A study of 126 children. J Bone Joint Surg 63B:83–88, 1981.

20. Ryoppy, S. Characteristics of the growing skeleton from the traumatological point of view, in Chapchal, E. (ed): *Fractures in Children.* New York, Thieme-Stratton, 1981, pp 6–7.

21. Salter, R. *Textbook of Disorders and Injuries of the Musculoskeletal System.* Baltimore, Williams & Wilkins, 1983.

22. Salter, R.B., and Harris, R.W. Injuries involving the epiphyseal plate. J Bone Joint Surg 45A:587–622, 1963.

23. Seharli, A.F. General observations, in Chapchal, G. (ed): *Fractures in Children.* New York, Thieme-Stratton, 1981, pp 1–2.

24. Sharrard, W.J.W. *Paediatric Orthopaedics and Fractures,* vol II. London, Blackwell Scientific, 1979.

25. Smith, D.G., Geist, R.W., and Cooperman, D.R. Microscopic examination of a naturally occurring epiphyseal plate fracture. J Paediatr Orthop 5:306–308, 1985.

26. Staheli, L.T. Femoral and tibial growth following femoral shaft fracture in childhood. Clin Orthop 55:159–163, 1967.

27. Tachdjian, M.O. *Paediatric Orthopaedics.* Philadelphia, Saunders, 1972.

28. Weber, B.G. Fracture healing in the growing bone and in the mature skeleton, in Weber, B.G., Brunner, C.H., and Freuler, F. (eds): *Treatment of Fractures in Children and Adolescents.* New York, Springer-Verlag, 1980.

29. Yao, J., and Huurman, W.W. Tomography in juvenile Tillaux fractures. J Paediatr Orthop 6:349–351, 1986.

PART III

General Considerations in Orthopaedics

CHAPTER 19

Rheumatologic Disorders

Raymond J. Dattwyler, Marc G. Golightly, Peter Gorevic, Avron Ross,
Esther Lipstein-Kresch, Robert Greenwald, A. P. Kaplan,
Lee Kaufman, and Roger Dee

SECTION A

Laboratory Tests

Raymond J. Dattwyler and
Marc G. Golightly

The clinical immunology laboratory is playing an increasingly important role in the diagnosis of many diseases. This is especially true of the rheumatologic diseases. Some of the most important tests available are those which detect autoantibodies, and an understanding of these tests can be a great aid in the diagnosis and treatment of many types of arthritis.

FLUORESCENT ANTINUCLEAR ANTIBODY TEST

The assay most often thought of when one thinks of autoantibodies is the fluorescent antinuclear antibody test, the so-called ANA, or FANA. Historically, this test dates back to the work of Hargraves, who in 1948 described the lupus erythematosus (LE) cell phenomenon associated with systemic lupus erythematosus.[3] Friou developed the fluorescent antinuclear antibody (ANA) test in 1957, and today[2] the ANA has made the LE cell prep almost totally obsolete since the ANA is easier, cheaper, and faster.

The ANA is an indirect immunofluorescent test in which patient serum is incubated with a tissue substrate, allowing any antinuclear antibodies in the patient's serum to bind to antigens in the nuclei of the cells in the substrate. The antinuclear antibodies are then detected with fluorescein-labeled antibodies directed against human antibodies.

A positive ANA is usually associated with systemic lupus erythematosus (SLE) in most physicians' minds. Although almost all patients with SLE have a positive ANA, there are other diseases in which the patient's serum can contain antinuclear antibodies. Among the connective tissue diseases,

progressive systemic sclerosis (PSS), rheumatoid arthritis (RA), mixed connective tissue disease (MCTD), juvenile rheumatoid arthritis (JRA), and some of the vasculitides, in addition to SLE, can and frequently do have high-titer positive ANAs.[1] An understanding of the various patterns and the association of a specific disease with these patterns can be a great aid in diagnosis.

There are four basic patterns of ANA positivity: homogeneous, peripheral (rim), speckled, and nucleolar. Each of the patterns is caused by an autoantibody directed against a different nuclear antigen. Antibodies to deoxyribonucleoprotein (DNP), the DNA-histone complex of the nucleus, give a uniform or homogeneous pattern. These same antibodies produce the LE cell phenomenon and are associated with SLE, but they can also be found in RA in lower titers. As expected, DNP is sensitive to the enzymes DNase and trypsin. It is not extractable in saline. Antibodies to double-stranded DNA classically produce a peripheral pattern, and their presence is highly suggestive of SLE. The antibodies that produce a speckled pattern are more varied. They are directed against a group of antigens known as extractable nuclear antigens (ENA) because of their ability to dissolve in saline and other aqueous buffers. The speckled pattern is classic for MCTD. However, it is also the most common pattern seen in patients with SLE, and can be seen in patients with RA, PSS, and JRA.[1] When a speckled pattern is found, it requires further investigation since definition of the antibody specificity can be highly diagnostic. This definition can be carried out using immunodiffusion, counterimmunoelectrophoresis, or hemagglutination. Antibody against Smith antigen (anti-Sm), a nuclear glycoprotein resistant to RNase and DNase, is virtually diagnostic of SLE.[13] The other major extractable nuclear antigens are ribonucleoprotein (RNP), a RNA–protein complex sensitive to RNase digestion.[12] Antibodies against RNP are found in high titer in almost all patients with MCTD (to the exclusion of other autoantibodies); they are present in some SLE patients; and they appear only very rarely in other diseases. Antibodies causing a nucleolar pattern are directed against a low-molecular-weight RNA-protein complex (4-6S); such antibodies are highly associated with PSS and Raynaud's phenomenon as well as drug-induced SLE (e.g., hydralazine, procainamide).

It should be noted, especially in SLE but also in some of the other connective tissue diseases, that multiple autoanti-

TABLE 19-1 Clinical Indications in the Use of the Fluorescent Antinuclear Antibody Test (FANA)

Disease	Positive, percent	Patterns
Systemic lupus erythematosus	98	Speckled Homogeneous Peripheral
Mixed connective tissue disease	100	Speckled Homogeneous
Progressive systemic sclerosis	70	Speckled Homogeneous Nucleolar
Rheumatoid arthritis	45	Speckled Homogeneous
Juvenile rheumatoid arthritis	23	Speckled

bodies can and do occur. This gives rise to the finding of more than one pattern being observed for the ANA. It is therefore critical that all positive ANAs should be titered out to their end point and that the pattern and any changes in the pattern be reported. It is also important to know one's own clinical laboratory since the titer where one considers the ANA to be truly positive varies significantly from lab to lab. Generally, any ANA below 1 to 80 may be nondiagnostic.

Even in SLE, the ANA is not always positive. In the 1960s and 1970s investigators found that some patients who clinically had classic SLE were ANA-negative. This led to the finding that there are cytoplasmic antigens which can be the target for autoantibodies in patients with SLE and SLE-like diseases. Two antigens, RO and LA, have been well-defined. RO is a cytoplasmic antigen, and unlike LA it is sensitive to RNase and trypsin. It is now recognized that RO is the same antigen as SS-A and that LA is identical to SS-B or HA.[6] The finding of anti-RO or anti-LA can be very helpful in defining ANA-negative SLE or an SLE-like illness. The test can be carried out using either immunodiffusion or counterimmunoelectrophoresis. Also important in the prognosis is that patients with both anti-RO and anti-LA are less prone to nephritic involvement than those without it.

COMPLEMENT

The determination of total hemolytic complement activity (CH_{50}) and/or some of the components of the complement cascade (most commonly C3, C4, and properdin factor B) has permitted a greater understanding of immunologically mediated diseases. In fact, the measurement of complement has become a valuable screen for certain diseases and is of aid in the prognosis and successful treatment of others.

The CH_{50} test measures the overall functional adequacy of the entire classical complement system. The procedure involves the ability of the complement system in the serum of fluid tested to lyse sheep erythrocytes coated with subagglutinating amounts of antisheep antiserum. The results are expressed as the inverse dilution of the amount of sample required to produce 50 percent hemolysis (CH_{50} Units). It must be stated that each performing laboratory sets its own standards and normal ranges according to the technique employed. Therefore, interlaboratory comparison is difficult. The determination of the functional ability of individual complement components is possible, but to date it is generally done only as a research procedure. On the other hand, quantitation of certain individual components (C3, C4, and properdin factor B) is routinely performed in the clinical laboratory and can be quite useful.

The list of diseases in which complement levels are altered is very long (Table 19-2). CH_{50}, C3, and C4 levels indicate the status of the classical pathway, whereas C3 and properdin factor B levels can indicate the status of the alternate complement pathway. This is important in various infectious diseases where the alternate pathway is preferentially activated. In SLE, classical complement depletion correlates with the active phases of the disease, especially in patients with immune complex deposition disease in the kidneys.[8] In contrast, since complement behaves much like an acute-phase reactant, it is occasionally above normal in patients with the acute, or active, phase of joint disease due to RA, JRA, or rheumatic fever.[1] In the synovial fluid, however, complement levels in seropositive RA patients are usually reduced to less than one-third of the serum values[11] owing to local activation of complement. Rheumatoid factor seronegative fluids tend to have complement reductions to a lesser extent. Pleural effusions associated with RA and SLE serositis also have decreased complement levels. Although the majority of RA

TABLE 19-2   Diseases Associated with Altered Complement Levels

Increase	Decrease
Acute rheumatoid arthritis	Systemic immune complex diseases
Polyarteritis nodosa	Systemic lupus erythematosus with glomerulo-nephritis
Dermatomyositis	Rheumatoid arthritis vasculitis
Gout	Acute serum sickness
Diabetes	
Acute rheumatoid fever	Glomerulonephritis
Others	Mesangiocapillary
	Poststreptococcal
	Infectious diseases
	Infectious hepatitis with arthritis
	Gram-negative infections
	Subacute bacterial endocarditis
	Hereditary deficiencies
	Hereditary angioedema
	Various deficiencies of complement components
	Severe combined immunodeficiency

patients do exhibit normal serum complement levels, hypocomplementemia may occur during severe disease activity and may precede the onset of vasculitis.[10] Patients with hypocomplementemic RA are especially prone to pyogenic infections and are therefore treated aggressively in order to bring the disease under control and avoid this complication.

RHEUMATOID FACTORS

The diagnosis of rheumatoid arthritis is largely based on clinical findings; however, the demonstration in the serum of rheumatoid factors is one of the diagnostic criteria listed by the American Rheumatism Association. *Rheumatoid factors are immunoglobulins, usually IgM, that react with various antigens on the Fc portion of IgG.* The serum may contain other immunoglobulin classes such as IgA and IgG which also have anti-IgG activity, but detection of these immunoglobulins is not in general clinical use because of the difficulty in assaying them and also because their significance is questionable. The presence of rheumatoid factors is detected by agglutination procedures using latex coated with IgG or sheep erythrocytes coated with rabbit antisheep RBC antibodies. The latex tests are more sensitive tests (80 to 90 percent) for rheumatoid factor than the sheep cell agglutination test (70 percent). However, the sheep cell agglutination test is more specific for rheumatoid arthritis.

The presence of rheumatoid factors is by no means diagnostic since they may be present in many different diseases (Table 19-3). However, at high titer such factors are discriminating for RA and carry the implication of a less favorable response to therapy and a greater risk of rheumatoid vasculitis and lung disease complications.[8] The practice of follow-

ing the titer as an indication of remission or of therapeutic response is advanced by some. However, rheumatoid factors often remain at constant levels irrespective of the patient's clinical status.[5] The laboratory assessment of disease activity can be better followed by CRP levels and the erythrocyte sedimentation rate. It should also be noted that from 1 to 5 percent of a normal healthy population are rheumatoid-factor-positive, and this percentage increases with age to as high as 25 percent in those over the age of 70, although the titer is typically low (1:128 or less). The significance of this is not

TABLE 19-3   Disease Occurrence of Rheumatoid Factors

Rheumatic diseases
   Rheumatoid arthritis
   Sjögren syndrome (with or without arthritis)
   Progressive systemic sclerosis
   Polymyositis/dermatomyositis

Infectious diseases
   Subacute bacterial endocarditis
   Viral infections
   Tuberculosis/leprosy
   Syphilis
   Schistosomiasis

Noninfectious diseases
   Diffuse interstitial pulmonary fibrosis
   Pulmonary silicosis
   Waldenström macroglobulinemia
   Cirrhosis, chronic active hepatitis
   Sarcoidosis
   Normal individuals, especially elderly

known. However, twice the number of healthy false-positive individuals subsequently go on to develop RA clinically as compared to healthy seronegative individuals. In seronegative RA patients who exhibit disease activity for two or more years, it is of little benefit to carry out more than two rheumatoid factor determinations in one or two laboratories as the number of the patients that convert to seropositivity after that time is small. Of this group of seronegative RA patients, a portion of them do have rheumatoid factors binding to autologous IgG and subsequently unavailable to bind to the IgG in the test. These "hidden rheumatoid factors" can be assayed by dissociating the IgM-IgG complex, fractionating the material, and reassaying for rheumatoid factors. A seronegative finding in a clinical RA patient may also be attributed to the fact that occasionally rheumatoid factors are found in synovial fluid and not in the serum. Since synovial fluid is not commonly tested, a patient could be incorrectly labeled as being "seronegative."[7]

ERYTHROCYTE SEDIMENTATION RATE

The erythrocyte sedimentation rate (ESR) is one of the oldest tests in medicine, and although it is not diagnostic, it remains one of the most useful tests in that it reflects degrees of inflammation and tissue damage. In the past there was considerable debate as to which method to use for the ESR. However, there is now general agreement that the Westergren method should be the standard. In any case, it is mainly a test of acute-phase reactants, especially fibrinogen.

As performed in most labs, the ESR is simply a measurement of how far a 200-mm column of citrated venous blood in a cylindrical tube will fall in 1 h. Basically, the ESR measures erythrocyte aggregation. Erythrocyte aggregation is a function of three things: van der Waal's forces, which attract one cell to another; the force of similarly charged particles repelling one another (the zeta potential), pushing the cells apart; and the charge dispersion characteristics of the plasma, causing changes in the relative relationship of the first two to each other. The addition of any asymmetrical molecules to the plasma causes a decrease in the repulsive force of the zeta potential, allowing the erythrocytes to aggregate more easily and thus producing a higher ESR. Of the acute-phase reactants, fibrinogen has the greatest effect on the ESR because of its extreme degree of asymmetry. The other acute-phase reactants are less asymmetrical, and much larger concentrations are required to produce the same effect on the ESR as modest increases in fibrinogen concentration. An example of where this can occur is multiple myeloma and other lymphoproliferative diseases where large concentrations of immunoglobulin cause increased erythrocyte aggregation and an elevated ESR.

Clinically, if it is not a diagnostic test, then what is the ESR useful for? It is useful as a crude screening test, as long as one remembers that a normal ESR does not absolutely rule out an illness and that a high ESR does not guarantee one. For example, pregnancy and oral contraceptives can both also raise the ESR. The test is, however, most useful for following a patient with either an inflammatory disease or a lymphoproliferative disease. The test is reliable and easy enough to do in an office setting.

C-REACTIVE PROTEIN

C-reactive protein (CRP) is the classic acute-phase protein seen with infection, inflammation, and tissue damage. Since its discovery in 1930, the test for it has seen a somewhat limited use owing to the insensitive and semiquantitative assays for its determination. However, with the advent of modern immunological methods such as nephelometry and fluoroimmunoassays, CRP can now be sensitivity-quantitated, and it is seeing a renewed widespread use. CRP, like the ESR, is an entirely nonspecific response. However, precise CRP quantitation can provide useful insight for initial evaluations, diagnostic problems, and monitoring of response to therapy.

CRP's rate of synthesis by hepatocytes increases within hours of an acute injury, inflammation, or infection. The serum concentration may rise 3000-fold in response to any of these assaults. The magnitude of the increase correlates well with the severity of the tissue damage, and following resolution of the inciting cause, the CRP level rapidly returns to normal.

Most patients with rheumatoid arthritis (> 90 percent) have an elevated CRP. In mild to severe disease the reading may be at levels of about 5 mg/dl (about 0.8 mg/dl is normal). In following these patients, CRP correlates with disease activity more closely than ESR, rheumatoid factor, or immune complexes.[4] Furthermore, CRP fluctuations correlate with serum amyloid A (involved in reactive systemic or secondary amyloidosis) fluctuations, which is a consideration in longstanding RA patients.[10] There is a rough correlation of CRP levels with the degree of erosive disease.[5] CRP levels have also been used to determine the presence of intercurrent infection in those conditions which on their own do not elicit large increases in CRP (e.g., SLE and certain malignancies); it is less well documented in myocardial infarction and major surgery.[4] Furthermore, it has been suggested the CRP levels are of value in distinguishing pyelonephritis from cystitis, bacterial pneumonia from acute bronchitis, acute bronchitis from uncomplicated acute or chronic obstructive pulmonary disease, and bacterial meningitis from aseptic meningitis.[7]

SECTION B

Rheumatoid Arthritis

Peter Gorevic

Rheumatoid arthritis (RA) is, worldwide, the most common inflammatory articular disease afflicting humans, exceeded only by osteoarthritis as a cause of joint symptoms in the general populace. RA affects about 3 percent of women and 1 percent of men, with very little variation in prevalence when

TABLE 19-4   American Rheumatism Association (ARA) Diagnostic Criteria for Rheumatoid Arthritis*[1]

1. Morning stiffness ⎫ In at least one joint
2. Pain on motion or tenderness ⎭
3. Soft tissue swelling
4. Swelling in at least one other joint within 3 months
5. Symmetrical joint swelling with simultaneous involvement of the same joint on both sides
6. Subcutaneous nodules
7. Typical x-ray changes:
   - *Stage I (early):* Juxtaarticular osteoporosis
   - *Stage II (moderate):* Osteoporosis plus evidence of subchondral bone destruction
   - *Stage III (severe):* Osteoporosis *plus* marginal erosions; cartilage, bone destruction; joint space narrowing; joint deformity
   - *Stage IV (terminal):* Fibrous or bony ankylosis
8. Rheumatoid factor (RF)
9. Characteristic synovial fluid findings:
   - Poor mucin clot
   - Group II, III fluid, predominantly polymorphonuclear leukocytes
   - "RA cells"
   - Hypocomplementemia
   - Immune complexes (IgM RF, IgG RF, etc.)
10. Characteristic histological changes in synovial membrane:
    - Villous hypertrophy
    - Hyperplasia of superficial cells
    - Palisading subsynovial focal collections of small lymphocytes (predominantly T cells), mononuclear and plasma cells
    - Few polymorphonuclear leukocytes
    - Fibrin deposition on the synovial surface or interstitially
    - Multinucleated giant cells
11. Characteristic histological changes in nodules:[2]
    - Necrotic central zone with evidence of vascular proliferation
    - May show positive immunofluorescence for IgG, RF, or complement
    - Palisade zone of elongated histiocytes and giant cells
    - Surrounding zone of granulation tissue

Categories	Number of criteria required	Minimum duration of continuous symptoms
Classic	7 of 11	6 weeks (symptoms 1–5)
Definite	5 of 11	6 weeks (symptoms 1–5)
Probable	3 of 11	6 weeks (1 of symptoms 1–5)

*Revised criteria proposed in 1958 updated to include newer information regarding synovial fluid and immunohistological studies.
Source:
[1] Ropes, M.W., et al, Bull Rheum Dis 9:175–176, 1958.
[2] Sokoloff, L., et al, Arth Rheum 5:323, 1962.

different populations are sampled.[76] The term actually encompasses a heterogeneous group of disorders that may in turn reflect common pathogenic mechanisms occurring in the settings of different etiologies and genetic backgrounds. An infectious etiology has been suspected for many years[6] and is the basis for the older designation of "chronic infectious arthritis," but actual person-to-person transmission has never been documented. The *exact* incidence of this disease is unknown, largely because criteria for its definition remain inexact. Criteria adopted by the American Rheumatism Association (ARA)[100] have been widely used for clinical retrospective studies (Table 19-4). They have been utilized primarily to

distinguish RA from other rheumatic diseases and from the so-called "rheumatoid variants" (see Sect. F, this chapter, on the spondyloarthropathies). Relevance of the ARA criteria to clinical practice is limited because (1) some criteria (e.g., specific histological findings in synovium) are not available for most patients, (2) a large group of patients with inflammatory joint disease who do not have (and may not develop) the distinctive features of RA (i.e., nodules, x-ray changes, seropositivity, etc.) are ignored, (3) the disease can be intermittent and may even remit, and (4) with the exception of subcutaneous nodules (criterion 6 in Table 19-4) extraarticular manifestations are not included.

ETIOLOGY OF RA

Considerable evidence has implicated an immune pathogenesis for rheumatoid arthritis, although the agent inciting the development of synovitis remains obscure. A viral etiology has been suggested by analogy to known examples of synovitis resulting from viral infection in humans (e.g., hepatitis B virus, Ross River virus, rubella) and on the basis of animal models of chronic arthritis due to viral infection.[31] A recent report of the transmission of chronic arthritis in mice via a parvovirus cultured from rheumatoid synovium[111] has renewed interest in this possibility. Other studies have shown that RA patients mount an unusual host reponse to, and may in fact have an increased body burden of, Epstein-Barr virus (EBV).[25] This immunologic defect may be a secondary phenomenon, however, and insignificant in the pathogenesis of joint disease. Furthermore, 15 percent of rheumatoids with "classic" disease show no evidence of EBV infection.

Animal models that have been widely used to investigate mechanisms of joint injury, include adjuvant,[65] streptococcal cell wall, and collagen-induced arthritides.[120] A persistent or recurrent polyarthritis is induced (usually in rats) in susceptible strains by immunization with Freund's adjuvant (Wax D); streptococcal cell walls (peptidoglycan-carbohydrate complex); or soluble, native type II collagen. The resultant synovitis resembles RA in the presence of marginal erosions, pannus, and mononuclear cell infiltrates, but differs in that no rheumatoid factor activity is detectable in serum and in the frequent progression of joint lesions to bony ankylosis. More than eight distinct types of collagen are now recognized.[40] Types I to V are found in articular tissue.

Only immunization with type II collagen will elicit chronic arthritis in experimental animals (rats, mice). Although antibodies to all types of articular collagen have been demonstrated in the sera of a significant percent of RA patients,[86] and specific cellular stimulation of peripheral blood lymphocytes has been found, these findings have also been seen in patients with other rheumatic diseases and thus may also be secondary phenomena.[120]

Rheumatoid Factors

Rheumatoid factors (RFs) are antiglobulins with antibody activity directed primarily against antigenic determinants on the Fc portion of the IgG molecule. IgM RFs are found in the sera of about three-quarters of patients with "definite" or "classic" RA, circulating in blood as high-molecular-weight (22 S) complexes with IgG[37] (Fig. 19-1). Many of these antibodies have enhanced reactivity if the IgG is aggregated or complexed to antigens (i.e., immune complexes). The former reaction is the basis for the standard latex fixation test,[112] which measures the ability of various dilutions of a test serum to agglutinate latex beads coated with IgG. The incidence of RF positivity increases with the duration of active synovitis, and may be present in as few as a third of RA patients within 3 months of the onset of their disease.[63] Up to a quarter of patients with "classic" RA remain consistently seronegative even though many have disease as severe as the seropositive patients. Among the seropositive patients, high titers of IgM

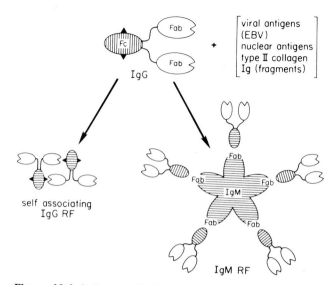

Figure 19-1 Antigen-antibody systems in rheumatoid arthritis.

RF correlate in a general way with long-standing disease, sustained activity, nodules, erosions, and extraarticular manifestations.[83,87] These correlations are inexact, however, and vary from patient to patient. IgM RF may also be found in the sera of patients with a variety of chronic inflammatory and infectious diseases, many of which have in common hyperimmunization and hyperglobulinemia (see Table 19-5). Among noninfectious clinical associations, it should particularly be noted that IgM RF may be a serological marker present in various chronic liver diseases, that it may be seen incidentally in the blood of elderly persons, and that it is an antibody activity found among 5 to 10 percent of IgM paraproteins occurring largely in patients with lymphoproliferative disorders.

RFs are heterogeneous both with respect to antigenic specificity and in that antiglobulin activity may be seen in all five classes of immunoglobulin.[15] Reactivity with a variety of determinants on IgG (including both heavy and light chain, as well as determinants only revealed following limited proteolytic digestion)[90] have been found when IgM RFs have been broken down as to specificity. A subset of these antibodies appears to cross-react with specific nuclear proteins[67] and thus might properly be considered a type of antinuclear antibody. Standard serologies do not, however, detect IgG or IgA RF activity. IgG RF preferentially self-associates (Fig. 19-1),[95] it can activate complement, and it correlates in titer with depressed levels of complement in joint fluid.[133] Self-associating IgG RF appears to be also responsible for so-called "intermediate" complexes (7 S to 22 S) that have been found in the sera of some RA patients who may also have pulmonary disease, systemic vasculitis, or hyperviscosity syndrome.[95]

RF is synthesized locally in the germinal centers of subsynovial tissue, and is demonstrable in plasma cells by immunofluorescence studies of rheumatoid synovium[90] as well as in the supernatants of synovial explants[113] or cultured lymphocytes. Immunoglobulin production by rheumatoid synovium may equal that of spleen or lymph node. In spite of 25 years of sustained research, however, the biological significance of this major antibody activity remains obscure. De-

TABLE 19-5   Clinical Incidence of IgM Rheumatoid Factor

Disease	Percent
Rheumatic diseases	
Juvenile chronic polyarthritis	20
Lupus erythematosus	30
Scleroderma	15
Polymyositis	10
Mixed cryoglobulinemia	100
Infectious diseases	
Subacute bacterial endocarditis	40
Tuberculosis	10
Syphilis	10
Leprosy	10
Rubella	(a)
Epstein-Barr virus or cytomegalovirus mononucleosis	(a)
Noninfectious diseases	
Cirrhosis; chronic hepatitis	10
Sarcoidosis	10
Macroglobulinemia	5–10
Aging	(b)

(a) Isolated case reports.
(b) Increasing incidence with age in otherwise healthy individuals over 60 years old.

spite correlations with severe extraarticular RA noted above, high-titer IgM RF may be present without significant synovitis. Infusion of RF-enriched plasma to volunteers does not produce joint disease, and some evidence has accrued for a protective function in viral infection.[91] Consequently, RF activity should be viewed as a marker rather than a specific pathogenic mechanism.

Amplification Systems in Synovial Fluid

The presence of large amounts of immune complexes, including RFs and collagen-anticollagen antibodies, in rheumatoid joint fluid has been demonstrated by various specific assays (Fig. 19-2).[16,51] The phlogistic potential of these complexes is

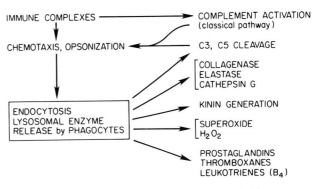

Figure 19-2 Amplification systems in synovial fluid.

mirrored in depressed levels of complement proteins,[93] representing both classical and alternative pathway activation, and the generation of complement split products. In contradistinction to the synovial membrane, in which polymorphonuclear leukocytes (PMNs) are relatively sparse, RA synovial fluid contains PMNs predominantly, often with inclusions (so-called RA cells or ragocytes) which can be shown by immunofluorescence studies or by direct extraction to contain IgM, IgG, and complement.[128] Ingestion of immune complexes by PMNs leads in turn to the release of elastase, cathepsins, myeloperoxidases, glycosidases, and collagenase.[130] Inhibitors of these enzymes normally present in joint fluids are saturated at white blood cell counts greater than 50,000 cells per millimeter.[50] Also released are prostaglandins, leukotrienes, free oxygen radicals, and platelet activating factor, leading in turn to further activation of complement, clotting, kinin, and fibrinolytic cascades.[130] The generation of potent chemotactic factors (C3a, C4a, leukotriene B4) explains in part the huge influx of PMNs into the joint space.

Proliferative Phase in Synovium

Pathological studies of the early synovial lesions in biopsy material,[104] as well as careful histological studies of established synovitis[74] and the rheumatoid nodule,[115] have shown vascular injury and proliferation to be a dominant feature early on (Fig. 19-3). This suggests an initiating event originat-

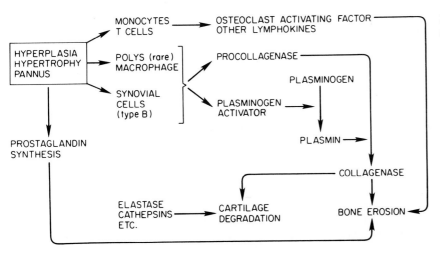

Figure 19-3 Proliferative phase in synovium.

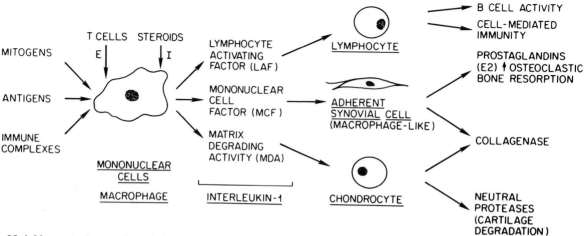

Figure 19-4 Monocyte-(macrophage-) dependent activation of synovial cells.

ing in the vascular space. The early pathological lesion in synovium is nonspecific, but manifests increasing cellular heterogeneity as the disease progresses. PMNs become more and more sparse with the establishment of synovial hyperplasia, vascular proliferation, and germinal centers. In the latter, lymphocytes and plasma cells mount a local immune response, producing IgM and IgG RF.[113] Monocytes release elastase, various monokines, and prostaglandins (mostly PGE_2) as a response to the ingestion of immune complexes. Mononuclear cells also release factors that activate chondrocytes and osteocytes and cause release of collagenase and PGE_2 by synovial cells (Fig. 19-4).[66,73] Several of these monokines have been shown to have molecular properties of interleukin 1 (I1-1), a generic term used to describe a single molecule or a group of molecules produced by activated macrophage. I1-1 has been shown to have diverse biological effects related to the acute-phase response, mediated in turn by different cell types including fibroblasts, osteoclasts, and chondrocytes.[27] I1-1-like activity has been demonstrated in rheumatoid effusions.

Proteoglycan is depleted early and collagen breaks down in a narrow zone between cartilage and the pannus.[5] The term *pannus* has been variously applied to the proliferative synovitis, ingrowth of granulation tissue, or resultant fibrosis. Pannus exhibits cellular heterogeneity, consisting of synovial, plasma and endothelial cells, lymphocytes, macrophage (accessory cells), fibroblasts, and dendritic cells.[54] Dendritic cells have been identified as an adherent cell in synovial cultures and as a distinct cell population in synovial membrane and synovial effusions. These cells produce large amounts of collagenase and PGE_2 in vitro, and are presumed to be responsible for the quantities of these substances that can be demonstrated in rheumatoid synovium, both immunohistologically and by direct extraction.[23,135]

Genetic Factors

The incidence of clinical disease among first-degree relatives of RA patients is disputed, but has been reported in some large series to be about twice that expected by chance. The prevalence of seropositivity in unaffected family members may be even greater than that of clinical disease. Concordance of RA among monozygotic twins is about 30 percent, compared to 9 percent among dizygotic twins, one of whom is affected by the disease. This suggests weak genetic influences on the expression of RA.[77] By comparison, the concordance of lupus among monozygotic twins with one affected twin is about 60 percent.

Several series have shown a relative risk (RR) of approximately 2 to 4 times that expected among seropositive RA patients who have the DW4 (DR4) histocompatibility (HLA) locus.[116] This is a relatively weak association, however, by comparison to the RR of ankylosing spondylitis in persons carrying the B27 locus, which is about 90. Although the precise reason for this weak, but significant, genetic association in RA is still obscure, several immunologic mechanisms suggest themselves from the known functions of histocompatibility antigens in experimental animals.[105] One possible locus could be genetic factors controlling the nature, degree, and duration of the humoral or cellular immune response, or Ir, genes) to defined antigens (e.g., autologous immunoglobulin). It may thus be significant that only some strains of rats or mice develop arthritis in response to adjuvant, bacterial cell wall products or type II collagen, this susceptibility being linked in part to specific histocompatibility loci. The MRL/1 mouse strain of murine lupus is of interest in this regard because these animals develop chronic arthritis, rheumatoidlike nodules, and IgG and IgM RFs,[52] i.e., proliferative synovitis associated with a RF response.

In humans, the DW4 (DR4) locus does not appear to be significantly linked to IgM RF production in the absence of arthritis.[33] The possibility remains, however, that the RF response in RA patients may be restricted, and some evidence has been advanced for shared RF idiotypes inherited in families in which more than one individual has developed RA.[92] Lastly, it should be noted that these genetic associations do not hold for seronegative RA patients, providing further evidence for the heterogeneous nature of the disease and the existence of different subsets of patients.[3]

Alternative possibilities for the association of RA and

DW4 include linkage to a third gene within, or close to, the HLA locus and a more general immunologic defect consequent to the important function of D locus products as cell surface glycoproteins. The latter are expressed on T cells, macrophage, and other (including endothelial, synovial lining, and adherent) cell types that regulate antigen presentation and cell-cell (macrophage-T or B-T) interactions.[105] The relevance of this potential mechanism to abnormalities of suppressor cell function (e.g., to EBV-driven B cell transformation, mixed lymphocyte culture, and lymphokine production) that have been identified in RA patients is unclear.

CLINICAL FEATURES

Most patients present to the physician with the insidious onset of disease. Typical symptoms include morning stiffness, "gelling" of joints following prolonged periods of inactivity, easy fatigability, weight loss, malaise, and polyarthritis.[30,110] The joint involvement may initially be asymmetric, but usually becomes more symmetrical with time.[63] The most common sites of presentation are the hands (metacarpophalangeal, carpal, proximal, interphalangeal joints) and the feet (metatarsophalangeal joints). The knees, elbows, shoulders, ankles, and neck are also often affected. By contrast, hip involvement is uncommon and distal interphalangeal joints are almost never inflamed.

About 10 percent of patients experience an abrupt onset of disease, with striking constitutional signs. A variant of this presentation is so-called adult Still's disease, in which patients may present with fever, rash, adenopathy, splenomegaly, and visceral involvement. These symptoms sometimes precede and overshadow articular complaints.[75] Patients with insidious onset and systemic disease may be evaluated for presumed malignancy before the true nature of their complaints becomes apparent. Other unusual presentations of RA include monoarticular or oligoarticular disease and palindromic rheumatism.

The activity of disease at diagnosis is evaluated by assessing objective and subjective evidence of inflammatory synovitis. This includes duration of morning stiffness, time of onset of fatigability, fever, weight loss, and the amount of medication required for control of symptoms. The history should yield some assessment of functional capacity often graded as I, no handicap; II, discomfort or limited mobility but still able to maintain normal activities; III, performs a few normal activities; IV, largely or wholly incapacitated.[117] Synovitis may be reflected in warmth, stiffness, swelling, pain, and limitation of motion. The rheumatoid joint is never red unless there is coincidental gout or a secondary septic arthritis. Considerable variation of pain threshold is seen between patients. Consequently, this specific complaint should be separated out by the clinician from objective signs of disease, individualized, and monitored longitudinally rather than assessed entirely by comparison to other patients. Objective evidence of inflammatory synovitis includes soft tissue swelling due to synovial hypertrophy and/or effusion, functional or anatomical deformity, and limitation of motion. An articular index may be constructed by grading individual joints and

assessing symmetry. A number of such indices have been employed, largely for clinical trials, and adapted for practice by rheumatologists.[10]

Additional measurements include grip strength (maximum rise in millimeters of mercury of a standard sphygmomanometer cuff starting at 20 mmHg) ring size (may be measured with a jeweler's loop) and 50-ft walking time. A careful search for nodules, particularly on the extensor surface of the forearm, may suggest the diagnosis before confirmatory tests return.

The initial laboratory evaluation should include a complete blood count, urinalysis, SMA-23, and erythrocyte sedimentation rate (ESR). Patients with severe disease may be anemic and have a mild leukocytosis, eosinophilia, and thrombocytosis, all of which may correct with appropriate therapy.[7] Elevation of the ESR, as well as the presence in blood of significantly elevated levels of other acute-phase reactants such as C-reactive protein, may help to distinguish RA from metabolic joint disease or osteoarthritis. Objective evidence of inflammatory joint disease merits blood testing for RF activity and, especially in women of child-bearing age, antinuclear antibodies.

The diagnosis may be further suggested by radiographs of affected joints, looking for juxtaarticular osteoporosis, joint space narrowing, subchondral cysts or marginal erosions. Radiographs are rarely diagnostic by themselves but may provide additional objective evidence of disease. Good prognostic features include male sex, under 40 years of age, duration of disease less than 1 year, and acute onset. Poor prognostic features include the presence of bone erosions, high-titer RF, continuous disease activity, nodules, and extraarticular disease.[81] Overall, as many as 20 percent of affected individuals may experience complete remission, some 25 percent may undergo remission with mild residual effects, 45 percent will have persistent disease, about 20 percent may be unable to work, and 10 percent will become severely disabled.[110]

Extraarticular Manifestations

In spite of early speculation to the contrary (see first section of chapter), RA may be a strikingly para- and extraarticular disease.[61] The involvement of both tendon sheaths and bursae contributes to soft tissue swelling, the development of localized soft tissue masses, functional abnormalities (e.g., swan neck and boutonniere deformities) and tenosynovitis. The latter may be the presenting symptomatology in some patients, mimicking the enthesopathy characteristic of the spondyloarthropathies and causing diagnostic confusion between the two. Synovial cysts are distended bursae which, in certain locations, may herniate or rupture. Specifically, popliteal (Baker's) cysts may dissect into the gastrocnemius muscle, producing calf pain and giving a clinical picture resembling thrombophlebitis.[69]

Striking extraarticular disease may develop in some patients, involving any of a variety of organ systems (Table 19-6). With the advent of more effective therapy for the articular manifestations of disease, extraarticular involvement has become an increasingly important cause of morbidity and

TABLE 19-6 Extraarticular Manifestations of RA

1. Nodules (20–25% of patients)

2. Eye[1]
   - Keratoconjunctivitis sicca (10% of patients)
   - Episcleritis (nodular, diffuse)
   - Scleritis (anterior, posterior)
   - Scleromalacia perforans

3. Pulmonary[2]
   - Pleuritis; pleural effusions (most common)
     1000 to 3000 cells per cubic millimeter (mostly mononuclear cells)
     Glucose less than 40 mg/dl
     Decreased complement level in pleural fluid
     Pleural RF titer greater than in serum, due to local synthesis
     "RA" cells in pleural space
   - Pulmonary nodules (granuloma)
     Isolated subpleural nodules
     Caplan's syndrome (rheumatoid pneumoconiosis)
   - Interstitial pneumonitis and fibrosis
   - Airway obstruction (upper, lower)
   - Pulmonary vasculitis

4. Cardiac[3]
   - Pericarditis (common and present in 1–2% of patients)
     Effusion (clinical cardiac manifestation present in 2% of patients)
       Decreased complement level in pericardial fluid
       950–28,000 cells per cubic millimeter in pericardial fluid
       Glucose less than 40 mg/dl
     Also present in pericardial fluids are:
       Immune complexes
       Lymphokines (MIF) macrophage inhibitory factor
       Cholesterol crystals
     Hemopericardium may occur but tamponade is rare
     Constrictive pericarditis can also occur
   - Myocardium
     Conduction system (granulomas), heart block
     Myocarditis (rare)
   - Valve leaflets involved
   - Coronary arteritis

5. Skin
   - Vasculitis (bland, necrotizing, acute, subacute)
   - Purpura (vasculitis, cryoglobulinemia, amyloidosis)
   - Leg ulcers (arteritic, gravitational, breakdown of nodules, agranulocytic, pyoderma gangrenosum)
   - Rash (adult Still's disease)
   - Vasomotor (livedo, Raynaud's phenomenon), usually mild

6. Neuromuscular
   - Cervical subluxations (especially C1–2)
   - Peripheral entrapment neuropathies
     Carpal tunnel (may be presenting symptom)
     Other (ulnar, radial, sciatic, etc.)
   - Peripheral neuropathy[4]
     Distal sensory
     Sensorimotor
     Autonomic
     Mononeuritis multiplex
   - Cerebral (rare)
     Vasculitis
     Dural nodules
   - Myositis/myopathy[5]

TABLE 19-6 (*continued*)

7. Osteoporosis (may occur unrelated to steroid administration)

8. Secondary amyloidosis

9. Vasculitis[6]

10. Hematologic[7]
    - Anemia (common)
    - Thrombocytosis
    - Eosinophilia (correlates with severe extraarticular disease)
    - Hyperviscosity syndrome (intermediate-size complexes; IgG RF)

11. Felty syndrome[8]
    - Rheumatoid arthritis; seropositive (high-titer)
    - Disease is extraarticular with nodules, neuropathy, infections, and vasculitis
    - Hypersplenism, splenomegaly, and erythrocyte sequestration may occur
    - Neutropenia
        Occasional myeloid metaplasia and mild thrombocytopenia
        Leg ulcers (25% of patients)
    - Circulating immune complexes
        22 S (IgM RF); 11–15 S
        Cryoprecipitates, complement
    - Antinuclear antibodies (some specific for polymorphonuclear leukocytes)

12. Sjögren syndrome[9]
    - Keratoconjunctivitis sicca consisting of xerophthalmia and xerostomia occurs and is diagnostic
    - The *primary* syndrome: No underlying disease
    - The *secondary* syndrome: This is associated with RA (30–55% of patients) and lupus (5% of patients)
    - Those patients with RA may show generalized autoimmune exocrinopathy (bronchitis, pancreatitis, etc.)
    - Plus lymphocyte (B cell) infiltrates in various organs, pseudolymphoma or lymphoma
    - Other manifestations include interstitial nephritis and renal tubular acidosis, also circulating immune complexes, vasculitis, chronic liver disease or biliary cirrhosis and antinuclear antibodies

Source:
[1] Hazleman, B. L., and Watson, P. G., Clin Rheum Dis 3:501–526, 1977.
[2] Turner-Warwick, M., and Evans, R. C., Clin Rheum Dis 3:549–564, 1977.
[3] Khan, A. H., and Spodick, D. H., Sem Arth Rheum 1:327–337, 1972.
[4] Cromartie, W. J., et al, J Exp Med 146:1585–1602, 1977; Jasin, H. E., et al, Fed Proc 32:147–155, 1973.
[5] Schmid, F. R., et al, Amer J Med 30:56–82, 1961.
[6] Scott, D. G., et al, Medicine (Balt) 60:288–297, 1986.
[7] Bennett, R. M., Clin Rheum Dis 3:433–465, 1977; Mowat, A. G., Sem Arth Rheum 1:195–219, 1971.
[8] Goldberg, J., and Pinals, R.S., Sem Arth Rheum 10:52–65, 1980.
[9] Mason, A. M. S., et al, Sem Arth Rheum 2:301–331, 1973; Montsopoulos, H. M., Am Int Med 92:212–226, 1980; Shearn, M. A., in Smith, L. H. (ed): *Major Problems in Internal Medicine,* Philadelphia, Saunders, 1971; Strand, V., and Talal, N., Bull Rheum Dis, 30:1046–1052, 1979–1980.

mortality. Extraarticular RA is statistically associated with long-standing erosive disease, nodules, and high-titer IgM RF,[44] though exceptions to each association are being increasingly recognized. In many patients (notably including those that develop neuropathy), the basic pathological process appears to be a systemic vasculitis,[107] with positive indirect immunofluorescence for IgM, IgG, and complement in vessel walls.[19] These patients frequently are found to have large amounts of circulating immune complexes and may be hypocomplementemic.[86] A specific association between hypocomplementemia, necrotizing vasculitis, and recurrent infection has been noted in about 5 percent of hospitalized patients with RA.[87]

Clinical Vasculitis

The exact incidence of vasculitis is unknown. Older series reported it in 20 to 25 percent of severe rheumatoid cases coming to autopsy.[76] More recent studies have placed the incidence of clinical vasculitis at about 8 percent among outpatients attending rheumatology clinics[87] and at 15 to 20 percent when hospitalized patients with RA are retrospectively reviewed.[44] At least two distinct types of vasculitis have been described pathologically: a bland obliterative endarteritis, primarily involving digital vessels, and an inflammatory vasculitis that is often focal and segmental, ranging from leukocytoclastic to frankly necrotizing arteritis.[114] The former manifests primarily as nailbed or periungual hemorrhages or erythema; it is usually self-limited, and does not require treatment.[26] The latter may be associated with major-vessel involvement, causing, in turn, infarction and gangrene which may be rapidly fatal.[13,103] Necrotizing vasculitis is significantly associated with neuropathy (75 percent) pericardial or pulmonary involvement, positive ANAs, 7 S IgM RF, IgG RF, eosinophilia, low complement levels systemically, and cryoglobulinemia.[107]

Felty Syndrome

Felty syndrome refers to subsets of RA patients that develop leukopenia with evidence of hypersplenism and splenomegaly.[42] Usually, though not invariably, these patients have severe long-standing RA with other evidence for extraarticular and immune-complex disease (Table 19-6). Distinctive features of the syndrome are a tendency to develop recurrent infections (75 percent), leg ulcers (25 percent), and evidence of hepatic dysfunction (25 to 50 percent). The leukopenia and splenomegaly appear to be qualitatively distinct from that found among RA patients without other clinical features of the syndrome.[12] Multiple mechanisms account for this leukopenia, including splenic sequestration, leukocyte-specific antibodies, circulating immune complexes, T suppressors and cytotoxic T cells that may suppress granulopoiesis and kill polymorphonuclear leukocytes (PMNs), and serum factors that may decrease production of PMNs by the bone marrow. Evidence for each mechanism has been developed by different investigators, varying in significance in clinical series. This suggests in turn that there may be considerable heterogeneity among this group of patients. Leukopenia may be accompanied by lymphopenia (33 percent), anemia, and thrombocytopenia (40 percent).

Sjögren Syndrome

Sjögren syndrome refers to the keratoconjunctivitis sicca complex (xerophthalmia, xerostomia), which may exist in primary or secondary forms, the latter most commonly associated with RA.[84,109,110] RA occurring in this setting is distinctive immunologically[36,88] in that there is often striking B-cell hyperactivity. This may be reflected in (1) polyclonal hyperglobulinemia, (2) multiple autoantibodies in blood [including IgM RF (75 to 90 percent) antinuclear (50 to 80 percent) and organ-specific (e.g., salivary duct) antibodies], (3) frequent clinical manifestations of immune-complex disease (e.g., vasculitis, mononeuritis multiplex), and (4) evidence of extraglandular lymphoproliferation (Table 19-6).[4] Lymphocytes may infiltrate various organs to produce (1) exocrinopathy (salivary, lacrimal glands, bronchial mucosa, GI tract),[119] (2) distinctive renal involvement (interstitial nephritis, renal tubular acidosis, diabetes insipidus),[123] and (3) hepatic disease (chronic active hepatitis, primary biliary cirrhosis). Some patients develop pseudolymphoma and a minority of patients frank lymphoma.

TREATMENT: GENERAL PRINCIPLES

Three major goals of therapy for the patient with active synovitis are reduction of inflammation and pain, maintenance of joint function, and the prevention of deformities.[59] Achieving the first requires an appreciation of the importance of providing analgesia as well as anti-inflammatory medication[14] for therapy. It is also important to recognize the need of many patients to adjust their lifestyle and to use bed rest judiciously. Achieving the last two goals requires an interdisciplinary approach that combines use of the medications described below with surgical intervention as indicated and adequate physical and other rehabilitative therapy.[59] Surgery and rehabilitation of RA are discussed elsewhere in this volume. An overview of modalities of drug therapy currently available and under study follows.

Salicylates and Other Nonsteroidal Anti-inflammatory Drugs (NSAIDs)

The efficacy of aspirin and other NSAIDs has traditionally been measured in terms of inhibition of prostaglandin synthetase activity (Fig. 19-5). Aspirin irreversibly inhibits this enzyme by acetylating it, other NSAIDs inhibit it reversibly.[127,99] The basis for this assumption as to the mechanism of action of these drugs is the observation that some prostaglandins (e.g., PGE_2) are proinflammatory, that they can potentiate the effect of mediators such as histamine and bradykinin, that they are present in increased amounts in rheumatoid synovium, and that there is a general correlation between the clinical effectiveness of NSAIDs and their relative potency as inhibitors of prostaglandin synthetase.[57] Two major caveats, however, must be recognized. These are the facts that some cyclooxygenase metabolites are in fact anti-inflammatory and that some potent experimental inhibitors of prostaglandin synthetase have little effect on inflammation. Indeed, the anti-inflammatory effect of nonacetylated salicylates (e.g., Disalcid, Dolobid) cannot be entirely explained on the basis of inhibition of synthetase activity.[34] Consequently, other effects of NSAIDs, including direct effects on leukocyte function[2] or on the immune system,[43] have been suggested to be equally or more important. Also, products of the lipoxygenase pathway, notably leukotriene B4, have multiple biological effects that may potentiate inflammation (chemotactic activity, hypalgesia),[102] and the generation of these mediators is not inhibited by classic NSAIDs. Considerable effort is thus being directed toward the development of safe lipoxygenase inhibitors that may have utility for the control of synovitis.

The great majority (50 to 70 percent) of RA patients can be managed by judicious use of aspirin, the nonacetylated salicylates, or other NSAIDs. The decision as to which to start first, however, remains controversial. Advantages of aspirin

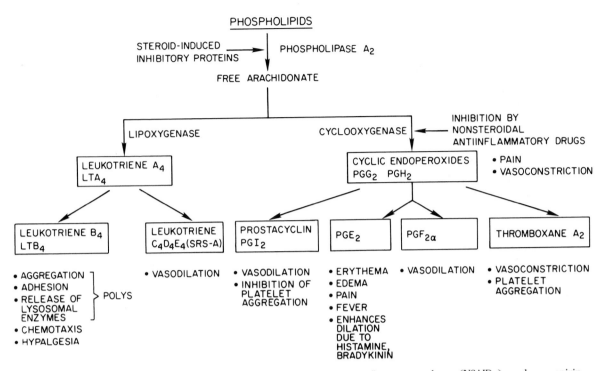

Figure 19-5 The inhibition of prostaglandin synthetase by nonsteroidal anti-inflammatory drugs (NSAIDs), such as aspirin.

include its established efficacy and low cost; a major disadvantage is significant variability between aspirin preparations and between patients in terms of absorption and blood levels attained.[11,29] Need to monitor salicylate levels may negate any savings in the cost of medications. Additionally, gastritis and gastric ulcerations occur in up to 20 to 40 percent of patients given soluble aspirin, requiring periodic monitoring for GI blood loss. The incidence of this side effect is reduced in patients on enteric-coated aspirin or nonacetylated salicylate preparations.

The relative efficacy of the various NSAIDs currently available compared to aspirin is in fact unknown.[32,68,97,98,108,126,134] This is because most newer NSAIDs have been tested against low-dose (fewer than 8 tablets per day) aspirin, with few controlled trials comparing these drugs to enteric-coated or complexed (salicylate) aspirin preparations. Like aspirin, all the NSAIDs are analgesic at the recommended starting dose and require high doses for effective anti-inflammatory action. Each can be advanced (cautiously) beyond the maximum recommended dose. Any gastrointestinal toxicity may occur with each, although the clinical impression is that some are associated with a lower incidence of serious GI side effects than others (Table 19-7). All are relatively contraindicated in a patient who has active ulcer disease or who has a recent history of it. All may cause fluid retention and must be monitored carefully in patients being treated for congestive heart disease, renal failure, or hypertension. Several distinct forms of nephrotoxicity have recently been delineated[18,39] (Table 19-8). Cross-reactions between toxicities (e.g., GI side effects, skin rash, etc.) among

different classes of, or even between individual drugs within a class of, NSAIDs are extremely variable. An exception to this rule is the development of an immediate hypersensitivity reaction (urticaria, acute bronchospasm, anaphylaxis) in a patient given aspirin or a NSAID. Here considerable cross-reactivity has been shown,[121] and resort to a nonacetylated salicylate or alternative therapy may be necessary.[118] Generally, the absolute incidence of toxicities increases with the age of the patient.

Many rheumatologists will begin with a proprionic acid derivative[108] (Motrin, naproxen), gradually advancing the dosage to maximum or toxicity if the clinical response is not satisfactory. Lack of response or toxicity is followed by trial of 1 or 2 members of different classes of NSAIDs (acetic acid derivatives, mefenamates, piroxicam),[32,97,134] and each patient should probably be tried on at least three or four different drugs before resort to a second-line drug. Indomethacin is generally reserved as a late alternative because of its potency and toxicities.[98] The morning stiffness of some patients is benefited, however, by a nightly dose of slow-release (75 mg) indomethacin in addition to the daytime use of other NSAIDs.[96]

Second-Line Drugs

Plaquenil, gold salts, and d-penicillamine are also referred to as "remittive" or "disease-modifying" drugs because a minority of patients who take these drugs *appear* to have the progression of their disease (erosions, nodules) arrested and

TABLE 19-7   Relative Efficiency of Available NSAIDs Compared to Aspirin

1. *Aspirin*[1]
   - Regular aspirin (acetylsalicylic acid)

   Acetylsalicylic acid (aspirin)

   Start at 6–8 tablets (1800–2400 mg) per day; q 4 h
   Increase by 2 tablets 4–6 h until a therapeutic salicylate level is achieved (20–30 mg/dl) or tinnitus
   Important variability between patients as well as between preparations (i.e., disintegration, deaggregation, dissolution of tablets)

   - Enteric-coated aspirin (Ecotrin)
     Same dosage as regular aspirin; about 4 times as expensive
     Lag time to absorption, bypassing stomach, increased by food; absorption may be erratic
   - Microencapsulated aspirin (Easprin)
     3900 mg/day; 1950 mg bid; about 4 times as expensive
     Matrices of wax, resins, plastics, polymers; flattens peak level after a single dose

2. *Nonacetylated salicylates*
   - Choline salicylate (Arthropan)

   Choline salicylate

   5–10 ml qid; about 9 times as expensive as aspirin
   Rapid peak (10 min); useful in children

   - Choline magnesium salicylate (Trilisate)
     1000–1500 mg bid
   - Salicylsalicylic acid (Disalcid)

   Salicylsalicylic acid

   1000–1500 mg bid (500 mg tablets)
   May be soluble in the small intestine

   - Diflunisal* (Dolobid)[2]

   Diflunisal

   1000 mg loading dose, then 500 mg bid
   About 11 times as expensive as aspirin
   Rapidly absorbed; half-life of 6 h

3. *Proprionic acids*
   - Ibuprofen (Motrin, Rufen)[3]

   Ibuprofen

   400–600 mg qid; up to 3600 mg/day
   Half-life of 2 h
   Said to have fewer GI side effects; may be used if there is a history of ulcer disease

   - Naproxen (Naprosyn)[4]

   Naproxen

   250 mg bid → 500 mg bid
   Half-life of 12–15 h
   GI bleeding, sometimes severe and occasionally fatal, has been reported

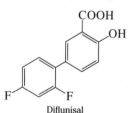

---

*The maximal daily dose prescribed by many rheumatologists exceeds that recommended by the PDR. This reflects the fact that most NSAIDs were underprescribed in early studies. At these higher dosages, close monitoring for toxicities is especially important.

Sources:
[1] Buchanan, W.W., et al, Clin Rheum Dis 5:499–539, 1979; Dromgoole, S.H., et al, Sem Arth Rheum 11:257–283, 1981.
[2] Van Winzum, C., and Verhaest, L., Clin Rheum Dis 5:707–731, 1979.

TABLE 19-7 (*continued*)

- Fenoprofen (Nalfon)

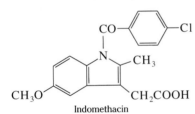

Fenoprofen (Nalfon)

4. *Indoleacetic Acids*
   - Sulindac (Clinoril)[5]

150 mg bid → 400 mg bid
Half-life of 18 h; difficult to titrate
Active form is sulfide metabolite
Low ulcerogenicity compared to indomethacin; does not share CNS side effects
Significant lower GI toxicity

Sulindac (Clinoril)

- Tolmetin (Tolectin)[6]

400 mg tid → 400 mg qid
Half-life of 60–90 min
No severe CNS effects, but GI upset common
Approved for use in children

Tolmetin (Tolectin)

- Indomethacin (Indocin)[7]

25–50 mg qid; 75 mg slow-release (SR) tablets, useful as an hs dosage for
  morning stiffness
Half-life of 2 h; $t_{1/2}$ increased in obstructive jaundice
Poorly tolerated by older patients
May be the most effective of all NSAIDs in terms of effect on prostaglandin synthetase
20% develop headaches, CNS changes
GI toxicities in 10–20%; ulcers usually symptomatic; dyspepsia, bleeding, lower GI
  tract ulcers

Indomethacin

5. *Fenemates*
   - Meclofenamate sodium (Meclomen)   100 mg qid ⎫
   - Mefenamic acid (Ponstel)   250 qid   ⎬ Diarrhea a problem with long-term use

6. *Oxicams*
   - Piroxicam (Feldene)[8]

20 mg once a day
Rapid onset: 80% peak plasma concentration in 1 h
Half-life of 45 h; can omit a day's dosage and take at anytime of day
Plateaus in 3–5 days; absorption unaffected by food, iron, antacids or coadministration of
  aspirin
Major side effect is GI toxicity

Piroxicam

[3]Kantor, T.G., Ann Int Med 91:877–882, 1979.
[4]Segre, E.J., Clin Rheum Dis 5:411–426, 1976.
[5]Rhymer, A.R., Clin Rheum Dis 5:553–568, 1979.
[6]Ehrlich, G.E., Clin Rheum Dis 5:481–497, 1979.
[7]Rhymer, A.R., Clin Rheum Dis 5:541–552, 1979.
[8]Wiseman, E.H., and Boyle, J.A., Clin Rheum Dis 6:585–613, 1980.

TABLE 19-8   Nephrotoxicity of NSAIDs

1. Reversible oliguric renal failure in a patient
   - With congestive heart failure
   - On diuretic therapy
   - With cirrhosis and ascites
   - With severe sodium depletion
   - With nephrotic syndrome
   - With high renin and/or decreased renal function
   - With basal renal blood flow

   e.g., Acetic acid derivatives (e.g., indomethacin)

2. Interstitial nephritis
   - Heavy proteinuria
   - Tubulointerstitial nephritis; minimal changes of glomeruli
   - Nonoliguric
   - May have flank pain, hematuria, eosinophilia
   - Rapid deterioration in renal function; steroids may be useful
   - Onset variable (weeks to months)
   - Idiosyncratic

   e.g., Fenoprofen

3. Hyperkalemia
   - Prostaglandin and renin release
   - Hyporeninemic hypoaldosteronism
   - May also develop in diabetics

   e.g., Indomethacin

4. Sodium and water retention (edema)
   Prostaglandins are natriuretic and induce a water diuresis

Sources: Cline, D.M., and Stuff, J.S., N Engl J Med 310:563–572, 1984; Garella, S., and Matarese, R.A., Medicine (Balt) 63:165–181, 1984.

even go into remission (Table 19-9).[78] Most patients, however, experience only a partial response, and it is not clear that disease progression is *truly* affected.[62] Each of these drugs is an example of the important role of serendipity in the development of new therapies for RA, as each was initially used for other diseases (tuberculosis, malaria, Wilson disease), and the original rationale for their usage has proved unfounded. All are slow-acting, taking weeks to months to effect any significant clinical response in most patients. This appears to reflect a long-term effect as immunosuppressive agents, acting to inhibit mononuclear (gold, Plaquenil)[101,125] or T-lymphocyte (D-penicillamine)[79] function. All are usually reserved for use in the patient with active disease who has not responded to a program of NSAID, rest, and physical therapy. The optimal point at which to use these agents, as well as the identification of which subsets of patients are most likely to respond or develop toxicities, is still unclear.

The major limitation to the use of second-line drugs is side effects (Table 19-4). Each must be supervised by a physician familiar with their toxicities who is able to adjust dosages and who will discontinue the drug if necessary. Each requires periodic monitoring of blood counts, liver functions,

and urinalysis in addition to parameters of disease activity outlined above. Because of the relative incidence of toxicities, Plaquenil and gold salts are often used before D-penicillamine. However, the efficacy of each compared to the others under optimal conditions of administration has not been established. Lastly, these drugs may be used sequentially, and possibly also in combination, as there is little evidence for synergism either as to therapeutic effects or toxicities.

An oral gold preparation (Auranofin, Ridaura) has recently been licensed for use as an alternative second-line drug for the treatment of RA.[9] This form of gold may work by mechanisms distinct from injectable gold salts and has a much lower incidence of renal toxicity. The most prevalent side effects are gastrointestinal. Relative efficacy and the place of oral gold in drug treatment sequencing is not yet clear.

Steroids

In principle, corticosteroids should be the most useful therapeutic modality for the treatment of RA because of their profound inhibitory effect on collagenase and plasminogen activator production by synovial cells,[131] their inhibitory effect on both the cyclooxygenase and lipoxygenase pathways (Fig. 19-5),[8] and their effects on mononuclear cell function.[22] They are limited in utility, however, by their acute and chronic side effects.[17] Intraarticular steroids are a mainstay of the therapy of RA, being particularly useful for the control of monoarticular or oligoarticular flares.[46] The role of parenteral corticosteroids, on the other hand, is problematical. Steroids are often used to "buy time" in patients being induced on a second-line drug. In this setting, the dose should probably not exceed 15 mg/day of prednisone by mouth, or its equivalent. It is also likely that low-dose (i.e., 5 mg/day), or even alternate day, steroids may have a place in the chronic management of elderly patients, many of whom are unable to tolerate most NSAIDs.[80] A commitment to long-term corticosteroid therapy requires that both patient and physician realize that the drug cannot be withdrawn suddenly, that periods of stress be covered with additional doses of steroids, and that there is provision for administration of calcium and vitamin D replacement to minimize acceleration of osteoporosis and the risk of pathologic fractures.[38]

Third-Line Drugs

Cytotoxic agents are generally reserved for the 5 to 10 percent of RA patients who have progressive disabling synovitis and who do not respond to, or cannot tolerate, antimalarials, gold, or D-penicillamine. Three of these immunosuppressive agents are currently used in the United States: azathioprine,[58] cyclophosphamide,[72] and methotrexate[132] (Table 19-10). Chlorambucil has been used with good results in France, but has not been widely accepted in this country.

Each of these agents has produced striking clinical improvements in 50 percent or more patients in whom they have been used, in some cases appearing to halt erosive disease. There is little correlation between the clinical effect

TABLE 19-9 Second-Line (Remittive, Disease-Modifying) Drugs

1. *Antimalarials*[1]

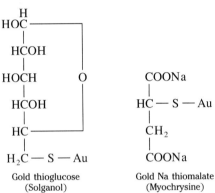

Hydroxychloroquine

Improved benefit-to-risk ratio over other second-line drugs
Up to 70% effective; only 3–7% drop out *if* properly monitored
Lowest toxicity
Less expensive (visits, lab monitoring)

- *Toxicity* 1° eye, usually after 2–3 years of treatment, ophthalmological evaluations q 4–6 months, GI toxicity (early), CNS symptoms, rash, neuromuscular symptoms

2. *Chrysotherapy*[2]

Gold thioglucose (Solganol)

Gold Na thiomalate (Myochrysine)

15–20% remit during treatment; 40–60% have good-to-excellent results; 20–30% fail or develop toxicity
May arrest progression of disease (disputed)
Intramuscular route inconvenient; cost of weekly follow-up
Loading schedule of 20 weeks of 50 mg/week; maintenance of 50 mg q 2–4 weeks

- *Toxicity*[3]
  Cutaneous: reversible, may reinstitute if mild; most common
    Pruritus
    Maculopapular rashes (50%)
    Stomatitis (metallic taste)
    Exfoliative dermatitis
    Lichen planuslike (30%)
    Pityriasis rosea (10%)
    Eosinophilia ↑ IgE
  Hematologic
    Leukopenia
    Agranulocytosis (rare)
    Thrombocytopenia (most common; 1%–3%)
    Aplastic anemia (rare)
  Renal
    Proteinuria (common, reversible; 3–7%)
    Nephrotic syndrome
    Membranous glomerulonephritis (two-thirds recover)
  GI
    Enterocolitis (rare, usually fulminant)
    Cholestatic jaundice
  Pulmonary
    Hypersensitivity pneumonitis (rare)
  Ocular

3. D-*Penicillamine*[4]

D-Penicillamine

Oral; once daily 125–250 mg → 1000 mg/day (or more)
Take on an empty stomach
60% improvement; 20–50% toxicity
May be particularly effective for extraarticular disease (vasculitis, pulmonary manifestations)
Toxicities minimized by starting at low dose and advancing slowly

(continued on next page)

TABLE 19-9 (*continued*)

- *Toxicity*
  Dysgeusia (early; ~10%)
  GI distress (early, most common)
  Rashes (~10%)
    Erythematous (early)
    Pruritic, scaling macules (late)
  Stomatitis
  Thrombocytopenia (any time; ~5%) > leukopenia (early)
  Proteinuria (6–9%); reversible, discontinue drug if > 1–2 g/day
    Nephrotic syndrome
    Rapidly progressive glomerulonephritis (rare)
  Autoimmune syndromes (1–2%)
    Myasthenia gravis
    Polymyositis
    Lupus erythematosus
    Goodpasture syndrome
    Pemphigus

Sources:
[1] Robinson, D.R., DM December 1983, 1–46; Schumacher, H.R., Ann NY Acad Sci 256:39–64, 1975.
[2] Carson, D.A., in Kelley, W.N., et al (eds): *Textbook of Rheumatology,* 2d ed, Philadelphia, Saunders, 1985, pp 664–679; Lipsky, P.E., in Utsinger, P.D., et al: *Rheumatoid Arthritis,* Philadelphia, Saunders, 1985, pp 601–634.
[3] Gibbons, R.B., Arch Int Med 139:343–346, 1979.
[4] Jaffe, I.A., Bull Rheum Dis 28:948–952, 1977-1978; Lipsky, P.E., in Utsinger, P.D., et al: *Rheumatoid Arthritis,* Philadelphia, Saunders, 1985, pp 601–634.

seen and the degree of suppression of immune function. Each must be monitored carefully for resulting marrow suppression and gastrointestinal toxicity, and each predisposes to infections such as herpes zoster. All are contraindicated for use in individuals with childbearing potential. Both azathioprine and cyclophosphamide are associated with a significantly increased risk of carcinoma,[29] by extrapolation from the experience with renal transplant patients treated long-term with these drugs. Consequently, none should be employed until other alternatives are exhausted and only with fully informed consent.

Alternative Forms of Therapy

A number of alternative therapies that have been shown to be effective in preliminary and often uncontrolled trials are currently under investigation. Many are being considered for use in patients not responding to, or unable to tolerate, first- or second-line drugs, but their optimal place in treatment sequence strategies is unclear. They include:

Intraarticular Therapies Therapeutic potential of arthroscopy (intraarticular lavage); improved and sustained drug delivery by use of carriers (e.g., liposomes); and intraarticular radiotherapy (synoviorthesis).[47]

Depletion of Lymphoid Cells This approach to therapy is based on experimental data suggesting an important role of cellular immunity in the pathogenesis of chronic synovitis. Early trials of thoracic duct drainage showed an ameliorative effect on synovitis. Two modalities under active current investigation are total lymphoid irradiation[35] and lymphoplasmapheresis.[129]

Immunomodulatory Agents Levamisole was the first group of immunologic agents that appeared to affect RA by way of the immune system. Recent studies have suggested cyclosporine may have some efficacy in this and other forms of synovitis.[28]

Combination Therapies This category embraces concomitant use of two different nonsteroidals or second-line drugs; combinations of second-line drugs with low-dose cytotoxic agents; combination chemotherapy.[85]

SUMMARY

There have been no controlled trials evaluating the efficacy of various treatment modalities for extraarticular disease. Consequently, current approaches to therapy are based largely on anecdotal experience. Systemic vasculitis (excepting the bland digital variety) is often managed acutely with 40 to 60 mg of prednisone in divided doses.[107] There has been some interest also in the use of "pulse" steroids (500 to 1000 mg of methylprednisolone given daily for 1 to 3 days) for the critically ill patient. Cryoglobulinemia or hyperviscosity provides a rationale for the use of plasmapheresis as a means of reducing the load of immune complexes, and some have advocated a regimen of apheresis and cytotoxic agents in patients who develop severe vasculitis.[1,106] Currently, cyclophosphamide is

TABLE 19-10 Third-Line Drugs

1. *Azathioprine* (Imuran)

Start at 50 mg/day; increase to 1.5–2.5 mg/kg per day over 4–6 weeks
Purine analogue
Must be taken at reduced dosage in patients on allopurinol
Specific toxicities:
    Hypersensitivity reactions (systemic, hepatitis)
    Agranulocytosis

2. *Cyclophosphamide* (Cytoxan)[2]

Start at 50 mg/day; increase to 1.5–2.5 mg/kg per day over 4–6 weeks; may need to titrate to mild leukopenia
Alkylating agent
Specific toxicities:
    Bladder (cystitis, carcinoma)
    Sterility

3. *Methotrexate*[3]

Start at 2.5 mg weekly, advancing in 2.5–5 mg increments as tolerated to 10 to 15 mg/week
May be given intramuscularly or orally; often given in divided doses for cell-cycle effect
Folic acid antagonist

- *Specific toxicity:* hepatic dysfunction, fibrosis, cirrhosis
- Appears to be well tolerated and effective as low-dose therapy; no information as yet as to the incidence of permanent sterility or increased incidence of carcinoma

Sources:
[1]Huskisson, E.C., Clin Rheum Dis 10:325–332, 1984.
[2]Korarsky, J., Sem Arth Rheum 12:359–372, 1983.
[3]Wilkens, R.F., Amer J Med (suppl) 73:19–25, 1983.

the preferred drug for such patients, based on a favorable experience with other forms of systemic vasculitis. This agent can be given orally or by intermittent intravenous bolus (e.g., in the patient with GI bleeding or intestinal vasculitis), but the relative efficacy of each is not yet clear.

The long-term management of extraarticular disease and Felty syndrome may include steroids, gold salts,[94] or a trial of D-penicillamine. Important considerations in the management of patients with Felty syndrome include the exclusion of bleeding or drug effects as the basis of hematological abnormalities observed and rapid prophylaxis for infection. For patients with recurrent infections, splenectomy has been found to benefit in 60 to 80 percent of cases, at least temporarily.[42] Persistent symptomatic neutropenia or leg ulcers may warrant a trial of lithium salts to stimulate granulopoiesis.[48] Lastly, steroids and cytotoxic agents have been used with disputed efficacy in refractory cases.

SECTION C

Juvenile Arthritis and Arthralgia

Avron Ross and Roger Dee

As the several types of arthritis affecting children have become better-defined in recent years, it has become possible to distinguish between them with increasing accuracy. Some of the conditions which are important in the differential diagnosis are shown in Table 19-11.

TABLE 19-11 Differential Diagnoses for Juvenile Rheumatoid Arthritis (JRA)

I. Systemic JRA (Still's disease)
II. Pauciarticular JRA (including those cases with spondyloarthropathy)
III. Polyarticular JRA
   A. Lyme arthritis
   B. Other connective tissue diseases (acute rheumatic fever, systemic lupus erythematosus, and dermatomyositis
   C. Reactive arthritis, septic arthritis (bacteria, virus, and fungal infection)
   D. Transient synovitis
   E. Hematologic disorders (Henoch-Schönlein purpura, hemophilia, sickle cell disease)
   F. Kawasaki disease
   G. Malignancy (leukemia, neuroblastoma)
   H. Nonrheumatic orthopaedic conditions, e.g., slipped epiphysis, osteochondritis
   I. Hypermobility syndromes
   J. Nocturnal leg pains
   K. Malingering

JUVENILE RHEUMATOID ARTHRITIS (JRA)

This condition is the principal and most familiar cause of chronic arthritis in childhood.[27] It may resolve fully or lead in 10 percent of patients to permanent disability.

Diagnostic Criteria

Juvenile refers to onset before the sixteenth birthday. The use of the word *arthritis* must be reserved for those joints which show unequivocal evidence of effusion or synovial proliferation either by clinical examination or by x-ray findings or which show damage to cartilage or bone resulting from the disease process. Or, in the absence of these, it must be reserved for those joints which show a decrease in the full range of motion in the presence of heat, tenderness, and/or pain. If arthritis persists in a joint or joints for 6 weeks or more, a diagnosis of JRA can certainly be entertained if no other cause has been found. The diagnosis is often made by exclusion. If the objective signs of arthritis are not present, even if there is a limp or some disability, the term *arthralgia* is preferable, and these patients should not be labeled as arthritic.

Incidence

About three children in a thousand develop JRA between early infancy and 15 years of age. The sexes are affected in a ratio of girls to boys of 1.5:1. It is seen most often in white children, next in Hispanic, and least often in blacks. In recent years cases similar to JRA have been recognized in the adult.

Pathogenetic Mechanism

Although the pathogenetic mechanism has not as yet been fully clarified, modern studies support the concept that there is a genetic predisposition. Family histories disclose an increased frequency of rheumatoid arthritis or other rheumatologic and immunologic disorders in close relatives. In monozygotic twins, a concordance of 30 percent has been reported. HLA studies reveal a decrease in DW4, the reverse of the situation of adults with rheumatoid arthritis, and increases in the frequency of DW7, DW8, and TMo in the subsets. The recognition that juvenile rheumatoid arthritis in children is often different from the adult disease has led to the suggestion, particularly in Europe, that these subsets and also the chronic arthritis associated with reactive arthritis, spondyloarthropathies, and systemic lupus erythematosus in children be referred to as *juvenile chronic arthritis.*

The musculoskeletal pathology is similar to that seen in adult rheumatoid arthritis. There is synovial hyperplasia and in severe cases, pannus formation, with erosion of articular cartilage and adjacent bone. Bony erosions and joint space loss are often, however, late manifestations of the disease by contrast with adult disease. The end result is often ankylosis of the joint which may become complete bony fusion. This is particularly likely in the dry type of arthritis with little synovial fluid which is seen in some patients with chronic disease and can lead to crippling loss of function. The hyperemia in the region of the epiphyses is responsible for growth disturbances which are commonly seen in this disease. There may be overgrowth with characteristic ballooning of the epiphyses; asymmetrical or symmetrical growth stimulation will cause leg lengthening, whereas selective medial or lateral stimulation may produce deformity, particularly in the region of the knee. Fractures may occur because the bone is osteopenic, and compression fractures of the epiphysis, particularly in the weight-bearing joints, lead to deformity.[1,25,26]

Soft tissue contractures are common and these may affect the iliotibial band causing an external rotation deformity of the tibia and an abduction deformity of the hip.[15] Adduction contractures of the hip may also occur and lead to joint subluxation unless corrected.

In the knee, in addition to varus valgus deformity, flexion contracture can also occur with posterior subluxation of the tibia. In the subtalar joint, spastic flatfoot can occur during the phase of joint irritability, and fusion often occurs in a position of cavovarus deformity.[15,19]

In the upper limb, flexion contractures of the elbows are common, and stiffness of the wrist with limited dorsiflexion also occurs. The metacarpophalangeal joints infrequently develop ulnar drift, such as is seen in adult disease. Instead they develop radial deviation, and limitation of flexion also occurs. Similar stiffness occurs in the proximal phalangeal joints which may develop flexion contractures rather than the swan neck and boutonniere deformities seen in adults.[15]

Involvement of the cervical spine is a frequent accompaniment of the polyarthritis. Atlantoaxial subluxation may occur, or there may be fusion of segments of the spine with a portion remaining unfused. These complications together with the involvement of the temporomandibular joint makes anesthesia extremely hazardous.[19]

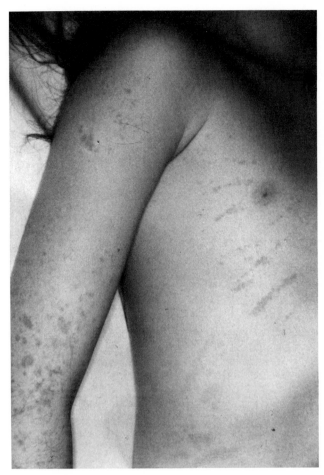

Figure 19-6 Rash of juvenile rheumatoid arthritis (JRA) and Koebner's phenomenon.

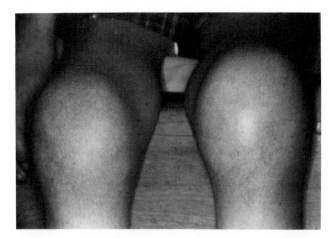

Figure 19-7 Bilateral synovitis of the knees in juvenile rheumatoid arthritis (JRA).

The Subsets of Juvenile Rheumatoid Arthritis

The disease has been divided into three distinctive subtypes, each of which appears to represent the different disease mechanisms (Table 19-11).

Systemic Onset JRA

This is the classic form of JRA known as *Still disease.*[31] This subtype can often be recognized or suspected clinically as early as a few days after the first signs and symptoms, because of its unique characteristics. However, the accepted criteria are the "general criterion" as above, plus a fever of $\geq 103°F$ or higher persisting for 2 weeks or more.

Distinctive Findings

1. Spiking intermittent fever which may range from as low as 96°F to as high as 106°F in a single day.
2. Painful arthralgia and/or myalgia at the height of daily fever, which may be reduced or absent at fever low point. The patient may be immobilized by pain when febrile, but active and playful when the temperature drops.
3. A rash which, in combination with the fever and musculoskeletal pains, may be diagnostic. (Fig. 19-6) This consists of generalized, pale pink, evanescent, erythematous macules mostly of 2 to 5 mm diameter, concentrated on the cheeks, neck, lateral thorax, and extensor aspects of the extremities. It is typically nonpruritic, becoming pruritic with high fever, warm baths, or heavy clothing. It is accompanied by the Koebner's phenomenon, an isomorphic response to scratching or stroking appearing as linear chains of macules similar to the above.
4. Arthritis, which may be present at onset, or delayed for weeks, months, or more than a year. Large joints may predominate, often symmetrically (Fig. 19-7) with knees and ankles most frequent, then wrists, elbows, hips, and shoulders. At other times small joints are involved, often only single PIP joints of fingers or toes. The cervical spine and the temporomandibular joints are less frequently but very characteristically involved and also the costochondral joints. Arthritis may be transient with complete remission in some, but in 25 percent it will go on to a chronic relentlessly destructive process (Fig. 19-8A and B) with a complete fusion of joints and severe deformity (Fig. 19-9). Joints likely to be spared are the thoracolumbosacral spine, and sacroiliac joints. In chronic cases, the joints remain swollen, cool, and nontender; they become restricted in the range of motion more by synovial hypertrophy and effusion than by pain.
5. Carditis occurs in 5 percent of cases as pericarditis, pericardial effusion, or even as myocarditis with failure. This may be present within days or weeks of onset, or may occur during relapses.
6. Generalized lymphadenopathy, discrete and nontender.
7. Hematologic changes. Most striking when it occurs is a polymorphonuclear leukocytosis of 12,000 to 50,000/mm^3 with increased percentage of band forms. An elevated ESR is usually present, at times rising to well above 100 mm/h. Mild anemia and thrombocytosis are also common.
8. There is often hepatosplenomegaly with a predisposition to infection and amyloidosis, which may be fatal.

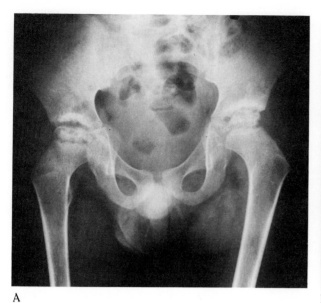
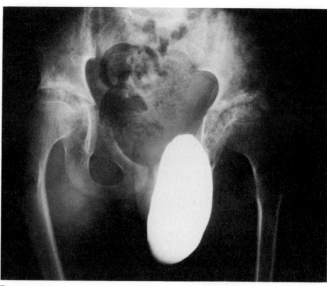

A   B

Figure 19-8 A. Early erosive hip disease in systemic onset JRA. **B.** Advanced hip joint destruction in the same patient.

Pauciarticular Onset JRA

Pauciarticular onset JRA, including spondyloarthropathy, refers to four or fewer joints involved with arthritis in the first 6 months of disease, in the absence of signs of systemic onset.

Salient Features

1. Abrupt occurrence of joint swelling, often monarticular.
2. No history or evidence of significant trauma.
3. Predilection for fingers, toes, knees, or ankles.
4. Chronicity of joints, swelling from time of onset.
5. Joints warm, of normal skin color, often not tender or painful. Child may show distinct loss of range of motion without complaints.
6. Iridocyclitis, chronic or recurrent, is the principal serious manifestation, with 20 percent overall incidence. Early phase is detectable only by biomicroscopy (slit lamp examination) by an ophthalmologist.
7. Female early childhood group, onset at about 2 to 4 years of age, have a frequent laboratory feature of importance: positive ANA, at a titer of $1:40$ to $1:320$, which raises the risk of iridocyclitis to about 40 percent. Unlike the male subset described next, they do not tend to have HLA-B27.
8. Male midchildhood group, onset at about 5 to 9 years of age. There is a substantial subset of male children who in fact fit clinical criteria for early ankylosing spondylitis (AS). They have arthritis of the large joints of the lower extremities, early sacroiliitis, and acute anterior uveitis; they are positive for HLA-B27. Unlike the female subset, they tend not to have serum antinuclear antibody. With the passage of time they fit in best with the spondyloarthropathies and show some response to NSAIDs other than aspirin. Ultimate lumbosacral spinal damage and aortic disease are variable, but they may not progress with the severity of the adult type.[7]

Polyarticular Onset JRA

The term polyarticular onset JRA is reserved for JRA involving five or more joints. This is the least common form, but may include destructive features in common with the systemic onset variety.

Distinctive Findings (1) Usually a rapid onset of arthritis in several joints; (2) two principal groups, depending upon rheumatoid factor seropositivity or seronegativity. The group with positive rheumatoid factor tends to have a progressive, destructive course.

Differential Diagnosis It is essential to differentiate JRA from the conditions listed in Table 19-11 and, in particular, from systemic lupus erythematosus, reactive arthritides,

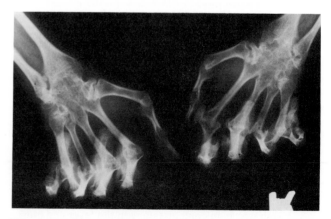

Figure 19-9 Hand and wrist ankylosis and deformity in polyarticular juvenile rheumatoid arthritis (JRA).

septic arthritis (including tuberculous arthritis), and viral arthritides.

Treatment of JRA

An individualized program of care is necessary for each child. Such a program must concern itself with social, recreational, and educational activity, the prescription of medication and physical therapy, the assessment of the need for orthotics or other specialized rehabilitation services, and the provision of surgical intervention if appropriate.

Wherever possible children should be encouraged to be active in play and sports and to attend school and gym with minimal restrictions. All the assessments should consider the possibility of future eye complications or amyloidosis.[1] Slit lamp examination is imperative at three monthly intervals in active JRA.

Drug Therapy

Ansell and Swann recommend that a nonsteroidal anti-inflammatory analgesic agent be given even in the absence of pain if there is clinically obvious muscle spasm.[1] They recommend ibuprofen (30 mg/kg) or Naproxen (10 mg/kg). The initial drug treatment is either aspirin 60 to 90 mg/kg per day (not to exceed 5 g daily) or, because of concern with aspirin and Reye syndrome, tolmetin sodium (20 mg/kg per day). Ansell and Swann believe that pauciarticular arthritis responds better to Naproxen and indomethacin than to aspirin. When these drugs fail, steroid therapy may be necessary for disabling attacks or for mild cardiac failure. Occasionally they have been used for pauciarticular arthritis in a young child unable to obtain relief from muscle spasm sufficient enough to allow physiotherapy.[1] When there is progressive joint damage, systemic or polyarticular JRA, the immunosuppressive drugs such as methotrexate may be justified in controlled conditions.

Rehabilitation

Goals of rehabilitation are to preserve good function and muscle strength while preventing deformity and eventually to enable the child to participate, if possible, in the normal activities of life. The physiotherapist will be involved in the routine management of these patients, preventing deformity by suitable splintage of affected joints and by range-of-motion exercises. Corrective orthotics and serial casting may be required to gently correct established deformities. Such a program may be interrupted during the acute phase by the need to rest the painful joint in a simple immobilization splint during the painful episode. Protective splints may also be required at night. Complete bed rest is rarely required for these children; the indications are acute pain in a lower limb joint for the patient with severe systemic disease or as part of a program of traction prior to surgical correction of severe deformity.[1] It goes without saying that during any period of rest, particularly bed rest, affected joints must not become stiff in a deformed position. The child should be encouraged therefore to lie clothed extending the hips and knees on a daily basis[1] when the disease is active. Prolonged sitting in the same position can be as dangerous as bed rest in promoting the development of contractures.

Surgical Treatment

Disease of the hip is the most common cause of limited mobility in juvenile chronic arthritis.[16,32]

Arthroscopy Halgersson and co-workers[16] have described their technique for arthroscopy of the hip in juvenile chronic arthritis and consider it to be valuable as a diagnostic procedure since it gives better information about the articular cartilage than does the x-ray examination. It can also be used to inspect the synovium. They consider that arthroscopy gives information which can be used to classify the disease and permit more rational selection of those cases which might benefit from synovectomy than from radiological findings alone. Synovial biopsy is valuable in excluding causes of arthritis other than JRA, but there is only limited correlation between the histological findings and the subsequent course of the disease.[16] Synovial biopsy is particularly helpful in excluding tuberculosis in monarticular joint disease.[6]

Synovectomy The results of joint synovectomy in JRA were reviewed by Granberry and Brewer.[15] These investigators concluded that the most consistent benefit from this procedure is relief of pain. The procedure is best done early in the disease, but in selective cases considerable benefit is occasionally obtained from the procedure even when done later on. They recommend that the operation be considered for patients with monarticular and pauciarticular arthritis because of proven results with these conditions. They observed that when the sedimentation rate was elevated, when the rheumatoid test was positive, when the disease had its onset in the small joints, or when x-ray films revealed periostitis and erosions, the prognosis following synovectomy was poor. Funk has observed however, that no patient with pauciarticular arthritis in his series ever developed a permanent deformity so that he abandoned synovectomy in such patients. He also observed that some degree of joint motion was also lost after surgery in his series.[13] Synovectomy seems to be particulary contraindicated in those patients with indolent dry disease and is tantamount then to performing an arthrodesis.[15,19]

Lower Limb Release of contracted soft tissue structures such as the iliotibial band and the adductors is of great benefit when associated with fixed deformity.[32] The release of the psoas tendon combined with adductor tenotomy may be required.[32]

For major joint deformity in the lower limb, osteotomy may occasionally be necessary. A subluxating hip joint may be stabilized by performing a varus osteotomy. Total joint replacement has been extensively performed in some centers,[1] and there is no doubt that functional improvement in the short term is dramatic. Nevertheless, the durability of these joints is so poor in this age group (see Chap. 71, Sect. A) that a cemented implant is better avoided. There may be an occasional indication for mold (cup) arthroplasty or a cementless implant.

Ansell and Swann recommend a mainly conservative approach to the hindfoot and midfoot, anticipating and correcting deformities by gentle manipulation and casting. However, triple arthrodesis may be necessary for a malpositioned cavovarus foot with subtalar pain.[19]

Upper Limb Total joint replacement should also be avoided in the upper limb. Fascial and cutis and other forms of interposition arthroplasty can often be used to satisfactorily mobilize the joint.[13] Excision arthroplasty may produce instability and should be avoided.

Deformities of the digits and metacarpophalangeal joints will benefit from soft tissue release. It may be necessary to arthrodese the wrist, particularly if it is subluxed. It is important to avoid fusing the wrist in dorsiflexion. The position of choice is neutral or slight palmar flexion because this is a better functional position for children with stiff elbows and shoulders.[19] Synovectomy of the tendons around the wrist may be valuable, as in the adult rheumatoid patient, to prevent destruction by erosion.

Cervical Spine When operative procedure on the cervical spine is necessary, the use of a halo cast and tracheotomy prior to surgery has been recommended.[19] Ansell and Swann recommend that atlantoaxial subluxation should be treated initially with a well-fitting collar which may result in stabilization provided there is no neurological deficit. They reserve fusion for those who develop progressive signs.[1]

Treatment of Growth Problems Rydholm and his co-workers[26] note that in patients with unilateral disease, symmetrical leg length inequality commonly occurs, whereas in patients with polyarticular disease, a valgus deformity is common. In the latter group, any leg length discrepancy often corrects within 2 years, probably because the arthritis also involves the contralateral knee. Valgus deformity of the knee joint also usually decreases with age.[26] They recommend that, when only one knee joint is involved, synovectomy is valuable in reducing the hypervascularity around the femoral physis. If this treatment fails however, stapling of the femoral and tibial physes is a minor procedure that in their hands has been successful. They note, however, that careful timing and supervision are important because of the inconsistency of both local and general growth patterns in patients with juvenile chronic arthritis. Stapling of the distal medial femoral or proximal tibial physis was performed successfully for progressive valgus deformity, and correction to within 5 degrees was obtained in the majority of joints.[26]

Finally, one should be aware that these patients have often been on steroids so that steroid replacement will be required to cover the surgical procedure. Further, as a consequence of this therapy the bones will be extremely porotic, and there may be hypervascularity and difficulty in obtaining purchase with screws and other implants.[1] Also, remember that the bones are usually very small. The anesthetic difficulties have already been described.

LYME DISEASE

Lyme disease (LD) is a tick-borne spirochetosis, first recognized in 1975 in Old Lyme, Connecticut. It is capable of causing fever, rash, neurological signs, cardiac symptoms, and arthritis.[30] It is a prominent cause of pauciarticular arthritis with recurrent brief attacks.

Incidence

In endemic areas, which now include 24 states, with concentrations on the northeastern and western coastal areas of the United States, reporting of Lyme disease has rapidly risen to 1498 cases in 1984. Male-female ratio is about 1:1. Patients younger than 21 years comprise over 30 percent of all cases.

Etiology

The causative spirochete, *Borrelia burgdorferi,* is transmitted by the bite, usually unobserved, of tiny nymphal deer ticks, *Ixodes dammini,* which abound in wooded areas or weedy seashore in the spring and appear as very small adults in the fall.

Diagnostic Signs

1. Early, swiftly expanding, pink ringlike, solid, or bull's-eye-shaped rash at the bite site termed erythema chronicum migrans (ECM). This may not occur or be recognized and treated.
2. There may be transient neurological signs.
3. Cardiac arrhythmia or myocarditis may occur.
4. Within a few weeks, in 50 percent of untreated patients a conspicuous effusion in a joint such as the knee occurs, with later involvement of other large or small joints.

The arthritis may be accompanied by fever, and the attack usually ends within a week. It then may recur at intervals of weeks or months, or eventually become chronic, with synovial changes similar to RA. The orthopaedist who obtains a purulent yellow joint fluid with 50,000 to 100,000 cells per cubic millimeter and finds no organisms with a Gram stain or culture should consider this among the principal diagnoses in children in endemic areas who play in the woods or at the seashore.

The diagnostic test for LD is the antispirochetal antibody titer performed by enzyme-linked immunosorbent assay (ELISA). The spirochete has recently been detected in joint synovium. This may account for the apparent response of the arthritis to substantial amounts of antibiotics.

Differential Diagnosis

The symptoms of LD are often confused with those of JRA or septic arthritis.

Treatment

Most effective in the ECM stage. Give phenoxymethyl penicillin 50 mg/kg per day for 30 days, or in children sensitive to penicillin, tetracycline 50 mg/kg per day (if over nine years of age). This may eradicate the arthritis, though prevention at the ECM stage is more successful. For severe manifestations newer IV cephalosporin antibiotics such as ceftriaxone are now in use.

In an established chronic arthritis medical therapy alone may not suffice and synovectomy has been used with success.[23]

ACUTE RHEUMATIC FEVER

Acute rheumatic fever (ARF), the most prominent cause of childhood arthritis in the United States until the antibiotic era began in the early 1940s, is an autoimmune reactivity to an untreated infection with a group A beta hemolytic streptococcus. Fever, migratory arthralgia and arthritis, rash, carditis, and/or nodules are the acute signs.

Incidence

With routine use of antibiotics for streptococcal sore throat ARF has become uncommon in our society. Nonetheless rheumatic fever appears at low frequency each year on any active pediatric service, most often as a sequel to an untreated or undertreated streptococcal pharyngotonsillitis.

Diagnosis

The modern disease is milder, with arthralgia and arthritis predominating. Carditis is less frequent, and erythema marginatum, subcutaneous nodules, and chorea are rarely seen. The modified Jones criteria for diagnosis are well known.[8]

Distinctive Findings

1. Transient and migratory nature of the arthralgia and arthritis.
2. Excruciating pain, redness and tenderness in affected joints, in contrast to the rheumatoid joint with its chronic indolent course, normal skin color, and lack of tenderness or pain other than at onset.
3. Evidence of antecedent streptococcal infection through a rising, and later, falling antistreptolysin O or streptozyme titer.
4. The rheumatic joint more than any other responds dramatically and in a sustained fashion to aspirin therapy.

Differential Diagnosis

It sometimes takes a few weeks in atypical cases to distinguish ARF from JRA. An attack similar to ARF, with migratory polyarthritis, may follow *Mycoplasma pneumoniae* infection.

Treatment

Once the diagnosis is established the patient must be

1. Put on phenoxymethyl penicillin 50 mg/kg up to 2.0 g/day for 2 weeks to eliminate streptococci.

2. Given long-term prophylaxis of 250,000 units of penicillin G twice daily. Alternatives for penicillin-sensitive persons are sulfadiazine 1.0 g daily for patients >60 lb, 0.5 g daily for patients <60 lb, or erythromycin 250 mg twice daily.
3. Closely observed for carditis in continued follow-up.

TRANSIENT SYNOVITIS OF THE HIP

Transient synovitis of the hip, is also known as "irritable hip" or "observation hip." It affects children under 10 years of age; boys are more commonly affected than girls and comprise 80 percent of cases.[18] The child presents with acutely irritable hip with muscle spasm, although pain is sometimes referred to the knee. Physical examination reveals a positive Thomas test (fixed flexion deformity of the hip joint). All motion is restricted.

Etiology

Harding studied 257 children with this condition. He failed to establish any infective etiology either by bacteria or virus, and there was no direct correlation with an allergic or traumatic etiology.[18] Several authors have noted that the condition is a precursor to Perthes' disease in a small proportion of cases. A survey of the literature by Spock[29] observed late radiological changes which varied from coxa magna to broadening of the neck, and in some cases osteoarthritic change. These changes were seen in approximately half of his series at long term follow up, indicating that the condition is not always totally benign.

Radiological Findings

There may be an effusion into the joint in this condition which is recognized radiologically by lateral displacement of the femoral head.[24] Persistence of this sign identified by widening of the medial compartment of the joint compared with the normal side is more likely to indicate Perthes' disease, however, than transient synovitis. Capsular thickening with lateral bulging and swelling of the surrounding muscles are variable and inconsistent findings.[9,18]

Clinical Course and Management

The diagnosis is established by exclusion: by the failure to develop characteristic radiological changes of other diseases and by the benign clinical course. The child is admitted to the hospital and treated in traction, a few pounds of skin traction usually producing relief in a few days. As the muscle spasm is relieved, hip motion returns. If ambulation and full activity are recommended too early, there may be a brief recurrence of the condition, but recurrence usually indicates some other diagnosis and a more serious condition. If resolution does not occur rapidly, or if there are persistent physical signs or positive laboratory tests, hip aspiration and a full workup for other conditions such as septic arthritis or Perthes disease may be required. The sedimentation rate is usually not elevated in transient synovitis, but this is not invariably the case.[9]

HENOCH-SCHÖNLEIN PURPURA

Henoch-Schönlein (anaphylactoid) purpura (HSP) is a form of necrotizing vasculitis causing manifestations in the skin, gastrointestinal tract, joints, and kidneys.[33]

Incidence

Not established, but it is seen in small numbers on a pediatric service, chiefly in the spring. Age range: chiefly children 6 months to 11 years of age, although it may occur at any age. Sex: males and females similarly affected.

Etiology

There is evidence of hypersensitivity, possibly to an antecedent bacterial or viral upper respiratory infection. Individuals with a homozygous C2 deficiency have an increased incidence of HSP.[14]

Pathological Findings

A leukocytoclastic vasculitis, with deposits of immunoglobulin A, C3, fibrin, and fibrinogen in blood vessels of affected skin and in the kidney glomeruli, suggesting that HSP may proceed through the alternative complement pathway.[10]

Differential Diagnosis

Polyarteritis nodosa and other collagen-vascular disorders must be ruled out.

Diagnosis

Presenting signs are usually rash, abdominal pain, and arthritis.

1. The skin lesions are striking, and are at first erythematous macules, concentrated largely on the lower extremities, buttocks, and distal upper extremities.
2. These evolve in a few days into purpuric lesions which then become papular and palpable.
3. These areas as well as unaffected areas may become edematous.
4. Abdominal pains are severe, and the most distressing complaint for the child.
5. Bowel signs range from bloody stools to hemorrhage to intussusception, which must be watched for.
6. The large joints, particularly knees and ankles, may develop warm, tender effusions, which are generally self-limited.
7. Renal involvement, although mild in most instances, may evolve into a chronic and serious form of nephritis.

Occasionally other organ system complications may be seen, including neurological. Most patients recover fully in 6 weeks to 4 months, and there is less than 10 percent relapse rate within a few months, among which patients are those with major renal problems.

Treatment

1. Supportive therapy.
2. Corticosteroids, while they do not suppress the overall clinical course, are useful in controlling severe abdominal pain and bleeding.
3. Joint swelling subsides in a few days. If therapy is needed, aspirin or other NSAIDs, such as tolmetin, may be helpful.

KAWASAKI DISEASE/MUCOCUTANEOUS LYMPH NODE SYNDROME

Kawasaki disease (KD), or mucocutaneous lymph node syndrome is an acute vasculitis similar to polyarteritis nodosa which is prevalent in Japan and which occurs or is being recognized more often in infants and children of all races in the United States.[21] It is of particular importance because of the incidence in about 20 percent of patients of coronary artery aneurysm formation.

Incidence

Infrequent in the United States. Between August 1984 and January 1985, 187 cases were reported. The male to female ratio is 1.5:1. Seen in all races in the United States.[4]

Diagnosis

Febrile illness of five or more days duration, and at least four of the following:

1. Bilateral conjunctival injection.
2. Fissured or injected lips, pharyngeal erythema, or strawberry tongue.
3. Erythematous or scarlatinaform rash.
4. Swelling of the hands or feet, erythema of palms or soles, or generalized or periungual desquamation.
5. Cervical lymphadenopathy with at least 1 node $\geq 1.5\,cm$ in diameter.

The arthritis or arthralgia usually occurs during the second or third week, in about 25 percent of patients. The arthritis is generally pauciarticular, involving the knees, ankles, or hips. Arthralgia may be present earlier with swelling of the digits.

The orthopaedic surgeon may be called, and should have little difficulty in recognizing this distinctive array of signs. Although there are no definitive laboratory tests, several tests are consistent with KD: leukocytosis, elevated ESR, mild proteinuria and pyuria, and a gradually increasing thrombocytosis that reaches 800,000 to 1 million platelets per cubic millimeter within a few weeks.

Cardiovascular complications occur in approximately 20 percent of those afflicted, and include coronary artery aneurysms 2 to 8 weeks after onset which may lead to thrombosis and sudden death during the acute, subacute, or postacute phases, and myocarditis with failure. Overall mortality in KD with modern management is less than 1 percent.

Treatment

1. Cardiac supervision with bidimensional echocardiography.
2. Aspirin at 100 mg/kg per day during the febrile period.
3. Low-dosage aspirin at 5 mg/kg per day when postfebrile and for an extended period while thrombocytosis is present.
4. Recent studies support the use of intravenous gamma globulin infusions in high dosage.

MALIGNANCY

The most unfortunate patient to be seen by the orthopaedist because of unexplained musculoskeletal pains is the infant or child with malignancy, most often neuroblastoma or leukemia-lymphoma, occasionally of the CNS, who presents because of disability, especially in the lower extremities.[11,27,28]

Diagnosis

1. Weight bearing may be intolerable in those with bone marrow infiltrates or metastases. The infant or child may crawl in place of previous ambulation.
2. Constitutional signs: fever, weight loss, anorexia, insomnia, irritability.
3. Anemia, high erythrocyte sedimentation rate, and elevated C-reactive protein.
4. Dysfunction out of proportion to visible joint pathology.

Once malignancy is suspected, the child should be immediately and intensively investigated by a oncologist.

HYPERMOBILITY SYNDROME

Hypermobility syndrome (HMS) is a common form of migratory polyarthralgia in children with marked ligamentous laxity.[22] Its recognition eliminates a source of false diagnosis of juvenile rheumatoid arthritis, with its attendant health, psychological, and economic costs.

Incidence

About 5 percent of patients seen in a pediatric rheumatology setting. Ratio of females to males is about 3:1. Age of onset is usually about 12 to 16 years, occasionally much younger. There is an expected increase in familial cases.

Etiology

This is a normal inborn variation in ligamentous structure permitting a wide range of motion at joints throughout the body.[12]

Diagnosis

1. Arthralgia in one or more joints lasting for only a few hours or up to 1 or 2 days, usually up to several times per month for an indefinite period of time.
2. Exclusion of other causes of arthritis or chronic disability is necessary. However in a series of children with HMS referred to a pediatric rheumatology service 20 percent were found to have concurrent JRA.[5] This is probably a high figure due to screening for referral, but it does underscore the need to occasionally consider the possibility of coexistence of the two.
3. Absence of secondary gain.
4. Normal ESR, CRP, ANA, and rheumatoid factor.
5. Accepted criteria for diagnosis of hypermobility are the performance of three or more of these five demonstrations of excessive ligamentous laxity: *(a)* Extension of wrists and metacarpophalangeal joints so that the fingers are parallel to the dorsum of the forearm. *(b)* Passive apposition of thumbs to the flexor aspect of the forearms. *(c)* Hyperextension of elbows 10 degrees or more. *(d)* Hyperextension of knees 10 degrees or more. *(e)* Flexion of trunk with knees extended so that palms rest on the floor.

Differential Diagnosis

Ehlers-Danlos and Marfan syndromes should be excluded.

Treatment

1. Reassurance concerning the benign nature of this condition is the most important therapeutic measure.
2. Therapeutic doses of aspirin or other nonspecific antiinflammatory drugs (NSAIDs) may be helpful, but patients are often more concerned about the nature of the condition than about therapy.
3. There should be no enforced restriction of physical education activity; specific exercises found to be aggravating may be omitted.

NOCTURNAL LEG PAINS

A traditional term for this common nonspecific benign entity of childhood is *growing pains* (GP). It is best defined as a very painful, self-limited muscle spasm, usually in the lower extremities, which tends to occur late in the day or at night.

Diagnosis

1. Very common childhood complaint starting between 2 and 5 years of age.
2. Seen in both sexes, more often in boys.
3. Often familial, in siblings or parents.
4. Occurs abruptly especially at bedtime, or awakening child from sleep.
5. Symmetrical or unilateral pain, behind knees, or in calves, shins, or soles of feet. Less often in thighs, and infrequently in upper extremities.
6. Often precipitated by exertion, cold weather, or minor illness.

7. Causes child to cry out in pain.
8. Stops in about 20 to 30 min with no sequelae whatsoever the next day.

Etiology

GP are probably caused by muscle cramps in the hamstrings, calves, anterior tibials, peroneals, or small muscles of the feet. Pain has been ascribed to stress from poor leg and foot posture, but this is undocumented.

Treatment

Relief can be obtained at once by manually stretching the spastic muscles. For example, calf pain is relieved by forcibly dorsiflexing the foot.

Differential Diagnosis

Diagnoses of rheumatic fever or rheumatoid arthritis are often made in these children in disregard of the accepted criteria. GP often occur in combination with other musculoskeletal conditions, such as JRA. Growing pains are a separate problem and not a feature of JRA, and can be relieved by being treated in their own right.

BEHAVIORAL DISORDER: PARENT AND CHILD

Bizarre complaints of arthralgia not fitting a recognizable disease entity, and with disability out of proportion to the physical findings, can alert to the likelihood of this etiology. Also no verifiable arthritis will be found on physical or radiologic examination.

It is important to recognize this type of behavioral disorder, so that the physician, family, and psychological counselor may help the child back to a normal social environment.[20]

SECTION D

Crystal Deposition and Disease

Esther Lipstein-Kresch and Robert Greenwald

Several chemically distinct types of crystal deposition disease have been identified as causes of arthritis or periarthritis. Monosodium urate, the most phlogistic of all, is associated with gouty arthritis, while calcium pyrophosphate dihydrate (CaPPi) crystals are responsible for pseudogout. Most re-cently, calcium hydroxyapatite and calcium orthophosphate have been identified in menisci of knees and in other periarticular structures (tendons, ligaments) where bursitis is the predominant clinical manifestation. Steroid crystals injected into joints have also been shown to cause an inflammatory synovitis and should be listed among the crystal deposition diseases that cause arthritis. Gout and pseudogout are the prototype crystal diseases which deserve major discussion.

GOUT

Asymptomatic Hyperuricemia

Asymptomatic hyperuricemia refers to elevated serum uric acid level (greater than 7 mg/dl) in the absence of complications of hyperuricemia, i.e., gouty arthritis, tophi, or renal stones. Asymptomatic hyperuricemia may last for decades without any untoward consequences. Prior to purberty, the serum urate concentration is approximately 3.6 mg/dl in both boys and girls; after puberty, the levels rise more in males than in females, and with menopause the serum urate level in women rises and approaches that in men. Differences in urate clearance may result from hormonal influences of androgens and estrogens, but this is unproven at this time. The variations in serum urate levels help to explain why men develop gout between the third and fifth decades whereas women rarely develop spontaneous primary gout prior to the fifth decade.

Many physicians unnecessarily treat asymptomatic hyperuricemia for fear that renal function will be compromised or gouty arthritis may develop if the biochemical abnormality is left untreated. However, current data suggests that renal function is not necessarily adversely affected by an elevated serum urate concentration. Berger and Yu followed 524 gouty patients over 12 years and found that renal function deterioration was predominantly associated with renal vascular disease attributed to hypertension and nephrosclerosis, not with the presence of hyperuricemia or gout.[4] Furthermore, correction of hyperuricemia with antihyperuricemic agents has no apparent effect on renal function.[25] Therapy in our opinion should therefore be directed toward the control of other associated conditions such as hypertension, obesity, and hyperlipidemia.

Types of Gout

There are primary and secondary forms of gout. Of the primary forms of gout, approximately 99 percent appears related to polygenic inheritance. In this group, 90 percent of the patients show normal or reduced urinary excretion of uric acid and are deemed underexcretors, although some may overproduce as well. Most gouty patients have a lower renal clearance of uric acid than nongouty individuals.[45] In the 10 percent of patients that are overproducers rather than underexcretors, there is a marked acceleration in the rate of purine biosynthesis. In particular, there may be one of three specific enzyme defects which can cause uric acid overproduction: (1) hypoxanthineguanine phosphoribosyl transferase (HGPRT) deficiency; (2) phosphoribosyl pyrophosphate synthetase overactivity; or (3) increased production of ribose-5-phosphate. Complete HGPRT deficiency patients have the Lesch-Nyhan syndrome, a secondary form of gout. Individuals with partial HGPRT deficiency, for the most part, lack the neurological dysfunction (choreoathetosis, spasticity, self-mutilation) and mental and growth retardation seen with complete HGPRT deficiency. They do, however, manifest hyperuricemia, hyperuricaciduria, and gouty arthritis.

In addition to complete HGPRT deficiency, there are other secondary forms of gout, including glucose-6-phosphatase deficiency. Increased nucleic acid turnover, as may occur with chemotherapy of myeloproliferative diseases, will produce hyperuricemia, as will decreased uric acid clearance either as a consequence of reduced functional renal mass or inhibition of secretion and/or enhanced reabsorption of uric acid. Drugs, toxins, or endogenous metabolic products, e.g., lactic acid and ketoacids, can inhibit urate reabsorption or secretion and thereby elevate serum uric acid.

Gouty Arthritis

Gout is an intensely inflammatory joint disorder caused by the deposition of monosodium urate crystals in the joint space. Urate crystals have been associated with attacks of gout as far back as 1899.[19] The identification of urate crystals in synovial fluid is based on their characteristic needle-shaped structure and their location within polymorphonuclear neutrophils. They can be appreciated with light microscopy, but, more definitively, they show negative birefringence with polarizing microscopy. The combination of an acutely inflamed joint with the finding of synovial fluid monosodium urate crystals provides sufficient evidence for the diagnosis of gout.

Several factors may trigger an acute episode. In particular, trauma, alcohol ingestion, surgery, dietary indiscretion, lactic acidosis, ketoacidosis, and infection are the most common culprits in inducing an acute episode of gout. Several of these factors will be discussed further in discussion of the management of gout.

Gouty attacks typically begin with monoarticular disease, although 5 percent of patients may present with polyarticular involvement as an initial manifestation. In at least one-half of the initial attacks, the first metatarsophalangeal joint will be the site of involvement *(podagra)*, and podagra will ultimately occur in 90 percent of gouty patients sometime in the course of their disease. The insteps, ankles, heels, knees, wrists, fingers, and elbows (in decreasing order of frequency) may be involved in initial attacks of gout. The joint involved is typically warm, swollen, erythematous, and exquisitely painful. Hyperesthesia may be present as well. A severe attack may resemble cellulitis with accompanying lymphangitis. Fever, an elevated erythrocyte sedimentation rate, and leukocytosis may be present. An acute episode may last several hours or as long as 3 to 4 weeks, but the average is 3 to 6 days.

When the attack of gout subsides, the patient enters an asymptomatic interval known as *the intercritical period,* which may last several months to years. Some patients never develop a second attack. In Gutman's series,[14] 62 percent of patients had recurrences within the first year, 16 percent in 1 to 2 years, 11 percent in 2 to 5 years, 4 percent in 5 to 10 years, and 7 percent no recurrences in 10 or more years. In untreated patients, as attacks recur, the intercritical period shortens and attacks may become polyarticular; they may have a longer duration, and may be of increased severity. In polyarticular gout, 83 percent of all joints involved are in the lower extremity. With increased frequency of attacks and increased duration, the patient may enter a phase of chronic polyarticular gout without pain-free intervals and with advancing articular disease.

Chronic tophaceous gout may evolve from 3 to 42 years[19] after the initial attack. In Hench's series[19] 72 percent of untreated patients had tophaceous deposits 20 years after their initial attack. The principal determinant of the rate of urate deposition in joints and soft tissue is the serum urate level and the duration of the hyperuricemia. Gutman[13] noted that while patients with tophaceous deposits had serum concentrations greater than 11.0 mg/dl, 722 gouty patients without tophi had a mean serum urate concentration of 9.1 mg/dl.

Urate crystals may deposit in the synovium, in the cartilage, or in the subcutaneous and tendinous tissues of the elbow, hand, foot, knee, and ulnar aspect of the forearm.[43] A classic location for tophi is the helix of the ear. Tophi may be identified by their asymmetry and irregularity; they are hard masses which may produce ulceration of the overlying skin with chalky extrusions (urate crystals). Severe tophaceous gout of the hands, fingers, and feet may produce disabling gross deformities which can progress to crippling by causing extensive destruction of bone and joints.

Prior to the institution of antihyperuricemic drugs, tophi were found in up to 70 percent of patients with gout[19] and destructive joint changes were thus more common. Yu[48] found a 17 percent incidence of tophi in 289 cases reviewed from 1969 to 1973, demonstrating the impact of antihyperuricemic drugs first introduced in 1950.

Roentgenographic Findings

Fusiform soft tissue swelling is found commonly with the initial acute attacks of gout. The swelling is due to synovial effusion and may be seen in the knee, ankle, or small joints of the feet and hands. When tophi are present, soft tissue swelling becomes asymmetrical and permanent (unless there is dissolution of tophi with the use of medications). Tophi are generally not calcified and may cause erosion of the opposing bone or joint. The erosions are usually round or oval-shaped and have a "punched out" appearance with a sclerotic border.[42] The typical location for punched-out lesions is the medial aspect of the head of the first metatarsophalangeal joint. An overhanging edge of bone at the margin of an erosion is characteristic of gout, and is known as Martell's sign.[22] Extensive osteoporosis is not a feature of the disease, although with long-standing gout, osteoporosis occurs most likely from disuse of painful joints. The joint space is remarkably preserved in width until late in the course of articular disease. Erosions, with contiguous soft tissue masses and normal joint spaces, characterize the early stage of tophaceous disease; in later stages, the joint space narrows and bony ankylosis, although rare, may result.[17] With appropriate medications, substantial repair of lytic lesions may occur. Of note is that aseptic necrosis has been reported in a few patients with gout and hyperuricemia.[25]

Associated Conditions

Several associated conditions have been identified with hyperuricemia and gout. Emerson and Knowles noted that subjects with primary gout were an average of 17.8 percent overweight.[10] Obesity may predispose to hyperglycemia in addition to hyperuricemia, and abnormal glucose tolerance tests have been noted in up to 70 percent of patients with gout.[5,7,31,33] Hypertriglyceridemia has been reported in 75 to 84 percent of patients with gout.[2,3,5] Although individual gouty subjects are frequently hypercholesterolemic,[19] several studies have been unable to show a correlation between serum urate and cholesterol values.[3,11] Hypertension is present in one-fourth to one-half of patients with gout.[19,38] Hyperuricemia has been proposed by some as a risk factor for coronary heart disease. It should be noted, however, that in the Tecumseh study,[35] there was no clear association between levels of blood pressure, blood sugar, or serum cholesterol with serum urate concentration when adjustments were made for the effects of age, sex, and relative weight.

The Kidney in Gout

In addition to the aforementioned studies by Berger and Yu on patients with hyperuricemia and renal dysfunction, it should be noted that significant urate nephropathy with urate deposits in the renal interstitial tissue is extremely rare in the absence of gouty arthritis. Uric acid nephropathy, however, may be found in conditions other than gout such as the acute renal failure that may occur in patients with leukemia who receive aggressive chemotherapy. An increased uric acid excretion through the tubules in combination with a low urine pH provides the setting for the precipitation of uric acid in the collecting tubules, which may produce an obstructive uropathy. Anuria may occur with bilateral obstruction.

Gutman and Yu found that the prevalence of uric acid stone formation increased with elevation of the serum urate concentration[15,49]; renal stones may precede the development of gouty arthritis in 40 percent of patients, in some by as much as a decade. For this reason, a history of nephrolithiasis should be sought when a patient presents with the first episode of gouty arthritis.

Treatment of Gout

During an acute attack of gout, when the joint is hot and swollen, rest and appropriate anti-inflammatory agents are indicated. The preferred anti-inflammatory agent is indomethacin, 50 mg three to four times a day until the attack markedly subsides (1 to 2 days), to be followed by tapering doses over the next 3 to 4 days. Active peptic ulcer disease is a contraindication to the use of indomethacin.

Colchicine Colchicine, which had been the "gold standard" up until 1963 when the effectiveness of indomethacin came to light, still has its place in the treatment of the acute attack. Oral colchicine, as traditionally given for acute gout (one tablet every 60 to 90 min), is limited in use by its gastrointestinal toxicity (nausea, vomiting, diarrhea) in as many as 50 to 80 percent of patients, and the preferred route of administration is intravenous. An initial dose of 2 to 3 mg is followed by prompt relief within 12 to 24 h provided that the acute attack was only of several hours duration. Once the treatment is delayed beyond the first 24 h, the response rate decreases. The dose of intravenous colchicine should not exceed 5 mg in a 24-h period since it may cause bone marrow suppression particularly in the presence of liver or renal disease. Intravenous colchicine remains useful as a diagnostic tool when the diagnosis of gout is in question; however, there have been reports of favorable responses to colchicine in pseudogout,[23] calcific tendinitis (hydroxyapatite),[46] sarcoid arthritis, serum sickness, and other inflammatory conditions.

Phenylbutazone Phenylbutazone, which has been used for the treatment of acute gouty arthritis since the early 1950s, is 75 to 90 percent effective in aborting an acute attack. Although lethal bone marrow suppression may occur, it is rare with short-term use of the drug and with doses not exceeding 600 mg/day (200 mg, three times a day). However, sodium retention is a major problem, and in view of the substantially lesser toxicity of newer nonsteroidal anti-inflammatory drugs, this agent should be considered archaic in the current era. Active ulcer disease also contraindicates its use. In addition, caution must be exercised when the drug is used with oral anticoagulants or oral hypoglycemic agents since phenylbutazone may displace these compounds from albumin and potentiate their effect.

Other Anti-inflammatory Drugs Other nonsteroidal anti-inflammatory drugs including naproxen, ibuprofen, and fenoprofen have been used with good results. Systemic corticosteroids are not generally indicated in acute gout. Intraarticular steroids, although useful in relieving pain, should be reserved for the patient with a contraindication to the use of NSAIDs and colchicine, or for the patient who fails on these medications. ACTH injection has also been used in patients for whom no other therapy is acceptable.

Prophylaxis

Prophylaxis of gouty episodes with daily colchicine has been advocated by several authors.[19,26] Colchicine prophylaxis is essential in the patient who has frequent attacks of gout. The dose is 0.6 mg once or twice a day. Indomethacin has been used prophylactically in doses of 25 mg two to four times a day with some success, and can be used for the patient who fails on the colchicine regime or who is intolerant to it.

Once a patient is diagnosed as having gout, some physicians treat the patient only with colchicine prophylaxis and ignore the hyperuricemia, whereas others believe that the first gouty attack is the endpoint of 20 to 30 years of hyperuricemia and that the patient must be treated with uric acid–lowering agents, either the uricosurics (probenecid, sulfinpyrazone) or allopurinol. Uricosuric agents reduce the serum urate by enhancing the renal excretion of uric acid, and are indicated in patients with primary gout who excrete less than 700 mg/day of uric acid in their urine. (A 24-h urine collection for uric acid, with the patient following a purine-restricted diet for 3 days in advance as well as on the day of the collection, is generally recommended for initial evaluation of all new cases of primary gout.) Serum urate is lowered in 75 to 80 percent of patients on these drugs. The uricosuric agents are known to be safe after more than 30 years of clinical use and should be first-line therapy for gouty patients with hyperuricemia, good renal function, and no history of renal calculi who excrete less than 700 mg/day of uric acid in the urine.

Uric acid synthesis is decreased by allopurinol, an inhibitor of the enzyme xanthine oxidase which catalyzes the conversion of xanthine to uric acid. The indications for allopurinol include (1) gouty individuals with a history of renal calculi, (2) patients with tophaceous disease, (3) failure of uricosuric drugs to produce a serum urate less than 7 mg/dl, (4) patients intolerant to the uricosuric agents, (5) patients with renal insufficiency and glomerular filtration rate under 30 ml/h, and (6) patients with myeloproliferative disorders prior to the initiation of chemotherapy for prophylaxis against uric acid nephropathy.

Several adjuvant therapies can be advocated for gouty patients. Weight reduction may have a role in reducing the serum urate concentration. The gouty patient should avoid foods with excessively high purine content such as organ meats, sardines, yeast, and anchovies. A restricted purine diet will reduce urinary excretion of uric acid by 200 to 400 mg/ day and lower the serum urate by 1 mg/100 ml. Intense dietary restriction of red meats and other moderate purine content foods is no longer recommended in an era of powerful pharmacological agents. Binges of alcohol produce a lactic acidemia which exacerbates hyperuricemia and may provoke an acute gouty episode. In addition, chronic alcohol use may result in increased hyperuricemia and hyperuricaciduria by stimulating increased purine production.[21] Finally, gouty attacks are seen in association with trauma and are not infrequent as postoperative complications.

The hypertriglyceridemia associated with gout may be treated by a combination of weight reduction and medications (clofibrate or nicotinic acid). Hypertension should be treated, and thiazide diuretics may be given despite their hyperuricemic effect. Through a combination of weight reduction, low purine diet, avoidance of alcohol, and the appropriate use of medications for hypertension, hypertriglyceridemia, and hyperuricemia, the gouty patient can preserve renal function, mitigate the pain of arthritic episodes, and perhaps even reduce chances of a cardiovascular or cerebrovascular event.

PSEUDOGOUT

Calcium pyrophosphate deposition disease (CPDD) is an inflammatory joint disorder caused by the deposition of CaPPi (calcium pyrophosphate dihydrate crystals). These crystals are typically rhomboid in shape and may vary in size. Under polarizing microscopy they appear pale-blue and positively birefringent (unlike the needle-shaped crystals of gout that are negatively birefringent). Like gout, an attack of CPDD may be triggered by trauma, medical illness, surgery, and other conditions of metabolic imbalance. CPDD may cause a spectrum of rheumatologic diseases with varying clinical manifestations.

Pseudogout and Chondrocalcinosis

Pseudogout (type A CPPD) is a clinical pattern of disease consisting of acute episodes of arthritis affecting predominantly the large joints associated with the deposition of CaPPi crystals. The term was coined in 1962 by McCarty et al. who were investigating patients with goutlike attacks whose synovial fluid contained nonurate crystals.[23,29,30] These crystals were identified subsequently as CaPPi by their x-ray diffraction powder pattern.[20] Of interest is the fact that the same clinical entity had been described 5 years earlier by Zitnan and Sitaj who named it chondrocalcinosis polyarticularis (familiaris).[42,50] These Czechoslovakian workers noted calcific deposits within the cartilage of the knee in 27 patients with a goutlike pattern of arthritis.

To date, several other crystals including calcium oxalate, calcium hydroxyapatite, dicalcium phosphate dihydrate, and as yet undefined crystals have been associated with cartilage calcification (chondrocalcinosis). It is therefore incorrect to equate pseudogout with chondrocalcinosis, as not only may the chondrocalcinosis be due to crystals other than CaPPi, but, in turn, the clinical picture of pseudogout with the presence of CaPPi crystals may not be associated radiographically with cartilage calcification.

The pseudogout pattern makes up approximately 25 percent of the clinical spectrum of CPDD. The attacks are generally self-limited, lasting between 1 and 28 days. The joints involved are typically the knees (by far the most common), hips, shoulders, elbows, ankles, and wrists. As in gout, the joints may be swollen, warm, and painful with occasional polyarticular and/or asymmetric involvement. Surgery or severe medical illness may provoke attacks. Systemic signs of inflammation including a moderate degree of leukocytosis, a high erythrocyte sedimentation rate, and a low-grade fever may be found.

Pseudorheumatoid Arthritis

Pseudorheumatoid athritis (type B CPDD) accounts for 5 percent of CPDD disease. It is characterized by almost continuous acute attacks of arthritis in a number of joints. They may last weeks to months affecting the wrists, metacarpophalangeal joints, elbows, knees, and shoulders. The features simulating rheumatoid arthritis include morning stiffness, fatigue, synovial thickening, with eventual development of flexion contractures, and an elevated ESR.

Pseudoosteoarthritis

Pseudoosteoarthritis (type C CPDD) with episodic attacks accounts for 25 percent of CPDD disease. It is marked by a chronic progressive arthritis with superimposed acute or subacute attacks. Joints commonly involved include the knees, wrists, metacarpophalangeal joints, hips, shoulders, elbows, and ankles. The joint involvement is symmetrical with flexion contractures of the knees and elbows often noted. The features of osteoarthritis include chronicity and osteophytosis seen on radiological examination.

Pseudoosteoarthritis

Pseudoosteoarthritis (type D CPDD) without acute attacks accounts for another 25 percent of the patients with CPDD disease. The joint distribution is as in type C, but without acute exacerbations. Women predominate in this classification.

Lanthenic, or Asymptomatic, CPDD disease

Lanthenic CPDD disease (type E) accounts for 20 percent of CPPD cases. This group of patients may become symptomatic and enter one of the other four classifications, or they may stay asymptomatic for life. The incidence of chondrocalcinosis has varied in different series from less than 0.5 percent[42,43] to 30 percent. The incidence of CPDD accounting for the chondrocalcinosis, however, is closer to 5 percent.[27] The number of patients in the asymptomatic group with CPDD may be underestimated. Ellman and Levin's series[9] of 58 patients whose mean age was 83 showed a 27 percent incidence of chondrocalcinosis with the majority of patients being asymptomatic, again reinforcing the fact that the mere presence of calcium in cartilage is not enough to cause clinical disease, and a large asymptomatic group of patients exists.

Other Presentations of CPDD Disease

There are less common presentations of CPDD, described as pseudotabes or destructive arthropathy where osteonecrosis is a prominent feature. Such presentations may involve the knees, wrists, shoulders, or ankles. A neurological deficit need not be present. Menkes[32] analyzed 15 patients, of whom 14 were women. Knees and shoulders were afflicted most frequently, and the arthropathy had the appearance of severe osteoarthritis, with exuberant osteophyte formation, and large subchondral bone cysts on radiological examination. In the shoulder, tendon avulsions and rotary cuff tears occurred. CaPPi crystals were found in the synovial fluid. Indistinguishable from this arthropathy is that reported by Jacobelli et al.[18] where four patients with evidence of latent syphilis or tabes dorsalis had CaPPi deposition in the damaged knee joints. A relationship between traumatic injury to a joint and pseudogout or chondrocalcinosis has been reported by several authors.[1,24,44]

Types A through E and the pseudotabes form of CPDD are sporadic or idiopathic forms of the disease which rarely occur prior to the sixth decade. They are to be distinguished from the hereditary group of CPDD and the secondary forms of CPDD associated with metabolic and degenerative disorders which may present as early as the second decade.

Hereditary Forms of CPDD

Three major studies have revealed a familial nature of CPDD. Zitnan and Sitaj[51] in the Czechoslovakian series followed 33 patients for 10 years. A severe form of disease was noted to start at a younger age, with more intense episodes of synovitis and eventual crippling leading to contractures of the wrists, knees, and elbows. Radiological findings were consistent with severe osteoarthritis (large spurs, cartilage destruction, and subchondral cyst formation) and chondrocalcinosis.

Nyulassy et al[36] found a probable association of chondrocalcinosis with the haplotype HLA-A2,w5; whether the haplotype is representative of inbreeding or an actual marker of chondrocalcinosis is debatable. The Chiloe Islands series[39–41] of patients similarly showed aggressive CPDD in young patients in the third and fourth decades with very active synovitis. In some patients, the joint calcification and cartilage destruction led to bony ankylosis. No HLA associations were found by Reginato et al. A milder form of hereditary CPDD in the Dutch was reviewed by Vanderkorst.[49] Patients in this series had mild attacks which were infrequent but associated with CaPPi crystals. The hereditary cases appearing early in life are accompanied by much more inflammatory and destructive disease.

Associated Conditions

There are a number of diseases that have been associated with CaPPi crystal deposition. The most commonly associated disease is osteoarthritis. The incidence of patients with both CPDD and degenerative disease in different series has varied from 40 to 70 percent.[16] It is possible, however, that what is being called osteoarthritis is a result of CPDD and its arthropathy. Gout coexisting with CPDD has been reported frequently,[6] although other studies have not substantiated an increased incidence of gout.[12] There is no definite established association between diabetes mellitus and CPDD. Although Moskowitz found a 28 percent incidence of rheumatoid arthritis in patients with CPPD,[34] others have found no increased association.[12]

Hyperparathyroidism and hemochromatosis are strongly associated with CPDD. The increased incidence of hyperparathyroidism in CPDD has been substantiated by several studies.[16] The study by McCarty et al found a 15 percent increase of hyperparathyroidism in 45 cases of CPDD.[30] Of interest, Phelps and Hawker found elevated immunoreactive parathyroid hormone levels in 10 of 26 patients with CPDD,[37] and McCarty et al found elevated parathyroid hormone levels in osteoarthritis. Of 61 patients with hemochromatosis, 41 percent were shown to have chondrocalcinosis.[16] The most striking feature about the arthropathy in these patients is the involvement of the second and third metacarpophalangeal joints. Calcification of the knees, wrists, hips, and symphysis pubis were also affected. The arthropathy correlated with the degree of overall hyaline cartilage calcification. Hypothyroid joint effusions may contain CaPPi crystals, but attacks occur typically after initiation of thyroid replacement.[8] Other conditions with a probable association with CPDD are hypophosphatasia, ochronosis, Wilson disease, and hypomagnesemia.[30]

Radiographic Findings

Radiologically, the arthropathy of CaPPi crystals simulates degenerative joint disease with narrowing of the articular space, osteophytosis, bony sclerosis, and subchondral cyst formation. Several features of CPDD, however, differ from primary osteoarthritis: (1) the location of the arthropathy is atypical for primary osteoarthritis with calcifications of the triangular ligament of the wrist, elbow, and glenohumeral joints; (2) the cysts associated with CPDD may lead to large radiolucent areas in the subchondral bone which have been mistaken for bony tumors; (3) bone changes may be rapidly progressive in CPDD as depicted by the neuroarthropathy or Charcot pattern of disease that is seen predominantly in the knees, shoulders, and hips. Primary osteoarthritis is more of an indolent disease.

Calcifications related to CaPPi may be located in articular cartilage, fibrocartilage, hyaline cartilage, synovium, or fibrous capsules and ligaments. Fibrocartilage is most densely calcified in the meniscus of the knee, triangular ligament of the wrist, symphysis pubis, and the glenoid and acetabular labra. Tendon and ligament calcifications are most frequently apparent in the Achilles tendon, triceps, quadriceps, and supraspinatus tendon.[43] Severe patellofemoral compartment involvement should suggest the diagnosis of CPDD. There is an unusual predilection for the radiocarpal compartment of the wrist, the most common site of abnormality radiographically. Involvement of the glenohumeral joint is another common site for CPDD.

Treatment

Anti-inflammatory agents are the mainstay of treatment of CPDD. Indomethacin in doses of 50 mg three to four times a day for the acute exacerbation with gradual tapering is accepted therapy. Other NSAIDs may be beneficial. The diagnostic aspiration itself may be beneficial. Although systemic steroids are not indicated, intraarticular treatment may be used sparingly for acute exacerbations of one or two joints. Intravenous colchicine has been reported to have an 80 percent response rate, although there is no role for prophylactic oral colchicine therapy. Rest of the acutely inflamed joint is indicated for any acute inflammatory process. When there is an associated disease (e.g., hyperparathyroidism, hemochromatosis, ochronosis, hypothyroidism, etc.), treatment of the underlying disease in conjunction with NSAIDs is indicated.

SECTION E

Systemic Lupus Erythematosus and Other Vasculitides

Allen P. Kaplan

SYSTEMIC LUPUS ERYTHEMATOSUS

Epidemiology

Incidence

The incidence of systemic lupus erythematosus is said to be between 6.4 to 7.6 cases per 100,000 in population.[23] The disease affects individuals of all races, but it is clearly more prominent in women, black women in particular.[68] For women between the ages of 15 to 64 years, the incidence can be as high as 1 in 700, and if restricted to black women, it is about 1 in 300. The peak age of onset is 15 to 25 years with a mean of about 30.

Etiology

Systemic lupus erythematosus (SLE) is a disease of unknown origin which causes inflammation in virtually any organ of the body and is characterized by the synthesis of a wide variety of autoantibodies and the formation of circulating immune complexes. Considerations regarding etiology have, in recent years, focused on the possibility that it is a chronic viral illness and there is some evidence to support this theory, but no proof. Electron microscopic observations from patients with lupus glomerulonephritis revealed inclusion bodies resembling viral particles,[28] but further studies demonstrated that these tubuloreticular structures are nonspecific manifestations of cell injury. In a dog model of systemic lupus, type C RNA coronaviruses have been found, and in some studies such viral antigens have been reported in the tissues of patients with systemic lupus.[48] But these studies have represented sporadic observations, and there is nothing to suggest that the viruses or viral antigens seen *caused* the disease. Further, human serum normally has low titers of "natural" antibody to mammalian type C retroviruses, thus complicating interpretation of results regarding specificity of any immune response seen to the inciting antigen.

Animal Studies Studies of mice that spontaneously get systemic lupus have frequently been used as a model of the human disease, and such studies also suggest a viral etiology as well as genetic predisposition and hormonal effects.[70] The best-studied is a cross between the New Zealand Black and New Zealand White mouse (NZB/NZW) which dies of SLE in about 1 year, usually due to glomerulonephritis. These mice harbor a variety of viruses, one of which stimulates a marked antibody response to a viral envelope protein. An antigen-antibody complex of this protein can be identified in renal deposits and appears to be pathogenic for the nephritis.[74] But the virus cannot be demonstrated to be etiologic in terms of the immune abnormalities seen or perpetuation of the auto-immune process. Like the human disease, the mice do make all sorts of autoantibodies including those to red cells (to cause hemolytic anemia), antinuclear antibody (ANA), antibody to double-stranded DNA (anti–ds DNA), etc. Virtually all the mice which develop clinically significant disease are female. Yet other mouse strains can get lupus; in some, one cannot consistently demonstrate viral particles in tissues, and in others there is no sex predilection, and there is at least one strain in which male mice get lupus. Thus, no unifying theme emerges from animal studies that can be applied to the human disease in terms of etiology other than the fact that only certain strains acquire it, and for a given strain, there are strong sex influences. The genetic element could be a function of viral susceptibility or viral transmission, or both.

Genetic Influences A genetic predisposition can certainly be extended to humans. There is an association of systemic lupus with certain histocompatibility types, particularly those associated with the D locus which deals with immune responsiveness and is located on chromosome 6 in humans. HLA-DR3 and -DR2 are strongly associated with SLE, and familial aggregation of cases has been described which is suggestive of a genetic predisposition.[56] Moreover, relatives of SLE patients have an incidence of autoantibody formation even if clinically significant disease is not evident. When monozygotic and dizygotic twins are compared, there is close to a 50 percent concordance for SLE in the monozygotic tissues whereas dizygotic tissues are no more likely to get it than the population at large. This suggests a definite genetic factor.

Hormonal Influences Hormonal influences are certainly one susceptibility factor since the female-male ratio for SLE in man is about 10:1 in most studies. In animal models that are sex-associated, any manipulation that alters the animals hormonal status affects the disease in a predictable manner. For example, NZB and NZW mice that get SLE are virtually all female. Giving estrogen worsens the disease, whereas castration or administration of testosterone decreases the severity and prolongs life span. Estrogen increases autoantibody and immune complex formation, whereas testosterone prevents it.[60]

Environmental Influences There are also environmental influences that affect the disease process but are not really etiologic. Exposure to sunlight (ultraviolet) can exacerbate the skin lesions of systemic lupus and at times, induce systemic attacks. There is also a syndrome of drug-induced lupus, most commonly caused by the antihypertensive agent hydralazine, the cardiac antiarrhythmic, procainamide or isoniazid.[3] In each case, there is an association with the inability of patients to rapidly inactivate these compounds by acetylation. Patients with this acquired form of lupus have low levels of the enzyme acetyl transferase which increases their likelihood to have a lupuslike disorder.[24,25] In most cases (but not

all) the syndrome is reversible when the drug is stopped and the disorder, when present, tends to be milder, usually with little or no CNS or renal disease and absence of anti-DNA antibodies. In those few patients who do not remit within 1 or 2 months after stopping the drug, there may have been true induction of the systemic disorder by a drug.

Pathogenesis

Systemic lupus erythematosus can be viewed as a prototype of immunologic-mediated tissue injury or more specifically one of the major disorders whose manifestations are largely (but not exclusively) caused by circulating immune complexes. Patients are characterized by the synthesis of abnormal quantities of antibody that are directed against normal body constituents, i.e., autoantibodies. The combination of such antibodies with circulating antigenic material (circulating immune complexes) or reaction of antibodies with cells or tissues leads to tissue injury, inflammation, and clinical symptoms. The formation of such antibodies implies an abnormality of immunoregulation, the cause of which is presently unknown. As can be seen in Fig. 19-10, the synthesis of immunoglobulin is performed by plasma cells, cells that are derived from B lymphocytes. The B lymphocyte possesses surface immunoglobulin, but is not secretory and becomes so only after differentiating to a plasma cell. The specificity of the immunoglobulin on the surface of B cells is in general the same as the immunoglobulin it is destined to eventually secrete. It is now known that there are subpopulations of B cells (clones) that possess on their surface autoantibodies, i.e., immunoglobulin capable of reacting with normal body constituents that is normally not expressed to a significant degree. But the potential to do so is present and somehow limited by normal control mechanisms. For synthesis of most antibodies when an immunization occurs, a three-cell system is needed. Accessory cells (e.g., macrophages, dendritic cells,

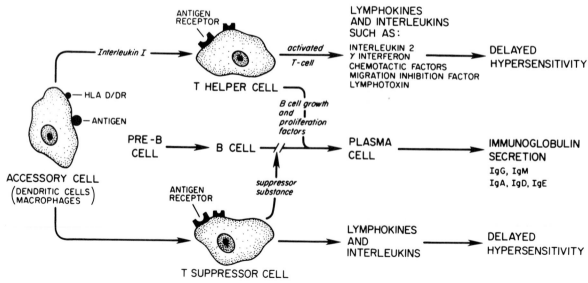

Figure 19-10 Requirements for cellular immunity and antibody production demonstrating the interactions among accessory cells, T lymphocytes, and B cells.

TABLE 19-12 Autoantibodies and Clinical Associations in Systemic Lupus Erythematosus

Antibody	Common or laboratory manifestation
Anti-double-stranded DNA	Nephritis, skin disease, rim or peripheral pattern ANA
Anti-single-stranded DNA	—
Anti-nucleohistone	(+) LE prep, homogeneous pattern ANA
Anti-Sm antigen	SLE pattern ANA
Antiribonucleoprotein (RNP)	Mixed connective tissue disease
Antihistone antibodies (hydralazine, procainamide)	Drug-induced lupus syndrome
Anticardiolipin	False-positive serology
Antiplatelet lipid (exogenous) paradoxical predisposition to thrombosis	Lupus anticoagulant
Anti-RBC (Rh) antibodies	Coombs' test positive, autoimmune hemolytic anemia
Antiplatelet antibody	Thrombocytopenia
Anti-WBC antibody, leukoagglutinins	Leukopenia
Anti-basement membrane	Lupus band test, skin disease
Antilymphocyte antibody (cross-reaction with neurons)	Decreased T suppressor cells (?)
Antineuronal antibody	CNS lupus
Anti-SS-A (anti-RO)	ANA negative or subacute cutaneous lupus
Antithyroid antibodies (thyroglobulin, microsomal)	Hashimoto thyroiditis

cutaneous Langerhans cells) interact with antigen, process it (mechanism as yet unclear), and "present" modified antigen to lymphocytes. Usually this includes a T (thymic-derived) cell which is termed a *T helper cell* since it cooperates with B cells, leading to proliferation and differentiation of the B cells into plasma cells. At the same time, other types of T cells are also activated which dampen either the T helper cell and/or the B cell; these are called *T suppressor cells.* In a normal immune response there is a proper balance between helper and suppressor influences; antibody combines with antigen and clears the antigen; and if no further antigen is supplied, immunity results. An example would be measles infection in which the measles virus acts as the stimulus to antibody formation. Gradually the titer rises, the antibody combines with the virus, and immune complexes lodge in the skin; at this time the characteristic maculopapular rash is seen. Then the virus is cleared, a residual antibody remains, and synthesis of antibody continues at a low but slowly diminishing rate unless virus is again contacted. Then with exposure, a booster response with rapid elevation of IgG antibody occurs so that the virus is eliminated (or at least prevented from reproducing) and no clinical illness is observed, i.e., immunity. However, in autoimmune diseases such as SLE, there appears to be protracted immunoglobulin formation, antigen remains present (or is continually reformed), and immune complex–mediated tissue injury is ongoing.

As can be seen in Fig. 19-10, the types of imbalance that could cause augmented antibody formation would include (1) an increase in T cell help, (2) a decrease in T cell suppression, (3) autonomous hyperactivity of B cells not properly regulated by T-cell influences. A multitude of studies bearing on this issue have been published and the consensus is that patients with SLE have evidence of mechanisms 2 and 3. That is, their B cells are hyperfunctional, and they also have a diminished number and function of T suppressor cells.[14,21,62] Both of these would contribute to excessive immunoglobulin production, and the hypergammaglobulinemia one sees in SLE patients is likely the result. However, within this generalized (called polyclonal) augmented response there is concomitant synthesis of increased immunoglobulin directed against a host of specific antigens. Among these are those antibodies directed against nuclear antigens, i.e., the antinuclear antibodies that are so frequently associated with SLE. Table 19-12 shows the wide variety of identified autoantibodies made by patients with SLE and some of their clinical consequences, where identifiable.

ANA-Negative SLE One of the hallmarks of SLE has been the positive ANA or antinuclear antibody. This is present at some point in time in 85 to 90 percent of patients with SLE. A small number of patients have so-called ANA-negative SLE, which differs somewhat from the more typical presentation of SLE and appear to be a distinctive subpopulation with particularly prominent cutaneous manifestations.[69] ANA testing is performed by immunofluorescence and represents many antigen-antibody systems having different fluorescent patterns. Some patterns are associated with more serious disease manifestations, but a significant titer ($> 1:64$) of any would be reported as a positive ANA.

Immunologic Reactions Two types of immunologic reactions are seen in patients with SLE. One type has specificity for a cell or tissue, e.g., anti-RBC antibodies that are associated with hemolytic anemia or antithyroid antibodies that can be associated with clinical thyroiditis. On the other hand, there can be circulating complexes of antigen and antibody (e.g., DNA–anti-DNA complexes) which deposit in tissue and cause inflammation.[2,53] These complexes have no specificity for the organ or tissue involved and are the prototype reaction of the immune complex–mediated disorder. Alternatively, it is possible to have antigen first bind to some specific component of an organ and then have circulating antibody combine with antigen, thus forming the immune complex in situ; the net result is, in general, the same.

The causes of inflammation and tissue destruction in SLE can be summarized as follows: (1) immune complexes lodge in vessel walls or within tissues (e.g., glomerular basement membrane) and fix complement; (2) vasodilation occurs due to anaphylatoxin-induced histamine release from tissue mast cells; (3) neutrophils plus monocytes or macrophages are recruited to the site of inflammation via C5a chemotactic factor; (4) neutrophils are then activated; they phagocytose immune complexes, secrete proteolytic enzymes, and initiate local blood coagulation by release of tissue thromboplastin; (5) tissue is enzymatically degraded; fibrin forms and is then partially degraded by plasmin due to activation of local fibrinolytic mechanisms. The combination of partially degraded fibrin and the necrotizing inflammatory reaction is termed *fibrinoid necrosis.*[43] If such a process is not rapidly reversed, healing occurs, but not without significant tissue damage and resultant organ impairment.

Clinical Features (Table 19-13)

At the onset or during acute exacerbation of systemic lupus erythematosus, a variety of nonspecific symptoms may be present. A feeling of fatigue is evident in 70 to 80 percent of patients, and the incidence of febrile reactions is high.[59] All such patients are, of course, evaluated for possible infection and any found is treated. But it is not unusual for SLE patients to present with fever, either alone or in association with organ involvement, and the incidence of infection in SLE is no higher than that of the general population. Any increased incidence of infection seen has been due to therapy, i.e., corticosteroids and immunosuppressive agents.

Joint Involvement

One of the most common clinical manifestations of SLE is joint involvement. Acute arthritis with redness, tenderness,

TABLE 19-13   Manifestation of Symptoms Associated with Systemic Lupus Erythematosus and Therapy

Manifestation	Therapy
Skin rash, malar rash	No therapy
Maculopapular rashes or discoid lesions	Hydroxychloroquine, topical corticosteroids
Vasculitis	Systemic corticosteroids
Bullous lesions	Systemic corticosteroids
Arthralgias	NSAIDs; systemic steroids if arthritis is unresponsive
Raynaud's phenomenon	Nifedipine, avoidance of cold and vasoconstrictor
Pleuritis	NSAIDs; systemic steroids for prominent effusion
Pericarditis, myocarditis	Systemic corticosteroids
Fever	Aspirin, other NSAIDs
Renal disease	Systemic steroids and azathioprine or Cytoxan
CNS lupus-diffuse cerebritis	High-dose corticosteroids; focal vasculitis: short-term plasmapheresis, Cytoxan
Thrombosis, hemorrhage	Cytoxan
Hemolytic anemia	Corticosteroids
Autoimmune thrombocytopenia	Corticosteroids
Aplastic anemia	Corticosteroids, plasmapheresis
Circulatory anticoagulants	Plasmapheresis, steroids, Cytoxan

and swelling most commonly affects the proximal interphalangeal joints, the metacarpophalangeal joints, and the knees and wrists, although virtually any joint can be involved. Arthralgias and/or myalgias in the absence of overt arthritis is even more common. Although deforming arthritis is occasionally seen in SLE, most commonly there is absence of significant deformity or radiographic evidence of erosive disease. The synovium in SLE has synovial lining cell proliferation, perivascular mononuclear cell reaction, and scattered areas of fibrinoid necrosis of small vessels. There is absence of pannus formation; thus the invasion of cartilage, bone, and surrounding connective tissue is far less than is seen in rheumatoid arthritis.

Cutaneous Disease

The skin is one of the major organ systems affected in SLE. The typical transient erythematous blush over the cheeks and bridge of the nose is the "butterfly" rash (Fig. 19-11). This rash does not scar and is often induced by sun exposure. An erythematous maculopapular rash may also be seen that is photosensitive and can occur in virtually any part of the body. These may or may not heal with scarring or with some residual hyperpigmentation. Lesions of discoid lupus may also be present. This rash occurs in isolated form in many patients who never develop serological or systemic manifestations of disease. In a small number of patients, the systemic disease begins after 25 or 30 years of discoid lesions. On the other hand, discoid lesions can occur concomitantly or during the course of SLE. These lesions start as papules or plaques typically located on the face, scalp, or upper thorax. The lesion enlarges; it has a central atrophic and often depressed area surrounded by an elevated, erythematous, and often hyperkeratotic periphery. The lesion is reminiscent of a fungus infection (tinea). By immunofluorescence one can demonstrate the presence of immune complexes and complement (C3) along the basement membrane in involved and uninvolved skin in systemic lupus. This is called a positive *lupus band test.* In discoid lupus, similar findings are seen in lesional skin but uninvolved skin is negative.[31,65]

Vasculitic cutaneous lesions can be seen by inflammation of small- and medium-sized vessels. These may ulcerate and heal very slowly. They are commonly seen on the extensor surfaces of the forearm, or the fingertips, and in the lower leg near the malleoli. In some, these lesions are associated with cryoglobulinemia.[34,72] Other cutaneous lesions may also be a manifestation of the underlying disease. These include chronic urticaria (which is seen in 5 to 10 percent of patients), angioedema, bullous lesions (subepidermal with antibasement membrane antibodies as is seen in pemphigoid), purpura [due to thrombocytopenia, vasculitis (palpable purpura), or steroid therapy], mucosal ulcerations, particularly of the mouth and nose, and nail deformities. Alopecia is commonly seen and can be diffuse or patchy, particularly when new hair growth commences as symptoms remit. However, discoid LE scalp lesions cause permanent hair loss due to atrophy and loss of cutaneous appendages.

Renal Disease

Renal disease can be focal (usually mild) proliferative glomerulonephritis, diffuse proliferative glomerulonephritis (severe), membranous lupus nephritis, and mesangial lupus nephritis. These, of course, are categorizations by biopsy,[5] yet it has been shown that one cannot accurately predict the biopsy pattern based upon the clinical presentation. In general, the presentation is with hematuria, proteinuria, and pyuria in varying combinations, nephrotic syndrome if proteinuria is severe (most common in diffuse proliferative and membranous), and red cell casts if a diffuse nephritis is acute. These can occur either with or without evidence of renal failure as assessed by BUN and creatinine. Interstitial nephritis is also common with inflammation surrounding the tubules. In each of these, immunofluorescent studies reveal immune complex

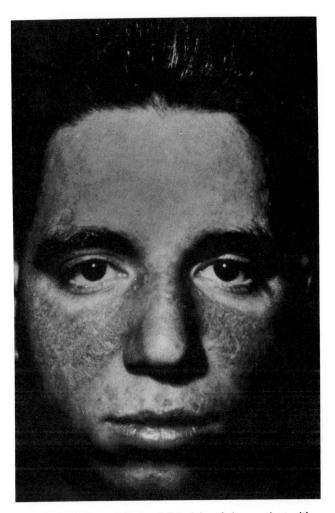

Figure 19-11 Typical "butterfly" facial rash in a patient with systemic lupus erythematosus. *(From The American Rheumatism Association slide collection. Reproduced with permission of The Arthritis Foundation.)*

deposition and complement (Clq, C4, C3) in the glomerulus (subendothelial, intrabasement membrane, or subepithelial), mesangium, and along renal tubule basement membrane in varying degrees depending on the type and distribution of inflammation seen. Biopsy specimens can be further categorized as to indices of activity and sclerosis. High-activity lesions include evidence of cellular proliferation, fibrinoid necrosis, nuclear debris, wire-loop lesions, hyaline thrombi, etc., and are more likely to be responsive to anti-inflammatory therapy (steroids or immunosuppression). More sclerotic patterns suggest lack of reversibility and an increased likelihood of progressive or fixed renal failure.[7]

Gastrointestinal Effects

Abdominal pain is common and can be nonlocalized as evidence of a serositis (peritonitis); ascites, although uncommon, can be seen. Bowel infarction due to mesenteric vasculitis must be considered; then an acute abdomen with localizing signs and guaiac-positive stools may be seen. An associated hepatitis, which can be acute or chronically active, may be seen as part of systemic lupus. Liver enlargement is commonly associated, but jaundice and progression to a cirrhotic picture is rare. Splenomegaly, however, is present in 20 percent of patients with SLE, and lymphadenopathy is similarly seen in 15 to 20 percent.

Cardiac Disease

The most frequent cardiac manifestation of SLE is pericarditis, which is seen in 25 percent of patients.[37] It can present with chest pain, cardiac enzyme elevations, and characteristic ST-T changes with elevated ST segments having a "scooped" appearance and inverted T waves. Pericardial fluid accumulation typically occurs and can be discovered by echocardiogram, but cardiac tamponade is rare.

Myocardial involvement that is clinically significant is less common than pericarditis, although the enzyme elevations typically seen with the latter imply an associated superficial myocarditis in virtually all cases. In some, however, inflammation throughout the myocardium can lead to arrhythmias, heart block of varying degree, and congestive heart failure. Coronary arteritis can also be seen and can present as a myocardial infarction.[10]

Valvular disease is commonly manifest but rarely is of clinical significance. The endocarditis of Libman and Sacks[49] is characterized by vegetations made up of fibrin and platelet thrombi seen along the valve edge and occasionally along the chordae tendineae and papillary muscles. Lesions are most often seen on the mitral and tricuspid valves, and a murmur of mitral insufficiency is commonly heard. Flow murmurs due to anemia are also common.

Pulmonary Effects

Pleuritic pain is commonly seen in patients with systemic lupus, and about one-third have a pleural effusion during the course of their disease. The fluid is due to a pleuritis, and the effusion has the characterization of an exudate. Parenchymal lung disease is less common and can be present as a pneumonitis (which is difficult to distinguish from infection upon initial presentation) or a diffuse interstitial pneumonitis.[35] The latter presents primarily with dyspnea or exertion; it is often a chronic process, and can lead to a restrictive lung picture with diminished volumes and abnormal diffusion capacity. Less common is the occasional patient with pulmonary vasculitis.

Hematologic Findings

Anemia, leukopenia, and thrombocytopenia can all be seen in patients with systemic lupus. The anemia is typically normocytic normochromic and can be simply the anemia seen with "chronic disease" with diminished iron utilization and marrow red cell release. More severe is hemolytic anemia (as diagnosed with positive direct and indirect Coombs tests) caused by IgG antibody directed toward red blood cell antigens. Coated red cells are sequestered in the spleen to mark-

edly shorten their half-life, thus the hemolysis is extravascular. Leukopenia is very common in SLE patients with active disease. This may be due to antibodies directed to neutrophils, and leukoagglutinins can sometimes be demonstrated. Thrombocytopenia is also common and can be an autoimmune phenomenon that is indistinguishable from idiopathic thrombocytopenia purpura. An IgG antibody directed to platelet surface antigens is made, and platelets are destroyed as they traverse the splenic sinusoids. Hypersplenism, in the absence of antibody directed to any blood element, can cause a pancytopenia and may be present alone or in combination with any of the aforementioned manifestations. Finally, severe pancytopenia can be due to a marrow aplasia; in some cases this has been shown to be due to autoantibodies directed to marrow stem cells or early precursors of blood cells. A bone marrow test performed on patients with pancytopenia can help distinguish marrow arrest from peripheral destruction. In the latter circumstances, compensatory marrow hyperplasia would be anticipated.

Abnormalities of blood coagulation are common in patients with systemic lupus but most do not lead to bleeding. The "lupus anticoagulant" is due to an autoantibody directed to the phospholipid used to perform the partial thromboplastin time (PTT).[64,67] The PTT can be markedly prolonged, the prothrombin time less so, and the thrombin time is normal. The antibody does not appear to be directed to platelet phospholipid and in vivo coagulation is normal. It does cross-react with cardiolipin,[51] and DNA and may be responsible for the false-positive serology[18] seen in lupus patients. Paradoxically, the presence of this autoantibody seems to be associated with an increased incidence of thrombosis.[12] Of course, vasculitis is also a predisposing factor to thrombosis.[4] True anticoagulants directed against factors VIII or IX (and less commonly other coagulation factors) have been described; these can be associated with severe bleeding as is seen in hemophiliacs.[57]

Effect on Nervous System

Systemic lupus commonly affects the peripheral or central nervous system, and CNS lupus has now replaced renal disease as the most common cause of fatalities. Approximately 10 percent of patients have a peripheral neuropathy, most commonly sensory, but combined sensory and motor involvement can be seen.[22] A Guillain-Barré syndrome with an acute motor ascending paralysis is an uncommon presentation. Cranial nerve involvement is less common than peripheral nerve involvement, but virtually any nerve can be affected.

A diffuse encephalopathy is the most common presentation of central nervous system lupus.[41,44] Seizures (most commonly grand mal), manic-depressive psychosis, and an organic brain syndrome are the most common manifestations. The patient may have altered consciousness and impaired orientation, memory, and intellectual functions. Less commonly, focal CNS lesions can be seen due to either thrombosis or hemorrhage. The latter appear to be manifestations of a CNS vasculitis. The pathogenesis of diffuse encephalopathy is less clear. At postmortem, a clear small-vessel vasculitis is usually *not* seen. Other possible causes are (1) inflammation caused by antibodies directed to neural tissue or antilymphocyte antibodies cross-reactive with neurons[11,13] or (2) vasculopathy due to agglutinated cells (white cell thrombi or aggregated platelets).[1]

Severe headaches are a frequent complaint in SLE patients, and occurrences that are atypical or unusually severe can be the predecessors of more severe manifestations. Migraine headaches can also be seen as an isolated symptom. Subarachnoid hemorrhage (often heralded by severe headache) is another possible CNS manifestation of SLE. The spinal fluid findings of cerebral thrombosis, cerebral hemorrhage, or subarachnoid hemorrhage reveal nothing unusual when they occur in the setting of SLE. The various manifestations of diffuse cerebritis may have a mild pleocytosis and an elevated protein. The latter consists primarily of IgG, and oligoclonal banding indistinguishable from that seen in multiple sclerosis can be seen. Of course, a glucose determination, culture, Gram stain, and cryptocococal antigen determination are critical to rule out infection, particularly in patients who are immunosuppressed or taking corticosteroids.

Therapy

The treatment of systemic lupus depends upon the particular manifestation and can vary from watchful waiting, administration of mild analgesics, to anti-inflammatory therapy with corticosteroids or immunosuppressive agents. Counseling must be provided to patients to caution them regarding environmental or functional occurrences that may exacerbate the disease. Some patients not only have a photosensitive rash, but also have systemic exacerbations temporally associated with sun exposure, and for them, minimizing exposure, use of sunscreens, a wide-brimmed hat, etc., can be critical. Exercise is encouraged but must not proceed to the point of exhaustion and is, of course, modified depending on prior organ involvement (joints, cardiac, etc.). Pregnancy can present particular problems in systemic lupus patients, particularly in those with a history of renal disease or cardiac disease. Although the incidence of spontaneous abortion is high in lupus patients, term births are usually normal, but the offspring may transiently have abnormal autoantibodies due to maternal IgG crossing the placenta. Neonatal thrombocytopenia and congenital heart block associated with anti-SS-A (anti-RO)[50] are of particular note. Particular caution must be taken in the postpartum period in which an increased incidence of maternal disease exacerbation is seen.

The drugs utilized to treat SLE include nonsteroidal anti-inflammatory agents, such as aspirin or indomethacin; antimalarial drugs, such as hydroxychloroquine, and corticosteroids; and immunosuppressive agents. The nonsteroidal agents are utilized to treat symptoms of fever, arthralgias, arthritis, and in some cases pleuropericarditis. Hydroxychloroquine in doses of 200 to 400 mg/day may be useful in controlling the aforementioned symptoms. It is also particularly efficacious in a subpopulation of patients in whom rash and arthralgias are particularly troublesome. Topical corticosteroids can be used to treat acute maculopapular rashes, or

discoid lupus. More severe pulmonary or cardiac involvement (arrhythmias, myocarditis, etc.) requires systemic corticosteroids as does the presence of autoimmune hemolytic anemia, autoimmune thrombocytopenia, severe cutaneous vasculitis, or other major organ involvement such as peripheral neuropathy, cerebritis, or nephritis. Patients who are toxic, e.g., with high fevers and acute arthritis without visceral involvement, may require corticosteroids, but usually for a brief course only, until symptoms abate. Joint pain, in a steroid-dependent lupus patient may, of course, represent aseptic necrosis due to steroids, and this must be checked. Replacement of the hip is a not-uncommon sequela to steroid therapy in SLE patients.

Renal disease presents particular difficulty in terms of prognosis and long-term therapy. Clearly preservation of renal function is the goal irrespective of abnormalities seen in the sediment or other serological evidence of disease activity. The kidney biopsy can yield some useful information regarding therapy. For example, local focal, mesangial, and membranous disease have a better prognosis than diffuse proliferative or membrane-proliferative disease.[8] Yet, with time, the renal picture for a patient may change, and so therapy must be individualized.[76] Recently criteria for active renal inflammation in contrast to sclerotic "burned-out" disease[7] have been developed; the former is predictive of response to anti-inflammatory therapy. At present, severe lupus nephritis is best-treated with a combination of corticosteroids and an immunosuppressive agent such as cyclophosphamide (Cytoxan).[9,15] The steroids are tapered, and maintenance Cytoxan is then utilized. The latter combination, irrespective of potential side effects, is likely superior to high-dose corticosteroids in terms of risk of infection with some increase in efficacy. Cytoxan has been administered as a monthly bolus as maintenance, with good effect.

Therapy of central nervous sytem involvement rests on less sound scientific support and usually consists of high-dose corticosteroid therapy for 2 to 3 weeks and the addition of an immunosuppressive agent if improvement is not evident. Plasmapheresis is an experimental mode of therapy for systemic lupus patients. It may have efficacy in acute nephritis or central nervous system lupus, the rationale being the elimination of circulatory immune complexes and reversal of reticuloendothelial clearance abnormalities.[27,42] Nevertheless, to date, there is no evidence to support its use chronically as a form of maintenance therapy.

VASCULITIS

Vasculitis is the general term used to signify systemic inflammatory disease involving blood vessels. Numerous classifications of these disorders have been proposed[19,75] and subdivided as to disorders involving large as opposed to small blood vessels (Table 19-14), focusing primarily on systemic disorders of large vessels. Systemic lupus erythematosus, described in the previous section, has vasculitis as one of its manifestations and involves primarily medium- and small-sized arteries or arterioles.

TABLE 19-14 Classification of Vasculitis

Large-vessel disorders
  Polyarteritis nodosa
  Wegener's glomerulomatosis
  Giant cell (temporal) arteritis and polymyalgias rheumatica
  Takayasu's arteriopathy

Small-vessel disorders (excluding SLE)
  Serum sickness
  Henoch-Schönlein purpura
  Cryoglobulinemia
  Hypocomplementemic vasculitis
  Idiopathic cutaneous vasculitis

POLYARTERITIS NODOSA

Polyarteritis nodosa is a relatively uncommon disease in which there is diffuse inflammation of the arterial tree involving primarily medium to large vessels, although small vessels can also be involved. It affects males predominantly with a male-female sex ratio of $2:1$. It occurs most commonly in the 40- to 60-year-old age group.

Etiology and Pathogenesis

The disorder is an immune complex–mediated disease in which there is deposition of complexes within blood vessel walls and transmural inflammation. In approximately one-third of cases, the antigenic material contained within the immune complex contains hepatitis B surface antigen (HBsAG),[29] and there is concomitant diminution of serum complement (C4 and C3) indicative of activation of the classical pathway.[66] In most cases that are HBsAG-negative, immune complexes can be identified and complement levels are diminished, although an etiologic agent is not identifiable. Study of involved vessels have demonstrated transmural inflammation, fibrinoid necrosis, and a prominent inflammation with neutrophils and variable numbers of lymphocytes and eosinophils. The inflammatory reaction is often eccentric; i.e., it involves one side of a vessel wall, and weakness of such involved vessels can lead to aneurysmal dilation. Pathologically, known organs involved are the kidney in 70 to 80 percent, the heart in 60 to 70 percent (coronary arteritis), the peripheral nerves in 50 percent, the skeletal system in 30 percent, and the central nervous system in 10 percent. However, it is important to note that virtually any organ can be affected by this systemic disorder. The eccentric inflammation seen in the walls of large vessels is due to vasculitis of the vasa vasorum nutrient vessels; likewise neuritic involvement, i.e., infarction of major nerves, is due to vasculitis of vasa nervosum.

Clinical Features

Patients may have systemic symptoms of fever, malaise, and weight loss. Common organs involved are the kidneys (often with hypertension), peripheral nerves, skin, joints, and abdo-

men. The cutaneous manifestations can be varied, e.g., maculopapular rash, ulceration, distal digital ischemia, or palpable purpura (cutaneous vasculitis). An asymmetric nondeforming polyarthritis most commonly affecting the large joints of the lower extremities may be seen. Asymmetrical peripheral neuropathy is seen in 50 to 70 percent of patients with both sensory and motor changes in involved nerves. This is mononeuritis multiplex and involvement of the sural nerve is most common. Less often seen is a distal diffuse sensory neuropathy. Renal disease is likewise seen in about 70 percent of patients and presents as an acute glomerulonephritis. Abdominal pain is a common symptom and may represent mesenteric artery involvement. Bowel infarction is a not-infrequent consequence involving superior or inferior mesenteric vessels. Liver involvement is most commonly seen in HBsAg-positive cases, i.e., with evidence of hepatitis, but hepatic infarction secondary to hepatic artery thrombosis can occur in any such patient. This is one of the only causes of a hepatic friction rub heard over the right upper gradient with deep inspiration. Cardiac involvement, although common pathologically, is uncommon clinically but can include myocardial infarction or sequelae of severe hypertension. There may also be diffuse muscle tenderness, cerebral thrombosis, retinal artery thrombosis, granulomatous pulmonary disease, or pulmonary infarction, again due to vessel involvement.

The combination of asthma, eosinophilia, vasculitis, and extravascular granulomas has been termed *allergic angiitis,* or *Churg-Strauss* syndrome, because it was thought to be allergic in origin.[45] In some analyses, this is grouped with polyarteritis nodosa and may, in fact, be polyarteritis in an allergic individual with a history of asthma for several years.

Diagnosis

There is typically a markedly elevated sedimentation rate, leukocytosis and neutrophilia (shift to left), positive HBsAg in one-third, diminished C4 and C3 levels, and elevated levels of circulating immune complexes. Skin and muscle biopsies can be informative in suspected cases when such involvement is seen, although blind biopsy of suspected cases is positive in a low percentage. A sural nerve biopsy is most useful when mononeuritis is evident. A celiac-axis angiogram may reveal aneurysmal dilation of renal, mesenteric, or hepatic arteries and, when seen, is diagnostic (Fig. 19-12). A renal biopsy may reveal diffuse glomerulonephritis with prominent vessel involvement but may not be distinguishable from other types of diffuse glomerulonephritis.

Therapeutic Steps

Corticosteroids are utilized to treat active inflammation of major organ symptoms. For long-term therapy, Cytoxan is utilized and over a 1- or 2-year period frequently leads to remission.[20] With the advent of cytotoxic agents, the 5-year survival is now perhaps as high as 80 or 90 percent, whereas in the past the survival rate was at best 50 percent with corticosteroids alone.[61] Steroids are tapered off as acute manifestations come under control.

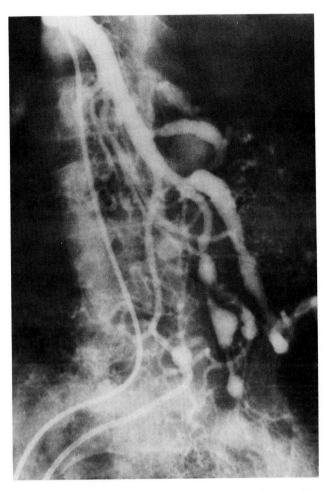

Figure 19-12 Aneurysmal dilatation of vessels (celiac arteriogram) in polyarteritis nodosa. *(From The American Rheumatism Association slide collection. Reproduced with permission of The Arthritis Foundation.)*

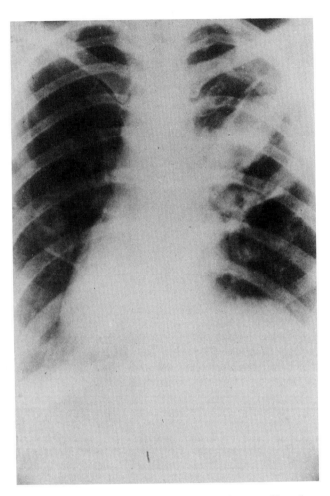

Figure 19-13 Cavitary lesion and infiltrates in x-ray film of patient with Wegener's granulomatosus. *(From The American Rheumatism Association slide collection. Reproduced with permission of The Arthritis Foundation.)*

WEGENER'S GRANULOMATOSIS

Wegener's granulomatosis is a multisystem disorder typically consisting of necrotizing granulomatous inflammation of the nasal-sinus passages, the lung, a segmental glomerulonephritis, and vasculitis.[73]

Etiology and Pathogenesis

No etiologic agent has been identified; however, elevated levels of circulating immune complexes or evidence of immune complex deposition in organs is seen variably and in fewer than half of cases. Pathologically, necrotizing granulomatous lesions of the upper airways is seen in conjunction with vasculitis of small arteries and veins. The granulomas have a central area of necrosis with a typically surrounding "palisade" layer containing lymphocytes, fibroblasts, and multinucleated giant cells. Depending on the organ involved, there may be a typical vasculitis or necrotizing granulomas. The kidney, for example, typically has a focal necrotizing glomerulonephritis, but granulomas per se are rarely seen.

Clinical Features

Most common are chronic rhinitis and sinusitis manifested as nasal congestion, rhinorrhea, facial pain, nasal ulceration, and septal perforation. A "saddle nose" due to septal necrosis may be seen. There is x-ray evidence of pansinusitis, mucosal thickening, and destruction of surrounding bone. Secondary bacterial infection may be present, and distinction from other cases of chronic sinusitis can be difficult. Pulmonary involvement may consist of cough, dyspnea, chest pain, and/or hemoptysis, and x-ray films typically reveal granulomas, often with cavitation (Fig. 19-13). Renal involvement with red cell casts, proteinuria, hematuria, and, at times, renal insufficiency can be seen, but renal disease is less common, in general, than pulmonary disease. Hypertension, in contrast to polyarteritis nodosa or systemic lupus, is seen only infrequently. Arthralgia is common, but synovitis presenting as obvious arthritis is not often seen. Other organs involved, albeit less often, are the skin (necrosis secondary to vasculitis, palpable purpura, or granulomatous nodules), nervous system (mononeuritis multiplex or peripheral neuropathy), and optic apparatus (e.g., uveitis, episcleritis, or retinal artery occlusion).

Diagnosis

There is a moderate leukocytosis, elevated sedimentation rate, and hypergammaglobulinemia. Like polyarteritis nodosa, tests for ANA, rheumatoid factor, and other autoantibodies are typically negative. Biopsy of nasal or sinus tissue is simplest but is often not diagnostic—i.e., not clearly distinguishable from other forms of sinusitis—but an open lung biopsy has a high yield. Renal biopsy can be suggestive but can be confused with other causes of a focal nephritis. It must be distinguished from other forms of granulomatous lung disease including tuberculosis, sarcoidosis, and fungal infections. It must also be distinguished from an atypical lymphoma,[40] designated lymphomatoid granulomatosis, as well as midline granuloma,[71] a similar but very aggressive disorder confined to the upper respiratory tract including the nose, sinuses, palate, and nasopharynx.

Therapy

Like polyarteritis nodosa, corticosteroids are utilized to treat acute organ inflammation, but cyclophosphamide is utilized for long-term therapy. Whereas before 1960, the disorder was often fatal, most patients remit with aggressive therapy when the diagnosis is made at an early stage.[63,73]

GIANT CELL (TEMPORAL) ARTERITIS

Giant cell arteritis is a disorder of an aging population and only rarely occurs prior to the age of 50. It is an inflammatory disease involving vessels emanating from the aortic arch characterized by proliferation of giant cells. In some cases a more generalized arteritis may be seen. Polymyalgia rheumatica is, by comparison, a benign disorder presenting as pain in the proximal musculature (shoulders and hips) without true weakness whose pathogenesis appears similar to giant cell arteritis. It is also at least three times as common.[38]

Etiology and Pathogenesis

The inflammatory reaction seen is caused by segmental involvement of large vessels with giant cell proliferation within the submucosa and destruction of the internal elastic lamina. This may be due to elastase secretion by these activated cells. The cause is unknown. At times the infiltrate may appear granulomatous, and when severe, all levels of the vessel wall may be affected. It is important to note that the inflammation is eccentric, i.e., upon biopsy it typically is evident along the side of a vessel wall but it is not circumferential (Fig. 19-14). It is also segmental in that if a biopsy is taken, serial sections must be done since the inflammatory reaction skips areas along the length of a vessel.[32] In postmortem studies of patients who died during the active phase, the highest incidence of severe involvement was noted in the superficial temporal artery (the only one usually biopsied), the vertebral arteries, and the ophthalmic and posterior ciliary arteries.

Clinical Features

Headache is the most common symptom of giant cell arteritis and is often bitemporal and throbbing. There may be redness and scalp tenderness along the superficial temporal artery. Visual symptoms can include diplopia and partial or complete sudden onset of blindness in one eye; these manifestations are due to ischemia or infarction of the optic nerve or tracts secondary to arteritis of the ophthalmic or posterior ciliary arteries. The involved fundus will show ischemic optic neuritis with slight pallor and edema of the optic disc. There may be intermittent claudication of the jaw muscles exacerbated by chewing. Although less common, the disorder can involve any vessel along the aorta including the internal carotid system, renal, coronary, and iliac arteries. Arthralgias or synovitis may also be seen. Polymyalgia rheumatica occurs in the same age group with a mean age of onset of about 65 years. There is severe malaise, fatigue, and myalgias of the neck, shoulder, and upper arms, as well as the hips and thighs. Such symptoms are frequently seen as part of temporal arteritis. Conversely, in patients with polymyalgia rheumatica having no symptoms or signs of arteritis, temporal artery biopsy may show evidence of giant cell arteritis. The percentage of positive biopsies has varied from 10 to 15 percent in some studies to as high as 66 percent in others.[36] There is, however, no good evidence to suggest that the severe myalgia is due to arteritis of vessels supplying the musculature.

Diagnosis

Patients may have a mild anemia, a normal leukocyte count and differential, and a markedly elevated sedimentation rate, often exceeding 100 mm/h. Diagnostic arterial biopsy should be performed in all patients suspected of having giant cell arteritis. Aortic angiography is indicated in those patients

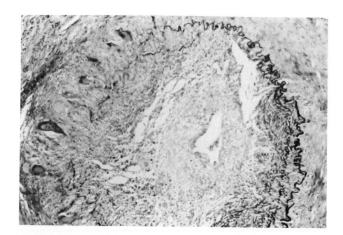

Figure 19-14 Temporal artery biopsy of patients with giant cell arteritis. The elastic fiber stain shows disruption of the internal elastic lamina on one side of the vessel wall where giant cells are clearly visible. *(From The American Rheumatism Association slide collection. Reproduced with permission of The Arthritis Foundation.)*

who appear to have a more diffuse arteritis. Polymyalgia rheumatica can be distinguished from polymyositis by the absence of true weakness and normal muscle enzymes. Other than nonspecific elevations of plasma proteins such as $alpha_2$ globulins, tests for autoantibodies are negative.

Therapy

Corticosteroids are the mainstay of therapy of giant cell arteritis, and ocular involvement is considered an emergency. It is treated with high doses of daily steroids; at least 60 mg/day of prednisone. The starting dose is continued until all reversible symptoms are gone and laboratory tests (sedimentation rate) is normal. This may take between 2 and 4 weeks. Then the dose is gradually decreased. Giant cell arteritis tends to run a self-limited course lasting a year or two, so that eventually steroids are discontinued. Patients with polymyalgia rheumatica are given low-dose corticosteroids, and they are exceedingly sensitive to such therapy. As little as 10 mg/day may ameliorate symptoms and return the sedimentation rate to normal. This too can be self-limited, often lasting only a few months or up to 1 year.[16] However, in some cases it may be present for years.

TAKAYASU ARTERIOPATHY

Takayasu disease, or aortic arch arteritis, is a chronic granulomatous arteritis that can involve any of the branches of the aortic arch and is associated with secondary occlusive thrombosis.[58] It primarily affects children and young women often between the age of 10 and 30. It is particularly common in Japanese. There is patchy or continuous involvement of the aorta, innominate, carotid, and subclavian vessels.[17] In addition, it can also affect the celiac, mesenteric, pulmonary, renal, coronary, or iliac arteries. Granulomatous inflammation throughout the vessel wall is seen often beginning along the adventitial outer layer with infiltration of lymphocytes, plasma cells, macrophages, and multinucleated giant cells. The vasa vasorum may show endothelial proliferation and obliteration of the lumen.

Clinical Features

Low-grade fever, fatigue, and weight loss is common and arthralgias or a mild arthritis is seen in about half of cases. There may be absence of pulses (e.g., radial, brachial, carotid) due to thrombosis, and for this reason it has been called "pulseless disease."[58] Vascular insufficiency may be apparent, and bruits over involved vessels may be heard. Decreased lower extremity pulses and bruits may also be seen. Hypertension may be caused by involvement of thoracic or abdominal vessels as is seen in a coarctation or may be due to renal arterial disease.[33] With progression, there may be ischemic changes of the head, e.g., atrophic facial skin, loss of teeth and hair, ulcers on the lips or tip of the nose, as well as central nervous system involvement. Many symptoms are associated with physical activity, e.g., abdominal pain, angina pectoris, or myocardial infarction and seizures.

Diagnosis

There is typically mild normocytic normochromic anemia, a normal leukocyte count, mildly elevated globulins, and a high sedimentation rate. It can present similarly to giant cell arteritis but affects a completely different age group. Aortography is essential to make the diagnosis, and it may sometimes be confused with uncommon hematologic disorders in which thrombosis is prominent. These include absence of inhibitors of coagulation factors or abnormalities of factors needed for normal fibrinolysis.

Therapy

Corticosteroids in high doses are utilized in the early stages of the disease and may have to be continued at low to moderate dosage for a protracted period.[26] The disorder is less responsive than giant cell arteritis, and the mortality is significantly greater. Death has been most commonly due to congestive heart failure or a cerebrovascular accident. Use of immunosuppressive agents in unresponsive patients plus vascular reconstructive surgery has significantly improved the prognosis.[39]

SMALL-VESSEL DISORDERS

Vasculitis of small vessels (arterioles, venules) include serum sickness, cryoglobulinemia, Henoch-Schönlein purpura, hypocomplementemic vasculitis, and idiopathic cutaneous vasculitis. All have in common prominent cutaneous symptoms, most typically petechiae and palpable purpura. There may be urticarial lesions in serum sickness, hypocomplementemic vasculitis,[54] and idiopathic cutaneous vasculitis, and in the last two, these may occur along with petechiae and palpable purpura. In general, these disorders are not associated with the sort of multiorgan involvement seen with large vessel vasculitides but, with the exception of cutaneous vasculitis, each may be associated with a diffuse glomerulonephritis.

Serum Sickness

Serum sickness is a self-limited disease typically consisting of fever, urticarial skin lesions, arthralgias or mild arthritis, lymphadenopathy, and, in some instances, glomerulonephritis. It can be caused by diverse agents such as adverse reaction to penicillin or as a prodrome to serum hepatitis. It is associated with circulating immune complexes, low C4 and C3 levels when symptoms are in an accelerating phase, and deposition of immune complexes in the above tissues.

Henoch-Schönlein Purpura

Henoch-Schönlein purpura is most commonly seen in children and is characterized by purpuric lesions predominating about the buttocks and lower extremities in association with a polyarthritis or with gastrointestinal bleeding, or both. In addition, there may be a diffuse glomerulonephritis. It is often seen after infections and is associated with an elevated IgA level, the presence of immune complexes in which IgA is the antibody, and evidence of activation of the alternative complement pathway. This is discussed in more detail in the chapter on rheumatic disorders of children.

Cryoglobulinemia

Cryoglobulinemia is the most severe of the vasculitides categorized as involving small vessels. It is a disease of middle age in which huge levels of circulating immune complexes are present having the property of precipitating in the cold.[52] Most are mixed cryoglobulins consisting of IgM antibody reactive against IgG.[55] Thus, patients have a high-titer rheumatoid factor, and the immune complexes lead to prominent activation of the classical complement pathway with markedly diminished C4 and C3 levels. In some patients there is evidence of infection with hepatitis virus, and they are positive for HBsAg. There is a widespread cutaneous vasculitis with petechiae, purpura, ulceration, and digital infarction. These can be markedly exacerbated with cold exposure with its attendant cryoprecipitation of protein, leading to occlusion of small vessels. Patients may also have a diffuse proliferative glomerulonephritis, arthralgias or a mild arthritis, lymphadenopathy, and hepatosplenomegaly. Those with positive HBsAg may have evidence of chronic active hepatitis.[47] It can be confused with systemic lupus erythematosus, but it lacks the autoantibodies seen in systemic lupus, and it does not have evident immunoglobulin deposition along the dermal-epidermal junction. There is no really effective therapy. Some patients respond to corticosteroids. Immunosuppressive agents may be tried. Likewise, although experimental, aggressive plasmapheresis lowers the immune complex load and can be used along with one or more of the above drugs.[30]

SECTION F

Spondyloarthropathies

Lee Kaufman

Ankylosing spondylitis (AS) is well recognized as a distinct entity that is prototypic of a group of rheumatologic diseases referred to collectively as the seronegative spondyloarthropathies (SNSA). Pathologically these individual diseases are typified by inflammation at the sites of insertion of tendons and ligaments into bone (enthesis) and are therefore known as the *enthesopathies*.[6] From a clinical, serological, and immunogenetic standpoint these disorders are common and distinctly different from classical rheumatoid arthritis with which they can be frequently confused.

The SNSA are characterized by both axial disease in the form of spondylitis and/or sacroiliitis as well as appendicular involvement presenting as lower extremity, asymmetrical oligoarticular arthritis. In addition, a spectrum of extraarticular features involving the heart, lungs, eyes, and skin provide evidence of a systemic disease.

These diseases should be considered in the differential diagnosis of any patient with mono- or oligoarticular joint disease and progressive low back pain. The unifying concept of the SNSA was initially proposed by Wright.[105] This places "primary" AS in a central position and the related spondyloarthropathies with "secondary" spondylitis and sacroiliitis peripherally. The discussion to follow is subdivided as follows: (1) ankylosing spondylitis, (2) Reiter syndrome or reactive arthritis, (3) psoriatic arthritis, and (4) enteropathic arthritis.

ANYKYLOSING SPONDYLITIS
Epidemiology and Etiopathogenesis

Ankylosing spondylitis is considered to be primary when features of other SNSA are lacking. As such, it is a disease of antiquity, having been described in Egyptian mummies.[95] In modern times it has been referred to by numerous eponyms such as Marie-Strümpell disease and misleadingly as rheumatoid spondylitis. The true prevalence of AS is uncertain but is felt to be between .05 and 1.5 percent.[103,100,19,20] This range is based on U.S. white populations in which the incidence of HLA-B27 is approximately 8.0 percent. In Native American Indians (HLA-B27 incidence, approximately 18 to 50 percent) and American blacks (HLA-B27 incidence, 3 to 4 percent) SNSA are found with a higher and lower prevalence, respectively. Recognition that the disease has been underestimated in women has led to the realization that the male-female ratio of 10:1 observed in the late 1940s[103] is not correct and approaches values closer to equality.[93]

It has been known for some time that AS tends to occur with increased frequency in families.[38] Since the recognition in 1973 that AS is associated with the major histocompatibility complex antigen HLA-B27,[12] the entire group of SNSA has assumed increasing importance in clinical rheumatology as an experimental model of immunogenetics and human disease expression. Based on epidemiological studies utilizing the HLA-B27 genetic marker, a risk factor for disease of between 10 and 20 percent was initially calculated for HLA-B27-positive individuals.[22] This relative risk has been subsequently demonstrated to be considerably lower.[24,101,59] In that regard, it has been shown that B27-positive relatives of B27-positive patients are significantly more likely to have disease (10.6 percent) than are B27-positive relatives of healthy B27-positive (2.0 percent) controls.[24]

The conceptual pathogenetic model for AS and the closely related spondyloarthropathy Reiter syndrome (or reactive arthritis) is similar. It has evolved from various epidemiological and immunologic studies utilizing the HLA-B27 genetic marker as a probe. The information elucidated from this work supports clinical disease expression resulting from a genetically predisposed host exposed to an environmental insult acting as the arthritogenic "trigger."[23,79,80] In the case of Reiter syndrome (RS), postvenereal (gonococcal and non-gonococcal urethritis) and postenteric (*Shigella, Salmonella, Yersinia,* and *Campylobacter*) triggering events are described.[1] With regard to AS, recent work has suggested an increased carriage of *Klebsiella* in the stools during clinical exacerbation.[35,36] In addition, culture filtrates of certain *Klebsiella* serotypes derived from fecal isolates of AS patients contain a "modifying factor" capable of immunologically altering HLA-B27-positive lymphocytes from asymptomatic controls.[45] Antibodies to a specific strain of *Klebsiella* which can lyse lymphocytes from HLA-B27-positive patients but not from HLA-B27-positive controls will lyse the latter cells after exposure to the modifying factor. This cross-reactivity between *Klebsiella* and HLA-B27 lymphocytes from AS patients has also been demonstrated with certain other enteric organisms (i.e., specific strains of *Salmonella, Shigella,* and *Escherichia coli*).[83]

Recent studies extend the role of *Klebsiella* in the pathogenesis of AS. Serum IgA immunoglobulin levels have been demonstrated to correlate with disease activity, elevation of C-reactive protein (CRP), and the erythrocyte sedimentation rate (ESR).[28] The primary source of this IgA is the plasma cell gut-associated lymphoid tissue which has presumably been activated by an enteric organism. The elevated serum IgA can be adsorbed out with a specific *Klebsiella* species and IgA-specific anti-*Klebsiella* antibodies fluctuate with disease activity.[99]

From these clinical and experimental observations the following potential mechanisms of etiopathogenesis can be deduced: (1) cross-reactive antigens could exist between an infectious agent and a host structure, and (2) direct interaction could occur between a cell surface structure (HLA-B27 marker) and the infectious agent or its products ("modifying factor"). This could then yield an altered molecular structure. Indirect evidence in favor of the latter postulate is the finding in AS of beta antibodies to beta$_2$ microglobulin, which is an integral part of the HLA cell surface structure.[30] It is conceivable that this antibody production resulted from structural alteration of an HLA subunit.

One might then imagine a potential sequence of events whereby lymphocyte activation occurs in the gut via a variety of enteric bacilli. This could then induce an inflammatory response in axial structures draining regions of the gastrointestinal and genitourinary tracts by means of lymphatics and the paravertebral venous plexus of Batson.[34,42]

Unfortunately, explanations for the presence of disease in HLA-B27-negative patients and the absence of disease in most HLA-B27-positive patients is lacking. To help explain the former situation, it has been noted that a certain subset of patients with RD have HLA antigens which cross-react with the HLA-B27 determinant. These include HLA-Bw22, -Bw42, and -B7.[3] With regard to the lack of disease in most patients who are HLA-B27-positive, the following are possible theories: (1) An immune response gene (HLA-DR) is in linkage dysequilibrium (occurring with a class I antigen HLA-A, -B, or -C more frequently than by chance alone) with HLA-B27 and

is necessary for disease expression. To date this has not been detected. (2) Furthermore, given that the HLA-B27 antigen when analyzed with monoclonal antibodies is heterogeneous and consists of at least two subpopulations, one could propose that certain subtypes are associated with clinical disease, whereas others are not.[50]

Despite the enormous understanding that has been gained with the HLA-B27 marker in the pathophysiology of these disorders, its usefulness for the diagnosis, management, and treatment of the SNSA is rather limited.

Pathological Findings

The early histology of AS appears to be a modest cellular infiltration accompanied by fibrous proliferation, chondrocyte metaplasia, and endochondral ossification. In the areas of enthesis, mast cells are numerous.[94] These mast cells are surrounded by lymphocytes, and it is possible that products of activated lymphocytes (from gut lymphatic drainage) induce mast cells to release vasoactive amines and proteolytic enzymes. Furthermore, an intimate association between mast cell granules and fibroblasts potentially leading to fibrosis has been described.[4]

Clinical Features

The typical patient with AS is below the age of 40 years and presents with insidious low back pain of greater than 3 months duration. Morning stiffness is present and improves with exercise. This aspect is more characteristic of inflammatory disease than mechanical low back pain, which often is worsened by exercise and improves with rest. Paresthesias radiating to the buttocks may occur but are usually diffuse and not well delineated anatomically. This contrasts with mechanical abnormalities associated with distinct neurological findings.[26]

The hallmark of AS is axial disease beginning in the thoracolumbar spine. This may progress to involve the cervical spine giving rise to a stiff and rigid column. As a result of this inflexibility, fractures following minor trauma are common and occur most often in the lower cervical column (C6–7).[52] In addition to prominent axial involvement, approximately one-third to two-thirds of patients will develop peripheral joint disease as well.[46] This is most common in the hip followed by the shoulders and asymmetrical oligoarticular arthritis of the lower extremities. Severe peripheral arthritis may occur at any time during the clinical course. Patients may also complain of peripheral periarticular manifestations of disease related to the enthesopathic pathology. Insertional tendinitis involving the Achilles tendon and plantar fascia may give rise to both superior and inferior calcaneal spurs. Involvement of intercostal muscle insertions can induce chest pain that is confusingly "pleuritic" in nature. Temporomandibular joint arthritis is not uncommon,[31] and C1-2 subluxation can occur as it does in rheumatoid arthritis.

AS is also considered a multisystem disease with many extraarticular manifestations.[70] Patients may present with nonspecific complaints such as low-grade fever, anorexia, and fatigue. Ocular disease is common (25 percent) and takes

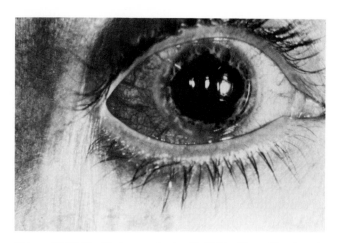

Figure 19-15 Uveitis in a patient with SNSA. *(From The American Rheumatism Association slide collection. Reproduced with permission of The Arthritis Foundation.)*

the form of anterior uveitis[20] (Fig. 19-15). Idiopathic uveitis also has a high association with HLA-B27 (50 percent) and may be a *forme fruste* of a SNSA.[13] Pulmonary involvement may be the result of chest wall abnormalities causing restrictive lung disease, or in long-standing disease it may be related to apical pulmonary fibrosis.[37] The latter occurs in 1 or 2 percent of patients and is associated with fibrocystic disease simulating tuberculosis.[90] The cavities are often superinfected with atypical mycobacteria and/or *Aspergillus.* Cardiac disease may take the form of significant aortic insufficiency and/or atrioventricular conduction disturbances requiring permanent pacemaker insertion.[84,7,8] The valvular disease has been well described pathologically and extends above and below the aortic valve ring, differentiating it from rheumatoid arthritis, rheumatic heart disease, aortic dissection, and syphilitic aortitis.[14] Recent studies with 2-D echocardiography indicate that early preclinical aortic root involvement may be identified.[61] Renal function in uncomplicated AS appears to be normal.[21] However, patients with IgA nephropathy[54] and patients with amyloidosis[16] have been described. Neurological catastrophes with cord compression may occur at any level secondary to fracture following even minor trauma.

Diagnostic Evaluation

The physical exam is not very specific with regard to the sacroiliac joints (SIJ). Many clinical maneuvers which have been described to help define the site of pain can be misleading (i.e., pelvic compression and forcible range of motion of the hips). The anatomically important part of the SIJ in the SNSA is the lower one-third. This area can best be palpated, if at all, by having the patient flex forward with the upper torso resting on the examining table (approximately 90 degrees of flexion). Probably the single best clinical measurement is the Schober test. This is an objective measurement of anterior flexion of the lumbar spine. It does not measure SIJ motion and correlates well with the radiographic angle of movement of the lumbar spine on the sacrum.[72] False-positive tests

occur with degenerative joint disease. To execute the Schober maneuver, two points are made along a line perpendicular to the midpoint of the posterior superior iliac spines. The inferior point is at the lumbosacral junction. The superior point is 10 cm above. Following maximum flexion, the distance between the two points is remeasured. A normal value is an increase in flexion by at least 5 cm. Normal anterior spinal flexion varies widely at each decade and may be reduced by about 25 percent with advanced age alone.[78] The manifestations and treatment of spinal lesions is dealt with further in Chap. 55.

Of critical importance in the evaluation of the SIJ is the demonstration by a plain film of the pelvis that radiographic sacroiliitis exists. This is an essential part of the New York ARA criteria for the diagnosis of AS.[9] It should be emphasized that the upper portion of the articulation is ligamentous and the lower one-third synovial. Although both portions can be affected, the predominant involvement is the inferior compartment. Inflammatory synovitis has a predilection for the iliac side and is radiographically characterized by a poorly outlined subchondral bone plate. Various grades of radiological sacroiliitis are described; the outcome is frequently bony fusion.

Sacroiliitis and spondylitis can vary radiologically among the SNSA. In primary AS and the axial disease of inflammatory bowel disease, the findings differ from that of Reiter syndrome and psoriatic arthropathy. The former two are more typically characterized by bilateral sacroiliitis, symmetrical syndesmophytes, facet joint involvement, and flowing delicate ossification of the annulus fibrosus of the intervertebral disc. The end product of this process is the classical "bamboo spine" (see Chap. 55). Patients with Reiter syndrome and psoriasis, however, tend to have more asymmetrical sacroiliitis, random syndesmophytes which are larger and nonmarginal, and less often have classical ascending disease.[75]

Routine laboratory procedures have revealed nonspecific abnormalities indicative of an inflammatory disorder. Typical findings include mild anemia and an elevated ESR which may not correlate with disease activity.[20] Rheumatoid factors are characteristically absent. Elevated serum IgA levels have been seen as discussed above and are of theoretical importance in the development of nephropathy in some patients. Lymphocyte studies have shown that T-cell subsets are normal and that both the number and functional activity of natural killer cells are elevated.[60] The diagnosis of AS is ultimately dependent upon the radiographic demonstration of sacroiliitis.[9] This is most effectively accomplished by an adequate review of an anteroposterior view of the pelvis. More elaborate studies (oblique views of the sacroiliac joints, CT scanning, and scintigraphy) are rarely required and should not by any means be considered routine.[20] Although it has been argued that HLA typing is useful in selective clinical situations,[58] it has essentially no role to play as a diagnostic test in the routine patient with AS or other SNSA.[17,18] It should be further emphasized that one cannot confirm or refute a diagnosis of AS with HLA-B27 typing. A potential clinical use of HLA typing might be in predicting which patients with inflammatory bowel disease or psoriasis have a greater likelihood of developing axial disease and in relatives of patients with AS in whom disease is clinically suspected.

TABLE 19-15   Differential Diagnosis of Sacroiliac Disease

General disease category	Specific disease
Seronegative spondyloarthropathy (lower one-third of sacroiliac joint)	1° Ankylosing spondylitis 2° Ankylosing spondylitis • Inflammatory bowel disease • Psoriatic arthropathy • Reactive arthritis: *Yersinia, Shigella flexneri, Salmonella, Campylobacter, Brucella* • Whipple disease • Behçet syndrome • Postintestinal bypass syndrome • Hidradenitis suppurativa
Metabolic disease	• Hyperparathyroidism • Tophaceous gout • Calcium pyrophosphate deposition disease • Paget disease
Immunologically mediated rheumatic syndromes	• Relapsing polychrondritis • Giant cell arteritis • Familial Mediterranean fever • SLE
Neoplastic disease	• Primary or metastatic lesion
Infection	• Pyogenic (*Staphylococcus aureus*, enteric gram-negative bacilli) • Mycobacterial • Fungal • Brucella
Miscellaneous	• Gaucher disease (bone infarction) • Hemoglobinopathies • Tuberous sclerosis • Acroosteolysis associated with polyvinyl chloride • Sarcoidosis • Osteitis condensans ilii • Degenerative joint disease

Differential Diagnosis

There are various other disorders which can affect the SI joints in addition to those belonging to the related SNSA (Table 19-15). Unilateral sacroiliitis should always raise the suspicion of infection which requires confirmation with fluoroscopically guided aspiration when clinically indicated. In particular, intravenous drug abusers and elderly patients with urinary tract infections are susceptible to gram-negative infections of the SIJ.

Treatment

The mainstay of treatment is physical therapy in conjunction with the nonsteroidal anti-inflammatory drugs (NSAIDs) to achieve maximum mobility and function while diminishing pain and local areas of inflammation. The role of rehabilitation medicine in the management of AS patients cannot be overemphasized. The most effective NSAID is phenylbutazone. In view of the potential for severe bone marrow toxicity and granulocytopenia, other NSAIDs such as indomethacin are generally chosen. As in other clinical situations, the decision to use one NSAID over another should be weighed against the potential toxicity related to concurrent medical problems and medications (e.g., liver or renal disease and Coumadin therapy). There is not extensive evidence to support a role for NSAIDs in delaying disease progression. To date there is no evidence supporting the use of remittive agents such as gold and D-penicillamine as in rheumatoid arthritis. Oral corticosteroids have no role for articular disease. Local corticosteroids may be useful for enthesopathic-related flares or for intraarticular injection.

Surgical intervention has been helpful for correcting axial defects with vertebral wedge osteotomy.[97] Occasionally hip ankylosis requires total hip arthroplasty. This, unfortunately, has been associated with a high incidence of postoperative ectopic paraarticular ossification and reankylosis.[10,86]

A new approach to the treatment of AS involves diet manipulation to help modify the enteric flora. Preliminary studies indicate that simple sugars are better substrates for bacterial growth than are amino acids. On that basis patients were given, in an open trial, a high-protein–low-carbohydrate diet. This was associated with a fall in IgA levels and ESR. Further work is clearly needed to support or refute the role of dietary protein in altering the clinical course of AS.

REITER SYNDROME, OR REACTIVE ARTHRITIS

Reactive arthritis is the presently preferred term used to describe inflammatory poly- or oligoarticular arthritis in a genetically susceptible host following an infectious ("triggering") event. Although given the eponym of Reiter syndrome following a report in 1916 of the association of arthritis with urethritis and conjunctivitis, there is ample evidence to support an association between genital infection and subsequent arthritis prior to that date. In fact it was Hippocrates that noted "a youth does not suffer from gout until after sexual intercourse."[69] It is now well-recognized that reactive arthritis can occur following dysenteric and venereal infection.

About 80 percent of whites presenting with reactive arthritis will be HLA-B27-positive. This may vary, depending upon the associated environmental insult, and is greatest in sexually acquired diseases.[57] Therefore, despite the fact that a genetic predisposition is detectable in the majority of patients, as in AS, there are still patients who will be HLA-B27-negative. Any theoretical approaches to etiopathogenesis will need to explain this latter group (as reviewed in the discussion of AS).

Preliminary criteria for Reiter disease (RD) have been established by an ARA subcommittee.[104] The diagnosis of RD by those guidelines includes arthritis lasting longer than 1 month in association with urethritis or cervicitis. Furthermore, evidence for primary AS, psoriasis, or inflammatory bowel disease should be excluded. It is also noteworthy that both gonococcal and nongonococcal septic arthritis may be followed by a sterile "postinfectious" arthritis that is not associated with HLA-B27.[47] Reactive arthritis has also been described with brucellosis,[2] certain intestinal parasites,[11] sup-

purative hidradenitis or acne conglobata,[92] and the postintestinal bypass syndrome.

It is commonly felt that the postvenereal form of RD is associated primarily with nongonococcal urethritis (NGU).[1] The prevalence of arthritis in this setting is approximately 1 percent,[57] and recent evidence supports an etiologic role for this agent: (1) 15 to 20 percent of heterosexual men and 25 to 60 percent of heterosexual women with gonococcal urethritis are simultaneously infected with *Chlamydia trachomatis.* This explains the high failure rate when penicillin is used to treat gonococcal urethritis as well as the inability of penicillin to prevent arthritis.[98] (2) Patients with acute nondiarrheal RD have higher mean antibody titers to *Chlamydia trachomatis* and greater in vitro lymphocyte transformation than patients with NGU alone. In addition, *Chlamydia trachomatis* has been isolated from the urethra of a significant number of patients with sexually acquired RD.[73]

The postenteric form of RD has been described primarily with *Shigella (flexneri,* not *sonnei), Salmonella, Campylobacter,* and *Yersinia.* The prevalence of disease in infected patients being approximately 3.3 percent for *Yersinia* and 2.0 to 3.0 percent collectively for the others. The male-female ratio approximates 1.0. The interval between infection and rheumatic symptoms is less for the venereal form (usually 7 days) than for the dysenteric form. In more than 80 percent of patients this is less than 1 month. Potential mechanisms for enteric-mediated diseases in HLA-B27-positive hosts have already been discussed as per AS.[57]

Pathological Findings

Pathologically, the synovitis of RD is divided into acute and chronic forms. Early on there is increased vascular permeability and a predominance of polymorphonuclear leukocytes. This is followed by mononuclear cell infiltrates resembling rheumatoid arthritis with lymphocytic aggregates.[102] Extrasynovial periarticular disease is explained by the enthesopathy affecting sites of tendinous insertion, whereas rheumatoid arthritis is primarily a synovial disease. Hence, dactylitis and plantar fasciitis develop as in the other SNSA.

Clinical Features

Clinically, RD is characterized by asymmetrical oligoarticular (or polyarticular) joint disease involving predominantly the knees, ankles, hips, metatarsophalangeal joints, and wrists. Lesions related to enthesopathic pathology occur in 10 to 20 percent of patients (tendinitis, dactylitis, and fasciitis). These are most frequent in the postvenereal group. Sacroiliitis occurs more often after chronic disease (50 to 70 percent) than after acute disease (16 percent). Spondylitis, although well described to resemble classic AS, is rare (10 to 20 percent) in follow-up studies.[57]

Extraarticular lesions help differentiate RD from other SNSA. Ocular involvement most commonly occurs as a conjunctivitis (10 to 35 percent).[57] Anterior uveitis may also occur. Mucocutaneous disease is manifested by painless oral ulcers (3 to 33 percent); circinate balanitis, painless erosions

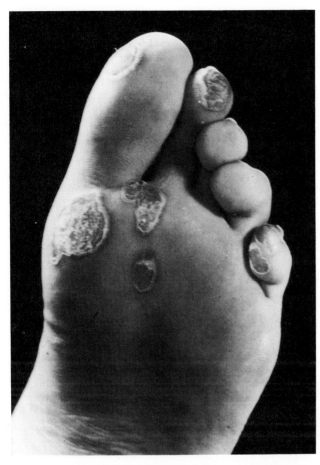

Figure 19-16 Keratoderma blennorrhagicum in association with Reiter's disease. *(From The American Rheumatism Association slide collection. Reproduced with permission of The Arthritis Foundation.)*

on the penis (25 to 50 percent); and keratoderma blennorrhagicum (1 to 31 percent) on the palms, soles, extremities, and trunk (Fig. 19-16). These lesions resemble psoriatic plaques clinically and histologically.[21] Patients with *Yersinia* may also have lesions of erythema nodosum (5 percent).[57] Nail changes, without pitting, also resemble psoriasis and include onycholysis, ridging, and subungual hyperkeratosis. It is of significant interest that AS, which is immunogenetically so similar to RD and which has similar articular manifestations, lacks this extensive cutaneous pathology.

More unusual systemic involvement includes: (1) cardiovascular disease (conduction disturbances, transient pericarditis and aortic insufficiency); (2) pulmonary disease (transient pleuritis); (3) neurological manifestations (peripheral and cranial neuropathies); and (4) amyloidosis.[29,48,57,61,81,84]

Diagnostic Evaluation

Radiological findings are primarily the consequence of enthesopathic involvement. These appear sequentially as areas of osteoporosis and erosions at sites of insertional tendinitis as well as new bone formation occurring as periostitis and plantar spurs. As noted above, the sacroiliitis and spondylitis resemble psoriatic arthritis and differ from AS.[75]

Laboratory abnormalities reflect a nonspecific acute-phase response. With regard to humoral and cellular immune mechanisms, a few relevant aspects can be delineated. On the humoral side, as with AS, serological abnormalities such as rheumatoid factors and antinuclear antibodies are characteristically absent. Serum complement levels may be normal or elevated. Recent studies have revealed the presence of circulating immune complexes in as many as two-thirds of patients with RD and AS alike.[67] Cellular abnormalities with enhanced lymphocyte proliferation to *Chlamydia trachomatis* in acute nondiarrheal RD has already been mentioned. In addition, synovial lymphocytes from patients with postenteric RD undergo significant proliferation in vitro when exposed to specific enteric antigens.[41]

The synovial fluid is most often inflammatory (or type II) in nature. Early studies indicated that elevated complement components in synovial fluid might be helpful in distinguishing RD from other forms of inflammatory synovitis. These findings, however, are variable and nonspecific. Furthermore, there has been some evidence for complement activation with a reduced synovial fluid–serum complement level,[109] and immunohistological studies have documented immunoglobulin (predominantly IgM) and complement (C3) deposition.[5] The latter studies support potential mechanisms of immune-mediated tissue destruction.

The polymorphonuclear leukocyte also appears to play an important role. Early studies suggested characteristic macrophages containing intracellular polymorphonuclear inclusions.[82] These findings, however, were subsequently demonstrated to be nonspecific.[96] Recent work in patients with reactive arthritis associated with *Yersinia* purports to show an augmented polymorphonuclear response in patients who are HLA-B27-positive but not those who are HLA-B27-negative.[85] These investigators found that, irrespective of *Yersinia* arthritis, HLA-B27-positive zymosan-activated serum was significantly more chemokinetic (random migration) than serum that was HLA-B27-negative as determined by migration in a modified Boyden Chamber assay. It follows from these experiments that in HLA-B27-positive patients with reactive arthritis potentially "hyperreactive" polymorphonuclear leukocytes accumulating in areas of inflammation could lead to tissue destruction.

Treatment

Therapy is similar to AS. NSAIDs, physical therapy, and emotional support form the basic approach. In view of the recent work linking *Chlamydia trachomatis* to exacerbating flares in patients with acute nondiarrheal RD, an argument for antibiotic therapy has been made.[73] Cytotoxic drugs (azathioprine, methotrexate)[15,40] may have a role in recalcitrant cases. In a recent open trial of patients with HLA-B27-related pauciarticular arthritis and enthesopathies resistant to NSAIDs, 11 out of 15 patients had long-lasting remission with sulfasalazine.[76] Controlled studies are awaited.

In recent years it has been clearly recognized that RD is often not a self-limited acute illness. Rather it tends to be chronic and associated with severe disability. A long-term follow-up study by Calin et al of 131 patients revealed that polyarthritis (83 percent), low back pain and heel pain (50 percent),[50] eye disease (30 percent), urethritis-cervicitis (42 percent), and mucocutaneous disease (25 percent) persist after a mean of 5.6 years.[43] Furthermore, greater than 25 percent of patients were unemployed or forced to change occupation. Of interest, this disability was equal among HLA-B27-positive and HLA-B27-negative patients.

PSORIATIC ARTHROPATHY

Psoriatic arthritis (PA) is the occurrence of inflammatory arthritis in patients with psoriasis and usually in the absence of rheumatoid factor. The prevalence of psoriasis in the population is about 1.6 percent, and the incidence of arthritis in patients with psoriasis is 6.8 percent. The overall prevalence of psoriatic arthritis in the population is estimated to be 0.1 percent. These figures are applicable to whites.[106]

Pathological Findings

Genetic predisposition to disease is not as clearly delineated as current HLA associations for AS and RD would suggest. A number of different loci have been linked to disease susceptibility. Those best-established are HLA-A1, -B13, -B17 (subset Bw57), and -Cw6, the main association with psoriasis being the HLA-C locus antigen. Furthermore, the immune response (Ir) gene DR7 has been variably associated with psoriasis and is in linkage dysequilibrium with HLA-Cw6, -Bw57, and -B13. HLA-B27 is found in 60 to 80 percent of patients with psoriasis who have sacroiliitis and/or spondylitis. It is not found in increased frequency in patients with only psoriatic peripheral arthritis.[32]

The polymorphonuclear leukocyte appears to be important in the skin lesion in which this cell type predominates. However, the infiltrates in the synovium are predominantly mononuclear after the initial acute stage. Histologically this resembles rheumatoid arthritis with the exception that typical granulomas or lymphoid follicles are absent. Lymphocyte abnormalities are conflicting, and there are no clear-cut differences between patients with and without arthritis.

Histologically the synovium differs from RA in that the lining cells are less hyperplastic. Vascular abnormalities are prominent with thickening of blood vessel walls and occasionally necrosis with cellular infiltrates in the media and adventitia.[39] Fibrosis with fibroblast proliferation can be prominent in erosive disease producing a proliferative component. In a small group of patients immunohistological studies revealed immune deposits predominantly of IgG and IgA contrasting with a control group of rheumatoid arthritis patients in who IgM and C3 were found.[44]

Clinical Features

Clinical presentation may vary considerably. The male-female ratio approaches 1.0 overall. It is greater than 1.0 in patients with spondylitis and less than 1.0 in patients with polyarticular disease simulating RA.[55] Females tend to develop disease at an earlier age than males. The mean age of onset is about 40 years; those patients who have deforming disease generally develop arthritis prior to the age of 20.[55,89]

In the overwhelming majority of cases the skin disease precedes joint disease (75 percent). In 10 to 15 percent the arthritis may predate the appearance of cutaneous lesions and in 10 to 15 percent, the two may be synchronous in onset. The severity of skin disease and arthritis may parallel each other.[72] However, the pattern of arthritis does not correlate with a clinical type of skin disease. Cutaneous involvement can be very subtle and involve only the scalp, perineum, or umbilicus in a patient with an undiagnosed mono- or oligoarticular arthritis.

Nail changes occur more commonly in patients with arthritis (80 percent) than in patients with psoriatic skin involvement alone (20 percent).[33] Clinically this can manifest with subungual hyperkeratoses, onycholysis, ridging, and pitting. Although nail pitting is generally considered characteristic of psoriasis, it can occur alone in 70 percent of the normal population. The association of two or more abnormalities is more consistent with psoriasis. Pitting helps to distinguish psoriasis from Reiter syndrome when other similar changes coexist (Fig. 19-17). Distal interphalangeal (DIP) involvement may parallel severe nail involvement.[55]

The patient with PA can present with any of five recognized subsets.[105,65] It is a misconception that PA implies DIP disease and nail pitting. This particular group, on the contrary, is a much rarer form of the disease. The most common variety is *oligoarticular arthritis* and represents about 80 percent of patients. Typically, small joints of the hands and feet are involved with evidence of dactylitis ("sausage digits"). It is not unusual for asymmetrical polyarticular progression to occur. A form of *symmetric polyarthritis* occurs in about 15 percent of patients and in many cases has been clinically mistaken for seronegative rheumatoid arthritis. *DIP involvement alone* is unusual (approximately 5 percent) despite the fact that DIP involvement overall in PA is in the 60 to 70 percent range. The classically described *arthritis mutilans* also involves approximately 5 percent of patients. These patients include those with significant deformities and frank osteolysis of small bones. The "opera glass" deformity is a manifestation of this process. Finally, 5 percent of patients with PA present with *isolated spondylitis.*

Axial disease in association with peripheral disease is not uncommon and in the majority is asymptomatic. Sacroiliitis occurs in 20 to 40 percent of patients.[64] Males and females are affected equally and there is no relationship to skin disease or peripheral arthritis. Spinal involvement may be asymmetric and random, and there is a predilection for cervical disease including the C1–2 articulation.[56]

Inflammatory eye disease can complicate PA as it can the other SNSA. Conjunctivitis is the most common form. In patients with axial disease, anterior uveitis may predominate.[62]

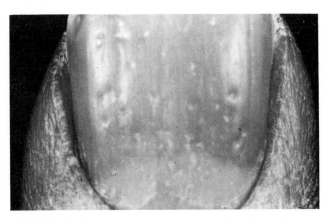

Figure 19-17 Nail pitting in psoriatic arthritis. *(From The American Rheumatism Association slide collection. Reproduced with permission of The Arthritis Foundation.)*

Diagnostic Evaluation

Laboratory abnormalities demonstrate an acute-phase response. The ESR and C-reactive protein readings are both elevated in patients with PA but are normal with psoriasis alone.[66] Quantitative IgA is frequently elevated but does not correlate with the degree of joint inflammation. Rheumatoid factor may occasionally be positive and confuse the clinical picture. Although initially felt to be associated with hyperuricemia, uric acid levels measured after discontinuing all medications were similar in patients with PA and a control group with rheumatoid arthritis.[63]

Radiographically one can see evidence of bone resorption and formation. Resorption progresses centrally producing massive destruction and whittling to frank osteolysis ("mutilans"). Erosions at sites of tendinous insertion (calcaneus) occur as in the other SNSA. Proliferative disease exists around erosions ("pencil-in-cup" deformity of middle phalanx into distal phalanx) (Fig. 19-18). Proliferative abnormalities also exist as "fluffy" periostitis on the shaft of phalanges of the hands and feet.

Treatment

Therapy is initially approached with NSAIDs and physical therapy. In patients with destructive inflammatory disease remittive agents are appropriate and useful. Gold has been shown to be effective.[88] The antimalarials have also been efficacious[55] but can be associated with severe exfoliating skin disease.[71] Cytotoxic drugs such as methotrexate are also quite beneficial and decrease skin involvement as well. Treatment of the skin lesions with PUVA (psoralens and UVA light) has helped the arthritis. Axial disease has not been shown to respond to these modalities.

Surgical intervention with arthroplasty and synovectomy may be associated with greater complications than with rheumatoid arthritis. These include potential postoperative infection, due to increased bacterial colonization of psoriatic skin,

and postoperative fibrosis with ankylosis resulting from the proliferative bone response.

A final note of caution: In patients given intraarticular corticosteroids or tendon sheath injections, the injecting needle should never traverse a psoriatic plaque because of the potential for suppurative sequelae.

ENTEROPATHIC ARTHRITIS

The various forms of gastrointestinal disease associated with rheumatologic syndromes include the following: (1) Inflammatory bowel disease (IBD), Crohn's disease (CD), and ulcerative colitis (UC); (2) reactive arthritis due to enteric pathogens (*Salmonella, Shigella, Campylobacter,* and *Yersinia*); (3) Whipple's disease; (4) postintestinal bypass surgery; (5) primary biliary cirrhosis (PBC); (6) hepatitis; and (7) parasitic disease. The present discussion will be limited to the arthritis of CD and UC. IBD has a very close relationship with the SNSA.

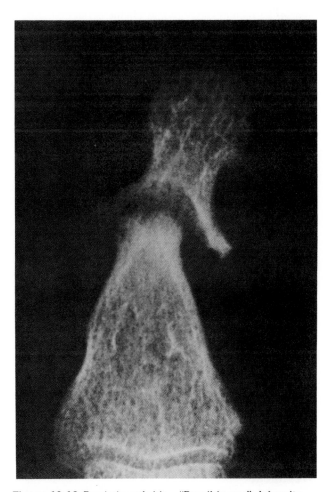

Figure 19-18 Psoriatic arthritis—"Pencil-in-cup" deformity. *(From Wright, V., in Kelly, W. N., et al: Textbook of Rheumatology, 2d ed. Reproduced with permission.)*

It resembles AS more closely than RD or PA.[75] However, there is an increased incidence of CD and UC in relatives of patients with psoriatic arthritis.[105]

Clinical Features

Clinically, patients can have peripheral or axial joint disease. The male-female ratio is equal in peripheral arthritis and greater than 1.0 with spondylitis. Peripheral joint involvement occurs in 10 to 20 percent of patients with both CD and UC. It is usually large joint, asymmetrical and lower more than upper extremity in distribution. The small joints of the hands and feet may be affected but are rarely presenting features. The arthritis is generally nondeforming and most often has its onset following established bowel diseases. In CD it may sometimes precede bowel symptoms.[49,51,107]

The peripheral arthritis in UC parallels the course of the colitis and is found more frequently in patients with bowel complications as well as those with more systemic disease (skin lesions, e.g., erythema nodosum, oral mucosal lesions, and uveitis). Arthritis presents three times more frequently in patients with diffuse colitis than in patients with disease limited to the rectum (proctitis). In CD the peripheral arthritis also follows the course of the bowel disease, however, there is no relationship to eye disease, oral lesions, or skin involvement. Furthermore, bowel complications such as fistulas do not worsen articular prognosis.[49,51,77,107]

Diagnostic Evaluation

Synovial fluid analysis most often reveals type II fluid with about 10,000 white blood cells per cubic millimeter (predominately polymorphonuclear leukocytes). Protein and complement levels are normal. Synovial biopsy has revealed granulomas in some patients with CD. The synovial lining has a mononuclear cellular infiltrate. Radiographically there may be mild osteoporosis related to the inflammatory process and cystic changes resembling the peripheral joint disease in AS. Acute attacks involve most commonly the knees, ankles, elbows, shoulders, wrists, and metacarpophalangeal joints. Approximately 75 percent of attacks resolve in 2 months.[74]

The incidence of axial disease in UC has varied from 1.3 to 25.6 percent. In CD, the range is 2.0 to 6.9 percent.[77] Spondylitis may have its onset at any time in the course of the bowel disease. It may precede bowel involvement in both CD and UC for many years. Sacroiliitis in IBD is frequently asymptomatic. Unlike spondylitis it occurs equally often in males and females. Axial disease does not correlate with the course of clinical colitis. The HLA-B27 marker is positive in 50 to 70 percent of patients with IBD and spondylitis. There is not an increased frequency in sacroiliitis alone.[53,77,108]

Treatment

Surgical treatment of bowel disease is associated with marked improvement in the peripheral arthropathy of UC. Results with CD are not as rewarding. Bowel resection does not improve axial disease in UC or CD.[107]

Associated Syndromes

Additional rheumatic syndromes associated with IBD include: (1) avascular necrosis of bone from corticosteroid usage, (2) septic arthritis of the hip related to fistulous tracts in CD, (3) psoas abscess in CD, and (4) clubbing and/or periostitis, usually asymptomatic.

SUMMARY

It is clear from the above discussion that the SNSA as a group are relatively common diseases. They appear to all be linked by varying degrees of spondylitis, sacroiliitis, and oligo- or polyarticular, asymmetrical, lower-extremity peripheral arthritis. Association with the HLA-B27 genetic marker is primarily with the axial disease, and its incidence may vary with each entity.

Misdiagnosis of these disorders is not uncommon for the following reasons:

1. Low index of suspicion because of asymptomatic axial disease with only peripheral arthropathy.
2. Transient or occult symptoms (i.e., conjunctivitis; cervicitis in females).
3. Lack of recognition of disease in females.
4. Suppression of venereal history.
5. Forgotten enteric symptoms that preceded articular complaints.

It follows from these potentially evanescent features that many patients diagnosed as "seronegative rheumatoid arthritis" may well have a SNSA.[25] It is therefore important in the patient with oligoarticular disease involving primarily the lower extremities that a high index of suspicion for these disorders be maintained. Radiographic examination of the pelvis should be considered even in the absence of low back pain in order to confirm the diagnosis. In addition, careful attention should be given to even subtle aspects of the history and exam. Rational management can then be appropriately instituted.

REFERENCES

Section A: Laboratory Tests

1. Bloch, K., and Salvaggio, J. Use and interpretation of diagnostic immunologic laboratory tests. JAMA 248:2734–2758, 1982.
2. Friou, G.J. Clinical application of lupus serum-nucleoprotein reaction using fluorescent antibody technique. J Clin Invest 36:890–898, 1957.
3. Hargraves, M.N., Richmond, H., and Morton, R. Presentation of two bone marrow elements: The "tart" cell and "L.E." cell. Proc Staff Meet Mayo Clin 23:25–28, 1948.
4. Hind, C., and Pepys, M. The role of serum C-reactive protein (CRP) measurement in clinical practice. Int Med 5:112–151, 1984.
5. Horwitz, C. Laboratory diagnosis of rheumatoid diseases. Postgrad Med 67:195–203, 1980.
6. Lerner, M.R., Boyle, J.A., Hardin, J.A., and Steitz, J.A. Two novel classes of small RNA proteins detected by antibodies associated with lupus erythematosus. Science 211:400–403, 1981.

7. Masi, A., and Feigenbaum, S. Is seronegative rheumatoid arthritis a valid clinical diagnosis? Int Med 5:56–69, 1984.
8. McKenna, C. Symposium on the role of the laboratory in orthopedic practice. Orthop Clin North Am 10:307–318, 1979.
9. Morley, J., and Kushner, I. Serum C-reactive protein levels in disease. NY Acad Sci 389:406–418, 1982.
10. Nakamura, R. *Immunopathology—Clinical Laboratory Concepts and Methods.* Boston, Little, Brown, 1974, p 125.
11. Rodman, G., and Schumacher, R. (eds): *Primer on the Rheumatic Diseases,* 8th ed. Atlanta, Arthritis Foundation, 1983, pp 38–46.
12. Sharp, G.C., Irvin, W.S., Tan, E.M., Gould, R.G., and Holman, H.R. Mixed connective tissue disease. An apparently distinct rheumatic disease syndrome associated with a specific antibody to extractable nuclear antigen. Am J Med 52:148–159, 1972.
13. Tan, E.M., and Kunkel, H.G. Characteristics of a soluble nuclear antigen precipitating with sera of patients with systemic lupus erythematosus. J Immunol 96:464–471, 1966.

Section B: Rheumatoid Arthritis

1. Abel, T., Andrews, B.S., Cunningham, P.H., Brunner, C.M., Davis, J.S., IV, and Horwitz, D.A. Rheumatoid vasculitis: Effect of cyclophosphamide on the clinical course and levels of circulating immune complexes. Ann Int Med 93:407–413, 1980.
2. Abramson, S., Edelson, H., Kaplan, H., Given, W., and Weissmann, G. The neutrophil in rheumatoid arthritis: Its role and the inhibition of its activation by nonsteroidal antiinflammatory drugs. Semin Arthritis Rheum 13:148–153, 1983.
3. Alarcon, G.S., Koopman, W.J., Acton, R.T., and Barger, B.O. Seronegative rheumatoid arthritis: A distinct immunogenetic disease? Arthritis Rheum 25:502–507, 1982.
4. Anderson, L.G., and Talal, N. The spectrum of benign to malignant lymphoproliferation in Sjögren's syndrome. Clin Exp Immunol 10:199–221, 1972.
5. Barrett, A.J. The possible role of neutrophil proteases in damage to articular cartilage. Agents Actions 8:11–17, 1978.
6. Bennett, J.C. The infectious etiology of rheumatoid arthritis. Arthritis Rheum 21:531–538, 1978.
7. Bennett, R.M. Hematological changes in rheumatoid disease. Clin Rheum Dis 3:433–465, 1977.
8. Blackwell, G.J., Carnuccio, R., DiRosa, M., Flower, R.J., et al. Suppression of arachidonate oxidation by glucocorticoid-induced antiphospholipase peptides. Adv Prostaglandin Thromboxane Leukotriene Res 11:65–71, 1983.
9. Blodgets, R.C., Jr., Hever, M.A., Pietrusko, R.G. Auranofin: A unique oral chrysotherapeutic agent. Semin Arthritis Rheum 13:255–273, 1984.
10. Buchanan, W.W., and Tugwell, P. Traditional assessments of articular diseases. Clin Rheum Dis 9:515–529, 1983.
11. Buchanan, W.W., Rooney, P.J., and Rennie, J.A.N. Aspirin and the salicylates. Clin Rheum Dis 5:499–539, 1979.
12. Bucknall, R.C., Davis, P., Bacon, P.A., and Jones, J.V. Neutropenia in rheumatoid arthritis: Studies on possible contributing factors. Ann Rheum Dis 41:242–247, 1982.
13. Bywaters, E.G.L., and Scott, J.L. The natural history of vascular lesions in rheumatoid arthritis. J Chronic Dis 16:905–914, 1963.
14. Calin, A. Pain and inflammation. Am J Med 77(suppl):9–16, 1984.
15. Carson, D.A. Rheumatoid factor, in Kelley, W.N., Harris, E.D., Jr., Ruddy, S., and Sledge, C.B. (eds): *Textbook of Rheumatology,* 2d ed. Philadelphia, Saunders, 1985, pp 664–679.
16. Clague, R.B., and Moore, L.J. IgG and IgM antibody to native type II collagen in rheumatoid arthritis serum and synovial fluid. Evidence for the presence of collagen-anticollagen immune complexes in synovial fluid. Arthritis Rheum 27:1370–1377, 1984.
17. Claman, H.N. Glucocorticosteroids. I. Antiinflammatory mechanisms. II. The clinical responses. Hosp Pract 18:123–134, 143–151, 1983.
18. Clive, D.M., and Stuff, J.S. Renal syndromes associated with nonsteroidal antiinflammatory drugs. N Engl J Med 310:563–572, 1984.
19. Conn, D.L., McDuffie, F.C., and Dyck, P.I. Immunopathologic study of sural nerves in rheumatoid arthritis. Arthritis Rheum 15:135–143, 1972.
20. Cooke, T.D.V. The interactions and local disease manifestations of immune complexes. Bath, Pitman Press.
21. Cromartie, W.J., Craddock, J.G., Schwab, J.H., Anderle, S.K., and Yang, C.H. Arthritis in rats after systemic injection of streptococcal cells or cell walls. J Exp Med 146:1585–1602, 1977.
22. Cupps, T.R., and Fauci, A.S. Corticosteroid-mediated immunoregulation in man. Immunol Rev 65:133–155, 1982.
23. Dayer, J.M., Krane, S.M., Russell, R.G.G., and Robinson, D.R. Production of collagenase and prostaglandins by isolated adherent rheumatoid synovial cells. Proc Natl Acad Sci 73:945–949, 1976.
24. Decker, J.L. Azathioprine and cyclophosphamide as slow-acting drugs for rheumatoid arthritis. Am J Med 75(suppl):74–78, 1983.
25. Depper, J.M., and Zvaifler, N.J. Epstein Barr virus: Its relationship to the pathogenesis of rheumatoid arthritis. Arthritis Rheum 24:755–761, 1981.
26. DeQueker, J., and Rosberg, G. Digital capillaritis in rheumatoid arthritis. Acta Rheum Scand 13:299–307, 1967.
27. Dinarello, C.A. Interleukin-l. Rev Infect Dis 6:51–95, 1984.
28. Dougados, M., and Amor, B. Cyclosporine in rheumatoid arthritis. Arthritis Rheum 28:536, 1985.
29. Dromgoole, S.H., Furst, D.E., and Paulus, H.E. Rational approaches to the use of salicylates in the treatment of rheumatoid arthritis. Semin Arthritis Rheum 11:257–283, 1981.
30. Duthie, J.J.R., Brown, P.E., Truelove, L.H., et al. Course and prognosis in rheumatoid arthritis. Ann Rheum Dis 23:193–204, 1964.
31. Editorial. The viral etiology of rheumatoid arthritis. Lancet 1:772–774, 1981.
32. Ehrlich, G.E. Tolmetin sodium: Meeting the clinical challenge. Clin Rheum Dis 5:481–497, 1979.
33. Engelman, E.G., Sponzilli, E.E., Batey, M.E., et al. Mixed lymphocyte reaction in healthy women with rheumatoid factor lack of association with HLA Dw4. Arthritis Rheum 21:690–693, 1978.
34. Fereira, S.H. Prostaglandins and nonsteroidal drugs, in Berti, F. Samuellson, B., and Velo, G. *Prostaglandins and Thromboxanes.* New York, Plenum, 1976, pp 353–361.
35. Field, E.H., Strober, S., Hoppe, R.T., Calin, A., Engleman, E.G. Kotzin, B.L., Tanay, A.S., Calin, H.J., Terrell, C.D., and Kaplan, H.S. Sustained improvement of intractable rheumatoid arthritis after total lymphoid irradiation. Arthritis Rheum 26:109–118, 1983.
36. Fox, R.I., Howell, F.V., Bone, F.C., and Michelson, P. Primary Sjogren syndrome: Clinical and immunopathologic features. Semin Arthritis Rheum 14:77–105, 1984.
37. Franklin, E.C., Holman, H.R., Muller-Eberhard, H.J., and Kunkel, H.G. An unusual protein component of high molecular weight in the serum of certain patients with rheumatoid arthritis. J Exp Med 105:425–438, 1957.
38. Garber, E.K., Fan, P.T., and Bluestone, R. Realistic guidelines of corticosteroids therapy in rheumatic disease. Semin Arthritis Rheum 11:231–256, 1981.
39. Garella, S., and Matarese, R.A. Renal effects of prostaglandins and clinical adverse effects of nonsteroidal antiinflammatory agents. Medicine (Balt) 63:165–181, 1984.
40. Gay, S., Gay, R. E., and Miller, E.F. The collagens of the joint. Arthritis Rheum 23:937–941, 1980.
41. Gibbons, R.B. Complications of crysotherapy. Arch Int Med 139:343–346, 1979.
42. Goldberg, J., and Pinals, R.S. Felty's syndrome. Semin Arthritis Rheum 10:52–65, 1980.

43. Goodwin, J.S., and Cueppens, J.L. Effect of nonsteroidal antiinflammatory drugs on immune function. Semin Arthritis Rheum 134–143, 1983.

44. Gordon, D.A., Stein, J.L., and Broder, I. Extraarticular features of rheumatoid arthritis. A systematic analysis of 127 cases. Am J Med 54:455–452, 1973.

45. Gottlieb, N.L. Crysotherapy. Bull Rheum Dis 27:912–917, 1976–77.

46. Gray, R.G., Tenebaum, J., and Gottlieb, N.L. Local corticosteroid injection treatment in rheumatic disorders. Semin Arthritis Rheum 10:231–254, 1981.

47. Gumpel, J.M. Radiosynoviorthesis. Clin Rheum Dis 4:311–326, 1978.

48. Gupta, R.C., Robinson, W.A., and Kurnick, J.E. Felty's syndrome: Effect of lithium on granulopoiesis. Am J Med 61:29–32, 1976.

49. Hadler, N.M. A pathogenetic model for erosive synovitis. Lessons from the animal arthritides. Arthritis Rheum 19:256–266, 1976.

50. Hadler, N.M., Johnson, A.M., Spitznagel, J.K., and Quimet, R.J. Protease inhibitors in inflammatory synovial effusions. Ann Rheum Dis 40:55–59, 1981.

51. Halla, J.T., Volanakis, J.E., and Schrohenloher, R.E. Immune complexes in rheumatoid arthritis sera and synovial fluids. A comparison of three methods. Arthritis Rheum 22:440–448, 1979.

52. Hang, L., Theofilopoulos, A.N., and Dixon, F.J. A spontaneous rheumatoid arthritis-like disease in MRL/1 mice. J Exp Med 155:1690–1701, 1982.

53. Harris, J., and Vaughan, J.H. Transfusion studies in rheumatoid arthritis. Arthritis Rheum 4:47–55, 1961.

54. Harris, E.D., Jr. Pathogenesis of rheumatoid arthritis, in Kelley, W.N., Harris, E.D., Jr., Ruddy, S., and Sledge, C.G. (eds): *Textbook of Rheumatology,* vol 1, 2d ed. Philadelphia, Saunders, 1985, pp 886–915.

55. Hart, F.D., and Golding, J.R. Rheumatoid neuropathy. Br Med J 1:1594–1603, 1960.

56. Hazleman, B.L., and Watson, P.G. Ocular complications of rheumatoid arthritis. Clin Rheum Dis 3:501–526, 1977.

57. Higgs, G.A., Harvey, E.A., Ferreira, S.H., and Vane, J.R. The effects of antiinflammatory drugs on the production of prostaglandins in vivo. Adv Prostaglandin Thromboxane Res 105–110,

58. Huskisson, E.C. Azathioprine. Clin Rheum Dis 10:325–332, 1984.

59. Hunder, G.G., and Bunch, T.W. Treatment of rheumatoid arthritis. Bull Rheum Dis 32:1–6, 1982.

60. Hunder, G.G., and McDuffie, F.C. Hypocomplementemia in rheumatoid arthritis. Am J Med 54:461–472, 1973.

61. Hurd, E.R. Extraarticular manifestations of rheumatoid arthritis. Semin Arthritis Rheum 8:151–176, 1977.

62. Ianuzzi, L., Dawson, N., Zein, N., and Kushner, I. Does drug therapy slow radiographic deterioration in rheumatoid arthritis? N Engl J Med 309:1023–1028,

63. Jacoby, R.K., Jayson, M.V., and Cosh, J.A. Onset, early stages and prognosis of rheumatoid arthritis. A clinical study of 100 patients with 11 year follow-up. Br Med J 2:96–100, 1973.

64. Jaffe, I.A. D-penicillamine. Bull Rheum Dis 28:948–952, 1977–78.

65. Jasin, H.E., Cooke, T.D., Hurd, E.R., Smiley, J.D., and Ziff, M. Immunologic models used for the study of rheumatoid arthritis. Fed Proc 32:147–155, 1973.

66. Jasin, H.E., and Dingle, J.T. Human mononuclear cell factors mediate cartilage matrix degradation through chondrocyte activation. J Clin Invest 68:571–581, 1981.

67. Johnson, P.M. Molecular nature and cross reactions of rheumatoid factor. Clin Immunol Allergy 1:103–115, 1981.

68. Kantor, T.G. Ibuprofen. Ann Int Med 91:877–882, 1979.

69. Katz, R.S., Zizic, T.M., Arnold, W.P., and Stevens, M.B. The pseudothrombophlebitis syndrome. Medicine (Baltimore) 50:151–164, 1977.

70. Kemper, J.W., Baggenstoss, A.H., and Slocumb, C.H. The relationship of therapy with cortisone to the incidence of vascular lesions in rheumatoid arthritis. Ann Int Med 46:831–851, 1957.

71. Khan, A.H., and Spodick, D.H. Rheumatoid heart disease. Semin Arthritis Rheum 1:327–337, 1972.

72. Kovarsky, J. Clinical pharmacology and toxicology of cyclophosphamide: Emphasis on use in rheumatic diseases. Semin Arthritis Rheum 12:359–372, 1983.

73. Krane, S.M., Goldring, S.R., and Dayer, J.M., Interactions between lymphocytes, monocytes and other synovial cells in the rheumatoid synovium. Lymphokines 7:75–136, 1982.

74. Kulka, J.P., Bocking, D., Ropes, M.W., and Bauer, W. Early joint lesions of rheumatoid arthritis. Arch Pathol 59:129–150, 1955.

75. Larson, E.B. Adult Stills disease. Medicine 63:82–91, 1984.

76. Lawrence, J.S., Bremner, J.M., Ball, J., Burch, T.A. Rheumatoid arthritis in a subtropical climate. Ann Rheum Dis 25:59–66, 1966.

77. Lawrence, J.S. Rheumatoid arthritis—Nature or nurture? Heberden Oration, 1961. Ann Rheum Dis 29:357–379, 1970.

78. Lipsky, P.E. Disease-modifying drugs, in Utsinger, P.D., Zvaifler, N.J., Ehrlich, G.E. (eds): *Rheumatoid Arthritis.* Philadelphia, Lippincott, 1985, pp 601–634.

79. Lipsky, P.E., and Ziff, M. Inhibition of human helper T cell function in vitro by D-penicillamine and $CuSO_4$. J Clin Invest 65:1069–1076, 1980.

80. Lockie, L.M., Gomez, C., and Smith, D.M. Low dose adrenocorticosteroids in the management of elderly patients with rheumatoid arthritis. Selected examples and summary of efficacy in the long-term treatment of 97 patients. Semin Arthritis Rheum 12:373–381, 1983.

81. Lukkainen, R., Isomaki, H., and Kajander, A. Prognostic value of the type of onset of rheumatoid arthritis. Ann Rheum Dis 42:274–275, 1983.

82. Mackensie, A.H. Antimalarial drugs for rheumatoid arthritis. Am J Med 75(suppl):48–58, 1983.

83. Masi, A.T., Maldonado-cocco, J.A., Kaplan, S.B., Feingenbaum, S.L., and Chandler, K.W. Prospective study of the early course of rheumatoid arthritis in young adults: Comparison of patients with and without rheumatoid factor positivity at entry and identification of variables correlating with outcome. Semin Arthritis Rheum 5:299–326, 1976.

84. Mason, A.M.S., Gumpel, J.M., and Golding, P.L. Sjogren's syndrome—A clinical review. Semin Arthritis Rheum 2:301–331, 1973.

85. McCarty, D.J., and Carrera, G.F. Intractable rheumatoid arthritis. J Am Med Assoc 248:1718–1723, 1982.

86. Michael, D., and Fudenberg, H.H. The incidence and antigenic specificity of antibodies against denatured human collagen in rheumatoid arthritis. Clin Immunol Immunopathol 2:153–159, 1974.

87. Mongan, E., Cass, R., Jacox, R., and Vaughan, J.H. A study of the relation of seronegative and seropositive rheumatoid arthritis to each other and to necrotizing vasculitis. Am J Med 47:23–35, 1969.

88. Moutsopoulos, H.M. Sjogren's syndrome (Sicca syndrome): Current issues. Ann Int Med 92:212–226, 1980.

89. Mowat, A.G. Hematological abnormalities in rheumatoid arthritis. Semin Arthritis Rheum 1:195–219, 1971.

90. Munthe, E., and Natvig, J.B. Immunoglobulin classes, subclasses and complexes of IgG rheumatoid factor in rheumatoid plasma cells. Clin Exp Immunol 12:55–70, 1972.

91. Notkins, A.L. Infectious virus-antibody complexes: Interaction with antiglobulins, complement and rheumatoid factor. J Exp Med 134:415–515, 1971.

92. Pasquali, J.L., Fong, S., Tsoukas, C., Vaughan, J.H., and Carson, D.A. Inheritance of IgM rheumatoid factor idiotypes. J Clin Invest 66:863–866, 1980.

93. Pekin, T.J., Jr., and Zvaifler, N.J. Hemolytic complement in syno-

vial fluid. J Clin Invest 43:1372–1382, 1964.

94. Percy, J.S. Gold in the treatment of Felty's syndrome J Rheumatol 8:878–879, 1981.

95. Pope, R.M., Teller, D.C., and Mannik, M. The molecular basis of self-association of antibodies to IgG (rheumatoid factors) in rheumatoid arthritis. Proc Natl Acad Sci 71:517–521, 1974.

96. Raman, D., Laycock, T., and Haslock, I. Comparison of two indomethacin treatments as night medication in rheumatoid arthritis. Eur J Rheumatol Inflamm 3:194, 1980.

97. Rhymer, A.R. Sulindac. Clin Rheum Dis 5:553–568, 1979.

98. Rhymer, A.R., and Dengos, D.C. Indomethacin. Clin Rheum Dis 5:541–552, 1979.

99. Robinson, D.R. Prostaglandins and antiinflammatory drugs. DM December:1–46, 1983.

100. Ropes, M.W., Bennett, G.A., Cobbs, S., Jacox, R., and Jessar, R.A. Revision of diagnostic criteria for rheumatoid arthritis. Bull Rheum Dis 9:175–176, 1958.

101. Salmeron, G., and Lipsky, P.E. The immunosuppressive potential of antimalarials. Am J Med 75:19–24, 1983.

102. Samuelsson, B. Leukotrienes: Mediators of immediate hypersensitivity reactions and inflammation. Science 220:568–575, 1983.

103. Schmid, F.R., Cooper, N.S., Ziff, M., and McEwen, C. Arteritis in rheumatoid arthritis. Am J Med 30:56–82, 1961.

104. Schumacher, H.R. Synovial membrane and fluid morphologic alterations in early rheumatoid arthritis: Microvascular injury and virus-like particles. Ann NY Acad Sci 256:39–64, 1975.

105. Schwartz, B.D. The human major histocompatability HLA complex, in Stites, D.P., Stobo, J.D., Fudenberg, H.H., Wells, J.V. (eds): *Basic and Clinical Immunology,* 5th ed. Los Altos, CA, Lange, 1984, pp 55–68.

106. Scott, D.G.I., Bacon, P.A., Bothamley, J.E., Allen, C., Elson, C.J., and Wallington, T.B. Plasma exchange in rheumatoid vasculitis. J Rheumatol 8:433–439, 1981.

107. Scott, D.G., Bacon, P.A., and Tribe, C.R. Systemic rheumatoid vasculitis. A clinical and laboratory study of 50 cases. Medicine (Balt) 60:288–297, 1981.

108. Segre, E.J. Naproxen. Clin Rheum Dis 5:411–426, 1971.

109. Shearn, M.A. Sjögren's syndrome, in Smith, L.H. (ed.): *Major Problems in Internal Medicine.* Philadelphia, Saunders, 1971.

110. Short, C.L. Rheumatoid arthritis: Types of course and prognosis. Med Clin North Am 52:549–557, 1968.

111. Simpson, R.W., Smith, C.A. et al. Association of parvoviruses with rheumatoid arthritis of humans. Science 223:1425–1428, 1984.

112. Singer, J.M., and Plotz, C.M. The latex fixation test I. Application to the serologic diagnosis of rheumatoid arthritis. Am J Med 21:888–896, 1956.

113. Smiley, J.D., Sachs, C., and Ziff, M. In vitro synthesis of immunoglobulin by rheumatoid synovial membrane. J Clin Invest 47:624–632, 1968.

114. Sokoloff, L. The pathophysiology of peripheral blood vessels in collagen diseases. Int Acad Pathol Monogr No 4:297, 1963.

115. Sokoloff, L., and Bartiner, H. A three dimensional reconstruction of the early subcutaneous nodule in rheumatoid arthritis. Arthritis Rheum 5:323, 1962.

116. Stastny, P. The HLA-D region and the genetics of rheumatoid arthritis. Adv Inflam Res 3:41–48, 1982.

117. Steinbrocker, O., Traeger, C.H. and Batterman, R.C. Therapeutic criteria in rheumatoid arthritis. JAMA 140:689–662, 1949.

118. Stevenson, D.D. Diagnosis, prevention, and treatment of adverse reactions to aspirin and nonsteroidal antiinflammatory drugs. Am J Med 74:617–622, 1984.

119. Strand, V., and Talal, N. Advances in the diagnosis and concept of Sjögren's syndrome (autoimmune exocrinopathy). Bull Rheum Dis 30:1046–1052, 1979–80.

120. Stuart, J.M., Townes, A.S., and Kang, A.H. Collagen autoimmune arthritis. Ann Rev Immunol 2:199–218, 1984.

121. Szczeklik, A., Gryglewski, R.J., and Czerniawska-Mysik, G. Clinical patterns of hypersensitivity to nonsteroidal antiinflammatory drugs and their pathogenesis. J Allergy Clin Immunol 60:276–284, 1977.

122. Trentham, D.E., Dynesius, R.A., Rocklin, R.E., and David, J.R. Cellular sensitivity to collagen in rheumatoid arthritis. N Engl J Med 299:327–332, 1978.

123. Tu, W.H., Shearn, M.A., Lee, J.C., and Hopper, J. Interstitial nephritis in Sjögren's syndrome. Ann Int Med 69:1163–1170, 1968.

124. Turner-Warwick, M., and Evans, R.C. Pulmonary manifestations of rheumatoid disease. Clin Rheum Dis 3:549–564, 1977.

125. Ugai, K., Ziff, M., and Lipsky, P.E. Gold-induced changes in the morphology and functional capabilities of human monocytes. Arthritis Rheum 22:1352–1360, 1979.

126. Van Winzum, C., and Verhaest, L. Diflusinal. Clin Rheum Dis 5:707–731, 1979.

127. Vane, J.R. Prostaglandins and the aspirin-like drugs. Hosp Pract March:61–71, 1972.

128. Vaughan, J.H., Brunett, E.V., Sobel, W.V., and Jacox, R.F. Intracytoplasmic inclusions of immunoglobulins in rheumatoid arthritis and other diseases. Arthritis Rheum 11:125–134, 1968.

129. Wahl, S.M., Wilder, R.L., Katona, I.M., Wahl, L.M., Allen, J.B., Scher, I., and Decker, J.L. Leukapheresis in rheumatoid arthritis. Arthritis Rheum 26:1076–1084, 1983.

130. Weissman, G. Activation of neutrophils and the lesions of rheumatoid arthritis. J Lab Clin Med 100:322–332, 1982.

131. Werb, Z., Mainardi, C.L., Vater, C.A., and Harris, E.D., Jr. Endogenous activation of latent collagenase by rheumatoid synovial cells. Evidence for a role of plasminogen activator. N Eng J Med 296:1017–1023, 1977.

132. Willkens, R.F. Reappraisal of the use of methotrexate in rheumatic disease. Am J Med 73(suppl):19–25, 1983.

133. Winchester, R.J., Agnello, V., and Kunkel, H.G. Gamma globulin complexes in synovial fluids of patients with rheumatoid arthritis: Partial characterization and relationship to lowered complement levels. Clin Exp Immunol 6:689–706, 1970.

134. Wiseman, E.H., and Boyle, J.A. Piroxicam (Feldene). Clin Rheum Dis 6:585–613, 1980.

135. Wooley, D.E., Crossley, J.M., and Evanson, J.M. Collagenase at sites of cartilage erosion in the rheumatoid joint. Arthritis Rheum 20:1231–1239, 1977.

Section C: Juvenile Arthritis and Arthralgia

1. Ansell, B.M., and Swann, M. The management of chronic arthritis of children. J Bone Joint Surg 65B:536–543, 1983.

2. Arden, G.P., and Ansell, B.M. (eds). *Surgical Management of Juvenile Chronic Arthritis.* London, Academic Press, 1978.

3. Barry, P.E., and Stillman, J.S. Characteristics of juvenile rheumatoid arthritis; its medical and orthopedic management. Orthop Clin North Am 6(3):641–651, 1975.

4. Bell, D.M., Brink, E.W., Nitzkin, J.L., et al. Kawasaki syndrome: Description of two oubreaks in the United States. N Engl J Med 304:1568–1575, 1981.

5. Biro, F., Gewanter, H.L., and Baum, J. The hypermobility syndrome. Pediatrics 72:701–706, 1983.

6. Blockey, N.J., et al. Monarticular juvenile rheumatoid arthritis. J Bone Joint Surg 62B:368–371, 1980.

7. Bywaters, E.G.L. Ankylosing spondylitis in childhood. Clin Rheum Dis 2:387–396, 1976.

8. Council on Rheumatic Fever and Congenital Heart Disease of the American Heart Association. Jones criteria (revised) for guidance in the diagnosis of rheumatic fever. Circulation 32:644–668, 1965.

9. De Valderrama, J.A.F. The observation hip syndrome and its late sequelae. J Bone Joint Surg 45B:462–470, 1963.

10. Emery, H., Larter, W., and Schaller, J.G. Henoch-Schonlein vascu-

litis. Arthritis Rheum 20:385–388, 1977.

11. Fink, C.W., Windmiller, J., and Sartain, P. Arthritis as the presenting feature of childhood leukemia. Arthritis Rheum 15:347–349, 1972.

12. Finsterbush, A., and Pogrund, H. The hypermobility syndrome: Musculoskeletal complaints in 100 consecutive cases of generalized joint hypermobility. Clin Orthop 168:124–127, 1982.

13. Funk, J.F., Jr. Orthopaedic management of juvenile rheumatoid arthritis. Instr Course Lect. 28:311–325, 1979.

14. Giangiacomo, J., and Tsai, C.C. Dermal and glomerular deposition of IgA in anaphylactoid purpura. Am J Dis Child 131:981–983, 1977.

15. Granberry, W.M., and Brewer, E.J., Jr. Early surgery in juvenile rheumatoid arthritis. Instr Course Lect 23:32–37, 1974.

16. Halgerson, S., et al. Arthroscopy of the hip in juvenile chronic arthritis. J Pediatr Orthop 1:273–278, 1981.

17. Hanson, V., Kornreich, H.K., Bernstein, B., King, K.I., Singsen, B.H., et al. Three subtypes of juvenile rheumatoid arthritis: Correlations of age at onset, sex and serologic factors. Arthritis Rheum 20:184–186, 1977.

18. Hardinge, K. The etiology of transient synovitis of the hip in childhood. J Bone Joint Surg 52B:100–107, 1970.

19. Isaacson, A.S. Operative procedures on patients with juvenile rheumatoid arthritis. Instr Course Lect 23:37–40, 1974.

20. Jacobs, J.C. *Pediatric Rheumatology for the Practitioner.* New York, Springer-Verlag, 1982, pp 18–19 and 162–165.

21. Kawasaki, T., Kosaki, F., Okawa, S., Shigematsu, I., and Yanagawa, H. A new infantile acute febrile mucocutaneous lymph node syndrome (MLNS) prevailing in Japan. Pediatrics 54:271–281 1974.

22. Kirk, J.A., Ansell, B.M., and Bywaters, E.G.L. The hypermobility syndrome. Musculoskeletal complaints associated with generalized joint hypermobility. Ann Rheum Dis 26:419–425, 1967.

23. McLaughlin, T.P., Zemel, L., Fisher, R.L., and Gosling, H.R. Chronic arthritis of the knee in Lyme disease. J Bone Joint Surg 68A:1057–1061, 1986.

24. Murray, R.O., and Jacobson, H.G. *The Radiology of Skeletal Disorders,* vol. 1, 2d ed. New York, Churchill Livingstone, 1977, p 350.

25. Resnick, D., and Niwayama, G. Juvenile chronic arthritis, in Resnick, D., and Niwayama, G. (eds): *Diagnosis of Bone and Joint Disorders,* vol 2. Philadelphia, Saunders, 1981, pp 1009–1039.

26. Rydholm, U., et al. Stapling of the knee in juvenile chronic arthritis. J Pediatr Orthop 7:63–68, 1987.

27. Schaller, J., Resnick, D., and Wedgwood, R.J. Juvenile rheumatoid arthritis: A review. Pediatrics 50:940–953, 1972.

28. Schaller, J. Arthritis as a presenting manifestation of malignancy in children. J Pediatr 81:793–797, 1972.

29. Spock, A. Transient synovitis of the hip joint in children. Pediatrics 24:1042, 1959.

30. Steere, A.C., Malawista, S.E., Snydman, D.R., Shope, R.E., Andiman, W.A., Ross, M.R., and Steele, F.M. Lyme arthritis: An epidemic of oligoarticular arthritis in children and adults in three Connecticut communities. Arthritis Rheum 20:7–17 1977.

31. Still, G.F. On a form of chronic joint disease in children. Arthritis Dis Child 16:156–165, 1941. Reprinted from Med-Chir Trans 80:47, 1987.

32. Swann, M., and Ansell, B.M. Soft tissue release of the hips in children with juvenile chronic arthritis. J Bone Joint Surg 67B:404–408, 1986.

33. West, R.J. Acute polyarthritis: Diagnosis and management. Clin Rheum Dis 2:305, 1976.

Section D: Crystal Deposition and Disease

1. Altman, R.D. Arthroscopic findings of the knee in patients with pseudogout. Arthritis Rheum 19:286–292, 1976.

2. Barlow, K.A. Hyperlipidemia in primary gout. Metabolism 17:289–299, 1968.

3. Benedek, T.G. Correlation of serum uric acid and lipid concentrations in normal, gouty, and atherosclerotic men. Ann Intern Med 66:851–861, 1967.

4. Berger, L., and Yu, T-F. Renal function in gout. IV: An analysis of 524 gouty subjects including long-term follow-up studies. Am J Med 59:605–613, 1975.

5. Berkowitz, D. Gout, hyperlipidemia and diabetes inter-relationships. JAMA 197:77–80, 1966.

6. Bjelle, A., and Sunder, G. Pyrophosphate arthropathy: A clinical study of fifty cases. J Bone Joint Surg 56B:246, 1974.

7. Denis, G., and Launay, M.P. Carbohydrate intolerance in gout. Metabolism 18:770–775, 1969.

8. Dorwart, B.B., and Schumacher, H.R. Joint effusions, chondrocalcinosis, and other rheumatic manifestations in hypothyroidism. A clinicopathologic study. Am J Med 59:780–790, 1975.

9. Ellman, M.H., and Levin, B. Chondrocalcinosis in elderly persons. Arthritis Rheum 18:43–47, 1975.

10. Emmerson, B.T., and Knowles, B.R. Triglyceride concentrations in primary gout of chronic lead nephropathy. Metabolism 20:721–729, 1971.

11. Feldman, E.B., and Wallace, S.L. Hypertriglyceridemia in gout. Circulation 29:508–513, 1964.

12. Good, A.E., and Rapp, R. Chondrocalcinosis of the knee with gout and rheumatoid arthritis. N Engl J Med 277:286–290, 1967.

13. Gutman, A.B. The past four decades of progress in the treatment of gout, with an assessment of the present status. Arthritis Rheum 16:431–445, 1973.

14. Gutman, A.B. Gout, in Beeson, P.B., and McDermott, W. (eds): *Cecil's Textbook of Medicine,* 15th ed. Philadelphia, Saunders, 1979, vol 2, pp 2029–2041.

15. Gutman, A.B., and Yu, T-F. Uric acid nephrolithiasis. Am J Med 45:756–000, 1962.

16. Hamilton, E.B.D. Diseases associated with calcium pyrophosphate dihydrate deposition disease. Arthritis Rheum 19:353–357, 1976.

17. Hughes, G.R., Barnes, C.G., and Mason, R.M. Bony ankylosis in gout. Ann Rheum Dis 27:67–70, 1968.

18. Jacobelli, S., McCarty, D.J., Silcox, D.C., and Mall, J.C. Calcium pyrophosphate dihydrate crystal deposition in neuropathic joints. Four cases of polyarticular involvement. Ann Intern Med 79:340–347, 1973.

19. Kelley, W.N., Harris, E.D., Ruddy, S., and Sledge, C.B. *Textbook of Rheumatology.* Philadelphia, Saunders, 1981, pp 1398–1421.

20. Kohn, N.N., Hughes, R., McCarty, D.J., Jr., and Faires, J.S. The significance of calcium phosphate crystals in the synovial fluid of arthritis patients: The pseudogout syndrome. II Identifications of crystals. Ann Intern Med 56:738–745, 1962.

21. MacLachlan, M.J., and Rodnan, G.P. Effect of food, fast, and alcohol on serum uric acid and acute attacks of gout. Am J Med 42:38–57, 1967.

22. Martel, W. The overhanging margin of bone: A roentgenologic manifestation of gout. Radiology 91:755–756, 1968.

23. McCarty, D.J., Jr. Crystal induced inflammation: Syndromes of gout and pseudogout. Geriatrics 18:467, 1963.

24. McCarty, D.J. Calcium pyrophosphate dihydrate crystal deposition disease 1975. Arthritis Rheum 19:275–285, 1976.

25. McCarty, D.J. *Arthritis and Allied Conditions. A Textbook of Rheumatology,* 9th ed. Philadelphia, Lea & Febiger, 1979, pp 1208–1209.

26. McCarty, D.J. *Arthritis and Allied Conditions. A Textbook of Rheumatology,* 10th ed. Philadelphia, Lea & Febiger 1985, pp 1507.

27. McCarty, D.J., Jr., and Haskin, M.E. The roentgenographic aspects of pseudogout (articular chondrocalcinosis): Analysis of 20 cases. AJR 90:1248, 1963.

28. McCarty, D.J., and Hollander, J.L. Identification of urate crystals in gouty synovial fluid. Ann Intern Med 54:452–460, 1961.

29. McCarty, D.J., Jr., Kohn, N.N., and Faires, J.S. The significance of

calcium phosphate crystals in the synovial fluid of arthritis patients. The pseudogout syndrome. Ann Intern Med 56:711, 1962.

30. McCarty, D.J., Silcox, D.C., Coe, F., Jacobelli, S., Reiss, E., Genant, H., and Ellman, M. Diseases associated with calcium pyrophosphate dihydrate crystal deposition. Am J Med 56:704–714, 1974.

31. McKechnie, J.K. Gout, hyperurecemia and carbohydrate metabolism. S Afr Med J 38:182–185, 1964.

32. Menkes, C.J., Simon, F., Delrieu, F., Forest, M., and Delbarre, F. Destructive arthropathy in chondrocalcinosis articularis. Arthritis Rheum 19:329–348, 1976.

33. Mikkelsen, W.M. The possible association of hyperuricemia and/or gout with diabetes mellitus. Arthritis Rheum 8:853–864, 1965.

34. Moskowitz, R.W., and Garcia, P. Chondrocalcinosis articularis. Arch Intern Med 132:87–91, 1973.

35. Myers, A., Epstein, G.H., Dodge, J.H., et al.: The relationship of serum uric acid to risk factors in coronary heart disease. Am J Med 45:520–529, 1969.

36. Nylassy, S., Stefanovic, J., Sitaj, S., and Zitnan, D. HLA system in articular chondrocalcinosis. Acta Rheumatol 19:391, 1975.

37. Phelps, P., and Hawker, C.D. Serum parathyroid hormone levels in patients with calcium pyrophosphate crystal deposition disease. Acta Rheumatol 16:590, 1973.

38. Rapado, A. Relationship between gout and arterial hypertension, in Speling, O., DeVries, A., and Wyngaarden, J.B. (eds): *Purine Metabolism in Man,* vol 41B. New York, Plenum, 1974, p 451.

39. Reginato, A.J. Articular chondrocalcinosis in the Chiloe islanders. Arthritis Rheum 19:395–404, 1976.

40. Reginato, A.J., Fuates, C., Galdamez, M., Zmyjiwsky, C., and Schumacher, H.R. *HLA Antigen and ankylosing chondrocalcinosis,* abstract 230. VII Pan American Congress of Rheumatology, Bogota, Colombia, June 18–23, 1978, pp 977.

41. Reginato, A.J., Hollander, J.L., Martinez, V., et al. Familial chondrocalcinosis in the Chiloe islands, Chile. Ann Rheum Dis 34:260–268, 1975.

42. Resnick, D., and Niwayama, G. *Diagnosis of Bone and Joint Disorders.* Philadelphia, Saunders, 1981, pp 1474–1503.

43. Resnick, A., Niwayama, G., Goergen, T.G., Utsinger, P.D., Shapiro, R.F., Haselwood, D.H., and Weisner, K.B. Clinical, radiographic, and pathologic abnormalities in calcium pyrophosphate dihydrate deposition disease: Pseudogout. Radiology 122:1–15, 1977.

44. Rubinstein, H.M., and Shah, D.M. Pseudogout. Semin Arthritis Rheum 2:259, 1972–73.

45. Snaith, M.D., Scott, J.T. Uric acid clearance in patients with gout and normal subjects. Ann Rheum Dis 30:285–289, 1971.

46. Thompson, G.R., Ming Ting, Y., Riggs, G.S., et al. Calcific tendonitis and soft tissue calcification resembling gout. JAMA 203:464–472, 1968.

47. VanderKorst, J.K., and Geerands, J. Articular chondrocalcinosis in a Dutch pedigree. Arthritis Rheum 19:405–409, 1976.

48. Yu, T-F. Milestones in the treatment of gout. Am J Med 56:676–685, 1974.

49. Yu, T-F., and Gutman, A.B. Uric acid nephrolithiasis in gout. Predisposing factors. Ann Intern Med 67:1133–1148, 1967.

50. Zitnan, D., and Sitaj, S. Chondrocalcinosis articularis. 1: Clinical and radiologic study. Ann Rheum Dis 22:142, 1963.

51. Zitnan, D., and Sitaj, S. Natural course of articular chondrocalcinosis. Arthritis Rheum 19:363–390, 1976.

Section E: Systemic Lupus Erythematosus

1. Abramson, S.B., Given, W.P., Edelson, H.S., and Weissmann, G. Neutrophil aggregation induced by sera from patients with active systemic lupus erythematosus. Arthritis Rheum 26:630–636, 1983.

2. Agnello, V., Koffler, D., Eisenberg, J.W., and Kunkel, H.G. Immune complex systems in the nephritis of systemic lupus erythematosus. Kidney Int 3:90–99, 1973.

3. Alarcon-Segovia, D. Drug-induced systemic lupus erythematosus and related syndromes. Clin Rheum Dis 1:573, 1975.

4. Angles-Curo E., Sultan, Y., and Clanvel, J.P. Predisposing factors to thrombosis in systemic lupus erythematosus. J Lab Clin Med 94:312–323, 1979.

5. Appel, G.B., Silva, F.G., Pirani, C.L., Meltzer, J.I., and Estes, D. Renal involvement in systemic lupus erythematosus (SLE): A study of 56 patients emphasizing histologic classification. Medicine 57:371–410, 1978.

6. Arnett, F.C., and Schulman, L.E. Studies in familial systemic lupus erythematosus. Medicine 55:313–322, 1976.

7. Austin, H.A., III, Muenz, L.R., Joyce, K.M., Antonovych, T.A., Kullick, M.E., Klippel, J.H., Decker, J.L., and Balow, J.E. Prognostic factors in lupus nephritis. Contribution of renal histologic data. Am J Med 75:382–391, 1983.

8. Baldwin, D.S., Lowenstein, J., Rothfield, N.F., Gallo, G., and McCluskey, R.T. The clinical course of the proliferative and membranous forms of lupus nephritis. Ann Intern Med 73:929–942, 1970.

9. Balow, J.E., Austin, H.A., III, Muenz, L.R., Joyce, K.M., Antonovych, T.T., Klippel, J.H., Steinberg, A.D., Plotz, P.H., and Decker, J.L. Effect of treatment on the evolution of renal abnormalities in lupus nephritis. N Eng J Med 311:491–495, 1984.

10. Bonfiglio, T.A., Botti, R.E., and Hagstrom, J.W.C. Coronary arteritis, occlusion and myocardial infarction due to lupus erythematosus. Am Heart J 83:153–158, 1972.

11. Bluestein, H.G. Neurocytotoxic antibodies in serum of patients with systemic lupus erythematosus. Proc Natl Acad Sci 75:3965–3969, 1978.

12. Boey, M.L., Colaco, C.B., Gharavi, A.E., Eikon, K.B., Loizou, S., and Hughes, G.R.V. Thrombosis in systemic lupus erythematosus: Striking association with the presence of circulating lupus anticoagulant. Br Med J 287:1021–1023, 1983.

13. Bresnihan, B., Oliver, M., Crigor, R., and Hughes G.R.V. Brain reactivity of lymphocytotoxic antibodies in systemic lupus erythematosus with and without cerebral involvement. Clin Exp Immunol 30:333–337, 1977.

14. Budman, D.R., Merchant, E.B., Steinberg, A.D., Deft, B., Gershwin, M.E., Lizzio, E., and Reeves, J.P. Increased spontaneous activity of antibody forming cells in the peripheral blood of patients with severe SLE. Arthritis Rheum 20:829–833, 1977.

15. Carette, S., Klippel, J.H., Decker, J.L., Austin, H.A., Plotz, P.H., Steinberg, A.D., and Balow, J.E. Controlled studies of oral immunosuppressive drugs in lupus nephritis. Ann Intern Med 99:1–8, 1983.

16. Chuang, KT.Y., Hunder, G.G., Ilstrup, D.M., and Kurland, L.T. Polymyalgia rheumatica. A 10 year epidemiologic and clinical study. Ann Intern Med 97:672–680, 1982.

17. Cipriano, P.R., Silverman, J.F., Perlroth, M.G., Griepp, R.B., and Wexler, L. Coronary arterial narrowing in Takayasu's aortitis. Am J Cardiol 39:744–750, 1977.

18. Colaco, C.B., and Elkon, K.B. The lupus anticoagulant. A disease marker in antinuclear antibody negative lupus. Arthritis Rheum 28:67–74, 1985.

19. Fauci, A.S., Haynes, B.F., and Katz, P. The spectrum of vasculitis: Clinical, pathologic, immunologic, and therapeutic considerations. Ann Intern Med 89(part I):660–676, 1978.

20. Fauci, A.S., Katz, P., Haynes, B.F., and Wolff, S.W. Cyclophosphamide therapy of severe systemic necrotizing vasculitis, N Engl J Med 301:235–238, 1979.

21. Fauci, A.S., Steinberg, A.D., Haynes, B.F., and Whalen, G. Immunoregulatory aberrations in systemic lupus erythematosus. J Immunol 121:1473–1479, 1978.

22. Feinglass, E.J., Arnett, F.C., Dorsch, C.A., Zizic, T.M., and Stevens, M.C. Neuropsychiatric manifestations of systemic lupus erythematosus: Diagnosis, clinical spectrum, and relationship to other features of the disease. Medicine 55:323–339, 1976.

23. Fessel, W.J. Systemic lupus erythematosus in the community. Arch Intern Med 134:1027–1035, 1974.

24. Fishbein, E., and Alarcin-Segovia, D. Phenotypically low acetyl transferase activity: A characteristic of systemic lupus erythematosus (SLE). Arthritis Rheum 19:796. Abstract. 1976.

25. Foad, B., Litwin, Z., Zimmer, H., and Hess, E.B. Acetylator phenotype in systemic lupus erythematosus. Arthritis Rheum 20:815–818, 1977.

26. Fraga, A., Mintz, G., Valle, L., and Flores-Izquierdo, G. Takayasu's arteritis. Frequency of systemic manifestations (study of 22 patients) and favorable response to maintenance steroid of therapy with adrenocorticosteroids (12 patients). Arthritis Rheum 15:617–624, 1972.

27. Frank, M.M., Hamburger, M.I., Lawley, T.J., Kimberly, R.P., and Plotz, P.H. Detective reticuloendothelial system Fc-receptor function in systemic lupus erythematosus. N Engl J Med 300:518–523, 1979.

28. Fresco, R. Viral-like particles in SLE. N Engl J Med 283:1231–1233, 1970.

29. Fye K.H., Becker, M.J., Theofilopoulos, A.N., Moutsopoulos, H., Feldman, J.L., and Talal, N. Immune complexes in hepatitis B antigen-associated periarteritis nodosa. Am J Med 62:783, 1977.

30. Geitner, D., Kohn, R.W., Gorevic, P., and Franklin, E.C. The effect of combination therapy (steroids, immunosuppressives, and plasmapheresis) on 5 mixed cryoglobulinemia patients with renal, neurologic and vascular involvement. Arthritis Rheum 24:1121, 1981.

31. Gillian, J.N., Cheatum, D.E., Hurd, E.R., Stastny, P., and Ziff, M. Immunoglobulin in uninvolved skin in systemic lupus erythematosus. Association with renal disease. J Clin Invest 53:1434, 1974.

32. Goodman, B.W., Jr. Temporal arteritis. Am J Med 67:839–000, 1979.

33. Grossman, E., Morag, B., Nussinovitch, N., Boichis, H., Knecht, A., and Rosenthal, T. Clinical use of Captopril in Takayasu's disease. Arch Intern Med 144:95, 1984.

34. Hanauer, L.B., and Christian, C.L. Studies of cryoproteins in systemic lupus erythematosus. J Clin Invest 46:400, 1967.

35. Haupt, H.M., Moore, W.G., and Hutchins, G.M. The lung in systemic lupus erythematosus. Analysis of the pathologic changes in 120 patients. Am J Med 71:791, 1981.

36. Hainrin, B., Jonsson, N., and Hellsten, S. Polymyalgia arteritica. Further clinical and histopathological studies with a report of six autopsy cases. Ann Rheum Dis 27:397, 1968.

37. Hejmancik, M.R., Wright, J.C., Quint, R., and Jennings, F.F. The cardiovascular manifestations of systemic lupus erythematosus. Am Heart J 68:119, 1964.

38. Hunder, G.G., and Hacleman, B.L. Giant cell arteritis and polymyalgia rheumatica, in Kelley, W.N., Harris, E.D., Jr., Ruddy, S., and Sledge, C.B. (eds): *Textbook of Rheumatology.* Philadelphia, Saunders, 1981, pp 1189–1196.

39. Ishikowa, K. Natural history and classification of occlusive thromboaortopathy (Takayasu's disease). Circulation 15:27, 1978.

40. Israel, H.L., Patchefsky, A.S., and Saldana, M.J. Wegener's granulomatosis, lymphoid granulomatosis, and benign lymphocytic angiitis and granulomatosis of lung. Recognition and treatment. Ann Intern Med 87:691, 1977.

41. Johnson, R.T., and Richardson, E.P. The neurological manifestations of systemic lupus erythematosus. Medicine 47:337, 1968.

42. Jones, J.V., Robinson, M.F., Parciany, R.K., Layfer, L.F., and McLeod, B. Therapeutic plasmapharesis in systemic lupus erythematosus. Effect on immune complexes and antibodies to DNA. Arthritis Rheum 24:1113, 1951.

43. Kaplan, A.P. Immune complexes, vasoactive mediators, and fibroid necrosis in connective tissue diseases, in Guptol, S., and Galal, N. (eds): *Immunology of Rheumatic Diseases.* New York, Rheum. Medical, 1985, pp 581–618.

44. Klippel, J.H., and Zwaifler, N.J. Neuropsychiatric abnormalities in systemic lupus erythematosus. Clin Rheum Dis 1:621, 1975.

45. Lanham, J.G., Elkon, K.B., Pusey, C.D., and Hughes, G.R. Systemic vasculitis with asthma and eosinophilia: A clinical approach to the Churg-Strauss syndrome. Medicine 63:65, 1984.

46. Leonhardt, T. Family studies in systemic lupus erythematosus. Acta Med Scand 416:51, 1964.

47. Levo, Y., Gorevic, P.D., Kassab, H.J., Tobias, H., and Franklin, E.C. Liver involvement in the syndrome of mixed cryoglobulinemia. Ann Intern Med 87:287, 1977.

48. Lewis, R.M., Tannenberg, W., Smith, C., and Schwartz, R.S. C-type viruses in SLE. Nature 252:78, 1974.

49. Libman, E., and Sacks, B. A hitherto undescribed form of valvular and mural endocarditis. Arch Intern Med 33:701, 1924.

50. Lockshin, M.D., Gibofsky, A., Peebles, C.L., Gigli, I., Fotino, M., and Hurwitz, S. Arthritis Rheum 26:210, 1983.

51. Lockshin, M.D., Druzin, M.L., Goei, S., Quimar, T., Magid, M.S., Jovanovic, L., and Ferenc, M. Antibody to cardiolipin as a prediction of fetal distress or death in pregnant patients with systemic lupus erythematosus. N Engl J Med 313:152, 1985.

52. Lospalluto, J., Dorward, B., Miller, W., Jr., and Zitt, M. Cryoglobulinemia based on interaction between a gamma macroglobulin and 75 gamma globulin. Am J Med 32:142, 1962.

53. Lloyd, W., and Scher, P. Immune complexes, complement, and anti DNA in exacerbations of systemic lupus erythematosus. Medicine 60:208, 1981.

54. McDuffie, F.C., Sams, W.M., Jr., Maldonado, J.E., Andreini, P.H., Conn, D.L., and Samayoa, E.A. Hypocomplementemia with cutaneous vasculitis and arthritis: Possible immune complex syndrome. Mayo Clin Proc 48:340, 1973.

55. Meltzer, M., Franklin, E.C., Elias, K., McCluskey, R.T., and Cooper, N. Cryoglobulinemia—A clinical and laboratory study. II. Cryoglobulins with rheumatoid factor activity. Am J Med 40:837, 1966.

56. Reveille, J.D., Bias, W.B., Winkelstein, J.A., Provost, T.J., Dorsch, C.A., and Arnett, F.C. Familial systemic lupus erythematosus: Immunogenetic studies in eight families. Medicine 62:21, 1983.

57. Rick, M.E., and Hoyer, L.W. Hemostatic disorders in systemic lupus erythematosus. Clin Rheum Dis 1:583, 1975.

58. Ross, R.S., and McKusick, V.A. Aortic arch syndromes: Diminished or absent pulses in arteries arising from arch of aorta: Aortic arch syndrome. Arch Intern Med 92:701, 1953.

59. Rothfield, N. Clinical features of systemic lupus erythematosus, in Kelley, W.N., Harris, E.D., Jr., Ruddy, S., and Sledge, C.B. (eds): *Textbook of Rheumatology.* Philadelphia, Saunders, 1981, pp 1106–1132.

60. Roubinian, J.R., Talal, N., Greenspan, J.S., Goodman, J.R., and Siiteri, P.K. Effect of castration and hormone treatment on survival, anti-nucleic acid antibodies and glomerulonephritis in NZB/NZW-Fl mice. J Exp Med 147:1568, 1978.

61. Sack, M., Cassidy, J.T., and Boleg, G. Prognostic factors in polyarteritis. J Rheumatol 2:411, 1975.

62. Sakane, T., Steinberg, A.D., and Green, I. Studies of immune functions of patients with systemic lupus erythematosus. I. Dysfunction of suppressor T cell activity related to impaired generation of, rather than response to, suppressor cells. Arthritis Rheum 21:657, 1978.

63. Schechter, S.L., Bole, G.G., and Walker, S.E. Midline granuloma and Wegener's granulomatosis: Clinical and therapeutic considerations. J Rheumatol 3:241, 1976.

64. Schleider, M.A., Nachman, R.L., Jaffe, E.A., and Colman, M. A clinical study of the lupus anticoagulant. Blood 48:499, 1976.

65. Schrager, M.A., and Rothfield, N.F. The lupus band test. Rheum Dis 1:597, 1975.

66. Sergent, J.S., Lockshin, M.D., Christian, C.L., and Gocke, D.J. Vasculitis with hepatitis B antigenemia: Long term observations in nine patients. Medicine 55:1, 1976.

67. Schapiro, S.S., and Hultin, M. Acquired inhibitors to the blood coagulation factors. Semin Thromb Hemost 1:336, 1975.

68. Siegel, M., Lee, S.L., Widelock, D., Reilly, E.B., Wise, G.J., Zingale, S.B., and Fuerst, H.T. The epidemiology of systemic lupus erythematosus: Preliminary results in New York City. J Chronic Dis 15:131, 1962.

69. Sontheimer, R.D., Maddison, P.J., Reichlin, M., Jordon, R.E., Stastny, P., and Grilliam, J.N. Serologic and HLA associations in subacute cutaneous lupus erythematosus, a clinical subset of lupus erythematosus. Ann Intern Med 97:664, 1982.

70. Steinberg, A.D., Raveche, E.S., Laskin, C.A., Smith, H.R., Santoro, T., Miller, M.L., and Plotz, P.H. Systemic lupus erythematosus. Insights from animal models. Ann Intern Med 100:714, 1984.

71. Tsokos, M., Fauci, A.S., and Costa, J. Idiopathic midline destructive disease (IMDD). A subgroup of patients with the midline granuloma syndrome. Am J Clin Pathol 77:162, 1982.

72. Winfield, J.B., Koffler, D., and Kunkel H.G. Specific concentration of polynucleotide immune complexes in the cryoprecipitates of patients with systemic lupus erythematosus. Clin Exp Immunol 19:399, 1977.

73. Wolff, S.M., Fauci, A.S., Horn, R.G., and Dale, D.C. Wegener's granulomatosis. Ann Intern Med 81:513, 1974.

74. Yoshiki, T., Mellors, R.C., Strand, M., and August, J.T. The viral envelope glycoprotein of murine leukemia virus and the pathogenesis of immune complex glomerulonephritis of New Zealand mice. J Exp Med 140:1011, 1974.

75. Zeek, P.M. Periarteritis nodosa: A critical review. Am J Pathol 22:777, 1952.

76. Zimmerman, S.W., Jenkins, P.J., Shelp, W.D., Bloodworth, J.M.B., Jr., and Burkholder, P.M. Progression from minimal or focal to diffuse proliferative lupus nephritis. Lab Invest 32:665, 1975.

Section F: Spondyloarthropathies

1. Aho, K., Leirisalo-Repo, M., and Repo, H. Reactive arthritis. Clin Rheum Dis 11:25–40, 1985.

2. Alarcon, G.S., Bocanegra, T.S., Gotuzzo, E., et al. Reactive arthritis associated with brucellosis: HLA studies. J Rheumatol 8:621–625, 1981.

3. Arnett, F.C., Hochberg, M.C., and Bias, W.B. Cross reactive HLA antigens in B27 negative Reiter's syndrome and sacroiliitis. Johns Hopkins Med J 141:193–197, 1977.

4. Atkins, F.M., Friedman, M.M., Rao, P.V.S., et al. Interactions between mast cells, fibroblasts, and connective tissue components. Int Arch Allergy Appl Immun 77:96–102, 1985.

5. Baldassare, A.R., Weiss, T.O., Tsai, C.C., et al. Immunoprotein deposition in synovial tissue in Reiter's syndrome. Ann Rheum Dis 40:281–285, 1981.

6. Ball, J. The Heberden oration, 1970: Enthesopathy of rheumatoid and ankylosing spondylitis. Ann Rheum Dis 30:213–223, 1971.

7. Bergfeldt, L. HLA-B27 associated rheumatic diseases with severe cardiac bradyarrhythmias. Am J Med 75:210–215, 1983.

8. Bergfeldt, L., Edhag, O., Vedin, L., et al. Ankylosing spondylitis: An important cause of severe disturbances of the cardiac conduction system. Am J Med 73:187–191, 1982.

9. Bennett, P.H., and Burch, T.A. New York symposium on population studies in the rheumatic diseases: New diagnostic criteria-ankylosing spondylitis. Bull Rheum Dis 17:453, 1967.

10. Bisla, R.S., Ranawat, C.S., and Inglis, A.E. Total hip replacement in patients with ankylosing spondylitis with involvement of the hip. J Bone Joint Surg 58A:233, 1976.

11. Bocanegra, T.S., Espinosa, L.R., Bridgeford, P.H. et al. Reactive arthritis induced by parasitic infestation. Ann Intern Med 94:207–209, 1981.

12. Brewerton, D.A., Caffrey, M., Hart, F.O., et al. Ankylosing spondylitis and HLA-27. Lancet 1:904–907, 1973a.

13. Brewerton, D.A., Caffrey, M., Nicholls, A., et al. Acute anterior uveitis and HLA-27. Lancet 2:994–998, 1973b.

14. Bulkley, B.H., and Roberts, W.C. Ankylosing spondylitis and aortic regurgitation. Description of the characteristic cardiovascular lesion from study of eight necropsy patients. Circulation 18:1014–1027, 1973.

15. Burns, T.M., Marks, S.H., and Calin, A. *A Double-Blind, Placebo-Controlled, Crossover Trial of Azathioprine in Refractory Reiter's* Syndrome. Abstract. ARA Annual Scientific Meeting, San Antonio, TX, June 1983.

16. Bywaters, E.G.L. A case of early ankylosing spondylitis with fatal secondary amyloidosis. Br Med J 2:412–416, 1968.

17. Calin, A. HLA B27: To type or not to type? Ann Intern Med 92:208–211, 1980.

18. Calin, A. HLA-B27 in 1982. Reappraisal of a clinical test. Ann Intern Med 96:114–115, 1982.

19. Calin, A. Patterns of the spondyloarthropathies. Adv Inflamm Res 9:237–248, 1985.

20. Calin, A. Ankylosing spondylitis. Clin Rheum Dis 11:41–60, 1985.

21. Calin, A. Ankylosing spondylitis, in Kelley, W.N., et al (eds): *Textbook of Rheumatology,* 2d ed. Philadelphia, Saunders, 1985.

22. Calin, A., and Fries, J.F. The striking prevalence of ankylosing spondylitis in "healthy" W27 positive males and females. A controlled study. N Engl J Med 293:835–839, 1975.

23. Calin, A., and Fries, J.F. An "experimental" epidemic of Reiter's syndrome, revisited. Follow-up evidence on genetic and environmental factors. Ann Intern Med 84:564–566, 1976.

24. Calin, A., Marder, A., Becks, E, et al. Genetic differences between B27 positive patients with ankylosing spondylitis and B27 positive healthy controls. Arthritis Rheum 26:1460–1464, 1983.

25. Calin, A., and Marks, S.H. The case against seronegative rheumatoid arthritis. Am J Med 70:992–994, 1981.

26. Calin, A., Porta, J., and Fries, J.F. The clinical history as a screening test for ankylosing spondylitis. JAMA 237:2613, 1977.

27. Clegg, D.O., Samuelson, C.O., Williams, H.J., et al Articular complications of jejuno-ileal by pass surgery. J Rheumatol 7:65–70, 1980.

28. Cowling, R., Ebringer, R., and Ebringer, A. Association of inflammation with raised serum IgA in ankylosing spondylitis. Ann Rheum Dis 39:545–549, 1980.

29. Csonka, G.W., Litchfield, J.W., Oates, J.K., et al. Cardiac lesions in Reiter's disease. Br Med J 1:243–247, 1961.

30. Curry, R., Thoen, J., Shelborne, C., et al. Antibodies to and elevations of beta-2 microglobulin in the serum of ankylosing spondylitis patients. Arthritis Rheum 25:375–380, 1982.

31. Davidson, C., Wojtulewski, J.A., Bacon, P.A., et al. Temporomandibular joint disease in ankylosing spondylitis. Ann Rheum Dis 34:87–91, 1975.

32. Eastmond, C.J., and Woodnow, J.C. The HLA system and the arthropathies associated with psoriasis. Ann Rheum Dis 36:112–120, 1977.

33. Eastmond, C.J., and Wright, V. The nail dystrophy of psoriatic arthritis. Ann Rheum Dis 38:226–228, 1979.

34. Ebringer, A., Barnes, M., Childerstone, M., et al. Etiopathogenesis of ankylosing spondylitis and the cross-tolerance hypothesis. Adv Inflam Res 9:101–128, 1985.

35. Ebringer, R.W., Cawdell, D.R., Cowling, P., and Ebringer, A. Sequential studies in ankylosing spondylitis: Association of *Klebsiella pneumoniae* and active disease. Ann Rheum Dis 37:146–151, 1978.

36. Ebringer, R., Cooke, D., Cawdell, D.R., et al. Ankylosing spondylitis: *Klebsiella* and HLA-B27. Rheumatol Rehabil 16:190–196, 1977.

37. Editorial. The lungs in ankylosing spondylitis. Br Med J 3:492–493, 1971.

38. Emery, A.E., and Lawrence, J.S. Genetics of ankylosing spondylitis. J Med Genet 4:239–244, 1967.

39. Espinoza, L.R., Vasey, F.B., Espinoza, C.G., et al. Vascular changes

in psoriatic synovium. A light and electron microscopic study. Arthritis Rheum 25:677–684, 1982.

40. Farber, G.A., Forshner, J.G., and O'Quinn, S.F. Reiter's syndrome, treatment with methotrexate. JAMA 200:171–000, 1967.

41. Ford, D.K. Synovial lymphocyte responses in the spondyloarthropathies. Adv Inflam Res 9:189–202, 1985.

42. Fournier, A.M., Denizet, D., and Delagrange, A. La lymphographie dans la spondylarthrite ankylosante. J Radiol Electrol 50:773–784, 1969.

43. Fox, R., Calin, A., Gerber, R.C., et al. The chronicity of symptoms and disability in Reiter's syndrome: An analysis of 131 consecutive patients. Ann Intern Med 91:190–193, 1979.

44. Fyrand, O., Mellbye, O.J., and Natvig, J.B. Immunofluorescence studies for immunoglobulins and complement C_3 in synovial joint membranes in psoriatic arthritis. Clin Exp Immunol 29:422–427, 1977.

45. Geczy, A.F., Alexander, K., Bashir, H.V., et al. A factor(s) in *Klebsiella* culture filtrates specifically modifies an HLA-B27 associated surface component. Nature 283:782–784, 1980.

46. Ginsburg, W.W., and Cohen, M.D. Peripheral arthritis in ankylosing spondylitis: A review of 209 patients followed up for more than 20 years. Mayo Clin Proc 58:593–596, 1983.

47. Goldenberg, D.L. "Postinfectious" arthritis. New look at an old concept with particular attention to disseminated gonococcal infection. Am J Med 74:925–928, 1983.

48. Good, A.E. Reiter's disease: A review with special attention to cardiovascular and neurologic sequelae. Semin Arthritis Rheum 3:253–286, 1974.

49. Greenstein, A.J., Janowitz, H.D., and Sachar, D.B. The extra intestinal complications of Crohn's disease and ulcerative colitis: A study of two patients. Medicine 55:401–412, 1976.

50. Grumet, F.C., Calin, A., Engleman, E.G., et al Studies of HLA-B27 using monoclonal antibodies: Ethnic disease associated variants. Adv Inflam Res 9:41–53, 1985.

51. Haslock, I., and Wright, V. The musculoskeletal complications of Crohn's disease. Medicine 52:217–225, 1973.

52. Hunter, T., and Dubo, H. Spinal fractures complicating ankylosing spondylitis. Ann Intern Med 88:546–549, 1978.

53. Hyla, J.F., Frank, W.A., and Davis, J.S. Lack of association of HLA-B27 with radiographic sacroiliitis in inflammatory bowel disease. J Rheumatol 3:196–200, 1976.

54. Jennette, J.C., Ferguson, A.L., Moore, M.A., et al. IgA nephropathy associated with seronegative spondyloarthropathies. Arthritis Rheum 75:144–149, 1982.

55. Kammer, G.M., Soter, N.A., Gibson, D.J., et al. Psoriatic arthritis: A clinical, immunologic and HLA study of 100 patients. Semin Arthritis Rheum 9:75–97, 1979.

56. Kaplan, D., Plotz, C.M., Nathanson, L., et al. Cervical spine in psoriasis and in psoriatic arthritis. Ann Rheum Dis 23:50–56, 1964.

57. Keat, A. Reiter's syndrome and reactive arthritis in perspective. N Engl J Med 309:1606–1615, 1983.

58. Khan, M.A., and Khan, M.K. Diagnostic value of HLA-B27 testing in ankylosing spondylitis and Reiter's syndrome. Ann Intern Med 96:70–76, 1982.

59. Khan, M.A., and Van der Linden, S.M. The risk of ankylosing spondylitis in HLA B27 positive individuals: A reappraisal. J Rheumatol 11:727–728, 1984.

60. Kinsella, T.D., Fritzler, M.J., and Ryan, J.P. Cell-mediated cytotoxicity in ankylosing spondylitis. Adv Inflam Res 9:231–236, 1985.

61. LaBresh, K.A., Lally, E.V., and Sharma, S.C. Two dimensional echocardiographic detection of preclinical aortic root abnormalities in rheumatoid variant diseases. Am J Med 78:908–912, 1985.

62. Lambert, J.R., and Wright, V. Eye inflammation in psoriatic arthritis. Ann Rheum Dis 35:354–356, 1976.

63. Lambert, J.R., and Wright, V. Serum uric acid levels in psoriatic arthritis. Ann Rheum Dis 36:264–267, 1977.

64. Lambert, J.R. and Wright, V. Psoriatic spondylitis a clinical and radiological description of the spine in psoriatic arthritis. Q J Med 96:411–425, 1977.

65. Laurent, M.R. Psoriatic arthritis. Clin Rheum Dis 11:61–85, 1985.

66. Laurent, M.R., Panayi, G.S., and Shepherd, P. Circulating immune complexes, serum immunoglobulins and acute phase proteins in psoriasis and psoriatic arthritis. Ann Rheum Dis 40:66–69, 1981.

67. Leirisalo, M., Gripenberg, M., Julkunen, I., et al. Circulating immune complexes in *Yersinia* infection. J Rheumatol 11:365–368, 1984.

68. Leonard, D.G., O'Putty, J.D., and Rogers, R.S. Prospective analysis of psoriatic arthritis in patients hospitalized for psoriasis. Mayo Clin Proc 53:511–518, 1978.

69. Lloyd, G.E. (ed): *Hippocratic Writings* (translated by Chadwick, J., and Mann, W.N.). New York, Pelican Books, 1978, p 229.

70. Luthra, H.S. Extra-articular manifestations of ankylosing spondylitis. Mayo Clin Proc 52:655–656, 1977.

71. Luzar, L.J. Hydroxychloroquine in psoriatic arthropathy: Exacerbations of psoriatic skin lesions. J Rheumatol 9:462–464, 1982.

72. Macrae, I.F., and Wright, V. Measurement of back movement. Ann Rheum Dis 28:584, 1969.

73. Martin, D.H., Pollock, S., Cho-Chou, K., et al. *Chlamydia trachomatis* infections in men with Reiter's syndrome. Ann Intern Med 100:207–213, 1984.

74. McEwen, C. Arthritis accompanying ulcerative colitis. Clin Orthop 57:9–17, 1968.

75. McEwen, C., Ditata, D., Lingg, C., et al. Ankylosing spondylitis accompanying ulcerative colitis, regional enteritis, psoriasis and Reiter's disease. Arthritis Rheum 14:291–318, 1971.

76. Mielants, H., and Veys, E.M. HLA-B27 related arthritis and bowel inflammation. I: Sulfasalazine (salazopyrin) in HLA-B27 related reactive arthritis. J Rheumatol 12:287–293, 1985.

77. Moll, J.M.H. Inflammatory bowel disease. Clin Rheum Dis 11:87–111, 1985.

78. Moll, J.M.H., and Wright, V. Normal range of spinal mobility: An objective clinical study. Ann Rheum Dis 30:381–386, 1971.

79. Noer, H.R. An "experimental" epidemic of Reiter's syndrome. JAMA 198:693–698, 1966.

80. Paronen, I. Reiter's disease; a study of 344 cases observed in Finland. Acta Med Scand 131 (suppl 212):1–114, 1978.

81. Paulus, H.E., Pearson, C.M., and Pitts, W. Aortic insufficiency in five patients with Reiter's syndrome. Am J Med 53:464–472, 1972.

82. Pekin, T.J., Malinin, T.I., and Zvaifler, N.J. Unusual synovial fluid findings in Reiter's syndrome. Ann Intern Med 66:677–684, 1967.

83. Prendergast, J.K., Sullivan, J.S., Geczy, A.F., et al. Possible role of enteric organisms in the pathogenesis of ankylosing spondylitis and other seronegative arthropathies. Infect Immun. 41:935–941, 1983.

84. Qaiyumi, S., Hassan, Z.U., and Toone, E. Seronegative spondyloarthropathies in lone aortic insufficiency. Arch Intern Med 145:822–824, 1985.

85. Repo, H., Leirisalo, M., Tiilikainen, A. et al. Chemotaxis in *Yersinia* arthritis. In vitro stimulation of neutrophil migration by HLA-B27 positive and negative sera. Arthritis Rheum 25:655–661, 1982.

86. Resnick, D., Dwosh, I.L., Georgen, T.G., et al. Clinical and radiographic "re-ankylosis" following hip surgery in ankylosing spondylitis. Am J Roentgenol 126:1181–1188, 1976.

87. Resnick, D., and Niwayama, G. Ankylosing spondylitis, in Resnick, D., and Niwayama, G. (eds): *Diagnosis of Bone and Joint Disorders.* Philadelphia, Saunders, 1981.

88. Richter, M.B., Kinsella, P., and Corbett, M. Gold in psoriatic arthropathy. Ann Rheum Dis 39:279–280, 1980.

89. Roberts, M.E.T., Wright, V., Hill, A.G.S., et al. Psoriatic arthritis. Follow-up study. Ann Rheum Dis 35:206–212, 1976.

90. Rosenow, E.C., Strimlan, C.V., Muhm, J.R., et al. Pleuropulmonary manifestations of ankylosing spondylitis. Mayo Clin Proc 52:641–649, 1977.

91. Rosenbaum, J.T., Theofilopoulos, A.N., McDevitt, H.D., et al. Presence of circulating immune complexes in Reiter's syndrome and ankylosing spondylitis. Clin Immunol Immunopathol 18:291–297, 1981.

92. Rosner, I.A., Richter, D.E., Huettner, T.L., et al. Spondyloarthropathy associated with hidradenitis suppurativa and acne conglobata. Ann Intern Med *97*:520–525, 1982.

93. Russell, M.L. Ankylosing spondylitis: The case for the underestimated female. J Rheumatol 12:4–6, 1985.

94. Shichikawa, K., Tsujimoto, M., and Nishioka, J. Histopathology of early sacroiliitis and enthesitis in ankylosing spondylitis. Adv Inflam Res 9:15–24, 1985.

95. Short, C.L. The antiquity of rheumatoid arthritis. Arthritis Rheum 17:193–205, 1974.

96. Spriggs, A.I., Boddington, M.M., and Mowat, A.G. Joint fluid cytology in Reiter's disease. Ann Rheum Dis 371:557–560, 1978.

97. Scudese, V.A., and Calabro, J.J. Vertebral wedge osteotomy—Correction of rheumatoid (ankylosing) spondylitis. JAMA 186:105–109, 1963.

98. Stamm, W.E., Guinan, M.E., Johnson, C., et al. Effect of treatment regimens for *Neisseria gonorrhoeae* on simultaneous infection with *Chlamydia trachomatis*. N Engl J Med 310:545–549, 1984.

99. Trull, A., Ebringer, R., Panayi, G.S., et al. IgA antibodies to *Klebsiella pneumoniae* in ankylosing spondylitis. Scand J Rheum 12:249–253, 1983.

100. Van der Linden, S.M., Valkenburg, H.A., and Cats, A. Risks for the development of ankylosing spondylitis in HLA-B27 positive individuals: Consensus, conflicts, and questions. Adv Inflam Res 9:83–89, 1985.

101. Van der Linden, S.M., Valkenburg, H.A., De Jough, B.M., and Cats, A. The risk of developing ankylosing spondylitis in HLA-B27 positive individuals. A comparison of relatives of spondylitis patients with the general population. Arthritis Rheum 27:241–249, 1984.

102. Weinberger, H.W., Ropes, M.W., Kulka, J.P. et al. Reiter's syndrome: Clinical and pathological observations—A long term study of 16 cases. Medicine 41:35–91, 1962.

103. West, F.H. The etiology of ankylosing spondylitis. Ann Rheum Dis 8:143–148, 1949.

104. Wilkins, R.F., Arnett, F.C., Bitter, T., et al. Reiter's syndrome: Evaluation of preliminary criteria for definite disease. Arthritis Rheum 24:844–849, 1981.

105. Wright, V. Seronegative polyarthritis: A unified concept. Arthritis Rheum 21:619–633, 1978.

106. Wright, V. Psoriatic arthritis, in Kelly, W.N. et al (eds): *Textbook of Rheumatology,* 2d ed. Philadelphia, Saunders, 1985.

107. Wright, V., and Watkinson, G. The arthritis of ulcerative colitis. Br Med J 2:670–675, 1965a.

108. Wright, V., and Watkinson, G. Sacroiliitis and ulcerative colitis. Br Med J 2:675–680, 1965b.

109. Yates, D.B., Maini, R.N., Scott, J.T., et al. Complement activation in Reiter's syndrome. Ann Rheum Dis 34:468, 1975.

CHAPTER 20

Generalized Metabolic Disorders of the Skeleton

Ashok Vaswani, John F. Aloia, Daniel O'Neill, Antoni Goral, and Roger Levy

SECTION A

The Osteopenias, Rickets, and Allied Disease

Ashok Vaswani and John F. Aloia

HYPERCALCEMIA

Hypercalcemia is a common metabolic abnormality which may be entirely asymptomatic or may present as an acute emergency. Some of the symptoms include polyuria, constipation, lethargy, and disorientation. If the patient has symptoms of hypercalcemia and the serum calcium is greater than 15 mg/dl, treatment is begun promptly. Malignant disease is the commonest cause of hypercalcemia in a hospital setting, whereas primary hyperparathyroidism is most often diagnosed incidentally on routine blood testing.

Since about 50 percent of the circulating calcium is protein-bound, changes in serum protein may affect serum calcium. In order to exclude factitious hypercalcemia due to hyperproteinemia or prolonged venous stasis during blood collection, a correction factor may be necessary. A general guideline is to adjust the observed serum calcium level by 0.8 mg/dl for each increase or decrease of 1 g of albumin outside the normal range. Ideally, the serum calcium should also be adjusted for the blood pH, but in practice this is not done.

Primary Hyperparathyroidism

The incidence of hyperparathyroidism in the general population is approximately 1 in 1000 subjects. More cases are now detected due to the increased availability of automated laboratory techniques which detect hypercalcemia, a diagnostic feature of hyperparathyroidism.[48]

Pathogenesis

Under physiological conditions, ionized calcium is the most important regulator of parathyroid hormone secretion. Other substances which affect plasma calcium levels, such as calcitonin, 1,25-dihydroxy vitamin D_3 and beta-adrenergic catecholamines also play a role in the secretory control of parathyroid hormone (PTH). In primary hyperparathyroidism, there is overproduction of hormone, leading to elevated and nonsupressible levels of PTH. Excessive production of parathyroid hormone may be due to the presence of an adenoma (80 percent), hyperplasia (19 percent), or parathyroid carcinoma (1 percent). Certain nonparathyroid tumors may produce excessive PTH or PTH-like peptides.

Excessive parathyroid hormone enhances the urinary loss of phosphate and bicarbonate, leading to hypophosphatemia and mild hyperchloremic metabolic acidosis. The hypercalcemia may be associated with hypercalciuria, which occurs due to increased filtration of calcium. Bone resorption is enhanced by osteoclastic stimulation, raising serum calcium and increasing calcium excretion. Parathyroid hormone increases the synthesis of 1,25-dihydroxy vitamin D_3 which enhances intestinal absorption of calcium and may contribute to hypercalcemia.

Clinical Features

In its mildest form, primary hyperparathyroidism may be entirely asymptomatic and may be detected incidentally during routine laboratory screening. Symptomatic hyperparathyroidism may develop insidiously and present as renal colic. Hyperparathyroidism may also occur rapidly, presenting with weight loss, bone pain, fractures, and hypercalcemia. Other symptoms may include depression, emotional lability, and proximal muscle weakness.[29] Although there are no classical physical findings, there may be fasciculations of the tongue, muscle weakness, and hyperreflexia. Other causes of hypercalcemia must be excluded before the diagnosis of hyperparathyroidism can be established (Fig. 20-1).

Laboratory Findings

Hypercalcemia is a hallmark of hyperparathyroidism, although in the early stages it may be intermittent. Hypophos-

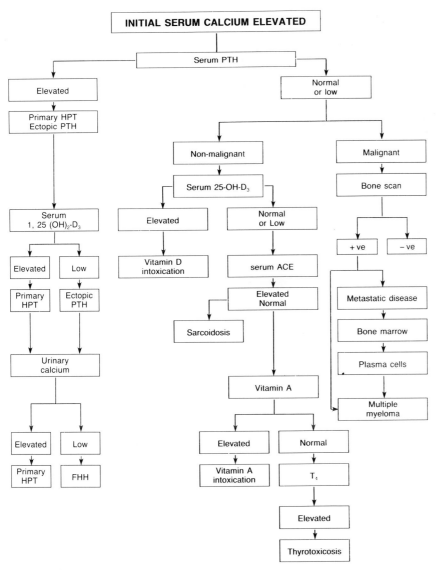

Figure 20-1 An algorithm which may be used for the diagnosis of hypercalcemic disorders.

ACE = Angiotensin converting enzyme;
HPT = Hyperparathyroidism;
T_4 = Thyroxine
FHH = Familial hypocalciuric hypercalcemia

phatemia in the presence of hyperphosphaturia is an important clue to the excessive production of PTH. Since the effect of parathyroid hormone is mediated by activation of the adenylate cyclase system, elevated levels of urinary cyclic AMP are commonly encountered in primary hyperparathyroidism. The finding of an elevated blood level of either the C-terminal or N-terminal PTH is required to establish the diagnosis of primary hyperparathyroidism in the presence of hypercalcemia. Since PTH activates the renal 1α-hydroxylase, elevated blood levels of 1,25-dihydroxy vitamin D_3 are often seen in hyperparathyroid patients with renal stones or colic.[9]

In long-standing hyperparathyroidism, bone changes of osteitis fibrosa cystica may be readily apparent radiographically (Fig. 20-2). There may also be generalized osteopenia or localized bone resorption at the terminal phalanges or distal clavicles, or changes in the skull (Fig. 20-3). Subcortical bone resorption in the jaw may produce characteristic "brown tumor," which may resolve spontaneously after correction of the hyperparathyroidism. Chondrocalcinosis may be seen in primary hyperparathyroidism. Osteoclastic bone resorption, reactive osteoblastic activity, and peritrabecular fibrosis are commonly seen histologically (Fig. 20-4).

Differential Diagnosis

The differential diagnosis of hyperparathyroidism includes all the causes of hypercalcemia (Table 20-1). Primary hyperparathyroidism must be distinguished from familial hypercalcemic syndromes and hypercalcemia of non-PTH causes.

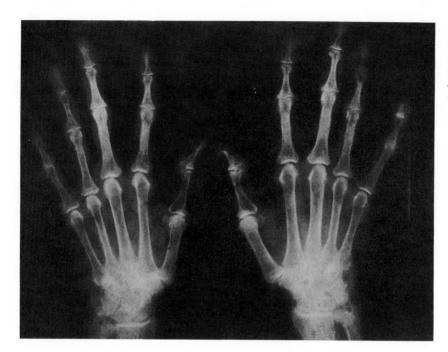

Figure 20-2 Extensive bone resorption in hyperparathyroidism. Note the cystic appearance of the proximal phalanges. (*From Greenfield, G.B., ed: Radiology of Bone Disease, 3d ed. Philadelphia, Lippincott, 1979. Reprinted with permission.*)

Familial Syndromes

Hypercalcemia may occur as a distinct entity in three familial syndromes. In multiple endocrine neoplasia type I (MEN-I), there may be associated pituitary or pancreatic adenomas. Serum gastrin may be elevated. Increased levels of calcitonin or catecholamines along with the hypercalcemia are usually seen in multiple endocrine neoplasia type II. Familial hypocalciuric hypercalcemia (FHH) is a distinct syndrome which can be diagnosed by a low calcium/creatinine clearance (<0.01) in the urine and high serum magnesium level.[31] In all the above syndromes, there may be hyperplasia of the parathyroid glands and there is usually a poor response to surgery. For this reason, the syndromes of familial hypercalcemia must be carefully excluded before neck exploration.

Non-PTH-Related Hypercalcemia

Although there are a number of causes within this group (Table 20-1), malignant disease is by far the most important in the differential diagnosis of non-PTH-related hypercalcemia.[34] Weight loss, anorexia, constipation, and depression, although nonspecific, should heighten the suspicion for malignant disease. If malignant disease is suspected, a search for bony metastases or myelomatosis must be instituted with appropriate diagnostic procedures.

A thorough history and physical examination is usually sufficient to diagnose hyperthyroidism, which can be confirmed by thyroid function tests (T_4, T_3 uptake, and free thyroxine index or equivalent test) and a radioisotope scan. Hypercalcemia is often an associated electrolyte abnormality in Addison disease. The presence of hyperpigmentation and hypotension along with other electrolyte abnormalities such as hyperkalemia and hyponatremia suggests the diagnosis. Drugs, such as thiazides and absorbable antacids as well as excessive ingestion of vitamin A and D, taken individually or in combination, may precipitate hypercalcemia.

Hypercalcemia is frequently reported in patients with granulomatous diseases, particularly sarcoidosis.[51] An increased synthesis of vitamin D (1,25-dihydroxy vitamin D_3) is believed to cause the hypercalcemia. Similar alterations in

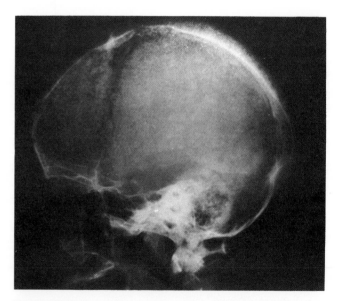

Figure 20-3 Characteristic "hair on end" appearance of the skull in primary hyperparathyroidism. (*From Greenfield, G.B., ed: Radiology of Bone Diseases, 3d ed. Philadelphia, Lippincott, 1975. Reprinted with permission.*)

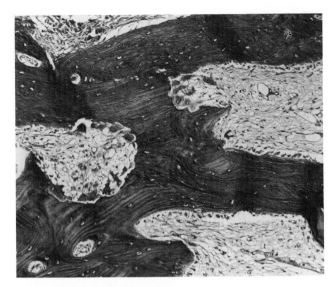

Figure 20-4 Photomicrograph of hyperparathyroidism showing "tunneling" resorption by two groups of osteoclasts, reactive osteoblastic activity, and peritrabecular fibrosis. (*Courtesy of Peter G. Bullough, The Hospital for Special Surgery, New York.*)

vitamin D metabolism have been reported in patients with tuberculosis.[21] Adrenal gland destruction by tuberculosis should be considered if clinical symptoms are suggestive of Addison disease.

Immobilization from any cause, particularly in patients with active bone turnover, may be an important cause of hypercalcemia.[53] There is typically increased bone reabsorption, presumably unrelated to PTH, which leads to hypercalciuria. If renal function is impaired, rapid hypercalcemia may ensue.

Treatment

No treatment may be necessary in asymptomatic subjects with minimal (less than 11.2 mg/dl) elevations in serum calcium. Bony involvement or abnormalities of renal function must be carefully sought and followed up at 6- to 12-month intervals. In addition, a detailed family history must be obtained to exclude familial or multiple endocrine neoplasia, before contemplating surgery. Surgery may be indicated in case of primary hyperparathyroidism with symptomatic disease or in any asymptomatic individual in whom renal or bone abnormalities are detected.

During hypercalcemic crisis, intravenous therapy will be necessary to correct the dehydration. As much as 4 to 6 liters of fluid may be given intravenously, depending on the age of the patient and on the severity of the hypercalcemia or coexisting diseases. Calcium excretion may be more effectively accomplished by the addition of a nonthiazide or loop diuretic.

Salmon calcitonin (Calcimar) may be used in doses of 50 to 100 units every 6 h to control hypercalcemia. Its effect may be transient. Mithramycin, an inhibitor of RNA synthesis, may

be used as a single dose (25 μg/kg IV bolus). The effect of a single dose usually lasts between 24 and 48 h. The use of IV phosphates should only be entertained when all other measures have failed, since this route of administration is often accompanied by ectopic soft tissue calcification. Oral phosphate may be less toxic and can be used in doses of 2 to 3 g of elemental phosphate daily. Serum calcium and phosphate must be monitored closely during therapy with phosphates.

Specific therapy for hypercalcemia is directed toward the known or established cause of the disease. Discontinuation of excess vitamin D may not immediately lower the serum calcium, since the drug is fat-soluble. The use of steroids is indicated, since glucocorticoids antagonize the gastrointestinal effect of vitamin D. Glucocorticoid therapy will improve hypercalcemia in patients with Addison disease, sarcoidosis, multiple myeloma, and certain lymphomas. Glucocorticoids should not be used in untreated tuberculosis.

TABLE 20-1 Differential Diagnosis of Hypercalcemia

Etiology	Differentiating features
Factitious	High-serum proteins
Primary hyperparathyroidism	High-PTH, low-phosphate mild metabolic acidosis
Familial hypercalcemia:	
Multiple endocrine neoplasia, type I	Pituitary and pancreatic endocrine hyperfunction
Multiple endocrine neoplasia, type II	Catecholamine and calcitonin excess
Hypocalciuric hypercalcemia	Low urinary calcium excretion, elevated serum magnesium
Malignant diseases:	
Multiple myeloma	Proteinuria, anemia, plasma cells in bone marrow
Lymphomas	Lymph node biopsy
Other causes:	
Thyrotoxicosis	Symptoms, elevated T_4, low PTH
Addison disease	Low cortisol, high ACTH, hyponatremia, hyperkalemia
Sarcoidosis	Chest x-ray; usually negative PPD, increased ACE levels
Tuberculosis	Chest x-ray; usually positive PPD
Paget disease (during immobilization)	High alkaline phosphatase
Drugs:	
Vitamin D intoxication	Serum 25-hydroxy vitamin D
Vitamin A intoxication	Serium levels of vitamin D
Thiazide diuretics	History of drug use
Antacids	Excessive use of milk or calcium-containing antacids

Key—T_4: thyroid function tests; ACE: angiotensin-converting enzyme; ACTH: adrenocorticotropin; PPD: tuberculin tests

TABLE 20-2 Differential Diagnosis of Hypocalcemia

Etiology	Differentiating features
Factitious	Low serum protein (albumin)
Primary hypoparathyroidism	Low to absent PTH, calcified basal ganglia
Pseudohypoparathyroidism (PHP)	Normal to high PTH, shortened metacarpals
Pseudopseudohypoparathyroidism (PPHP)	Phenotype of PHP, usually normal serum calcium
Magnesium deficiency	Low PTH, low serum Mg^{2+}
Chronic renal failure	Markedly elevated PTH, renal function abnormal
Vitamin D deficiency	Low phosphate, high PTH, low 25-hydroxy vitamin D
Pancreatitis	Diarrhea, malabsorption
Neonatal hypocalcemia	Maternal diabaetes mellitus

Drugs:
  Intravenous phosphates
  Citrate
	Ectopic calcification during blood transfusions

HYPOCALCEMIA

This condition occurs as a result of deficiency or inadequate function of parathyroid hormone or vitamin D (Table 20-2). It is not caused by dietary deficiency of calcium alone because this is corrected by the secondary hyperparathyroidism which increases bone resorption and corrects the hypocalcemia. Increased synthesis of $1,25(OH)_2D_3$ also helps correct low calcium levels.

Clinical Features

The symptoms of hypocalcemia include neuromuscular irritability, seizures, and tetany. Patients may have positive Chvostek's or Trousseau's signs. In the former there is irritability of the masseter muscle to percussion, and in the latter the characteristic position of the hand occurs with flexion of the thumb and wrist and extension of the fingers. Physical examination may reveal lenticular cataracts or fungal infections of the nails, or there may be the obvious phenotypytic features of pseudohypoparathyroidism described below. In this condition, x-ray films will reveal short fourth metacarpals and metatarsals. Routine radiographs of the abdomen may reveal pancreatic calcification indicating a malabsorption syndrome as an etiologic factor in the hypocalcemia. The electrocardiogram may show a prolonged Q interval.

Hypoparathyroid Syndromes

Hypoparathyroidism may be defined as an absolute or relative deficiency or inadequacy of parathyroid hormone func-

tion. There is associated hypocalcemia and hyperphosphatemia associated with diminished action of PTH. Since PTH mediates its action by the adenylate cyclase system, any receptor abnormalities or lack of cofactors (particularly magnesium) at the target cell can render the hormone ineffective.[46] Consequently, in these syndromes there may be normal or even high levels of PTH. There may also be diminution in $1,25(OH)_2D_3$ production, which in turn affects calcium balance. Severe magnesium deficiency, which may be seen in chronic alcoholism, may mimic hypoparathyroidism. Hypoparathyroidism may be idiopathic, or it may occur as part of an autoimmune polyglandular dysfunctional syndrome.[35] Hypoparathyroidism may occur as a complication of thyroid or parathyroid surgery.

Clinical Features

The decrease in ionized serum calcium leads to neuromuscular irritability and tetany. Symptoms range from mild circumoral tingling, paresthesia, or tetany. Chronic hypocalcemia leads to elevated CSF pressure, papilledema, and occasionally seizures. Lenticular cataract is an important feature of long-standing hypoparathyroidism.[8]

When the condition occurs as part of the pluriglandular syndrome, there may be associated thyroid and gonadal hypofunction with occasional pernicious anemia. When hypoparathyroidism occurs early in life, there may be delayed dentition or dental hypoplasia. Hypoparathyroidism may be associated with mucocutaneous candidiasis.

Hypoparathyroidism Associated with Parathyroid Hormone Resistance

Some patients with the typical biochemical features of hypoparathyroidism present with the characteristic physical appearance indicating a syndrome of parathyroid hormone resistance, sometimes termed *pseudohypoparathyroidism (PHP)*, or Albright hereditary osteodystrophy.

In PHP, PTH levels are elevated in the presence of hypocalcemia and hyperphosphatemia, this being consistent with hormone resistance. Recent evidence suggests that the guanine nucleotide regulatory components of the membrane-bound adenylate cyclase system may be defective, accounting for the deficiency in parathyroid hormone function.[19] Thus, after injection of PTH there may be no increase in cyclic AMP. However, in some affected family members cyclic AMP response to an injection of PTH is normal. These subjects also have the characteristic familial type of PHP, however, and are classified as a separate subtype of hormone resistance known as *pseudopseudohypoparathyroidism (PPHP)*.

Clinical Features

The symptoms of PTH resistance are indistinguishable from those of idiopathic hypoparathyroidism. The characteristic familial type of short stature and bony abnormalities helps to distinguish the two. Bony abnormalities include shortening of the metacarpal and metatarsals (particularly the fourth metacarpal), brachydactyly, and exostoses. The patients are obese with a round face and usually have diminished intelligence.

Patients with PHP may have coexistent hypothyroidism and subcutaneous calcification.

Differential Diagnosis

The history, physical examination, and appropriate laboratory tests usually permit an appropriate diagnosis (Table 20-2). The presence of a neck scar is suggestive of postsurgical hypoparathyroidism, whereas monilial infection of the nails, alopecia, or vitiligo is more commonly associated with autoimmune or idiopathic hypoparathyroidism. Detectable or low levels of serum PTH will usually confirm the diagnosis of hypoparathyroidism, whereas higher levels suggest a parathyroid hormone resistance syndrome. A history of alcoholism may suggest hypomagnesemia which may cause impaired secretion of PTH from the gland and may decrease the effect of PTH at its target cells in the bone and kidney. A history of chronic diarrhea, abdominal pain, or chronic alcohol abuse should heighten the suspicion of pancreatitis or other malabsorption syndromes, particularly if there is pancreatic calcification. Reabsorption of vitamin D and calcium can be affected by malabsorption, worsening the problem of hypocalcemia.

The phenotype of PHP is characteristic, and there is no history of neck surgery. The bony exostoses of PHP are typical and do not occur in idiopathic hypoparathyroidism. Brachydactyly may also be seen in PHP. Factitious hypocalcemia can easily be excluded by correcting for abnormal serum albumin levels; serum phosphate is usually normal. All the causes of hypoparathyroid dysfunction should be considered in the differential diagnosis of hypocalcemia. Hypocalcemia with hyperphosphatemia and a markedly elevated level of PTH usually indicates the secondary hyperparathyroidism of chronic renal failure. Abnormal renal function tests will confirm the diagnosis.

Serum calcium levels must be determined in any newborn infant with a seizure disorder. Neonatal hypocalcemia is often seen in premature infants as well as infants of diabetic mothers. Massive blood transfusion in premature infants or adults with hepatic insufficiency may induce hypocalcemia due to the chelating effect of citrate on calcium. Intravenous phosphate therapy for hypercalcemic crises also carries a risk of inducing acute hypocalcemia. Mithramycin and calcitonin, used for correction of hypercalcemia, rarely produce hypocalcemia. Hypocalcemia can occasionally occur following surgical treatment of long-standing hyperparathyroidism. Chronic suppression of the normal remaining parathyroid tissue and a delayed release of PTH may be the cause of the transient hypocalcemia following surgery.

Treatment of Hypocalcemia and Hypoparathyroidism

Acute tetany requires immediate correction with intravenous calcium. A 10% solution of calcium gluconate (10 to 20 ml) can be given slowly over a period of several hours. Vitamin D therapy is required, with supplemental calcium, in the management of hypoparathyroidism of all types discussed. If the condition is due to magnesium deficiency, replacement of magnesium either orally or intravenously is sufficient to correct the biochemical abnormality; 1–2 g of elemental calcium

will correct the hypocalcemia. The goal of therapy is to maintain serum calcium in the normal range so that the patient is free of symptoms of hypoparathyroidism and does not develop significant hypercalciuria or hypercalcemia.

Renal Osteodystrophy

Renal osteodystrophy is a complex bone disorder in patients with chronic renal failure. The renal impairment leads to an inability to excrete phosphate, with a compensatory reduction in serum calcium.[23]

Clinical features

The hallmark of this syndrome is hyperphosphatemia, hypocalcemia, and markedly elevated blood levels of PTH. Bone histomorphometry reveals a mixture of both osteoporosis and osteomalacia. Radiographically, the changes may resemble hyperparathyroidism. X-ray films of the spine may reveal the typical rugger jersey appearance associated with sclerosis in the region immediately beneath the vertebral end plates (Fig. 20-5).

RICKETS

Rickets includes several diseases of different etiologies (Table 20-3), all of which severely affect normal skeletal development.

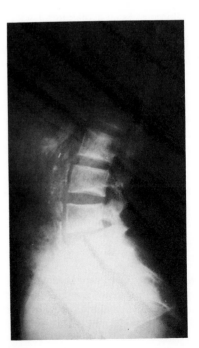

Figure 20-5 Rugger jersey spine seen in renal osteodystrophy. There is sclerosis near the vertebral end plates. (*Courtesy of Radiology Department, Winthrop University Hospital, Mineola, N.Y.*)

TABLE 20-3 Differential Diagnosis of Rickets

Etiology	Differentiating features
Vitamin D deficiency	Tetany, carpopedal spasms, bowing of legs, craniotabes low 25-hydroxy vitamin D_3
Hereditary vitamin D– dependent rickets:	
Type I	Seizures, low $1,25(OH)_2D_3$
Type II	Alopecia, normal or high $1,25(OH)_2D_3$
Familial hypophosphatemia	No tetany or myotonia, low serum phosphate, minimally elevated PTH
Hypophosphatasia	Low alkaline phosphatase, high urinary phosphorylethanolamine

Vitamin D Deficiency Rickets

At the turn of the century, dietary deficiency of vitamin D was by far the commonest cause of rickets in this country. This public health problem has been eliminated by the fortification of dairy products with vitamin D. Dietary sources of vitamin D includes fish oils and vitamin D_2 (ergocalciferol) present in plants. Vitamin D is also synthesized in the skin from 7-dehydrocholesterol by untraviolet irradiation.[13] In countries, such as the United Kingdom, where vitamin D is not added to dairy products, rickets is occasionally seen, particularly in the children of Asian immigrants. Lack of exposure to sunlight can also pose an additional health hazard in the perpetuation of rickets. Premature infants, receiving prolonged therapy with total parenteral nutrition may exhibit radiographic changes of rickets.[59]

A reduction in the absorption of calcium and phosphorus occurs in the vitamin D–deficient state. There is a compensatory increase in parathyroid hormone when the serum calcium levels decline. Increased bone resorption is initially able to maintain serum calcium levels in the normal range. Continued unavailability of vitamin D intensifies the secondary hyperparathyroidism, leading to a loss of phosphorus and decreased ability to maintain a normal serum calcium. At the skeletal level, deficient mineralization may be most evident in the regions of rapid bone turnover.

Clinical Features

In the first year of life, there may be delayed closure of the fontanelles, leading to widened cranial sutures. Flattening of the occiput (craniotabes) and thickening of the skull (frontal bossing) are also common. In the thorax, bulging and enlargement of the costochondral junction (rachitic rosary) may be an early indication of vitamin D deficiency. Other thoracic abnormalities include a posterior displacement of the sternum and the appearance of Harrison's groove, which mani-

fests itself as an indentation of the lower ribs at the site of diaphragmatic insertion.

Bony deformities, such as genu varum or genu valgum, may appear as soon as the child is able to stand or walk. Long-standing disease may lead to coxa vara, saber shin, or lordosis of the spine. In addition to the skeletal deformities, there is weakness and hypotonia of the muscles, resulting in a peculiar waddling gait. If the hypotonia of muscles is profound, it may lead to a delay in standing or walking. Dental enamel may be hypoplastic, and there may be delayed eruption of teeth.

In older children, vitamin D deficiency may manifest as short stature, or an increased tendency to pathologic fractures of the long bones. In premature infants, symptoms of vitamin deficiency may occur in the first few months of life, due to delayed maturation of the hepatic enzyme systems.

Laboratory Findings

Since serum calcium levels are usually in the low normal range, tetany is uncommon. However, serum calcium is maintained in the low normal range by an increase in the circulating level of parathyroid hormone, leading to the classic manifestations of secondary hyperparathyroidism, i.e., increased phosphaturia, low serum phosphate and mild hyperchloremic acidosis. Plasma level of alkaline phosphatase is usually elevated. The plasma concentration of the metabolites of vitamin D is low, in particular 25-OH-D_3. Inability to absorb sufficient calcium in the absence of vitamin D, usually leads to a decrease in urinary calcium excretion. There may be a tendency to aminoaciduria.

Radiographically, the poorly mineralized, but abundant, cartilage creates cupped metaphyses. The physis appears enlarged with increased height and width. The bone appears demineralized, with a thin cortex and few trabeculae. Features of secondary hyperparathyroidism, such as subperiosteal erosion of metaphyses of long bones, may be present. Radiography of the rachitic bone depends, to some extent, on the severity of the metabolic defect. Histologically, the growth plate in a rachitic child shows irregular widening, disrupted maturation, and delayed endochondral ossification (Fig. 20-6). There is irregularity of calcification and vascular invasion in the zone of provisional calcification, and the osteoid in the primary spongiosa remains uncalcified.[14] There is peripheral splaying of cartilage cells, and the physis herniates into microfractures in the primary spongiosa, causing the cupped appearance of the metaphysis. The mineralization front may be absent or decreased. There is deficient mineralization of osteoid in cortical and trabecular bone. In some areas of the bone, osteoclastic activity may be increased, if secondary hyperparathyroidism supervenes.

Differential Diagnosis

In addition to dietary deficiency of vitamin D, malabsorption syndromes and renal and hepatic diseases must be considered.

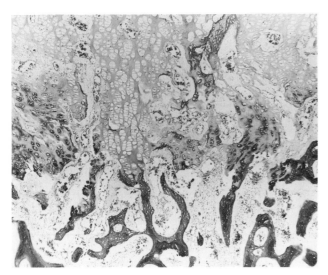

Figure 20-6 Photomicrograph of the growth plate in a rachitic child, showing irregular widening, disrupted maturation, and delayed endochondral ossification. (*Courtesy of Peter G. Bullough, The Hospital for Special Surgery, New York.*)

Treatment

Correction of bony abnormalities must be attempted only after the vitamin deficiency has been adequately treated. This can be satisfactorily achieved by giving 5000 units of vitamin D (as ergocalciferol) daily. In the early stages of treatment, since bone mineralization may be rapid, the serum calcium level may decrease, giving rise to hypocalcemia. Supplemental calcium, up to 3 g daily, may be required to avoid symptoms of hypocalcemia. In an emergency, 15 mg/kg of calcium chloride may be infused intravenously, slowly, over a few hours, in order to maintain serum calcium in the normal range.

Calcification in the unmineralized osteoid may begin after 1 week of treatment with vitamin D and calcium supplements. Serum alkaline phosphatase may increase above the baseline levels. As the vitamin and mineral deficits are corrected, mild to moderate bony abnormalities may resolve spontaneously. If a severe deformity persists after growth is complete, an osteotomy may be indicated.

Hereditary Vitamin D–Dependent Rickets

This condition has been called *pseudo-vitamin D deficiency*. As the name implies, this variety of rickets is unresponsive to the usual physiological replacement doses of vitamin D. Hereditary vitamin D dependency, which is inherited as an autosomal recessive trait, can be categorized into two groups, distinguished only by low (type I) or normal (type II) levels of 1,25-dihydroxy vitamin D_3.

Pathogenesis

Vitamin D dependency may represent a defect in the renal 1α hydroxylation of 25-hydroxy vitamin D_3. The resultant decrease in the synthesis of $1,25(OH)_2D_3$ will impair calcium absorption, leading to the typical features of low serum calcium, secondary hyperparathyroidism, and clinical manifestations of vitamin D deficiency.[50]

Clinical Features

The clinical characteristics of this syndrome are identical to that of nutritional vitamin D deficiency, although the disease may be more florid. Occasionally, the child may present with tetany or convulsions as the initial manifestation of this disease. Alopecia totalis, which is a distinctive feature of the type II syndrome, has been reported in several kindreds with this disorder. In the adult, pseudo-vitamin D deficiency may present as osteomalacia.

Laboratory Findings

Serum calcium may be low, owing to the relatively low levels of 1,25-dihydroxy vitamin D_3. Serum phosphate may be decreased and the urinary phosphate increased as a result of the secondary hyperparathyroidism. The plasma level of alkaline phosphatase is usually elevated. The plasma concentration of 1,25-dihydroxy vitamin D_3 is low in the type I syndrome and normal or elevated in the type II vitamin D–dependent rickets. The radiographic abnormalities are similar to those seen in vitamin D deficiency rickets.

Differential Diagnosis

Nutritional vitamin D rickets is characterized by extremely low levels of circulating $25\text{-}OH\text{-}D_3$ and can be readily distinguished from the pseudodeficiency syndromes by the therapeutic response to lower levels of vitamin D therapy. The presence of alopecia totalis can be helpful in diagnosing the type II syndrome. Moreover, patients with alopecia are often the most resistant to treatment with vitamin D.

Treatment

High doses of vitamin D (ergocalciferol) are required to correct the metabolic abnormalities. The usual doses for therapy of this disorder range from 20,000 to 100,000 units of vitamin D daily. Normalization of serum calcium can be achieved by physiological doses of an analogue of $1,25(OH)_2D_3$ (Rocaltrol), thereby suggesting a defect in the 1α-hydroxylase system as the potential pathogenic mechanism for this syndrome.[28] Therapy with these potent compounds should be carefully monitored in order to prevent hypercalcemia. Frequent (weekly) serum and urine calcium determinations may be necessary in the initial phase of therapy. If surgical correction of the skeletal deformities is necessary and prolonged immobilization is anticipated, appropriate reductions in the vitamin D dosage is required to prevent hypercalcemia and hypercalciuria. Normalization of the biochemical parameters can be expected in 1 to 6 months. The maintenance dosage of Rocaltrol may vary from 0.25 to 2.0 μg daily.

Familial Hypophosphatemic Rickets (Vitamin D–Resistant Rickets)

This familial disease is transmitted via an abnormal gene on the X chromosome. Accordingly, an affected male will transmit this disease to all his daughters but to none of his sons, and half the children of an affected female will be normal.

Pathogenesis

The most characteristic abnormality present in all the affected individuals is hypophosphatemia and decreased renal tubular reabsorption of phosphate. There may be an associated abnormality in the intestinal absorption of phosphate. Physiologically, low phosphate should stimulate the synthesis of $1,25(OH)_2D_3$. However, these individuals also have a low normal or depressed concentration of $1,25(OH)_2D_3$, which is inappropriate for the circulating level of phosphate.[50] Hereditary hypophosphatemic rickets has recently been reported in one kindred with normal serum calcium, marked hypercalciuria, and elevated levels of 1,25-dihydroxy vitamin D_3.[57]

Clinical Features

Short stature in childhood and osteomalacia in adults are the commonest manifestations of this disorder. Tetany and myotonia are typically absent. If there is a family history of this disease, recognition of the characteristic features in childhood is not difficult. Within the families, female members have a lower incidence of the bone disease. Calcification of joint capsules, ligaments, and tendons without inflammatory or degenerative disease has recently been reported.[39]

Laboratory Findings

In the typical syndrome, hypophosphatemia may be the only manifestation in some family members; these individuals may be entirely asymptomatic. Serum calcium is usually normal. The alkaline phosphatase may be elevated. Urinary phosphate excretion is high, whereas calcium excretion is low in the untreated individuals. The serum PTH may be slightly elevated.

Radiographically, the features of familial hypophosphatemic rickets may be indistinguishable from those of vitamin D deficiency. There may be bowing of the lower extremities and occasionally genu varum or genu valgum. Calcium deposits in the hand and sacroiliac joints were observed in 50 to 60 percent of the patients in one kindred. Histomorphometry of bone in hypophosphatemic rickets indicates a marked decrease in the calcification rate and a reduction in the bone formation rate.[30]

Differential Diagnosis

Absence of tetany or seizures and normal muscle strength and tone are features of hypophosphatemic rickets which are uniquely different from symptoms of vitamin D–deficient or –dependent rickets. Hypophosphatemia with only minimal elevation of PTH can also serve to distinguish this disease from the marked secondary hyperparathyroidism seen in D-deficient rickets.

Treatment

Large doses of vitamin D usually result in incomplete healing of bone, with little or no effect on the hypophosphatemia. Satisfactory treatment of this disease requires the addition of phosphate to correct the specific biochemical abnormality of low serum phosphate. The usual dose for phosphate replacement is 1 to 4 g of neutral phosphate daily, in divided doses, given orally. It should be recalled that phosphate therapy alone, i.e., without vitamin D, can initiate bone mineralization. The process of remineralization, however, may be patchy or incomplete, with phosphate alone. Therefore a combination of phosphate with vitamin D, such as 1,25-dihydroxy vitamin D_3, is most beneficial and can prevent some of the complications encountered with high dose phosphate therapy.[11,41] These include the development of secondary hyperparathyroidism, since increasing serum phosphate is a stimulus for parathyroid hormone release. Once the doses of vitamin D and oral phosphate have been finely titrated, an accelerated growth can be achieved in children, with remission of the rachitic changes in bone (radiographic and histological). Genu valgum deformity may be surgically corrected.[18] If a new proband has been identified, skeletal and biochemical abnormalities should be sought in other members of the family. Genetic counseling may be necessary.

Hypophosphatasia

Hypophosphatasia is probably an autosomal recessive disorder, which may present in its more severe form as childhood rickets, and is less severe in adults.

Pathogenesis

Alkaline phosphatase is required for bone mineralization, in addition to the vitamin D, calcium, and phosphate. The enzyme, alkaline phosphatase, is present in vesicles in the matrix; it hydrolyzes pyrophosphate to yield inorganic phosphate. This step is believed to be necessary to initiate apatite formation in the matrix. Hypophosphatasia is characterized by a low alkaline phosphatase, the lack of which gives rise to the typical features of rickets.[40]

Clinical Features

In infancy, the disease is invariably severe and may present with rickets and hypercalcemia. A less severe variety of this disorder in childhood and in adults is characterized by premature loss of deciduous teeth and a tendency to fracture.

Laboratory Findings

A low serum alkaline phosphatase is the hallmark of this disease. Substrates from the enzyme, such as phosphorylethanolamine, are typically excreted in increased quantities in the urine. Serum calcium and urinary calcium may be elevated in the severe form of the disease. Radiographically, the epiphyses appear irregular and notched. Other features of rickets may be common.

Differential Diagnosis

The laboratory finding of a low alkaline phosphatase in the presence of rickets is an important consideration for differentiating this disease from the other types of rickets discussed above. Hypercalcemia or hypercalciuria are unusual in untreated rickets.

Treatment

There is no satisfactory treatment for this disorder, although phosphate therapy has been tried with some success. Surgical correction of pathologic fractures may be difficult to achieve.[5]

Hyperphosphatasia

In this uncommon disease (also called *juvenile Paget disease*) there is elevation of alkaline phosphatase and also acid phosphatase of bone origin. The disease is autosomal recessive in hereditary transmission and resembles Paget disease in children.

OSTEOMALACIA

Clinically and histologically, osteomalacia may be considered as an adult counterpart of rickets. Many of the hereditary or familial disorders discussed under the heading of rickets are equally applicable in this section and may be considered in the differential diagnosis of osteomalacia.

The primary underlying defect seen in osteomalacia in adults is a disproportionately large amount of unmineralized osteoid associated with a failure of mineralization. This can be quantified using the technique of histomorphometry (Table 20-4).

Etiology

A low 25-hydroxy vitamin D_3 level causing osteomalacia is commonly seen in patients with malabsorption, hepatic, or pancreatic disease. Impaired fat absorption, such as occurs in steatorrhea, reduces calcium and vitamin D absorption. Gastric bypass surgery also has this effect. Celiac disease occasionally will induce osteomalacia. Phosphate-binding antacids (aluminum hydroxide) if used in excess may also induce osteomalacia. Parathyroid hormone levels will be typically increased, in an attempt to maintain the serum calcium in the normal range. Anticonvulsant drugs (e.g., phenobarbitone, phenytoin) may induce the hepatic microsomal hydroxylase enzyme systems which enhance 25-hydroxy vitamin D_3 degradation. The clinical and biochemical profile will be identical to that of hepatic disease.

Renal tubular acidosis (multiple causes) should be suspected if there is hypophosphatemia and phosphaturia accompanied by glycosuria, aminoaciduria, or bicarbonate excretion.[7] In patients with chronic renal failure, there is hyperphosphatemia along with low or undetectable levels of 1,25-dihydroxy vitamin D_3. Aluminum toxicity may present as osteomalacia in patients with chronic renal failure undergoing hemodialysis. Bone morphometry in these patients suggests that aluminum may inhibit mineralization directly.[16]

Tumor-induced osteomalacia should be considered if rickets or hypophosphatemia is not responsive to treatment, since surgical correction of a benign tumor may reverse the osteomalacia.[38]

Diagnosis

Laboratory studies Serum calcium may be low or normal, whereas the phosphate is usually low. Serum alkaline phosphates is generally elevated in all types of osteomalacia. Indices of renal and hepatic function are necessary.

TABLE 20-4 Histological and Histomorphometric Hallmarks of Classical Metabolic Bone Disorders

Disorder	Histological feature(s)	Histomorphometry
Osteoporosis	Decreased bone mass	↓ TBV, ↓ MTW
Osteomalacia	Increased osteoid (poorly mineralized bone) Smudged, irregular tetracycline uptake	↑ TOS, ↑ TOV, ↑ MOSW ↓ CR, ↑ MLT
Hyperparathyroidism	Increased osteoclasts Osteoclastic tunneling resorption Bone spicules with "punched-out" holes	↑ TRS, ↑ ORS ↓ MTW
Paget disease	Woven bone of variable thickness Increased osteoclasts Large, bizarre osteoclasts	↑ TRS, ↑ ORS

Key—TBV: trabecular bone volume; MTW: mean trabecular width; TOS: trabecular osteoid surface; TOV: trabecular osteoid volume; MOSW: mean osteoid seam width; CR: calcification rate; MLT: mineralization lag time; TRS: trabecular resorptive surface; ORS: osteoclastic resorptive surface; ↑: increased; ↓: decreased.
Source: From: Vigorita, V. J., Orthop Clin North Am 15:4, 1984. Reproduced with permission.

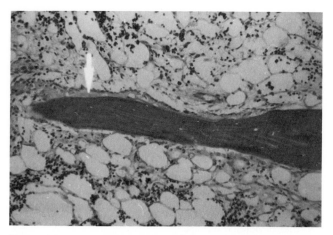

Figure 20-7 Osteomalacia, showing increased mineralized osteoid (arrow). (*From Mishriki, Y., Histopathology for Medical Students Series, part VII: Bone and Joints System, New York, Medcom, 1986. Reprinted with permission.*)

Bone Biopsy Histologically, osteomalacia is characterized by an increased width of unmineralized bone as well as blurred or discontinuous mineralization (Figs. 20-7 and 20-8).

An increase in the osteoid width is demonstrated using double tetracycline labeling (Table 20-4), but may also be seen in other diseases associated with an accelerated synthesis of matrix, such as Paget disease and thyrotoxicosis. The rate of mineralization, however, is normal in these disorders.[32] Thyrotoxicosis is readily recognized by its specific symptoms and can be confirmed by finding elevated thyroid function tests. Serum PTH in both these conditions is low or normal, unless primary hyperparathyroidism coexists.

Radiological Diagnosis Radiology in osteomalacia may be normal, but Looser's zones, also known as *pseudofractures,* may be seen and confirmed by bone scan. These are radiolucencies occurring as bands at right angles to the cortex (Fig. 20-9). They occur at points of stress on the cortex of long bones; they are often symmetrical and tend to occur on concave surfaces of long bones as well as on flat bones. They may become complete fractures and are also seen in Paget disease and osteogenesis imperfecta.[47]

Treatment

Initially the primary cause of the osteomalacia must be treated. Anticonvulsant osteomalacia can be treated with vitamin D in doses sufficient to overcome the biochemical abnormalities. Patients with chronic renal failure usually respond to treatment with 1,25-dihydroxy vitamin D_3 or other synthetic analogues of vitamin D. Hypophosphatemic syndromes may require supplemental phosphate, in addition to the vitamin D.

When treating osteomalacia, serum calcium and phosphate should be monitored frequently, particularly if the more potent forms of vitamin D are used. During treatment,

serum calcium may decrease at first due to rapid remineralization of bone. Supplemental calcium should be provided.

VITAMIN C DEFICIENCY (SCURVY)

Ascorbic acid, which is a low-molecular-weight water-soluble vitamin, is an essential nutrient since it cannot be synthesized by humans. Ascorbic acid is required for the normal repair and growth of collagen as well as for the absorption of iron. It is derived from rapidly growing fresh fruits and vegetables. The recommended allowance for this vitamin is about 60 mg daily, an amount readily available in the average American diet. When ascorbic acid is consumed in large quantities, the percent of absorption of ascorbic acid is reduced. Moreover, excretion of ascorbic acid is enhanced above a certain renal threshold. If an individual is fed a diet deficient in vitamin C, symptoms or signs of scurvy may not appear for at least 2 months.[22]

Clinical Features

Deficiency of vitamin C may manifest itself as generalized fatigue, bleeding gums, perifollicular hemorrhage, or ecchymoses. There may be pain in the joints and occasional joint effusions. Bone pain and deformities at the costochondral junction may mimic rickets.

Diagnosis

Iron deficiency anemia may occur, but this is a nonspecific finding. Serum ascorbic acid determinations may not be help-

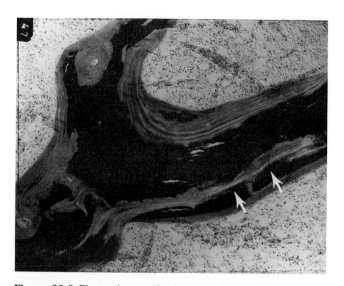

Figure 20-8 Photomicrograph of osteomalacic trabeculum demonstrating the increased amount of unmineralized bone ("osteoid") with blurred mineralization fronts (arrows) and discontinuous mineralization. (*Courtesy of Peter G. Bullough, The Hospital for Special Surgery, New York.*)

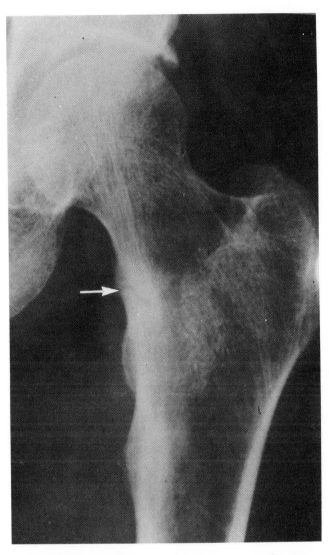

Figure 20-9 Osteomalacia: pseudofracture seen on the superior medial aspect of the lesser trochanter. (*From Greenfield, G.B., ed: Radiology of Bone Disease, 3d ed. Philadelphia, Lippincott, 1975. Reprinted with permission.*)

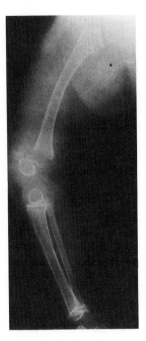

Figure 20-10 Radiographic findings in scurvy. (*From Greenfield, G.B., ed: Radiology of Bone Disease, 3d ed. Philadelphia, Lippincott, 1975. Reprinted with permission.*)

ful, since depletion of vitamin C may take 2 or 3 months. Radiographically, the cortices may be thin and the trabeculae may be poorly defined. As the disease progresses, spurs and zones or rarefaction may develop. Metaphyseal clefts (corner sign) are characteristic of scurvy (Fig. 20-10). There may be generalized subperiosteal hemorrhage.

The typical clinical presentation, normal serum calcium, and PTH will readily distinguish scurvy from vitamin D deficiency.

Treatment

Initially, vitamin C should be given in doses of 100 mg three times daily. This is usually sufficient dosage to replenish tissue stores within a week with marked improvement of symptoms. Massive doses of vitamin C are unnecessary.

PITUITARY, THYROID, AND STEROID HORMONE DYSFUNCTION: THEIR EFFECT ON BONE

Endocrine Hyperfunction

Pituitary, thyroid, and gonadal hormones are required for somatic growth at the time of puberty. The effect of each of these hormones is varied, however, under physiological conditions, they being required for accelerating linear growth spurt. Overproduction of any of these hormones will disrupt normal growth and produce abnormalities specific to each hormone.

Pathophysiology

Growth hormone exerts its effect on somatic growth indirectly by increasing synthesis of insulinlike growth factors (IGF), or somatomedins. Chromophobe or eosinophilic adenoma of the pituitary, which produces excessive growth hormone, present in a child as gigantism and as acromegaly in an adult. Thyroid hormone enhances bone resorption, and thyroid hormone production, e.g., in Graves' disease, leads to demineralization of bone rather than alterations in height. Glucocorticoids directly inhibit bone growth and affect collagen synthesis.[56]

Clinical Features

Headache, changes in visual field (hemianopsia), and excessive somatic growth are symptoms and signs of growth hormone excess. If the disorder develops before puberty, tall stature is the rule. There is laxity of ligaments and joints.

Arthritis, enlargement of the hands and feet, and carpal tunnel syndrome also occur in acromegaly. Encroachment of the tumor onto the normal pituitary gland may cause hypofunction of other pituitary hormones.

A history of weight loss, tremors, nervousness, and heat intolerance is highly suggestive of thyroid hyperfunction. The gland is usually palpable and enlarged in Graves' disease, whereas symptoms of thyroid hormone excess and no glandular enlargement is compatible with factitious thyrotoxicosis. There may be proximal muscle weakness on physical examination. Bone pain, fracture, and osteoporosis occur in hyperthyroidism with significant bone loss in the axial and appendicular skeleton.[55] There may be intracortical striations in the phalangeal hands and feet.

Glucocorticoid excess, e.g., Cushing syndrome, is highlighted by truncal obesity, "moon facies," supraclavicular fat pad, hypertension, and occasionally glucose intolerance or overt diabetes mellitus. Short stature is a hallmark of excess glucocorticoid production in childhood. Glucocorticoid excess may also present as osteoporosis, and diminished bone density may be seen with photon absorptiometry.

Diagnosis

Growth hormone and somatomedin C levels are elevated in acromegaly and gigantism. Serum phosphate is usually elevated, whereas the serum calcium and PTH are normal unless hyperparathyroidism is associated as in multiple endocrine neoplasia. Thyroid function tests are diagnostic in thyrotoxicosis of any cause. Twenty-four hour urinary collection for cortisol is the best test to diagnose Cushing syndrome. Dexamethasone suppression tests may be necessary to further define the exact cause of the excess cortisol production (adrenal versus pituitary tumor).

Radiography of the hands may reveal cortical thickening or tufting of the distal phalanges in acromegaly. On skull x-ray films, the sinuses may be enlarged and there may be a thickened mandible with its characteristic underbite. Computed tomography of the sella turcica should be done in patients suspected of having growth hormone excess. Cushing syndrome and thyrotoxicosis may present as osteoporosis or demineralization of bone. The characteristic features of the various hormonal excess syndromes should not pose any difficulty in the diagnosis of specific disorders.

Treatment

Growth hormone excess can be treated by transsphenoidal hypophysectomy or bromocriptine (Parlodel). Thyrotoxicosis can be managed by the use of antithyroid drugs or ablation with radioactive iodine. Adrenal or pituitary adenomas as a cause of the Cushing syndrome, should be treated surgically. Patients receiving prednisone in high doses may not improve bone mass even with supplements of calcium and vitamin D.

Endocrine Hypofunction

Hypofunction of growth hormone or thyroid hormone usually manifests itself as short stature in a child.[45] In an adult, dis-

order of hypofunction of endocrine glands may appear insidiously over a number of years. The presentation is usually less dramatic and therefore more often missed.

Pathogenesis

Surgical ablation of endocrine glands to treat hormonal excess may lead to an endocrine hypofunction syndrome. Pituitary gonadal deposits of excess iron may occur in patients receiving chronic blood transfusion and may impair the release of any of the pituitary or gonadal hormones. Eating disorders, such as anorexia nervosa, produce changes in the hypothalamic-pituitary axis and present as hypofunction of gonadal hormones.

Clinical Features

Symptoms of hypofunction of any hormone may occur insidiously, depending upon the severity of initial inciting events. In disorders such as thalassemia which require repeated blood transfusions symptoms of iron overload may occur before those of hormonal inadequacy. Patients with hemochromatosis may exhibit diabetes mellitus, a bronze discoloration of the skin, and hepatic or cardiac abnormalities. Pain and stiffness of the metacarpophalangeal (MCP) joints are not uncommon.[6]

There may be no musculoskeletal manifestation in early anorexia nervosa. Chronic deficiency of estrogen due to the impaired pituitary gonadal axis, eventually leads to osteopenia. Fatigue is a common symptom of many of these disorders and hypofunctioning thyroid or adrenal function should be suspected. There may be no history of weight loss or salt craving in primary hypopituitary disease. Amenorrhea and diminished bone mass may be seen in athletes.[15]

Diagnosis

In general, hypofunction of endocrine glands is not easily diagnosed by single measurements of the hormones believed to be deficient. Repeat testing or dynamic testing is often necessary (see differential diagnosis). A complete blood count, hepatic function tests, serum iron, and ferritin assays are also required to distinguish the disorders of iron overload.

A low normal thyroid test may be due to primary thyroid or primary pituitary hypofunction. A TRH [hypothalamic thyroid-stimulating hormone (TSH) releasing hormone] test may be required to establish the diagnosis of hypopituitary disease. In the primary hypothyroidism, the TSH level is markedly elevated. Low levels of luteinizing hormone (LH) and follicle-stimulating hormone (FSH) may be seen in hypopituitary disease or anorexia nervosa. The history and physical findings are usually sufficient to distinguish the two disorders. Growth hormone is typically elevated in anorexia nervosa, whereas it may be deficient in hypofunction of the pituitary.

The radiographic features of hemochromatosis are quite characteristic. The initial swelling of the MCP joints should not be confused with rheumatoid arthritis, since the characteristic ulnar deviation is not present. Chondrocalcinosis is a characteristic finding on x-ray examination in hemochromatosis. There is irregularity of the articular surfaces and loss of joint space with sclerosis, typically affecting the second and third metacarpophalangeal joints. Osteopenia may be the only manifestation of disorders of the hypothalamic-pituitary axis.

Treatment

Treatment of the primary cause of endocrine hypofunction is necessary.

OSTEOPOROSIS

Osteoporosis is characterized by diminution in bone mass. There is a tendency for the bone to fracture. An estimated 15 to 20 million persons in the United States may be afflicted with osteoporosis, accounting for over a million fractures annually at an estimated cost of about \$4 billion.[37] Osteoporotic fractures commonly occur at sites of a large volume of trabecular bone, such as the proximal femur, the distal radius, and the vertebral body.

Pathogenesis

At maturity, bones change their anatomical dimensions by gradually increasing their periosteal and endosteal diameters. In menopausal women, a net loss of cortical bone results, and endosteal diameter begins to increase more rapidly than the periosteal diameter. Most elderly women have a calcium-deficient diet and a poor adaptation to low-calcium intake due to deficient production of $1,25(OH)_2D_3$. Similar changes occur only gradually in elderly men.[26] It appears that there is decreased renal conversion of 25-hydroxy vitamin D_3 to $1,25(OH)_2D_3$ in response to PTH in elderly patients with osteoporosis.[52]

The accelerated loss of calcium typical of postmenopausal osteoporosis, which can reach a rate of over 1 percent annually, is believed to occur as a consequence of the loss of estrogen.[3] Subdivisions of primary osteoporosis have been proposed on the basis of age on onset of the fracture and the site of the fracture.[44]

Risk Factors

The multifactorial nature of osteoporosis has led to the risk factor approach. Men have a greater bone mass than women at maturity, and blacks have a greater bone mass than whites. Clinical osteoporosis, which is rare in black women, is common in fair-complexioned whites with blonde or reddish hair, freckles, and a northwestern European background.[27] Other risk factors are an early menopause, chronic smoking, and use of alcohol.[2] Lack of exercise may prove to be extremely important in influencing bone mass, particularly during the growth phase.

Associated Diseases

A number of hormonal diseases such as hyperparathyroidism, hyperthyroidism, diabetes, and hypercortisolism have all been associated with the development of generalized osteoporosis. Infiltrative disorders, such as thalassemia, multiple myeloma, and leukemia may produce localized areas of osteoporosis as they expand the marrow cavity at the expense of trabecular bone.[27] Localized osteoporosis at the site of metastatic bone disease may be associated with the production of osteoclast-activating factors in neoplasia.[34]

Clinical Presentation

The presence of kyphosis giving rise to the typical dowager's hump may be the only finding on physical examination. This deformity may occur rapidly or following surgically induced menopause without estrogen replacement. The commonest presentation, however, is a fracture. Although kyphoscoliosis and blue sclera in the child or young adult suggest osteogenesis imperfecta, the tarda II variety of this condition may present undiagnosed in an adult with no deformity of the lower extremities and with normal height and appearance. This disease, characterized by abnormal collagen production, may be diagnosed by bone biopsy.

Laboratory Findings

Initial laboratory tests should include serum and urine calcium, serum protein, inorganic phosphorus, alkaline phosphatase, and a complete blood count. Renal function tests, 24-h urinary calcium creatinine, and hydroxyproline will give information about mineral and collagen turnover disorders.[27] Studies of plasma cortisol, 25-hydroxy vitamin D_3, the level of $1,25(OH)_2D_3$, as well as PTH and thyroid levels are recommended in all cases.

Additional Investigations in Vertebral Fractures

Investigation of a vertebral crush fracture should take into account whether there was a significant injury. In osteoporosis, spontaneous collapse will often follow no trauma or the mildest stress to the dorsal spine. A convenient algorithm to differentiate osteoporosis from other disorders is shown in Fig. 20-11. Scintigraphy may be helpful in differentiating crush fractures due to osteoporosis from the multiple foci of metastatic disease. It should be recalled that at least 30 percent of the bone mass from the vertebra must be removed before there is significant radiological abnormality.[24] In the spine, since the small horizontal trabeculae disappear first, there is a characteristic prominence of the vertically oriented trabeculae, which appear as vertical striation.[47] In addition, the vertebral end plates appear more prominent due to the resorption of the trabeculae. There is biconcavity due to the intervertebral pressure against the weakened bone (Fig. 20-12). Compression fractures occur most frequently at T12 followed by T11 and then L1. Vertebrae above T3 are rarely involved, and the cervical spine is not involved. There is no destruction of the pedicles, which would indicate other pathological processes.

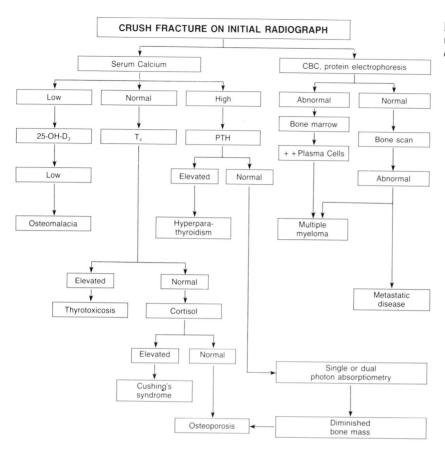

CBC = complete blood count; T_4 = thyroxine

Figure 20-11 An algorithm which may be used for differential diagnosis of vertebral crushed fractures.

Measurement of Bone Mass Techniques to determine bone mass are increasingly available and are valuable aids in establishing the diagnosis or in following the course of therapy. Bone density of the radius and the spine can be determined by single and dual photon absorptiometry, respectively.[47] In the former technique the absorption by bone of a monoenergetic gamma ray from radioisotopes such as iodine 125 is measured when the bone is surrounded by a soft tissue equivalent, such as water. In the latter the use of two photons of different energies allows measurement of bone where there may be prominent soft tissue cover, such as the hip and spine. Quantitative computed tomography of the vertebra has also been used to determine bone mass.[20] Other techniques, such as neutron activation analysis, which can detect the calcium content of the whole body, are only available in special centers and for research purposes.

The Bone Biopsy Occasionally a bone biopsy is necessary to distinguish between the osteopenia of osteoporosis and osteomalacia. The technique has now been relatively standardized.[60] The biopsy is performed 1.5 in. inferior and posterior to the anterior superior iliac spine, using a cutting needle with a diameter in excess of 5 mm (Fig. 20-13). Bone biopsy is

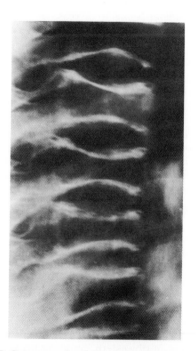

Figure 20-12 Osteoporosis of the spine showing marked loss of density of the vertebral bodies. There is relative density of the end plate. Note some wedging and marked bioconcavity. *(From Greenfield, G.B., ed: Radiology of Bone Disease, 3d ed: Philadelphia, Lippincott, 1975. Reprinted with permission.)*

recommended after double labeling of the skeleton is performed by the administration of tetracycline approximately 2 weeks apart, the first label being tetracycline and the second being a different tetracycline, Declomycin. The definition of some of the histomorphometric measurements that are available and their standard reference values are shown in Table 20-5.

Histologically, bone mass is reduced and there is characteristic reduction in trabeculae (Fig. 20-14). Histological distinction between osteoporosis and osteomalacia can be made by bone biopsy. There is, however, no uniform metabolic picture, and variations are seen histologically from little, to no active remodeling, to greatly increased bone turnover.[62] In osteogenesis imperfecta, although routine chemistry is normal, histologically the bone appears immature with a high ratio of woven to lamellar structure. This condition must be differentiated from other diseases with hypermobility of the joints, such as the Ehlers-Danlos and Marfan syndromes. In all these conditions, the calcium and phosphorus levels are normal in serum and urine.[10]

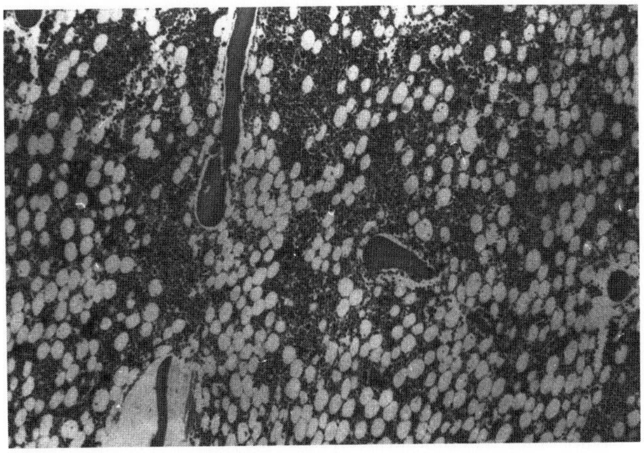

Figure 20-14 Osteoporotic bone, characterized by reduced bone mass (and brittle trabeculae). (*From Mishriki, Y.: Histopathology for Medical Students Series, part VII: Bone and Joints System, New York, Medcom, 1986. Reprinted with permission.*)

Differential Diagnosis

The generalized osteoporosis of hyperthyroidism, primary hyperparathyroidism, and Cushing syndrome should be detected in the endocrine screen. Cushing syndrome has characteristic stigmata. A history of weight loss, anorexia, and anemia are suggestive of malignant disease, and diagnosis of multiple myeloma can be established by the finding of Bence Jones protein in the urine, increased plasma cells in the bone marrow, and appropriate plasma protein electrophoretic patterns. Often there is associated hypercalcemia which responds to a course of steroid therapy. A technetium bone

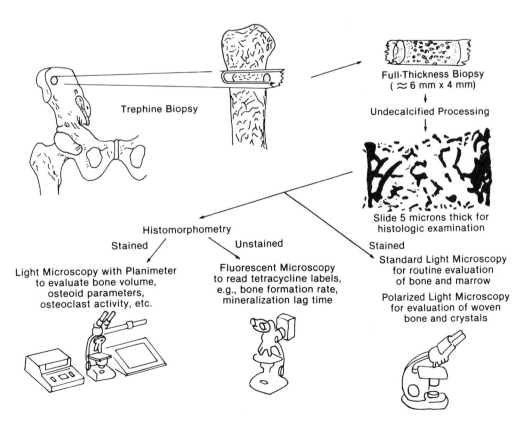

Figure 20-13 Outline of bone biopsy and evaluation procedure. (*From Vigorita, V.J. Orthop Clin North Am 15:616, 1984. Reprinted with permission.*)

TABLE 20-5 Histomorphometric Definitions and Literature Reference Values for Iliac Trabecular Bone

Terms	Definitions	Reference values (mean = standard deviations)
Indices of bone mass:		
Trabecular bone volume (TBV) (%)	The percentage of the medullary cavity occupied by mineralized and unmineralized bone	$22.5 \pm 3.5\%$
Mean trabecular width (MTW) (μm)	The average width of all trabecular bone spicules	$213 \pm 65\ \mu$m
Mean cortical width (MCW) (μm)	The mean thickness of both cortices	$909 \pm 98\ \mu$m
Indices of osteoid (unmineralized bone):		
Trabecular osteoid surface (TOS) (%)	The percentage of bone surface covered by osteoid	$18.9 \pm 5.0\%$
Trabecular osteoid volume (TOV) (%)	The osteoid area expressed as a percentage of trabecular bone area	$1.9 \pm 0.4\%$
Mean osteoid seam width (MOSW) (μm)	The osteoid area divided by the millimeters of bone surface covered by osteoid	$9.7 \pm 0.4\ \mu$m
Indices of resorption:		
Trabecular resorptive surface (TRS) (%)	The percentage of bone surface showing Howship's lacunae	$5.1 \pm 0.6\%$
Osteoclastic resorptive surface (ORS) (%)	The percentage of bone surface lined by osteoclasts	$0.13 \pm 0.6\%$
Osteoclasts per mm^2 of medullary space	The number of osteoclasts per medullary space area	0.11 ± 0.04
Osteoclasts per mm of trabecular perimeter	The number of osteoclasts per millimeter of bone perimeter	0.03 ± 0.01
Osteoclasts per mm^2 of trabecular area	The number of osteoclasts per bone area	0.20 ± 0.14
Indices of mineralization activity:		
Calcification (apposition) rate (CR) (μm/day)	The distance between the middle of all double tetracycline labels divided by the number of days between the administration of two labels	$0.64 \pm 0.10\ \mu$m/day
Mineralization lag time (MLT) (days)	The mean osteoid seam width divided by the bone formation rate	29.0 ± 3.0 days
Bone formation rate (BFR) (μm/day)	The calcification rate times the percentage of trabecular surface labeled	$0.44 \pm 0.04\ \mu$m/day
Percentage of trabecular surface labeled	The percentage of bone surfaces labeled by tetracycline labels	$12.8 \pm 2.3\%$
Percentage of osteoid labeled	The percentage of bone surfaces covered by osteoid that take up a tetracycline label	$73.4 \pm 26.5\%$

Source: Adapted from Vigorita, V. J., Orthop Clin North Am 15:4, 1984. Reproduced with permission.

scan will show increased uptake in bone in numerous conditions including spontaneous and pathologic fractures, infections, malignancies, and metastatic disease. It can be seen that the diagnosis of primary osteoporosis is primarily made by exclusion.

Treatment

Treatment is directed to the specific etiology. A period of analgesia and bed rest should be prescribed for the patient with compression fracture. Bracing should be provided only for minimal periods since physical activity should be recommenced as soon as possible to prevent further bone loss.

Drug Treatment The treatment of osteoporosis with a combination of calcium supplements and sodium fluoride has been shown to increase bone mass and to decrease the fracture rate in postmenopausal osteoporosis.[43] Treatment with fluoride increases trabecular thickness and volume. Sodium fluoride promotes transformation of lining cells to osteoblasts, bypassing the normal remodeling mechanism. Additional osteoid is produced, which has to be mineralized, and hence there is a need for calcium supplements. Adverse reactions reported with the use of fluoride have included gastrointestinal upset and arthritic type symptoms. Radiographic changes resembling fluorosis have also been reported, including increased bone density and trabeculation and partial obliteration of the medullary cavity.[17] Skeletal scintigraphy has been used to evaluate the skeletal response to fluoride treatment.[49] Lane and his co-workers in their study[25] found that 66 percent of patients suffered no fractures following the onset of this treatment, and in over 90 percent no more fractures developed in the spine after 18 months of treatment. Hip fracture rates were not influenced during the first 2 years of treatment but then seemed to diminish somewhat, although these changes were not statistically significant.[25]

Calcimar (salmon calcitonin) has been used with some success in preventing bone loss in postmenopausal osteoporosis.[4] The drug can be given intramuscularly or subcutaneously 25 units three times a week. Side effects are minimal and include nausea, flushing, and a mild diuretic effect. These effects may be transient. Hypocalcemia does not develop with Calcimar therapy. Calcitonin induces osteoclast quiescence and attempts are now being made to stimulate bone remodeling with other agents such as PTH. These experimental regimens are termed ADFR (activation-depression-free-release), a protocol during which there is alternate activation and depression of bone cells to promote maximal bone growth.

Preventive Therapy Women at risk for development of osteoporosis should consider preventive measures. Recommended preventive therapy is to increase physical activity (weight-bearing), ensure a calcium intake of 1000 to 1500 mg of elemental calcium daily, and in some cases, judicious use of estrogens.[2]

Therapy in Endocrine Disorders The osteoporosis associated with hormonal diseases, such as thyrotoxicosis, does not improve once the thyroid disease has been treated.[58] Similarly, bone mineral content does not improve in patients on long-term steroid therapy, even when a combination of fluoride, calcium, and vitamin D are used.[42]

Heterotopic Calcification

Dystrophic Calcification

Calcification is common in necrotic or infarcted tissue, e.g., following kidney infarcts. Calcium is also deposited in the region of injured muscle in hematomas and in chronic hematoma. Its deposition in the injured or degenerated rotator cuff of the shoulder can be acutely painful. Calcification can also occur in long-standing chronic abscesses, and its presence is helpful in the diagnosis of tuberculosis abscess in the psoas muscle. In all these circumstances it is unusual for there to be abnormalities in the blood chemistry, the changes being typically due to local abnormalities rather than systemic effects. Therefore, this type of calcification is conveniently called *dystrophic calcification.*

Metastatic Calcification

If there is an increase in the level of calcium or phosphate in the blood then calcium deposition can occur ectopically. This is conveniently called *metastatic calcification.* Such calcification may occur in the kidney and in the subintimal layer of the arteries in many conditions causing hypercalcemia. In chronic renal disease, the serum phosphate is elevated and the serum calcium is low. However, there are elevated levels of PTH. Symptoms of renal disease are invariably present before the onset of calcification.[23]

When oral or intravenous phosphate is used in the treatment of hypercalcemia, metastatic calcification may occur. The presenting features in this instance are those of hypercalcemic disorders. Metastatic calcification may also occur after tumor lysis. A patient receiving chemotherapy for lymphoma may release phosphate from a large mass of cells. This could produce an endogenous hyperphosphatemia which may in turn cause acute precipitation of calcium phosphate in the kidney.

Miscellaneous Causes

Calcification of basal ganglia is typically seen in primary hypoparathyroidism. Calcification of the posterior spinal ligaments in the cervical spine is an affliction more common in the Japanese. Associated glucose intolerance may occur in these patients, suggesting that this calcification may be of metastatic type.[33] Ectopic calcification is not uncommon also in collagen vascular diseases, such as dermatomyosites or scleroderma.

Tumoral Calcinosis

Tumoral calcinosis is a disease in which calcific deposits occur in the region of the buttocks and on the extensor aspect of the elbow also around other joints. These collections of calcific material can be large and may require surgical excision, but unfortunately they do recur. The disease is more common in blacks.

Treatment

Treatment of the primary cause, if possible, can prevent further worsening of the calcification, as long as the metabolic abnormalities are kept in control. Surgical decompression may be necessary to relieve symptoms of calcification or those from ossification of the posterior longitudinal ligament.[1]

In dystrophic calcification, the calcification often represents an end point in the process of healing of an area of damaged tissue. In the rotator cuff, the soft calcium deposits can be excruciatingly painful and the clinical presentation may resemble an acute arthritis. Injection of steroids may increase the discomfort; the material should be leached out between two large needles inserted into the deposits. If this is unsuccessful, the toothpastelike material can be extruded through a small incision.

SECTION B

Heterotopic Ossification

Daniel O'Neill

Heterotopic, or *ectopic, ossification* is the formation of mature bone in soft tissues that accompanies many disease processes. It occurs commonly in the periarticular areas after trauma, CNS injury, and total hip arthroplasty. It has also been described following tetanus, burns, polio, and some forms of carcinoma.[15] Mature lamellar bone is deposited in this condition which should not be confused with calcification of soft tissues. Induction of bone in soft tissues is a complex and multifaceted process which requires osteogenic precursor cells, inducing agents, and a permissive environment.[5] Such agents as bone morphogenetic protein, bone chemotactic factor (BCF), osteonectin, and chondrocalcin may be involved (see Chap. 7).

The initiating agent can be surgery itself, with disruption of soft tissues and periosteum, leaving bone debris, hematoma, damaged muscle, and an environment of uncommitted fibroblasts. However, there may be no history of surgical intervention. It is unclear why the hip and elbow are most often affected or why abnormal neurological function, with spasticity, often seems to accompany the formation of heterotopic bone.

A common form of ectopic ossification is *traumatic myositis ossificans* which follows direct injury. This type of heterotopic bone formation is frequently seen in the thigh and brachialis muscle following localized trauma in young athletes, usually in the region of the diaphysis. Myositis ossificans is also common following dislocation of joints, especially knees, elbows, and hips. In rabbits, repeated forcible passive exercising for 5 min daily of joints otherwise immobilized produced muscle necrosis which later (2 to 5 weeks) produced heterotopic ossification. If the joints were immobilized in extension—not flexion—the extensor muscles suffered, and vice versa. Denervation did not exert a protective effect.[17]

Myositis ossificans progressiva is a rare genetic disease which begins in early childhood affecting first the back and neck muscles and then progressing inexorably to almost complete immobility in early life.

INCIDENCE

The reported incidence of ectopic bone following primary total hip arthroplasty varies from 5 to 50 percent, but only a small percentage form a significant amount of bone to interfere with motion.[21,25] Less than 1 percent of hip arthroplasty patients require reoperation due solely to ectopic bone.[16] Morrey reported that the posterior approach had the lowest risk (22 percent) compared with 29 percent for the anterolateral and 28 percent for the transtrochanteric approach.[19] An increased incidence has been observed after trochanteric osteotomy by other authors[8]: up to 32 percent in high-risk patients (see below) compared with 22 percent without osteotomy.

Traumatic paraplegics seem susceptible to ectopic bone formation as are patients with spastic involvement of any limb.[15] An incidence of 20 to 25 percent is reported in spinal cord–injured patients with resultant restriction in joint motion observed in about one-third of these patients. In paraplegics those areas most often affected have a nerve supply which originates from the spine below the lesion.[32] Head-injured patients are noted to have a somewhat lower incidence of involvement, with the upper extremity most often involved.[13]

CLINICAL FEATURES

Heterotopic bone formation usually begins approximately 2 weeks after injury or neurological insult. Patients may complain of pain and swelling with local tenderness. A decreased range of motion and low-grade fever may be present. These early signs may mimic other common complications including infection or venous thrombosis.

Diagnosis

Laboratory Tests Orzel and Rudd found an acute rise in serum alkaline phosphatase concomitant with heterotopic bone formation, i.e., just over 2 weeks after the insult.[20] The rise was followed by positive findings on nuclear scan and plain radiographic studies. They therefore recommended monitoring the alkaline phosphatase level during periods of increased risk of bone formation and then using bone scans to confirm the diagnosis. This scheme is not applicable when the increased alkaline phosphatase level may be due to healing fractures. Even such "early" diagnosis, however, may be too late to initiate effective treatment.

Although tests for alkaline phosphatase, urine hydroxyproline, and serum calcium levels may have some value during development and maturation of ectopic bone, no adequate prophylactic screening test has been established. Measurement of serum alkaline phosphatase has been shown to be of little clinical value when used as a routine screening test.[18]

Conventional Radiology Detection by standard radiographs is not possible until mineralization has occurred. This is too late for effective preventive treatment.

CT Scan CT may aid in the diagnosis of ectopic ossification and is particularly valuable in delineating the extent of involvement. A CT scan is also of benefit since it may show a clear space between normal and ectopic bone and thus provide differentiation from primary bone tumors.[22]

Angiography Angiography will show increased vascularity and is occasionally useful if malignancy is suspected since arteriovenous shunting, venous lakes, or amputated vessels will be absent.[22]

Scintigraphy Nuclear scans are useful for early diagnosis. Increased vascularity is noted on three-phase bone scan at about 24 h after insult with roentgenogram evidence visible approximately 1 week later.[20]

TREATMENT

Prophylactic Treatment

Prophylactic treatment has been used principally in two groups of patients. The first consists of those identifed as high-risk for heterotopic bone formation undergoing hip arthroplasty, i.e., those with previous ectopic ossification, previous hip surgery or injury, ankylosing spondylitis,[31] diffuse idiopathic skeletal hyperostosis syndrome (DISH), and makes with osteoarthritis.[2,3,25,30] The second group of patients are those undergoing excision of heterotopic bone in an effort to prevent recurrence. Use has been made of diphosphonates, nonsteroidal anti-inflammatory medications, irradiation, and physical therapy.

Diphosphonates

These drugs have an inhibitory effect on the mineralization of osteoid. They can inhibit formation and growth of crystals of calcium hydroxyapatite in bone by chemisorption to calcium phosphate surfaces. They also have some osteoclastic inhibitory effect, making them particularly useful in Paget disease (see Sect. C). The use of 10 to 20 mg/kg per day beginning 2 weeks preoperatively in total hip arthroplasty patients resulted in a decreased incidence of ossification compared to placebo-treated groups.[9] Treatment may be extended up to 9 months. At completion of treatment, calcification of any ectopic nonmineralized matrix will occur, resulting in some bone formation, although this is not believed to be as extensive as in untreated patients.[10] The delay in bone formation may allow the patient to develop an adequate range of motion.[29] Similar results follow its use in patients with spinal cord injury. It seems to have no value if given after heterotopic ossification has appeared and does not halt the progression observed radiologically. Its prophylactic effect in these spine-injured cases is debatable.[12] A recent study found no improvement in range of motion or function following use of diphosphonates in hip arthroplasty patients treated for 3 months postoperatively.[30] This conflicts with previous studies.

Side effects of diphosphonate treatment include gastrointestinal upsets. Extended periods of treatment are required, and systemic dose-related effects may occur that can produce osteomalacia with long-term use.[16,21]

Indomethacin

Indomethacin used prophylactically in dosages of 25 mg tid for 2 months postoperatively has also proved successful in total hip replacement patients.[23,24] No cases of disabling ossification were reported even in high-risk patients. No increased incidence of trochanteric nonunion was described.

Preliminary favorable results following use of ibuprofen prophylaxis are also now being reported.[7]

Irradiation

The results of prophylactic irradiation are documented in a number of studies.[6,21] Irradiation arrests the initial step in osteoid formation by altering the DNA transcription period. Osteocytes already present, however, are seemingly unaffected and remain active for bone healing and remodeling. As with other forms of treatment, irradiation should begin within the first week after injury. The recommended dosage is a total of 2000 rad through anterior and posterior portals for over 10 days. No cases of induced neoplasm have been reported using this dosage regimen.[6,21]

Coventry reported no evidence of significant heterotopic ossification after early postoperative irradiation in 48 hip patients.[6] This study included seven patients who underwent excision of bone for ankylosis following previous hip surgery. The only untoward effect was an increased rate of trochanteric nonunion in irradiation-treated hip arthroplastic patients.[16] Irradiation is of doubtful value once ossification is noted on roentgenograms.

Physical Therapy

Physiotherapy may have an important role in preventing heterotopic ossification in the CNS-injured patient. In patients with spinal cord injury who are progressing toward ankylosis, some motion can be maintained with a program of daily joint ranging. Overenthusiastic physiotherapy, particularly passive motion, had been believed to initiate such changes, particularly in the elbow joint. However, no increased incidence of ectopic bone was observed in a series of neurologically impaired patients who underwent such treatment even when performed during periods of high risk for ectopic ossification.[26]

The use of physical therapy in CNS-injured patients should be distinguished from its use in patients with myositis ossificans. In the presence of myositis ossificans, passive motion or massage is condemned. The injury should be treated conservatively with ice and elevation during the acute stages (7 to 14 days) and progress very gradually to active and resistance exercises.

Surgical Treatment

Surgical excision has been recommended in the rare case when ossification causes important limitation of function, pressure effects, or other complications. Much controversy exists, however, on exactly when the bone is mature and thus ready for excision without inviting recurrence. Since it is known that areas of apparently mature bone may coexist with developing new bone, roentgenograms alone are inadequate to confirm maturity. One study using serum alkaline phosphatase measurements and biopsy data concluded that one should wait a minimum of 14 months before surgical intervention.[4] However, isolated determination of alkaline phosphatase levels are of little prognostic value and even normal levels do not necessarily indicate stabilization of the pathological process.[27]

In the head injured patient, the neurological status is the most useful prognostic indicator for recurrence of new bone

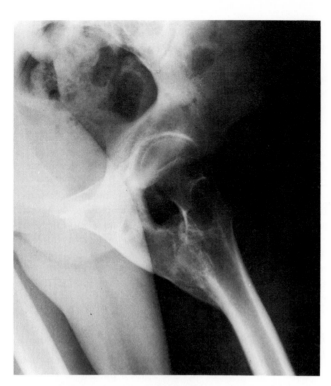

Figure 20-15 Heterotopic ossification in a 24-year-old female with hemiplegia following severe head injury. Ossification occurred in the spastic lower limb. (*Courtesy of Roger Dee.*)

SECTION C

Paget Disease

Ashok N. Vaswani and Antoni Goral

NATURE OF THE DISEASE

Although the clinical description of osteitis deformans was first published in 1877 by Sir James Paget, the skeletal defects of this disease have been well-recognized in archaeological finds.[28] The incidence of Paget disease from autopsy studies is about 3 percent, which has been corroborated by surveys of radiographs.[31,37] The incidence of the disease increases with age, and is probably equally common in men and women.

Pathophysiology

Pagetoid bone is characterized by increased osteoclastic bone resorption which is coupled to irregular bone formation, leading to focal areas of structurally impaired bone. The ce-

following surgical removal. Surgery at around 18 months is recommended provided there is a normal or only slightly elevated alkaline phosphatase level and there has been good functional recovery. Surgery may possibly be performed a little earlier in the nonfunctional patient to prevent ankylosis and permanent joint contracture.[14]

Serial bone scans have been used to assess maturity of ectopic bone. A progressively decreased uptake on serial radionuclide scans, even if still greater than adjacent normal bone, probably indicates that a good prognosis will follow surgical excision.[27] Again, a single bone scan is of little value in determining maturity.

Surgical excision of heterotopic bone has a better prognosis when coupled with one of the adjuvant drug therapies described.[6,9,21,24,25] The bone is noted to be in the fascial connective tissue with intramuscular extensions, and may be attached to the periosteum. Ossification does not involve the joint surfaces (Figs. 20-15 and 20-16).[26,27] Tendon and muscle masses may remain uninvolved but produce grooves or tunnels in the bone. Muscle fibers and blood vessels have been noted incorporated within the bony mass, however.[27] Major nerve branches are often encountered abutting, but only rarely coursing through, the ectopic bone.[29] Because of the variety of anatomical patterns, surgical removal is challenging and the approach is carefully planned after CT scan and possibly arteriography.

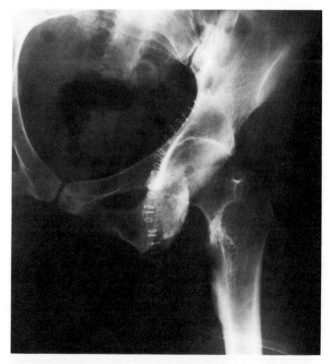

Figure 20-16 Bone has been removed through posterior approach after identifying the sciatic nerve, which did not traverse the bone. Excellent range of hip motion recovered. No recurrence 4 years postoperatively. (No prophylaxis used against recurrence except wide excision and early physiotherapy.) (*Courtesy of Roger Dee.*)

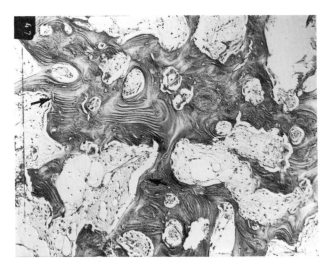

Figure 20-17 Paget disease. This H&E section illustrates the irregular mosaic pattern of lamellar bone. Characteristically immature woven bone is also present (arrows). (*Courtesy of Peter Bullough.*)

ment lines are more frequent, and there is an irregular mosaic pattern. On bone histomorphometry, osteoclasts are multinucleated and found within the haversian system as well as on trabecular surfaces (Fig. 20-17). Ultrastructure of osteoclasts have demonstrated cytoplasmic and nuclear inclusions resembling nucleocapsids of the respiratory syncytial virus and the measles virus.[24] Osteoblasts typically appear in areas where bone resorption has occurred, laying down the matrix for eventual mineralization. There is usually no abnormality in the mineralization of bone, although occasionally wide osteoid seams, representing unmineralized bone, may be observed.

Clinical Features

Paget disease may be asymptomatic, especially if it is localized to one bone. Common sites of bone involvement include the sacrum, spine, femur, and cranium. The skull changes are commonly osteocytic in the vault (osteoporosis circumscripta). As the disease progresses, osteoblastic activity may predominate, leading to an increase in the size of the skull (Fig. 20-18).

Bone pain may be present during the osteolytic phase of the disease, although the severity of the pain may be unrelated to the extent of the bony involvement. Enlargement of the skull is commonly associated with hearing loss in about 50 percent of the patients. Hearing loss may be sensorineural due to cochlear dysfunction or conductive loss due to ankylosis of the ossicles.[39] Advanced disease of the skull may lead to life-threatening complications of spinal cord compression or impingement of the brainstem.

Involvement of the long bones may be present symptomatically as pain, deformity, or fracture; occasionally, there may be osteoarthritis of the hip joint (Fig. 20-19). Headache, hydrocephalus, or symptoms of spinal cord compression may occur with advanced disease of the skull. Increased vascularity and arteriovenous shunting in the bones may lead to high output cardiac failure, particularly in the elderly individual.

Osteosarcoma, which may occur in less than 1 percent of patients with Paget disease, may present as a pathologic frac-

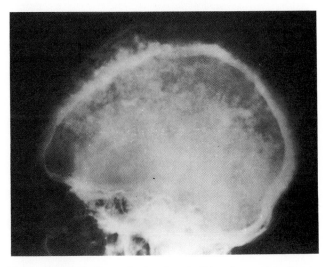

Figure 20-18 Radiograph showing skull involvement in Paget disease. (*From Greenfield, G.B., ed: Radiology of Bone Disease, 3d ed. Philadelphia, Lippincott, 1975. Reprinted with permission.*)

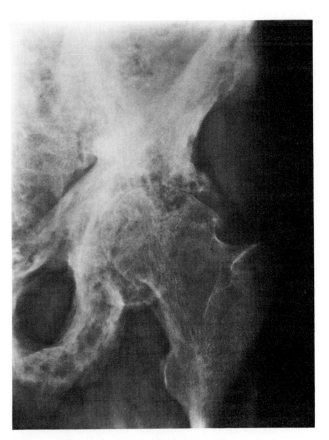

Figure 20-19 Secondary osteoarthritis of the hip joint in Paget disease.

TABLE 20-6   Stages of Paget Disease

Stage	Most common sites	Appearance
Active:		
Osteolytic	Cranial vault	Osteoporosis circumscripta
	Long tubular bones	Subchondral location; advancing wedge of radiolucency
Osteolytic	Cranial vault	Osteoporosis circumscripta, focal radiodensities
and/or	Pelvis	Patchy radiolucency and radiodensity
osteosclerotic	Long tubular bones	Diaphyseal radiolucency; epiphyseal and metaphyseal radiodensity
Inactive:		
Osteosclerotic	Cranial vault	"Cotton-wool" appearance; thickened cranial vault; basilar invagination; "picture frame" vertebral body; "ivory" vertebral body
	Pelvis	Thickening of pelvic ring; focal or diffuse radiodensity
	Long tubular bones	Epiphyseal predilection; coarse trabeculae; widened and deformed bone

Source: Resnick, R., and Nawiyama, G.: *Paget's Disease in Diagnosis of Bone and Joint Infections,* vol 2.
Philadelphia, Saunders, 1981. Reproduced by permission.

ture. Hypercalcemia is not a usual feature in Paget disease, unless the patient has been immobilized by a fracture or unless the patient has metastatic disease.

Radiological Findings

Changes in the axial skeleton include areas of sclerosis and radiodensity (Table 20-6). Vertebrae may be densely sclerotic (ivory vertebrae) and must be differentiated from metastasis. They may show the pathognomonic "picture frame" appearance (Fig. 20-20). Occasionally compression fractures may occur.

Thickening of the iliopectineal line (Brim sign) and widening of the pubic ischial bone are characteristic findings in the pelvis. Tibial bowing is common.

Laboratory Findings

Elevated alkaline phosphatase in the serum is a hallmark of active Paget disease. Minor elevations in the serum alkaline phosphatase may occur if the disease is localized. A rapid increase in the serum alkaline phosphatase may indicate the presence of a sarcoma. Measurement of urinary hydroxyproline excretion, which is an index of bone resorption, is useful to determine the extent and progress of the disease. There is usually no alteration in calcium metabolism, although there is rapid bone turnover. Hypercalcemia and hypercalciuria may occur in an immobilized patient with Paget disease. However, primary hyperparathyroidism should be considered in the differential diagnosis. Serum uric acid may be elevated, and may lead to clinical gout.

Other Tests

Localization of sites of activity can be accomplished by the use of technetium 99–labeled compounds.[33] A bone biopsy may be necessary to diagnose localized Paget disease.

Differential Diagnosis

The markedly high values of serum alkaline phosphatase are uncommon in any other disease. Hydroxyproline excretion may be increased in patients with acromegaly. However, prognathism, enlarged sella turcica, and elevated growth hormone are diagnostic of acromegaly.

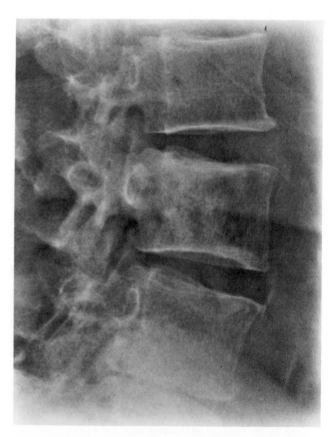

Figure 20-20 Vertebrae showing pathognomonic "picture frame" appearance with sclerosis at margins of the vertebral centrum.

Osteolytic lesions of the skull may be confused with multiple myeloma. Anemia, monoclonal gammopathy, and plasma cells in a bone marrow aspirate will distinguish the two disorders. Hypercalcemia may also be present in patients with multiple myeloma.

The sclerotic vertebral lesion must be differentiated from sclerotic metastasis, e.g., from prostate or lymphoma. Occasionally biconcavity of vertebrae may occur and resemble osteomalacia. Generally speaking, the radiological appearance of trabecular thickening is diagnostic. However, renal osteodystrophy, fluorosis, and fibrous dysphasia can cause confusion.

Treatment

Treatment of Paget disease is directed against the disordered osteoclastic activity. Calcitonin (salmon calcitonin, Calcimar) is a potent inhibitor of osteoclastic activity and inhibits bone resorption. The drug must be given subcutaneously three times a week, and can produce symptomatic relief in 1 to 2 weeks.[9] Nausea and flushing are common, but transient, side effects of the drug. Antibodies against calcitonin may interfere with the clinical response. Hypocalcemia does not occur with calcitonin treatment. The effect of treatment with calcitonin is an improvement in pain, and a reduction of hydroxyproline and alkaline phosphatase level, indicating inhibition of bone resorption.

Diphosphonates, which are analogues of pyrophosphate, have also been used in the treatment of Paget disease.[41] Disodium etidronate [ethane-1, hydroxy-1, 1 diphosphonate (EHDP)] can be given orally, 5 mg/kg per day. However, at this dose there is inhibition of bone resorption due to the osteoclast inhibitory activity whereas in higher doses there may be impairment of bone formation. EHDP, because of its action to inhibit the mineralization of osteoid, should be given only intermittently.[1] The drug will reduce by about 70 percent the excess levels of serum alkaline phosphatase and total 24-h urinary hydroxyproline. There is no increase in the incidence of fractures occurring in these patients.[17] There may be hyperphosphatemia and secondary hyperparathyroidism associated with the use of diphosphonates. A combination of calcitonin and diphosphonates has also been shown to be effective. Mithramycin (Plicamycin) should not be used except in the most refractory cases.

SURGICAL MANAGEMENT

Complications of Paget disease requiring surgical intervention include fracture, deformity, degenerative joint disease, spinal cord compression, and tumor. Operative intervention, especially in those patients requiring open reduction and internal fixation for fracture or hip arthroplasty, carries the risk of significantly increased intraoperative bleeding. Preoperative suppression of the activity of the disease with such agents as calcitonin may have effect in reducing hemorrhage in elective surgery.[21,22]

Fractures in Paget Disease

Fractures through pagetoid bone have been reported to occur most commonly in long bones involving the femur, tibia, humerus, radius, and ulna. Less frequently reported are cases of spine and hand fractures.[8] A pathologic fracture of pagetoid bone may be the initial sign of the disease in as many as two-thirds of all patients.[25] Surgical management of these fractures is frequently complicated by the presence of deformity and abnormal bone quality which makes internal fixation difficult.

The closed treatment of these fractures yields varying results depending upon the activity of the disease and location.[12,26]

Fracture of the Femur

The most common site of fracture is the femur. Trivial violence to the diseased bone is frequently sufficient to fracture this bone, which may already be laterally bowed (the tibia characteristically bows anteriorly). Fractures are generally transverse with disruption of the periosteal sleeve and comminution. Although union may be achieved by conservative management in shaft fractures, operative intervention is frequently employed to avoid the complications of immobilization (deep venous thrombosis, pneumonia, decubiti, and the hypercalcemia and acidosis to which these patients may be particularly predisposed). Although only 7 percent of femoral fractures are intracapsular, nonunion rates in these patients approach 100 percent despite adequate internal fixation.[2] Grundy[12] and Nicholas,[26] however, both reported poor results in those patients treated with primary endoprosthetic replacement. Grundy even suggested acceptance of the risk of nonunion by treating those patients nonsurgically by early mobilization, noting that not all patients had significant pain despite nonunion.[12] Primary total hip arthroplasty is an option especially if there is associated hip joint involvement with the disease.[42,43]

Subtrochanteric and intertrochanteric femoral fractures occur more commonly and generally go on to union after internal fixation. Short intramedullary rod fixation or compression plates have been described, with union achieved in over 50 percent by 6 months.[8] Fracture of the femoral shaft is often associated with a preexisting varus deformity and a sclerotic intramedullary canal which will make intramedullary rod fixation technically difficult. Osteotomy at the time of internal fixation whether with an intramedullary rod or plate is recommended.[13] Fixation devices should be left in place after union is achieved to maintain correction of the deformity as a prophylaxis for refracture. Several authors describe satisfactory results with conservative management of femoral shaft fractures and in addition were able to correct the contributory deformity while in Thomas splintage.[12,26] Nonunion was seen in conservatively treated femoral shaft fractures in 10 to 15 percent, whereas operatively managed fractures had a nonunion rate of 20 to 30 percent.[7,8,26] Hypercalcemia and acidosis can occur in an immobilized patient with Paget disease but is relatively uncommon.[12] Those patients with femoral shaft fractures may require a longer-than-average length of hospital stay whether treated by either open or closed methods.[26]

Fracture of Other Bones

Fracture of the tibia commonly will show stress fractures on the convex aspect of the apex of the bowed bone (by contrast with Looser's zones seen on the concave aspect in osteomalacia). Complete fractures are treated along the same lines as femoral fractures.[3] The few reported cases of metacarpal fractures through pagetoid bone have been traumatic in origin and generally achieve union by conservative means.[16,27]

Osteotomy

Surgical treatment of the deformities seen in Paget disease (coxa vara, femoral and tibia vara) has a high risk of producing nonunion, but in selective cases may be recommended as prophylaxis for changes in joint mechanics and fracture.[3,10,19,21]

Associated coxarthropathy occurs in 10 percent of patients with Paget disease (Fig. 20-19). They show acetabular protrusion, medial joint or concentric space narrowing, and coxa vara deformity.[21] Intertrochanteric osteotomy with bone grafting may be the surgical procedure of choice if the joint space is well preserved.[43] Roper reported an improved postoperative range of motion in patients treated by intertrochanteric osteotomy for Paget coxarthropathy as compared to those treated for primary osteoarthritis.[33] Surprisingly, union is achieved in virtually all such osteotomized patients.[32]

Total Hip Arthroplasty

The indications for total hip arthroplasty are similar to nonpagetoid degenerative joint disease. Care must be taken to be certain that the pain is in the joint and not associated with the bony changes remote from the articular surfaces. The procedure may also be justified for subcapsular fracture with displacement and associated acetabular disease.

Bony deformity, particularly coxa vara, may make total hip arthroplasty technically difficult. Preoperative medical management with calcitonin and diphosphonates is recommended[21,42] but Merkow found that in 66 percent of patients the disease was already relatively quiescent at the time of hip arthroplasty.[21] Intraoperative bleeding does not seem to be excessive, whether or not preoperatively treated with calcitonin or EHDP.[14,21,22,42] However, heterotopic new bone formation occurs in as many as 52 percent of patients undergoing total hip arthroplasty for Paget disease as compared to 5 percent in routine hip arthroplasty.[20,21] Another concern has been the fear that the underlying bone disease may predispose the patient with Paget disease to early prosthesis loosening, but this has not been substantiated to any degree.[14,19b,42]

Spinal Stenosis

Spinal stenosis secondary to Paget disease is discussed in Chap. 59, Sect. C. Characteristically this problem is encountered in the middle-aged male with the gradual onset of paresis over a year's time.[14] More fulminant courses have been reported, and in those sarcoma must be suspected.[36] Compression may occur at a single level, most commonly thoracic, or at multiple vertebral bodies.

Malignant Degeneration

Malignant degeneration in Paget disease has been reported in 6.5 percent of documented cases.[35] The most frequent sites of malignant change include the femur, humerus, pelvis, and tibia in that order of frequency. Vertebral tumors do occur, but rarely. Tumors generally take the more common forms of osteogenic sarcoma and fibrosarcoma as well as reticulum cell sarcoma, giant cell sarcoma, and a mixed, anaplastic type. The occurrence of tumor at the site of previous fracture has been reported, but there is no direct correlation.[4] Sarcomatous degeneration is generally seen in patients with the polyostotic form of the disease. Treatment consists of palliative resection or amputation along the lines outlined in Chap. 23, Sect. A. Surgery may be combined with chemotherapy, but the latter is not well tolerated in these patients, who are often elderly. Most of these patients are dead within two years.[4,35] Long-term survival greater than 2 years is a rarity.

SECTION D

Gaucher Disease

Roger Levy

NATURE OF THE DISEASE

Gaucher disease is a rare familial disorder. The disease is more frequent in Ashkenazic Jews, but not restricted to that group. There is an inborn error of metabolism with consequent deposition of glucosyl ceramides in the reticuloendothelial system. The bone marrow, liver, and spleen are among the areas affected.

General Clinical Features

The sedimentation rate may be chronically elevated in late disease. A bleeding diathesis may occur with complications in the skin, conjunctivae, and gums. Splenomegaly is common and often of extensive degree.

For these reasons, splenectomy is required in many patients with Gaucher disease. A clinical impression exists that bone manifestations worsen after splenectomy, but no study has ever documented this as fact.

Hepatomegaly is also common, and many patients ultimately suffer from severe hepatic dysfunction, which can add further risk to surgery.

Occasional reports in the literature suggest that patients with Gaucher disease are more prone to myeloma,[16] Hodgkin

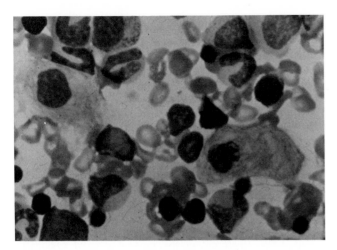

Figure 20-21 Lipid-laden "foamy" macrophages; the typical Gaucher cell.

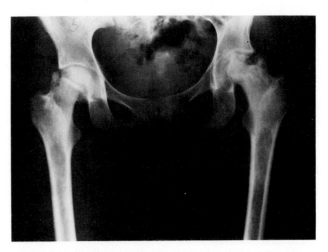

Figure 20-22 Pathologic fracture of femoral neck following bilateral ischemic necrosis due to Gaucher bone disease.

disease,[5] and leukemia.[10] Serum acid phosphatase is ordinarily elevated in these patients.

Orthopaedic Aspects of Gaucher Disease

As with the viscera, the reticuloendothelial macrophage cells of the bone marrow become progressively laden with the ceramide in the intracellular lysosomal bodies (Fig. 20-21). A variety of major bone changes takes place in a somewhat sequential manner. However, these changes may all be present in different bones of the same patient at the same time. Furthermore, these osseous manifestations do not correlate with factors such as the degree of enzyme deficiency, level of circulating ceramide, or the degree of visceral involvement. Circulatory embarrassment on either the arterial or venous side secondary to marrow packing with these cells may well play a role in the development of bone changes, but other cellular mechanisms may also be important. Macrophages may play an indirect role in the production of osteoclast-activating factor (OAF),[4] and studies in our own laboratory have suggested high collagenase levels in tissues obtained from the proximal femur at the time of surgery.[12]

Virtually any bone can be involved symptomatically, pathologically, and radiographically. Most clinical problems have involved the proximal femur with hip disability (Fig. 20-22). However, other clinical problems may include the distal femur and proximal tibia with thigh and knee symptoms and the proximal humerus with shoulder symptoms, and especially the vertebrae with problems ranging from back pain to cord compression.

Radiological Changes (Table 20-7)

Most of the radiographic changes occur within the marrow space and on the endosteal surface of the cortex. However, periosteal bone formation is also common. Important bony manifestations may be enumerated as follows:

TABLE 20-7   Radiological Stages of Skeletal Lesions in Gaucher Disease

Stage	Nature of lesion	Appearance
0	Normal	Normal
1	Diffuse osteoporosis	Coarse trabecular pattern of osteoporosis
2	Medullary expansion	Loss of normal concavity above femoral condyles; erlenmeyer flask deformity
3	Localized destruction (osteolysis)	Small erosions, well-defined or moth eaten; cortex rarefied and endosteally notched; ground glass veiling
4	Ischemic necrosis of long bones; sclerosis; osteitis	Patchy densities and erosions; serpiginous sclerotic streaks; layered periostitis; sequestra
5	Diffuse destruction; epiphyseal collapse; osteoarthrosis	Flattening or irregular destruction of femoral heads, with mixed lytic and sclerotic foci. Larger "soap bubble" pattern

Osteopenia

A diffuse osteopenia is often present in many of the bones of patients with Gaucher disease. The bone density is diminished, but our CT studies consistently demonstrate a positive attenuation coefficient ($+15$ to $+80$ Hounsfield units)[9] measured from pathologic bone marrow. Normal bone marrow, like fat, has a negative attenuation coefficient. Cortices are thinned and trabecular markings are reduced.

Localized Areas of Bone Erosion

These can be seen and may be major or minor. We have observed several cases of apparent soft tissue extension through transcortical defects, but biopsy has revealed only red blood cells.

These general and localized areas of bone loss create stress risers within bone and when located in a vertebra or long bone can lead to pathologic fracture following trivial trauma.

Osteosclerosis

Sclerotic areas are often noted within the medullary cavity with serpiginous streaks and islands of sclerosis touching the endosteal surface or isolated from them. These areas are generally considered to be the sequelae of prior infarcts or Gaucher "crises" within the medullary cavity.

Medullary Expansion

The term *medullary expansion* has been used to describe the radiological "enlargement" of the metaphyseal portion of bones in patients with Gaucher disease. Especially involved is the distal femur leading to the characteristic erlenmeyer flask deformity. The cause for such metaphyseal deformity must doubtless be due to a primary failure of remodeling. CT scan,^{99m}Tc MDP, and ^{99m}Tc SC scans reveal an equal incidence of distal femoral and proximal tibial involvement.

Complications

Osteonecrosis

This is one of the most serious of the complications of Gaucher disease of bone. It may affect an articular area of bone such as a femoral head, a humeral head, or a condyle at the knee. Alternatively it may present as an infarct involving the shaft of a long bone. Children may present with moderate symptoms and a limp or show a silent course mimicking a case of Perthes disease. Adolescents and adults often have an acute onset of extremely severe hip, groin, or thigh pain. Weight bearing is extremely painful as is any movement of the limb. ^{99m}Tc MDP scans performed very early have revealed avascularity of the femoral head. A small number of patients treated by immediate core decompression have had rapid pain relief, and no further evidence of pathological progression of head deformity. Femoral head collapse and secondary degenerative joint changes have occurred in most, but not all, cases where the diagnosis was made later or early surgical treatment refused. Examples exist of patients treated nonsurgically with acceptable results.

Gaucher "Crisis"

The term *Gaucher "crisis"* is applied to the sudden onset of intractable pain involving a joint or shaft of a long bone in afflicted individuals. The clinical problem is to distinguish this from osteomyelitis. Early radionuclide scans may be helpful, showing decreased activity with Gaucher crisis and increased activity with osteomyelitis.

Treatment

Much of the treatment of the musculoskeletal system in Gaucher disease is symptomatic and supportive. The correct diagnosis is imperative to avoid harm. Crises are managed with rest, analgesics, and external support. Acute episodes of osteonecrosis may be managed surgically or nonsurgically. Our experience with core decompression in the early acute phase has been uniformly successful, but numbers are limited. Late problems of secondary degenerative joint disease, especially at the hip, can be managed by joint replacement. Such an endeavor requires care and considerable experience since often the bone anatomy is atypical and the patients young. Bleeding and infection hover as threats to success. With considerable attention to detail results can be encouraging.[13] Unusually high failure rates have also been reported in these patients.[1,11] The treatment of pathologic fractures can be challenging. Because of the paucity of bone cells, delay or failure of union may occur. Inadequate periods of immobilization or premature weight bearing may lead to malunion.[9a] Internal fixation devices must be carefully selected if surgical treatment is elected. Pathologic fracture in the spine can lead to neurological compression syndromes and may require vertebrectomy and stabilization with spinal rods.

REFERENCES

Section A: The Osteopenias, Rickets, and Allied Disease

1. Abe, H., Tsuru, M., and Ito, T. Anterior decompression for ossification of the posterior longitudinal ligament of the cervical spine. Neurosurgery 55:108–116, 1981.
2. Aloia, J.F., Cohn, S.H., Vaswani, A.N., et al. Risk factors for postmenopausal osteoporosis. Am J Med 78(1):95–100, 1985.
3. Aloia J.F., Ross, P., Vaswani, A.N., et al. Rate of bone loss in postmenopausal and osteoporotic women. Am J Physiol 242:E82–E86, 1982.
4. Aloia, J.F., Vaswani, A.N., Kapoor, A., et al. Treatment of osteoporosis with and without growth hormone. Metabolism 34:124–129, 1985.
5. Anderton, J.M. Orthopedic problems in adult hypophosphatasia: A report of two cases. J Bone Joint Surg 61B:82–84, 1979.
6. Bellamy, R.E. The orthopedic surgeon and hemochromatosis. Orthopedics 3(5):419–423, 1980.
7. Brenner, R.J., Spring, D.B., Sebastian, A., et al. Incidence of radiographically evident bone disease, nephrocalcinosis and nephroli-

thiasis in various types of renal tubular acidosis. N Engl J Med 307:217–221, 1982.

8. Breslau, N.A., and Pak C.Y.C. Hypoparathyroidism. Metabolism 28:1261–1276, 1979.

9. Broadus, A.E., Horst, R.L., Lang, R., et al. The importance of circulating 1,25 dihydroxy vitamin D in the pathogenesis of hypercalciuria and renal stone disease in primary hyperparathyroidism. N Engl J Med 302:421, 1980.

10. Burtis, W.J., and Lang, R. Chemical abnormalities. Orthop Clin N Am 15:653–669, 1984.

11. Chesny, R.W., Mazess, R.B., Rose, P., et al. Long term influence of calcitriol (1,25 dihydroxy vitamin D) and supplemental phosphate in X-linked hypophosphatemic rickets. Pediatrics 71:559–567, 1983.

12. Coventry, M.B., and Scanlon, P.W. The use of radiation to discourage ectopic bone: A nine year study in surgery about the hip. J Bone Joint Surg 63A:201–208, 1981.

13. De Luca, H.F. Metabolism and mechanism of action of vitamin D, in Peck, W.A., (ed): *Bone and Mineral Research,* annual 1. Excerpta Medica, 1983, pp 7–73.

14. Doppelt, S.H. Vitamin D, rickets and osteomalacia, in *Symposium on Metabolic Bone Disease.* Orthop Clin North Am 15:671–686, 1984.

15. Drinkwater, B.L., Nilson, K., Chestnut, C.H., et al. Bone mineral content of amenorrheic and eumenorrheic athletes. N Engl J Med 311:277–280, 1984.

16. Dunstan, C.R., Evans, R.A., Hills, E., et al. Effect of aluminum and parathyroid hormone on osteoblasts and bone mineralization in chronic renal failure. Calcif Tissue Int 36:133–138, 1984.

17. El-Khoury, G.Y., Moore, T.E., Albright, J.P., et al. Sodium fluoride treatment of osteoporosis: Radiologic findings. AJR 139:39–43, 1982.

18. Evans, G.A, Arulanantham, K., and Gage, J.R. Primary hypophosphatemic rickets: Effects of oral phosphate and vitamin D on growth and surgical treatment. J Bone Joint Surg 62A:1130–1137, 1980.

19. Farfel, Z., Brickman, A.S., Kaslow, H.R., et al. Defect of receptor cyclase coupling protein in pseudohypoparathyroidism. N Engl J Med 303:237–242, 1980.

20. Genant, H.K., Cann, C.E., Ettinger, M.B., et al. Quantitative computed tomography of vertebral spongiosa: A sensitive method for detecting early bone loss after oophorectomy. Ann Intern Med 97:699–705, 1982.

21. Gnokos, P.J., London, R., and Hendler, E.D. Hypercalcemia and elevated 1,25 dihydroxy vitamin D levels in a patient with end-stage renal disease and active tuberculosis. N Engl J Med 311:1683–1685, 1984.

22. Hodges, R. Ascorbic acid, in Goodhart, R.S., and Shils, M.E. (eds): *Modern Nutrition in Health and Disease,* 6th ed. Philadelphia, Lea & Febiger, 1980, pp 259–273.

23. Klein, K.L., and Maxwell, M.H. Renal osteodystrophy. Orthop Clin North Am 15:687–695, 1984.

24. Lachman E. Osteoporosis: The potentialities and limitations of its roentgenologic diagnosis. AJR 74:712–715, 1955.

25. Lane, J.M., Healey, J.H., Schwartz, E., et al. Treatment of osteoporosis with sodium fluoride and calcium: Effects on vertebral fracture incidence and bone histomorphometry. Orthol Clin North Am 15(4):729–745, 1984.

26. Lane, J.M., and Vigorita, V.J. Osteoporosis, in *Symposium on Metabolic Bone Disease.* Orthol Clin North Am 15:711–727, 1984.

27. Lane, J.M., and Vigorita, V.J. Current concepts review: Osteoporosis. J Bone Joint Surg 65A(2):274–278, 1983.

28. Liberman, U.A., Eil, C., Marx, S.J. Resistance to 1,25 dihydroxy vitamin D: Association with heterogenous defects in skin fibroblasts. J Clin Invest 71:192–200, 1982.

29. Mallette, L.E., Bilezikian, J.P., Heath, D.A., and Aurbach, G.D. Primary hyperparathyroidism: Clinical and biochemical features. Medicine 53:127–146, 1974.

30. Marie, P.J., and Glorieux, F.H. Histomorphometric study of bone remodeling and hypophosphatemic vitamin D-resistant rickets. Metab Bone Dis Relat Res 3:31–38, 1981.

31. Marx, S.J., Stock, J.L., Attie, M.F., et al. Divalent cation metabolism; familial hypocalciuric hypercalcemia versus typical primary hyperparathyroidism. Am J Med 65:235–242, 1978.

32. Meunier, P.J. Bone biopsy in diagnosis of metabolic bone disease, in Cohn, D.V., Talmage, R.V., and Matthews, J.L. (eds): *Hormonal Control of Calcium Metabolism.* Proceedings of the Seventh International Conference on Calcium Regulating Hormones. Excerpta Medica, 1980.

33. Miyasaka, K., Kaneda, K., and Ito, T. Ossification of spinal ligaments causing thoracic radiculomyelopathy. Radiology 143:463–468, 1982.

34. Mundy, G.R., Ibbotson, K.J., D'Souza, S.M., et al. The hypercalcemia of cancer: Clinical implications and pathogenic mechanisms. N Engl J Med 310:1718–1727, 1984.

35. Neufield M., McLaren, N.K., and Blizzard R.M. Two types of autoimmune Addison's disease associated with different polyglandular autoimmune syndromes. Medicine 60:355–362, 1981.

36. Ogilvie-Harris, D.J., and Fornasier, V.L. Pseudomalignant myositis ossificans: Heterotopic new bone formation without a history of trauma. J Bone Joint Surg 62A:1274–1282, 1980.

37. *Osteoporosis.* National Institutes of Health Consensus Conference. JAMA 252:799, 1984.

38. Parker, M.S., Klein, I., Haussler, M.R., et al. Tumor-induced osteomalacia: Evidence of a surgically correctable alteration in vitamin D metabolism. JAMA 245(5):492–493, 1981.

39. Pollison, R.P., Martinez, S., Khoury, M., et al. Calcification of entheses associated with X-linked hypophosphatemic osteomalacia. N Engl J Med 313:1–6, 1985.

40. Rasmussen, H. Hypophosphatasia, in Stanbury, J.B., Wyngaarden, J.B., Fredrickson, D.S., et al. (eds): *The Metabolic Basis of Inherited Disease,* 5th ed. New York, McGraw-Hill, 1983, pp 1497–1507.

41. Rasmussen, H., Pechet, M., Anast, C., et al. Long term treatment of familial hypophosphatemic rickets with oral phosphate and 1-alpha-hydroxy vitamin D. J Pediatr 99(1):16–25, 1981.

42. Rickers, H., Deding, A., Christiansen, C., et al. Mineral loss in cortical and trabecular bone during high dose prednisone treatment. Calcif Tissue Int 36:269–273, 1984.

43. Riggs, B.L., Seeman, E., Hodgson, S.F., et al. Effect of the fluoride calcium regimen on vertebral fracture occurrence in postmenopausal osteoporosis. N Engl J Med 306:446–450, 1982.

44. Riggs, B.L., Wahner, H.W., Dunn, R.B., et al. Differential changes in bone mineral density of the appendicular and axial skeleton with aging. J Clin Invest 67:328–335, 1981.

45. Rimoin, D.L., and Horton, W.A. Short stature, part I. J Pediatr 92:523, 1978.

46. Rude, R.K., Oldham, S.B., Sharp, C.F., Jr., et al. Parathyroid hormone secretion in magnesium deficiency. J Clin Endocrinol Metab 48:800–806, 1978.

47. Schneider, R. Radiologic methods of evaluating generalized osteopenia. Orthop Clin North Am 15(4):631–651, 1984.

48. Scholz, D.A., and Purnell, D.C. Asymptomatic primary hyperparathyroidism. 10 year prospective study. Mayo Clin Proc 56:473–478, 1981.

49. Schulz, E.E., Libanti, C.R., Farley, S.M., et al. Skeletal scintigraphic changes in osteoporosis treated with sodium fluoride: Concise communication. J Nucl Med 25(6):651–655, 1984.

50. Scriver, C.R., Frazer, D., and Kooh, S.W. Hereditary rickets, in Heath, D.A., and Marx, S.J. (eds): *Calcium Disorders.* Boston, Butterworth Scientific, 1982, pp 1–46.

51. Sharma, O.P. Hypercalcemia in sarcoidosis. Arch Intern Med 145(4):26–627, 1985.

52. Slovik, D.M., Adams, J.S., Neer, R.M., et al. Deficient production of 1,25 dihydroxy vitamin D in elderly osteoporotic patients. N Engl J Med 306:1136, 1981.

53. Stewart, A.F., Adler, M., et al. Calcium homeostasis in immobilization. N Engl J Med 306:1136, 1982.

54. Stover, S.L., Niemann, K.L.W., and Miller, J.M., III. Disodium etidronate in the prevention of postoperative recurrence of heterotopic ossification in spinal cord injury patients. J Bone Joint Surg 688, 1976.

55. Stulberg, B.N., et al. Hyperparathroidism, hyperthroidism and Cushing's disease. Orthop Clin North Am 15:697–710, 1984.

56. Thompson, J.S., Palmieri, G.M.A., and Crawford, R.L. The effect of porcine calcitonin on osteoporosis induced by adrenal cortical steroids. J Bone Joint Surg 54A:1490–1496, 1972.

57. Tieder, M., Modai, D., Samuel, R., et al. Hereditary hypophosphatemic rickets with hypercalciuria. N Engl J Med 312:611–617, 1985.

57. Tieder, M., Modai, D., Samuel, R., et al. Hereditary hypophosphatemic rickets with hypercalciuria. N Engl J Med 312:611–617, 1985.

58. Toh, S.H., Claunch, B.C., and Brown, P.H. Effect of hyperthyroidism and its treatment on bone mineral content. Arch Int Med 145:883–890, 1985.

59. Toomey, F., Hoag, R., Batton, D., et al. Rickets associated with cholestasis and parenteral nutrition in premature infants. Radiology 142(1):85–86, 1982.

60. Vigorita, V.J. The tissue pathologic features of metabolic bone disease. Orthop Clin North Am 15:613–629, 1984.

61. Wharton, G.W. Heterotopic ossification. Clin Orthop 112:142–149, 1975.

62. Whyte, M.P., Bergfield, M.A., Murphy, W.A., et al. Postmenopausal osteoporosis—A heterogenous disorder as assessed by histomorphometric analysis of iliac crest bone from untreated patients. Am J Med 72:193–202, 1982.

Section B: Heterotopic Ossification

1. Ackerman, L.V. Extraosseous localized non-neoplastic bone and cartilage formation (so-called myositis ossificans). J Bone Joint Surg 40A:279–298, 1958.

2. Blasingame, J.P., Resnick, D., Coutts, R.D., and Danzig, L.A. Extensive spinal osteophytosis as a risk factor for heterotopic bone formation after total hip arthroplasty. Clin Orthop 161:191–197, 1981.

3. Bundyck, T.J., Cook, D.E., and Resnick, C.S. Heterotopic bone formation in patients with DISH following total hip replacement. Radiology 155:595, 1985.

4. Buring, K. On the origin of cells in heterotopic bone formation. Clin Orthop 110:293–302, 1975.

5. Chalmers, J., Gray, D.H., and Rush, J. Observations on the induction of bone in soft tissues. J Bone Joint Surg 57B:36–45, 1975.

6. Coventry, M.B., and Scanlon, P.W. The use of radiation to discourage ectopic bone. Bone Joint Surg 63A:201–208, 1981.

7. Elmstedt, E., Lindholm, T.S., Nilsson, O.S., and Tornkvist, H. Effect of ibuprofen on heterotopic ossification after hip replacement. Acta Orthop Scand 56(1):25–27, February 1985.

8. Errica, T.J., Fetto, J.F., and Waugh, T.R. Heterotopic ossification. Incidence and relation to trochanteric osteotomy in 100 total hip arthroplasties. Clin Orthop 190:138–141, 1954.

9. Finerman, G.A., Brooker, A.F., Coventry, M.B., Krengel, W.F., McRoberts, R.L., Salvati, E.A., and Volz, R.G. Symposium: heterotopic ossification following total hip replacement. Contemp Orthop 5:95, 1982.

10. Finerman, G.A. The role of diphosphonate on heterotopic ossification after total hip arthroplasty. J Bone Joint Surg 59B:501, 1977.

11. Finerman, G.A., Krengel, W.F., Lowell, J.D., Murray, W.R., Volz, R.G.,

Bowerman, J.W., and Gold, R.H. Role of diphosphonate (EHDP) in the prevention of heterotopic ossification after total hip arthroplasty: A preliminary report. Hip 5:222–234, 1977.

12. Garland, D.E., Alday, B., Venos, K.G., and Vogt, J.C. Diphosphonate treatment for heterotopic ossifications in spinal cord injury patients. Clin Orthop 176:197–200, 1983.

13. Garland, D.E., Blum, C.E., and Waters, R.L. Periarticular heterotopic ossification in head-injured adults. J Bone Joint Surg 62A:1143–1146, 1980.

14. Garland, D.E., et al. Resection of heterotopic ossification in the adult with head trauma. J Bone Joint Surg 67A:1261–1269, 1985.

15. Hait, G., Boswick, J.A., and Stone, N.H. Heterotopic bone formation secondary to trauma (myositis ossificans traumatica). J Trauma 10:405, 1970.

16. Jowsey, J., Coventry, M.B., and Robins, P.R. Heterotopic ossification: Theoretical consideration, possible etiologic factors, and a clinical review of total hip arthroplasty patients exhibiting this phenomenon. Hip 5:210, 1977.

17. Michelsson, J.E., and Rauschnig, W. Pathogenesis of experimental heterotopic bone formation following temporary forcible exercising of immobilized limbs. Clin Orthop 176:265–272, 1983.

18. Mollan, R.A.B. Serum alkaline phophatase in heterotopic paraarticular ossification after total hip replacement. J Bone Joint Surg 61B:432–434, 1979.

19. Morrey, B.F., Adams, O.P.A.-C, and Cabenela, M.E. Comparison of heterotopic bone after anterolateral transtrochanteric and posterior approaches for total hip arthroplasty. Clin Orthop 188:160–161, 1983.

20. Orzel, J.A., and Rudd, T.G. Heterotopic bone formation: Clinical laboratory and imaging correlation. J Nuclear Med 26:125, 1985.

21. Parkinson, J.R., Evarts, C.M., Hubbard, L.F. Radiation therapy in the prevention of heterotopic ossification after total hip arthroplasty. Hip 10:211, 1982.

22. Ray, M.J., and Basset, R.L. Myositis ossificans. Orthopedics 7:532, 1984.

23. Ritter, M.A., and Gide, T.J. Effect of indomethacin on para-articular ectopic ossification following total hip arthroplasty. Clin Orthop 167:113–117, 1982.

24. Ritter, M.A., and Sieber, J.M. Prophylactic indomethacin for the prevention of heterotopic bone formation following total hip arthroplasty. Clin Orthop 196:217–225, 1985.

25. Ritter, M.A., and Vaughan, R.B. Ectopic ossification after total hip arthroplasty. J Bone Joint Surg 59A:345–351, 1977.

26. Roberts, J.B., and Pankratz, D.G. Surgical treatment of heterotopic ossification at the elbow following long-term coma. J Bone Joint Surg 61A:760–763, 1979.

27. Rossier, A.B., Bussat, P., Infante, F., Zender, R., Courvoisier, B., Muheim, G., Donath, A., Vasey, H., Taillard, W., Lagier, R., Gabbiani, G., Baud, C.A., Pouezat, J.A., Very, J.M., and Hachen, H.J. Current facts on para-osteo-arthropathy (POA). Paraplegia 11:36, 1973.

28. Spielman, G., Gennarelli, T.A., and Rogers, C.R. Disodium etidronate: Its role in preventing heterotopic ossification in severe head injury. Arch Phys Med Rehabil 64:539, 1983.

29. Stover, S.L., Niemann, K.M.W., and Miller, J.M. Disodium etidronate in the prevention of post-op recurrence of heterotopic ossification in spinal-cord injured patients. J Bone Joint Surg 58A:683–688, 1976.

30. Thomas, B.J., and Amstutz, H.C. Results of administration of diphophonate for the prevention of heterotopic ossification after total hip arthroplasty. J Bone Joint Surg 67A:400–403, 1985.

31. Williams, E., Taylor, A.R., Arden, G.P., and Edwards, D.H. Arthroplasty of the hip in ankylosing spondylitis, J Bone Joint Surg 59B:393–397, 1977.

32. Wharton, G.W. Heterotopic ossification. Clin Orthop 112:142–149, 1975.

Section C: Paget Disease

1. Alexandre, C.M., et al. Treatment of Paget's disease of bone with ethane-1, hydroxy-1, diphosphonate (EHDP) at a low dosage (5 mg/kg/day). Clin Orthop 174:193–205, 1983.
2. Barry, H.C. Fractures of the femur in Paget's disease of bone in Australia. J Bone Joint Surg 49A:1359–1370, 1967.
3. Berruex, P. Traitement par plague des fractures et deformations axicles des membres dans la maladie de Paget. Rev Chir Orthop 64:123–129, 1978.
4. Brice, C.H.G., and Goldie, W. Paget's sarcoma of bone. J Bone Joint Surg 51B:205–224, 1969.
5. Buchman, J. Total femur and knee joint replacement with a vitallium endoprosthesis. Bull Hosp Jt Dis 21–34, 1965.
6. Cartlidge, N.E.E., McCollum, J.P.K., and Ayyar, R.D.A. Spinal cord compression in Paget's disease. J Neurol Neurosurg Psychiatry 35:825–828, 1972.
7. Cruess, R., and Rennie, W. *Adult Orthopedics,* vol. New York, Churchill Livingstone, 1984, pp 449–457.
8. Debeyre, J., and Bovcker, C. Maladie de Paget et Chirurgie. Rev Rheum 43:93–96, 1976.
9. DeRose, J., Singer, F.R., Avramides, A., et al. Response of Paget's Disease to porcine and salmon calcitonins. Am J Med 56:858, 1974.
10. Direkze, M., and Milnes, J.N. Spinal cord compression and Paget's disease. Br J Surg 57:239, 1970.
11. Graham, J., and Harris, W.H. Paget's disease involving the hip joint. J Bone Joint Surg 53B:650–659, 1971.
12. Grundy, M. Fractures of the femur in Paget's disease of bone: Their etiology and treatment. J Bone Joint Surg 52B:252–263, 1970.
13. Haddad, J.G.J. Paget's disease of bone: Problems and management. Orthop Clin North Am 3:775–780, 1972.
14. Ha'Erie, G.B., and Schatzker, J. Total replacement of the hip joint affected by Paget's disease. Can J Surg 21:370–372, 1978.
15. Handy, R.C. Paget's disease of bone. Endocrinol Metab 1:167, 1981.
16. Haverbush, T.S., Wilde, A.H., and Phalen, G.S. The hand in Paget's disease of bone. J Bone Joint Surg 54A:173–175, 1972.
17. Johnston, C.C., Jr., et al. Review of fracture experience during treatment of Paget's disease of bone with etidronate disodium (EHDP). Clin Orthop 172:186–194, 1983.
18. Lentle, B.C., Russell, A.S., Heslip, P.G., and Percy, J.S. The scintigraphic findings in Paget's disease of bone. Clin Radiol 26:129–135, 1976.
19. Louyot, P., Purel, J., Delagoute, J.P., and Zanetti, A. Quelques aspects inhabituels de fracture des pagetique. Rev Rheum 42:653–660, 1975.
19a. McDonald, D.J., and Sim, F.H. Total hip arthroplasty in Paget's disease. J Bone Joint Surg 69A:766–772, 1987.
20. *Mercer's Orthopedic surgery,* 8th ed. Baltimore, University Press, 1983, pp 279–290.
21. Merkow, R.L., Pellicci, P.M., Hely, D.P., and Salvati, E. Total hip replacement for Paget's disease of the hip. J Bone Joint Surg 66A:752–757, 1984.
22. Milgram, J.W. Orthopedic management of Paget's disease of bone. Clin Orthop 127:63–69, 1977.
23. Miller, S.W., Castronovo, F.P. Jr., Pendegrass, H.P., et al. J Roentgenol Rad Therapy Nucl Med 121:177, 1974.
24. Mills, B.G., Singer, F.R., Weinger, L.P., et al. Evidence for both syncytial virus and measles virus antigens in the Clin Orthop 183:303, 1984.
25. Mitchell, D.C. Fractures in brittle bones. Orthop Clin North Am 3:787–790, 1972.
26. Nicholas, J.A., and Hilloram, P. Fracture of the femur in patients with Paget's disease: Results of treatment in 23 cases. J Bone Joint Surg 47A:450–461, 1965.

27. Oglivie-Harris, D.J., and Formasier, V.L. Pathologic fractures of the hand. Clin Orthop 143:168–170, 1979.
28. Paget, J. On a form of chronic inflammation of bones (osteitis deformans). Med Chir Trans 60:37, 1877.
29. Plaut, M. Paget's disease of the vertebrae. J Neurosurg 40:791–792, 1974.
30. Postel, M., and Senley, G. Correction des courbures diaphysaires pagetiques. Rev Chir Orthop 64:667–676, 1978.
31. Pygott, F. Paget's disease of bone. The radiological incidence. Lancet 1:1170, 1957.
32. Roper, B.A. Paget's disease at the hip with osteoarthrosis: Results of intertrochanteric osteotomy. J Bone Joint Surg 53B:660–662, 1971.
33. Roper, B.A. Paget's disease involving the hip joint: A classification. Clin Orthop 80:33–38, 1971.
34. Sadar, E.S., Walton, R.J., and Gossman, H.H. Neurological dysfunction in Paget's disease of the vertebral column. J Neurosurg 37:661–665, 1972.
35. Schajawicz, F. *Tumors and Tumorlike Lesions of Bone and Joint.* New York, Springer-Verlag, 1981, pp 399–407.
36. Schmidek, H.H. Neurologic and neurosurgical sequelae of Paget's disease of bone. Clin Orthop 127:70–77, 1977.
37. Schmorl, G. Uber osteitis deformans Paget. Virchows Arch [Pathol Anat Physiol] 283:694, 1957.
38. Shenoy, B.V., and Scheithauer, B.L. Sir James Paget, F.R.S. Mayo Clin Proc 58:51–55, 1983.
39. Singer, F.R. Paget's disease of bone, in Avioli, L.V. (ed): *Topics in Bone and Mineral.* New York Plenum, 1977.
40. Siris, E.S., and Canfield, R.E. Paget's disease of bone: Current concepts as to its nature and management. Orthop Rev 11:43–49, 1982.
41. Smith, R., Russell, R.G.G., and Bishop, M. Diphosphonates and Paget's disease of bone. Lancet 1:945, 1971.
42. Stauffer, R.N., and Sim, F.H. Total hip arthroplasty in Paget's disease of the hip. J Bone Joint Surg 58A:476–478, 1976.
43. Turek, S.L. *Orthopedics,* vol, 4th ed. Philadelphia, Lippincott, 1984, pp 734–743.

Section D: Gaucher Disease

1. Amstutz, H.C. The hip in Gaucher's disease. Clin Orthop 90:83–89, 1973.
2. Bentler, E., and Krihl, W. The diagnosis of the adult type of Gaucher's disease and its carrier state by demonstration of deficiency of beta glucosidase activity in peripheral blood leukocytes. J Lab Clin Med 76:747–755, 1970.
3. Brady, R.O., Kanfer, J.N., and Shapiro, D. Metabolism of glucocerebrosides. II. Evidence of an enzymatic deficiency in Gaucher's disease. Biochem Biophys Res Commun 18:221–225, 1964.
4. Brady, R.O., and Barranger, J.A. Glucosylceramide lipidosis: Gaucher's disease, in Stanbury, J.B., Wyngaarden, J.B., Frederickson, S.D., Brown, M.S., and Goldstein, J.L. (eds): *The Metabolic Basis of Inherited Disease,* 5th ed. New York, McGraw-Hill, 1983, pp 842–856.
5. Bruckstein, A.H., Karanas, A., and Dire, J.J. Gaucher's disease associated with Hodgkin's disease. Am J Med 68:610–613, 1980.
6. Desnick, R.J., Gatt, S., and Grabowski, G. (eds). *Gaucher's Disease: A Century of Delineation and Research.* New York, Alan R. Liss, 1982.
7. Fried, K. Population study of chronic Gaucher's disease. Isr Med J Sci 9:1396–1398, 1973.
8. Gaucher, P.C.E. *De l'epithelioma printif de la rate, hypertrophe idiopathique de la rate sans lucemie.* Paris, Octave Doin, 1882.
9. Hermann, G., Goldblatt, J., Levy, R.N., Goldsmith, S.J., Desnick, R.J.,

and Grabowski, G.A. Assessment of bone marrow and bone involvement in Gaucher disease type I by computed tomographic and radionuclide scans.

9a. Katz, K., Cohen, I.J., Ziv, N., Grunebaum, M., Zaizov, R., and Yosipovitch, Z. Fractures in children who have Gaucher disease. J Bone Joint Surg 69A:1361–1370, 1987.

10. Krause, J.R., Bures, C., and Lee, R.E. Acute leukemia and Gaucher disease. Scand J Haematol 23:115–118, 1979.

11. Lachiewicz, P.F., Lane, J.M., and Wilson, P.D., Jr. Total hip replacement in Gaucher's disease. J Bone Joint Surg 63A:602–608, 1981.

12. Levy, R.N., Oronsky, A.L., Guzman, N.A., Grabowski, G.A., and Desnick, R.J. *Collagen Biosynthesis and Degradation in Gaucher's Disease.* New York, Petrie Arthritis Research Laboratory, Department of Orthopaedics, Mount Sinai School of Medicine, 1984.

13. Levy, R.N. *Orthopaedic Aspects of Gaucher Disease.* Jackson, WY Association of Bone and Joint Surgeons, July, 1984.

14. Mundy, G.R., and Yoneda, T. Monocytes: Interaction with bone cells and lymphocytes during bone resorption, in Cohn, D.V. (ed): *Hormonal Control of Calcium Metabolism.* Proceedings of the Seventh International Conference on Calcium. Amsterdam. Excerpta Medica, 1981, p 178.

15. Patrick, D.A., A delinquency of cerebrosidase in Gaucher's disease. Biochem J 95:170, 1965.

16. Pinkhas, J., Djaldetti, M., and Yaron, M. Coincidence of multiple myeloma with Gaucher disease. Isr J Med Sci 1:537–540, 1965.

CHAPTER 21

Hematologic Disorders

David Westring, Michael Ries, and Roger Dee

Conditions which lead to pathological bleeding may be inherited or acquired and may result from defects in the platelets, coagulation proteins, vascular wall, or any combination of these.

Of the inherited disorders *hemophilia* is the most important, but not the most common form encountered. Far more common are the *acquired or inherited bleeding tendencies* from platelet and vascular disorders; as causes, always to be considered first are drugs including salicylates, other nonsteroidal anti-inflammatory agents, warfarin (Coumadin), and heparin. *Vitamin K deficiency* is not an uncommon cause of bleeding in patients receiving antibiotics or prolonged intravenous therapy.

THE HEMOPHILIAS

Hemophilias most commonly encountered in an orthopaedic practice are listed in Table 21-1. Von Willebrand's disease (VWD) has been included with the hemophilias because of the similar clinical expression in many victims. In each case the surgeon must be prepared to act appropriately before, during, and after operative intervention. The presence of ineffective factors VIII and IX, producing what is hereafter called hemophilias A and B, respectively, results in bone and joint lesions. However, factor XI deficiency and VWD may present in similar ways.

Hemophilias A and B

Hemophilia A is the commonest of the variants, with estimates of its incidence between 1 in 20,000 and 1 in 10,000 people. The remaining clinical experience occurs in diminishing order of frequency in VWD, hemophilia B (factor IX deficiency), and factor XI deficiency (plasma thromboplastin antecedent deficiency, or PTA). The hemophilias are a result of genetic mutations, which may result in two basic defects: an abnormal protein, which produces functional impairment, or the complete absence of a protein factor, a true functional deletion. In hemophilias A and B there is convincing evidence of an abnormal protein, while in VWD and in factor XI deficiency qualitative defects have not been demonstrated. Table 21-2 lists the essential differences in the pathophysiology of these three hemophilias and VWD.

Von Willebrand's Disease

VWD is known to surgeons for its clinical subtleties rather than for specific or predictable manifestations. Confusion results from its many names, which include vascular hemophilia and pseudohemophilia, and from the long uncertainty about its nature. Many patients in whom the diagnosis is made state that they have "hemophilia" or are "bleeders." The incidence of the disorder is unknown because of the variable presentation and manifestations, but it is probably a common inherited bleeding disorder. In VWD, factor VIII pro-

TABLE 21-1 Common Hemophilias

Disorder	Biosynthesis	Inheritance	Affected persons	Clinical manifestation	Laboratory screening
Hemophilia A	Abnormal factor VIII	Sex-linked recessive	Male children, in alternate generations	Spontaneous bleeding, hemarthrosis, crippling	PTT prolonged. Bleeding time usually normal
Hemophilia B	Abnormal factor IX	Sex-linked recessive	Male children, in alternate generations	Spontaneous bleeding, hemarthrosis, crippling	PTT prolonged. Bleeding time usually normal
Factor XI deficiency	Probable abnormal factor XI	Autosomal recessive	Male or female children or adults, usually Jewish	Hemorrhage after trauma or surgery, occasional hemarthrosis	PTT prolonged. Bleeding time usually normal
Von Willebrand's disease	Abnormal or absent VWD multimers plus deficient factor VIII	Autosomal dominant	Males and females, often adults; generations may be skipped	Usually mild, but may be severe	Bleeding time prolonged

coagulant may be normal in quantity and function, decreased in quantity, or virtually absent. The von Willebrand factor, inherited independently by an autosomal mechanism, is a group of subunits (*mers*) which form multimers of various sizes that bind factor VIII. Type I disease is mild; the basic defect is in the decreased amounts of von Willebrand factor. Type II disease commonly lacks large multimers of von Willebrand factor. Type III VWD is the most severe, the rarest, and the most difficult to treat.[57]

Epidemiology

That a bleeding disorder is inherited may be entirely unsuspected. Such is commonly the case with hemophilia A because of the sex-linked recessive pattern which omits clinical expression in the female carrier generation, and because of a relatively high percentage of new mutations associated with this disease. A clinical diagnosis of clotting disorder must be confirmed by identification of the specific lesion.

TABLE 21-2 Clinical Diagnosis of Common Inherited Bleeding Disorders

Disease	Usual manifestation	Preliminary Laboratory Findings				Specific therapeutic approach
		PT	PTT	Platelet count	Bleeding time	
Hemophilia A	Spontaneous bleeding, into joints and intense pain. Bleeding may arise, anywhere, however.	Normal	Prolonged	Normal	Normal	Factor VIII concentrate
Hemophilia B	Same	Normal	Prolonged	Normal	Normal	Prothrombin complex (factors II, VII, IX, and X)
Factor XI deficiency	Hemorrhage after trauma or surgery. Spontaneous bleeding rare.	Normal	Prolonged	Normal	Normal	Prothrombin complex if volume is a consideration. Fresh frozen plasma is often adequate to terminate bleeding
Von Willebrand's disease	Types I and II: variable, usually post traumas or operative. Type III: may be spontaneous hemarthrosis.	Normal	Usually prolonged	Normal	Prolonged	Fresh frozen plasma. Desmopressin except in types II and III.

Laboratory Findings

Laboratory identification of the specific hemophilias requires specialized studies which are not readily available at all times or in all hospitals. Many take more than one day to accomplish, and frequently additional steps are required to ascertain the precise diagnosis. For the surgeon who must make prompt clinical decisions, it is best to establish the broadest range of possibilities so that risks and benefits may be assessed. This can be done with the platelet count, the prothrombin time (PT), the activated partial thromboplastin time (PTT), the bleeding time, and the plasma fibrinogen content. Table 21-2 indicates distinctions between VWD and the hemophilias on the basis of the results of these few studies and clinical presentation.

When factor VIII activity is found to be diminished, clinical correlation with the laboratory results and further in vitro and in vivo investigations are needed to exclude VWD. Prolonged bleeding time is a critical and useful bedside test of platelet functions. Early judgments about the inaccuracy of this test have been reversed since the introduction of the template method. The test is performed best by someone with experience.[19] The template allows a blade to make in the forearm dermis a superficial cut of standard depth and length under controlled capillary pressure. Timed measurements of clot formation are based on filter paper blotting of the lesion. The method is highly sensitive, safe, and reliable and when positive identifies qualitative defects in platelet function.

VWD is further defined by laboratory assessment of ristocetin cofactor, platelet aggregation, and immunologic studies to identify the aberrant or absent molecule. Such definition is critical to the patient's future care since the management of type III VWD may be quite different from that for types I and II. It is necessary to refer all patients with an abnormal bleeding time to a center where such a laboratory exists.

Treatment

Treatment for inherited bleeding disorders depends on whether the problem arises in the preoperative, intraoperative, or postoperative period.

The Preoperative Period

Strategy depends on the time available before surgery and whether the diagnosis of the bleeding disorder is known. Unknown blood specimens should be submitted to the laboratory while measures are taken to delay surgery. In most elective situations this is possible, but in multiple trauma cases in which life is threatened, intervention cannot be delayed. The infusion of fresh frozen plasma provides the greatest opportunity for correction of the bleeding time. In the male patient with undiagnosed excessive bleeding, addition of cryoprecipitate infusion is reasonable. Further augmentation of hemostasis with 1-deamino-8-D-arginine vasopressin (desmopressin) may be accomplished if the patient has mild factor VIII deficiency, but at the risk of inducing platelet aggregation and a disseminated intravascular coagulation-like picture.

While awaiting the platelet count, fibrinogen level, PT, and PTT, a simple bleeding time which gives significant diagnostic guidance can be determined. If it is longer than 12 min, it is reasonable evidence of VWD. A bleeding time less than 12 min does not exclude VWD but increases the probability of other causes. Also, if the patient is female, the likelihood of factor VIII and IX deficiency is exceedingly low.

Specific replacement therapy cannot begin until initial coagulation assessment is complete. When the platelet count and the PT are normal and the PTT is prolonged beyond the control value, factor analysis must be done.

Drug Therapy Desmopressin was licensed in 1984 for the treatment of mild hemophilia (factor VIII blood levels above 5 percent; see Table 21-3). Originally produced for the treatment of diabetes insipidus by intranasal instillation, it is now known to produce two to threefold increases in plasma levels of factor VIII and related proteins when given by intravenous infusion. It is thought to cause release of factor VIII from endothelial storage sites but also may increase platelet adhesion and spreading at injury sites. Desmopressin is contraindicated in patients with type II VWD and pseudo-VWD, a platelet disorder, because it may precipitate extensive immediate platelet aggregation and thrombocytopenia. It is ineffective in type III VWD. For this reason it cannot be used until a diagnosis has been established.[29]

When the diagnosis of the bleeding disorder is already known and surgery is needed immediately, the infusion of specific factors should be instituted before anesthesia is induced. Appropriate therapy must be determined by a hematologist who is experienced with treating hemophilia. In general, concentrates are superior to plasma and plasma fractions because of their small volume. There is no indication in modern infusion therapy for whole blood.

Intraoperative Bleeding

Unexpected abnormal bleeding during surgery requires immediate attempts at diagnoses. In the hemophiliac patient the usual cause is inadequate levels of factor VIII, but this cannot be assumed since these patients are subject to the same disorders experienced in surgical patients without inherited coagulopathies. In addition they have a greatly increased risk for developing plasma inhibitors. New blood specimens for determining the platelet count, PT, PTT, and fibrinogen level should be obtained from an extremity or line free of heparin contamination and fluid infusions. Additional history may be sought from the patient's chart and, if necessary, from the family.

Postoperative Bleeding

Postoperative bleeding generally arises from the same causes as intraoperative bleeding. Delayed bleeding in factor VIII and IX deficiencies is not unusual, and transient increased doses of the depleted factor should be given when it occurs. Another cause of late recurrence is prothrombin deficiency, which can result from liver dysfunction, malabsorption, lack of dietary fat, and large doses of antibiotics. This should be treated with oral vitamin K whenever possible since intra-

TABLE 21-3   Classification and Manifestations of Hemophilias A and B

VIII or IX blood level, %	Category	Characteristic bleeding patterns
0–1	Severe	Spontaneous muscle and joint bleeding; crippling usual
1–5	Moderate	Severe bleeding after minor injuries; occasional spontaneous bleeding
5–25	Mild	Severe bleeding after surgery or injury
25–50	Mild	Prolonged bleeding after major injury

muscular administration may cause hematomas and intravenous therapy has been associated with cardiovascular complications. If the intravenous route is necessary, the drug should be diluted and given slowly. Regardless of the route of administration, correction of prothrombin deficiency in patients with normal liver function takes at least 24 h; the intravenous route does not shorten this response rate.

Postoperative bleeding often arises in association with antibiotic administration when serum vitamin K levels are adequate. The antibiotics most often implicated are penicillin in dosage of 10 to 40 million units per day, carbenicillin (20 to 40 g/day), and ticarcillin (16 g/day), but other beta-lactam antibiotics have been reported to cause bleeding. The mechanism by which these antibiotics inhibit platelet function is unclear, and more than one defect is probably involved. Hematologists seem to agree that the potential for bleeding should not be a consideration for antibiotic selection.[10]

Complications of Replacement Therapy

Complications of replacement therapy occur early and late. Dilution of clotting factors by excessive transfusion of bank blood may be prevented by infusion of fresh frozen plasma at a ratio of 1 unit after each 4 units of packed red cells. Although platelet counts may fall by the same mechanism, it is not necessary to replace platelets unless the count falls below 80,000/dl. Replacement of a patient's functionally inadequate platelets may also be required, such as in VWD, polycythemia vera, uremia, and the uncommon thrombasthenias.

Volume overload from the infusion of large amounts of replacement factors can be avoided by treating with concentrates. If these are not available, simultaneous use of diuretics such as furosemide is advised. Transfusion reactions rarely occur as a complication of plasma component replacement therapy. However, when red cells are administered for blood loss, transfusion reactions are a possibility. Allergic reactions from replacement therapy are not uncommon and most frequently manifest as skin rash or fever. Anaphylaxis is the most serious of this category and is detected by an otherwise unexplained sudden fall of blood pressure, edema of the oral

mucous membranes, pruritus and/or rash, and tachycardia. Immediate therapy with epinephrine, antihistamines, and steroids should be commenced and a hematologist consulted.

Some investigators have reported an increased risk of local or widespread thrombosis when the lyophilized prothrombin complex is used to treat factor IX deficiency; the use of slow infusion and saline flush are adequate to prevent this complication.

Late complications of replacement therapy include at least two serious diseases. Hepatitis, despite greatly improved methods of detection among blood donors, remains a threat to hemophilic patients and other recipients of multiple or massive transfusions. There are few patients with hemophilia who do not demonstrate prior or chronic infection with hepatitis B virus. Presently, however, most hepatitis resulting from transfusion is non-A, non-B. Patients treated with cryoprecipitate are at increased risk since this material cannot be treated to inactivate virus and is usually given in multiple units.

Acquired immunodeficiency syndrome (AIDS) is a more recently described disorder caused by infection with the human immunodeficiency virus (HIV). The mortality is very high and no effective therapy currently exists. Hemophilic patients have an increased risk for this disease if they have received factor VIII which has not been treated with heat or other virus inactivating procedure, or is from a pool of unscreened donors.

PATHOLOGICAL INHIBITORS OF COAGULATION

Patients occasionally present with acquired bleeding disorders that appear to be deficiencies in one or more coagulation factors. These disorders are due to pathological inhibitors of coagulation. The inhibitors are broadly defined as abnormal endogenous components of blood that inhibit normal blood coagulation.[42] Some have been clearly identified as antibodies, and it is expected that most if not all act as antibodies. They may appear as single, specific inhibitors or as groups. The commonest is probably an antibody to factor VIII; this antibody is found in patients with severe hemophilia A who have received extensive exogenous factor VIII replacement therapy. Up to 21 percent of patients with hemophilia may develop anti-factor VIII.

Treatment

Hemophilia A patients who develop factor VIII antibody represent a serious challenge to hematologists and to blood banks. Surgery of any sort is rarely possible when the patient becomes refractory to replacement therapy. When an inhibitor is suspected, the level of anti-factor VIII should be measured and followed during the course of the patient's illness. Treatment with massive doses of factor VIII concentrates is sometimes effective but frequently is not.

In the remainder of patients with acquired factor inhibitors, the condition is rarely as severe and may not need therapy. Some patients experience spontaneous remission. Lupus erythematosus patients may develop inhibitory factors but seldom require corrective therapy and may be prepared for elective, and even emergency, surgery with corticosteroids or immunosuppressant drugs. For those who develop thrombosis (about 10 percent of patients with the lupus inhibitor), chronic warfarin anticoagulation has been recommended.[35]

ORTHOPAEDIC ASPECTS OF HEMOPHILIA

Table 21-3 correlates disease manifestations with plasma levels of factors VIII and IX. Therapeutic plasma levels recommended in patients with severe disease vary from 20 percent in mild disease and minor injuries to greater than 100 percent in any disease category with life-threatening bleeding such as in the CNS or throat.

Hemophilic Arthropathy

Repeated hemarthroses eventually lead to the development of hemophilic arthropathy. The number of joint hemorrhages does not necessarily correlate with the severity of the arthropathy. Hemophilic arthropathy begins with an early phase characterized by synovitis and progresses to a later phase of cartilage destruction and joint deformity.[15]

Hemarthroses may be separated into acute, subacute, and chronic categories. Acute hemorrhages may occur with minimal or no trauma. Approximately one-half of hemarthroses in hemophiliac patients occur at the knee.[51] The elbow is also commonly involved, while hemarthroses of the shoulder, spine, and hand occur less frequently.[18] Subacute hemarthropathy generally develops after at least three hemorrhages into the same joint within 6 weeks after the last joint hemorrhage.[14] Joint motion is slightly restricted. The joint swelling is mainly due to synovial hypertrophy. Chronic hemarthropathy is characterized by synovial thickening, cartilage destruction, and fibrosis leading to progressive joint deformity, pain, and stiffness.

Radiological Classification

Early radiographic changes after repeated joint hemorrhage include soft tissue swelling, osteoporosis, and epiphyseal enlargement. Epiphyseal enlargement may be overestimated on routine anteroposterior views of the knee if a flexion contracture is present, and correlation with the lateral view should be noted.[25] Later radiographic changes such as squaring of the patella, widening of the intercondylar notch of the knee, widening of the trochlear notch of the ulna, and subchondral cysts are characteristic. Finally joint space narrowing and osteophyte formation occur.

Arnold and Hilgartner have described a radiographic classification of hemophilic arthropathy as follows[3]:

Stage I. No skeletal abnormalities, but soft tissue swelling is present.

Stage II. Osteoporosis and overgrowth of the epiphysis. No joint space narrowing or bone cysts.

Stage III. Subchondral bone cysts, squaring of the patella, widening of the intercondylar notch of the knee, and widening of the trochlear notch of the ulna. Joint space is not narrowed.

Stage IV. Narrowing of joint space with progression of changes in stage III.

Stage V. Fibrous contracture, loss of joint space, extensive enlargement of epiphysis, and substantial disorganization of joint structures.

Stages I and II are associated with a 90 percent of normal or greater range of motion at the elbow, knee, and ankle with a progressive decrease in motion with advanced stages.[25] Loss of joint space appears to be the most important radiographic finding related to loss of motion.

Pettersson et al developed a radiographic classification based on a point system (Table 21-4).[37] No radiographic changes were seen before age 3, while all patients demonstrated some radiographic changes beyond age 6. The increase in score with age was fairly constant until the late teens, when changes progressed more slowly. This method of assessing the severity of the arthropathy appears to correlate well with clinical findings.[37]

Nonoperative Management of Hemophilic Arthropathy

The management of orthopaedic problems associated with hemophilia involves concomitant care by the orthopaedic and hematologic services. Adequate clotting factor levels must be achieved to control acute bleeding and are required prior to an arthrocentesis or surgical procedure. The presence of an inhibitor is a contraindication to an elective surgical procedure.

Acute Hemarthroses

Acute hemarthroses may be managed with transfusion to achieve factor levels of 30 to 50 percent of normal, immobilization with splints or compressive dressings, ice, and analgesics. One unit of factor VIII or IX is the amount of activity in 1

TABLE 21-4 Radiologic Classification of Hemophilic Arthropathy

Radiologic change	Finding	Score, points
Osteoporosis	Absent	0
	Present	1
Enlargement of epiphysis	Absent	0
	Present	1
Irregularity of subchondral surface	Absent	0
	Present	1
	Pronounced	2
Narrowing of joint space	Absent	0
	<50%	1
	>50%	2
Subchondral cyst formation	Absent	0
	1 cyst	1
	>1 cyst	2
Erosions at joint margins	Absent	0
	Present	1
Incongruence between joint surfaces	Absent	0
	Slight	1
	Pronounced	2
Deformity coagulation and/or displacement of articulating bones	Absent	0
	Slight	1
	Pronounced	2

Source: Pettersson, A.H.: Clin Orthop 149:153–159, 1980.

ml of fresh normal pooled plasma.[18] One unit of factor VIII per kilogram of body weight should raise the plasma level by 2 percent, while 1 unit of factor IX per kilogram of body weight raises the plasma level by 1.5 percent, since more factor IX goes into the extravascular space.[18] The development of factor concentrates permits transfusions to increase plasma clotting factor levels without overloading the patient from transfusion of plasma.

Although the role of joint aspiration in acute hemarthroses remains controversial, this may be required for the management of severe hemorrhages with a very tense hematoma. A second transfusion may be required 48 h after a major joint hemorrhage and a third at 72 h to help prevent the development of hypertrophic synovitis.[14]

Subacute Hemarthropathy

The nonoperative management of subacute hemarthropathy involves factor replacement, splinting, and muscle-strengthening exercises. Green and Wilson recommend 3 weeks of cast immobilization with 6 weeks of prophylactic transfusion therapy, and muscle-strengthening exercises if no joint space narrowing is present.[14] If synovitis persists, a 1 week course of steroids is given and the joint is protected with an orthosis.

Chronic Hemarthropathy

Management of chronic hemarthropathy is directed toward maintaining range of motion and muscle strength. Once a fixed flexion deformity of the knee occurs, correction by wedging casts may be accompanied by posterior subluxation of the tibia.[33] Stein and Dickson used a modified balanced Thomas traction with a Pearson attachment to correct knee flexion contractures.[48] A padded sling is passed over the thigh at the level of the suprapatellar pouch and underneath the metal bars on both sides of the Thomas splint. This is attached by pulleys to a 2.8-kg weight to force the distal femur posteriorly while longitudinal skin traction is applied to the lower leg. The Pearson attachment is then gradually extended.

The Quengel cast, which consists of a short hip spica cast attached to an outrigger extending over the anterior tibia, and a short leg cast attached to the outrigger at both the proximal and distal tibia, enables the knee to be slowly extended while lifting the proximal tibia anteriorly.[14,26] Significant flexion deformities can be corrected by either method, although one disadvantage of the Quengel cast is a longer hospitalization. Greene and Wilson noted an average hospital stay of 38.2 days for the Quengel cast method,[14] while Stein and Dickson reported an average of 14.1 days for the modified traction method.[48]

Surgical Management of Hemophilic Arthropathy

The presence of an inhibitor is a contraindication to any elective surgical procedure. Adequate factor replacement should be available. Multiple procedures under one anesthetic are recommended to minimize the complications of repeated clotting factor transfusions.[38,39] Tourniquet should be released prior to closure. Vessels should be ligated rather than cauterized. Precautions such as double gloves and plastic aprons are advised to help protect the surgical team from exposure to hepatitis and AIDS.[53]

Synovectomy

Synovectomy can decrease the occurrence of recurrent hemarthroses,[31,49,50] although radiographs may demonstrate progression of joint destruction with time.[39] The synovium that regenerates is relatively fibrous and avascular.[18] After synovectomy of the knee, there is frequently some loss of motion, particularly terminal flexion;[7,16] in the elbow, by contrast, motion may be improved.[28a] Indications for synovectomy are generally recurrent hemarthroses for at least 6 months associated with persistent synovial hypertrophy not controlled with conservative means in early (stage I or II) arthritis.[16,31,53] Factor levels of 75 to 100 percent for the first postoperative week, 50 to 75 for the second, and 25 to 50 percent for the third are recommended.[53]

Chemical synovectomy (synoviorthesis) with osmic acid or radioactive gold have been used with variable results. Osmic acid treatment can decrease the number of hemarthroses, although less effectively than surgical synovectomy, and joint function can be reduced.[49] The results of radioactive gold treatment are less reliable, 1 year follow up discloses.[30]

Osteotomy

Osteotomy may be of benefit in selected patients with more advanced arthropathy. Smith et al in a small series reported that patients with stage IV or V disease treated with high tibial osteotomy for varus deformity showed no progression of the arthropathy at an average follow-up of 18 months.[44]

Total Joint Arthroplasty

Total joint replacement is generally reserved for end-stage arthropathy. Factor levels of 100 percent on the day of surgery, followed by 75 to 100 percent for the first postoperative week, 50 to 75 percent for the second, and 25 to 50 percent for the third are recommended.[53] McCullough et al reported pain improvement in 10 total knee arthroplasties in 8 patients, although there was an average loss of flexion of 15° with a 6.5° gain of extension.[31] In a series of 13 total knee arthroplasties in 10 patients, Goldberg et al noted complications of intramuscular or intraarticular bleeding in 3 patients, and 1 posterior tibial and 3 peroneal nerve palsies.[13] The nerve palsies were attributed to correction of long-standing flexion contracture at surgery putting tension on the neurovascular structures.

Total knee arthroplasty appears useful in the treatment of advanced hemophilic arthroplasty. Lachiewicz et al reported on 24 total knee arthroplasties with a 2- to 9- year follow-up.[28] Pain was markedly reduced and function was markedly improved. Some knees required manipulation, and this was eventually performed routinely during the third postoperative week.

Arthrodesis

Arthrodesis is indicated after failed total joint replacement or as an alternative to joint replacement. Arthrodesis utilizing compression techniques has been used successfully in hemophilia.[36] It is preferred to total joint replacement in the case of the ankle.[53,56] The results of interposition arthroplasty of the elbow may offer an advantage over the less predictable results of total elbow replacement and functional limitations of arthrodesis of this joint.[45]

Fractures

Fractures can occur after minor trauma and are seen more frequently in patients with severe hemophilia.[5,11,27,46,55] This has been attributed to the combination of osteoporosis, muscle weakness, and limited joint motion associated with hemophilia. Fracture healing occurs at a normal rate.[27] Orthopaedic management should be similar to that for non-hemophiliacs. Care should be taken to avoid neurovascular compromise from expanding hematomas. Splints or bivalved casts are preferred to circumferential casts.

For conservative management of fractures, Boardman and English recommend factor levels of 30 percent for the first 2 to 7 days. In the surgical treatment of fractures, a factor level of 60 percent should be maintained for 2 weeks or until the wound has healed.[5]

Skeletal traction has been avoided in the past because of the risk of recurrent bleeding from pin tracks. However, since the advent of effective replacement therapy, skeletal traction[2] and compression arthrodesis utilizing the Charnley technique[18,36] have been employed successfully.

Hemorrhage in Muscle

Bleeding in muscle may occur after minimal trauma. Pain is less intense than in a joint hemorrhage[53] and becomes severe as the hematoma distorts fascial layers.[22] Neurological complications are not uncommon, particularly femoral nerve with iliopsoas hemorrhages.[6,21] The muscle heals by fibrosis, and limb contractures occur in approximately 20 percent of severe calf and forearm hemorrhages.[21] Characteristic sites of muscle hemorrhages in the lower limb are the iliopsoas, quadriceps, and calf. In the upper limb, the deltoid, and the forearm flexors brachioradialis and biceps, are most frequently involved.[40a]

Treatment

Treatment is directed toward prompt clotting factor replacement to 30 to 40 percent of normal levels until bleeding has stopped.[4,40a,53] The joints affected by the involved muscle should be splinted comfortably in the acute phase rather than forcing correction which can accentuate bleeding. Physical therapy after the acute bleeding has subsided should then be employed to prevent contractures. Diagnostic ultrasound can usefully monitor resolution or recurrence of bleeding and give guidance during such therapy.[53a]

The role of surgical decompression is controversial. Houghton and Duthie indicated that aspiration or surgical decompression is not likely to be beneficial and may introduce infection.[22] They reported on 170 patients with muscle hemorrhages, 43 of which had nerve lesions. Nerve lesions were usually due to neuropraxia and recovered. Mintzer et al noted that if compartment pressures exceed 40 mmHg, consideration should be given to fasciotomy.[34] Handelsman advocates surgical decompression if there is not a rapid reduction in the size of the muscle over 8 h.[18]

Pseudotumor

A hemophilic pseudotumor is a progressive cystic swelling involving muscle and results from recurrent hemorrhage. Pseudotumors are a rare manifestation of hemophilia involving approximately 1 percent of patients with severe hemophilia.[1] These lesions are found in association with the long bones, pelvis, and small bones of the hand and foot. Most commonly pseudotumors are found around the femur and pelvis. These usually occur in mature patients. Those occurring in the hand and foot are found more frequently in young patients with open epiphyses.[12] Radiologically a pseudotumor appears as a calcified or ossified mass in proximity to bone. There may be areas of bone erosion and new bone formation. The mass can increase in size at regular intervals and may be associated with nerve compression, or pressure necrosis of skin.

Treatment

Conservative treatment consists of clotting factor replacement and immobilization. Hilgartner and Arnold reported a case of a pseudotumor in the distal femur successfully treated by irradiation and factor replacement.[20] Aspiration is not advocated since this may lead to chronic sinus formation and infection.[17]

If conservative measures fail and the pseudotumor continues to increase in size or neurovascular structures are compromised, surgical excision should be considered. Further delay in treatment may lead to soft tissue necrosis and infection.[47]

PLATELET DISORDERS

Circulating platelets, numbering between 150,000 and 400,000/ml in the healthy state, are a major contributor to normal blood clotting.

Epidemiology

Platelet disorders may be quantitative, qualitative, or both. The severity of bleeding is proportional to the degree of thrombocytopenia but appears to be less when the condition is chronic. Platelet counts below 90,000 to 100,000/dl may result in bleeding from trauma, and spontaneous bleeding becomes a threat when the count falls below 50,000/dl. Thrombocytopenia is evaluated by examination of the bone marrow megakaryocytes. When these are present in normal or increased numbers, conditions causing destruction of platelets in the circulation are considered. When they are greatly diminished, absent, or morphologically abnormal, diseases affecting bone marrow production must be sought. Sustained thrombocytosis of greater than 1 million platelets/dl also requires evaluation of the bone marrow. Qualitative defects which may lead to abnormal bleeding or clotting are also associated with some conditions producing thrombocytosis. Finally, abnormal distribution of platelets sometimes occurs in patients whose bone marrow megakaryocytes are intact and in whom no pathological destruction of platelets can be demonstrated.

Clinical Significance

Thrombocytopenia, if sustained, must be explained. This is, of course, especially true in patients for whom surgery is contemplated. When the need for surgical intervention is urgent, even a mild reduction in platelet numbers can be catastrophic if the underlying nature of the condition is not understood. A patient with chronic idiopathic thrombocytopenic purpura and a platelet count of 90,000/dl will tolerate surgery satisfactorily because in the immune thrombocytopenias a disproportionately high number of young, potent platelets are present, but the same platelet count in a uremic patient may result in serious intraoperative and postoperative bleeding.

In addition to uremia, impaired platelet function may result from drugs, paraproteinemias, the myeloproliferative disorders, excessive fibrinogen degradation, and a variety of mechanisms that occur in systemic lupus erythematosus, leukemia, pernicious anemia, and scurvy.

Drug impairment of platelet function is commonly used therapeutically, especially in cardiovascular disease; in other drug therapy the antiplatelet effect is an unwanted side effect. Nonsteroidal anti-inflammatory drugs with an antiplatelet effect include aspirin, phenylbutazone, sulfinpyrazone, indomethacin, and ibuprofen. Dipyridamole, also used as an antiplatelet agent, is effective through another mechanism. Antidepressants such as chlorpromazine, reserpine, imipramine, promethazine, and the tryptophans all have diminishing effect on platelet function, and a third, miscellaneous group includes diphenhydramine, dextrans, ethyl alcohol, nialamide, carbenicillin and related antibiotics, heparin, papaverine, and clofibrate. In most individuals the drugs in this third group cause no symptoms or findings to suggest platelet dysfunction, but when taken by surgical patients with other impairment of the coagulation process, they can cause serious problems.

Among the acquired disorders, uremia represents the most common obstacle to adequate coagulation in surgical patients.[40] Clinical bleeding in these patients leads to generalized oozing. Similar problems are seen with polyclonal hyperglobulinemia resulting from cirrhosis, rheumatoid arthritis, or amyloid or chronic infections, and in patients who have the monoclonal disorders such as multiple myeloma or Waldenström's macroglobulinemia.

Treatment

The availability of platelets for transfusion has greatly increased the survival of these patients when surgical conditions arise, but careful selection of candidates is needed to avoid dangerous complications and to preserve valuable resources. Correction of the underlying cause of thrombocytopenia or platelet dysfunction is the treatment of choice if surgery may be delayed accordingly.

Fibrinogen Degradation Products

Fibrinogen degradation products (FDPs) are protein fragments which result from the proteolytic action of plasmin on fibrin and fibrinogen. These fragments impair both the aggregation and the release reactions. FDPs are elevated in patients with cirrhosis or other decompensated liver disease who are bleeding, and in disseminated intravascular coagulation and fibrinogenolysis. The only effective treatment is the management of the underlying disorder.

DISSEMINATED INTRAVASCULAR COAGULATION (DIC)
Epidemiology

The mechanism of this abnormal form of coagulation is diffuse rather than localized and consumes clotting factors to such a degree that their concentration in the plasma becomes low, and diffuse bleeding may occur. DIC manifests itself clinically as generalized bleeding from many sites and from needle punctures. There may be nosebleeds or gastrointestinal hemorrhage. In addition to the consumption coagulopathy, there is widespread tissue damage due to the formation of fibrin from fibrinogen in the circulation. There is a characteristic sequence of changes in the coagulation mechanism. Initially there is a decrease in circulating levels of platelets, fibrinogen, prothrombin complex, and factors V, VII, VIII, X, XI, XIII. These substances are consumed during the coagulation, and intravascular clotting and fibrinolysin activation occur simultaneously. After the decrease in their concentration, these substances may recover and indeed rise to above normal values so that laboratory interpretation of the data requires a skilled hematologist. Important clinical manifestations include hypotension (shock) in addition to the bleeding tendency. There may be renal shutdown, dyspnea, and cyanosis. In addition there may be abdominal or back pains, nausea, vomiting, and diarrhea.[32] The major categories of etiologic factors in the acute syndrome include intravascular hemolysis, bacterial endotoxin, anoxia and anoxemia, activated complement or antigen-antibody complexes, endothelial damage, virus infection, and release of tissue thromboplastin.[32] The condition is common during certain obstetric emergencies. It may occur during treatment of multiple injuries and in asso-

ciation with acute respiratory distress syndrome or fat embolism.[43] It has also been described accompanying toxic shock syndrome (see below).

Laboratory Findings

Platelet count usually varies from 30,000 to 120,000 cells/mm^3. The activated PTT may be prolonged to as much as 100 s. Abnormalities in fibrinogen metabolism may be shown by the presence of fibrin monomers detected by the protamine sulfate test or the ethanol gelation test. The latex agglutination test or the staphylococcal clumping test may demonstrate by immunologic techniques the increase in FDPs in the circulation.[52] The prolonged PT and PTT may be due to vitamin K deficiency, and a trial of vitamin K should be made.[52] The use of heparin is controversial. It may effectively stop the coagulopathy and so control bleeding, but it may make matters worse.[8] Since the antithrombin III (AT III) levels in DIC are decreased, the administration of AT III concentrates in DIC has been used with some success.

TOXIC SHOCK SYNDROME

Dysfunction of multiple systems associated with fever, hypotension, and a diffuse, erythematous rash may indicate this lethal postoperative complication.

Recent studies have implicated *Staphylococcus aureus* phage group I, types 29 and 52. The F enterotoxin produced by these organisms is considered the most likely cause of the syndrome. The wound may not look infected but organisms may be cultured from the wound or joint aspirate.[24] Blood cultures are negative.[41]

The features of this syndrome are outlined in Table 21-5. When the diagnosis is suspected, material for cultures and Gram's stain should be obtained from the wound and intravenous antistaphylococcal antibiotics administered. The antibiotics have no effect on circulating toxin but remove the incriminating infecting organisms. Debridement may be indicated.

Treatment

Aggressive treatment of the systemic manifestations is essential to save life. Fluid therapy for the hypotension is usually required. Acute respiratory distress syndrome, thrombocytopenia, renal dysfunction, and electrolyte abnormalities may occur and require sophisticated management. The mortality may be as high as 100 percent.[24,41]

REFERENCES

1. Ahlberg, A.K. On the natural history of hemophilic pseudotumor. J Bone Joint Surg 57A:1133–1135, 1975.
2. Ahlberg, A.K., and Nilsson, I.M. Fractures in haemophiliacs with special reference to complications and treatment. Acta Chir Scand 133:293 1967.

TABLE 21-5 Toxic Shock Syndrome

Characteristics

1. Fever [temperature $\geq$ 38.9°C (102°F)]
2. Rash (diffuse macular erythroderma)
3. Desquamation, 1–2 weeks after onset of illness, particularly of palms and soles
4. Hypotension (systolic blood pressure $\leq$ 90 mmHg for adults or < 5th percentile by age for children < 16 years of age, or orthostatic syncope)
5. Involvement of 3 or more of the following organ systems:
    A. Gastrointestinal (vomiting or diarrhea at onset of illness)
    B. Muscular (severe myalgia or creatinine phosphokinase level $\geq$ 2 × ULN*)
    C. Mucous membrane (vaginal, oropharyngeal, or conjunctival hyperemia)
    D. Renal (BUN† or Cr‡ $\geq$ 2 × ULN or $\geq$ 5 white blood cells per high-power field—in the absence of a urinary tract infection)
    E. Hepatic (total bilirubin, SGOT§, or SGPT¶ $\geq$ 2 × ULN)
    F. Hematologic (platelets $\leq$ 100,000/mm^3)
    G. Central nervous system (disorientation or alterations in consciousness without focal neurological signs when fever and hypotension are absent)
6. Negative results on the following tests, if obtained:
    A. Blood, throat, or cerebrospinal fluid cultures
    B. Serologic tests for Rocky Mountain spotted fever, leptospirosis, or measles

*Twice upper limits of normal for laboratory.
†Blood urea nitrogen level.
‡Creatinine level.
§Serum glutamic oxaloacetic transaminase level.
¶Serum glutamic pyruvic transaminase level.
Source: MMWR:

3. Arnold, W.D., and Hilgartner, M.N. Hemophilic arthropathy. J Bone Joint Surg 59A:287–305, 1977.
4. Aronstam, A., Browne, R.S., Wassef, M., and Hamad, Z. The clinical features of early bleeding into the muscles of the lower limb in severe haemophilics. J Bone Joint Surg 65B:19–23, 1983.
5. Boardman, K.P., and English, P. Fractures and dislocations in hemophilia. Clin Orthop 148:221–232, 1980.
6. Brower, T.D., and Wilde, A.H. Femoral neuropathy in hemophilia. J Bone Joint Surg 48A:487–492, 1966.
7. Clark, M.W. Knee synovectomy in hemophilia. Orthopaedics 1:285–290, 1978.
8. Collen, D. Treatment of disseminated intravascular coagulation. Bibl Haematologica 49:295–303, 1983.
9. De Valderrama, J.A.F., and Matthews, J.M. The haemophilic pseudotumor or haemophilic subperiosteal haematoma. J Bone Joint Surg 47B:256–265, 1965.
10. Editorial. Antimicrobials and haemostasis. Lancet 1:510–511, 1983.
11. Feil, E., Bentley, G., and Rizza, C.R. Fracture management in patients with haemophilia. J Bone Joint Surg 56B:643–649, 1974.
12. Gilbert, M.S. Characterizing the hemophilic pseudotumor. Ann Acad Sci 240:311–315, 1975.
13. Goldberg, V., Heiple, K.G., Ratnoff, C.D., Kurczynski, E., and Arvan, G. Total knee arthroplasty in classic hemophilia. J Bone Joint Surg 63A:695–701, 1981.
14. Greene, W.B., and Wilson, F.C. Nonoperative management of hemophilic arthropathy and muscle hemorrhage. Instr Course Lect 32:223–233, 1983.
15. Greene, W.B., and Wilson, F.C. Pathophysiologic and roentgenographic changes in hemophilic arthropathy. Instr Course Lect 32:217–223, 1983.
16. Greer, R.B. Operative management of hemophilic arthropathy. An overview. Orthopaedics 3:135–138, 1980.
17. Hall, M.R.P., Handley, D.A., and Webster, C.U. The surgical treatment of haemophilic blood cysts. J Bone Joint Surg 44B:781–789, 1962.
18. Handelman, J.E. The knee joint in hemophilia. Orthop Clin North Am 10:139–172, 1979.
19. Harker, L.A., and Slechter, S.J. The bleeding time as a screening test for platelet function. N Engl J Med 287:155–159, 1972.
20. Hilgartner, M.W., and Arnold, W.D. Hemophilic pseudotumor treated with replacement therapy and radiation. J Bone Joint Surg 57A:1145–1146, 1975.
21. Hoskinson, J., and Duthie, R.B. Management of musculoskeletal problems in the hemophilias. Orthop Clin North Am 9:455–480, 1978.
22. Houghton, G.R., and Duthie, R.B. Orthopaedic problems in hemophilia. Clin Orthop 138:197–216, 1979.
23. Insall, J., Scott, W.N., and Ranawat, C.S. The total condylor knee prosthesis. A report of two hundred and twenty cases. J Bone Joint Surg 61A:173–180, 1979.
24. Irvine, G.W., Kling, T.F., Jr., and Hensinger, R.N. Postoperative toxic shock syndrome following osteoplasty of the hip. J Bone Joint Surg 66A:955–958, 1984.
25. Johnson, R.P., and Babbitt, D.P. Five stages of joint disintegration compared with range of motion in hemophilia. Clin Orthop 201:36–42, 1985.
26. Jordan, H.H. *Orthopaedic Appliances,* 2d ed. Springfield, IL., Thomas, 1963.
27. Kemp, H.S., and Matthews, J.M. The management of fractures in haemophilia and christmas disease. J Bone Joint Surg 50B:351–358, 1968.
28. Lachiewicz, P.F., Inglis, A.E., Insall, J.N., Sculco, T.P., Hilgartner,

M.W., and Bussel, J.B. Total knee arthroplasty in hemophilia. J Bone Joint Surg 67A:1361–1366, 1985.

28a. LeBalc'h, T., Ebelin, M., Laurian, Y., Lambert, T., Verroust, F., and Larrieu, M.J. Synovectomy of the elbow in young hemophilic patients. J Bone Joint Surg 69A:264–268, 1987.

29. Mannucci, P.M., Canciani, M.T., Rota, L., and Donovan, B.S. Response of factor VIII/von Willebrand factor in healthy subjects and patients with hemophilia A and von Willebrand's disease. Br J Haematol 47:283–293, 1981.

30. Martin-Villar, S. Long term evaluation of 4 cases of haemophilic arthropathy treated with synoviorthesis with 198 Au. *Symposium on the Coordinated Management of Musculoskeletal Manifestations of Haemophilia: Current Concepts.* London, 1981.

31. McCullough, N.C., Enis, J.E., Levitt, J., Lian, E.C.Y., Nieman, K.W., and Laughlin, E.C. Synovectomy or total replacement of the knee in hemophilia. J Bone Joint Surg 61A:69–75, 1979.

32. McKay, D.G. Clinical significance of intravascular coagulation. Bibl Hematologica 49:63–77, 1983.

33. Miller, E.H., Flessa, H.C., and Glueck, H.I. The management of deep soft tissue bleeding and hemarthrosis in hemophilia. Clin Orthop 82:92–106, 1972.

34. Mintzer, D.M., Cotler, J.M., and Shapiro, S.S. Compartment syndromes in hemophilia. Contemp Orthop 9:77–82, 1984.

35. Mueh, J.R., Herbst, K.D., and Rapaport, S.I. Thrombosis in patients with the lupus anticoagulant. Ann Intern Med 92:156–159, 1980.

36. Patel, M.R., Pearlman, H.S., and Lavine, L.S. Arthrodesis in hemophilia. Clin Orthop 86:168–174, 1972.

37. Petterson, H., Ahlberg, A., and Nilsson, I.M. A radiologic classification of hemophilic arthropathy. Clin Orthop 149:155–159, 1980.

38. Post, H. Hemophilic arthropathy of the hip. Orthop Clin North Am 11:65–77, 1980.

39. Post, M., and Telfer, M.C. Surgery in hemophilic patients. J Bone Joint Surg 57A:1136–1145, 1975.

40. Rabiner, S.F. Uremic bleeding. Prog Hemost Thromb 1:233–250, 1972.

40a. Railton, G.T. and Aronstam, A. Early bleeding into upper limb muscles in severe hemophilia J Bone Joint Surg 69B:100–102, 1987.

41. Rouner, R.A. Fatal toxic shock syndrome as a complication of orthopaedic surgery. J Bone Joint Surg 66A:952–954, 1984.

42. Shapiro, S.S., and Hultin, M. Acquired inhibitors to the blood coagulation factors. Semin Thromb Hemost 1:336–358, 1975.

43. Sharp, A.A. Diagnosis of disseminated intravascular coagulation. Bibl Haematologica 49:251–261, 1983.

44. Smith, M.A., Urquhart, D.R., and Savidge, G.F. The surgical management of varus deformity in haemophilic arthropathy of the knee. J Bone Joint Surg 63B:261–265, 1981.

45. Smith, M.A., Savidge, G.F., and Fountain, E.J. Interposition arthroplasty in the management of advanced haemophilic arthropathy of the elbow. J Bone Joint Surg 65B:436–440, 1983.

46. Solomon, C., Dvonch, V., and Dobozi, W.R. Difficult fracture in a patient with hemophilia. Orthopaedics 6:600–607, 1983.

47. Steel, W.M., Duthie, R.B., and O'Connor, B.T. Haemophilic cysts. J Bone Joint Surg 51B:614–625, 1969.

48. Stein, H., and Dickson, R.A. Reversed dynamic slings for knee-flexion contractures in the hemophiliac. J Bone Joint Surg 57A:282–283, 1975.

49. Storti, E., and Ascari, E. Surgical and chemical synovectomy. Ann NY Acad Sci 240:316–327, 1975.

50. Storti, E., Traldi, A., Tosatti, E., and Davoli, P.G. Synovectomy, a new approach to haemophilic arthropathy. Acta Haematol 41:193–205, 1969.

51. Stuart, J. Davies, S., Cummings, R.A., Girwood, R.H. and Darg, H. Haemorrhagic episodes in haemophilia: A 5-year prospective study. Br Med J 2:1624, 1960.

52. Wallerstein, R.O. Blood, in Krupp, M.A., and Chattmon, J.J. (eds): *Current Medical Diagnosis and Treatment.* Los Altos, CA, Lange, 1984, pp 343.

53. Wilson, F.C., Makew, D.E., and McMillen, C.W. Surgical management of musculoskeletal problems in hemophilia. Instr Course Lect 32:233–241, 1983.

53a. Wilson, D.J., McLardy-Smith, P.D., Woodham, C.H., and MacLarnon, J.C. Diagnostic ultrasound in hemophilia. J Bone Joint Surg 69B:103-107, 1987.

54. Wintrobe, M. *Clinical Hematology,* 8th ed. Philadelphia, Lea & Febiger 1981.

55. Wolff, L.J., and Lovrien, E.W. Management of fractures in hemophilia. Pediatrics 70:431–436, 1982.

56. Zimbler, S., McVerry, B., and Levine, P. Hemophilic arthropathy of the foot and ankle. Orthop Clin North Am 7:985–997, 1976.

57. Zimmerman, T.S., and Ruggeri, Z.M. Von Willebrand's disease. Clin Haematol 12:175–200, 1983.

CHAPTER 22

Bone and Joint Infections

Hormozan Aprin and Roger Dee

ACUTE HEMATOGENOUS OSTEOMYELITIS

Osteomyelitis is an infectious process of the bone and its marrow. The term *osteomyelitis* normally refers to infections caused by pyogenic microorganisms but can be used for granulomatous infections such as tuberculosis and syphilis, or specific viral or fungal infections.

Hematogenous spread from a primary source of infection is the commonest route of infection. Acute osteomyelitis can also be produced by extension of soft tissue infection adjacent to bone, or it can be initiated from an open fracture or a penetrating wound.

Organisms

The most commonly isolated organism in this condition in all age groups remains the hemolytic *Staphylococcus aureus*. This organism is responsible for between 50 and 70 percent of all such infections in children between 1 month and 5 years of age.[55] The second most common organism are hemolytic streptococci. Both group A and group B streptococci have been implicated in acute hematogenous osteomyelitis, the latter particularly within the first 2 months of life.[19,55,84] In neonates *Haemophilus influenzae* is an occasional cause of osteomyelitis but more commonly is a cause of septic arthritis. There is often an associated meningitis.[29,60] The wide variety of organisms seen in bone infection following a penetrating wound is not seen in hematogenous infection.

Pathophysiology

Nade quotes the unpublished observations of Emslie and co-workers, who have recently demonstrated that intravenous injection of bacteria may produce abscesses selectively in the bony metaphysis, sparing other organs.[84]

Blood Supply of Epiphysis and Metaphysis

It is believed that the vascular architecture of the metaphysis, where the nutrient capillaries form sharp loops, predisposes to the establishment of infection following bacteremia.

There are three possible patterns of vascularity.[101] In a child, the nutrient artery terminates in end arteries and capillaries adjacent to the growth plate. An infection of the metaphysis is usually prevented from crossing the growth plate but may progress to septic arthritis depending on the physeal anatomy (Fig. 22-1*A*). In an adult, the metaphysis and epiphysis are in continuity and hematogenous osteomyelitis may be primarily metaphyseal or epiphyseal. In an infant, some metaphyseal vessels may penetrate the open growth plate and ramify in the epiphysis. Thus, the infant infection may originate in the metaphysis and have epiphyseal extensions (Fig. 22-1*B*).[101] It is believed that there is probably a relation between the sites of predilection (proximal tibia, distal femur) and the relative contributions to growth of the physis in those areas.[91] Because of the epiphyseal involvement, secondary intrusion into the joint is more common in the infant and in the adult than in the child.[101]

The Infectious Process and Its Consequences

The infectious process is characterized by an inflammatory response and the formation of pus within the metaphysis. There is probably impairment of the capillary circulation some 48 h after the beginning of the infection.[10] Pus from the developing metaphyseal abscess gradually finds its way to the subperiosteal region by penetrating through the haversian systems and Volkmann's canals. If the infectious process continues, the subperiosteal abscess strips the periosteum over an extended portion of the diaphysis and circumferentially around the bone (Fig. 22-2). The periosteum may rupture, allowing pus to escape into the adjacent tissues (Fig. 22-1*A*).

Damage to the metaphyseal blood supply, caused by the release of bacterial toxins and the stripping of the periosteum, results in portions of the bone becoming necrotic. The inner portion of the cortex is supplied by the injured metaphyseal vessels.[101] These portions of dead bone which are separated from the surrounding viable bone by granulation tissue are called *sequestra*. The periosteal response is to lay down new bone called the *involucrum* which surrounds the infected bone and sequestra (Fig. 22-3). In a fully established infection, defects in the involucrum become cloacae through which drainage occurs, establishing sinus tracts. In an advanced case, a major portion of the diaphysis of a long bone may form one large sequestrum, bathed in a lake of subperiosteal pus extending the entire length of the bone. This florid picture is occasionally seen in neonates.

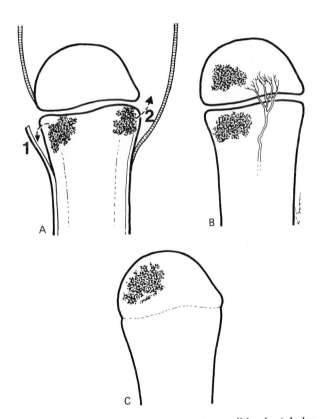

Figure 22-1 Sites of hematogenous osteomyelitis of a tubular bone in the child, the infant, and the adult. **A.** In the child a metaphyseal focus is frequent. From this site cortical penetration can result in a subperiosteal abscess in those locations in which the growth plate is extraarticular (1) or in a septic joint in those locations in which the growth plate is intraarticular (2). **B.** In the infant a metaphyseal focus may be complicated by epiphyseal extension owing to the vascular anatomy in this age group. **C.** In the adult a subchondral focus in an epiphysis is not unusual owing to the vascular anatomy in this age group. *(From Resnick, D., and Niwayama, G.: Diagnosis of Bone and Joint Disorders. Philadelphia, Saunders, 1981. Reproduced with permission.)*

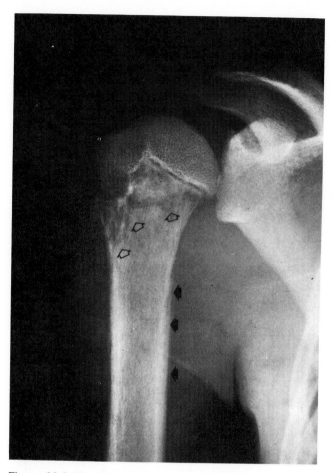

Figure 22-2 Metaphyseal focus in the proximal humerus (*hollow arrows*). Note the periosteal elevation in the diaphysis (*solid arrows*).

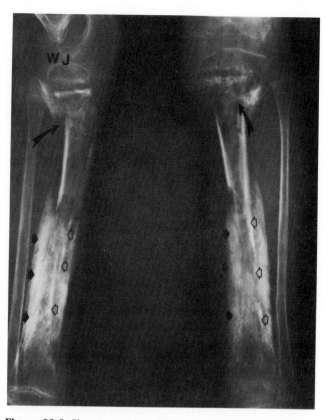

Figure 22-3 Chronic osteomyelitis in a child. The diaphyseal cortex is becoming sequestrated (*hollow arrows*). There is a prominent involucrum (*solid arrows*) and a pathologic fracture proximally (*curved arrows*).

Clinical Features

The first symptom is pain in the region of the infection; the pain is continuous and may be believed to be the result of some recent trauma. There is frequently an association with a recent traumatic injury to the metaphyseal area which may have predisposed to the infection. Unfortunately at this stage the child may be given an antibiotic because it is noticed that he or she is febrile. This will in all probability delay timely diagnosis by masking the systemic signs. If antibiotics are not administered the child will exhibit symptoms and signs consistent with a septic focus. There may be generalized aches and pains, a flushed appearance, and high fever.[84]

The diagnosis is more difficult in neonates and infants who are ill from other causes (e.g., meningitis in the case of *H. influenzae*). These children may be septicemic and have multiple foci of infection which may be life-threatening. They may need respiratory assistance, be immobile, and be connected to a ventilator. Sometimes the infection is not detected until a large soft tissue abscess is apparent.[19,31,78] They are then at risk for severe long-term complications due to damage to the physis.

Physical Examination

Physical examination shows loss of limb function in all cases. The neonate is observed not to use that limb, and the child holds the limb in a protective attitude. The child resists motion of the limb, but some movement of the joints can usually be produced with gentle encouragement; this is in contrast with septic arthritis, in which the slightest motion may be excruciating. Local bone tenderness usually points strongly to the diagnosis. It is unusual to be able to elicit fluctuation except in the very late case of untreated disease. There may well be an effusion in the joint, which may indicate a sympathetic reaction in the joint or the complication of coexistent septic arthritis. Soft tissue abscess is accompanied by the usual signs of redness, swelling, and local rise in temperature.

Laboratory Studies

The white blood cell count is raised and the differential shifted to the left, although the count is not as high as that seen in septic arthritis. A range of 7000 to 26,000 was reported by Sullivan et al.[112] A blood smear should be studied to rule out the possibility of leukemia. Mild anemia may be present. The erythrocyte sedimentation rate (ESR) may be normal within the first 48 h but then rises rapidly and may exceed 100 mm/h.[19] The ESR usually remains elevated for weeks. Its gradual decline is an indication of a successful response to treatment.

Blood culture is positive in about 50 to 75 percent of cases.[3,8,19,90,131] A positive blood culture can be obtained in 24 h, but more time is required for determining specific antibiotic sensitivity. Other tests which may occasionally be helpful include the antistreptolysin O titer and C-reactive protein. The anti-alpha hemolysin titer is normal in more than 50 percent of patients with staphylococcal osteomyelitis and so is of limited value as a test.[7] Although not a sensitive test for septic arthritis, the detection of antibodies to the teichoic acid cell wall of $S. aureus$ has been found valuable for detecting staphylococcal osteomyelitis, especially the acute variety. The test seems to be more sensitive in acute (82 percent) than in chronic (43 percent) osteomyelitis. Gel diffusion technique is used to determine the antibody titer in a specimen of serum that has been found to be positive by counterimmunoelectrophoresis.[120]

Radiographic Studies

Within the first 2 to 3 days, a careful evaluation may show some deep soft tissue swelling in the region of the bone adjacent to the metaphyseal lesion.[33] The soft tissue swelling is identified by displacement of the fat lines that normally parallel the bony surfaces between the muscle planes. Often comparison films are necessary for diagnosis.[11,84]

Radiographically detectable demineralization does not occur in less than 10 days and is usually first seen as single or multiple areas within the medullary canal, reflecting trabecular destruction. Penetration of the cortex leads to periosteal changes, which may be seen as early as 3 or as late as 6 weeks.[11]

Radionuclide Imaging

Confirmatory bone scan should not be necessary if the diagnosis is clinically obvious, and under no circumstances should appropriate treatment be delayed while awaiting such a test.[84] Technetium 99m-labeled methylene diphosphonate (^{99m}Tc-MDP) can be used to differentiate osteomyelitis from overlying soft tissue lesions. The three-phase bone scan shows a well-defined increase in uptake in the bone on both the blood-pool and the delayed scan. The blood-pool phase (phase 2) shows the relative vascularity of an area, whereas the delayed image phase (phase 3) obtained 3 to 4 h after the injection reflects increased uptake in the skeleton. By contrast with the well-defined bone uptake seen in osteomyelitis, there is rather diffuse uptake in cellulitis and septic arthritis, in the former case into the soft tissue and in the latter case into the region of the joint on blood-pool and delayed scans. Scintigraphy with technetium, although showing positive before the radiographs, nevertheless has only a 77 percent ac-

curacy rate in differentiating between cellulitis, osteomyelitis, and septic arthritis.[112] There may be preferential uptake in periosteal new bone of whatever cause and also in normal physis (which will tend to obscure an adjacent lesion). False positives can occur when changes in bone metabolism or vascularity from other causes cause increased uptake. Bone scanning often gives false positives in the hands and feet and has been pronounced to be valueless in neonatal osteomyelitis.[4,112]

Because ^{67}Ga-labelled gallium citrate uptake is due to the accumulation locally of white cells, particularly polymorphonuclear leukocytes (as well as various labeled serum proteins),[6] this isotope has been used sequentially following the technetium scan to increase the specificity of the test.[50,51,52,73] The technetium scan is followed by a 48-h [^{67}Ga] gallium citrate scan. An accumulation of both isotopes in the same region of bone is highly suggestive of infection, with an accuracy of 62 percent.[74] However, other conditions such as a local fracture can give the same appearance.[105] Septic arthritis patients show an increased periarticular uptake of ^{99m}Tc-MDP and diffuse gallium concentration around the joint. Patients with cellulitis show an abnormal concentration of gallium in the soft tissue with minimal uptake of the other isotope.

Gallium citrate has a high sensitivity to infectious inflammatory processes but a variable and unpredictable sensitivity to other inflammatory conditions which may be noninfective. The ^{67}Ga scan is therefore not helpful without the results being taken in conjunction with the use of technetium. A problem associated with the use of technetium is the occurrence of "cold spots." These are photopenic areas of diminished activity associated with damaged vascularity of portions of the bone or compression of the vasculature by elevated intraarticular pressures associated with joint effusions.[82] If misinterpreted they will be responsible for false negative diagnosis.

More recently a third radionuclide scanning method has been employed using ^{111}In-labeled leukocytes prepared from a sample of the patient's blood. This technique avoids the false positives seen with the technetium technique (which may be sensitive to fractures, bone tumors, heterotopic ossification, and arthritis) and the gallium technique (which may give false-positive results in tumors and other forms of inflammatory disease). The initial problem with the indium technique was the length of time that it took to prepare the white cells (not appropriate in a sick child). However, now it is possible to prepare and reinject ^{111}In-labeled leukocytes in a few hours.[74] This technique appears to be more accurate and easier to interpret than sequential Tc-Ga scanning.[74] It is too early to assess its role in the diagnosis of acute hematogenous osteomyelitis in children, but it certainly has great promise in the entire area of muscoloskeletal sepsis, with a reported sensitivity of 83 percent, specificity of 86 percent, and an accuracy of 83 percent.[74]

Magnetic Resonance Imaging (MRI)

In the early stage of osteomyelitis the MRI will show intraosseous and extraosseous changes. These changes are evident before any that may be seen on routine x-ray films.

Aspiration and Biopsy

Although aspiration in the early stage of disease may fail to obtain any fluid or pus, it is particularly valuable in obtaining the infecting organism in the presence of a subperiosteal abscess. There is danger that the pus may be so thick that aspiration even with a fairly large needle is not productive. A negative aspiration should not rule out the diagnosis. Even a small amount of pus is valuable for culture and Gram's stain. A needle biopsy is usually not appropriate in acute osteomyelitis unless there is reason to suspect the possibility of malignancy in the differential diagnosis.

Treatment

Resuscitation of a sick, dehydrated child, is commenced in the usual way with appropriate intravenous fluids. Blood is sent to the laboratory for the procedures already described.

Parenteral administration of bactericidal antibiotics in doses adequate to provide satisfactory local blood levels is the cornerstone of treatment.[40] It is reasonable to start the treatment with a combination of drugs active against *S. aureus* and also beta-hemolytic *Streptococcus.* When the organism is identified and antibiotic sensitivity is determined, treatment can be continued with a single appropriate drug.[19] Either nafcillin, cloxacillin, or oxacillin is satisfactory for the treatment of staphylococcal infections, and benzylpenicillin is recommended for *Streptococcus.*[19,84] Ampicillin may be indicated if there is reason to suspect *H. influenzae* (e.g., associated meningitis). Some authors recommend adding a drug such as chloramphenicol in a child of 6 months to 5 years because of a 15 to 30 percent incidence of *H. influenzae* resistance to ampicillin.[60] If available, counterimmunoelectrophoresis provides a rapid test for the *H. influenzae* type b organism; the test can give a result in 1 to 2 h and can also be used on patients who are already receiving antibiotic therapy.[60,75]

Nafcillin and oxacillin are given in a dosage of 100 to 200 mg/kg per day in four divided doses, and benzylpenicillin is given in a dosage of 1 to 4 million units every 6 h. If a child is allergic to penicillin, another antibiotic such as clindamycin or vancomycin is selected or a cephalosporin such as cephalothin is given parenterally in a dosage of 100 mg/kg per day. Some cross reactivity in patients who are allergic to penicillin is theoretically possible with cephalosporins. Cross reaction seems to be rare, but such patients should be skin-tested.[100]

In the early stage of disease, successful response to treatment is seen within 24 to 36 h, with a dramatic fall in temperature and improvement in local signs. The white blood cell count falls rapidly provided there is no abscess. The ESR will probably decline more slowly. Return of function in the infected limb is a good sign of positive response. After a period of intravenous therapy, a decision may be made to switch to oral antibiotics. There is no uniform opinion concerning the best time to do this. A necessary prerequisite is identification of the causative organism. Also the patient must have achieved a satisfactory response to intravenous antibiotics and laboratory facilities must be available for measuring

bactericidal levels of antibiotics in the patient's blood after oral administration. Levels are measured after dilution of serum drawn before and after ingestion of oral antibiotic. If bactericidal levels are present in a postdose dilution of 1:8, the dose is thought to be adequate.[60]

Role of Oral Antibiotics

Several papers have documented the treatment of acute osteomyelitis using only oral antibiotics.[87,114] The criteria outlined above must be met, particularly the ability to measure minimal inhibitory and bactericidal concentrations of antibiotic in the blood and a certain identification of the appropriate organism. The use of large doses of cephalexin to treat staphylococcal osteomyelitis following only 1 week of parenteral therapy is a regime that offers many advantages if it can be shown over the long term that the results are as satisfactory as more traditional methods.[114,118] There is no role for oral antibiotics in gram-negative infections with the exception of infection with *H. influenzae, Escherichia coli,* and *Proteus mirabilis.*[24]

Immobilization

During treatment the affected limb is immobilized to diminish pain. A well-padded posterior mold can be used. Occasionally some form of skin traction is required. For ambulant therapy, a cast brace or one leg hip spica enables the patient to ambulate with the aid of a walker or a pair of crutches. Protective splintage is continued in the upper limb until antibiotic therapy is terminated. In the lower limb it is continued for an additional 4 to 6 weeks. The average overall length of time for antibiotic therapy is 6 weeks.

Surgical Procedures

Failure to respond to treatment after 36 h probably means that pus is present in the metaphysis and possibly in the subperiosteal region. Occasionally the patient presents late with osteomyelitis which has been ineffectively treated. Radiological examination may show areas of bony change and abscess formation. Surgical drainage of any intramedullary or subperiosteal abscess is required in these patients without further delay.

With the patient under general anesthesia, a pneumatic tourniquet is applied on the affected limb; the tourniquet should be inflated only if absolutely necessary. The extremity should not be exsanguinated with an elastic bandage, as this procedure may release showers of bacteria into the systemic circulation.

If the adjacent joint is swollen, it is aspirated before any surgical incision since it may be involved and require drainage. Otherwise its contamination must be scrupulously avoided. The bone is exposed at the site of maximum tenderness and swelling, and the periosteum is incised longitudinally. Pus is evacuated, and specimens are obtained for a

Gram stain, cultures, and tests for antibiotic sensitivity. Any devitalized soft tissue is excised, and the entire area then irrigated with several liters of normal saline. Some authors do not recommend drilling the cortex to explore the metaphysis since it is their view that pus under pressure is rarely found inside the medulla.[19] They believe that the concept of decompressing the medulla and improving the blood flow is unlikely to be of much benefit since any bone death has already occurred in the presence of a large subperiosteal abscess. It is, however, worthwhile drilling any obviously soft areas in the cortex.

The skin may be loosely closed but provision made for free drainage through appropriate surgical drains. The value of closed suction drainage with continuous intramedullary irrigation remains to be proved.[2,61] This technique consists of inserting a perforated plastic catheter through a large hole in the medullary canal; the tip of the catheter is then brought up through a separate hole so that its major portion, which is perforated, lies within the medullary cavity. The periosteum is left open, and an additional outflow catheter is placed in the subperiosteal space. The inflow and outflow tubes are brought out through separate stab incisions in the skin, and the skin is closed around these incisions to prevent leakage of fluid. A supply of irrigating fluid is connected to the inflow tube, which provides continuous flow under gravity at a rate of 500 ml each 8-h period. This irrigation is continued for 4 to 5 days. If the outflow tube becomes plugged by debris, however, it is discontinued. In spite of careful precautions, this technique seems to invite the possibility of secondary infection. For this reason it is probably not applicable in acute osteomyelitis, though it certainly may have a place in the treatment of more chronic infections. It is important that the limb be immobilized during this treatment in such a way that the wound may be frequently observed.

Prognosis and Complications

Acute hematogenous osteomyelitis is curable provided there is early diagnosis and prompt treatment with the correct antibiotic for the correct period of time. Any other course of action negatively affects prognosis. Features such as host resistance and virulence of the infecting organism also play their part.[84]

The risk of recurrence depends on the site of the infection and the time interval between the onset of symptoms and the beginning of appropriate treatment.[114] Metatarsal lesions have the highest rate of failure, with a 50 percent recurrence rate.[40] Failure rates of 20 to 30 percent have been cited for involvement of the metaphysis in distal femur and proximal and distal tibia, with a more favorable outcome for lesions involving the lower end of the fibula and bones of the upper extremity and spine.[40] Cole and co-workers observed that the prognosis for cure is much worse in patients diagnosed late (25 percent) than in patients diagnosed early, in whom the cure rate was 92 percent in their series. The risk of recurrence is below 4 percent 1 year following treatment.[40]

Involvement of an adjacent joint is common in the proximal humerus and shoulder joint in neonates because of the anatomy of the vasculature in this age group and also because of the intracapsular position of the physis. Irreversible damage to the physis and joint may result.[19,31,78] Damage to the physis can result in overgrowth as well as growth retardation.[41,104] Leg length discrepancy and angular deformity can result. Bowing of the forearm or leg may result because of retardation of growth in an affected bone with relative overgrowth of its parallel companion.

Pathologic fracture may be caused by resorption of bone either in the acute phase or following surgery and decompression by drill holes through the cortex. A preventive splint or cast for an appropriate period of 2 to 3 months is indicated. This complication is seen more often in chronic osteomyelitis.

SUBACUTE OSTEOMYELITIS

In subacute osteomyelitis the patient may present with a painful limp and radiological examination unexpectedly reveals a well-established lesion visible in the bone. The patient is not systemically ill and often has had no previous complaints. There may be no local signs of infection.[44,106] Alternatively there may be clinical signs of subperiosteal pus, synovitis, or pus within a joint.[106] There may be an elevation of the white blood cell count and the ESR, but in half the cases laboratory results are normal.[44] The femur and the tibia are by far the commonest bones affected.

Radiographic Findings: Brodie's Abscess

Certain localized radiolucencies in the tibia, developing silently without any systemic signs and without previous febrile illness, were described by Brodie in 1836.[13] They are common in metaphyses of tubular bones, particularly the tibia, but may also occur occasionally in flat bones, vertebral bodies, and even the diaphysis (Fig. 22-4). They are usually manifestations of subacute osteomyelitis classified by Gledhill into four types depending on location and radiographic manifestation.[42] A type I lesion is a solitary metaphyseal-area lesion which may communicate with the epiphysis.[20] The lesion consists of a solitary cavity which has been walled off so that a ring of sclerotic reactive new bone is seen. A type II lesion is a radiolucent lesion located in the metaphysis not surrounded by reactive sclerotic bone but with adjacent loss of the cortex. A type III lesion is a diaphyseal lesion associated with cortical hypertrophy and periosteal or endosteal new bone. Radiolucent zones within such an area of hyperostosis can be detected by tomography. These lesions may be confused with osteoid osteoma. A type IV lesion is associated with layers of subperiosteal new bone formation which on x-ray views give an onionskin appearance such as that seen in early Ewing's sarcoma. There is cortical hyperostosis, and careful evaluation of the x-ray film may show intramedullary radiolucency.

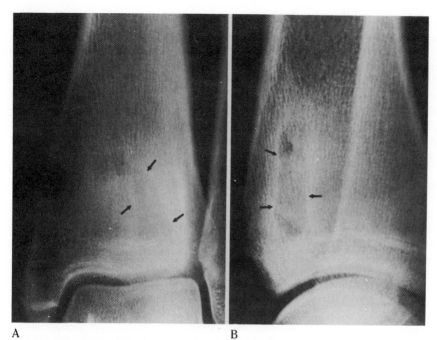

A   B

Figure 22-4 **A** and **B.** Anteroposterior and lateral radiographs outline a typical appearance of an abscess of the distal tibia due to staphylococci. Observe the elongated radiolucent lesion with surrounding sclerosis (*arrows*). This extends to the closing growth plate. The channel-like shape of the lesion is important in the diagnosis of this condition. *(From Resnick, D., and Niwayama, G.: Diagnosis of Bone and Joint Disorders. Philadelphia, Saunders, 1981. Reproduced with permission.)*

SUBACUTE EPIPHYSEAL OSTEOMYELITIS

Green, Beauchamp, and Griffin believe that there is an entity called *primary subacute epiphyseal osteomyelitis.*[44] They point out that the blood supply of the epiphysis has hemodynamic features, including sluggish blood flow and vascular loops, which make it equivalent to the metaphysis in its susceptibility to infection (Fig. 22-5). They identified lesions of the epiphysis which did not communicate with the metaphysis either radiologically or when examined with a probe during surgery. They pointed out that when a subacute metaphyseal lesion crosses the physis, the communication is always apparent. Ross and Cole also identified some cavities confined to the epiphysis and noted that these were eccentric and were either circular or oval.[106] Half of them had a fine sclerotic margin. Such lesions were occasionally found in the talus, where they occasionally eroded the subchondral bone plate of the ankle joint. Other presentations of this disease identified by these authors were patients with cavities communicating between metaphysis and epiphysis and other patients with aggressive lesions which had clinical, radiological, and hematologic features indistinguishable from those of primary malignant bone tumors such as Ewing's sarcoma.[106] They stressed the need to exclude such lesions as simple bone cysts, aneurysmal bone cysts, fibrous cortical defect, chondroblastoma, or chondromyxoid fibroma.

Staphylococcus aureus is the only organism causing this pathological entity. The recommended treatment for these patients without signs of pus in the subperiosteal layer or in the joint is administration of antibiotics such as cloxacillin or floxacillin (Flucloxacillin) and immobilization without operation. Intravenous antibiotics for 48 h followed by oral drugs for 6 weeks is satisfactory.[106] However, in patients who have signs of pus the lesions should be surgically drained. Green and co-workers described a technique of locating the epi-

physeal lesion by using two-plane x-ray views.[44] They first inserted a needle into the lesion and then drilled it from within the joint capsule, avoiding the articular surface and the physis.

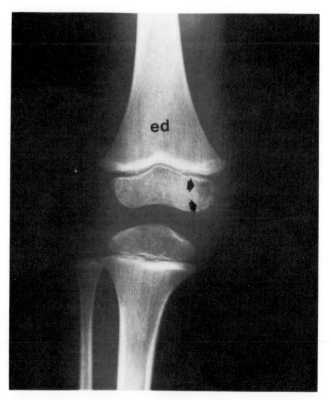

Figure 22-5 Primary epiphyseal subacute osteomyelitis. Note the sclerotic reaction around the lytic focus (*solid arrows*).

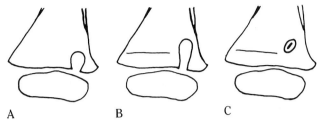

Figure 22-6 Diagrams to show possible outcomes of treatment of subacute osteomyelitic cavities in the lower end of the femur. **A.** Drawn from a typical preoperative x-ray view following the failure of conservative treatment. Possible sequelae include **B,** continuing enlargement of the metaphyseal cavity, the mouth of which remains open (there is a growth arrest line) or **C,** in which case the cavity has failed to heal completely but it no longer communicates with the physis. Failure to heal is here associated with presence of a sequestrum. *(From Ross, E.R., and Coel, W.G.: J Bone Joint Surg 67B:443–447, 1985. Reproduced with permission.)*

Ross and Cole reported that opening and gently curetting metaphyseal lesions was successful in healing these cavities. Although the curetted tissue showed the characteristic appearance of osteomyelitis, more than half the patients did not grow an organism. These authors believe that epiphyseal lesions heal without surgery.[106] They gave interesting information on the healing process, noting that there are two observed patterns. In the first the growth plate grows away from the entire metaphyseal cavity, indicating that it is functioning normally. In the second pattern of healing, the growth plate grows away from the body of the cavity, but a channel-like communication with the physis remains for several months (Fig. 22-6*B*). Occasionally a small sequestrum persists and prevents complete healing of the cavity (Fig. 22-6*C*). Growth arrest lines and defects in the epiphysis or metaphysis can result.[106]

CHRONIC OSTEOMYELITIS

Etiology

Acute hematogenous osteomyelitis inappropriately treated can become chronic in adults and children (Figs. 22-3 and 22-7). Pertinent factors include the degree of bone necrosis, the general nutritional status of the involved tissues, and the nature of the infecting organism. Certain risk categories of patients include the old, the debilitated, and intravenous drug users. Chronic osteomyelitis may also occur following surgery or penetrating trauma. The disease may be a sequel to an open fracture, which may then successfully unite or proceed to nonunion.[17]

The adjacent soft tissues are involved in all forms of osteomyelitis with the exception of the Brodie abscess. The etiologic term *contiguous focus infection* describes the occurrence of bone infection secondary to soft tissue breakdown.[17] This may occur in patients with vascular disease or other conditions such as diabetes. Steroid therapy, tobacco abuse, immune deficiency and malnutrition are other factors which

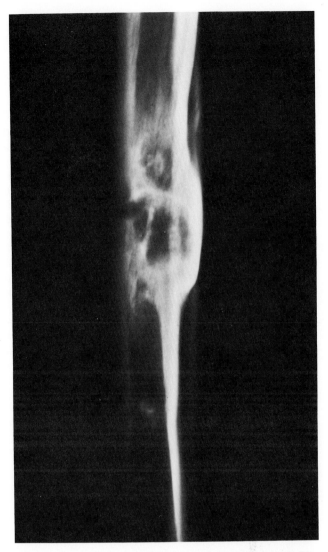

Figure 22-7 Chronic osteomyelitis in an adult tibia, stage IV (see also Fig. 22-8). Note that this multiloculated bony cavity has a sequestrum proximally lying within a separate sclerotic cavity. The separate area of sclerosis distally represents a pin track which was also infected with gram-negative organisms. Treatment required radical debridement and a free myocutaneous flap.

predispose to secondary osteitis following soft tissue lesions which do not initially affect the bone.[17] However chronic hematogenous osteomyelitis accounts for at least one-third of the cases of chronic osteomyelitis.[128]

Infecting Organisms

Penicillin-resistant *S. aureus* and gram-negative rods are common infecting organisms. With better collection techniques, anaerobic organisms (e.g., *Bacteroides*) are being cultured increasingly in up to 40 percent of cases.[17] *Pseudomonas aeruginosa, P. mirabilis, Enterobacter,* and *E. coli* have been found to be the most common gram-negative rods in chronic osteomyelitis.[62] Infection with *Salmonella* and fungi will be discussed separately.

Late Complications

Constant drainage in chronic osteomyelitis causes irritation and destruction of the adjacent skin and soft tissues. An eczematous reaction or neoplastic change may follow.[96,121] The skin may become thin, desquamate, and be easily traumatized. The epithelium of the skin edge grows inward into the margins of the sinus tract. Epidermoid carcinoma may develop at any point along the fistulous tract and is present in at least 0.5 percent of patients with long-term drainage.[101] Other tumors that may occur include fibrosarcoma, angiosarcoma, rhabdomyosarcoma and adenocarcinoma, basal cell carcinoma, and plasmacytoma.[101] Amyloidosis is a complication that now seems to be infrequent, probably because of improved treatment of this condition.[101]

The prognosis depends upon many factors. A continuously draining sinus and concomitant joint involvement or an infection that has been of long duration is a negative prognostic factor.[62] The sinus tract may close following the spontaneous discharge of a sequestrum, and the disease may be quiescent for a while. However, after a period of stability in the relationship between bacteria and host, following a deterioration in the patient's local resistance or some local trauma, another cycle of activity is initiated with the formation of another abscess or period of offensive discharge.

Management

Bacterial Investigation

Sinus tract cultures do not usually reflect the bacteria infecting the bone. The depths of the wound or sinus at the very least should be curetted, but bone biopsy is preferable.[81] Aerobic and anaerobic cultures are necessary. Superficial, subcutaneous biopsies may be performed on an ambulant basis. Additionally, material obtained during surgical debridement is invaluable. Histological preparations are useful. They identify secondary neoplasms and fungal and granulomatous infections. If the histological findings are consistent with chronic infection but the culture is negative, it may be that the organism was lost during the attempt at culture or it may be an anaerobe or there may have been some technical error. If the biopsy material and histological findings do not suggest infection, a positive culture on meat broth medium alone may well be the result of a contaminant.

Staging

The classification used at the University of Texas (Fig. 22-8) has much to recommend it.[17] The four stages described are stage I, which is medullary osteomyelitis; stage II, which is superficial osteomyelitis following primary breakdown in soft tissues with secondary involvement of the periosteum and cortex; stage III, which is a localized osteomyelitis involving

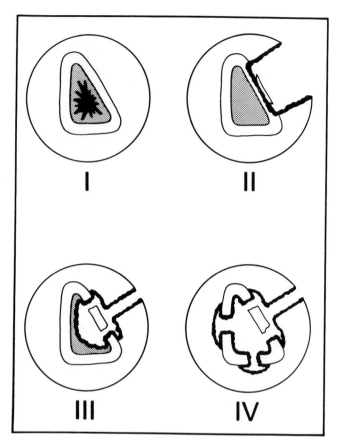

Figure 22-8 The four stages which may be used to classify osteomyelitis (for explanation see text). *(From Cierny, G., III, and Mader, J.T., Orthopaedics 7:10, 1984. Reproduced with permission.)*

the medulla of the bone and also the periosteal surface, and in which cloaca are present and there is a fistulous tract; and stage IV, which represents "through and through" osteomyelitis. In stage IV the bone is riddled with disease and may have to be excised en bloc to eradicate the disease.[17]

Antibiotic Therapy

Staphylococcus aureus was cultured in 72 percent of the cases reported by Damholt.[25] Antibiotics appropriate for the infecting organism are initiated after appropriate sensitivity results are available. The sensitivity of the organism is measured quantitatively, and minimum inhibitory concentrations (MICs) and minimum bactericidal concentrations of antibiotic are estimated.[17] Antibiotics are administered to maintain the serum level at least eight times above the MIC. Serum levels of bacteriostatic and bactericidal activity are monitored on a weekly basis, especially if antibiotics with side effects, such as aminoglycosides, are being used. The intravenous route gives a higher serum and tissue concentration of antibiotic, and this is valuable in chronic infections where the blood supply to the region may be limited.[118] With established osteomyelitis, at least 4 to 6 weeks of intravenous antibiotic therapy is usually necessary. In children a shorter period of intravenous antibiotics may be adequate, with treatment being continued with oral antibiotics as already described. In chronic osteomyelitis the total period of antibiotic administration may be as long as 3 months.[25]

Bone scans may help to indicate areas of osteoblastic activity, and both technetium and indium scans have been used in this disease.[17] If the patient is seriously ill some authors recommend commencing therapy with clindamycin, which is effective against anaerobic organisms such as *Bacteroides fragilis,* together with an aminoglycoside such as tobramycin against aerobic gram-positive bacilli, gram-negative cocci such as gonococci and meningococci, some species of *Haemophilus,* and also common infecting gram-negative bacilli such as *Pseudomonas* and *Serratia.* The risk factors for aminoglycoside nephrotoxicity include (1) preexisting renal disease, (2) hypokalemia, (3) dehydration, (4) obesity, (5) an inappropriately high dose, and (6) an overlong period of therapy.[129]

Third-generation cephalosporins (e.g., cefotaxime, ceftizoxime) have also proved useful against gram-negative osteomyelitis and may be used if the sensitivities are appropriate.[24,89] In *Pseudomonas* infections, success primarily depends on the quality of the surgical debridement and the local host resistance.[24]

Occasionally the best treatment is a combination of antibiotics. Beta-lactam antibiotics include two classes: the penicillins and the cephalosporins, both of which affect bacterial cell wall synthesis. A combination of aminoglycoside with beta-lactam drug acts synergistically and may prevent the emergence of resistance.[100]

Under certain circumstances closed irrigation suction methods may have their place in the treatment of this disease. Kawashima and Tamura recommend their use when septic emboli, thrombi, or necrosis have contributed to the infection.[56] They describe an 88.3 percent success rate. They measured the blood concentration levels of antibiotics during the procedure and observed that absorption of antibiotics from the wound was insignificant. Postoperative bleeding is, however, an important complication.[61] Continuous suction drainage removes exudate from the wound and does not have the complications of the local antibiotic irrigation treatments, which remain controversial.

Surgical Treatment

Without appropriate surgery, antibiotic therapy alone will not eradicate chronic osteomyelitis.

Debridement

The first stage in surgical treatment, following biopsy and culture and initiation of appropriate antibiotic treatment, is a thorough debridement to remove all devitalized and infective material. The surgery should be planned so that the intrusion does not further damage the local blood supply. Saucerization is performed by removing a generous piece of cortex. The medullary contents are exposed and curetted back to bleeding bone, all sequestra being removed. Following completion

of the debridement, the area is thoroughly irrigated. If there is instability perhaps made worse by an aggressive debridement, it may be necessary to stabilize with an external fixator, pins being placed in healthy bone at a distance from the infected area. Placement of antibiotic-impregnated polymethylmethacrylate beads into the defect has been used at this stage as a temporary measure before definitive bone grafting.

Closure of the Dead Space

Local Flaps A second procedure is required to repair the bone defect and close the dead space following debridement. It should be remembered that fracture through a large bone defect is an important late complication of chronic osteomyelitis. However, if the bony defect is small and does not compromise present or future stability, no additional bone work is required and the dead space may be obliterated with a soft tissue flap. Such techniques as the cross leg flap are not now recommended because they require prolonged immobilization of both lower extremities and expose the normal limb to the infected area. In recent years the techniques of local muscle flap and free vascularized muscle flap have changed the treatment of chronic osteomyelitis. A muscle flap enhances the healing of the lesion by bringing in a blood supply and can fill an irregularly contoured cavity.

Myocutaneous Flaps If a local muscle flap is inadequate, consideration may be given to bringing a free myocutaneous flap from a distant site and using microsurgical techniques to revascularize it locally. Integrity of the bony structure is a requirement for using either of these techniques. In general, lesions involving the middle and proximal third of the tibia are more suitable for coverage than those in the distal third of the tibia and regions of the ankle joint and foot. Coverage is easier in the thigh. The rate of success varies from 79 to 100 percent.[48,70,71,126] Complications include sloughing of the muscle flap,[43,56] persistence of infection in the cavity, and fracture of the bone through the saucerized area.[107]

Weiland and co-workers noted major complications in 41 percent of free tissue transfers performed for chronic osteomyelitis.[127] More than half the patients in whom this operation failed subsequently underwent amputation. Thus, although this procedure has advantages when it succeeds (a free latissimus dorsi flap can cover an area as large as 25 to 35 cm), the authors note that it is doomed to failure if the transfer is to tissue which is still infected.

When treating the infected unstable defect or one which is so large that future pathologic fracture and consequent instability seem likely, the techniques of open cancellous bone grafting, vascularized bone graft, and bypass graft have been utilized.

Open Cancellous Bone Grafting

Open cancellous bone grafting was first used by Rhinelander[102] and later by Papineau.[93,94] A careful description of the necessary protocol has been given by Sachs and Shaffer.[108]

After the debridement the defect in the bone is filled with autogenous cancellous iliac bone chips. The timing of surgery depends upon the appearance of the wound some 3 weeks following the initial debridement. If nonviable sclerotic bone remains, a second debridement precedes the bone graft procedure. Following the application of the graft, a Zenoform dressing is applied. This is changed every few days, whilst intermittently debriding any necrotic bone from the surface. This process is continued until the bone graft is covered with healthy granulation tissue. The defect is then ready for coverage. This can be achieved by allowing the wound to epithelize, but preferably flap coverage is achieved. Split skin coverage on the graft usually fails.[108] It is important that free drainage be permitted following the initial grafting procedure since pressure from retained infected tissue exudates may compress fine capillaries and prevent the cancellous bone chips from revascularizing. Contraindications include segmental defects greater than 4 cm, especially in the diaphyseal area. If the quality of the bone and soft tissue or its location is such that bony stabilization cannot be achieved, some other treatment must be used. If an external fixator is applied for stability, it is important that attention be paid to pin site care as well as to the grafted area.

Vascularized Bone Graft

The vascularized bone graft technique involves the isolation and transfer of a bony segment with its nutrient vascular pedicle. With this technique, the healing process is similar to that of a segmental fracture rather than the process of creeping substitution that occurs when the cancellous bone graft is used.[134] The vascularized bone graft provides immediate and adequate blood flow to the involved area; this is very important and may also increase local antibiotic penetration.

The procedure is usually indicated where there is a bony defect more than 6 cm long and minimal soft tissue loss.[116,124,125,126] However, the technique can be modified, and an appropriate bony segment can be transplanted with attached muscle or skin if there is also major soft tissue loss.[134] This procedure allows a generous resection of all suspicious or equivocally viable bone in patients having chronic and complex infection with extensive bony involvement. The procedure can be performed within 1 to 2 weeks after complete debridement without intervening wound closure, or it can be performed after completion of soft tissue wound healing.

The fibula and the iliac crest are the most common bones used for vascularized bone transfer. There are other bones which can be transferred with their vascular pedicle, but these are less useful in orthopaedic reconstruction. These other bones include rib, lateral scapula, metatarsal bone, and the lateral portion of the radius.[133] The technique of harvesting these grafts is well-described.[114,116,125,126] The fibula is the most useful bone for replacement of a long segment of bone. A length of 6 to 35 cm can be obtained with a fibular graft, while the iliac crest is most useful for the defects shorter than 8 cm.[133] The vascular supply to the fibula is from branches of the peroneal vessels which enter the bone in the middle third. The graft can be obtained in three ways: bone with a thin cuff of muscle, bone with a substantial muscular flap, or bone with a combined musculocutaneous flap. The segment of the iliac crest commonly used has multiple nutrient arteries, which are branches of the deep circumflex iliac vessels and enter the bone through the inner cortex.[117,126]

Complications The complications of free vascularized bone grafting include failure of vascularity in the graft, recurrence of infection, and delayed union or nonunion of the segment. Wood and Cooney reported their experience with patients who had vascularized bone transfer for an established chronic osteomyelitis. They had 1 patient with immediate vascular failure. Infection was controlled in 11 patients (84.6 percent) with no evidence of recurrence of the sepsis, but 5 patients (38.4 percent) developed nonunion which required further bone grafting.[133]

Bypass Grafts

Bypass grafting involves the establishment of cross union between the tibia and fibula proximal and distal to a defect (Fig. 22-9). This technique offers some protection to the reconstituting bone in a large defect that has been separately grafted and does not impair its blood supply.[17]

Amputation

Failure to successfully manage a limb with segmental bony defects, persisting instability, and infection leads to amputation. This is particularly unfortunate if such an outcome follows a long period of painful, expensive treatment during

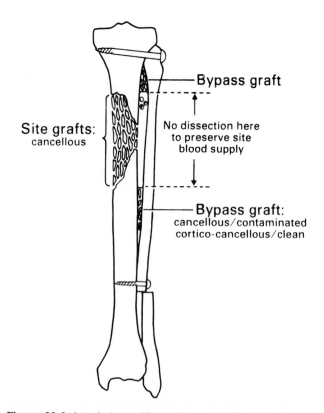

Figure 22-9 A technique of bone bypass grafting following open cancellous bone grafting to a large infected defect. This technique avoids further impairment of the blood supply to the vascularizing graft in the infected bony defect. *(From Cierny, G., III, and Mader, J.T., Orthopaedics, 7:10, 1984. Reproduced with permission.)*

which time the patient's morale may steadily deteriorate. It is important that all the options be placed before the patient and the possibility of failure be explained. In some cases the patient is wise to choose early oblation. A successful outcome, on the other hand, can be jeopardized without informed consent and the patient's determination to stay the course.

CHRONIC SCLEROSING OSTEOMYELITIS

Chronic sclerosing osteomyelitis was described by Garré in 1893. Patients have no necrosis or purulent exudate and little granulation tissue but show intense proliferation of the periosteum leading to bony deposition.[38,101] It is a condition that mainly affects children and young adults.[38,59,76] The average age at onset was 16 years in a series reported by Collert and Isacson.[21] The etiologic basis of sclerosing osteomyelitis is unclear, and routine aerobic cultures may not disclose any organism.[21,63] With more sophisticated techniques it is possible to incriminate anaerobic organisms such as *Propionibacterium acnes.*[21] Histological examination shows a nonspecific chronic inflammation with new bone formation and areas of necrosis.

The disease has an insidious onset with local pain and tenderness of the affected bone and moderately elevated ESR. The most common site of the involvement is the shaft of the long bones, but involvement of other bones such as the mandible has also been reported.[32,56,57] Fifty percent of the cases reported by Collert and Isacson developed similar lesions at a different site after an average of 5.5 years.[21] The roentgenograms show pronounced sclerosis with small cystic areas (Fig. 22-10).

The sclerosis may become progressively more dense even in patients who have not been symptomatic for a long period of time.[21] Clinically and radiographically, it is difficult to distinguish this lesion from osteogenic sarcoma.[21] There are other conditions which should also be differentiated. These include: Ewing's sarcoma, osteoid osteoma, osteoblastoma, and Paget disease. The symptoms recur at intervals for several years and then gradually subside. There is no satisfactory treatment to eradicate chronic sclerosing osteomyelitis. Fenestration and curettage provide temporary relief. Prolonged antibiotic therapy does not change the clinical course of the disease.[21]

OSTEOMYELITIS IN THE HANDS AND FEET

Osteomyelitis in the distal phalanx follows tardily treated pulp space infection, though such an outcome is uncommon in developed countries. Puncture wounds and human and animal bites, however, remain important sources of infection in the hand. Inappropriate suturing of a small laceration on the hand after it has delivered a blow to the mouth may result in the loss of a digit. The metacarpophalangeal joint is particularly vulnerable in the closed fist. Either septic arthritis or

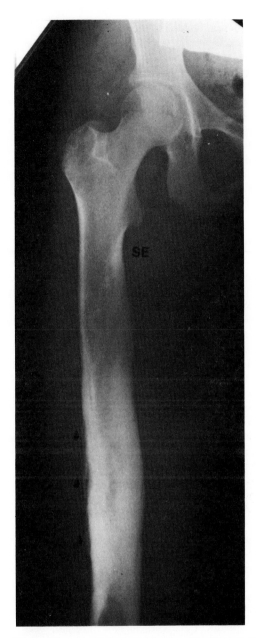

Figure 22-10 Chronic sclerosing osteomyelitis (Garré). Note the area of cortical irregularity and sclerosis (*solid arrows*).

osteomyelitis may occur with a whole variety of organisms including anaerobes being involved (see Chap. 45).

Puncture wounds of the foot by foreign bodies may inoculate bone or joint. Bacterial osteomyelitis may result. In many of the reported cases *Pseudomonas* species including *aeruginosa, maltaphilea,* and *cepacia* have been isolated.[12,47,58,103] Local pain and swelling persist, but there may be surprisingly few systemic symptoms. There is often delay in diagnosis.[45] Additional studies such as scintigraphy are helpful. Aspiration may produce diagnostic fluid.

The treatment consists of antibiotic therapy similar to that described for other areas of chronic osteomyelitis combined with appropriate radical debridement. These wounds are common in children. It is noteworthy that *P. aeruginosa* has an apparent propensity to infect cartilage as well as bone.[81] Parenteral antibiotic therapy for 3 to 6 weeks with aminoglycoside and a broad-spectrum penicillin effective against this organism is recommended.

The calcaneus has a firmly attached periosteum, and elevation and subperiosteal abscess formation is less likely. Extraosseous extension occurs usually by perforation of the periosteum. The principles of treatment are similar to those outlined for other bones. The approach through the plantar surface of the heel devised by Gaenslen is useful in extensive chronic osteomyelitis.[1,36]

PELVIC OSTEOMYELITIS

Osteomyelitis of the pelvis may simulate other disease processes. Acute septic arthritis or sciatica associated with discitis may be suspected in children. There may be an abdominal-type presentation resembling the acute abdomen.[35,80] Blood culture is positive in about 70 percent of acute cases. *Staphylococcus aureus* is again the most common organism.[54] Computed tomography and appropriate scintigraphy are helpful in this region. Because of the excellent blood flow to the pelvis, antibiotic therapy alone may be adequate to cure the infection if early diagnosis is made. The differential diagnosis of a cystic or sclerotic lesion may include such conditions as eosinophilic granuloma, metastatic neuroblastoma, leukemia, or Ewing's sarcoma.[54]

INTRAVENOUS DRUG USERS

Septic arthritis and osteomyelitis are well-recognized complications of intravenous drug abuse. *Pseudomonas aeruginosa* and *S. aureus* are common infecting agents. In addition *Serratia marcescens* may produce multifocal osteomyelitis in these patients. Some authors recommend co-trimoxazole as the antibiotic of choice for this organism if appropriately sensitive. Gentamicin and carbenicillin have also been recommended alone or in combination.[14,77] Areas commonly involved are in the axial skeleton, particularly the lumbar vertebrae and sacroiliac joints.[14]

OSTEOMYELITIS CAUSED BY OTHER ORGANISMS
Brucella Osteomyelitis

The various types of *Brucella* can involve the joints and also produce osteomyelitis (frequently chronic) of the flat bones or tubular bones. Sometimes secondary invasion by staphylococci follows.[101] Of the four *Brucella* species which affect human beings, *B. abortus* is the most common species seen in the United States, and it is the type most likely causing bone infection. Vertebrae, especially the lumbar spine, are the most common site of involvement; this is dealt with in Chap.

53.[67,135] The diagnosis requires a high index of suspicion. *Brucella* osteomyelitis is often an occupational disease of young adults in the meat trade.[28]

Treatment follows the general principles already outlined for other bone infections, with splintage antibiotics, and surgery when appropriate. Tetracyclines are effective antibiotics, but streptomycin or gentamicin with tetracycline may be more effective. Trimethoprim and sulfamethoxazole (TMP-SMX) in a dosage of 7 mg of TMP, 35 mg of SMX per kilogram per day has been recommended. Rifampin has also been used.

Nonvertebral brucellosis is rare in the United States. The incidence of brucellosis has been reduced by appropriate control in cattle and swine but still persists in the region of the Mexican border.[53]

Salmonella Osteomyelitis

Patients with major sickle cell hemoglobinopathies have a high incidence of *Salmonella* osteomyelitis, and when bone infection occurs in sickle cell disease, *Salmonella* is the causative organism in 74 percent of cases.[60] A photopenic area on bone scan, following the onset of pain, is more consistent with infarction than with infection. On the other hand, an early finding of increased uptake of ^{99m} Tc-MDP is much more likely to represent osteomyelitis.[60] Ampicillin is a satisfactory drug, and surgery is rarely necessary.[60] Other antibiotics used include TMP and SMX.

Infections with Anaerobic Organisms

Increasing numbers of cases of chronic osteomyelitis in which anaerobic bacteria are isolated reflect an increased recognition of the appropriate precautions that must be taken in collecting and transporting biopsy material. Cultures of drainage material of open wounds and sinus tracts are often contaminated and may give misleading results.[49,68] A surgical procedure may be performed to obtain bone or tissue biopsy, or a closed aspiration may obtain fluid. Fluid should be drawn into a syringe and handled rather like a blood gas specimen. The usual indications of anaerobic infections such as putrid exudate and foul odor are unfortunately not always present. Swabs are not recommended because of problems of inadequate sampling. If a few milliliters of pus or a piece of tissue or bone can be sent to the laboratory, avoidable loss of microorganisms due to exposure to oxygen can be prevented. If transportation is to be delayed more than 20 min, a specific transport system that will keep anaerobes viable for as long as 24 h should be used.[48]

In postsurgical infections, anaerobes are probably introduced into the surgical wound from the skin, where they form part of the normal flora.[35,43] Although clostridial rods may infect open wounds, anaerobic cocci, particularly the gram-positive peptostreptococci (*Peptococcus magnus*) are frequently isolated from wound cultures. *Bacteroides fragilis* may also be isolated from wounds, particularly in patients with debilitating conditions and vascular disease who develop bone or joint infection. These organisms are usually treated with clindamycin, cefoxitin, chloramphenicol, or metronidazole.[16] Because of the development of resistant strains, the effectiveness of these antibiotics has recently become less. This underlies the importance of appropriate sensitivity tests.[48,83,109]

GRANULOMATOUS INFECTIONS OF BONE

Fungal Infections

Blastomycosis

Blastomycosis is endemic to the southeast and the midwestern parts of the United States but not to the southwestern and western regions.

Most systemic infections are caused by hematogenous spread from pulmonary portals of entry. A proportion of these patients have involvement of bone and joint. Osseous lesions are multiple and involve the epiphyseal and metaphyseal ends of long bones. Lesions may also be seen in the small bones of the hands and feet and over bone prominences. Diagnosis is by organ culture from biopsy material, and successful treatment is with amphotericin-B. Without treatment the progress of the disease is rapid and the outcome may be fatal.[98]

Coccidioidomycosis

The fungus *Coccidioides immitis* is endemic to the southwestern United States and also to Central America and parts of South America. The infectious spores are inhaled, and the primary lung disease is accompanied by weight loss, eosinophilia, and skin lesions, and occasionally an associated arthritis. Osseous lesions resemble blastomycosis in their distribution (Fig. 22-11). Necrosis and caseation produces abscesses which may involve joints.

Skin tests are specific but may be negative in disseminated disease. Complement fixation tests are available; a titer of 1:64 or higher is positive for systemic disease.[90] Curettage, ablation, or fusion may be required combined with intravenous amphotericin B in doses of 1 to 1.5 mg/kg up to 2 to 4.6 mg/kg total. Renal and bone marrow function should be closely monitored. Aplastic anemia can occur as a complication of the drug. Synovectomy may be required for joint involvement.

Actinomycosis

In actinomycosis, involvement of mandible and the facial bones commonly occurs because the organism is usually introduced through the oral cavity. Bone involvement is a secondary event following the soft tissue infection. The extremities are infrequently involved. Actinomycotic colonies can be observed in granules called *sulfur granules* which may be recovered from the abscesses. The granulomas may be seen in biopsy material. Pencillin G is the drug of choice. Cephalothin, lincomycin, or tetracyclines are alternatives.

Cryptococcosis

Skeletal cryptococcosis tends to produce radiolucent lesions, and periosteal reaction is unusual.[90] All bones of the skeleton have been reported to be involved, and the disease has been reported from all parts of the world. Cryptococcal meningitis should be particularly suspected in a patient with leukemia, Hodgkin's disease, sarcoidosis, or diabetes who has a fever of unknown origin or central nervous system disorder.[98] Amphotericin B may be lifesaving. Surgery is rarely indicated in skeletal cryptococcosis except for diagnostic purposes. Other antifungal agents such as 5-flucytosine may also be effective in controlling these infections.[95]

Mycetoma

Cutaneous fungal infections can occur from direct implantation following a minor breach of the skin and lead to disseminated disease which may also affect bone. Sporotrichosis is a common example.[30] Amphotericin B and potassium iodide are commonly used for the treatment of this type of infection.[95]

Fungi may enter the body via an opening in the skin, such as compound fractures or a puncture wound.[95] These fungi may infect bone and soft tissues, producing tumoral enlarge-

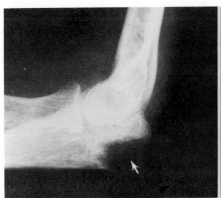
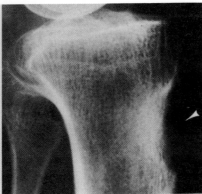

A B

Figure 22-11 Coccidioidomycosis: osteomyelitis. Involvement of bony protuberances such as the olecranon (*A*) and the tibial tubercle (*B*) is frequent. These are discrete lesions with surrounding sclerosis. (*From Resnick, D., and Niwayama, G.: Diagnosis of Bone and Joint Disorders. Philadelphia, Saunders, 1981. Reproduced with permission.*)

ments called *mycetoma.* There are two groups of organisms causing mycetoma; the higher bacterial species (causing actinomycetoma) and fungal species (causing eumycetoma).[95] The management depends on the type of the organism.

Actinomycetoma can be treated effectively with drugs such as sulfa or trimethoprim sulfate.[95] For most of the eumycetomas, however, surgery is indicated because of resistance to ordinary antibiotic therapy. Iodide and radiation therapy have not been effective.[64,72] Although amphotericin B, griseofulvin, miconazole, and ketoconazole have been effective against the systemic and cutaneous fungal infections[15] they are less effective or even ineffective for eumycetoma without aggressive surgical drainage.[64,72,92,95]

Once the diagnosis of osteomyelitis with eumycetoma, especially caused by *Petriellidium boydii* or *Madurella mycetomi,* has been established, a radical resection of all the infected bone and soft tissue is necessary. Any spores that remain in the wound will continue to grow and cause recurrence of the infection. Recurrent drainage and spread of the infection with decrease or loss of the function is an indication for amputation.[95]

Syphilis of the Bones

Bone syphilis may be congenital (intrauterine infection) or acquired (postnatal infection). Infection which is blood-borne is caused by the spirochete *Treponema pallidum.* The infection is localized in the metaphyseal and diaphyseal region and does not spread to the joints. With better prenatal supervision and the sensitivity of the spirochete to pencillin, syphilis of the newborn is now less common.

Congenital Syphilis

In early congenital syphilis, the infant is irritable and restless. The child may have a large, tender swelling around the involved joint. The limb is held immobile. Other signs of syphilis such as skin lesions, mucous patches, and keratitis may be present.

Radiographs demonstrate widening of the metaphysis with marginal density and an indentation on its epiphyseal border. The metaphysis looks osteoporotic or may have patchy areas of radiolucency. There is usually diffuse periostitis seen as periosteal elevation with layers of new bone formation (Fig. 22-12).

The affected bones may assume a spindle shape, and the medullary outlines become indistinct. With proper preparation, the spirochete can be identified in histological sections. It is important to remember that in an infant with congenital syphilis, the serological tests are not positive in the first 3 months because of the infant's inability to produce sufficient antibodies.

The infection responds rapidly to antibiotic therapy. If the child has an adequate defense mechanism and survives the early days after birth, there will be progressive signs of improvement with resorption of the exudate and healing of the bone within a few months. Following successful treatment of the infection, the bone architecture returns to normal.[113]

The late stage of congenital syphilis usually occurs in the second or the third year. It is characterized by osteoblastic activity producing a condensing osteitis which occurs mainly in the tibia, femur, and skull. Subperiosteal bone formation causes a prominent border along the anterior margin of the tibia without any bowing.

In an untreated patient or when the infection is particularly virulent, initially there may be erosion of the cortex which then progresses to the typical increased densities of osteoblastic activities on x-ray views. The child may eventually show other signs of syphilis such as interstitial keratitis, deformed incisor teeth, and auditory nerve palsy.[121]

Clutton's Joints In the late stage of congenital syphilis between the age of 8 and 18, patients may develop large bilateral painless effusion of the knee. This is called Clutton's joints. The condition is an intermittent recurrent effusion of the knees. The x-ray examination is negative, and the examination of the joint fluid reveals a high content of mononuclear cells.

Syphilis in Adults

In adults, involvement of bone and joint occurs in the late or tertiary stage of the disease. The patient manifests painless, nontender swelling of a long bone or the skull. Occasionally

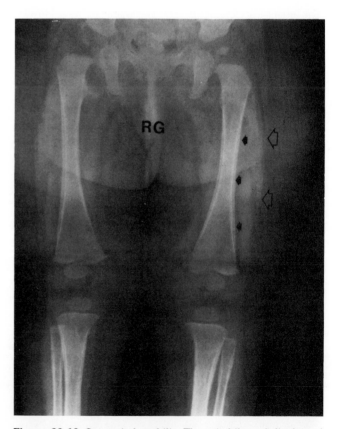

Figure 22-12 Congenital syphilis. There is bilateral diaphyseal periostitis (*solid arrows*). There is also swelling of the soft tissues (*hollow arrows*).

there are localized gummatous lesions of bones. These may be diffuse sclerosing periostitis suggesting Paget disease. Radiographs reveal soft tissue swelling in the region of the gummas which represents an extraosseous extension of the infection. The relative or absolute absence of pain is one of the characteristic features of syphilitic lesions due to peripheral neuropathic changes (Charcot's joints). Also normal motion of the joint is often preserved.[121]

Yaws

Another spirochete infection endemic in some tropical countries is yaws. It is common in equatorial Africa, India, and southeast Asia. The primary phase consists of maculopapular lesions. The secondary skin eruption of papillomas begins a few months later. The late tertiary stage, which not all patients develop, consists of nodular lesions which ulcerate, spread, and may penetrate deeply into underlying tissues involving muscles, joints, and bones. They cause gross deformities by producing contractures and ankylosis.[111] The lesions resemble the gummas seen in syphilis. The introduction of penicillin into affected areas has reduced the incidence of this serious infection.[111]

Viral Osteomyelitis

Viral osteomyelitis is a rare condition.[18,22,26] The most common type is osteomyelitis secondary to smallpox virus, normally manifesting itself 5 to 28 days after the onset of the disease in a child between 9 months and 14 years of age.[10] The disease has a slow course and is self-limiting. It may cause growth disturbance and bone and joint deformities. Surgery is not indicated, and antibiotics are not effective. Treatment consists of conservative measurements and protection of the extremity.[26]

Tuberculosis of Bones and Joints

Tuberculosis is a chronic granulomatous infection caused by *Mycobacterium tuberculosis.* Involvement of the bones and joints is secondary to the hematogenous spread or local extension from the lungs, kidneys, or lymph nodes. The spine is the most common site of bony involvement. The other sites of involvement in decreasing order of frequency are knee, hip, ankle, wrist, sacroiliac joint, pubic symphysis, and small bones of hand and foot (tuberculous dactylitis).[27]

The disease is slowly progressive, and the degree of local and general reaction depends on the intensity of the infection and the patient's general condition and resistance. Immunosuppression, which accompanies AIDS and some treatments for rheumatoid arthritis, predisposes to tuberculous infection.

Diagnosis

In the mild granular type of infection, the white blood cell count and ESR may be normal. In the exudative form, caseous material is produced, and there is leukocytosis and an elevated ESR accompanied by general symptoms.

The tuberculin skin test is an allergic inflammatory reaction to the purified protein derivative (PPD) antigen. It is positive in 80 to 90 percent of active cases. A positive reaction indicates that the patient has at some time been infected, but does not have diagnostic value for present activity of the disease. A positive reaction in a person who previously had a negative test has diagnostic importance.

Microscopic studies of a smear of material from infected bone or joint fluid usually shows the acid-fast bacilli. The culture of any pus obtained will be positive, but it requires 5 to 30 days to grow the organism. Intraperitoneal inoculation of the pus in guinea pigs will show tubercles in 5 to 8 weeks. A microscopic study of biopsy material or sometimes a local enlarged lymph node demonstrates typical tubercles showing epithelioid cells, an encircling ring of round cells and fibrous tissue, and the characteristic Langhans' giant cell. There may be central caseation.

Tuberculous Osteomyelitis Vertebral infection is dealt with in Chap. 55.

Tuberculous osteomyelitis rarely originates in a long bone, but metaphyseal foci can occur in children, and also the disease may originate in an epiphysis and spread into a neighboring joint.[101] It can be difficult if not impossible to differentiate radiologically between tuberculosis and ordinary pyogenic osteomyelitis of bone.

Tuberculous Dactylitis Tuberculous dactylitis presents with multiple soft tissue swelling of the digits and diffuse lytic areas of the phalanges and metacarpals associated with periostitis (Fig. 22-13).

Tuberculous Arthritis In joints, subchondral osteoporosis and cystic changes associated with narrowing of the joint space are common (Fig. 22-14). Differential diagnosis includes rheumatoid arthritis and pigmented villonodular synovitis. Occasionally the condition may be confused with reflex sympathetic dystrophy because of the patchy osteoporotic appearance of the bone. Marginal erosions at the corner of the articulating surface are common.[101]

Treatment

In the management of bone and joint tuberculosis, it is important to improve the patient's general condition and nutritional status.

The principles of the treatment of chronic osteomyelitis caused by tuberculosis are identical to those of other granulomas. Drainage of abscesses, debridement, and sequestrectomy assist antibiotic therapy. The chemotherapeutic drugs which are most effective include para-aminosalicylic acid (PAS), streptomycin, isonicotinic acid hydrazide (isoniazid), ethambutol, and rifampin. In drug therapy, one should consider the possible side effects and the possibility of the organism's resistance.[27,65]

Early Disease Early bone and joint involvement can be controlled with drug therapy, usually isoniazid and rifampin. The

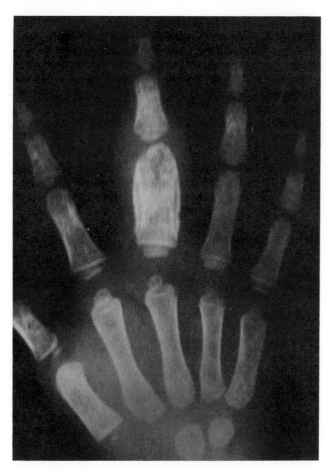

Figure 22-13 Tuberculous dactylitis. Radiographic findings in this child include soft tissue swelling of multiple digits, lytic lesions of several middle and proximal phalanges and metacarpals, and exuberant periostitis and enlargement of the proximal phalanx of the third finger. *(From Resnick, D., and Niwayama, G.: Diagnosis of Bone and Joint Disorders. Philadelphia, Saunders, 1981. Reproduced with permission.)*

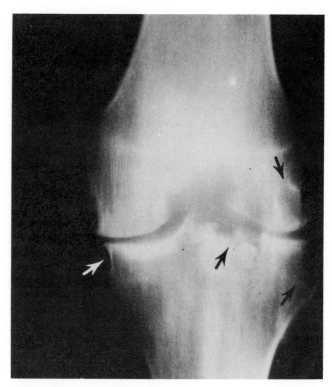

Figure 22-14 Tuberculous arthritis of the knee joint. This tomogram shows typical marginal and central osseous erosions (*arrows*). Osteoporosis is not prominent. *(From Resnick, D., and Niwayama, G.: Diagnosis of Bone and Joint Disorders. Philadelphia, Saunders, 1981. Reproduced with permission.)*

joints are splinted and gently mobilized as the disease abates and the local signs diminish. The result in early disease should be a mobile joint free from infection.

Surgical Joint Clearance Joint clearance is recommended for a joint which remains irritated with persisting effusion, thickened synovium, and other local signs of persisting activity. All debris and infected synovium are removed. This operation assists the antibiotics to penetrate and sterilize the joint and permits its eventual mobilization.

Arthrodesis Arthrodesis is now rarely required in tuberculous arthritis but performed extraarticularly was the standard operation prior to the discovery of antibiotics. It was considered that arthrodesis rendered a joint safe from repeated flare-ups of infection. Before antibiotic therapy was available, it was impossible to be certain that the organisms had been completely overcome and that a flare-up was not a possibility at some point in the future despite clinical remission. Nowadays with adequate treatment, joint infection can be cured without obliterating the joint. Indeed, total hip replacement

may be performed after a suitable interval in healed tuberculous arthritis. If arthrodesis is chosen, it is for mechanical and pain-relieving reasons rather than to assist in controlling the infection. Nevertheless, the earlier practice is worth remembering in the event of resistant organisms.

Arthroplasty Arthroplasty has no role in the treatment of active disease and is only performed as salvage surgery after the infection has been eradicated.

Atypical Mycobacterial Infections

Infection by atypical mycobacteria (e.g., *M. kansasii, M. fortuitium* and *M. intercellulare*) usually affects the tendon sheaths and spreads later to the joints of the knee, ankle, and elbows.[136]

Leprosy

Leprosy is caused by infection with *Mycobacterium leprae.* Arthritis is uncommon, and the skeletal lesions include interosseous granulomas, periostitis, and destructive changes in the foot and hand with loss of the phalanges and metatarsals. Occasionally there is disintegration of the mid foot.[101] The bone atrophy in the hands and feet may occasionally give to the resorbing bone a conical appearance which is characteristic and has been likened to a licked candy stick.[101]

SEPTIC ARTHRITIS

Septic arthritis can be produced by hematogenous spread to the synovium or by extension of osteomyelitis involving the epiphysis or an intracapsular metaphysis (Fig. 22-15). Direct contamination of the joint can follow diagnostic or therapeutic aspiration and has been described following venipuncture in the groin.

Clinical Features

The infection can occur at any age, but 50 percent of the cases occur in children under 3 years of age, and 30 percent of cases occur in children less than 2 years of age.[85,86,88] In infants the hip joint is most commonly affected, whereas in older children knee joint involvement is more common. Some 10 percent of childhood cases may have involvement of more than one joint.[85]

Adult Cases

In adults, infection, particularly tuberculous, may occur in a joint already involved with rheumatoid arthritis. The sterno-clavicular and sacroiliac joints are often affected in drug abusers.[97]

Septic Arthritis in Children

In the neonate, septic arthritis may occur in a child already seriously ill with septicemia and other focal infections. Alternatively the child may fail to thrive and run a pyrexia. It is only with a high index of suspicion and considerable clinical acumen that the area of infection is localized. Pain on motion of the affected joint, or lack of function, may be all that is apparent. Later in the disease the hip may become dislocated or in the case of other joints a soft tissue abscess may form. The diagnosis is then facilitated but unfortunately somewhat belated. Unilateral swelling of an extremity may also be a valuable clue. In an older child the presentation may be with an acutely painful joint held rigidly, permitting not even the slightest motion.[85] In the hip there may be a fixed flexion deformity associated with intense muscle spasm. In such cases bumping into the bed or cot inadvertently is sufficient to cause the child to cry out in pain since the joint is exquisitely sensitive to motion. The need to search for a skin lesion or a focus of infection elsewhere in the body should not be overlooked.

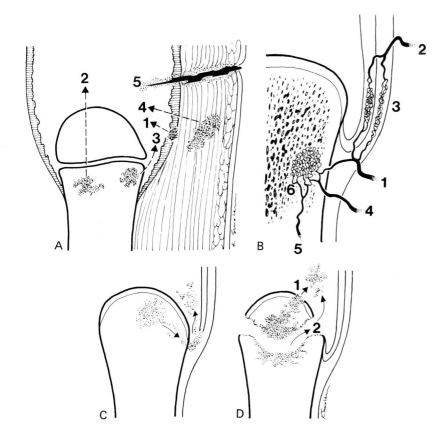

Figure 22-15 Septic arthritis: potential routes of contamination. **A.** Hematogenous spread of infection to a joint can result from direct lodgment of organisms in the synovial membrane (1). Spread into the joint from a contiguous source can occur from a metaphyseal focus that extends into the epiphysis and from there into the joint (2), from a metaphyseal focus with extension into the joint when the growth plate is intraarticular (3), or from a contiguous soft tissue infection (4). Direct implantation following a penetrating wound (5) can also lead to septic arthritis. **B** and **C.** Hematogenous spread of infection to a joint can also occur due to vascular continuity between the epiphysis and synovial membrane. In *B* the vessels shown include arterioles (1), venules (2), and capillaries (3) of the capsule; periosteal vessels (4); the nutrient artery (5); and metaphyseal-epiphyseal anastomoses (6). In this fashion, the synovial membrane may become infected from an osseous focus before the joint fluid is contaminated. In *C* this sequence of events is diagrammed. **D.** Spread from a contiguous osseous surface can result from penetration of the cartilage (1) or pathologic fracture with articular contamination (2). In this situation, synovial fluid may become infected before the synovial membrane. *(From Resnick, D., and Niwayama, G.: Diagnosis of Bone and Joint Disorders. Philadelphia, Saunders, 1981. Reproduced with permission.)*

Radiographic Studies

Displacement of the muscles around the joint may be seen as asymmetrical soft tissue shadows compared with the opposite side. In addition, lateral displacement, some upward subluxation of the femoral head, or even frank dislocation may be observed in the hip.

In adults, destruction of subchondral bone and articular cartilage may produce considerable subchondral osteoporosis and joint space narrowing at a relatively early stage of the disease.

Late radiological sequelae in children include infarction and sequestration of the epiphysis. Arthrography may be helpful in the unossified nucleus to ascertain whether or not it has been destroyed by the infective process. Lloyd-Roberts has pointed out that infants with previous knee joint infections may present with an established genu valgum deformity. This fact plus the x-ray appearance may lead one to believe that the physis and part of the distal femoral epiphysis have been permanently damaged. Under these circumstances, careful clinical examination and palpation will reveal the presence of the portion of epiphysis considered to have been destroyed. Similarly, the examination may indicate that the range of motion is well-preserved. This is not the case if a large portion of the intraarticular epiphysis has been destroyed and sequestrated.[65]

Lloyd-Roberts also points out that in the child's hip, areas of translucency appearing approximately 1 month following infection may resemble a pseudoarthrosis of the femoral neck. Provided the capital epiphysis still remains within the acetabulum, this does not, however, necessarily indicate a fracture, and recalcification of the area often follows with resolution of the illness. Delay in appearance of the ossific nucleus in these cases also does not mean that it has been destroyed, and arthrography is a valuable study in these hips.

Scintigraphic Studies

Although raised intraarticular pressure may occasionally cause a cold spot (photopenia) on the technetium scan, in most cases one may expect increased uptake in the region of the joint. Interpretation of this and the sequential scan with gallium has already been discussed in the section on osteomyelitis. The ^{99m}Tc-MDP scan is less specific for infection, but the ^{67}Ga-labeled gallium citrate scan may take considerably longer. Labeling leukocytes with ^{111}In requires a degree of laboratory technology which may not be available, but this test is the most specific and probably will detect infection at an earlier stage than the above-mentioned isotopes.[97] In general, bone scans are less useful than other tests and clinical diagnosis in septic arthritis. The MRI scan is valuable if available.

Diagnostic Aspiration

Synovial fluid analysis is required at the earliest possible moment, and fluid should be obtained by aspiration in all suspected cases. It is important that the needle be placed accurately within the joint, and fluoroscopic control may be necessary, with a light general anesthetic if necessary.

The joint fluid should be sent for bacteriologic studies and also for a white blood cell count and differential blood cell count. In well-established septic arthritis, an average of 100,000 cells/mm^3 (range 25,000 to 250,000) is commonly found. Septic arthritis is strongly suspected when there are more than 50,000 cells/mm^3 with 90 percent polymorphs even if there are no organisms grown on culture.[85,123] A Gram stain should also be performed and may give some guidance concerning the most effective antibiotic before the results from sensitivity tests are available. Blood cultures and cultures from other septic areas must be obtained prior to the commencement of any antibiotic therapy.

The glucose concentration in the synovial fluid is usually less than blood levels, and the protein concentration may be up to 6 or 8 g/dl with an electrophoretic pattern resembling that of plasma. Examination of the fluid for urate or calcium pyrophosphate crystals is important in differential diagnosis, particularly in adults. Additionally, if *Haemophilus influenzae* is suspected, techniques for directly detecting antigens in the fluid (counterimmunoelectrophoresis) may be valuable in establishing early diagnosis.[97]

Differential Diagnosis

It is unlikely that bacterial arthritis will be confused with a periarticular condition such as bursitis. In children, transient synovitis of the hip, which is the commonest cause of irritable hip in children under 10 years of age, may cause confusion. Children with this self-limiting aseptic inflammatory process may also present with a painful joint and a slight limp. Examination of the hip in these children also reveals a diminished range of motion with some fixed flexion deformity. However, the child is usually apyrexial and laboratory studies are normal. Aspiration of the joint usually settles the diagnosis. An MRI scan may be employed to exclude Perthes disease.

Acute osteomyelitis has to be differentiated from septic arthritis in the manner already described. Cellulitis similarly is unlikely to cause confusion, although it is important that any aspiration of the joint not be performed through such an infected area. Other conditions in the differential diagnosis include crystal deposition disease and chronic arthritis. In children, acute rheumatic fever, hemophilia, and Henoch-Schönlein purpura may occasionally be encountered. In adults with septic arthritis, consideration should also be given to the presence of associated infective conditions such as bacterial endocarditis.

Treatment

Treatment with parenteral antibiotics should be commenced immediately upon admission provided that all the necessary culture material has been obtained. The type of antibiotic chosen is based on the natural history of the disease, the age of the patient, and the result of the Gram stain.[97]

Haemophilus influenzae outnumbers *S. aureus* 3:1 as the organism most commonly causing septic arthritis in patients between 1 month and 5 years of age.[60] In patients over age 5, staphylococci are more common and *Haemophilus* infection is rare. If the Gram stain is negative but the evidence of infection is strong, it is appropriate whilst awaiting culture and sensitivity test results to treat with an antistaphylococcal drug such as methicillin or oxacillin, adding ampicillin in patients below age 5. Consideration should be given to the use of chloramphenicol in the high-risk group (that is, those between 6 and 24 months of age) in geographic areas where the incidence of ampicillin-resistant strains of *Haemophilus influenzae* is high.[85]

In adults a negative Gram stain is an indication to treat the patient with penicillin G (or tetracycline in allergic patients) since gonococci cause 60 percent of all cases of bacterial arthritis in adults under age 50. Staphylococci are responsible for only 15 percent of cases in the under-50 age group, but this is the probable infecting organism in older patients, who are consequently treated with nafcillin while awaiting the result of cultures. Patients who are sensitive to penicillin may be treated with a cephalosporin such as cefazolin.[97]

If the patient shows gram-negative cocci on the Gram stain, the likelihood of gonococcal infection is very high in the age group at particular risk. Similarly, if the Gram stain shows gram-negative rods, particularly in a patient such as a drug abuser, the patient is likely to have a *Pseudomonas* infection. A third-generation cephalosporin may be commenced. These drugs are superior to aminoglycosides in the treatment of *E. coli, Serratia,* and *Proteus* infections.

There is some evidence that although all cephalosporins have some value in the treatment of gram-negative septic arthritis, the third-generation cephalosporins (such as ceftazidime, cefsulodin, and aztreonam) are of particular value. Aminoglycosides may be less effective in joint fluid with a large number of polymorphs and an acid pH, but gentamicin is an acceptable alternative.[89] Once the results of synovial fluid or other cultures are available, it may be necessary to change to a more specific antibiotic. Antibiotics are administered parenterally at first. Oral antibiotics may be used when the infection is under control using the criteria already described for osteomyelitis. Therapy is monitored by measurement of bactericidal or bacteriostatic levels in the serum and maintaining levels eight times the minimal microbicidal concentration to ensure satisfactory kill rates.

Surgical Drainage

Although serial aspiration appropriately performed can be relatively pain free and accompanied by minimal risk of introducing additional contaminating organisms into the joint, nevertheless open drainage and surgical irrigation with large quantities of fluid is often preferred.

Controversy about surgical drainage of septic arthritis still continues, however. There are those who believe that open drainage should now rarely be used[97] and by contrast those who concur with Lloyd-Roberts that "the misguided conservation of the needle should yield to the conservation of the knife."[66]

In the hip joint, relief of the capsular distension produced by incision not only prevents lateral migration of the head, leading to dislocation, but has a profound and immediate beneficial effect on the patient's clinical status. By the anterolateral approach the hip joint can be exposed without cutting any muscle fibers. The proximal portion of this approach is relatively avascular, and the capsular distension enables one to find the hip joint rapidly so that the procedure lacks substantial morbidity. If the posterior approach is used, there is the advantage of gravitational drainage. Once the capsule is freely opened, it is not necessary to leave the wound open and the skin may be closed after appropriate irrigation. It is advisable to insert a subcutaneous drain through a separate stab incision following the surgical procedure. Similar principles are observed in surgical drainage of other involved joints. The authors have no experience with closed drainage systems using suction irrigation, and no control study has been performed with these methods. The problem with continuous irrigation of fluid into the joint remains the possibility of additional contamination.[10,23,85] All authorities agree that instilling antibiotics locally into the joint is not helpful and may be harmful.[10,23,85]

In superficial joints such as the knee, lavage using the arthroscope is an alternative which may effectively drain a joint and irrigate it without a large incision. However, there may be continuing anxiety that free drainage has not been established without incision of the joint capsule and synovium.

Immobilization

Although it is traditional to immobilize the joint to relieve pain during the acute phase of the disease, Salter believes that motion of the joint should be established as soon as possible. He advocates use of a continuing passive motion machine. From his experimental study on rabbits, he believes this improves nutrition of the cartilage, prevents adhesions, and enhances clearance of lysosomal enzymes and purulent exudate from the infected joint while at the same time stimulating the chondrocytes to synthesize matrix components.[110]

Complications

Lloyd-Roberts has pointed out that despite the alarming x-ray changes which may give a false impression of the extent of damage to the joint, the prognosis may in fact be relatively good and a favorable outcome predicted with confidence in many of these children.[65] He also points out that the final shape of the articulating surface is not dependent upon the degree of decalcification of the ossific nucleus (epiphysis) or even the metaphysis, but upon the damage caused to the physis. Such damage cannot be seen in an early radiograph. The same author suggests that the hip joint be manipulated and explored if the radiographic and physical signs suggest either that dislocation has occurred or that there is so much damage that dislocation may occur in the future. In favorable cases the hip may be relocated and thereby stabilized.[65]

With modern treatment, substantial mortality and morbidity no longer follow this disease. In general it can be said that growth disturbances such as coxa magna and those associated with destruction of the femoral capital epiphysis relate to the duration of symptoms before appropriate diagnosis and correct treatment were instituted.[85]

In cases of chronic septic arthritis, there may be an occasional indication for synovectomy as part of a general debridement. At the same time appropriate cultures may be obtained by biopsy of synovium and bone.[119] Biopsy is rarely required in pyogenic infections. The procedure would seem to be particularly indicated following traumatic injuries to joints and in those cases where the infection is superimposed upon an underlying chronic arthritis.

Fungal Arthritis

Fungal infections of joints associated with *Candida albicans,* although rare, are being reported with increasing frequency both in neonates and in drug users. They may be successfully treated with 5-flucytosine.[34,122] Arthritis can also be associated with coccidioidomycosis, cryptococcosis sporotrichosis, and blastomycosis, etc.

PROPHYLAXIS AGAINST INFECTION IN BONE AND JOINT SURGERY

Elective total joint surgery and open fractures are indications for prophylaxis. There is controversy about which antibiotic should be used, most authors recommending a first-generation cephalosporin.[130]

The current view is that there is no advantage in continuing intravenous prophylactic antibiotics beyond 24 h following surgery. The first dose should be administered intravenously immediately prior to the operation. Similar guidelines govern prophylaxis during dental procedures for patients with joint implants.

REFERENCES

1. Anderson, L.D. Infections, in Edmonson, A.S., and Crenshaw, A.H. (eds): *Campbell's Operative Orthopaedics,* 6th ed. St. Louis, Mosby, 1980, p 1051.
2. Anderson, L.D., and Horn, L.G. Irrigation suction technique in treatment of acute hematogenous osteomyelitis, chronic osteomyelitis and acute and chronic joint infections. South Med J 63:745, 1970.
3. Anderson, J.R., Orr, J.D., MacLean, D.A., and Scobie, W.G. Acute hematogenous osteitis. Arch Dis Child 55:953, 1980.
4. Ash, J.M., and Gilday. The futility of bone scanning in neonatal osteomyelitis: Concise communication. J Nucl Med 21:417, 1980.
5. Beaupre, A., and Carroll, N. The three syndromes of iliac osteomyelitis in children. J Bone Joint Surg 61A:1087–1095, 1979.
6. Berkowitz, I.D. Normal technetium bone scans in patients with osteomyelitis. Am J Dis Child 114:828–830, 1980.
7. Black, C.H., and Shelswell, J.H. A serological test in the diagnosis of staphylococcal infection. J Bone Joint Surg 37B:135–138, 1955.
8. Blockey, N.J., and Watson, J.T. Acute osteomyelitis in children. J Bone Joint Surg 52B:77–87, 1970.
9. Bobechko, W.P. Auto-immune reactions of articular cartilage. Orthop Surg Traumatol International Congress Series, SICOT, 1972, p 291.
10. Bobechko, W.P. Infections of bones and joints, in Lovell, W.W., and Winter, R.B. (eds): *Pediatric Orthopaedics.* Philadelphia, Lippincott, 1978.
11. Bonakdar-Pour, A., and Gaines, V.D. Orthop Clin North Am 14:21–37, 1983.
12. Brand, R.A., and Black, H. Pseudomonas osteomyelitis following puncture wounds in children. J Bone Joint Surg 56A:1637, 1974.
13. Brodie, Sir B. *Pathological and Surgical Observation on the Diseases of the Joints,* 4th ed. London, Longman, Rees, Orme, Brown, Green and Longman, 1836.
14. Chan, D.P.K., et al. Multifocal hematogenous serratia marcescens osteomyelitis in a drug user. Case report and review of the literature. Contemp Orthop 2:344–347, 1980.
15. Check, W.A. Oral antifungal agent effective even for widespread infections. JAMA 244:2019, 1980.
16. Chow, A.W., Montgomerie, J.Z., and Guze, L.B. Parenteral clindamycin therapy for severe anaerobic infections. Arch Intern Med 134:78, 1974.
17. Cierny, G., III, and Mader, J.T. Adult chronic osteomyelitis. Orthopaedics 7:1557–1564, 1984.
18. Cochran, W., Connolly J.H., and Thompson, I.D. Bone involvement after vaccination against smallpox. Br Med J 2:285, 1963.
19. Cole, W.G., Dalziel, R.E., and Leitl, S. Treatment of acute osteomyelitis in childhood. J Bone Joint Surg 64B:218–223, 1982.
20. Colville, J., Brady, P.G., and Regan, B.F. Acute hematogenous osteomyelitis in children with emphasis on treatment. J Ir Med Assoc 69:200, 1976.
21. Collert, S., and Isacson, J. Chronic sclerosing osteomyelitis (Garre). Clin Orthop 164:136–140, 1982.
22. Collip, P.J., and Koch, R. Cat-scratch fever associated with an osteolytic lesion. N Engl J Med 260:278, 1959.
23. Compere, E.L., Metzger, W.I., and Mitra, R.N. The treatment of pyogenic bone and joint infections by closed irrigation (circulation) with a non-toxic detergent and one or more antibiotics. J Bone Joint Surg 49A:614–624, 1967.
24. Cunha, B.A. The use of penicillins in orthopaedic surgery. Clin Orthop 190:36–49, 1984.
25. Damholt, V.V. Treatment of chronic osteomyelitis. Acta Orthop Scand 53:715–720, 1982.
26. Davidson, J.C., and Palmer, P.E.S. Osteomyelitis varioloso. J Bone Joint Surg 45B:687–693, 1963.
27. Davies, P.D.O., Humphries, M.J., Byfield, S.P., Nunn, A.J., Darbyshire, J.H., Citron, K.W., and Fox, W. Bone and joint tuberculosis: A survey of notifications in England and Wales. J Bone Joint Surg 66B:326–330, 1984.
28. Del Rio, M.D.L.A. Brucella osteomyelitis. Pediatr Infect Dis 2:50–52, 1983.
29. DiLiberti, J.H., and Tarlow, S. Bone and joint complications of haemophilus influenzae. Clin Pediatr 22:7–10, 1983.
30. Duran, R.J., Coventry, M.B., Weed, L.A., and Kierland, R.R. Sporotrichosis: A report of twenty-three cases in the upper extremity. J Bone Joint Surg 39A:1330–1342, 1957.
31. Ekengren, K., Bergdahl, S., and Eriksson, M. Neonatal osteomyelitis. Acta Radio [Diagn] 23:305, 1982.
32. Ellis, D.J., Winslow, J.R., and Indovina, A.A. Garre's osteomyelitis of the mandible. Oral Surg 44:183, 1977.
33. Ferguson, A.B. *Orthopaedic Surgery in Infancy and Childhood,* 4th ed. Baltimore, Williams & Wilkins, 1975.
34. Fitzgerald, E., Lloyd-Still, J., and Gordon, S.L. Candida arthritis. Clin Orthop 106:143–146, 1975.
35. Fitzgerald, R.H., Rosenblatt, J.E., Tenney, J.H., and Bourgault, A.M. Anaerobic septic arthritis. Clin Orthop 164:141, 1982.
36. Gaenslen, F.J. Split-heel approach in osteomyelitis of the os calcis. J Bone Joint Surg 13:759–772, 1931.
37. Gamble, J.G., Rinsky, L.A., and Bleck, E.E. Acetabular osteomyelitis in children. Clin Orthop 186:71–74, 1984.

38. Garré, C. Uber Besondere Formen und Folgerzustande der Akuten Infektiosen Osteomyelitis. Beitr Klin Chir Tubing 10:241–257, 1893.

39. Gelfand, M.J., and Silberstein, E.B. Radionuclide imaging: Use in diagnosis of osteomyelitis in children. JAMA 237:245, 1977.

40. Gillespie, W.J., and Mayo, K.M. The management of acute haematogenous osteomyelitis in the antibiotics era: A study of the outcome. J Bone Joint Surg 63B:126–131, 1981.

41. Gilmour, W.N. Acute haematogenous osteomyelitis. J Bone Joint Surg 44B:841, 1962.

42. Gledhill, R.B. Subacute osteomyelitis in children. Clin Orthop 96:57–69, 1973.

43. Gorbach, S., and Partlett, J.G. Anaerobic infections: Parts I, II and III. N Engl J Med 290:1177, 1237, 1289, 1974.

44. Green, N.E., Beauchamp, R.D. and Griffin, P.P. Primary subacute epiphyseal osteomyelitis. J Bone Joint Surg 63A:107–113, 1981.

45. Green, N.E. Pseudomonas infection of the foot following puncture wounds. Instr Course Lect 32:43, 1983.

46. Haberling, J.A. A review of 201 cases of suppurative arthritis. J Bone Joint Surg 23:917–921, 1941.

47. Hagler, D.S. Pseudomonas osteomyelitis: Puncture wounds of the feet. Pediatrics 48:672, 1971.

48. Hall, B.B., Fitzgerald, R.H., Jr., and Rosenblatt, J.E. Anaerobic osteomyelitis. J Bone Joint Surg 65A:30–35, 1983.

49. Hall, B.B., Rosenblatt, J.E., and Fitzgerald, R.H., Jr. Anaerobic septic arthritis and osteomyelitis. Orthop Clin North Am 15(3):505, 1984.

50. Handmaker, H. Acute hematogenous osteomyelitis: Has the bone scan betrayed us? Radiology 135:787, 1980.

51. Handmaker, H., and Giammona, A. The "hot-joint"—Increased diagnostic accuracy using combined 99mTc-phosphate and 67Ga citrate imaging in pediatrics. J Nucl Med 17:554, 1976.

52. Handmaker, H., and Leonards, R. The bone scan in inflammatory osseous disease. Semin Nucl Med 6:95, 1976.

53. Handow, G., and Lukop, M. Brucellosis. Clin Orthop 168:211–213, 1982.

54. Highland, T.R., and LaMont, R.L. Osteomyelitis of the pelvis in children. J Bone Joint Surg 65A:230–234, 1983.

55. Jackson, M.A., and Nelson, J.D. Etiology and medical management of acute suppurative bone and joint infection in pediatric patients. J Pediatr Orthop 2:313–323, 1982.

56. Jacobsson, S., Hollender, L., Lindberg, S., and Larsson, A. Chronic sclerosing osteomyelitis of the mandible. Scint Radiogr Find Oral Surg 45:167, 1978.

57. Johannsen, A. Chronic sclerosing osteomyelitis of the mandible. Acta Radio [Diagn] 18:360, 1977.

58. Johannsen, P.H. Pseudomonas infection in the foot following puncture wounds. JAMA 204:262,1968.

59. Jones, S.F. Sclerosing non-suppurative osteomyelitis as described by Garré. JAMA 24:985, 1921.

60. Kasser, J.R. Hematogenous osteomyelitis. Postgrad Med 76:79–86, 1984.

61. Kawashima, M., and Tamura, H. Topical therapy in orthopaedic infection. Orthopaedics 7:1592–1598, 1984.

62. Kelly, P.K. Osteomyelitis in the adult. Orthop Clin North Am 6:983–989, 1975.

63. Kopits, S.E., and Debuskey, M. Primary sclerosing osteomyelitis. Johns Hopkins Med J 140:241, 1977.

64. Lang, A.G., and Peterson, H.A. Osteomyelitis following puncture wounds of the foot in children. J Trauma 16:993, 1976.

65. Lloyd-Roberts, G.C. Suppurative arthritis in infants. J Bone Joint Surg 42B:706–720, 1960.

66. Lloyd-Roberts, G.C. Septic arthritis in infancy. Aust Pediatr J 15:41–43, 1979.

67. Lowbeer, L. Brucellotic osteomyelitis of the spinal column in man. Am J Pathol 24:723, 1948.

68. Mackowsiak, P.A., Jones, S.R., and Smith, J.W. Diagnostic value of sinus-tract cultures in chronic osteomyelitis. JAMA 239:2772, 1978.

69. Mantle, J.A. Brucellar spondylitis. J Bone Joint Surg 37B:456–461, 1955.

70. Mathes, S.J., Alpert, B.S., and Chang, N. Use of muscle flap in chronic osteomyelitis: Experimental and clinical correlation. Plast Reconstr Surg 69:815, 1982.

71. May, J.W., Jr., Gallico, G.G., III, and Lukash, F.N. Microvascular transfer of free tissue for closure of bone wounds of the distal lower extremity. N Engl J Med 306:253, 1982.

72. McCall, R.E. Maduromycosis allescheria boydii arthritis of the knee: A case report. Orthopaedics 4:1144, 1981.

73. Merkel, K.D., Fitzgerald R.H., Jr., and Brown, M.L. Scintigraphic evaluation in musculoskeletal sepsis. Orthop Clin North Am 15(3):401, 1984.

74. Merkel, K.D., Brown, M.L., Dewanjee, M.K., and Fitzgerald, R.H., Jr. Comparison of infections labelled leukocytes imaging with sequential technetium gallium scanning in diagnosis of low grade musculoskeletal sepsis. J Bone Joint Surg 67A:465–475, 1985.

75. Merritt, K. Counter immunoelectrophoresis diagnosis of septic arthritis caused by *Hemophilus influenzae.* J Bone Joint Surg 58A:414–415, 1976.

76. Meyerding, H.W. Chronic sclerosing osteitis (sclerosing non-suppurative osteomyelitis of Garré). Surg Clin North Am 24:762, 1944.

77. Meyrick-Thomas, J. Lowes, J.A., and Tabaqchali, S. *Serratia marcescens* in mixed aerobic infections of the bone. J Bone Joint Surg 62B:289–319, 1980.

78. Mok, P.M., Reilley, B.J., and Ash, J.M. Osteomyelitis in neonates: Clinical aspects and the role of radiography and scintigraphy in diagnosis and management. Radiology 145:677, 1982.

79. Moore, J.R., Weiland, A.J., and Daniel, R.K. Use of free vascularized bone graft in treatment of bone tumors. Clin Orthop 175:37, 1983.

80. Morgan, A., and Yates, A.K. The diagnosis of acute osteomyelitis of the pelvis. Postgrad Med J 42:74, 1966.

81. Munson, T.M., and Nelson, C.L. Microbiology for orthopaedic surgeons: Selected aspects. Clin Orthop 190:14–22, 1984.

82. Murray, I.P.C. Photopenia, skeletal scintigraphy of suspected bone and joint infection. Clin Nucl Med 7:13–29, 1982.

83. Murray, P.R., and Rosenblatt, J.E. Penicillin resistance and penicillinase production in clinical isolates of *Bacteroides melaninogenicus.* Antimicrob Agents Chemother 11:605, 1977.

84. Nade, S. Acute hematogenous osteomyelitis in infancy and childhood. J Bone Joint Surg 65B:109–119, 1983.

85. Nade, S. Acute septic arthritis in infancy and childhood. J Bone Joint Surg. 65B:234–251, 1983.

86. Nade, S., Robertson, F.W., and Taylor, T.K.J. Antibiotics in the treatment of acute osteomyelitis and acute septic arthritis in children. Med J Aust 2:703, 1974.

87. Nelson, J.D., Bucholz, R.W., Kuzmiesz, H., and Shelton, S. Benefits and risks of sequential parenteral-oral cephalosporin therapy for suppurative bone and joint infections. J Pediatr Orthop 2:255–262, 1982.

88. Nelson, J.D., and Koontz, W.C. Septic arthritis in infants and children: A review of 117 cases. Pediatrics 38:966, 1966.

89. Neu, H.C. Cephalosporin antibiotics as applied in surgery of bones and joints. Clin Orthop 190:50–63, 1984.

90. O'Brien, T., McManus, F., MacAuley, P.H., and Ennis, J.T. Acute hematogenous osteomyelitis. J Bone Joint Surg 64B:450–453, 1982.

91. Ogden, J.A. Pediatric osteomyelitis and septic arthritis: The pathology of neonatal disease. Yale J Biol Med 52:423–448, 1979.

92. Oyston, J.K. Madura foot: A study of twenty cases. J Bone Joint Surg 43B:259–267, 1961.

93. Papineau, L.J. L'excision-greffe avec fermeture retardée deliberée dans l'ostomyelite chronique. Nouv Presse Med 2:2753, 1973.

94. Papineau, L.J., Alfageme, A., Dalcourt, J.P., and Pilon, L. Osteomyelitie chronique: Excision et greffe de spongieuz a l'air libre apres mises a plat extensive. Int Orthop (SICOT) 3:165, 1979.

95. Peterson, H.A. Fungal osteomyelitis in children. Instr Course Lect 32:46, 1983.

96. Phemister, D.B. Chronic fibrous osteomyelitis. Ann Surg 90:756, 1929.

97. Philips, P.E. Bacterial arthritis: Uncovering the underlying cause. J Musculoskel Med 1:14–22, 1984.

98. Pritchard, D.J. Granulomatous infections of bones and joints. Orthop Clin North Am 6:1029–1047, 1975.

99. Propst-Proctor, S.L., Dillingham, M.F., McDougall, I.R., and Goodwin, D. The white blood scan in orthopaedics. Clin Orthop 168:157–165, 1982.

100. Quintiliani, R., and Nightingale, C. Principles of antibiotic usage. Clin Orthop 190:31–35, 1984.

101. Resnick, D., and Niwaya, G. Osteomyelitis, septic arthritis and soft tissue infection, in Resnick, D., and Niwayama, G. (eds): *Diagnosis of Bone and Joint Disorders,* vol III. Philadelphia, Saunders, 1981, pp 2042–2129.

102. Rhinelander, F.W. Minimal fixation of tibial fractures. Clin Orthop 107:188–220, 1975.

103. Riegler, H.F., and Rouston, F.W. Complications of deep puncture wounds of the foot. J Trauma 19:18, 1979.

104. Roberts, P.H. Disturbed epiphyseal growth at the knee after osteomyelitis in infancy. J Bone Joint Surg 52B:692–703, 1970.

105. Rosenthal, L. et al. Sequential use of radiophosphate and radio gallium imaging in the differential diagnosis of bone, joint and soft tissue infection: Quantitative analysis. Diagn Imaging 51:249–258, 1982.

106. Ross, E.R.S., and Cole, W.G. Treatment of subacute osteomyelitis in childhood. J Bone Joint Surg 67B:443–447, 1985.

107. Ruttle, P.E., Kelly, P.J., Arnold, P.G., Irons, G.B., and Fitzgerald, R.H. Chronic osteomyelitis treated with a muscle flap. Orthop Clin North Am 15(3):451, 1984.

108. Sachs, B.L. and Shaffer, B.W. A staged Papineau protocol for chronic osteomyelitis. Clin Orthop 184:256–263, 1984.

109. Salaki, J.S., Black, R., Tally, F.P., and Kislak, J.W. *Bacteroides fragilis* resistant to the adminstration of clindamycin. Am J Med 60:426, 1976.

110. Salter, R.B., Bell, R.S., and Keeley, F.W. The protective effect of continuous passive motion of living articular cartilage in acute septic arthritis: An experimental investigation in rabbit. Clin Orthop 159:223–247, 1981.

111. Sengupta, A. Musculoskeletal lesions in yaws. Clin Orthop 192:193–198, 1985.

112. Sullivan, J.A., Vasileff, T., and Leonard, J.C. An evaluation of nuclear scanning in orthopaedic infections. J Pediatr Orthop 1:73–79, 1981.

113. Tachdjian, M.O. *Pediatric Orthopaedics.* Philadelphia, Saunders, 1972, p 352.

114. Tatzlaff, T.R., et al. Oral antibiotic therapy for skeletal infections of children. J Pediatr Orthop 92:485, 1978.

115. Taylor, G.I. Microvascular free bone transfer: A clinical technique. Orthop Clin North Am 8:425, 1977.

116. Taylor, G.I., Miller, G.D.H., and Ham, F.J. The free vascularized bone graft. Plast Reconstr Surg 55:533, 1975.

117. Taylor, G.I., Townsend, P., and Corlett, R. Superiority of the deep circumflex iliac vessels as the supply for free groin flaps: Experiment work. Plast Reconstr Surg 64:595, 1979.

118. Thompson, R.L., and Wright, A.J. Anti-microbial therapy in musculoskeletal surgery. Orthop Clin North Am 15(3):547, 1984.

119. Tscherne, H., et al. Synovectomy as treatment for purulent joint infection. Arch Orthop Trauma Surg 103:162–164, 1984.

120. Tuazon, C.U. Teichoic acid antibodies in osteomyelitis and septic arthritis cause by *Staphylococcus aureus.* J Bone Joint Surg 64A:762–765, 1982.

121. Turek, S.L. Bone infections, in *Orthopaedics: Principles and Their Application.* Philadelphia, Lippincott, 1977, pp. 207.

122. Umber, J. Candida, pyoarthrosis. J Bone Joint Surg 56A:1520–1524, 1974.

123. Ward, J., Cohen, A.S., and Bauer, W. The diagnosis and therapy of acute suppurative arthritis. Arthritis Rheum 3:522, 1960.

124. Weiland, A.J. Current concepts review: Vascularized free bone transplant. J Bone Joint Surg 63A:166–169, 1981.

125. Weiland, A.J., Kleinert, H.E., Kutz, J.E., et al. Free vascularized bone graft in the surgery of the upper extremity. J Hand Surg 4:129, 1979.

126. Weiland, A.J., Moore, J.R., and Daniel, R.K. Vascularized bone autografts: Experience with 41 cases. Clin Orthop 174:87–95, 1983.

127. Weiland, A.J., Moore, J.R., and Daniel, R.K. The efficacy of free tissue transfer in the treatment of osteomyelitis. J Bone Joint Surg 66A:181–193, 1984.

128. West, W.F., et al. Chronic osteomyelitis: Factors affecting the results of treatment in 186 patients. JAMA 213:1837, 1970.

129. Whelton, A. The aminoglycosides. Clin Orthop 190:67–74, 1984.

130. Williams, D.N., and Gustilo, R.B. The use of preventive antibiotics in orthopaedic surgery. Clin Orthop 190:83–88, 1984.

131. Winters, J.L., and Cohen, I. Acute haematogenous osteomyelitis. J Bone Joint Surg 42A:691–704, 1960.

132. Wishner, J. Chronic sclerosing osteomyelits (Garré). J Bone Joint Surg 15:723, 1933.

133. Wood, M.B., and Cooney, W.P. Vascularized bone segment transfers for management of chronic osteomyelitis. Orthop Clin North Am 15(3):461, 1984.

134. Zammit, F. Undulant fever spondylitis. Br J Radiol 31:683, 1958.

135. Zvetina, J.R. *Mycobacterium kansasii* infection of the elbow joint. J Bone Joint Surg 61A:1099–1101, 1979.

CHAPTER 23

Principles of Orthopaedic Oncology

Martin M. Malawer, Barry M. Shmookler, Stephen Feffer, and David Westring

SECTION A

Musculoskeletal Oncology

Martin M. Malawer and Barry M. Shmookler

Neoplasms of the musculoskeletal system (sarcomas) are the least common of all tumors. Their diagnosis, management, and treatment have changed at a revolutionary pace within the past decade. Advances in radiographic imaging, chemotherapy, radiation therapy, and biotechnology, coupled with a better understanding of the biological behavior of mesenchymal neoplasms, have led to a rational basis of diagnosis, staging, and surgical treatment.[8-12,16,20,30,63,64,103]

NATURAL HISTORY OF BONE AND SOFT TISSUE TUMORS

Tumors arising in bone and soft tissue have characteristic patterns of behavior and growth that distinguish them from other malignant lesions.[24,30] These patterns, which form the basis of a staging system and current treatment strategies, are described here.[24]

Biology and Growth

Spindle cell sarcomas form a solid lesion that grows centrifugally. The periphery of this lesion is the least mature. In contradistinction to benign lesions, which are surrounded by a true capsule composed of compressed normal cells, the malignant tumor is generally enclosed by a pseudocapsule, which consists of compressed tumor cells and a fibrovascular zone of reactive tissue with a variable inflammatory component that interdigitates with the normal tissue adjacent and beyond the lesion. The thickness of the reactive zone varies with the degree of malignancy and histogenetic type.

High-grade sarcomas have a poorly defined reactive zone

that may be locally invaded and destroyed by the tumor. In addition, tumor nodules not in continuity with the main tumor may be present in tissue that appears to be normal (see Skip Metastasis). Low-grade sarcomas rarely form tumor nodules beyond the reactive zone.

Sarcomas respect anatomic borders and remain within one compartment. Local anatomy influences the growth by setting natural barriers to extension.[108] In general, bone sarcomas take the path of least resistance. The three mechanisms of growth and extension of bone tumors are compression of normal tissue, resorption of bone by reactive osteoclasts, and direct destruction of normal tissue. Benign tumors grow and expand by the first two mechanisms, whereas direct tissue destruction is characteristic of malignant bone tumors. Most benign bone tumors are unicompartmental; they remain confined and may expand the bone in which they arise. Most malignant bone tumors are bicompartmental; they destroy the overlying cortex and go directly into the adjacent soft tissue. Soft tissue tumors may start in one compartment (intracompartmental) or between compartments (extracompartmental).[29]

The determination of anatomic compartment involvement has become more important with the advent of limb preservation surgery.

Patterns of Behavior

Based on biological considerations and natural history, all bone and soft tissue tumors, benign and malignant, may be classified into five categories, each of which shares certain clinical characteristics and radiographic patterns and requires similar surgical procedures. The five general patterns of behavior are as follows:[24]

1. *Benign/latent* Lesions whose natural history is to grow slowly during normal growth of the individual and then to stop, with a tendency to heal spontaneously. They never become malignant and heal rapidly if treated by simple curettage.
2. *Benign/active* Lesions whose natural history is progressive growth: excision leaves a reactive zone with some tumor.
3. *Benign/aggressive* Lesions which are locally aggressive but do not metastasize. Pathologically there is tumor extension through the capsule into the reactive zone. Local

TABLE 23-1 Behavioral Classification of Bone and Soft Tissue Tumors

	Typical example	
Classification	**Bone**	**Soft tissue**
Benign/latent	Nonossifying fibroma	Lipoma
Benign/active	Aneurysmal bone cyst	Angiolipoma
Benign/aggressive	Giant cell tumor	Aggressive fibromatosis
Malignant/low-grade	Parosteal osteosarcoma	Myxoid liposarcoma
Malignant/high-grade	Classic osteosarcoma	Malignant fibrous histiocytoma

control can be obtained only by removing the lesion with a margin of normal tissue beyond the reactive zone.

4. *Malignant, low-grade* Lesions which have a low potential to metastasize. Histologically there is no true capsule but a pseudocapsule. Tumor nodules exist within the reactive zone but rarely beyond. Local control can be accomplished only by removal of all tumor and reactive tissue with a margin of normal bone. These lesions can be treated successfully by surgery alone; systemic therapy is not required.

5. *Malignant high-grade* Lesions whose natural history is to grow rapidly and to metastasize early. Tumor nodules are usually found within and beyond the reactive zone and at some distance in the normal tissue. Surgery is necessary for local control, and systemic therapy is warranted to prevent metastasis.

Examples of bone and soft tissue tumors in each of these categories are shown in Table 23-1.

Tumor Spread

Unlike carcinomas, bone and soft tissue sarcomas disseminate almost exclusively through the blood. Soft tissue tumors occasionally (5 to 10 percent) spread through the lymphatic system to regional nodes.[121] Hematogenous spread is manifested by pulmonary involvement in the early stages and by bony involvement in later stages.[8,9,15,70] Bone metastasis occasionally is the first sign of dissemination.

Skip Metastasis

The histological hallmark of malignant sarcomas is their potential to break through the pseudocapsule to form satellite lesions called *skip metastases.* A skip metastasis is a tumor nodule that is located within the same bone as the main tumor but not contiguous to it. Transarticular skip metastases are located in the joint adjacent to the main tumor (Fig. 23-1).[29] Skip metastases are most often seen with high-grade sarcomas. Skip lesions develop by the embolization of tumor cells within the marrow sinusoids; they are in effect local micrometastases that have not passed through the circulation. Soft tissue sarcomas similarly may be associated with noncontinuous tumor nodules away from the main tumor mass. These nodules are responsible for local recurrences

that develop in spite of apparently negative margins after a resection.

Local Recurrence

Local recurrence is due to inadequate removal and subsequent regrowth of either a benign or a malignant lesion. Adequacy of surgical removal is the main determinant of local control. The aggressiveness of the lesion determines the choice of surgical procedure. Ninety-five percent of all local recurrences, regardless of the histological findings, develop within 24 months of surgery.[24,29]

STAGING SYSTEM OF MUSCULOSKELETAL TUMORS

In 1980, the Musculoskeletal Tumor Society adopted a surgical staging system (SSS) for both bone and soft tissue sarcomas.[30] The system is based upon the fact that mesenchymal sarcomas of bone and soft tissue behave alike, irrespective of histogenetic type. The SSS is based on the GTM classification: Grade (G), location (T), and lymph node involvement and metastases (M). The stage accurately predicts overall survival.

1. *Surgical grade (G)* The letter *G* represents the histological grade of a lesion and other clinical data. A low-grade tumor is rated G1. A high-grade tumor is rated G2.

2. *Surgical site (T)* The letter *T* represents anatomic site, either intracompartmental (T1) or extracompartmental (T2). Compartment is defined as "an anatomic structure of space bounded by natural barriers of tumor extension." The clinical significance of T1 lesions is easier to define clinically, surgically, and radiographically than that of T2 lesions, and there is a higher chance of adequate removal by a nonamputative procedure.

3. *Lymph nodes and metastases (M)* When a bone or soft tissue sarcoma has metastasized through the lymphatic system (M1), the prognosis is extremely poor. Lymphatic spread is a sign of extensive dissemination. Regional lymphatic involvement is equated with distal metastases.

The SSS developed for surgical planning and assessment of bone sarcomas is summarized as follows:[30]

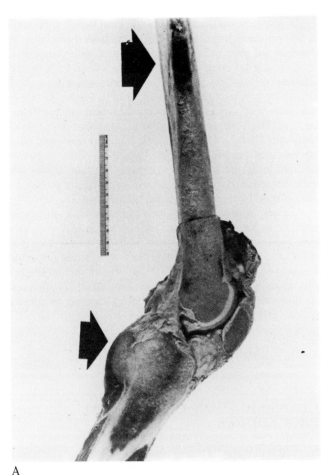
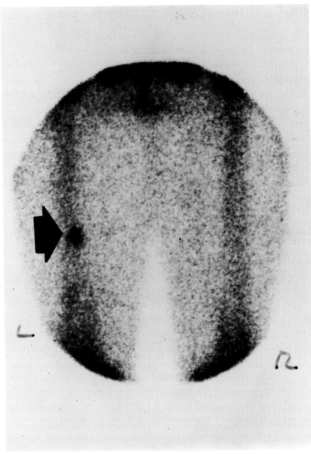

A

B

Figure 23-1 A skip metastasis from an osteosarcoma of the proximal tibia to the ipsilateral femur. Satellite nodules that occur from a bony sarcoma are termed *skip metastases*. These may occur within the same bone as the primary lesion or across the adjacent joint, termed a *transarticular skip metastasis*. **A.**

Gross specimen following an above-knee amputation, showing the primary tumor (*lower arrow*) and the skip metastasis (*upper arrow*). **B.** Bone scan of the same lesion (*solid arrow*), demonstrating a small well-defined area of uptake of the skip lesion.

Stage IA (G1, T1, M0) Low-grade intracompartmental lesion without metastasis

Stage IB (G1, T2, M0) Low-grade extracompartmental lesion without metastasis

Stage IIA (G2, T1, M0) High-grade intracompartmental lesion without metastasis

Stage IIB (G2, T2, M0) High-grade extracompartmental lesion without metastasis

Stage IIIA (G1 or G2, T1, M1) Intracompartmental lesion, any grade, with metastasis

Stage IIIB (G1 or G2, T2, M1) Extracompartmental lesion, any grade, with metastasis

PREOPERATIVE EVALUATION STAGING AND BIOPSY

If the clinical examination and/or plain radiographs suggest an aggressive or malignant tumor, staging studies should be performed before biopsy. All radiographic studies are influenced by surgical manipulation of the lesion, making interpretation more difficult.[24,107] Bone scintigraphy, computed tomography (CT), and angiography are required to delineate local tumor extent, vascular displacement, and compartmental localization.[3,20,22,29,37-43,65,75,99]

Radiographic Evaluation

Bone Scans

Bone scintigraphy is useful for evaluation of both bony and soft tissue tumors. It assists in determining metastatic disease, polyostotic involvement, intraosseous extension of tumor, and the relation of the underlying bone to a primary soft tissue sarcoma.[38,56,81] Malignant bone tumors may present with skeletal metastasis (1.6 percent).[3]

Computed Tomography

CT scanning allows accurate determination of intra- and extraosseous extension of skeletal neoplasms.[20,22,56,81,104] CT accurately depicts the transverse relations of a tumor. By varying window settings, one can study cortical bone, intramedullary space, adjacent muscles, and extraosseous soft tissue extension. The anatomic compartmental involvement by soft tissue sarcomas is easily determined.[29] CT evaluation must be individualized. To obtain the maximum benefit of image reconstruction, the surgeon should discuss the information desired with the radiologist. Magnetic resonance imaging (MRI), currently being investigated, is a promising modality.

Angiography

The arteriographic technique for bone and soft tissue lesions differ from that used for arterial disease. A minimum of two views (biplane) is necessary to determine the relation of the major vessels to the tumor.[43] Extraosseous extension is easily demonstrated by angiography. As experience with limb-sparing procedures has increased, surgeons have become more aware of the need to determine the individual vascular patterns prior to resection. This is especially crucial for tumors of the knee, where vascular anomalies are common.[66] The increasing preoperative use of intraarterial chemotherapy also has increased the need for accurate angiography.

CT (transverse data) combined with bone scans and angiography (longitudinal data) allows the physician to develop a three-dimensional construct of the local tumor area prior to surgery and to formulate a detailed surgical approach.

Biopsy Considerations

A biopsy should be performed *after* the staging studies are obtained. If a resection is to be performed, it is crucial that the location of the biopsy be in line with the anticipated incision for the definitive procedure. Extreme care should be taken *before* biopsy not to contaminate potential tissue planes or flaps that will compromise the management of the lesion. To minimize contamination, a needle biopsy of soft tissue masses or of extraosseous components should be attempted *prior* to an incisional biopsy whenever possible.

Needle or core biopsy of bone tumor often provides an adequate specimen for diagnosis.[86,105] Radiographs should be obtained to document the position of the trocar. Core biopsy is preferred if a limb-sparing option exists since it entails less local contamination than open biopsy does. Core biopsy is especially helpful in difficult areas such as the spine, pelvis, and hips. If a core biopsy proves to be inadequate, a small incisional biopsy is performed. A small incisional or needle biopsy is recommended for all soft tissue tumors.

Every possible precaution should be taken to avoid contamination when performing an open biopsy for either a bone or a soft tissue tumor.

A tourniquet is used if feasible. If a soft tissue component is present, there is no need to biopsy the underlying bone. To decrease subsequent hemorrhage, polymethylmethacrylate is used to plug a cortical window; Gelfoam is used for hemostasis in the soft tissue. The overlying pseudocapsule is carefully closed for maximum hemostasis. If it is necessary to biopsy the underlying bone, a small, rounded cortical window should be used. This is especially true for a tumor that requires primary radiotherapy. Large segments do not reossify and often fracture and require amputation. Regardless of the technique utilized, tumor cells will contaminate all tissue planes and compartments traversed. All biopsy sites must therefore be removed en bloc when the tumor is resected.

Frozen section analyses are performed on all biopsy specimens. Many bone tumors can be adequately sectioned with a microtome. The purpose of the first frozen section is to demonstrate if viable tumor has been obtained. If not, additional specimens must be obtained. Frozen section studies may also suggest that additional material should be obtained so that electron microscopy or special staining techniques may be carried out.

CLASSIFICATION OF SURGICAL PROCEDURES

Surgical removal—including curettage, resection, and amputation—is the traditional method of managing skeletal neoplasms. More recently, limb-sparing techniques have been introduced.[11,26,28,34,53,67,70,71,75,87,107,120]

A method of classification of surgical procedures based on the surgical plane of dissection in relation to the tumor and the method of accomplishing the removal has recently been developed. This system, summarized below, permits meaningful comparison of various operative procedures and gives surgeons a common language.[29,30]

1. *Intralesional* An intralesional procedure passes through the pseudocapsule and directly into the lesion. Macroscopic tumor is left, and the entire operative field is potentially contaminated.
2. *Marginal* A marginal procedure is one in which the entire lesion is removed in one piece. The plane of dissection passes through the pseudocapsule or reactive zone around the lesion. When performed for a sarcoma, it leaves macroscopic disease.
3. *Wide (intracompartmental)* This is commonly termed *en bloc* resection. A wide excision includes the entire tumor, the reactive zone, and a cuff of normal tissue. The entire structure of origin of the tumor is not removed. In patients with high-grade sarcomas, this procedure may leave skip nodules.
4. *Radical (extracompartmental)* The entire tumor and the structure of origin of the lesion are removed. The plane of dissection is beyond the limiting fascial or bony borders.

It is important to note that any of these procedures may be accomplished *either* by a local (i.e., limb-sparing) procedure or by amputation. Thus, an amputation may entail a marginal, wide, or radical excision, depending upon the plane through which it passes. An amputation is *not* necessarily an adequate cancer operation, but it is a method of achieving a specific margin. The local anatomy determines how a specific margin is to be obtained. Therefore, the aim of preoperative staging is to assess local tumor extent and relevant local anatomy in order to permit determination of how a desired margin is to be achieved, i.e., the feasibility of one surgical procedure versus another. In general, benign bone tumors are treated adequately either by an intralesional procedure (curettage) or by marginal excision. Malignant tumors require either a wide (intracompartmental) or a radical (extracompartmental) removal, be it an amputation or an en bloc procedure. Similarly, benign soft tissue tumors are treated by marginal excision, aggressive tumors by wide excision, and malignant tumors by wide or radical resection.

SOFT TISSUE SARCOMAS

Soft tissue sarcomas (STSs) are a heterogeneous group of tumors arising from the supporting extraskeletal tissues of the body, i.e., muscle, fascia, connective tissues, fibrous tissues, and fat. They are rare lesions, constituting less than 1 percent of all cancers. There is a wide morphological difference among these tumors, probably resulting from the different cells of origin. All STSs, like bone sarcomas, however, share certain biological and behavioral characteristics.

The clinical, radiographic, and surgical management of most STSs is identical, regardless of histogenesis. The surgical grading system developed by the Musculoskeletal Tumor Society applies to both bone sarcomas and soft tissue sarcomas.

Clinical Findings

Soft tissue sarcomas are a disease of adulthood, occurring in persons between 30 and 60 years of age. The sole exception is rhabdomyosarcoma, which occurs in young children. Approximately one-half of STSs are found in the extremities; the remainder arise in the head/neck and trunk. The lower extremity is the most common anatomic site; 40 percent of all STSs occur in this location.[102] The anterior thigh (quadriceps) is the most common compartment, followed by the adductors and hamstrings.[29,108]

Most STSs present as a painless mass. Systemic signs such as fever, weight loss, or anemia are rare. There are no laboratory screening examinations. Clinical suspicion is therefore crucial to diagnosis. Any adult presenting with an extremity mass must be presumed to have a sarcoma until proved otherwise and should be further evaluated. Unfortunately, a presumptive diagnosis of lipoma, ganglion, or hema-

toma is often made, thereby delaying definitive evaluation and treatment. Local examination reveals a well-localized, nontender mass that may be movable. The lesion may be firm or cystic. (The latter indicates that necrosis has occurred and is a sign of high-grade sarcoma.)

Biological Behavior and Natural History

The pattern of growth, metastasis, and recurrence of STSs is similar to that of spindle cell sarcomas arising in bone. The major distinctions are the tendency of STSs to remain intracompartmental and a significant incidence of lymphatic involvement in a few of the less common entities such as the epithelioid, synovial, and alveolar soft-part sarcomas. The prognosis of an STS is most closely related to its histological grade and the presence or absence of metastases.[29,30] Historically, high-grade STS had an overall survival rate of 40 to 60 percent.[30,41,58,82,108] In half of all cases, wide local excision was followed by local recurrence within 12 to 24 months, followed by pulmonary metastases resulting from hematogenous dissemination to the lungs. Enneking has noted that if a local recurrence develops, the risk of pulmonary metastases doubles.[31,41] Visceral and lymphatic involvement was rare. Pulmonary and/or local recurrence are the most common sites of relapse.

Pathology and Staging

Table 23-2 lists the various STSs. Individual grading is often difficult; in general, however, the extent of pleomorphism, atypia, mitosis, and necrosis correlates with the degree of malignancy. Notable exceptions are synovial sarcomas, which tend to behave like high-grade lesions even in the absence of these findings. The exact histogenesis of some soft tissue sarcomas often cannot be accurately defined, although the grade can be determined. The surgical stage is determined by grade, location, and the presence or absence of pulmonary or lymphatic metastases.[30] Staging studies must be done prior to treatment.

CT is the most useful study for evaluating STS of the extremities. Serial sections with contrast enhancement can delineate the anatomic compartment of the lesion; in addition, unicompartmental vs. bicompartmental involvement can be determined. Computed tomography is generally more helpful for proximal lesions than for those that are distal to the elbow or knee.

Biplane angiography is used to demonstrate the position of the major vessels. Although CT often shows the vessels, angiography is helpful in planning an operative approach, especially if displacement is noted on the CT scan. Bone scintigraphy is used to determine the relation of adjacent bony structures to the tumor. Increased contrast medium uptake by a bone in close proximity to an STS usually indicates a reactive rim of tumor near the periosteum, rather than direct intraosseous tumor extension. Such findings indicate that

TABLE 23-2 Histological Types and Grades of Soft Tissue Sarcomas

Histological Type	Grade*		
	1	2	3
Well-differentiated liposarcoma	X	—	—
Myxoid liposarcoma	X	—	—
Round cell liposarcoma	—	X	X
Pleomorphic liposarcoma	—	—	X
Fibrosarcoma	—	X	X
Malignant fibrous histiocytoma	—	X	X
Inflammatory malignant fibrous histiocytoma	—	X	X
Myxoid malignant fibrous histiocytoma	—	X	—
Dermatofibrosarcoma protuberans	X	—	—
Malignant giant cell tumor	—	X	X
Leiomyosarcoma	X	X	X
Malignant hemangiopericytoma	X	X	X
Embryonal rhabdomyosarcoma	—	—	X
Alveolar rhabdomyosarcoma	—	—	X
Pleomorphic rhabdomyosarcoma	—	—	X
Combined rhabdomyosarcoma	—	—	X
Chondrosarcoma	X	X	X
Mesenchymal chondrosarcoma	—	—	X
Myxoid chondrosarcoma	X	X	—
Osteosarcoma	—	—	X
Soft tissue sarcoma resembling Ewing's sarcoma	—	—	X
Synovial sarcoma	—	—	X
Epithelioid sarcoma	—	X	X
Clear cell sarcoma	—	X	X
Malignant superficial schwannoma	—	X	—
Neurofibrosarcoma	X	X	X
Epithelioid schwannoma	—	X	X
Malignant Triton tumor	—	—	X
Angiosarcoma	—	X	X
Alveolar soft part sarcoma	—	—	X
Malignant granular cell tumor	—	X	X
Kaposi's sarcoma	—	X	X

*The usual variation in grade is indicated for each recognized common histological type.
Source: Costa, J., Wesley, R.A., Glatstein, E., et al: Cancer 53:530–541, 1984. Reproduced with permission.

surgical resection of the underlying bony cortex or periosteum may be required.

Treatment

The treatment of high-grade STS has undergone fundamental changes within the past decade. Successful management requires cooperation of the surgeon, chemotherapist, and radiation oncologist. The appropriate role of each modality is continuously changing, but can be described in general as follows.

Surgery

Removal of the tumor is required for local control. This may be accomplished either by a nonablative resection or by an amputation. The procedure chosen depends on results of the preoperative staging studies.

Chemotherapy

Combination chemotherapy is effective in preventing pulmonary dissemination from high-grade sarcomas.[102] The most effective drugs are doxorubicin hydrochloride (Adriamycin), methotrexate plus cyclophosphamide, and cisplatin; these are also effective against bone sarcomas. The various combinations are given postoperatively and are presumed effective against clinically indetectable micrometastases. Preoperative chemotherapy is presently being evaluated in several institutions. Intraarterial chemotherapy has been shown to increase local control in several studies.

Radiation Therapy

Radiation in the range of 5000 to 6500 R is effective in an adjuvant setting in decreasing local recurrence following nonablative resection.[82] The degree to which the initial surgical volume should be decreased in these circumstances is controversial, although the local recurrence following a wide excision and postoperative radiotherapy is less than 51 percent. The technique of radiation therapy includes irradiating all the tissues at risk, shrinking fields, preserving a strip of unirradiated skin, and using filters and radiosensitizers. The local morbidity has been greatly decreased within the past decade.

Surgical Management

The majority of extremity sarcomas can be treated by a limb-sparing procedure. Enneking has shown that a radical resection for an STS has about a 5 percent local recurrence rate with surgery alone.[29,30] A wide excision (without adjuvant radiation or chemotherapy) had a 50 percent rate of local failure. More recently, investigators at the National Cancer Institute reported that local recurrence decreased to 5 percent following local excision (either a marginal or wide excision) combined with postoperative radiation therapy and chemotherapy. Others have reported similar good results from preoperative radiation, with or without preoperative chemotherapy. Contraindications to limb-sparing surgery are similar to those for the bony sarcomas. In general, nerve or major vascular involvement is a contraindication. Most stage IIA lesions can be treated by a limb-sparing procedure, whereas stage IIB lesions often require amputation to achieve negative margins.

Surgical Technique

The technique of resection for specific anatomic compartments is discussed in their respective anatomic sections. The general surgical and oncological principles are summarized as follows:

1. All tissue at risk should be removed with a wide en bloc excision. This includes the tumor with normal muscle and all potentially contaminated tissues. The entire muscle group need not be removed.
2. The biopsy site should be removed with 3 cm of normal skin and subcutaneous tissue en bloc with the tumor.
3. The tumor and/or pseudocapsule should never be visualized during the procedure. Contamination of the wound with tumor greatly increases the risk of local recurrence.
4. Distant flaps should not be developed at the time of resection. This may contaminate a noninvolved area.
5. All dead space should be closed, and there should be adequate drainage to prevent hematoma.

6. The surgical wound should be marked with hemoclips. This helps the radiotherapist determine the high-risk area.
7. A tourniquet should be used if possible. Although there is no evidence that this improves survival, it makes resection safer by preventing inadvertent violation of the tumor.
8. Perioperative antibiotics should be given. These procedures have a significant rate of postoperative infections, especially following preoperative adjuvant therapy.

Characteristics of Specific Soft Tissue Sarcomas

Malignant Fibrous Histiocytoma

Malignant fibrous histiocytoma (MFH), first described in 1963, is the most common STS.[109,122,123] MFH occurs in adults and is most common in the lower extremity. The histological grade is a good prognosticator of metastatic potential. The myxoid variant tends to have a more favorable prognosis than the other subtypes.[20]

Gross Characteristics The lesions may be solitary or multinodular and present well-circumscribed or ill-defined infiltrative borders. The size at the time of diagnosis often is directly related to the ease of clinical detection; superficial variants may be but a few centimeters in diameter, whereas those arising in the retroperitoneum often attain a diameter of 15 cm or greater. Color and consistency vary considerably and relate to the proportion of stromal and cellular elements. The myxoid variant contains a predominance of white-gray, soft mucoid tumor lobules, reflecting the high content of myxoid ground substance. Red-brown areas of hemorrhage and necrosis are not uncommon. Approximately 5 percent of MFHs undergo extensive hemorrhagic cystification, often leading to a clinical diagnosis of hematoma.[122]

Microscopic Characteristics The broad histological spectrum encompasses many variants which were formerly considered to be distinct clinicopathological entities. These variants, which are named according to the predominant cell type, include fibroxanthosarcoma, malignant fibroxanthoma, inflammatory fibrous histiocytoma, and malignant giant cell tumor of soft parts. The basic cellular constituents of all fibrohistiocytic tumors include fibroblasts, histiocyte-like cells, and mesenchymal cells. The proportion of these cellular elements and their degree of maturation account for the wide variety of histological patterns. The storiform type, which is the most common variant, is so named because the spindle and histiocytic cells form a storiform, that is, cartwheel, pattern. There can be a considerable degree of pleomorphism with the appearance of atypical and bizarre giant cells, often containing abnormal mitotic figures. Chronic inflammatory cells along with xanthoma cells often permeate the stroma. In the myxoid variant, the tumor cells are dispersed in a richly myxoid matrix. Diagnosis depends on the recognition of the cytological atypia and presence of mitotic figures. The less common giant cell type (malignant giant cell tumor of soft parts) is characterized by abundant osteoclast-like giant cells diffusely distributed among the fibrohistiocytic elements.

Fibrosarcoma

Fibrosarcoma used to be considered the most common STS. Following the identification of MFH as a distinct entity, fibrosarcoma is now quite rare. Clinical and histological difficulty occasionally arises in differentiating low-grade fibrosarcoma from fibromatosis and its variants. The anatomic site, age, and histological findings must be carefully evaluated.

Gross Characteristics This neoplasm usually arises from the fascial and aponeurotic structures of the deep soft tissues; superficial variants are rare. The smaller tumors present as partially to completely circumscribed masses. As the lesions enlarge, a more diffusely infiltrative pattern predominates.

Microscopic Characteristics The fundamental cell of this neoplasm is the fibroblast, a spindle cell capable of producing collagen fiber. The collagen matrix can be easily identified in the more differentiated fibrosarcomas; moreover, its presence can be confirmed with the application of Masson's trichrome stain. Well-differentiated fibrosarcoma is characterized by intersecting fascicles of relatively uniform spindle cells showing minimal atypical features and sparse mitotic figures. The fascicles often intersect at acute angles and form the typical herringbone pattern (Fig. 23-2). In contrast, poorly differentiated fibrosarcoma often has a barely discernible fascicular arrangement. Furthermore, the cells show increased

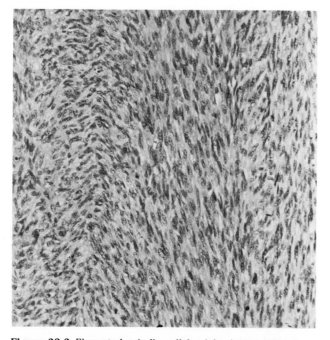

Figure 23-2 Elongated spindle cell fascicles intersecting at acute angles form the characteristic "herringbone" pattern of fibrosarcoma.

TABLE 23-3 Histological Classification of Liposarcoma

Well-differentiated liposarcoma
  Lipoma-like
  Sclerosing
  Inflammatory
  Dedifferentiated

Myxoid liposarcoma

Round cell liposarcoma

Pleomorphic liposarcoma

pleomorphism and nuclear atypia and often have a brisk mitotic rate. In the latter presentation, distinction from MFH may be exceedingly difficult.

Liposarcoma

Liposarcoma is a common STS. It has a wide range of malignant potential dependent upon the grade of the individual tumor. Determination of subtype and grade is essential to appropriate management. Grade I liposarcomas rarely metastasize. Unlike other sarcomas, liposarcomas may be multiple and occur in unusual sites within the same individual. Careful evaluation of other masses in a patient with a liposarcoma is mandatory. Occasionally, these lesions occur in children. Liposarcomas rarely arise from preexisting benign lipomas.

Gross Characteristics Liposarcomas, particularly those arising in the retroperitoneum, can become quite large; examples measuring 10 to 15 cm are not unusual. The tumors tend to be well-circumscribed and multilobulated. The color and consistency observed on cut section usually correlate with the histological type. Well-differentiated liposarcomas, containing variable proportions of relatively mature fat and fibrocollagenous tissue, vary from yellow to white-gray and can be soft, firm, or rubbery. A tumor which is soft and pink-tan and reveals a mucinous surface is typical of myxoid liposarcoma. The high-grade liposarcomas (round cell and pleomorphic) vary from pink-tan to brown and may disclose hemorrhagic and necrotic foci.

Microscopic Characteristics A current histological classification of liposarcoma recognizes four distinct types (Table 23-3). Regardless of the histological type, the identification of typical lipoblasts is mandatory to establish the diagnosis of liposarcoma. The lipoblast contains one, several, or multiple round, cytoplasmic fat droplets which form sharp, scalloped indentations on the central or peripheral nucleus.

Well-differentiated liposarcomas often contain a predominance of mature fat cells with a few, widely scattered lipoblasts. In the sclerosing subtype, delicate collagen fibrils that encircle fat cells and lipoblasts constitute a prominent part of the matrix (Fig. 23-3). A diagnosis of myxoid liposarcoma is based on the presence of a delicate plexiform capillary network associated with both primitive mesenchyme-like cells and a variable number of lipoblasts. The stroma contains a high proportion of myxoid ground substance (hyaluronic acid) which, in areas, may form microcyst-like collections. In round cell liposarcoma, the lipoblasts are interspersed within sheets of poorly differentiated roundcells. Pleomorphic liposarcoma is characterized by an admixture of bizarre, often multivacuolated, lipoblasts and atypical stromal cells, many of which contain highly abnormal mitotic figures. Areas of hemorrhage and necrosis are common.

Synovial Sarcoma

Synovial sarcomas are the fourth most common STS. They characteristically have a biphasic pattern which gives the impression of glandular formation and suggests a synovial origin. These tumors, however, do *not* arise from a joint and have a distribution similar to those of other STSs. Synovial sarcomas occur in a younger age group than other sarcomas; 72 percent of patients in one large study were below the age of 40 years. There is a propensity for the distal portions of extremities; hand (5 percent), ankle (9 percent), or foot (13 percent). The plain radiograph often shows small calcifications within a soft tissue mass; this should alert the physician to the diagnosis. Occasionally lymphatic spread occurs (5 to 7 percent). Virtually all synovial sarcomas are high-grade.

Gross Characteristics Typically the tumor presents as a deep-seated, well-circumscribed, multinodular firm mass. Actual contiguity with a synovium-lined space is rare. It is common to find solitary or multiple cysts on sectioning the lesion. The poorly differentiated variety is likely to present as an ill-defined, infiltrative lesion with a soft, somewhat gelatinous consistency.

Microscopic Characteristics The classic form of this tumor is a biphasic pattern (Fig. 23-4). This implies the presence of

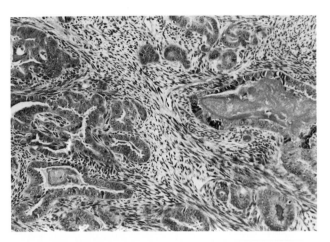

Figure 23-4 Typical synovial sarcoma in its biphasic form characterized by glandlike structures lined by cuboidal cells intimately associated with a spindle cell sarcomatous component.

two distinct cell populations; namely, spindle cells and epithelioid cells. The plump spindle cells, usually the predominant component, form an interlacing fascicular pattern. The epithelioid cells form either solid nests or glandlike structures. When constituting glandular spaces, the cells range from cuboidal to tall and columnar and rarely undergo squamous metaplasia. The application of special stains demonstrates that the lumina of these glandular spaces contain epithelial-type mucins. The neoplasm may contain extensive areas of dense stromal hyalinization, and focal calcification is common. The presence of extensive areas of calcification, sometimes with modulation to benign osteoid, deserves recognition, as this variant imparts a significantly more favorable prognosis. Within the spindle cell portion of the tumor, areas resembling the branching vascular pattern of hemangiopericytoma commonly occur. The existence of a monophasic spindle cell sarcoma is recognized, although distinction from fibrosarcoma can be exceedingly difficult.

Epithelioid Sarcoma

Epithelioid sarcoma was first described in 1970.[32] It is an unusually small tumor that is often misdiagnosed as a benign lesion. It occurs in the forearm and wrist one-half the time and is the most common sarcoma of the hand. This lesion has a propensity for eventual lymph node involvement. Unlike other sarcomas, it occurs predominantly in adolescents and young adults (average age 26 years). When it arises in the dermis, whereby it presents as a nodular or ulcerative process, it often simulates benign cutaneous diseases.

Gross Characteristics The tumor usually arises in the deep soft tissues, particularly in relation to tendons, fascia, and aponeuroses, and presents as a firm, often multinodular, mass. Central nodular hemorrhage and/or necrosis is occasionally encountered.

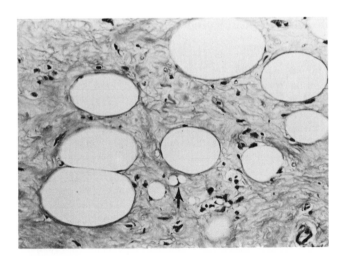

Figure 23-3 In the sclerosing type of well-differentiated liposarcoma, delicate collagen fibrils constitute a prominent part of the matrix. Note the bivacuolated lipoblast (*arrow*).

Microscopic Characteristics The typical low-power picture is that of nodules or granuloma-like collections of epithelioid cells. These are large cells with deeply eosinophilic cytoplasm and with nuclei which tend to be angulated and hyperchromatic. Mitotic figures are occasionally seen. The predominant epithelioid cells often transform to plump spindle cells. A characteristic feature of this tumor is the rather diffuse infiltration of tendinous and fascial structures by small elongated nests of tumor cells.

Clear Cell Sarcoma (Malignant Melanoma of Soft Parts)

Clear cell sarcoma is a small, unusual neoplasm that arises in conjunction with tendons or aponeuroses. Clear cell sarcomas occur most often around the foot and ankle (46 percent) and in persons between 20 and 40 years of age.[32] The histogenesis is unknown but is considered by some to be related to melanoma; 50 percent of these lesions contain melanin. Appropriate diagnosis depends on special histological stains—Fontana preparation for melanin, periodic acid Schiff (PAS) for intracellular glycogen, and reticulin stains to demonstrate a nesting pattern. Lymphatic as well as hematogenous spread occurs. One must examine the regional lymph nodes carefully. If there is any suggestion of enlargement, a lymph node dissection is recommended.

Gross Characteristics The neoplasm presents as a solitary or multinodular firm mass frequently attached to tendons or aponeuroses. The tumor infrequently exceeds 6 cm in diameter and varies from white to brown on cut surface.

Microscopic Characteristics The characteristic feature of this neoplasm is the formation of distinct fascicles and nests of spindle cells that are separated by well-defined collagenous trabeculae. The uniform spindle cells are often plump and contain pale to faintly eosinophilic cytoplasm. In addition, the cells contain a vesicular nucleus with a prominent solitary nucleolus. Frequently, bland-appearing multinucleated giant cells are found within the spindle cell fascicles. Application of special stains discloses that the clear spindle cells contain glycogen (PAS$^+$) and that melanin pigment is present in half of the tumors.

Neurofibrosarcoma (Malignant Schwannoma)

Neurofibrosarcomas (NFSs) are malignant tumors that arise from peripheral nerves. They represent about 10 percent of all sarcomas. A large percentage (25 to 67 percent) are associated with von Recklinghausen's disease.[32] In general, patients with von Recklinghausen's disease are at high risk (3 to 13 percent) for developing sarcomas, and the risk increases with each decade of life. Unlike other sarcomas, an NFS often presents with neurological symptoms (pain, paresthesia, and weakness), reflecting its relation to major peripheral nerves. An NFS not associated with neurofibromastosis tends to occur in an older age group. An extremity mass associated with neurological symptoms must be considered malignant and be evaluated by the appropriate staging studies.

Gross Characteristics This neoplasm presents as a fusiform or bulbous enlargement of a large nerve, usually within the deep soft tissues. As the tumor enlarges and infiltrates the adjacent soft tissues, its origin from and relation to the nerve structure is frequently obscured. On section, the gray to white neoplasm varies from firm to soft with areas of necrosis and hemorrhage.

Microscopic Characteristics The basic pattern consists of intersecting spindle cell fascicles, not unlike that observed with fibrosarcoma or leiomyosarcoma. However, the presence of certain differential features supports the diagnosis of a malignant nerve sheath tumor. The slender nuclei of the spindle cells tend to be wavy or buckled. A palisading pattern, although not pathognomonic, typifies this entity. In areas, the spindle cells may form a whorled or spiral arrangement. The rarely encountered epithelioid variant may closely resemble malignant melanoma or even carcinoma. Infrequently, heterologous elements, such as osteoid, chondroid, skeletal muscle, or glandular structures, arise within the spindle cell background.

BENIGN SOFT TISSUE TUMORS

All mesenchymal tissue can give rise to benign lesions. Occasionally they can be confused with malignant lesions, or they may become symptomatic due to their size, anatomic location, or both. Although these tumors are benign, local recurrence or difficult anatomic location can cause significant morbidity. Some, such as lipomas, are easily cured by simple removal, while others, most notably fibromatoses, require extensive resection. Thus, it is important to differentiate these lesions from their malignant counterparts, establish a correct diagnosis, and remove them surgically.

There are a large number of benign lesions. The more common lesions and their unique characteristics are described.

Benign Adipose Tumors

Simple Lipoma

Lipomas, the most common mesenchymal neoplasm, arise from normal fat and appear during adulthood. They may be single or multiple; the latter occur in only 5 percent of all patients. They are found either subcutaneously or deeply embedded. Eighty percent of all lipomas are of the simple type.[32] The shoulder girdle and proximal thigh are the two most common sites. Simple surgical excision is curative.

Gross Characteristics Superficial lipomas, arising within the subcutaneous layer, present as well-circumscribed, movable, round to ovoid masses. The lesions reveal, on cut section, a homogeneous pale- to bright-yellow tissue. Deep lipomas, which are much rarer than the superficial variety, may occur in an intermuscular space. The gross appearance of these lipomas is indistinguishable from that of the superficial type.

Microscopic Characteristics Both types of lipoma consist of monotonous sheets of mature fat cells which are ovoid to round and usually contain a single fat droplet which compresses the nucleus along the cell membrane. Capillary-like vessels occasionally appear between the fat lobules. Areas of myxoid change or dense fibrous trabeculae are sometimes encountered.

Spindle Cell Lipoma

This is a variant of lipoma consisting of benign spindle cells in addition to mature fat. The most common location is the neck and shoulder. Spindle cell lipomas are encapsulated and are easily removed by simple excision. It is essential to distinguish this lesion clinically from a well-differentiated (pleomorphic) liposarcoma.

Gross Characteristics Both these benign lipomatous tumors are similar to and usually indistinguishable from the ordinary lipoma. They invariably arise within the subcutis and are encapsulated with a delicate fibrous membrane. On sectioning, they vary from diffuse yellow to having foci of white firm fibrous tissue or even gray myxoid areas.

Microscopic Characteristics Spindle cell lipoma reveals a component of mature adipose tissue with rare to abundant clusters of spindle cells dispersed throughout the fat. The spindle cells are uniform and in parallel arrangement. Mitotic figures are rarely noted.

Pleomorphic lipomas also consist of mature fat cells, but they are more variable in size. Instead of spindle cells, both pleomorphic and distinctive multinucleated giant cells are found. These giant cells contain multiple peripheral overlapping nuclei. Occasionally, lipoblast-like cells occur.

Intramuscular and Intermuscular Lipoma

Lipomas occurring within (intramuscular) and between (intermuscular) muscle groups often become large, produce few symptoms, and present as a mass mimicking an STS. Clinical evaluation and staging are similar to those of any suspected sarcoma. The pathologist must be aware of the clinical setting, and an adequate sample must be obtained in order to differentiate a low-grade liposarcoma from a true benign lipoma. Unlike superficial lipomas, these lesions often do not have a capsule and tend to infiltrate the surrounding muscle. A marginal or wide resection is required to obtain local control. These lesions never become malignant.

Gross Characteristics This tumor presents either as a relatively well delineated yellow mass clearly distinguishable from the surrounding skeletal muscle or as an ill-defined infiltrative lesion that gradually blends into the adjacent muscle tissue.

Microscopic Characteristics The lesion is characterized by sheets and nests of mature adipose tissue insinuating between bundles and individual fibers of viable skeletal muscle. The fat cells lack features of cytological atypia, and lipoblasts never occur.

Benign Tumors of Peripheral Nerves

The two most common nerve tumors are neurilemmoma (schwannoma) and neurofibroma.

Neurilemmoma

These benign growths arise within a nerve and are surrounded by a true capsule composed of the epineurium. They are composed of Antoni A (cellular) and Antoni B (loose myxoid) components. These lesions generally are not associated with von Recklinghausen's disease. Surgical treatment entails opening the capsule and enucleating the growth from the nerve. "Ancient" neurilemmoma is cystic degeneration of a neurilemmoma. These lesions clinically present as a large mass with some cellular atypia. They must be differentiated from malignant lesions. Simple excision, done for diagnostic purposes or if the lesion is symptomatic, is curative.

Gross Characteristics These tumors are invariably encapsulated and range from fusiform to ovoid. It is usually possible to demonstrate the nerve of origin. The tissue varies from white to yellow. As the lesion increases in size, there is a greater likelihood of cystic degeneration and focal hemorrhage.

Microscopic Characteristics Reliable diagnosis depends on the identification of the two basic cell patterns, the so-called Antoni A and Antoni B areas. The Antoni A pattern, the more cellular of the two, is characterized by plump spindle cells arranged in fascicles, palisaded rows, or whorls (Fig. 23-5). The parallel alignment of two rows of nuclei has been called a *Verocay body*. An Antoni B area discloses a nonpatterned distribution of spindle cells in a loose, somewhat myxoid matrix (Fig. 23-6). There may be a sprinkling of chronic inflammatory cells and clusters of xanthoma cells.

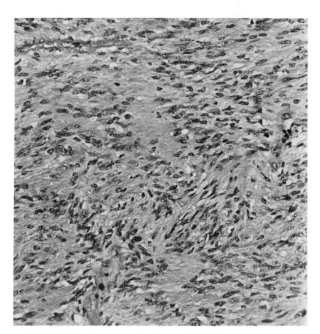

Figure 23-5 The solid, or Antoni A, portion of a neurilemmoma with an area of nuclear palisading.

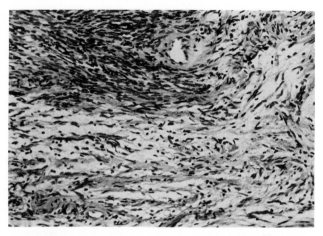

Figure 23-6 In contrast to the Antoni A pattern, the Antoni B region reveals a less organized cellularity dispersed in a loose myxoid matrix.

Neurofibroma

Neurofibromas may be solitary or multiple. Unlike the neurilemmomas, they are not encapsulated, often enlarge the nerves, and may undergo malignant degeneration. Histologically they consist of Schwann cells associated with collagen fibrils and myxoid material. Multiple neurofibromas are found in patients with von Recklinghausen disease (multiple neurofibromatosis). These lesions cannot be surgically detached from the underlying nerve. Surgery is indicated only if malignant degeneration is suspected. Between 20 and 65 percent of patients with neurofibromatosis ultimately develop a sarcoma.

Gross Characteristics These lesions may be encapsulated, although they usually infiltrate into adjacent soft tissues.

Microscopic Characteristics The tumor is characterized by individual or slender bundles of elongated wavy spindle cells closely apposed to dense fibers of mature collagen. Groups of these spindle cell–collagen units randomly intersect at variable angles. The matrix, which is rich in hyaluronic acid, can be sparse or present as a highly myxoid background; in the latter case they often obscure the nerve sheath origin of the lesion. The spindle cell nuclei occasionally appear hyperchromatic or pleomorphic, yet mitotic figures are exceedingly rare.

Benign Fibrous Tumors

There is a large variety of benign fibrous tumors.[32] Most are treated by simple excision. Aggressive fibromatosis is a benign but locally aggressive lesion deserving special consideration.

Aggressive Fibromatosis

This tumor, which appears harmless microscopically, is the most serious of all the benign soft tissue tumors. It does not have a capsule and tends to infiltrate far beyond its recognized boundaries. This lesion does not respect fascial borders and thus can attain a large size involving multiple anatomic compartments if left untreated. The most common locations are the neck, shoulder, and pelvic girdle. Death results from intrathoracic or retroperitoneal extension. The clinical history often reveals multiple recurrences despite "adequate" surgical removal. The appropriate surgical procedure is wide excision. Local recurrence uniformly follows excision with positive margins. Surgical staging studies should be performed prior to resection. Amputation is occasionally required. Radiation and chemotherapy have recently been utilized for unresectable fibromatosis.

Gross Characteristics The general category of fibromatosis can be split into two subtypes. The superficial fibromatoses encompass, among others, the palmar (Dupuytren's contracture) and plantar types. Among the deep fibromatoses (desmoids) are the abdominal and extraabdominal varieties. Palmar and plantar fibromatoses appear identical and range from foci of thickened fascia to individual or coalescent firm nodules. In contrast, the abdominal and extraabdominal fibromatoses present as firm, often multinodular, masses, which arise from fascial planes and infiltrate, to some extent, into the adjacent skeletal muscle. These lesions can attain a rather large size. They tend to be firm, and the cut surface reveals a white-gray tissue.

Microscopic Characteristics The hallmark of both the superficial and the deep varieties is the uniformity of the spindle cells and the regularity of the pattern. The cellularity can be focally increased, particularly in the superficial types, yet the arrangement of uniform spindle cells in a typical nodular or fascicular pattern is maintained. The matrix consists of a variable quantity of mature, dense collagen bundles. At the deep margin of the deep fibromatoses, infiltration of underlying skeletal muscle is characteristic and does not by itself serve as a valid basis for a diagnosis of fibrosarcoma.

Benign Vascular Tumors

Hemangioma

Benign tumors of the blood vessels consist of a variety of hemangiomas. It is not certain if these are true neoplasms, hamartomas, or vascular malformations. In general there are two types of hemangiomas, generalized and localized; localized are more common. Hemangiomas are classified based upon their pathological appearance—capillary, cavernous, venous, or arteriovenous. Capillary hemangiomas are the most common type. Most hemangiomas occur during childhood. Venous hemangiomas occur during adulthood and are often deeply situated. Intramuscular hemangiomas are rare and are occasionally difficult to differentiate from angiosarcomas. Evaluation requires angiography and venography. Surgery is indicated if symptoms develop. Hemangiomas rarely become malignant.

Gross Characteristics The gross characteristics depend in large part on the histological variety and anatomic distribu-

TABLE 23-4 Classification of Soft Tissue Vascular Tumors

I. Benign
   Localized hemangioma
      Capillary hemangioma
      Cavernous hemangioma
      Venous hemangioma
      Arteriovenous hemangioma
      Epithelioid hemangioma
      Deep soft tissue hemangiomas (synovial, intramuscular, neural)
   Diffuse hemangioma
      Angiomatosis

II. Borderline malignancy
   Epithelioid hemangioendothelioma

III. Malignant
   Angiosarcoma
   Kaposi's sarcoma

Source: Enzinger, F.M., and Weiss, S.W.: *Soft Tissue Tumors,* 1983.

tion of the hemangioma (Table 23-4). The localized types tend to appear as a well-circumscribed, red-to-purple mass, although examples with poorly defined, infiltrative borders, particularly in the deep-seated hemangiomas, are not uncommon. Intramuscular hemangioma (infiltrating angiolipoma) can present as a red highly vascular lesion or as a yellow-to-gray firm mass, depending on the proportion of the vascular component to the amount of accompanying adipose tissue and fibrous stroma.

Angiomatosis indicates a benign condition in which multiple types of tissue are involved. Large anatomic regions, even an entire limb, may be affected. These extensive vascular lesions, which are probably hamartomatous, can involve the skin, subcutaneous fat, skeletal muscle, fascia, and bone. Involvement of an entire extremity can cause hypertrophy of the limb.

Microscopic Characteristics Pure types of vascular tumors are uncommon; there tends to be some degree of admixture of small and large vessels. Capillary hemangioma consists of myriad small vascular channels lined by a flattened endothelial layer. Particularly in some juvenile types of capillary hemangioma, the vascular channels may be miniature and a highly cellular stroma predominates. Cavernous hemangioma, in contrast, is characterized by large, engorged vascular channels separated by fibrocollagenous septa.

The diagnosis of intramuscular hemangioma or angiomatosis usually requires clinical and gross pathological correlation. At the microscopic level, these entities are nonspecific, except that the identification of adjacent skeletal muscle or other soft tissue elements indicates the extensive involvement of the lesion. The vessels, as in the circumscribed hemangiomas, are well-formed and vary from capillary to venous size. There is a single flat endothelial layer. The extravascular stroma contains adipose tissue and sometimes fibromuscular fascicles.

Pigmented Villonodular Synovitis

Pigmented villonodular synovitis (PVS) is a rare primary disease of the synovium characterized by exuberant proliferation with the formation of villi and nodules. It presents with localized pain, joint swelling, a thickened synovium, and an effusion which on aspiration shows either a brownish or a serosanguineous discoloration. PVS commonly occurs between the second and the fifth decade of life. The knee is most commonly involved (75 to 90 percent), followed by the hip and ankle joint. Treatment is often delayed because PVS is not considered in the differential diagnosis. Clinical suspicion is the key to early diagnosis. PVS should be considered in the differential diagnosis of a monoarticular arthritis of the knee or hip joint. Simple aspiration is often suggestive, and a synovial biopsy is definitive. Plain radiographs demonstrate juxtacortical erosions of both sides of an affected joint and may show marked joint and/or bone destruction if the disease has been present for a long time. Arthrography and/or arthroscopy are helpful in establishing the correct diagnosis. Arthrography shows diffuse nodular masses, while arthroscopy shows a brownish, discolored synovium with large, flattened nodules and villous proliferation. Rarely, PVS may present as a primary bony or soft tissue tumor due to marked proliferation of the synovium with destruction of the adjacent joint and/or a soft tissue mass. The histological findings in this clinical situation may incorrectly suggest a MFH.

PVS is treated by surgical excision. Localized lesions require simple excision, while extensive involvement requires a synovectomy. The anterior and/or posterior compartments of the knee may be extensively involved. This necessitates a staged approach. The anterior joint is treated through a standard midline incision and arthrotomy. The posterior knee is best approached by a popliteal incision with complete exposure of the posterior capsule. In general, it is the author's preference first to proceed with the anterior synovectomy and regain knee motion, and secondarily to perform a posterior synovectomy. Joint manipulation is often required at 10 days. Recurrent disease should be retreated by surgical excision. If there is extensive bony destruction, arthrodesis or prosthetic replacement, combined with an extraarticular joint resection, is required.

Gross Characteristics The thick synovium is variegated tan-brown to yellow and ranges from villous to nodular.

Microscopic Characteristics The typical lesion consists of heterogeneous cells. The villi are lined by several layers of plump synovial cells (Fig. 23-7). Beneath the synovium are found sheets of histiocytes, xanthoma cells, hemosiderin-laden macrophages, and multinucleated giant cells, all in variable proportion. Occasionally, slitlike spaces are present within the more cellular areas.

Ganglion

Ganglia are among the most common soft tissue lesions treated by the orthopaedic surgeon. The wrist is the most common location; other sites include the metatarsophalangeal joints and the ankle and knee joints. When the lesions are

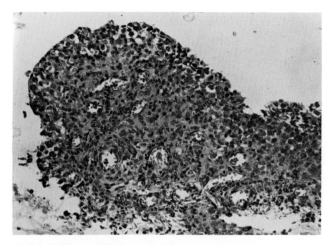

Figure 23-7 In pigmented villonodular synovitis, there is hyperplasia of the surface synovial cells and the stroma is filled with inflammatory cells, histiocytes, and hemosiderin-laden macrophages.

located in unusual sites, the diagnosis is often less obvious. Ganglia represent benign myxoid degeneration. It must be emphasized that all masses are not ganglia and should be critically evaluated. All too often a sarcoma of the hand or ankle is assumed to be a ganglion. Excision is undertaken, and the correct diagnosis is made only after extensive soft tissue contamination has occurred. This unfortunate circumstance leads to many lost limbs. Treatment of ganglia is simple excision or aspiration.

Gross Characteristics Ganglia are uniloculated or multiloculated cystic lesions arising in dense ligamentous tissue. The cysts contain a translucent gelatinous material the expression of which results in the partial collapse of the thin-walled cysts.

Microscopic Characteristics The cyst walls consist of a dense paucicellular collagenous tissue lacking an epithelial or synovial lining. The intercystic connective tissue often contains small foci of myxoid stroma with scattered spindle cells.

MALIGNANT BONE TUMORS

Malignant bone tumors consist of primary mesenchymal tumors, those arising from the bone marrow (multiple myeloma), and those resulting from metastasis of a carcinoma. Osteosarcoma and Ewing's sarcoma, the most common malignant mesenchymal bone tumors, usually occur during childhood and adolescence. Other mesenchymal tumors (MFH, fibrosarcoma, chondrosarcoma) also occur occasionally during childhood. Multiple myeloma and metastatic carcinoma commonly involve the skeletal system and occur in adults. This section describes the clinical, radiographic, and pathological characteristics and treatment of the primary bone sarcomas. Orthopaedic considerations of multiple myeloma and metastatic carcinoma are emphasized. Table 23-5 presents a general classification of the benign and malignant

TABLE 23-5   General Classification of Bone Tumors*

Histological type	Distribution, % [†]	Benign	Malignant
Hematopoietic	41.4		Myeloma
			Reticulum cell sarcoma
Chondrogenic	20.9	Osteochondroma	Primary chondrosarcoma
		Chondroma	Secondary chondrosarcoma
		Chondroblastoma	Dedifferentiated chondrosarcoma
		Chondromyxoid fibroma	Mesenchymal chondrosarcoma
Osteogenic	19.3	Osteoid osteoma	Osteosarcoma
		Benign osteoblastoma	Parosteal osteogenic sarcoma
Unknown origin	9.8	Giant cell tumor	Ewing's tumor
			Malignant giant cell tumor
			Adamantinoma
		(Fibrous) histiocytoma	(Fibrous) histiocytoma
Fibrogenic	3.8	Fibroma	Fibrosarcoma
		Desmoplastic fibroma	
Notochordal	3.1		Chordoma
Vascular	1.6	Hemangioma	Hemangioendothelioma
			Hemangiopericytoma
Lipogenic	<0.5	Lipoma	
Neurogenic	<0.5	Neurilemmoma	

*Classification based on Lichtenstein: Cancer 4:335–351, 1951.
†Distribution based on Mayo Clinic experience.
Source: Adapted from Dahlin, D.C.: *Bone Tumors: General Aspects and Data on 6,221 Cases*, 3rd ed. Springfield, IL, Charles C. Thomas, 1978.

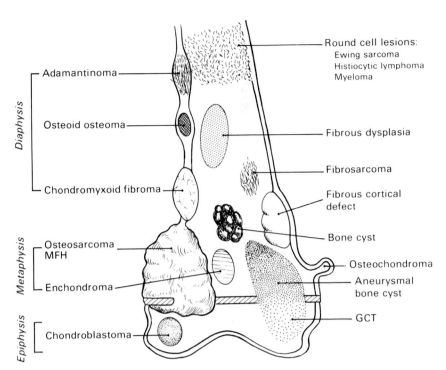

Figure 23-8 Common anatomic location of benign and malignant bone tumors with respect to the diaphysis, metaphysis, and epiphysis of the bone. *(From Madewell, J.E., Ragsdale, B.D., Sweet, D.E.: Radio Clin North Am 19:715–814, 1981. Modified and reproduced with permission.)*

bone tumor as described by Dahlin et al. Their characteristic locations within a bone are shown schematically in Fig. 23-8.

Classic Osteosarcoma

Osteosarcoma (OS) is a high-grade malignant spindle cell tumor arising within a bone. Its distinguishing characteristic is the production of "tumor" osteoid, or immature bone, directly from a malignant spindle cell stroma.[15,17,19,104]

Clinical Characteristics

OS typically occurs during childhood and adolescence. In patients over the age of 40, it is usually associated with a preexistent disease such as Paget disease, irradiated bones, multiple hereditary exostosis, or polyostotic fibrous dysplasia.[15,17] The most common sites are bones of knee joint (50 percent) and the proximal humerus (25 percent). Between 80 and 90 percent occur in the long tubular bones;[1,3,15,17,45,91,92,12] the axial skeleton is rarely affected.

With the exception of the level of serum alkaline phosphatase, which is elevated in 45 to 50 percent of patients, laboratory findings are usually not helpful.[33] Furthermore, an elevated alkaline phosphatase level per se is not diagnostic since it is also found in association with other skeletal diseases such as hyperparathyroidism (brown tumor), fibrous dysplasia, and Paget disease. Pain is the most common complaint. Incidence of pathologic fracture is less than 1 percent.[33] Systemic symptoms are rare. A mass is a common finding.

Radiographic Characteristics

Typical findings are increased intramedullary radiodensity (due to tumor bone or calcified cartilage), an area of radiolucency (due to nonossified tumor), a pattern of permeative destruction with poorly defined borders, cortical destruction, periosteal elevation, and extraosseous extension with soft tissue ossification.[25,124] This combination of characteristics is not seen in any other lesions. Wilner classified 600 radiographs of OS seen at New York's Memorial Sloan-Kettering into three broad categories:[124] sclerotic OS (32 percent), osteolytic OS (22 percent), and mixed (46 percent) (Fig. 23-9). Although there was no statistically significant difference among overall survival rates of these types, it is important to recognize the patterns. The sclerotic and mixed type offer few diagnostic problems. Errors of diagnosis most often occur with pure osteolytic tumors. The differential diagnosis of osteolytic OS includes giant cell tumor, aneurysmal bone cyst, fibrosarcoma, and MFH.[21]

Gross Characteristics

This tumor is central in origin, but at the time of diagnosis there is often already substantial cortical destruction. Continued growth of the lesion results in bulky involvement of the adjacent soft tissues. As the neoplasm extends through the cortex, the periosteum may be elevated; this stimulates reactive bone formation and accounts for the radiological features of the so-called Codman's triangle. Longitudinal sectioning of the involved bone often reveals wide extension within the marrow cavity. Rarely, skip areas can be demonstrated.[1] The consistency of the tumor varies greatly and generally reflects

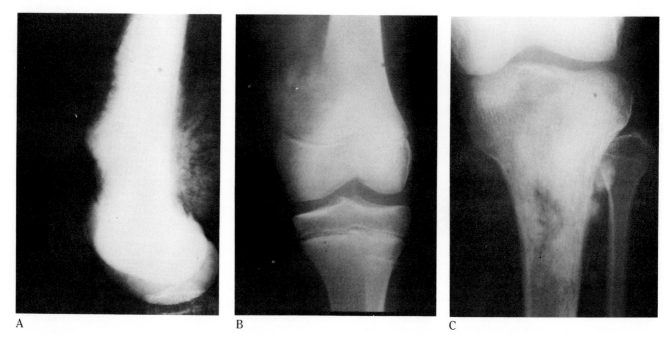

A   B   C

Figure 23-9 The three radiographic patterns of osteosarcoma. **A.** Sclerosing. **B.** Osteolytic. **C.** Mixed (osteolytic and osteoblastic). Mixed is the most common. There is no correlation between radiographic type and survival. All three show extraosseous new bone formation. This is pathognomonic of a bone-forming neo- plasm. *(From Malawer, M.M., Abelson, H.T., and Suit, H.D., in DeVita, V.T., Hellman, S., and Rosenberg, S.A., eds: Cancer: Principles and Practice of Oncology, 2d ed. Philadelphia, Lippincott, 1985. Reproduced with permission.)*

the predominant histological composition. There may be soft necrotic and hemorrhagic foci. Sclerotic and bony regions reflect a preponderance of fibrotic or osteoblastic elements, respectively. Occasionally, a lobulated cartilaginous appearance is observed.

Microscopic Characteristics

The diagnosis of OS is based on the identification of a malignant stroma which produces unequivocal osteoid matrix. The stroma consists of a haphazard arrangement of highly atypical cells. The pleomorphic cells contain hyperchromatic, irregular nuclei. Mitotic figures, often atypical, are usually easy to identify. Between these cells is a delicate, lacelike eosinophilic matrix, assumed to be malignant osteoid. Both malignant and benign osteoblast-like giant cells can be found in the stroma. An abundance of the latter type can create confusion with giant cell tumor of bone.

A predominance of one tissue type has resulted in a histological subclassification of OS.[57] The term *osteoblastic osteosarcoma* is utilized for those tumors in which the production of malignant osteoid prevails. The pattern is usually that of a delicate meshwork of osteoid, as noted above, although broader confluent areas can be present (Fig. 23-10). Calcification of the matrix is variable. Some tumors reveal a predominance of malignant cartilage production; hence, the term *chondroblastic osteosarcoma.* Even though the malignant cartilaginous elements may be overwhelming, the presence of a malignant osteoid matrix warrants the diagnosis of OS. Yet another variant is characterized by large areas of proliferating fibroblasts, arranged in intersecting fascicles. Such areas are

indistinguishable from fibrosarcoma, and thorough sampling may be necessary to identify the malignant osteoid component. The so-called telangiectatic type of OS contains multiple, blood-filled cystic and sinusoidal spaces of variable size. Identification of marked cytological atypia in the septa and in more solid areas rules out the diagnosis of aneurysmal bone cyst.

The advent of several successful chemotherapeutic regi-

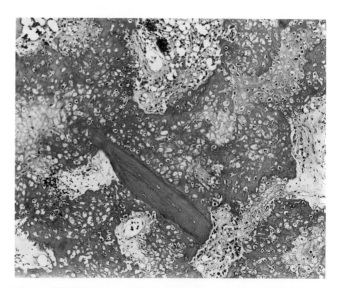

Figure 23-10 Broad coalescent sheets of malignant osteoid typify this osteoblastic osteosarcoma. The spicule of lamellar bone is a remnant of the normal medullary bone.

mens for OS has permitted the examination of multiple post-therapy radical resection specimens.[49] The degree of tumor necrosis is variable and ranges between 0 and 100 percent. The osteoid or osseous matrix remains, without its accompanying cellular component. There may be growth of a reparative type of connective tissue with fibroblastic proliferation and clusters of small vessels. The spindle cells may reveal a degree of cytological atypia.

Prognosis

Prior to adjuvant chemotherapy, treatment consisted of amputation. Metastasis to the lungs and other bones generally occurred within 24 months. Overall survival ranged from 5 to 20 percent at 2 years.[8,52,73] This pattern has been altered by adjuvant chemotherapy and aggressive thoracotomy for pulmonary disease.[16,38] Less common sites of metastases may now be involved, and disease-free intervals are longer.[8]

Localized Extremity OS The traditional procedure for localized OS has been amputation one joint above the tumor-containing bone or, in some cases, transmedullary amputation.[7,8,15,17,52,73,115] Within the past decade parallel developments in radiology, orthopaedics, and oncology have made nonamputative procedures an option in select patients.[11,26,28,34,53,64,67,70,71,75,87,107,120] A significant impetus for these developments was the introduction of effective chemotherapeutic agents in the early 1970s.[12,13,51,88,100,101] Today adjuvant chemotherapy is considered efficacious in the treatment of nonmetastatic OS. In general, high-dose methotrexate (HDMTX), doxorubicin hydrochloride, and cisplatin are the most effective agents. Several combinations and dosage schedules are recommended. Overall cures have increased from a range of 15 to 20 percent (historical controls) to a range of 40 to 80 percent (modern trials) because of the use of these adjuvants. Polydrug regimens are now recommended for all patients with OS.

The unique features of evaluation, management, and surgical resection of tumors of the most common anatomic areas are discussed in Chaps. 46, Sect. A, and 74. Guidelines and principles discussed in the following section are applicable to all bone sarcomas except round cell tumors.

Limb-Sparing Resection Limb salvage surgery is a safe operation in select individuals.[26,28,34,67,70,71,75,87,110] This technique may be utilized for all spindle cell sarcomas, regardless of histogenesis. The majority of OSs can be treated safely by a limb-sparing resection. The successful management of localized OS and other sarcomas requires careful coordination and timing of staging studies, biopsy, surgery, and preoperative and postoperative chemotherapy and/or radiation therapy. The site of the lesion is evaluated as previously described. Preoperative studies allow the surgeon to conceptualize the local anatomy and the volume of tissue to be resected and reconstructed. All patients can be considered candidates for limb-sparing procedures unless a surgical oncologist familiar with these procedures feels that a nonamputative option has little chance of success.

Successful limb-sparing procedures consist of three surgical phases.[63]

1. *Resection of tumor* Resection strictly follows the principles of oncological surgery. Avoiding local recurrence is the criterion of success and the main determinant of the amount of bone and soft tissue to be removed.
2. *Skeletal reconstruction* The average skeletal defect following adequate bone tumor resection measures 15 to 20 cm. Techniques of reconstruction (prosthetic replacement, arthrodesis, or allograft) vary and are independent of the resection, although the degree of resection may favor one technique over the other.
3. *Soft tissue and muscle transfers* Muscle transfers are performed to cover and close the resection site and to restore lost motor power. Adequate skin and muscle coverage is mandatory to decrease postoperative morbidity. Distal tissue transfers are not used because of the possibility of contamination.

Based on the above, the surgical guidelines and technique of limb-sparing surgery utilized by the author are summarized as follows:[63]

1. The major neurovascular bundle must be free of tumor.
2. Wide resection of the affected bone with a normal muscle cuff in all directions should be done.
3. All previous biopsy sites and all potentially contaminated tissues should be removed en bloc.
4. Bone should be resected 6 to 7 cm beyond abnormal uptake as determined by bone scan. This is a safe margin to avoid intraosseous tumor extension.
5. The adjacent joint and joint capsule should be resected. Extraarticular resection is preferred; it is mandatory in the presence of effusion.
6. A tourniquet should be placed proximal to the lesion if possible. This allows amputation to proceed proximal to the tourniquet without iatrogenic contamination of the amputation site if the tumor is found unresectable at the time of surgery.
7. Adequate motor reconstruction must be accomplished by regional muscle transfers. The type of transfer depends upon the anatomic site and the patient's functional requirements.
8. Adequate soft tissue coverage is needed to decrease the risk of skin flap necrosis and secondary infection.

Contraindications for Limb-Sparing Surgery[63] The contraindications of limb-sparing surgery are as follows:

1. *Major neurovascular involvement* Though vascular grafts may be utilized, the adjacent nerves are usually at risk, making the successful resection less likely. In addition, the magnitude of resection in combination with vascular reconstruction is often prohibitive.
2. *Pathological fractures* A fracture through a bone affected by a tumor spreads tumor cells via the hematoma beyond accurately determined limits. The risk of local recurrence increased following a pathologic fracture.
3. *Inappropriate biopsy sites* An inappropriate or poorly planned biopsy jeopardizes local tumor control by inadvertently contaminating normal tissue planes and compartments.
4. *Infection* Implantation of a metallic device or allograft to

an infected area is contraindicated. Sepsis jeopardizes the effectiveness of adjuvant chemotherapy.

5. *Immature skeletal age* In the lower extremity the predicted leg length discrepancy should not be greater than 6 to 8 cm. Upper extremity reconstruction is independent of skeletal maturity.

6. *Extensive muscle involvement* There must be enough muscle remaining for a functional extremity to be reconstructed.

Treatment Considerations

Four clinical scenarios may be encountered in the treatment of patients with classic OS. These and the general considerations are discussed below.

Localized Extremity Disease without Demonstrable Metastases Approximately 50 percent of these patients are cured with surgery alone. The aim of surgical treatment is removal of the primary tumor, by either amputation or resection. All patients are considered for limb-sparing resection. In general, surgery is combined with chemotherapy pre- and/or postoperatively. There is increasing interest in preoperative treatment in an effort to make limb-sparing surgery safer and to extend the surgical indications. The considerations of preoperative versus postoperative chemotherapy are summarized in Table 23-6. To date there is little data to favor either approach. The most effective agents are doxorubicin hydrochloride, cyclophosphamide (Cytoxan), methotrexate, and cisplatin.[88] Preoperative, intraarterial doxorubicin hydrochloride and postoperative chemotherapy have been shown to cause a median tumor necrosis of 90 percent.

Localized Extremity Disease with Synchronous Pulmonary Metastases Pulmonary metastatic disease does not preclude an attempt to cure a patient. In general there are two approaches. The first is treatment of the primary tumor by ablation (resection or amputation) and thoracotomy to remove all pulmonary disease with the goal of rendering the patient free of all known disease. Adjuvant chemotherapy follows. The second approach is chemotherapy followed by surgical removal of all disease; i.e., ablation of the primary tumor and pulmonary resection if a clinical response is noted. The choice must be individualized. In general, amputation should be avoided in the presence of unresectable pulmonary disease, though an amputation is often necessary for palliative reasons alone.

Pelvic Tumors and Unresectable Disease Most pelvic OS can be treated with standard or extended hemipelvectomy. Sacral involvement precludes this procedure. On rare occasions, vertebral and sacral resections have been attempted, although these tumors are usually unresectable and are best treated by radiotherapy and chemotherapy. Palliative decompression of the spine is often required to avoid neurological damage. Vertebral and paraspinal tumors are often unresectable and are best treated with radiation and chemotherapy.

Management of Patients with Pulmonary Relapse Treatment varies for patients with osteogenic sarcoma who subsequently develop pulmonary metastases. In general, aggressive resection of pulmonary nodules is recommended. Chemotherapy is generally begun or continued following pulmonary resection.

TABLE 23-6 Preoperative Versus Postoperative Chemotherapy Regimens

Adjuvant chemotherapy	Pro	Con
Preoperative chemotherapy	Early institution of systemic therapy against micrometastases	High tumor burden (not optimal for first-order kinetics)
	Reduction in tumor size increasing the chance of limb salvage	Increased probability of the emergence of drug-resistant cells
	Less chance of viable tumor being spread at the time of surgery	Delay in definitive control of bulk disease
	Individual response to chemotherapy allowing selection of different risk groups	Psychological trauma of returning tumor
Postoperative chemotherapy	Decreasing tumor burden and increasing growth rate of residual disease from radical removal of bulk tumor, making S-phase-specific agents more active and optimizing conditions for first-order kinetics	Delay of systemic therapy for micrometastases
		No preoperative in vivo assay of cytotoxic response
		Possible spread of viable tumor by surgical manipulation
	Delay in probability of selecting a drug-resistant clone in the primary tumor	

Variants of Osteosarcoma

There are 11 recognizable variants of the classic OS.[19] OS arising in the jaw bones is the most common of all variants. Parosteal and periosteal OS are the most common variants of the classic OS occurring in the extremities. In contrast to classic OS, which arises within (intramedullary) a bone, parosteal and periosteal OS arises on the surface (juxtacortical) of the bone.

Parosteal Osteosarcoma

Parosteal OS (POS) is a distinct variant (4 percent) of conventional OS.[1] It arises from the cortex of a bone and generally occurs in an older age group. It has a better prognosis than classic OS.

Clinical Characteristics Females are more commonly affected than males. Characteristically the distal posterior femur is involved; the proximal humerus and proximal tibia are the next most frequent sites. POS is a slow-metastasizing tumor with a high rate of survival; overall survival ranges from 75 to 85 percent.[1,117] The natural history is progressive enlargement and late metastasis. POS clinically presents as a mass and occasionally is associated with pain. In contrast with the duration of conventional OS symptoms, the duration of POS symptoms varies from months to years.[117] Size, location, and duration of symptoms do not correlate with survival.[1] Table 23-7 summarizes the radiographic and clinical differential of classic, parosteal, and periosteal OS.

Radiographic Findings Roentgenograms characteristically show a large, dense lobulated mass broadly attached to the underlying bone without involvement of the medullary canal (Fig. 23-11). If present long enough, the tumor may encircle the entire bone. The periphery of the lesion is characteristically less mature than the base. Despite careful evaluation, it is difficult to determine intramedullary extension from the plain radiographs.[1] In addition, tumors with high-grade foci do not usually alter the roentgenographic appearance.[117]

Diagnosis and Grading The diagnosis is difficult and must include evaluation of the radiographs, age of the patient, and location of tumor. Differential diagnoses are osteochondroma, myositis ossificans, and conventional OS. Cortical tumors of the posterior femur should always be suspected of malignancy; this is a rare location for a benign osteochondroma. In contrast to sarcoma, myositis ossificans is rarely attached to the underlying bone. In addition, the periphery is more mature, both radiographically and histologically, than in sarcoma.

POSs are graded from low- to high-grade: grade I (low-grade), grade II (intermediate), and grade III (high-grade).[1] The majority are grade I. It is important to evaluate the fibroblastic, cartilaginous, and osseous components independently. The survival rate of patients with grade III tumors is similar to that of patients with conventional OS. Intramedullary involvement does not necessarily imply a worse prognosis, although it may with high-grade lesions.

Gross Characteristics The tumor arises from the periosteal surface and presents as a protuberant multinodular firm mass. The surface may be covered in part by a cartilaginous cap, whereas the tumor in other areas may infiltrate into adjacent soft tissue. The tumor usually encircles, partially or even completely, the shaft of the underlying bone. Unlike the osteochondroma, in the POS the medullary canal of the bone is not contiguous with that of the neoplasm.

Microscopic Characteristics This neoplasm is generally of low grade. Irregularly formed osteoid trabeculae are surrounded by a spindle cell stroma containing widely spaced, bland-appearing spindle cells. There may be foci of atypical chondroid differentiation. (Infrequently, more cellular foci with appreciable atypia and mitotic activity are present.) A four-step grading system which is based on features of the fibrous and chondroid components has been proposed.[10] With the higher grades the likelihood of intramedullary involvement increases. This, in turn, correlates well with the occurrence of distant metastasis.

TABLE 23-7 Radiographic and Clinical Differential of Classic, Parosteal, and Periosteal Osteosarcoma

Type of tumor	Common anatomical site	Location	Radiographic appearance	Histology	Metastases
Classic	Distal femur Proximal tibia	Intramedullary	Destructive, osteoblastic/ osteolytic	High-grade (fibroblastic, chondroblastic, and osteoblastic)	Early
Parosteal	Posterior distal femur	Cortical	Dense, homogeneous new bone	"Mature" bone and fibroblastic stroma, low-grade	Late
Periosteal	Proximal tibia and humerus	Cortical	"Scooped-out" lesion with calcification	Chondroblastic high-grade	Intermediate

Source: Malawer, M.M., Abelson, H.T., and Suit, H.D., in DeVita, V., Hellman, S., and Rosenberg, S.A., eds: *Cancer, Principles and Practice of Oncology,* 2d ed. Philadelphia, Lippincott, 1985, pp 1293–1343.

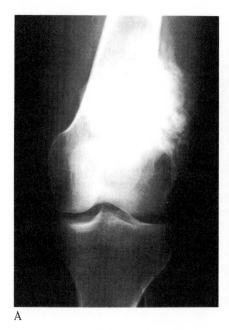
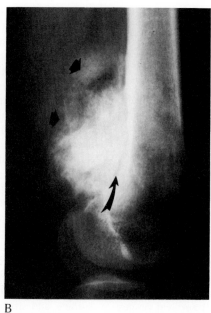

A

B

Figure 23-11 Parosteal osteosarcoma. **A** and **B**. Anteroposterior and lateral radiographs of a typical parosteal osteosarcoma. There is a dense, lobulated broad-based mass attached to the posterior aspect of the distal femur. Note that the periphery (*arrowheads*) is less mature than the center. There is a characteristic radiolucent line (*curved arrow*) at the base denoting an attempt of the tumor to surround the bone along the cortex. A large intramedullary extension found at surgery was not well-seen on these plain radiographs.

Treatment Wide excision of the tumor is the treatment of choice. This may be accomplished by either an amputation or a limb-sparing procedure. POSs are often amenable to limb preservation because of their distal location, low grade, and lack of local invasiveness. If the adjacent neurovascular bundle is free of tumor, resection is feasible. Vascular displacement is not a contraindication for resection. The major surgical decision usually is whether to remove the entire end of the bone and the adjacent joint or to perform a wide excision with preservation of the joint. If the medullary canal

is involved, the joint usually cannot be preserved. A second factor mitigating against joint preservation is extensive cortical involvement. Small lesions can be resected with joint preservation. Resection and reconstruction techniques are similar to those described for conventional OS. The major difference is that only a small amount of adjacent soft tissue usually needs to be resected; consequently, a good functional result is obtained. The high-grade (III) parosteal lesion may warrant systemic therapy due to the risk of metastasis.

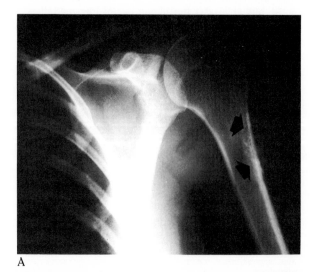
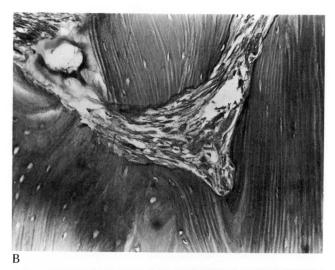

A

B

Figure 23-12 Periosteal osteosarcoma. **A.** Typical radiograph of a periosteal osteosarcoma of the humerus. Note the cortical location (*arrowheads*) with a scooped-out defect on the lateral shaft and the diaphyseal location. **B.** High-power photomicrograph of the underlying cortex demonstrating early extension of tumor within the cortex. Periosteal osteosarcomas most commonly in-

volve the humerus and tibia and are diaphyseal, in contrast to periosteal osteosarcomas, which arise from the posterior aspect of the distal femur. *(From Hall, R.B., Robinson, L.H., Malawer, M.M. et al, Cancer 55:165–171, 1985. Reproduced with permission.)*

Periosteal Osteosarcoma

Periosteal OS is a rare cortical variant of OS which arises superficially on the cortex, most often on the tibial shaft.[118] Radiographically, it is a small radiolucent lesion with some evidence of bone spiculation. The cortex is characteristically intact with a scooped-out appearance and a Codman's triangle (Fig. 23-12). POSs, by contrast, are large, broad-based, and radiodense. Periosteal OSs are relatively high-grade chondroblastic OSs composed of malignant cartilage with areas of anaplastic spindle cells and osteoid production. Periosteal OSs are one-third as frequent as the parosteal variant.[118] Treatment is similar to that of other high-grade lesions. En bloc resection should be performed when feasible; otherwise, amputation is indicated.

Gross Characteristics Like POS, this lesion arises from the periosteal surface. It projects as a well-circumscribed mass into the overlying soft tissues. On section, the tumor often reveals a chondroid consistency (Fig. 23-12A).

Microscopic Characteristics The features are essentially those of a chondroblastic OS. The cartilaginous lobules can contain markedly atypical chondrocytes. At the periphery of the lobule is situated a cellular spindle cell component, wherein a fine intercellular osteoid matrix is produced. Areas of malignant osteoid and chondroid can be seen to infiltrate into the cortical bone at the base of the neoplasm (Fig. 23-12B).

Small Cell Osteosarcoma

Small cell OS is a rare variant of OS. The cells are round,

The recommendations for treatment vary; radiation and chemotherapy are used at some institutions, while others choose primary surgical ablation with pre- and/or postoperative chemotherapy. Too few cases have been reported to make definitive recommendations.

Microscopic Characteristics The tumor consists of nests and sheets of small round cells separated by fibrous septa, a pattern reminiscent of Ewing's sarcoma. Occasionally, transition to spindle cells is noted. The cells have well-defined borders and a distinct rim of cytoplasm. The round nuclei disclose a delicate chromatin pattern. The presence of a characteristic delicate lacelike osteoid matrix, often surrounding individual or small nests of cells, confirms the diagnosis of OS.

Chondrosarcoma

Chondrosarcoma, the second most common primary malignant spindle cell tumor of bone,[15] is a heterogeneous group of tumors whose basic neoplastic tissue is cartilaginous without evidence of direct osteoid formation. Bone formation occasionally occurs from differentiation of cartilage. If there is evidence of direct osteoid or bone production, the lesion is classified as an OS. There are five types of chondrosarcoma: central, peripheral, mesenchymal, differentiated, and clear cell.[15,50,57,106] The classic chondrosarcomas are central (arising within a bone) or peripheral (arising from the surface of a bone). The other three are variants and have distinct histological and clinical characteristics. Their characteristics are summarized in Table 23-8.

TABLE 23-8   Classification and General Characteristics of Chondrosarcomas

Type	Size, location, grade	Primary* or secondary†
Central	Intramedullary Moderate to high-grade Small extraosseous component Little calcification	Usually primary
Peripheral	Cortical Usually low-grade, myxomatous Large soft tissue component Heavily calcified	Usually secondary
Mesenchymal	Intramedullary High-grade, may respond to radiotherapy Small round cells	Primary
Dedifferentiated	High-grade anaplastic (osteosarcoma, MFH) in association with recognizable low-grade chondrosarcoma	Primary
Clear cell chondrosarcoma	Low-grade Appears as a chondroblastoma Locally recurrent	Primary

*76% of primary chondrosarcomas are central.
†Usually from benign cartilage tumors, ex. osteochondromas.

rather than spindle-shaped. There is definite evidence of osteoid production; thus, the inclusion of this entity as an OS.

Both central and peripheral chondrosarcomas can arise as a primary tumor or secondary to underlying neoplasm. Seventy-six percent of primary chondrosarcomas arise centrally.[15,74,94,106] Secondary chondrosarcomas most often arise from benign cartilage tumors. The multiple forms of the benign osteochondromas or enchondromas have a higher rate of malignant transformation than the corresponding solitary lesions do.[35,68,94,104]

Central and Peripheral Chondrosarcomas

Clinical Characteristics Half of all chondrosarcomas occur in persons above the age of 40.[15,46] The most common sites are the pelvis, femur, and shoulder girdle.[46,74] The clinical presentation varies. Peripheral chondrosarcomas may become quite large without causing pain, and local symptoms develop only because of mechanical irritation. Pelvic chondrosarcomas are often large and present with referred pain to the back or thigh, sciatica secondary to sacral plexus irritation, urinary symptoms from bladder neck involvement, unilateral edema due to iliac vein obstruction, or as a painless abdominal mass. Conversely, central chondrosarcomas present with dull pain. A mass is rarely present. Pain, which indicates active growth, is an ominous sign of a central cartilage lesion. This cannot be overemphasized. An adult with a plain radiograph suggestive of a "benign" cartilage tumor but associated with pain most likely has a chondrosarcoma.

Radiographic Findings Central chondrosarcomas have two distinct radiological patterns.[23] One is a small, well-defined lytic lesion with a narrow zone of transition and surrounding sclerosis with faint calcification. This is the most common malignant bone tumor that may appear radiographically benign. The second type has no sclerotic border and is difficult to localize. The key sign of malignancy is endosteal scalloping. This type is difficult to diagnose on plain radiographs and may go undetected for a long period of time. In contrast, peripheral chondrosarcoma is recognized easily as a large mass of characteristic calcification protruding from a bone. Its differential diagnosis includes large benign osteochondroma, POS, and juxtacortical myositis ossificans. Correlation of the clinical, radiographic, and histological data is essential for accurate diagnosis and evaluation of the aggressiveness of cartilage tumor. In general, proximal or axial location, skeletal maturity, and pain point toward malignancy, even though the cartilage may appear benign.

Grading and Prognosis Chondrosarcomas are graded I, II, and III; the majority are either grade I or grade II.[15,46,74,104] The metastatic rate of moderate-grade versus high-grade is 15 to 40 percent versus 75 percent.[1,12,14,15,65,69,77,86,88,94,104,106] Grade III lesions have the same metastatic potential as osteosarcomas (Fig. 23-13).[68,74]

In general, peripheral chondrosarcomas are a lower grade than central lesions. Forty-three percent of the peripheral lesions are grade I, compared with 13 percent of the central lesions.[36] Ten-year survival rates among those with peripheral lesions are 77 percent compared with 32 percent among those with central lesions. Secondary chondrosarcomas arising from osteochondromas also have a low malignant potential; 85 percent are grade I.

Gross Characteristics Primary intraosseous (central) chondrosarcomas is an expansile lesion which eventuates in corti-

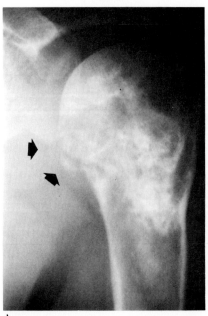

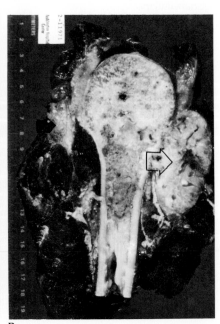

A   B

Figure 23-13 High-grade chondrosarcoma associated with enchondromatosis. **A.** Plain radiograph of a radiolucent lesion of the proximal humerus with little calcification. **B.** The gross specimen. The incidence of malignant degeneration associated with multiple enchondromas increases with each decade of life with an overall risk of 15 to 25 percent. Chondrosarcomas arising centrally tend to be high-grade.

cal destruction. Subsequent extension into soft tissue often occurs. Chondrosarcoma arising from a rib or from the pelvis may protrude, as a smooth-surfaced multinodular mass, into the pleural cavity or pelvic retroperitoneum, respectively.

Typically, the tumor consists of fused, variably sized nodules which on cut section are composed of a white-gray hyaline tissue. Areas of calcification and even ossification are common. There may be focal myxoid areas. The nodules occasionally contain degenerative cysts of various sizes.

Microscopic Characteristics The histological spectrum of this neoplasm varies tremendously: high-grade examples can be easily identified, whereas certain low-grade tumors are exceedingly difficult to distinguish from chondromas. Correlation of the histological features with both the clinical setting and the radiographic changes is therefore of utmost importance in avoiding serious diagnostic error. The grade of malignant cartilaginous tumors correlates with clinical behavior. Grade I tumors are characterized by an increased number of chondrocytes set in a matrix that is chondroid to focally myxoid. The cells contain hyperchromatic nuclei and occasionally binucleate forms and show minimal variation in size (Fig. 23-14).

Areas of increased cellularity with more marked variation in cell size, significant nuclear atypia, and frequent pleomorphic forms define a grade II lesion. Binuclear forms are more common in this group.

Grade III chondrosarcomas, which are relatively uncommon, disclose still greater cellularity, often with spindle cell areas, and reveal prominent mitotic activity. Chondrocytes may contain large, bizarre nuclei. Areas of myxoid change are common.

Areas of calcification and enchondral ossification can be observed in tumors of all grades. However, the presence of unequivocal malignant osteoid production, even in the face of chondrosarcomatous areas, dictates that the tumor be classified as OS.

Treatment The treatment of chondrosarcoma is surgical removal.[2,75,94,106] Guidelines of resection for high-grade chon-

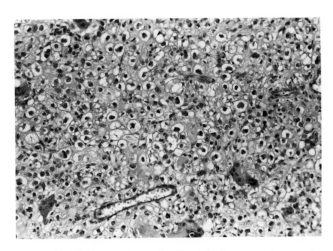

Figure 23-15 Sheets of round cells with clear cytoplasm and central nuclei point to a diagnosis of clear cell chondrosarcoma. Multinucleated giant cells, very rare in the usual chondrosarcoma, are common in this entity.

drosarcomas are similar to those for OSs. The sites of origin and the fact that chondrosarcomas tend to be low-grade make them amenable to limb-sparing procedures. The four most common sites are the pelvis, proximal femur, shoulder girdle, and diaphyseal portions of long bones.

Marcove pioneered the technique of cryosurgery for bone tumors. Cryosurgery involves thorough curettage and cryotherapy of the cavity with liquid nitrogen;[67,72,74,77] the major advantages are preservation of bone stock and the avoidance of resection. Cryosurgery has recently been used for central, low-grade chondrosarcomas.[69,77] High-grade chondrosarcomas warrant adjuvant chemotherapy. With increasing experience, Marcove has expanded the cryosurgery indications to low-grade intramedullary cartilage tumors as well as a few high-grade lesions. With these indications he has treated 30 chondrosarcomas with only one local recurrence.

Variants of Chondrosarcoma

Clear Cell Chondrosarcoma

Clear cell chondrosarcoma, the rarest form of chondrosarcoma, is a slow-growing, locally recurrent tumor resembling a chondroblastoma but with some malignant potential.[107,119] It generally occurs in adults. The most difficult clinical problem is early recognition (Fig. 23-15); it is often confused with chondroblastoma. Metastases occur only after multiple local recurrences. Primary treatment is wide excision. Systemic therapy is not required.

Gross Characteristics The neoplasm commonly presents as a solid expansile mass with focal cystic changes.

Microscopic Characteristics The diagnostic feature consists of sheets or vague lobules composed of round clear cells with a central nucleus. Occasional mitoses are observed. Variably sized foci that are typical of chondrosarcoma frequently occur. In addition, areas indistinguishable from other primary bone lesions can obscure the underlying clear cell neoplasm.

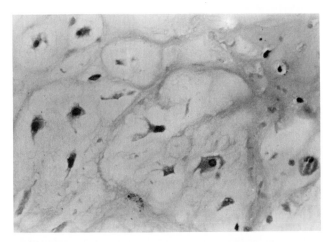

Figure 23-14 The presence of chondrocytes with central hyperchromatic nuclei is typical of chondrosarcoma, grade I. Binucleate forms are not uncommon. The matrix may vary from chondroid to myxoid.

Foci resembling aneurysmal bone cyst, OS, osteoblastoma, chondroblastoma, and giant cell tumor have been identified.[6]

Mesenchymal Chondrosarcoma

Mesenchymal chondrosarcoma is a rare aggressive variant of chondrosarcoma characterized by a biphasic histological pattern; i.e., small compact cells intermixed with islands of cartilaginous matrix.[42,48] This tumor has a predilection for flat bones; long tubular bones are rarely affected. It tends to occur in the younger age group and has a high metastatic potential. The 10-year survival rate is 28 percent.[48] This entity responds favorably to radiotherapy. Treatment is surgical removal combined with adjuvant chemotherapy. Radiotherapy is recommended if the tumor cannot be completely removed.[42]

Gross Characteristics The firm white-gray tumor usually contains hard calcified or ossified areas. Prominent cartilaginous features are unusual.

Microscopic Characteristics The hallmark of this neoplasm is the juxtaposition of foci of poorly differentiated round cells with islands of relatively mature chondroid tissue. The small round to slightly spindled cells are arranged in broad sheets and typically form a hemangiopericytoma-like pattern. Scattered islands of chondroid, which can be focally calcified or ossified, arise abruptly among the sheets of round cells.

Dedifferentiated Chondrosarcoma

Around 10 percent of chondrosarcomas may dedifferentiate into either a fibrosarcoma or an OS.[15,68,106] They occur in older individuals and are often fatal. Surgical treatment is similar to that described for other high-grade sarcomas. Adjuvant therapy is warranted.

Gross Characteristics The central region of the tumor is comparable to that of ordinary chondrosarcoma and is characterized by distinctly lobulated gray-white translucent tissue. Calcified foci are commonly found within this zone. Peripheral to this chondroid portion, but contiguous to it, is a firm to soft, often focally necrotic component which, after eroding the cortical bone, often extends into the adjacent soft tissue.

Microscopic Characteristics Two distinct components are identified. The central portion shows features of a low-grade chondrosarcoma (grade I or II), identical to that described elsewhere in this chapter. At the periphery of the lobules arises an anaplastic high-grade infiltrative sarcoma that can present features of MFH, OS, or fibrosarcoma.

Giant Cell Tumor of Bone

Giant cell tumor of bone (GCT) is an aggressive, locally recurrent tumor with a low metastatic potential.[18,37,44,46,54,55,116] Giant cell sarcoma of bone refers to a de novo, malignant GCT, not to the tumor which arises from the transformation of a GCT previously thought to be benign. These two lesions are separate clinical entities.

Clinical Characteristics

GCTs occur slightly more often in females than in males. Eighty percent of GCTs in the long bones occur after skeletal maturity; 75 percent of these develop around the knee joint.[15,37,57] An effusion or pathologic fracture, uncommon with other sarcomas, is common with GCTs. GCTs occasionally occur in the vertebrae (2 to 5 percent) and the sacrum (10 percent).[1–3,5,15]

Natural History

Although GCTs are rarely malignant de novo (2 to 8 percent),[20,46,89] they may undergo transformation and demonstrate malignant potential histologically and clinically after multiple local recurrences.[16–18,44,54] Between 8 and 22 percent of known GCTs become malignant following local recurrence.[18,44,46,54,89] This rate decreases to less than 10 percent if patients who have undergone radiotherapy are excluded. Approximately 40 percent of malignant GCTs became malignant at the first recurrence.[44] The remainder become malignant by the second and third recurrence; thus, each recurrence increases the risk of malignant transformation. A recurrence after 5 years is extremely suspicious for a malignancy. Primary malignant GCT generally has a better prognosis than secondary malignant transformation of typical GCT does, especially if the transformation occurs after radiation therapy. Local recurrence of a GCT is determined by the adequacy of surgical removal, not the histological grade.

Radiographic and Clinical Evaluation

GCTs are eccentric lytic lesions without matrix production (Fig. 23-16). They have poorly defined borders with a wide area of transition. They are juxtaepiphyseal with a metaphyseal component. Although the cortex is expanded and appears destroyed, at surgery it is usually found to be attenuated but intact. Periosteal elevation is rare; soft tissue extension is common. In the skeletally immature patient, aneurysmal bone cyst must be differentiated, although both lesions are closely related.

Gross Characteristics

The typical lesion presents as a large expansile mass in the region of the epiphysis. Cortical destruction of the adjacent bone is not uncommon. The periphery of the tumor is often partially surrounded by a thin, delicate rim of reactive bone. The soft, somewhat gelatinous tumor tissue varies from gray-tan to red-brown. (Areas of hemorrhage with hemosiderin deposition account for the color of the latter.) Small, cystlike foci frequently occur; however, occasionally the cystic degeneration can become so extensive that the tumor resembles an aneurysmal bone cyst. Firm fibrous or osteoid tissue can be associated with a site of pathologic fracture.

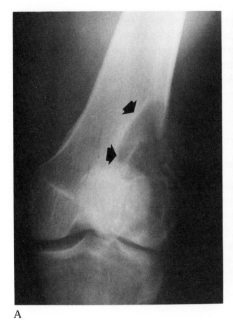

A

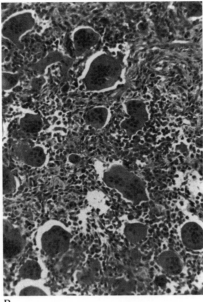

B

Figure 23-16 Aggressive giant cell tumor. **A.** Typical GCT of bone. GCTs are eccentric without matrix formation and are metaphyseal. They often have poorly defined margins with some sclerosis (*arrows*). Pathologic fracture is common. Cortical expansion and poorly defined margins are signs of aggressivity. **B.** Low-power photomicrograph showing a uniform distribution of giant cells in a benign stroma. The stroma cells tend to be ovoid. No mitoses are seen, but they are occasionally present. *(From Malawer, M.M., Abelson, H.T., and Suit, H.D., in DeVita, V.T., Hellman, S., and Rosenberg, S.A., eds: Cancer: Principles and Practice of Oncology, 2d ed. Philadelphia, Lippincott, 1985. Reproduced with permission.)*

Microscopic Characteristics

Two basic cell types constitute the typical GCT. The stroma is characterized by polygonal to somewhat spindled cells containing central round nuclei. Mitotic figures, sometimes numerous, are often noted, but they are not typical and do not warrant a malignant interpretation.

Scattered diffusely throughout the stroma are benign multinucleated giant cells. Small foci of osteoid matrix, produced by the benign stroma cells, can be observed; however, chondroid matrix never occurs. Extensive hemorrhage, pathologic fracture, or previous surgery can alter significantly the usual histological picture of GCT. These events must be recognized at the time of histological interpretation in order to prevent diagnostic errors. Cystic areas with surrounding hemosiderin pigment and xanthoma cells correspond to the grossly observed cysts.

Grading

The grading of GCTs into three groups in order to predict clinical behavior, as originally proposed by Jaffe,[50] has been generally abandoned. Recognition of the overtly malignant type (grade III), as described below, is valid; however, lesions rated as histologically benign (grade I or II) have been shown to metastasize.[57,97]

Malignant GCT contains areas of unequivocal sarcomatous transformation, usually typical fibrosarcoma or OS. The sarcomatous component is devoid of GCT features; thus, it is only by the recognition of foci of residual benign GCT or by the confirmation of preexisting benign GCT that an accurate diagnosis of malignant GCT can be established.

Treatment

Treatment of GCT of bone is surgical removal. Resection is

curative in 90 percent of these cases.[16–18,44,65,83] In contrast, curettage, with or without bone grafts, has a recurrence rate of 40 to 75 percent.[18,37,44,54] Johnson and Dahlin reported a recurrence rate of 29 percent within 1 year of curettage and of 54 percent within 5 years. Figure 23-17 summarizes the results of treatment of the various techniques. Though en bloc excision offers reliable results, routine resection is not recommended.[9] Primary resection of a joint has a significant morbidity. Primary resection is recommended for GCT of the proximal radius and fibula; distal ulna; tubular bones of hand and foot; coccyx; sacrum; and pelvic bones. Under certain situations it is reasonable to perform a curettage. In general, curettage does not rule out a later curative resection. Amputation is reserved for massive recurrence, malignant transformation, or infection. Because of the risk of malignant transformation and pathologic fracture, as well as the lack of effectiveness, radiation is used only for surgically inaccessi-

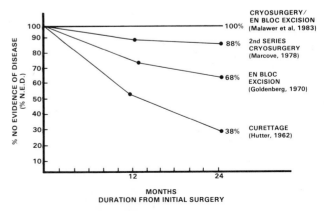

Figure 23-17 Reported cure rates of GCTs of bone treated by various modalities.

ble sites.[16,18,37,60] Treatment of GCTs of the vertebrae and sacrum is difficult and must be individualized. A combination of surgical excision, cryosurgery, and/or radiotherapy is required for tumor eradication and the prevention of neurological impairment.[78,112,113]

Cryosurgical Treatment Cryosurgery has been utilized more successfully for GCTs than for any other type of bone tumor.[65,69,72,76,77] Cryosurgery was developed by Marcove in an attempt to overcome the high recurrence rates after curettage and the significant risk of sarcomatous degeneration in GCTs treated by irradiation. Figure 23-18A shows the technique of cryosurgery. Marcove found cryosurgery effective in eradicating the tumor while preserving joint motion and avoiding resection or amputation. Recently he reported a 17-year experience of 100 GCTs treated by thorough curettage and cryosurgery.[69] He noted a recurrence rate of 16 percent in the first 50 cases and 2 percent in the following 50 cases. The major complications of cryosurgery are necrosis of the adjacent bones (Fig. 23-18B), which are liable to develop a late pathologic fracture, and delayed union. The rate of secondary pathologic fracture has been decreased by a combination of polymethylmethacrylate augmentation, bone graft, internal fixation of the cavity, and postoperative use of a long leg brace with a quadrilateral socket. Recently, curettage with methylmethacrylate augmentation of the bony defect has been performed with the intent of inducing thermal necrosis of regional tumor cells utilizing the heat of polymerization. This technique may provide better local control than curettage alone; however, few cases have been reported to date.[92]

Radiation Therapy Radiation is considered when surgical excision is not technically feasible. Most often this is the case when the tumor occurs in the vertebrae. Dahlin[18] reports from the Mayo Clinic a significant risk of radiation-induced sarcoma following radiation alone or in conjunction with surgery for the treatment of GCT of bone. More recently, successful surgical excision of vertebral GCTs have been reported,[78,112,113] thus avoiding the need for radiation. Neurological involvement secondary to cord compression requires a posterior and/or an anterior decompression.

Malignant Fibrous Histiocytoma

Clinical Characteristics

MFH is a high-grade bone tumor histologically similar to its soft tissue counterpart. Osteoid production is absent.[45,79,110] It is a disease of adulthood. The most common sites are the metaphyseal ends of long bones, especially around the knee. Alkaline phosphatase values are normal. Pathologic fracture is common. MFH disseminates rapidly. Lymphatic involvement, although rare for other bone sarcomas, has been reported.

Radiographic Characteristics

MFH is an osteolytic lesion associated with marked cortical disruption, minimal cortical or periosteal reaction, and no evidence of matrix formation.[45] The extent of the tumor routinely exceeds plain radiographic signs. MFH may be multicentric (10 percent) and associated with bone infarcts (10 percent).[79]

Gross Characteristics

The features are nonspecific and vary greatly. Firm, fibrouslike areas can alternate with soft necrotic foci. Some lesions are relatively homogeneous white-gray, whereas others are

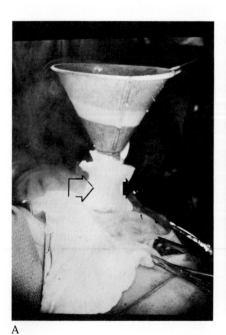

A

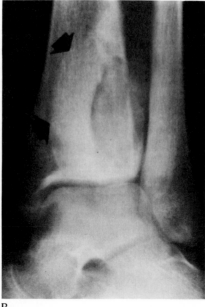

B

Figure 23-18 Cryosurgery. **A.** Intraoperative photograph demonstrating the direct-pour method of cryosurgery. After thorough curettage of the lesion, liquid nitrogen is poured directly into the cavity through a funnel. This ensures complete contact of the liquid nitrogen with the wall of the cavity in order to kill any remaining tumor cells. The temperature of the freeze is monitored by thermocouples (*solid arrow*); $-20°C$ to $-40°C$ is necessary for cryonecrosis. The base of the funnel is packed with Gelfoam to prevent leakage. **B.** GCT of the distal tibia treated by curettage and cryosurgery. Radiograph at 18 months demonstrates the typical "cryonecrotic" rim (*arrows*), an area of necrotic and reparative bone at the limit of the original freeze. Presumably any tumor cells remaining within the cavity or the bony interstices following curettage were killed by the liquid nitrogen. A radiograph at 2 years shows no evidence of recurrence, incorporation of the graft with a normal appearing joint space, and some persistence of the cryonecrotic rim.

more variegated with ill-defined brown-red and yellow regions.

Microscopic Characteristics

As in its soft tissue counterpart, primary MFH of bone reveals a remarkably broad histological spectrum. Plump histiocyte-like cells and spindled fibroblastic cells, in variable proportion, are the main elements. Characteristic is the storiform or pinwheel pattern, in which the fibroblasts radiate from a central focus. The histiocyte-like cells can form sheets or transform into markedly bizarre, often multinucleated, forms with atypical mitotic figures (Fig. 23-19). The spindle cell component may predominate, forming areas resembling fibrosarcoma. Chronic inflammatory cells and occasional osteoblast-like giant cells are usually scattered throughout the stroma. Occasionally small foci of osteoid matrix production by tumor cells can be observed. Metastatic pleomorphic carcinoma, particularly from the kidney, can closely mimic MFH, and such a possibility must be excluded in the differential diagnosis.

Treatment

Treatment is similar to that of other high-grade sarcomas.

Fibrosarcoma of Bone

Clinical Characteristics

Fibrosarcoma of bone is a rare entity characterized by interlacing bundles of collagen fibers (herringbone pattern) without any evidence of tumor bone or osteoid formation.[47] Fibrosarcoma occurs in middle age. The long bones are most affected. Fibrosarcomas occasionally arise secondarily in conjunction with an underlying disease such as fibrous dys-

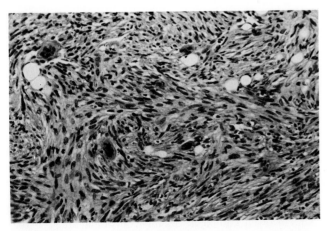

Figure 23-19 This example of malignant fibrous histiocytoma of bone demonstrates pleomorphic and bizarre tumor cells admixed with spindle cells and inflammatory cell infiltrates.

plasia, Paget disease, bone infarcts, osteomyelitis, postirradiation bone, and GCT.[47] Fibrosarcoma may be either central or cortical (termed *periosteal*). The histological grade is a good prognosticator of metastatic potential. Overall survival rate is 27 percent and 52 percent for central and peripheral lesions, respectively.[47] Late metastases do occur, and 10- and 15-year survival rates vary. In general, periosteal tumors have a better prognosis than central lesions do.

Radiographic Features

Fibrosarcoma is a radiolucent lesion which shows minimal periosteal and cortical reaction. The radiographic appearance closely correlates with the histological grade of the tumor.[47] Low-grade tumors are well-defined, whereas high-grade lesions demonstrate indistinct margins and bone destruction similar to those of osteolytic OS. Plain radiographs often underestimate the extent of the lesion. Pathologic fracture is common (30 percent) because of the lack of matrix formation.[125] Differential diagnosis includes GCT, aneurysmal bone cyst, MFH, and osteolytic OS.[47,125]

Gross Characteristics

The presentation correlates reasonably well with the histological grade. Low-grade lesions tend to be firm and white-gray and may appear encapsulated. With the higher-grade tumors, the tissue becomes soft, somewhat myxoid, and even necrotic. Transgression of the cortex with soft tissue extension is not uncommon.

Microscopic

The hallmark of this neoplasm is the formation of fascicles of elongated spindle cells containing tapered nuclei. The fascicles often intersect at acute angles, forming the so-called herringbone pattern. Intercellular collagen production may be abundant, especially in the low-grade examples. In contrast, high-grade fibrosarcoma is characterized by more of the pleomorphic spindle cells with atypical nuclear features. Mitotic activity is brisk. Collagen production may not be discernible. Differentiation of a grade I fibrosarcoma from a desmoplastic fibroma is frequently difficult.

Staging and Treatment

Staging and treatment are similar to those of other spindle cell sarcomas. Low-grade central and peripheral variants are treated by en bloc resection. Axial and fascial lesions should be treated by resection and local radiotherapy. Adjuvant chemotherapy is warranted for high-grade lesions.

Secondary Tumors

Secondary tumors are neoplasms arising from an underlying pathological process or from another tumor (Table 23-9).[17]

TABLE 23-9 Classification of Secondary Tumors

Primary disease	Secondary tumor
Osteochondroma	Peripheral chondrosarcoma
Enchondroma	Central chondrosarcoma
Fibrous dysplasia	MFH, fibrosarcoma
Paget disease	Paget's sarcoma (usually osteosarcoma), giant cell tumor (rare)
Irradiated tissue	Radiation-induced sarcoma of the bone* or soft tissue (osteosarcoma, MFH, fibrosarcoma)

*Approximately 200 cases. Average latent period is 10 to 12 years; range 4 to 30 years.

Though rare, this diverse group of lesions requires separate consideration. In general the management of each tumor is similar to that of its primary counterpart.

Paget's Sarcoma

Sarcomas arising in a bone affected with Paget disease have been termed Paget's sarcoma. These tumors develop with equal frequency in Paget patients of all ages. Histologically, OS is the most common; fibrosarcoma, chondrosarcoma, and MFH also have been described. The anatomic distribution is similar to that of uncomplicated Paget disease. The femur, pelvis, and humerus are most often involved. Increasing pain is the chief presenting complaint.

The diagnosis may be difficult because of the presence of the underlying Paget disease. Radiographic studies may show an area of increased destruction, with or without increasing sclerosis. Periosteal elevation may not be present. The level of alkaline phosphatase does not help in diagnosis. Paget's sarcoma often presents with a pathologic fracture. Any patient with Paget disease with increasing pain, a soft tissue mass, and/or pathologic fracture must be carefully evaluated for a secondary sarcoma. Prognosis is poor. There have been few long-term survivors among patients who received surgery alone. Hemipelvectomy is required for the pelvic and proximal femoral tumors. Adjuvant chemotherapy is warranted following surgical removal.

Radiation-Induced Sarcoma

Sarcomas rarely arise in previously irradiated bone. Approximately 200 cases have been reported. The average latent period is 10 to 12 years, with a range of 4 to 30 years.[46] Criteria for diagnosis of a radiation-induced sarcoma are as follows:

1. Histologically proven sarcoma
2. Tumor arising in documented previously radiated field
3. Asymptomatic latent period (minimum of 3 to 4 years)

Surgical management is similar to that of other high-grade sarcomas. Overall survival ranges from 25 to 35 percent. Adjuvant chemotherapy is warranted.

Small Round Cell Sarcomas of Bone

Round cell sarcomas of bone behave differently and require different therapeutic management than spindle cell sarcomas do.[96,114] Round cell sarcomas of bone consist of poorly differentiated small cells without matrix production. They present radiographically as osteolytic lesions. These lesions are best treated with radiation and chemotherapy; surgery is reserved for special situations. Non-Hodgkin's lymphoma and Ewing's sarcoma are the two most common small cell sarcomas. The differential diagnosis of all round cell sarcomas includes metastatic neuroblastoma, metastatic undifferentiated carcinoma, histiocytosis, small cell OS, osteomyelitis, and multiple myeloma.

Ewing's Sarcoma

Ewing's sarcoma is the second most common bone sarcoma of childhood; it is approximately one-half as frequent as OS. The lesion is characterized by poorly differentiated small round cells with marked homogeneity. The exact cell of origin is unknown. The clinical and biological behavior is significantly different from that of spindle cell sarcomas. Within the past 2 decades the prognosis of patients with Ewing's sarcomas has dramatically been improved by the combination of effective adjuvant chemotherapy, improved radiotherapy techniques, and the select use of limited surgical resection.[90,93,95,99]

Clinical Characteristics Ewing's sarcomas tend to occur in young children, though rarely in those below the age of 5 years. Characteristically the flat and axial bones (50 to 60 percent) are involved.[15,90] When a long (tubular) bone is involved, it is most often the proximal or diaphyseal area. In contrast, OSs occur in adolescence (average age 15), most often around the knees, and involve the metaphysis of long bones. Another unique finding with Ewing's sarcomas is systemic signs, i.e., fever, anorexia, weight loss, leukocytosis, and anemia.[93] All may be a presenting sign of the disease (20 to 30 percent); this is in contrast to the distinct absence of all systemic signs with OS until late in the disease process. In Ewing's sarcoma the incidence of pathologic fracture implies a poor prognosis. The most common complaint is pain and/or a mass. Localized tenderness is often present with associated erythema and induration. These findings, in combination with systemic signs of fever and leukocytosis, closely mimic those of osteomyelitis.

Radiographic Findings Ewing's sarcoma is a highly destructive radiolucent lesion without evidence of bone formation. The typical pattern consists of a permeative or moth-eaten destruction associated with periosteal elevation. Characteristically there is multilaminated periosteal elevation or a "sunburst" appearance (Fig. 23-20). When Ewing's sarcoma occurs in flat bones, however, these findings are usually absent. Tumors of flat bones appear as a destructive lesion with a large soft tissue component. The ribs and pelvis are most often involved. Pathologic fractures occur and are secondary to extensive bony destruction and the absence of tumor matrix. The differential diagnosis is osteomyelitis, osteolytic OS, metastatic neuroblastoma, and histiocytosis.

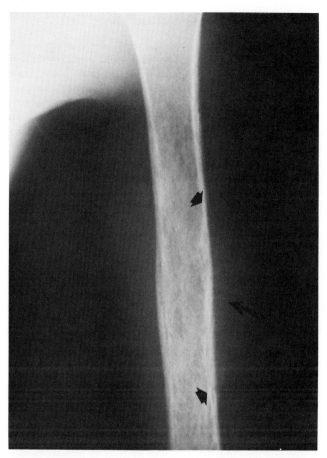

Figure 23-20 Ewing's sarcoma of the humerus. Typical permeative destruction associated with a sunburst appearance (*arrows*). Ewing's sarcoma is often diaphyseal, whereas osteosarcoma tends to be metaphyseal.

Natural History Ewing's sarcoma is highly lethal and rapidly disseminates. Historically, fewer than 10 to 15 percent of patients remained disease-free at 2 years.[15,98,99] Many patients present with metastatic disease. The most common sites are the lungs and other bones. It used to be thought that Ewing's sarcoma was a multicentric disease because of the high incidence of multiple bone involvement. Unlike other bone sarcomas, Ewing's sarcoma is associated with visceral, lymphatic, and meningeal involvement, and these must be searched for.

Evaluation and Staging There is no general staging system for Ewing's sarcoma. The musculoskeletal staging system does not apply to the round cell sarcomas of the bone. Because of the propensity of these lesions to spread to other bones, bone marrow, the lymphatic system, and the viscera, evaluation is more extensive than that for the spindle cell sarcomas. It must include a careful clinical examination of regional and distal lymph nodes and radiographic evaluation for visceral involvement. Liver-spleen scans and bone marrow aspirates are required in addition to CT of the lungs and the primary site. Angiography is required only if a primary resection is planned.

Biopsy Considerations Because of the frequent difficulty of accurate pathological interpretation and potential problems with bone healing, the following are guidelines for the biopsy of suspected round cell tumors:

1. Adequate material must be obtained for histological evaluation and electron microscopy. Frozen section analysis should be performed to assure adequate material for interpretation.
2. Routine cultures should be made to aid in the differentiation from an osteomyelitis.
3. Biopsy of the bony component is *not* necessary; the soft tissue component often provides adequate material. Bone biopsy should be through a *small* hole on the compressive side of the bone. Pathologic fracture through an irradiated bone often does not heal.

Gross Characteristics The tumor appears to arise in the medullary cavity, although permeation into cortical bone and into surrounding soft tissues occurs frequently. The mass is soft and gray-white and may contain areas of necrosis and hemorrhage.

Microscopic Characteristics Large nests and sheets of relatively uniform round cells are typical (Fig. 23-21). The sheets of cells are often compartmentalized by intersecting collagenous trabeculae. The cells contain round nuclei with a distinct nuclear envelope. Nucleoli are uncommon, and mitotic activity is minimal. There may be occasional rosettelike structures, although neuroectodermal origin has never been confirmed. In the vicinity of necrotic tumor, small pyknotic cells may be observed. Vessels in these necrotic regions often are encircled by viable tumor cells. The cells often contain cytoplasmic glycogen, although its presence or absence cannot be considered as the only criterion for the confirmation or exclusion, respectively, of Ewing's sarcoma. This neoplasm belongs to the category of small blue round cell tumors, a designation which also includes neuroblastoma, lymphoma, metastatic OS, and occasionally osteomyelitis and histiocytosis. When confronted with this differential diagnosis, the pa-

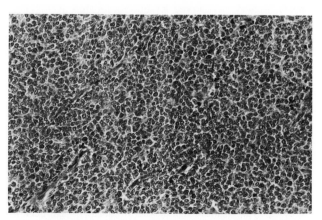

Figure 23-21 Ewing's sarcoma is characterized by sheets of small round uniform cells. Application of special stains may disclose cytoplasmic glycogen, although its presence in such cells is not diagnostic. Some cells reveal eccentric nuclei with a paranuclear clear zone, clues to plasma cell differentiation.

thologist may turn to electron microscopy or immunohistochemistry for additional information.

Treatment Ewing's sarcomas are generally considered radiosensitive. Radiation therapy to the primary site has been the traditional mode of local control. Within the past decade, surgical resection of selected lesions has become increasingly popular. Though detailed management is beyond the scope of this chapter, the following sections summarize some common aspects of the multimodality approach.[90-92,94,95,99]

Chemotherapy Doxorubicin, actinomycin D, cyclophosphamide, and vincristine are the most effective agents.[90,98] There are a variety of different combinations and schedules. All patients require intensive chemotherapy to prevent dissemination. Overall survival in patients with lesions of the extremities now ranges between 40 and 75 percent.

Radiation Therapy Radiation to the entire bone at risk is required. The usual dose ranges between 4500 and 6000 rad delivered in 6 to 8 weeks. In order to reduce the morbidity of radiation, it is recommended that between 4000 and 5000 rad be delivered to the whole bone, with an additional 1000 to 1500 rad to the tumor site.[90,91,98,99] Sophisticated techniques are required for optimal results: preservation of a strip of unirradiated skin, compensators and/or filters, and simulation and immobilization of the target area. Physical therapy of the affected part is begun during radiation to decrease stiffness and swelling.

There has been increasing concern regarding the development of secondary sarcomas within the irradiated fields in the patients now surviving. This is a valid concern that may favor reduced radiation dosage and increased use of limited surgery.

Surgical Treatment The role of surgery in the treatment of Ewing's sarcoma is currently undergoing change. The Intergroup Ewing's Study recommends surgical removal of expendable bones such as the ribs, clavicle, and scapula.[90,93] In general, surgery is reserved for tumors located in high-risk areas, e.g., ribs, ilium, and proximal femur. *Risk* is defined as an increased incidence of local recurrence and metastases. In general, surgery is considered an adjunct to the other treatment modalities. When surgical resection is performed, a marginal resection only is usually feasible, because of the extensive extraosseous component. Extensive bleeding must be anticipated. Morbidity of surgery is increased secondary to radiation and chemotherapy effects. Primary amputation is often required for lower extremity lesions in a child younger than 10 years because of predicted leg length shortening. Patients presenting with pathologic fractures also often require a primary amputation. Fractures occurring following adequate control of the tumor may heal following immobilization and/or internal fixation. It must be stressed that surgery in conjunction with high-dose radiation and chemotherapy entails significant local morbidity which in itself may necessitate amputation. There is a significant increase of infection, bleeding, late fracture, and flap necrosis following high-dose radiation and/or chemotherapy.

Lymphomas of Bone (Diffuse Large Cell Lymphoma)

Lymphoma of bone localized to bone is a rare primary tumor (5 percent).[89] In general, lymphoma of the bone is a sign of disseminated (stage IV) disease; only occasionally is it a true solitary lesion (stage IE).[114] The classification and treatment of lymphoma are dealt with in Chap. 22, Sect. B. The role of surgery is limited to obtaining adequate tissue for diagnosis, treating pathologic fracture, and possibly resecting an expendable bone. The technique of biopsy is important to avoid secondary fracture through potentially irradiated bone. If an extraosseous component exists, there is no need to biopsy the underlying bone. Biopsy of a suspected round cell tumor should always include a frozen section and additional material for electron microscopy, tissue cultures, and other special studies. Patients presenting with a pathologic fracture usually require a primary resection. To prevent late fracture, all patients treated with radiotherapy should be protected with a brace until reossification occurs.

Gross Characteristics

The tumor tends to fill the marrow cavity and extend through the cortex and into adjacent soft tissues. The soft gray-white mass often reveals areas of necrosis and hemorrhage.

Microscopic Characteristics

The histological features of large cell "histiocytic" lymphoma of bone are indistinguishable from those of its primary lymph node counterpart. The tumor cells are large with indistinct cytoplasmic borders and eosinophilic cytoplasm. The nuclei reveal characteristic folded or convoluted nuclear membranes and contain prominent nucleoli. Well-differentiated lymphocytic lymphoma and Hodgkin's lymphoma rarely present with primary bone involvement.

METASTATIC BONE DISEASE AND PATHOLOGIC FRACTURE

Approximately 100,000 patients a year in the United States develop metastatic disease. The exact incidence of skeletal metastasis and the fracture rate are unknown. The orthopaedic surgeon is commonly asked to manage patients with skeletal metastases. The operative and nonoperative treatment of metastatic disease is continuously evolving.

Diagnosis

Clinical Characteristics

Metastatic carcinoma is the most common bone tumor in patients over 40. Despite the wide variety of carcinomas, the hallmark of skeletal involvement is pain. A patient with a known cancer who develops skeletal pain must be assumed to have a bony metastasis until proved otherwise. Approximately 10 percent of cancer patients present with bony metastasis as the first sign of the disease. Plain radiographs may appear normal for weeks or months after the onset of pain. Thus, clinical suspicion is the key to accurate diagnosis. The most common primary sources of skeletal metastases are the lungs, breast, prostate, pancreas, and stomach.

Bone scans are highly accurate and demonstrate increased uptake of contrast medium. The most common sites of involvement are spine (thoracic, then lumbar), pelvis, femur, and ribs. This distribution reflects the pattern of hematogenous spread. Vertebral lesions are thought to be secondary to seeding via Batson's plexus, i.e., perivertebral via the valveless venous plexus that permits retrograde flow. The hip and femur are the most common sites of pathologic fracture. Spinal involvement presents with back pain or neurological deficit secondary to epidural compression. Laboratory data may show hypercalcemia, reflecting accelerated bone resorption. An elevated alkaline phosphatase level is less common and is due to a secondary osteoblastic attempt to repair the destructive lesion. An elevated acid phosphatase level is pathognomonic of metastatic prostate cancer.

Radiographic Findings

Most metastatic carcinomas tend to be irregularly osteolytic with some osteoblastic response. Characteristically, osteoblastic metastases occur in the breast, prostate, lung, or bladder. In general, most endocrine tumors tend to be osteoblastic, whereas nonendocrine tumors tend to be radiolucent or osteolytic. Between 75 and 90 percent of patients with metastatic disease have multiple lesions at initial presentation. Soft tissue extension is rare for metastatic disease; the major exceptions are hypernephroma and thyroid cancer. These two lesions characteristically present as a ballooning expansile lesion with a soft tissue component; both tend to be extremely vascular. Periosteal elevation is rare except with prostate cancer. Radiographic diagnosis of metastatic disease tends to be simple. Factors favoring metastasis are irregular osteolytic and/or mixed osteoblastic lesion, multiple lesions, and age above 40 years. A few metastatic lesions may mimic a primary sarcoma. Specifically, a metastatic prostate (osteoblastic) lesion may appear as a primary osteosarcoma and a solitary hypernephroma as an osteolytic sarcoma, e.g., MFH of bone.

Staging Studies

Staging studies are similar to those used in the evaluation of primary sarcomas. The information obtained is useful in local evaluation and in therapy.

Bone Scans

Bone scintigraphy is the most helpful study in evaluating metastatic disease. Presence of multiple lesions favors the diagnosis of metastatic carcinoma and often suggests that there is involvement of other anatomic areas not suspected from clinical examination. Intraosseous extension beyond the area indicated by the plain radiographs is not unusual; this is due to the propensity of carcinoma cells to permeate between the bony trabeculae. Occasionally, decreased uptake of contrast is noted in rapidly growing lesions, presumably because of tumor necrosis.

Computed Tomography

CT has become increasingly useful in patients with spinal, pelvic, and hip lesions. This study often demonstrates extraosseous tumor not suspected on the plain radiographs. If a bone scan is "hot" but the x-ray film is normal, CT often demonstrates marked bony destruction. Thus, CT is useful in preoperative evaluation.

Angiography

Angiography is useful in specific clinical situations when evaluating metastatic disease, most commonly for preoperative embolization for suspected vascular lesions and for planning preoperative resection of certain pelvic and shoulder girdle lesions. Hypernephromas are extremely vascular and should be embolized prior to surgery.

Biopsy

The principles and techniques of biopsy are similar to those described for primary bone tumors. If a metastatic lesion is strongly suspected, a needle biopsy is often sufficient (90 percent) for a correct diagnosis. Needle biopsies are most useful for confirming metastatic carcinoma in a patient with a known cancer.[14] Conversely, if the primary tumor is unknown, a larger range of material is required for special stains, culture, and electron microscopy. A small incisional biopsy is recommended. Material for hormonal receptor tests (approximately 1 g of tissue is required) must be immediately preserved by freezing in liquid nitrogen.

Gross Characteristics

Since essentially any viscus can be the origin of osseous metastasis, the gross presentation can be quite variable. The nodules are usually well-defined and can show a variable amount of hemorrhage and necrosis. A tan-brown or black lesion suggests melanoma.

Microscopic Characteristics

The primary site determines, to a large degree, the histological appearance of the metastatic focus. Unequivocal epithelial features such as acinar formation, papillae with epithelial lining, or keratin pearl formation indicate that the lesion is not primary in bone; furthermore, based on both the pattern and certain histochemical properties, a likely primary site can be suggested. For example, the presence of epithelial mucins within tumor cell vacuoles suggests lung, gastrointestinal tract, or pancreas, among others, as possible primary sites. The Fontana stain confirms the presence of melanin pigment, as would be expected in malignant melanoma. Immunohistochemical studies, as for thyroglobulin or prostate-specific acid phosphatase, offer an additional means of tumor identification. It can be difficult to determine whether a neoplasm is a metastasis or a primary lesion. Metastatic small cell carcinoma can be misinterpreted as primary bone sarcoma or lymphoma. At the other extreme are metastatic pleomorphic carcinomas, particularly from the kidney, which have been misdiagnosed as primary MFH of bone.

Treatment: General Considerations

Treatment considerations for patients with metastatic skeletal disease differ from those for patients with primary bone neoplasms. In general, overall survival is less than 1 year. The main goals of treatment are relief of bone pain, the prevention of fracture, continued ambulation, and the avoidance of cord compression from metastatic vertebral disease. The treatment for each patient must be highly individualized, but there are certain guidelines:

1. Bone pain can be relieved by analgesics and radiation therapy. Lesions of the lower extremity often require prophylactic fixation to avoid fracture. Closed intramedullary rodding reduces the local morbidity of diaphyseal lesions. Prophylactic fixation is recommended if the lesion is greater than one-third to one-half the width of the bone.
2. If multiple sites are involved, the lower extremity (especially the hips) should be treated early to permit ambulation.
3. Early spinal cord compression should be treated aggressively with radiotherapy. If symptoms persist, early decompression is required. Increasing back pain is an early sign of cord compression.
4. Intramedullary fixation is preferred over screw-and-plate fixation. Endoprosthetic replacement is preferred for the hip in lieu of nail or plate fixation. Polymethylmethacrylate is required to permit immediate stable fixation and to prevent loosening. Recurrent tumor, radiation, and poor bony stock are causes for failure if stable fixation is not obtained. Bone graft is never used for pathologic fractures.
5. Perioperative antibiotics are required because of the increased risk of infection.
6. Hematologic parameters should be carefully evaluated before, during, and after surgery because of the increased risk of bleeding in cancer patients. The platelet count, PT, and PTT are routinely obtained.

BENIGN BONE TUMORS

The orthopaedic surgeon is often called to treat benign bone neoplasms. Some benign bone tumors are difficult to differentiate from their malignant counterparts, have a significant rate of local recurrence, and may undergo malignant transformation. Some can be treated successfully by simple curettage (intralesional procedure), while others require extensive resection (marginal or wide). Treatment is based upon the natural history of the specific entity. Treatment must be individualized; preservation of function is important. The important

clinical aspects of these tumors are emphasized in this section. In general, the preoperative staging studies are extremely accurate and the plain radiographs often suggest the correct diagnosis. The biologic classification as discussed helps determine the ideal surgical procedure.

Solitary and Multiple Osteochondromas (Exostosis)

Osteochondromas are the most common benign bone tumor. They are characteristically sessile or pedunculated, arising from the cortex of a long tubular bone adjacent to the epiphyseal plate. Osteochondromas are usually solitary except in patients with multiple hereditary exostosis. Plain radiographs are usually diagnostic, and no further tests are required. Sessile osteochondromas present difficulty in diagnosis, especially when found in unusual sites such as the distal posterior femur, in which case they must be differentiated from a parosteal OS. Bone scintigraphy and CT are helpful in distinguishing between these two entities.

Osteochondromas grow along with the individual until skeletal maturity is reached; growth of an osteochondroma during adolescence therefore does not signify malignancy. Pain is not a sign of malignancy in children or adolescents, although in an adult it is a significant warning sign. Pain in a child may be due to a local bursitis, mechanical irritation of adjacent muscles, or a pathologic fracture.

Between 1 and 2 percent of solitary osteochondromas undergo malignant transformation; patients with multiple hereditary exostosis are at a higher (5 to 25 percent) risk.[45,50] Malignant tumors arising from a benign osteochondroma are usually low-grade chondrosarcomas. Proximal osteochondromas are at a higher risk to undergo malignant transformation than distal lesions are. In general, surgical removal is recommended only for symptomatic osteochondromas or for those arising along the axial skeleton and pelvic and shoulder girdle.

Gross Characteristics

The lesion presents as a protuberant mass which can range in shape from sessile to a long-stalked polyp with a cauliflower appearance. The polypoid portion is covered by a cartilaginous cap of relatively uniform thickness which becomes thinner in the adult years. Either persistence of a thick cartilage cap or the presence of irregular nodular chondroid foci in adults should raise the question of chondrosarcomatous transformation occurring within an osteochondroma.

On perpendicular section, the hyaline cartilage cap rests on cortical bone which blends into that of the underlying bone of origin. Furthermore, the marrow cavity of the osteochondroma is contiguous with that of the normal bone.

Microscopic Characteristics

The cartilage component consists of mature lacunar chondrocytes, often arranged in clusters or rows reminiscent of epiphyseal cartilage. In the growth phase during adolescence, occasional binucleate chondrocytes may be observed. The osseous element is formed by mature lamellar bone; foci of endochondral ossification can be observed. The marrow space may be predominantly composed of adipose tissue or be filled with hematopoietic elements. It is never fibroblastic.

Enchondromas

Enchondromas may be solitary or multiple (Ollier disease). They have been reported in most bones.[15,50,57] These lesions are often difficult to diagnose radiographically and histologically. The biological potential is often over- or underestimated. Malignant transformations do occur, but the rate is difficult to determine.[46] In general, lesions of the pelvis, femur, and ribs are at higher risk than more distal sites are.[74]

Enchondromas are rarely painful unless a pathologic fracture exists. Otherwise, pain is a sign of local aggressiveness and possible malignancy. Enchondromas of the hands and feet, irrespective of pathological findings, are benign,[15] whereas cartilage tumors of the pelvic or shoulder girdle are often malignant, despite a benign-appearing histological appearance. Plain radiographs may be helpful in this differentiation. Radiographic scalloping is a sign of local aggressiveness. Bone scintigraphy is not helpful in differentiating a low-grade chondrosarcoma from an active enchondroma. Age is an important indicator of possible malignancy. Enchondromas rarely undergo malignant transformation prior to skeletal maturity. Painful, benign-appearing, proximal enchondromas in an adult are often malignant, despite the histological findings. The correlation of symptoms, plain radiographs, and histological findings is crucial in assessing an individual cartilage tumor. The medical oncologist may be called to aid in this differentiation.

Curettage of enchondromas, with or without bone graft, in a child is usually curative. Pathologic fracture may require internal fixation in addition to curettage. In an adult, curettage has a significant rate of local recurrence; resection or curettage combined with cryosurgery has a high success rate.[77,79]

Gross Characteristics

When removed intact, the lesion consists of variably sized lobules of white-gray hyaline cartilage. The tumor usually appears to be well-circumscribed. Focal myxoid areas can be encountered. In addition, calcification and ossification, which impart a gritty consistency on cutting, frequently occur.

Microscopic Characteristics

When chondroid lesions are under evaluation, histological features must be correlated with both radiographic changes and clinical setting. There may be variable cellularity, but the chondrocytes tend to remain small and uniform. Nuclear atypia is minimal, and occasional binucleate forms are not inconsistent with the diagnosis of a benign lesion. As a rule, the chondrocytes are situated in individual lacunae. Correlating with the gross findings, foci of calcification and endochondral ossification can be observed. Features such as marked nuclear atypia, mitotic activity, and multiple cells in

individual lacunae should raise the strong suspicion of chondrosarcoma.

Chondroblastoma and Osteoblastoma

Chondroblastoma and osteoblastoma are characterized by immature but benign chondroid and osteoid production, respectively. Both may undergo malignant transformation in rare cases.[47,74] Chondroblastomas typically occur in the epiphysis of a skeletally immature child (Fig. 23-22). Although osteoblastomas may be found in any bone, the spine and skull account for 50 percent of all reported cases. The differential

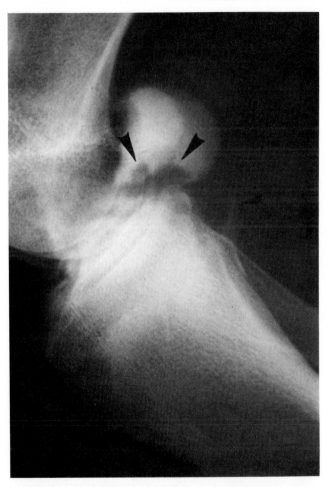

Figure 23-22 Chondroblastoma of the tibia. The contrast material in the radiograph was supplied for arthrography. Arrows outline an expansile lytic lesion of the proximal tibia. Chondroblastomas are always epiphyseal and radiolucent, and occur before skeletal maturity. Faint calcifications may be present but often are not seen despite histological evidence of calcification. The differential diagnosis includes giant cell tumor, aneurysmal bone cyst, and clear cell chondrosarcoma. *(From Malawer, M.M., Abelson, H.T., and Suit, H.D., in DeVita, V.T., Hellman, S., and Rosenberg, S.A., eds: Cancer: Principles and Practice of Oncology, 2d ed. Philadelphia, Lippincott, 1985. Reproduced with permission.)*

diagnosis of chondroblastoma includes GCT, aneurysmal bone cyst, and clear cell chondrosarcoma. Osteoblastoma n.ust be differentiated from osteosarcoma and osteoid osteoma. Clinical correlation of age, site, and histological finding often points to the correct diagnosis.

Chondroblastomas and osteoblastomas are aggressive benign lesions with a high recurrence rate following simple curettage.[15,46,50,57] Local control can be obtained by primary resection; however, routine resection cannot be recommended for tumors adjacent to a joint. Marcove reports a 5 to 10 percent local recurrence when curettage is combined with cryosurgery.[69] This method has avoided the need for resection and extensive reconstruction in select patients. It is generally difficult to obtain negative margins in osteoblastomas of the vertebrae. Radiotherapy may be required for axial lesions if there is recurrence. Osteoblastomas may metastasize following several recurrences.[84]

Osteoblastoma

Gross Characteristics These neoplasms have been reported as large as 10 cm and are unusually well circumscribed. This is often a highly vascular tumor which has areas of gritty osteoid formation. The overlying cortical bone can be bulging and minimally sclerotic.

Microscopic Characteristics The basic architecture of this lesion consists of a complex network of osteoid trabeculae which are lined by large but uniform osteoblasts (Fig. 23-23). A variable number of multinucleated giant cells are usually present, on occasion causing confusion with GCT. The intervening stroma, particularly in the younger lesions, is highly vascular. The extent of ossification varies from a few small foci to prominent confluent areas.

Chondroblastoma

Gross Characteristics The tumors are relatively small and almost invariably located in the epiphyseal region. They are

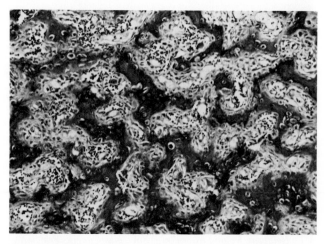

Figure 23-23 Interlacing network of irregular partially calcified bony trabeculae as seen in osteoblastoma.

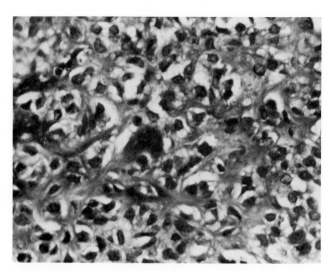

Figure 23-24 Chondroblastoma is characterized by polygonal chondrocytes and scattered multinucleated giant cells enmeshed in a lacelike chondroid matrix.

firm and vary in color from gray-white to red-brown. Irregular chondroid areas are occasionally present. On section, hemorrhagic foci and small cysts are encountered. Extension into adjacent soft tissue is rare.

Microscopic Characteristics These highly cellular neoplasms are composed of round to polygonal cells with large nuclei. Scattered mitotic figures are not uncommon. A variable number of giant cells are almost always present. Some zones demonstrate a characteristic lacelike chondroid matrix (Fig. 23-24). These chondroid strands become focally calcified.

Osteoid Osteoma

Osteoid osteoma is a small (less than 1 cm), benign bone-forming tumor that occurs throughout childhood and into the third decade of life.

Clinical Characteristics This lesion has classic symptoms and radiographic appearance in 80 percent of patients affected. Osteoid osteomas are extremely painful (equivalent to a severe toothache) and well-localized to the area of bony abnormality. Pain is often worse at night. The pain is relieved by salicylates; narcotics often are not helpful. The response to salicylates is dramatic, occurring in 20 to 30 min with a minimal dose of one or two tablets of regular aspirin. This pain pattern may exist for 6 to 9 months before the appropriate diagnosis is considered. Occasionally, the pain precedes the appearance of radiographic abnormalities and therefore leads to multiple incorrect diagnoses, including neuroses. The most common anatomic sites are the femur and/or tibia, although any bone, including the skull, spine, and small bones of the hands and feet, can be involved. When the lesion is located near a joint, the symptoms may mimic those of a monoarticular arthritis. Osteoid osteomas of the spine often present as a painful scoliosis mimicking a vertebral osteomyelitis, spinal cord tumor, or abdominal disease.

Radiographic Appearance and Evaluation The tumor can be found in any portion of a bone. The position relative to the cortex, periosteum, and spongiosa determines the radiographic appearance. The most common site is intracortical. Plain radiographs may show the nidus (lesion), which is radiolucent, but it is often obscured by a large amount of dense, white, reactive bone that is stimulated in response to the tumor. When the lesion is intramedullary, there is less sclerotic response. Detection and localization of the lesion are difficult. Bone scintigraphy is the most useful staging study and demonstrates markedly increased uptake of contrast medium. CT (in a transverse dimension) may demonstrate the nidus and is helpful in determining which portion of the bone is involved. This aids in determining the appropriate surgical approach and the section of bone to be excised. Occasionally CT does not demonstrate the lesion because of the lesion's small size and a partial volumning effect. In this case, linear tomography may be more useful. The authors recommend that all the above studies be performed because of the likely difficulty of accurate localization and need for complete surgical removal. In addition, intraoperative scanning of the specimen and the patient is required to assure localization and removal of the lesion.

Treatment Surgical removal of the nidus is required; the sclerotic, reactive bone need not be removed. Pain is dramatically resolved postoperatively if the nidus has been excised. A marginal excision is recommended. Curettage should *not* be performed because of the risk of leaving a portion or missing the lesion completely. Incomplete removal routinely results in a clinical recurrence. A wide excision of a portion of the reactive bone and area of presumed nidus is often required to accomplish successful removal.

Gross Characteristics Identification of the characteristic nidus is essential to establish a diagnosis of osteoid osteoma. The round, well-delineated nidus rarely measures greater than 1.0 to 1.5 cm. It is usually red and can vary from soft and friable to sclerotic.

Microscopic Characteristics The nidus is characterized by an interlacing network of osteoblast-lined trabeculae. Calcification of the osteoid may be prominent, particularly in the center, and cement lines are common. Scattered multinucleated giant cells are commonly noted. The intertrabecular stroma consists of a richly vascular connective tissue, devoid of hematopoietic elements (Fig. 23-25). The bone surrounding the nidus usually reveals nonspecific sclerotic changes. On occasion, it may be exceedingly difficult to differentiate a large osteoid osteoma from an osteoblastoma.

Unicameral (Simple) Bone Cysts

Unicameral bone cysts (UBCs) are benign lesions that occur during growth. They involve the metaphysis and/or diaphysis of a long bone (Fig. 23-26A). They are believed not to be true neoplasms.

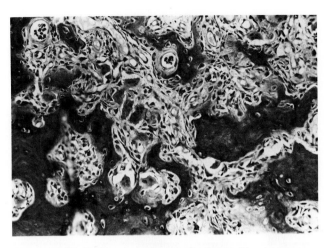

Figure 23-25 High-power micrograph of osteoid osteoma reveals osteoblast-lined trabeculae. Note the richly vascular stroma and scattered multinucleated giant cells.

The most common sites are the proximal humerus (67 percent) and proximal femur (15 percent).[62] UBCs are usually asymptomatic until a fracture occurs. Radiographically, UBCs are radiolucent and slightly expansile with well-defined margins. UBCs are rarely confused with other benign or malignant tumors. They are easily diagnosed by plain radiographs when found in the more common locations. Other preoperative staging studies are usually not required. Bone scintigraphy is the most useful study when the diagnosis is in doubt. The bone scan typically shows a photon-deficient area corresponding to detail on the plain radiograph (Fig. 23-26B). A small area of increased uptake of contrast reflects a typical hairline crack that initiates pain and radiographic investigation.

Treatment The traditional treatment has been curettage. Local recurrence rates have ranged from 35 to 70 percent. Recently, UBCs have been successfully treated by aspiration, flushing, and injection with methylprednisolone acetate. In one series of 40 patients, a second aspiration and injection was required in 27 percent of patients; 95 percent eventually healed.[62] In order to avoid erroneously injecting a bone lesion other than a UBC, four radiographic, nonhistological criteria have been established and are summarized as follows:[62]

1. Typical plain radiograph (and age and location)
2. Positive aspiration (yellow fluid)
3. Typical transduced "arteriolar" pressure curve (range 15 to 28 mmHg)
4. Complete filling of cyst with meglumine diatrizoate (Renografin) following aspiration

In general, UBCs should be treated by aspiration, high-pressure Renografin injection, and intracavitary methylprednisolone. Pathologic fractures should be allowed to heal *before* injection is performed. If the diagnosis is in doubt, a Craig needle procedure or small incisional biopsy should be performed. There may be radiographic recurrence; this can be successfully treated with repeat injections. UBCs should not be left untreated in the hope that they will spontaneously regress. Fewer than 1 percent of UBCs do so; the remainder

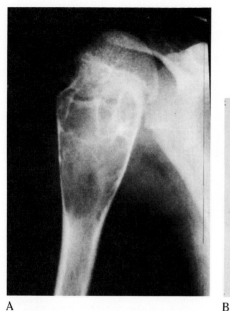

A

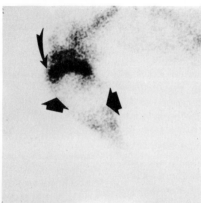

B

Figure 23-26 Unicameral bone cyst. **A.** Typical unicameral bone cyst of the proximal humerus. There is a slight expansion of the cortices without evidence of cortical destruction or periosteal elevation. **B.** Bone scintigraphy. Unicameral bone cysts are classically photon-deficient (cold) lesions (*solid arrows*). In contrast, GCTs and aneurysmal bone cysts routinely show increased uptake. Bone scans are recommended preoperatively only if the diagnosis is in doubt. The epiphyseal plate (*curved arrow*) is noted.

often become large before the appropriate treatment is undertaken, making definitive treatment more difficult.

Gross Characteristics On section, the UBC usually contains a clear or blood-tinged fluid. Occasionally, the cavity is empty. The wall of the cyst reveals protruding thin-walled septa of variable depth. The cyst lining may be thin and white-gray or may reveal foci of brown-red soft tissue. Prior fracture or hemorrhage substantially alters these basic features.

Microscopic Characteristics The cyst lining varies from a thin fibrocollagenous membrane to a thicker, more cellular tissue. The latter foci contain an admixture of giant cells, chronic inflammatory cells, and hemosiderin-laden macrophages. Areas with granulation tissue and reactive bone are occasionally noted.

Eosinophilic Granuloma

Eosinophilic granuloma (EG) is a solitary destructive lesion arising presumably from the reticuloendothelial system during the first decade of life. There is slight male predominance. Any bone may be involved. The most common sites are the long bones and commonly the periacetabular region. The skull, mandible, ribs, and vertebrae are frequent sites. Multiple bony involvement is common; between 10 and 50 percent of patients develop multiple lesions. Plain radiographs characteristically show a lytic, punched-out lesion with some evidence of cortical destruction; approximately 50 percent of patients have periosteal elevation. The differential diagnosis includes osteomyelitis, Ewing's sarcoma, and lymphoma. The diaphysis and the metaphysis are equally affected. Primary epiphyseal involvement or extension is rare. Leeson reviewed the literature in 1985 and reported three new cases. A total of 10 cases have been reported to date.

Good results have been achieved with the use of steroids to treat localized bony EG. The natural history of EG of bone is to spontaneously heal. Curettage or intralesional steroid is recommended for documented lesions, especially in a weight-bearing bone.

Gross Characteristics

The curetted tissue is soft and friable and can be pink or yellow.

Microscopic Characteristics

Sheets of large histiocytes (Langerhans cells) characterize this process. These cells have abundant amphophilic cytoplasm and a large vesicular nucleus which is usually folded or convoluted. There may be inflammatory cells in the background, although abundant eosinophils are almost always present. With this disease it is not possible to predict the extent of the visceral involvement based on the histomorphology of the bone lesions.

Desmoplastic Fibroma

Desmoplastic fibroma is an extremely rare bone tumor. Only 50 cases have been reported.[46] The tumor is characterized by abundant collagen formation and a fibrous stroma without evidence of mitosis or pleomorphism. Radiographically it presents as an osteolytic lesion with well-defined margins. The basic differential diagnosis is primary fibrosarcoma of bone. Adequate treatment is en bloc resection; curettage has a significant rate of local recurrence.

Gross Characteristics

The lesion consists of a homogeneous firm, white-gray whorled fibrouslike tissue.

Microscopic

The tumor is characterized by intersecting dense collagen bundles containing bland-appearing, uniform spindle cells. Mitotic activity is rare to absent. The histological picture is essentially indistinguishable from that of soft tissue fibromatosis (desmoid).

SECTION B

Other Malignancies Affecting Bone

Stephen Feffer and David Westring

Tumors which arise within the marrow and its related vascular and lymph channels not infrequently require orthopaedic attention for diagnosis or treatment. This is especially true for the reticuloendothelioses, a poorly understood group of tumors which range widely in their malignant behavior, location, and clinical expression. These and the more common malignancies of the bone marrow will be briefly described.

LYMPHOMA

Lymphomas are neoplasms of the immune system which, because of the wide distribution of lymphocytes in the body, may arise from virtually any site. Lymph nodes, tonsils, spleen, and bone marrow are the most frequent sites of origin, but commonly the malignant cells invade bone marrow or blood, making the diagnosis of lymphoma or leukemia one of tumor distribution.[36] Classification of these diseases has been confusing and in constant evolution, but the separation of Hodgkin's disease from the other lymphomas is widely accepted and useful. It is unfortunate that no better term than *non-Hodgkin's lymphoma* has become widely used for the other lymphomas; in this text *lymphoma* refers to lymphatic malignancies other than Hodgkin's disease and multiple myeloma unless qualified.

Classification

The clinical presentation, natural history, and response to therapy are heavily influenced by the pathological nature of lymphomas. The most commonly utilized classification was described by Rappaport,[37] and its usefulness was demonstrated in a report by Jones et al.[22] This classification recognizes five categories:

1. Lymphocytic, well-differentiated
2. Lymphocytic, poorly differentiated (formerly lymphosarcoma)
3. Histocytic (formerly reticulum cell sarcoma)
4. Mixed histiocytic and lymphocytic
5. Undifferentiated (stem cell)

All may present as nodular or diffuse types except 5, which presents only in the diffuse form.

Whether the malignant cell is distributed in the tissue in the nodular or diffuse pattern contributes more to the natural history of the illness than the description of the involved cell type does.

Treatment

When lymphoma appears to be limited to one extranodal site (stage I), treatment is usually local radiation therapy in curative doses; an overall 5-year disease-free survival of 41 percent of these patients has been reported in one series, with far better results in the more favorable cell and pattern variants.[40]

When lymphoma (non-Hodgkin's) presents as an isolated skeletal lesion, local radiation therapy can be curative if other potential sites of involvement have been systematically excluded. In the Mayo Clinic series, 90 percent of such patients complained of bone pain, 33 percent reported local swelling, and 9 percent presented with a pathologic fracture. Systemic symptoms such as fever and weight loss were unusual. Most frequently involved were the pelvis, femur, humerus, ribs, and tibia. Radiological examination revealed locally destructive lesions, not distinctively different from other malignant tumors. The mean age of the patients was 44 years, with a slight male predominance. When the patients were treated with local radiation therapy, a 5-year survival of 44 percent was obtained.[51] Other reports confirmed these favorable results,[9] while one described a poorer prognosis for patients presenting with pelvic rather than long bone involvement.[43]

These studies affirm the necessity of thorough staging evaluation of a patient whose presenting complaint relates to a focus of skeletal malignant lymphoma. Radiation therapy alone provides a respectable 5-year survival; if disease is found elsewhere, local radiation therapy is palliative only and systemic therapy is called for. Surgical intervention for pathologic fractures may be useful when it will hasten the patient's mobilization, but radiosensitive tumors of the bone may heal rapidly with radiation therapy alone.

Within the past decade, aggressive multidrug chemotherapy programs of relatively brief duration, usually 6 months, have produced extraordinarily high remission rates as well as long-term disease-free survivors in patients with disseminated lymphoma. Most regimens contain the anthracycline doxorubicin as well as alkylating agents, *Vinca* alkaloids, and corticosteroids. Toxicities include significant bone marrow suppression, gastrointestinal disturbance, and nearly universal alopecia. Response rates in some variants reach 80 percent, and cure rates of greater than 50 percent have been reported in some varieties of malignant lymphoma that were previously uniformly fatal.[3,27,39]

HODGKIN DISEASE

Hodgkin disease is a rare malignancy of lymph tissue first described in 1832;[21] each year approximately 7000 new cases are reported in the United States, with a male-female ratio of 3.6:2.6.[2] Etiology has not been determined.

Diagnosis

Hodgkin disease must be differentiated from other disorders presenting as widespread adenopathy, i.e., infections such as tuberculosis, syphilis, toxoplasmosis, or infectious mononucleosis, and other forms of malignant lymphoma. The diagnosis can never be made without a histological examination of a tissue biopsy. The hallmark is the presence of the Reed-Sternberg (RS) cell accompanied by the appropriate cellular reaction. The RS cell is a giant binucleate or multinucleate cell with one or more prominent nucleoli. It is believed to be derived from the mononuclear phagocyte line.[23] The pathological description of involved lymph nodes is predictive of disease response to treatment and of survival and forms the basis of the current classification of this disease; the two variables involved are the number of RS cells present and local cellular host response to those cells.[10]

Prognostic significance is attached to the presence of certain systemic symptoms: (1) fever, (2) night sweats, and (3) weight loss of greater than 10 percent of the patient's body weight over 6 months. The presence of any of these is designated stage B and denotes less favorable prognosis than their absence.

Bone Lesions

Bony involvement occurs in 15 percent of patients with advanced Hodgkin disease. The thoracic and lumbar vertebrae are most commonly involved. Deep localized pain is frequently described. Radiographs and bone scans are effective in making the diagnosis, while blood analyses including determination of alkaline phosphatase levels, are not helpful. The radiographic appearance of Hodgkin lesions is sclerotic, lytic, or mixed. Most often, osseous involvement occurs in patients with one or more of the stage B symptoms described above.[34]

Treatment

The treatment of Hodgkin disease is complex and is most effectively accomplished through multidisciplinary teams that are assembled on the basis of the findings during the pathological staging procedures. Team decisions are usually reached at interdepartmental or tumor board conferences at which surgical, radiotherapy, and medical oncologists are permanent members and other specialties are represented as consultants. The orthopaedist may be requested to attend when bone lesions are present or when other forms of therapy may threaten future musculoskeletal function.

Stages I, II, and III are most often treated by radiation therapy, while treatment for stages IIIB and IV requires systemic combination chemotherapy. The standard regimen uses nitrogen mustard, vincristine, procarbazine, and prednisone (MOPP).[15] In stage IV, 80 percent of patients with bone involvement treated with combination chemotherapy and radiation have a greater than 5-year survival probability.[34] Thus bone involvement does not appear to adversely alter response to therapy. Local bone pain or nerve compression syndromes can be palliated by local radiation therapy or surgery, but often respond to systemic therapy.

The prognosis for patients with Hodgkin disease has changed dramatically since the 1960s, when Kaplan reported curative radiation therapy[24] followed by introduction of the MOPP drug regimen. Continuing refinements in diagnosis and therapy promise further improvement in prognosis.

MULTIPLE MYELOMA

Multiple myeloma is a disease of uncontrolled proliferation of plasma cells in the bone marrow. Plasma cells are highly differentiated lymphocytes of the B cell series which are responsible for production of the five classes of immunoglobulins, the circulating antibodies of the human immune system. Although multiple myeloma is thus a malignancy of the immune system, it has not been classified conventionally with the lymphomas.

Clinical Features

Clinical manifestations commonly involve bone marrow suppression, bone destruction, hypercalcemia, hypoglobulinemia with recurrent infection, and renal failure. Bleeding tendencies and signs of hyperviscosity syndrome occur less frequently. Incidence increases with age, the mean age at diagnosis being 62 years, and is about equal in men and women.

Diagnosis

The diagnosis of multiple myeloma should be suspected in any patient presenting with bone pain and anemia, particularly if serum chemistry screening reveals an elevated serum globulin level. Serum protein electrophoresis should then be performed to confirm that the increased serum globulin level truly represents a monoclonal gammopathy, expressed as a "spike," usually in the gamma globulin region. In 20 percent of patients, no abnormal serum protein can be detected; in these, electrophoretic examination of the urine reveals increased light chain fragments of the pathological immunoglobulin. The Bence Jones method of identifying this protein has been abandoned in favor of this more sensitive test.

Finally, a bone marrow aspirate and biopsy must be performed to establish the diagnosis. The specimen should be cellular, with greater than 30 percent of the cells identified as plasma cells. These are usually arranged in clusters or "sheets" and often appear immature or with multiple nuclei. Failure to meet these criteria in a patient with otherwise convincing evidence justifies repeat biopsy, since the disease may be unevenly distributed.

The abnormal clone of plasma cells in the marrow usually causes diffuse osteoporosis of lytic lesions by eliciting activity of osteoclasts.[33] On rare occasions osteoblastic activity is predominant.[38] As a result, x-ray studies are more sensitive for evaluating extent of disease than the technetium bone scan[31] and show characteristic punched-out or expansile lesions without reactive borders (Fig. 23-27). This destruction can be a cause of symptomatic hypercalcemia.

Despite the presence of a significant increase in one class of intact immunoglobulin or of one of the light chain fragments, total effective immunoglobulin production is drastically reduced. As a result, patients are vulnerable to overwhelming infection by encapsulated bacteria, such as pneumococcus. Therapy with ionizing radiation, alkylating agents, or corticosteroids further impairs resistance to other opportunistic infections. Consequently, pneumonia and other infections are common complications of multiple myeloma.

The pathogenesis of renal failure with multiple myeloma is complex. Contributing factors may include immunoglobu-

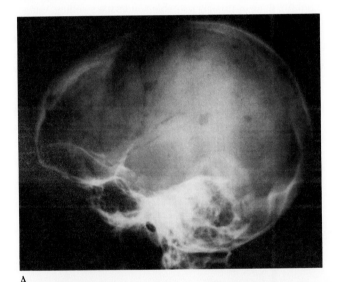

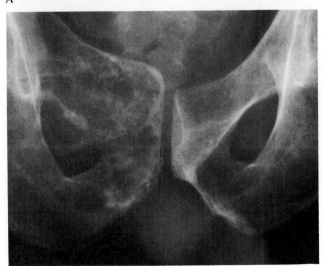

Figure 23-27 Multiple myeloma. **A.** Skull film showing round "punched out" lesions with sharp, nonsclerotic borders. **B.** Extensive expansile lesion of pubis and ischium. Serum alkaline phosphatase levels were normal.

lin light chains in the urine, hypercalcemia, hyperuricemia, renal infection, and amyloidosis. It is interesting that hypertension is infrequently found in the renal failure of multiple myeloma.

Occasionally, solitary masses composed of plasma cells (plasmacytomas) arise in patients with no evidence of multiple myeloma. These lesions may originate in bones, or in soft tissue such as in the head and neck region. They are best treated locally in an aggressive fashion, requiring either excision or ablative radiation therapy,[4,53] but despite local control, the bulk of these patients return with full-blown multiple myeloma within 5 years. This appears to be particularly true for those whose plasmacytomas arise in bone.[12,48]

Treatment

The standard systemic therapy for multiple myeloma was developed in the late 1960s and consists of an alkylating agent plus a corticosteroid. Clinical remissions, indicated by decreasing abnormal globulin levels in the serum, absence of bone pain (lesions rarely heal radiographically), and improvement in anemia and/or renal function, etc., occur in between 40 and 70 percent of patients.[1,6,13] Complete remissions are rare. Somewhat better response rates have been reported when additional agents are added, but the improvement appears to be modest.[1]

Symptoms of local bone lesions are usually effectively palliated by radiation therapy; frequently this requires 2000 to 3000 rad over 10 treatments. Pathologic fractures can usually be prevented by treating bony lesions before the destruction becomes extensive.[32] If fracture should occur, intramedullary fixation either followed or preceded by radiation therapy is generally recommended.[14,32] (The treatment of spinal lesions is discussed under Malignant Tumors of the Spine in Chap. 56.)

Treatment of the osteoporotic changes with sodium fluoride and calcium carbonate is controversial.[26,45] Meanwhile, dichloromethylene disphosphonate (DP), an osteoclast inhibitor, promises substantial improvement in calcium balance and reduction of bone pain.[45]

LEUKEMIA

Leukemia is a disease characterized by malignant proliferation of one or more of the blood-forming cells. Clinical manifestations reflect the developmental stage of the malignant cell, which is usually, but not always, morphologically immature; it is always dysfunctional, however, and when untreated inevitably leads to the death of the patient by progressive invasion of the marrow, blood, and tissues. The SEER program of the U. S. National Cancer Institute estimated that 26,400 new cases of leukemia would occur in 1987[44]; from 1973 to 1976 it was the leading malignant disease in children at a rate of 33.6 per 100,000 children. Modern therapy increased 5-year survival in Caucasians from 14 percent in 1960 to 1963 to 33 percent in 1976 to 1981.

Leukemias are most simply divided into chronic and acute varieties. Chronic leukemias are defined by consistently elevated white blood cell counts, usually with a large percentage of morphologically normal-appearing cells. Acute leukemias, on the other hand, have variable peripheral white blood cell counts and nearly always display a majority of immature forms. In all leukemias the bone marrow is heavily infiltrated with abnormal cells; replacement of normal hematopoietic elements is the rule, predisposing the patient to life-threatening episodes of infection and/or bleeding.

Sternal tenderness is often present. Tenderness of long bones occurs more often in children than in adults. Skeletal involvement by leukemia is most often manifested as diffuse bone or joint pain, reflecting rapid expansion of the marrow space by proliferating leukemic cells. In children, transverse radiolucent bands in the metaphyseal region may be seen. In adults, a wide variety of lytic lesions may be seen but the majority of adult patients show few skeletal changes. There have been reports of both acute and chronic leukemia causing diaphyseal radiolucency which in chronic granulocytic leukemia usually heralds the onset of the more aggressive and refractory accelerated phase of the illness.[8,46]

RETICULOENDOTHELIOSES

Histiocytosis X is a term coined by Lichtenstein in 1953 to define three clinically distinct disorders which share a common histological pattern; they are eosinophilic granuloma of bone, Hand-Schüller-Christian syndrome, and Letterer-Siwe syndrome.[29] The histological findings of each of these are characterized by a proliferation of histiocytes accompanied by an increased number of eosinophils. In the more advanced clinical states (particularly Letterer-Siwe syndrome) the histiocytes appear lipid-laden with variable amounts of fibrous reaction.[49]

At some time during the course of any of these diseases, bone tumors are found in nearly all patients. By conventional x-ray examination, the overwhelming majority of early lesions are sharply marginated round or oval rarefactions (Fig. 23-28A). Occasional radiodense lesions may be seen. Cystlike structures are formed as the tumor expands in flat bones; eventually irregularly marginated lucent lesions develop (Fig. 23-28D). As tumor grows in the medullary cavity of long bones, pressure atrophy leads to scalloping along the inner margin of the cortex. Finally, tumor eroding through the cortex may stimulate the periosteum to produce new bone, simulating Ewing's sarcoma or osteomyelitis. Continued growth often presents as grossly palpable soft tissue swelling. Lung is commonly involved in Hand-Schüller-Christian syndrome. The most frequent sites of osseous involvement are the flat bones of the skull, ribs, pelvis, and scapula. The long bones of the arms, legs, and dorsolumbar spine are also commonly involved.[49]

Clinical descriptions of the three entities which constitute histiocytosis X are summarized in Table 23-10. The triad of exophthalmos, diabetes insipidus, and cranial bone lesions said to be characteristic of Hand-Schüller-Christian syndrome in reality occurs only in 10 percent of patients considered to have that disorder.

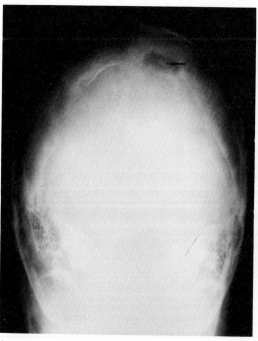

A   B

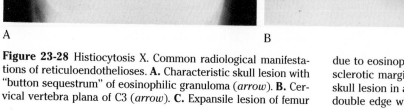

Figure 23-28 Histiocytosis X. Common radiological manifestations of reticuloendothelioses. **A.** Characteristic skull lesion with "button sequestrum" of eosinophilic granuloma (*arrow*). **B.** Cervical vertebra plana of C3 (*arrow*). **C.** Expansile lesion of femur due to eosinophilic granuloma. Note cortical thickening without sclerotic margins. **D.** Classic scalloping and beveled edges in a skull lesion in a case of eosinophilic granuloma. Arrows point to double edge which gives beveled appearance.

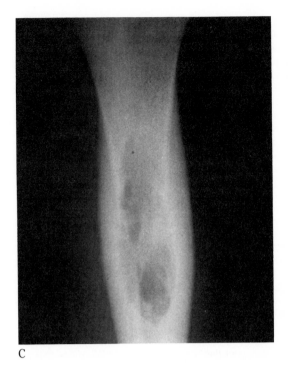

C

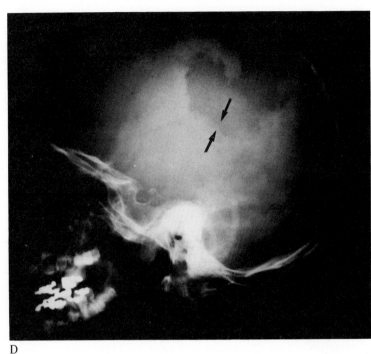

D

The etiology of these disorders remains unknown. One view is that the lesions in eosinophilic granuloma and Hand-Schüller-Christian syndrome are reactive and inflammatory, while those of Letterer-Siwe syndrome appear to be neoplastic.[49]

Forms of the illness confined to bone appear to have a favorable outlook; primary treatment is curettage with radiation therapy reserved for lesions incompletely ablated by curettage or in regions where surgical management is not feasible. The disseminated forms vary greatly in severity and prognosis. In a review of 50 cases of histiocytosis X in which two or more extraosseous organs were involved, the following negative prognostic indicators were identified: (1) age less than 2 years, (2) dyspnea and cyanosis due to pulmonary involvement of flat or spinal bones, and (3) severe anemia or thrombocytopenia.[35] All patients were divided into prognostic groups as shown in Table 23-11. The Southwest Oncology Group similarly reported that age and organ dysfunction are important in determining survival and added a third variable

TABLE 23-11 Prognostic Groups in Histiocytosis X

Group	Disease distribution	Mortality, %
I	Skeleton only	33
II	Skeleton, skin, visceral, lymphatic	43
III	Nonosteolytic, skin, visceral lymph nodes	62

for predicting survival: response to initial chemotherapy.[25]

Systemic corticosteroids usually provide immediate improvement in skin lesions, pain, and overall well-being; however, when they are discontinued, recurrence of cutaneous and visceral symptoms are frequent.[47] Another Southwest Oncology study used chlorambucil for systemic therapy and reported a remission rate of approximately 60 percent.[19] This

TABLE 23-10 The Clinical Syndromes of Histiocytosis X

Syndrome	Usual age of onset	Findings	Course
Eosinophilic granuloma	Children, young adults	Single or multiple osseous involvement	Recurrences common, rarely fatal
Hand-Schüller-Christian	5 years	Widespread visceral and bony involvement	Chronic course
Letterer-Siwe	2 years	Hepatosplenomegaly, adenopathy, fever, anemia, thrombocytopenia	Acute or subacute

and other reports confirm the utility of single agent or multiple drug chemotherapy in advanced cases of histiocytosis X, but survival advantage is yet to be confirmed.

REFERENCES

Section A: Musculoskeletal Oncology

1. Ahuja, S.C., Villacin, A.B., Smith, J., et al. Juxtacortical (parosteal) osteogenic sarcoma. J Bone Joint Surg [Am] 59:632–647, 1977.
2. Aprin, H., Riserborough, E.J. and Hall, J.E. Chondrosarcoma in children and adolescents. Clin Orthop 166:226–232, 1982.
3. Bacci, G., Picci, P., Calderoni, P., et al. Full-lung tomograms and bone scanning in the initial work-up of patients with osteogenic sarcoma. A review of 126 cases. Eur J Cancer Clin Oncol 18:967–971, 1982.
4. Bacci, G., Picci, P., Gitelis, S., et al. The treatment of localized Ewing's sarcoma. Cancer 49:1561–1570, 1982.
5. Bergsagel, D.E., and Rider, W.D. Plasma cell neoplasms, chap 47, in DeVita, V.T., Hellman, S., and Rosenberg, S.A. (eds): *Cancer, Principles and Practice of Oncology,* 2d ed. Philadelphia, Lippincott, 1985, pp 1753–1759.
6. Bjornsson, J., Unni, K.K., Dahlin, D.C., et al. Clear cell chondrosarcoma of bone. Observations in 47 cases. Am J Surg Pathol 8:223–230, 1984.
7. Brostrom, L-A. On the natural history of osteosarcoma. Aspects of diagnosis, prognosis and endocrinology. Acta Orthop Scand 183 (suppl):1–38, 1980.
8. Campanacci, M., Bacci, G., Bertoni, et al. The treatment of osteosarcoma of the extremity: Twenty years' experience at the Istituto Ortopedico Rizzoli. Cancer 48(7):1569–1581, 1981.
9. Campanacci, M., Giunti, A., and Olmi, R. Giant-cell tumors of bone: A study of 209 cases with long-term follow-up in 130. Ital J Orthop Traumatol 1:249–277, 1977.
10. Campanacci, M., Picci, P., Gherlinzona, F., et al. Parosteal osteosarcoma. J Bone Joint Surg 66B:313–321, 1984.
11. Chaos, E.Y.S., and Ivins, J.C. *Design and Application of Tumor Prosthesis for Bone and Joint Reconstruction—The Design and Application.* New York, Thieme-Stratton, 1983.
12. Cortes, E.P., and Holland, J.P. Adjuvant chemotherapy for primary osteogenic sarcoma. Surg Clin North Am 61:1391–1404, 1981.
13. Cortes, E.P., Holland, J.F., Wang, J.J., et al. Amputation and adriamycin in primary osteosarcoma. N Engl J Med 291:998–1000, 1974.
14. Craig, F.S. Metastatic and primary lesions of bone. Clin Orthop 73:33, 1970.
15. Dahlin, D.C. *Bone Tumors: General Aspects and Data on 6,221 Cases,* 3d ed. Springfield, IL, Thomas, 1978.
16. Dahlin, D.C. The problems in assessment of new treatment regimens of osteosarcoma. Clin Orthop 153:81–85, 1980.
17. Dahlin, D.C., and Coventry, M.B. Osteosarcoma, a study of 600 cases. J Bone Joint Surg 49A:101–110, 1967.
18. Dahlin, D.C., Cupps, R.E., and Johnson, E.W., Jr. Giant cell tumor: A study of 195 cases. Cancer 25:1061–1070, 1970.
19. Dahlin, D.C., and Unni, K.K. Osteosarcoma of bone and its important recognizable varieties. Am J Surg Pathol 1(1):61–72, 1977.
20. deSantos, L.A., Bernardino, M.E., and Murry, J.A. Computed tomography in the evaluation of osteosarcoma: Experience with 25 cases. AJR 132:535–540, 1979.
21. deSantos, L.A., and Edeiken, B. Purely lytic osteosarcoma. Skeletal Radiol 9:1–7, 1982.
22. Destouet, J.M., Gilula, L.A., and Murphy, W. Computed tomography of long bone osteosarcoma. Radiology 131:439–445, 1979.
23. Edeiken, J. Bone tumors and tumor-like conditions, in Edeiken, J. (ed): *Roentgen Diagnosis of Diseases of Bone,* 3d ed. Baltimore, Williams & Wilkins, 1981, pp 30–414.
24. Enneking, W.F. *Musculoskeletal Tumor Surgery,* vol 1. New York, Churchill Livingstone, 1983, pp 1–60.
25. Enneking, W.F. *Musculoskeletal Tumor Society,* vol 7. New York, Churchill Livingstone, 1983, pp 1021–1125.
26. Enneking, W.F., and Dunham, W.K. Resection and reconstruction for primary neoplasms involving the innominate bone. J Bone Joint Surg [Am] 60:731–746, 1978.
27. Enneking, W.F., and Kagan, A. Intramarrow spread of osteosarcoma, in *Management of Primary Bone and Soft Tissue Tumors.* Chicago, Yearbook, 1976, pp 171–177.
28. Enneking, W.F., and Shirley, P.D. Resection-arthrodesis for malignant and potentially malignant lesions about the knee using an intramedullary rod and local bone graft. J Bone Joint Surg [Am] 59:223–235, 1977.
29. Enneking, W.F., Spanier, S.S., and Malawer, M.M. The effect of the anatomic setting on the results of surgical procedure for soft parts sarcoma of the thigh. Cancer 47:1005–1022, 1981.
30. Enneking, W.F., Spanier, S.S., and Goodman, M.A. A system for the surgical staging of musculoskeletal sarcoma. Clin Orthop 153:106–120, 1980.
31. Enneking, W.F., Spanier, S.S., and Malawer, M.M. The effects of the anatomic setting on the results of surgical procedures for soft parts sarcoma of the thigh. Cancer 47(5):1005–1022, 1981.
32. Enzinger, F.M., and Weiss, S.W. *Soft Tissue Tumors.* St. Louis, Mosby, 1983.
33. Francis, K.C., Kohn, H., and Malawer, M.M. Osteogenic sarcoma. J Bone Joint Surg [Am] 55:754, 1976.
34. Francis, K.C., and Worcester, J.N., Jr. Radical resection for tumors of the shoulder with preservation of a functional extremity. J Bone Joint Surg [Am] 44:1423–1429, 1962.
35. Garrison, R.C., Unni, K.K., McLeod, R.A., et al. Chondrosarcoma arising in osteochondroma. Cancer 49:1890–1897, 1982.
36. Gitellis, S., Bertoni, F., Chieti, P.P., and Campanacci, M. Chondrosarcoma of bone. J Bone Joint Surg [Am] 63A(8):1248–1257, 1981.
37. Goldenberg, R.R., Campbell, C.J., and Bongfiglio, M. Giant cell tumor of bone. An analysis of two hundred and eighteen cases. J Bone Joint Surg [Am] 52:619–664, 1970.
38. Goldstein, H., McNeil, B.J., Zufall, E., et al. Changing indications for bone scintigraphy in patients with osteosarcoma. Radiology 135:177–180, 1980.
39. Gray, S.W., Singhabhandhu, B., Smith, R.A., and Skandalakis, J.E. Sacrococcygeal chordoma: Report of a case and review of the literature. Surgery 78(5):573–582, 1975.
40. Guterberg, B., Romanus, B., and Sterner, B.L. Pelvic strength after major amputation of the sacrum. An experimental study. Acta Orthop Scand 47:635–642, 1976.
41. Hajdu, S.I., Shiu, M.H., and Fortner, J.C. Tendosynovial sarcoma. A clinicopathological study of 136 cases. Cancer 39:1201, 1977.
42. Harwood, A.R., Krajbich, J.I., and Fornasier, V.L. Mesenchymal chondrosarcoma: A report of 17 cases. *Clin Orthop* 158:144–148, 1981.
43. Hudson, T.M., Hass, G., Enneking, W.F., and Hawkins, E.F. Angiography in the management of musculoskeletal tumors. Surg Gynecol Obstet 141:11–21, 1975.
44. Hutter, V.P., Worcester, J.N., Jr., Francis, K.C., et al. Benign and malignant giant cell tumor of bone. A clinicopathological analysis of the natural history of the disease. Cancer 15:653–690, 1962.
45. Huvos, A.G. Primary malignant fibrous histiocytoma of bone. Clinicopathologic study of 18 patients. NY State J Med 76:552–559, 1976.
46. Huvos, A.G. *Bone Tumors. Diagnosis, Treatment and Prognosis.* Philadelphia, Saunders, 1979.

47. Huvos, A.G., and Higinbotham, N.L. Primary fibrosarcoma of bone. A clinicopathologic study of 130 patients. Cancer 35:837–847, 1975.

48. Huvos, A.G., Rosen, G., Dabska, M., and Marcove, R.C. Mesenchymal chondrosarcoma: A clinicopathologic analysis of 35 patients with emphasis on treatment. Cancer 51:1230–1237, 1983.

49. Huvos, A.G., Rosen, G., and Marcove, R.C. Primary osteogenic sarcoma. Pathologic aspects in 20 patients after treatment with chemotherapy, en bloc resection and prosthetic bone replacement. Arch Pathol Lab Med 101:14–18, 1977.

50. Jaffe, H.L. *Tumors and Tumorous Conditions of the Bone and Joints.* Philadelphia, Lea & Febiger, 1958.

51. Jaffe, N., Link, M.P., Cohen, D., et al. High-dose methotrexate in osteogenic sarcoma. Natl Cancer Inst Monogr 56:201–206, 1981.

52. Jaffe, N., Smith, E., Abelson H.T., et al. Osteogenic sarcoma: Alterations in the pattern of pulmonary metastases with adjuvant chemotherapy. J Clin Oncol 1:251–254, 1983.

53. Janeck, C.J., and Nelson, C.L. En bloc resection of shoulder girdle: Technique and indications. Report of a case. J Bone Joint Surg [Am] 54:1754–1758, 1972.

54. Johnson, E.W., Jr., and Dahlin, D.C. Treatment of giant cell tumor of bone. J Bone Joint Surg [Am] 41:895–904, 1959.

55. Johnson, E.W., and Dahlin, D.C. Treatment of giant cell tumor of bone: An evaluation of 24 cases treated at the Johns Hopkins Hospital between 1925–1955. Orthopedics 62:187–191, 1969.

56. Levine, E. Computed tomography of musculoskeletal tumors. CRC Crit Rev Diagn Imaging 16:279–309, 1981.

57. Lichtenstein, L. *Bone Tumors,* 4th ed. St. Louis, Mosby, 1972.

58. Lindberg, R.D., Martin, R.M., and Rohmsdahl, M.M. Surgery and postoperative radiotherapy in the treatment of soft-tissue sarcomas in adults. AJR 123:123, 1976.

59. Localio, A.S., Eng, K., and Ranson, J.H.C. Abdominosacral approach for retrorectal tumors. Ann Surg 179:555–560, 1980.

60. Localio, A.S., Francis, K.C., and Rossano, P.C. Abdominosacral resection of sacrococcygeal chordoma. Ann Surg 166:394–400, 1967.

61. Malawer, M.M. Distal femoral osteogenic sarcoma, principles of soft tissue resection and reconstruction in conjunction with prosthetic replacement (adjuvant surgery), in Chao, E.Y.S. (ed): *Design and Application of Tumor Prothesis for Bone and Joint Reconstruction.* New York, Thieme-Stratton, 1983, pp 297–309.

62. Malawer, M.M. The diagnosis, treatment and management of unicameral bone cysts by percutaneous aspiration, hemodynamic evaluation and intracavitary methylprednisolone acetate. Orthopedic Update Series IV(26):1–7, 1986.

63. Malawer, M.M., Abelson, H.T., and Suit, H.D. Sarcomas of bone, chap 37, in DeVita, V.T., Hellman, S., and Rosenberg, S.A. (eds): *Cancer, Principles and Practice of Oncology,* 2d ed. Philadelphia, Lippincott, 1985, pp 1293–1343.

64. Malawer, M.M., Sugarbaker, P.H., Lambert, M., et al. The Tikhoff-Linberg procedure: Report of ten patients and presentation of a modified technique for tumors of the proximal humerus. Surgery 97(5) 518–528, 1985.

65. Malawer, M.M., and Zielinski, C.J. Giant cell tumor of bone: Surgical management-cryosurgery and en bloc resection. Analysis of 20 consecutive cases and recommendations for treatment. Presented at the American Academy of Orthopedic Surgeons, Anaheim, California, March 1983.

66. Malawer, M.M. Surgical management of aggressive and malignant tumors of the proximal fibula. Clin Orthop 186:172–181, 1984.

67. Mankin, H.J., Fogelson, F.S., Thrasher, A.Z., et al. Massive resection and allograft transplantation in the treatment of malignant bone tumors. N Engl J Med 294:1247–1255, 1976.

68. Marcove, R.C. Chondrosarcoma: Diagnosis and treatment. Orthop Clin North Am 8:811–819, 1977.

69. Marcove, R.C. A 17-year review of cryosurgery in the treatment of bone tumors. Clin Orthop 163:231–233, 1982.

70. Marcove, R.C., Lewis, M.M., Rosen, G., et al. Total femur and total knee replacement. A preliminary report. Clin Orthop 126:147–152, 1977.

71. Marcove, R.C., Lewis, M.M., and Huvos, A.G. En bloc upper humeral-interscapular resection, the Tikhoff-Linberg procedure. Clin Orthop 124:219–228, 1977.

72. Marcove, R.C., Lyden, J.P., Huvos, A.C., and Bullough, P.B. Giant cell tumor treated by cryosurgery. A report of twenty-five cases. J Bone Joint Surg [Am] 55:1633–1644, 1973.

73. Marcove, R.C., Mike, V., Hajack, J.V., et al. Osteogenic sarcoma under the age of twenty-one. J Bone Joint Surg [Am] 52:411–423, 1970.

74. Marcove, R.C., Mike, V., Hutter, R.V., et al. Chondrosarcoma of the pelvis and upper end of femur. J Bone Joint Surg [Am] 54:561–572, 1972.

75. Marcove, R.C., and Rosen, G. En bloc resection for osteogenic sarcoma. Cancer 45:3040–3044, 1980.

76. Marcove, R.C., Weiss, L., Vaghaiwall, M., and Pearson, R. Cryosurgery in the treatment of giant cell tumor of bone: A report of 52 consecutive cases. Clin Orthop 134:275–289, 1978.

77. Marcove, R.C., Stovell, P., Huvos, A.C., and Bullough, P. The use of cryosurgery in the treatment of low and medium grade chondrosarcoma: A preliminary report. Clin Orthop 122:147–156, 1977.

78. Martin, N.S., and Williamson, J. The role of surgery in the treatment of malignant tumors of the spine. J Bone Joint Surg [Br] 52:227–237, 1970.

79. McCarthy, E.F., Matsuno, T., and Dorfman, H.D. Malignant fibrous histiocytoma of bone: A study of 35 cases. Hum Pathol 10:57–70, 1979.

80. McKenna, R.J., Schwinn, C.P., Soong, K.Y., and Higinbotham, N.L. Sarcomata of the osteogenic series (osteosarcoma, fibrosarcoma, chondrosarcoma, parosteal osteosarcoma) and sarcomata arising in abnormal bone: An analysis of 552 cases. J Bone Joint Surg [Am] 48:1–26, 1966.

81. McKillop, J.H., Etcubanas, E., and Goris, M.L. The indications for and limitations of bone scintigraphy in osteogenic sarcoma: A review of 55 patients. Cancer 48:1133–1138, 1981.

82. McNeer, G.P., Cantin, J., Chu, F., and Nickson, J.J. The effectiveness of radiation therapy in the management of sarcoma of the soft somatic tissues. Cancer 22:391–397, 1968.

83. Madewell, J.E., Ragsdale, B.D., and Sweet, D.E. Radiographic and pathologic analysis of solitary bone lesions. Radiol Clin North Am 19:715–814, 1981.

84. Merryweather, R., Middlemiss, J.H., and Sanerkin, N.G. Malignant transformation of osteoblastoma. J Bone Joint Surg [Br] 62:381–384, 1980.

85. Mindell, E.R. Current concept review. Chordoma. J Bone Joint Surg [Am] 63:501–505, 1981.

86. Moore, T.M., Meyers, M.H., Patzakis, M.J., et al. Closed biopsy of musculoskeletal lesions. J Bone Joint Surg [Am] 61:375–380, 1979.

87. Morton, D.L., Eilber, F.R., Townsend, C.M., Jr., Grant, T.T., et al. Limb salvage from a multidisciplinary treatment approach for skeletal and soft tissue sarcomas of the extremity. Ann Surg 184:268–278, 1976.

88. Muggia, F., Catani, R., Lee, Y.J., et al. Factors responsible for therapeutic success in osteosarcoma, in Jones, S., and Salmon, S. (eds): *Adjuvant Therapy for Cancer,* 2d ed. New York, Grune and Stratton, 1979.

89. Nascimento, A.G., Huvos, A.C., and Marcove, R.C. Primary malignant giant cell tumor of bone. A study of eight cases and review of the literature. Cancer 44:1393–1402, 1979.

90. Nesbit, M.E., Perez, C.A., Tefft, M., et al. Multimodal therapy for the management of primary nonmetastatic Ewing's sarcoma of

bone: An intergroup study. Natl Cancer Inst Monogr 56:255–262, 1981.

91. Perez, C.A., Razek, A., Tefft, M., et al. Analysis of local tumor control in Ewing's sarcoma: Preliminary results of a cooperative intergroup study. Cancer 40:2864–2873, 1977.

92. Persson, B.M., and Wouters, H.W. Curettage and acrylic cementation in surgery of giant cell tumor of bone. J Bone Joint Surg [Am] 120:125–133, 1976.

93. Pritchard, D.J., Dahlin, D., Dauphine, R., et al. Ewing's sarcoma: A clinopathological and statistical analysis of patients surviving five years or longer. J Bone Joint Surg [Am] 57(1):10–16, 1975.

94. Pritchard, D.J., Lunke, R.J., Taylor, W.F., et al. Chondrosarcoma: A clinicopathologic statistical analysis. Cancer 45:149–157, 1980.

95. Razek, A., Perez, C.A., Tefft, M., et al. Intergroup Ewing's sarcoma study: Local control related to radiation dose, volume, and site of primary lesion in Ewing's sarcoma. Cancer 46:516, 1980.

96. Reimer, R.R., Chabner, B.A.C., Young, R.C., et al. Lymphoma presenting in bone. Results of histopathology, staging and therapy. Ann Intern Med 87:50–55, 1977.

97. Rock, M.G., Pritchard, D.J., and Unni, K.K. Metastases from histologically benign giant-cell tumor of bone. J Bone Joint Surg 66A:269–274, 1984.

98. Rosen, G., Caparros, B., Nirenberg, A., et al. Ewing's sarcoma: Ten-year experience with adjuvant chemotherapy. Cancer 47(9):2204–2213, 1981.

99. Rosen, G., Caparros, B., Mosende, C., et al. Curability of Ewing's sarcoma and consideration for future therapeutic trials. Cancer 41:888, 1978.

100. Rosen, G., Caparros, B., Huvos, A.C., et al. Preoperative chemotherapy for osteogenic sarcoma: Selection of postoperative adjuvant chemotherapy based upon the response of the primary tumor to preoperative chemotherapy. Cancer 49:1221–1230, 1982.

101. Rosen, G., Marcove, R.C., Caparros, B., et al. Primary osteogenic sarcoma. The rationale for preoperative chemotherapy and delayed survey. Cancer 43:2163–2177, 1979.

102. Rosenberg, S.A., Tepper, J., Glatstein, E., et al. Adjuvant chemotherapy for patients with soft tissue sarcomas. Surg Clin North Am 61:1415–1423, 1981.

103. Rosenthal, D.I. Computed tomography in bone and soft tissue neoplasms: Application and pathologic correlation. CRC Crit Rev Diag Imaging 18:243–278, 1982.

104. Sanerkin, N.G. The diagnosis and grading of chondrosarcoma of bone. A combined cytologic and histologic approach. Cancer 45:582–594, 1980.

105. Schajowicz, F., and Derqui, J.C. Puncture biopsy in lesions of the locomotor system. Review and results in 4050 cases, including 941 vertebral punctures. Cancer 21:5331–5487, 1968.

106. Shives, T.S., Wold, L.E., Dahlin, D.C., and Beaubout, J.W. Chondrosarcoma and its variants, in Sim, F.H. (ed): *Diagnosis and Treatment of Bone Tumors: A Team Approach.* Mayo Clinic Monograph. Thorofare, NJ, Slack Inc., 1983, pp 211–217.

107. Sim, F.H., Bowman, W.E., and Chao, E.Y.S. Limb salvage surgery and reconstructive techniques, in Sim F.H. (ed). *Diagnosis and Treatment of Bone Tumors: A Team Approach.* Mayo Clinic Monograph. Thorofare, NJ, Slack Inc., 1983, pp 75–105.

108. Simon, M.A., and Enneking, W.F. The management of soft-tissue sarcomas of the extremities. J Bone Joint Surg 58A:317, 1976.

109. Soule, E.H., and Enriquez, P. Atypical fibrous histiocytoma, malignant fibrous histiocytoma and epithelioid sarcoma. A comparative study of 65 tumors. Cancer 30:128–143, 1972.

110. Spanier, S.S., Enneking, W.F., and Enriquez, P. Primary malignant fibrous histiocytoma of bone. Cancer 36:2084–2098, 1975.

111. Springfield, D.S., and Goodman, M.A. Biopsy of musculoskeletal lesions. Orthopedics 3:868–870, 1980.

112. Sterner, B. Total spondylectomy in chondrosarcoma arising in the seventh thoracic vertebra. J Bone Joint Surg [Br] 288–295, 1971.

113. Sterner, B.L., and Johnson, O.E., Complete removal of three vertebrae for giant-cell tumor. J Bone Joint Surg [Br] 53:278–287, 1971.

114. Sweet, D.L., Moss, D.P., Simon, M.A., et al. Histiocytic lymphoma (reticulum-cell sarcoma) of bone. Current strategy for orthopedic surgeons. J Bone Joint Surg [Am] 63:79–84, 1981.

115. Sweetnam, R. Surgical management of primary osteosarcoma. Clin Orthop 111:57–64, 1975.

116. Uehlinger, E. Primary malignancy, secondary malignancy and semimalignancy of bone tumors, in Grundman, E. (ed): *Malignant Bone Tumors.* New York, Springer-Verlag, 1976, pp 109–119.

117. Unni, K.K., Dahlin, D.C., Beaubout, S.W., and Ivins, J.C. Parosteal osteogenic sarcoma. Cancer 37:2466–2475, 1976.

118. Unni, K.K., Dahlin, D.C., and Beaubout, S.W. Periosteal osteogenic sarcoma. Cancer 37:2476–2485, 1976.

119. Unni, K.K., Dahlin, D.C., Beaubout, J.W., and Sim, F.H. Chondrosarcoma: Clear-cell variant. A report of 16 cases. J Bone Joint Surg [Am] 57:676–683, 1976.

120. Watts, H.G. Introduction to resection of musculoskeletal sarcomas. Clin Orthop 153:31–38, 1980.

121. Weingrad, D.N., and Rosenberg, S.A. Early lymphatic spread of osteogenic and soft-tissue sarcomas. Surgery 84:231–240, 1978.

122. Weiss, S.W., and Enzinger, F.M. Malignant fibrous histiocytoma. An analysis of 200 cases. Cancer 41:2250, 1978.

123. Weiss, S.W., and Enzinger, F.M. Myxoid variant of malignant fibrous histiocytoma. Cancer 39:1672, 1977.

124. Wilner, D. Osteogenic sarcoma (osteosarcoma), in Wilner, D. (ed): *Radiology of Bone Tumors and Allied Disorders.* Philadelphia, Saunders, 1982, pp 1897–2095.

125. Wilner, D. Fibrosarcoma, in Wilner, D. (ed): *Radiology of Bone Tumors and Allied Disorders,* vol. I. Philadelphia, Saunders, 1982, pp 2291–2324.

Section B: Other Malignancies Affecting Bone

1. Alexanian, R., Bonnet, J., Gehan, E., Haut, A., Hewlett, J., Lane, M., Monto, R., and Wilson, H. Combination chemotherapy for multiple myeloma. Cancer 30:382–389, 1972.

2. American Cancer Society. Cancer statistics, 1985. CA 35:19–35, 1985.

3. Armitage, J.O., Fyfe, M.A., and Leuro, J. Long-term remission durability and functional status of patients healed for diffuse histiocytic lymphoma with the CHOP regimen. J Clin Oncol 2:898–902, 1984.

4. Bataille, R., and Sany, J. Solitary myeloma: Clinical and prognostic features of a review of 114 cases. Cancer 48:845–851, 1981.

5. Berard, C. A multidisciplinary approach to non-Hodgkin's lymphoma. Ann Intern Med 94:218–235, 1981.

6. Bergsagel, D., Bailey, A.J., Langley, G.P., MacDonald, R.M., White, D.F., and Miller, A.B. The chemotherapy of plasma cell myeloma and the incidence of acute leukemia. N Engl J Med 301:743–748, 1979.

7. Blacklock, H., Matthews, J., Buchanen, J., Ockelford, P., and Hill, R. Improved survival from acute lymphoblastic leukemia in adolescents and adults. Cancer 48:1931–1935, 1981.

8. Bos, G., Simon, M., Spiegel, P., and Moohr, J. Childhood leukemia presenting as a diaphyseal radiolucency. Clin Orthop 135:66–68, 1978.

9. Boston, H.C., Dahlin, D.C., Ivins, J.C., and Cupps, R.E. Malignant lymphoma of bone. Cancer 34:1731–1737, 1976.

10. Byrne, G. Histopathologic diagnosis of Hodgkin's disease. Semin Oncol 7:103–113, 1980.

11. Cline, M., Golde, D., Belling, R., Groopman, J., Zighelbaim, J., and Gale, R. Acute leukemia. Biology and treatment. Ann Intern Med 91:758–773, 1979.

12. Corwin, J., and Lindberg, R. Solitary plasmacytoma of bone vs. extramedullary plasmacytoma and their relationship to multiple myeloma. Cancer 43:1007–1013, 1979.

13. Costa, G., and Engle, R. Melphalan and prednisone: An effective combination for the treatment of multiple myeloma. Am J Med 54: 589–598, 1973.

14. Crenshaw, A. *Campbell's Operative Orthopedics*, 5th ed. New York, Mosby, 1971.

15. DeVita, V., Serpick, A.A., and Carbone, P.P. Combination chemotherapy in the treatment of advanced Hodgkin's disease. Ann Intern Med 73:881–895, 1970.

16. Drapkin, R., Gee, T., Dowling, M., Arlin, Z., McKenzie, S., Kempin, S., and Clarkson, B. Prophylactic heparin therapy in acute promyelocytic leukemia. Cancer 41:2484–2490, 1978.

17. Ezkinli, E.Z., Costello, W., Lenhard, R.E., Bakemeier, R., Bennet, J., Berard, C., and Carbone, P. Survival of nodular versus diffuse pattern lymphocytic poorly differentiated lymphoma. Cancer 41: 1990–1996, 1978.

18. Gale, R., Foon, K., Cline, M., and Zighelbaim, J. Intensive chemotherapy for acute myelogenous leukemia. Ann Intern Med 94:735–757, 1981.

19. Greenberger, J., Crocker, A.C., Jaffe, N., and Cassady, J.R. Treatment and end results in 139 patients with histiocytosis. Proc Am Soc Clin Oncol 19:399, 1978.

20. Gutensohn, N., and Cole, P. Epidemiology of Hodgkin's disease. N Engl J Med 304:135–140, 1981.

21. Hodgkin, T. On some morbid appearances of the absorbent glands and spleen. Med Chir Trans 17:68–114, 1832.

22. Jones, S., Fuks, Z., Bull, M., Kadin, M.E., Dorfman, R.F., Kaplan, H.S., Rosenberg, S.A., and Kim, H. Non-Hodgkin's lymphomas: IV. Clinicopathologic correlation in 405 cases. Cancer 31:806–823, 1973.

23. Kaplan, H. Hodgkin's disease: Unfolding concepts concerning its nature, management and prognosis. Cancer 45:2349–2374, 1980.

24. Kaplan, H. Long-term results of palliative and radical radiotherapy of Hodgkin's disease. Cancer Res 26:1250–1252, 1966.

25. Komp, D., Herson, J., Starling, K., Vietti, T., and Hoizdala, E. Prognostic variables in histiocytosis X. Proc Am Soc Clin Oncol 19: 390, 1978.

26. Kyle, R., and Jowsey, J. Effect of sodium fluoride, calcium carbonate, and vitamin D on the skeleton in multiple myeloma. Cancer 45:1669–1674, 1980.

27. Laurence, J., Coleman, M., Allen, S., Silver, R., and Pasmantier, M. Combination chemotherapy of advanced diffuse histiocytic lymphoma with the six-drug COP-BLAM regimen. Ann Intern Med 97: 190–195, 1982.

28. Lichtenstein, A., and Golde, D. Myeloma, heavy chain disease and macroglobulinemia, Chap. 66 in Haskell, C. (ed): *Cancer Treatment*, 2d ed. Philadelphia, Saunders, 1985, pp 740–757.

29. Lichtenstein, L. Histiocytosis X. Integration of eosinophilic granuloma of bone, "Letterer Siwe disease," and "Schuller-Christian disease" as related manifestations of a single nosologic entity. Arch Pathol 56:84–102, 1953.

30. Lister, T. Combination chemotherapy for acute leukemia in adults. Br Med J 1:199–203, 1978.

31. Loeffler, R.K., DiSimone, R.N., and Howland, W.J. Limitations of bone scanning in clinical oncology. JAMA 234:1228–1232, 1975.

32. Mill, W., and Griffith, R. The role of radiation therapy in the management of plasma cell tumors. Cancer 45:647–652, 1980.

33. Mundy, G.R., Raisz, L.G., Cooper, R.A., Schechter, G.P., and Salmon, S.E. Evidence for the secretion of an osteoclast stimulating factor in myeloma. N Engl J Med 291:1041–1046, 1974.

34. Newcomer, L., Silverstein, M., Cadman, E., Farber, L., Bertino, J., and Prosnitz, L. Bone involvement in Hodgkin's disease. Cancer 49:338–342, 1982.

35. Nezelof, C., Frileux-Herbet, F., and Cronier-Sachot, J. Disseminated histiocytosis X. Cancer 44:1824–1838, 1979.

36. Pangalis, G., Nathwani, B.N., and Rappaport, H. Malignant lymphoma, well-differentiated lymphocytic. Cancer 39:999–1010, 1977.

37. Rappaport, H. Tumors of the hematopoietic system, in *Atlas of Tumor Pathology*, sec III, fascicle 8. Armed Forces Institute of Pathology, Washington, DC, 1966, pp 97–156.

38. Rodriguez, A.R., Lutchen, C.L., and Coleman, F.W. Osteosclerotic myeloma. JAMA 236:1872–1874, 1976.

39. Rodriguez, V., Cabanilles, F., Burgess, M., McKelvey, E., Valdivieso, M., Bodey, G., and Freireich, E. Combination chemotherapy ("Chop-Bleo") in advanced (non-Hodgkin) malignant lymphoma. Blood 49:325–333, 1977.

40. Rudders, R.A., Ross, M.E., and DeLellis, R.A. Primary extra-nodal lymphoma. Cancer 42:406–416, 1978.

41. Sacks, E.L., Donaldson, S.S., Gordon, J., and Dorfman, R.F. Epithelioid granulomas associated with Hodgkin's disease. Clinical correlations in 55 previously untreated patients. Cancer 41:562–567, 1978.

42. Schimpff, S., Greene, W., Young, V., Fortner, C., Jepsen, L., Nusack, N., Block, J., and Wiernik, P. Infection prevention in acute nonlymphocytic leukemia. Ann Intern Med 82:351–358, 1975.

43. Shoji, H., and Miller, T.R. Primary reticulum cell sarcoma of bone. Cancer 28:1234–1344, 1971.

44. Silverberg, E., and Lubera, J. Cancer statistics, 1987. CA 37:1–19, 1987.

45. Siris, E.S., Sherman, W.H., Baquirau, D.C., Schlatterer, J.P., Osserman, G.F., and Canfield, R.E. Effects of dichloromethylene diphosphonate on skeletal mobilization of calcium in multiple myeloma. N Engl J Med 302:310–315, 1980.

46. Spengler, D. Rapid diaphyseal destruction. Clin Orthop 115:231–234, 1976.

47. Starling, K., Iyer, R., Silva-Sosa, M., Komp, D., Herson, J., and Trueworthy, R. Chlorambucil in histiocytosis X. A Southwest Oncology Group study. J Pediatr 96:266–268, 1980.

48. Tong, D., Griffin, T., Laramore, G., Kurtz, J.M., Russell, A.H., Groudine, M.T., Herron, T., Blasko, J.C., and Tesh, D.W. Solitary plasmacytoma of bone and soft tissues. Radiology 135:195–198, 1980.

49. Vogel, J., and Vogel, P. Idiopathic histiocytosis: A discussion of eosinophilic granuloma, the Hand-Schuller-Christian syndrome, and the Letterer-Siwe syndrome. Semin Hematol 9:349–369, 1972.

50. Wade, J., Schimpff, S., Hargaden, M., Fortner, C., Young, V., and Wiernik, P. A comparison of trimethoprim sulfamethoxazole plus nystatin with gentamycin plus nystatin in the prevention of infections in acute leukemia. N Engl J Med 304:1057–1062, 1981.

51. Wang, C.C., and Fleischlie, D. Primary reticulum cell sarcoma of bone. Cancer 22:994–998, 1968.

52. Wintrobe, M., Lee, G., Boggs, D., Bithell, T., Foerster, J., Athens, J., and Lukens, J. Chronic lymphocytic leukemia, Chap. 67 in Wintrobe, M. (ed): *Clinical Hematology*, 8th ed. Philadelphia, Lea & Febiger, 1981, pp 1631–1647.

53. Woodruff, R., Malpas, J., and White, F. Solitary plasmacytoma: II. Solitary plasmacytoma of bone. Cancer 43:2344–2347, 1979.

CHAPTER 24

Amputations and Prosthetics

Ernest M. Burgess, Drew A. Hittenberger, and Joan T. Gold

SECTION A

Amputations and Prosthetics in Adults

Ernest M. Burgess and Drew A. Hittenberger

AMPUTATION

General Considerations

Historically, trauma and infection have been responsible for most amputations. Pyogenic infections associated with open trauma, and in particular gas gangrene, required amputation as a lifesaving measure. War surgeons have measured their skill in terms of speedy and lifesaving limb ablation.

Congenital amputations and severe congenital limb deficits are recorded in the earliest medical history. They occur in all countries. The thalidomide experience provided a remarkable opportunity to observe the influence of exogenous agents as a cause of limb teratogenesis. A majority of these limb deficits can be fitted with appropriate prosthetic devices and do not require surgical revision. Surgical conversion or amputation when indicated often necessitates considerable ingenuity.

Tumors of the extremities continue to require amputations. While connective tissue malignancies of the limbs are few and with modern oncology management require amputation less frequently than in the past, they have continued to be responsible for a small percentage of limb loss.

As we approach the 21st century the profile of persons requiring amputation is radically changing in the developed countries. Several circumstances are responsible for the change. The first of these is the control of local and systemic infection. Gas gangrene, tuberculosis, leprosy, and other similar scourges are being effectively managed. Following trauma and tumor resection, highly refined limb salvage surgery involving microvascular reconstruction, composite tissue grafting, and prosthetic replacement techniques now saves many limbs that formerly would have come to amputation.

The most important factor changing the profile of limb loss in the population is increasing longevity with greater numbers of elderly patients developing limb ischemia. Circu-latory diseases are responsible for 80 percent or more of major amputations in civilian life today. Approximately half of these individuals suffer from diabetes.[1,16,20]

Revascularization can prolong viability of the ischemic limb with acceptable comfort and function. This treatment is, however, by its nature palliative—the underlying disease processes are not arrested or eliminated by vascular reconstruction, and most end-stage vascular disease requires amputation usually involving the lower limbs. The majority of these patients are 65 years old and older. The systemic nature of their vascular disease and associated chronic disease states make rehabilitation with restoration of a useful degree of pain-free mobility following amputation a challenge involving many health care disciplines.

The changing indications for amputation and remarkable improvements in surgical management have rendered obsolescent many time-honored concepts.[12,17] Long-established sites of election have become obsolete with improved understanding of limb viability,[4] the great progress in prosthetic limb substitutes, and scientific rehabilitation. Staged amputations in the presence of infection have been radically modified as a result of antibiotics. The amputation has become a reconstructive surgical exercise, the reconstruction of a terminal motor and sensory end organ which through a prosthetic substitute will interface with the environment.

Surgery

Amputation surgery has been considered dull, professionally unrewarding, and requiring modest technical skills. Surgical training programs often use amputation as a source of basic training in surgical technique to be performed by the most junior member of the house staff, often inadequately supervised. The surgery is further diminished by many surgeons' inadequate knowledge of prosthetic substitution. The surgeon's involvement must continue beyond the period of wound healing to effective rehabilitation. Not only is this a professional requisite, but it provides the surgeon the opportunity to see the patient relieved of pain, with mobility restored and an improved quality of life.

Preoperative Evaluation When the need for amputation has been established and the patient's condition is amenable to surgery, a level of amputation must be established. The tissues must be able to heal at the selected level, and the amputation site must be tolerant of its interface with the prosthesis. An additional requirement is the availability of a suitable prosthesis to fit the residual limb created by the level of amputation.

Detailed physical examination and objective limb viability measurements dictate the most distal level of amputation that can be expected to heal. A working knowledge of modern limb substitutes consolidates the decision.

Wound healing is particularly critical in determining the level of amputation for end-stage vascular disease. One of the most significant advances in amputation surgical technique for ischemia relates to an improved understanding of limb viability, allowing more accurate amputation level determination.[4,19] Consequently the number of more distal amputations in the lower limb, i.e., below the knee, has dramatically increased in the last decade and a half. This change is reflected in the improved performance of elderly amputees whose knee joint is preserved and who may thereby maintain functional independence.

The Operation With few exceptions, all prostheses today totally contact the residual limb. The basic principles of plastic and reconstructive surgery apply in the same manner that they are used in surgery of the hand and the foot. Since the amputation site becomes the end organ of the limb contacting the environment, each structure is carefully treated at surgery to permit uneventful healing. Surgical conservation of tissues is the rule. This means in most instances preservation of limb length.

The surgeon seeks a well-healed, nonadherent, painless scar. The surrounding skin should be healthy with retained sensation. Since the prosthetic socket totally contacts the stump, placement of the scar is relatively unimportant.[1,7]

Muscles make up the bulk of the limb at the site of major amputations. The contractile function of the muscle is lost when skeletal attachment has been severed. Under these circumstances muscles atrophy and residual limb function is diminished. Muscles can be stabilized at or near the site of amputation by suturing the muscle itself or its ligamentous and tendinous insertion into bone.[1] This technique (myodesis) is most effective in above-knee and through-knee amputations in the lower limb, and in above-elbow and through-elbow amputations in the upper limb. The suture of muscles to periosteum and distally to each other (myoplasty) is also effective provided the sutured muscle groups do not form a sling over the end of the severed bone. A fixed attachment is necessary to allow physiological muscle function and also to prevent the formation of painful bursae. In the presence of ischemia when primary wound healing is of critical importance, the added surgery for muscle stabilization can compromise wound healing. Fascial closure is used in these conditions.

The treatment of nerves sectioned by amputation has been controversial for centuries. All sectioned nerves form neuromas. Surgical attempts to minimize neuroma formation and to limit or diminish stump pain and/or phantom pain include burying the ends of the nerves in bone, cauterizing, crushing, injection with a variety of chemical agents, and ligation. Current practice dictates ligation only with the nerve moderately retracted to allow the sectioned end to retract into the soft tissues away from the site of prosthetic interface pressure. Ligation confines the neuroma and tends to prevent

outgrowth. Hemorrhage from the blood vessels contained within the nerve is also controlled by the ligation. Gentle handling of tissues is essential for minimal scar formation. Blood vessels are ligated and cautery is used on the small vessels only.

Proper surgical management of the bone is of great importance. With diaphyseal amputations the bone is divided with a sharp saw and the cortex is well-rounded using a saw or a file. Good soft tissue coverage is necessary to avoid pressure-sensitive skin problems. With children, the periosteum is removed 0.5 cm from its distal end to diminish or prevent bone regeneration and spur formation. With the adult, and particularly with the elderly, the periosteum should be left long to be drawn over the end of the sectioned bone and sutured, closing off the medullary canal.

A number of significant improvements and innovations in techniques of amputation surgery have been developed. Muscle stabilization, myodesis, and myoplasty were described above. Angulation osteotomy, tibiofibular synostosis, and cineplasty are among others.[1,12]

Immediate Postoperative Care Important recent improvements in postoperative wound management include the use of rigid dressings, controlled environment chambers, and early mobilizing systems.[6] The amputation presents a unique opportunity for postoperative physical wound management. The wound being terminal, the dressings can apply pressure to control edema. This permits the use of rigid dressings which allow quiet healing, protect the limb, and minimize pain and trauma. As wound healing progresses, the cast or other rigid dressing material can be used as a temporary socket to which is applied a terminal device for limited weight bearing in the lower limb and dexterous hand substitution in the upper limb. The skills required to apply appropriate rigid dressings are precise but are easily acquired. Immediate postoperative soft compression dressings are still extensively used but are less effective in providing an ideal wound healing environment than rigid dressings. They displace easily, and pressures are difficult to control, especially with elastic wrapping. Frequent reapplication is usually needed.

The Amputation Team The health care skills requisite for amputee rehabilitation are surgical, prosthetic, and rehabilitative. No single discipline encompasses these basic needs, and wartime experience suggests that dedicated amputation centers with an integrated team is the best approach.[16] Although the amputation team functions best in such a setting, it is possible to achieve good communication between the surgeon, the prosthetist, and the therapist operating independently. Absence of a fully integrated team need not preclude many of the benefits of team care.

Rehabilitation

Clinical rehabilitation following amputation is generally carried out by the physical therapist, corrective therapist, and others under the direction of the surgeon or physiatrist. Emphasis is on early, progressive restoration of function. As wound healing progresses, the initial or subsequent rigid dressings can serve as early, temporary prostheses. As soon as wound healing is sound, a provisional or preparatory limb is prescribed.[8,17] As the tissues mature and stabilize in size and pressure tolerance, a definitive limb can be provided. Early progressive rehabilitation has largely eliminated stump and phantom pain as sources of significant long-term disability.

Kinesiologists including those specializing in gait and a considerable number of people involved in rehabilitation research are contributing to improved, rapid amputee function. Amputee seminars, amputee recreation groups, and physical competition among amputees have combined to enhance social adjustment to achieve oftentimes remarkable performance levels.

Complications of Amputation Surgery

Complications following amputation are those generally related to wound healing observed in all types of limb surgery. These include primary wound infections, ischemic necrosis, wound dehiscence, pain, edema, and dysfunction and deformity of proximal structures, especially joints.[1,7]

As the amputation wound is terminal, there are no tissues beyond the site of the surgery to require postoperative management; the wound itself can be subjected to a controlled postoperative physical environment. This environment includes pressure gradients, wound immobilization, thermal and humidity parameters, and sterility.

Postoperative wound infections are handled in the usual manner of adequate drainage, debridement, and antibiotics. Secondary closure or reamputation may be required.

Wound complications secondary to ischemia may involve the skin or the deeper tissues or both. Ischemic wound dehiscence with or without infection is characteristically seen where determination of the level at which the limb is viable has been inadequate prior to surgery and the amputation is performed through tissues incapable of healing the surgical insult primarily. When local ischemia and necrosis are present, there is usually no chance for secondary healing with local or skin graft coverage. The ischemia related to the wound breakdown militates against there being sufficient healing capacity of those local tissues to close by secondary intent. Reamputation is usually required.

Postsurgical amputee pain is a phenomenon differing from the pain ordinarily experienced following limb surgery. When all structures of the limb including major and minor nerves are sectioned transversely, subsequent immediate and long-range pain phenomena are often unique to the amputation alone. This subject will be covered in more depth later in this chapter. Edema and ischemia result in pain. Early postsurgical wound management is directed toward minimizing these normal inflammatory responses following the trauma of surgery. Controlled and carefully monitored postsurgical pressure dressings, whether rigid or soft, are essential. Terminal edema by proximal constriction must be avoided. Skilled application of the rigid dressings, and proper bandaging of the stump postoperatively, are essential ingredients to management preventing these complications.

Hematomas can be a very serious complication, especially when the amputation has been performed for ischemia. They can be avoided by adequate hemostasis and careful closure of the dead space. Their prompt recognition postoperatively allows early evacuation of their contents.

Regional Considerations

The amputation is by nature destructive. The whole or a part of a functioning organ is removed and replaced by an inert artificial device, the prosthesis. Since the prosthesis is applied specifically to restore function, it is necessary to understand the functional characteristics of what has been removed and to duplicate them as completely as possible with the artificial limb, that is, functional substitution. This implies that the surgeon has a detailed working knowledge of the function which has been lost. The amputation carries with it the additional loss of body form. The social and psychological outcomes of this loss of body image are in many ways quite unique. The specifics of functional loss and the priorities related to prosthetic substitution will be covered when considering the levels of limb loss.

Amputation, Lower Limb

The basic physiological/mechanical function of the lower limb is to provide stability in stance and gait. This requirement carries over directly into prosthetic substitution. An amputee can stand on a well-secured rigid pylon with no intervening articulations. As sophistication of prosthetic design progresses, an enlarged range of functional capability and cosmesis are achieved. Today many unilateral lower-limb amputees, even including those with amputations at high, above-knee levels, can walk with little or no perceptible limp. Below-knee amputees, including those with Syme's amputations, not only may have a normal gait but can perform many complex functional activities including running.

Amputations through the Foot

The foot is an articulated platform providing us with important kinesthetic and proprioceptive information. Removal of any portion of the foot including the toes progressively decreases the size of the platform. The amputation also interferes with the motor leverage system, thus impairing gait. Sensory loss following amputation may affect postural balance.[1,21]

Removal of one or more of the lesser toes disturbs gait minimally if at all. No prostheses are required other than minor shoe adjustments and, on occasion, toe fillers for comfort. Amputation of the great toe is more disabling. Balance and push-off are appreciably affected. Loss of great toe function is especially noticeable when attempting to walk rapidly or run in ordinary shoes, particularly soft shoes. This deficit can be masked to some degree by firm shoes that have a rocker bar mechanism on the sole in the metatarsal region. As with the lesser toes, removal of the great toe does not require prosthetic substitution other than an insole with toe filler for comfort and attention to proper shoe mechanics.

Amputation of one or more toes is occasioned usually by trauma and/or peripheral vascular disease. The surgical techniques are standard. Amputations through the foot including the toes should be viewed as reconstructive plastic surgery. Scars are placed to avoid pressure on the weight-bearing surfaces. Tight skin closures specifically are avoided, and underlying rigid structures, i.e., bone and cartilage, are carefully tailored to avoid sources of pressure that could cause pain or overlying skin breakdown.

Like all amputations in the foot, transverse amputation through the metatarsals or resection of one or more rays requires careful planning to avoid painful scars. Plantar skin, which is anatomically designed for weight bearing, should be used to cover the plantar and distal surfaces where weight-bearing forces are concentrated. Bone surfaces should be free of irregularities, especially in the weight-bearing areas. Muscle rebalancing is not usually required since the leg muscles which control ankle and foot function are preserved and postsurgical deformities do not develop.

For amputations through the metatarsals, shoe modification and an insole with forefoot space replacement are satisfactory to improve gait and push-off. Most patients with such amputations can then walk well with little or no appreciable limp other than occasionally having a short stride. If the patient attempts to move from slow and average walking speeds to a fast walk and a run, the deficit becomes apparent.

Amputations through the midfoot have been described in past literature by proper names. Lisfranc's amputation is performed at the tarsometatarsal joints. Chopart's amputation is carried out through the midtarsal joints, and in Pirogoff's amputation the calcaneus is rotated forward to be fused to the tibia after vertical section through the midportion of the calcaneus. The Boyd amputation consists of talectomy and forward shift of the calcaneus with calcaneotibial arthrodesis. With present surgical and prosthetic management of amputations through the body of the foot, surgical modifications are often required so that it is now more appropriate to describe the level of amputation anatomically.

Amputations through the tarsometatarsal joints and through the area of the cuneiforms and distal cuboid bone significantly reduce the size of the foot platform. Major long tendon insertions are disturbed. When the blood supply is adequate for primary healing, muscle rebalancing can be ac-

complished by surgical section or transfer of tendon insertions. These procedures are designed to maintain a plantigrade, controlled residual foot without contractures or deformity.

The common deformity which develops is a fixed equinus and varus due to the overpull of the gastrocnemius—soleus and posterior tibial muscles. Loss of insertion of the peroneus longus and the long toe extensors additionally produces the deformity. Heel cord lengthening or section, transfer of the anterior tibial tendon insertion to the midline on the dorsum of the foot, and section of the tibialis posterior tendon may prevent fixed equinovarus deformity. Tibiocalcaneal arthrodesis, as with the Boyd and Pirogoff operations, provides a stable, direct weight-bearing surface covered by heel skin. In the presence of ischemia, questionable healing potential, and a tenuous skin envelope, this rebalancing surgery may not be justified. At this amputation level, dynamic imbalance with potential deformity is best managed in the presence of ischemia by simple tendon sectioning. As the surgeon is able to more accurately assess skin-healing potential throughout the foot, more through-foot amputations are being carried out with successful primary healing.

Proximal foot amputation with retention of the talus and calcaneus or preservation of the calcaneus alone is reserved principally for individuals who will not be fitted with a prosthesis and will be able to walk barefoot in a simple shoe or boot. This amputation is frequently used in the less developed countries where prosthetic services are limited. Proximal foot amputations eliminate those muscle insertions responsible for ankle and toe dorsiflexor power as well as inversion and eversion. Plantar flexion deformity can be prevented or corrected by heel cord section.

Prosthetic substitution for midfoot and hindfoot amputations is difficult. The degree of loss of the foot platform causes an unstable gait. Absence of the forefoot lever arm eliminates physiological push-off. The advantages of full limb length and a distal end-bearing residual limb can be weighed against the improved function available in more proximal level of amputations such as the Syme's amputations, where prosthetic components which functionally replace the ankle mechanism

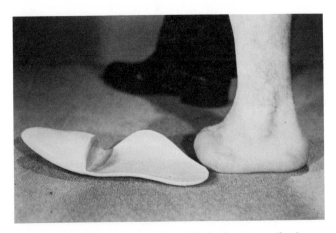

Figure 24-1 Midfoot amputation with the insert prosthesis.

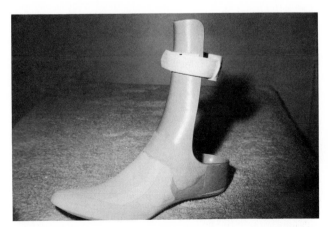

Figure 24-2 Ankle, foot orthosis for amputations through the hindfoot.

are available. Ingenuity is required when designing shoes and prostheses for the more proximal foot amputations (Figs. 24-1 and 24-2). If a combination insole support with anterior filler is fitted into a high boot with a stiff sole and an anterior rocker bar, it allows some gravity push-off as well as increasing stability. Retention of the partial foot in the proper position in the shoe can be a problem. With proper amputee rehabilitation, however, these individuals can enjoy long periods of comfortable function. Modifications of shoes using ski boot foaming techniques, and custom-type footwear, enhance function.

The most effective prosthesis for proximal foot amputations extends to just below the knee and blocks the ankle joint, preventing dorsiflexion. In this way gravity push-off gait is regained. Objections to the prosthetic appliance which encompasses the lower leg are outweighed by comfort and enhanced walking capability on the part of the amputee.

Good foot hygiene on the part of the patient is essential. Pressure of shoes and appliances on pressure-sensitive areas, maceration of the skin from retained moisture, and low-grade skin infection can be avoided with proper foot hygiene such as bathing and drying, avoidance of oily and greasy preparations, and the use of lamb's wool and antifungal powder. Individuals with insensitive feet should neither stand nor walk without a protective covering, i.e., shoe or slipper. The trimming of toenails and calluses is a particular source of acquired infection. Conforming footwear to include relief for pressure-sensitive areas is a necessity.

Amputations through the Ankle: Syme's Amputation

Amputation through the ankle joint as described in 1843[1,25] by the Scottish surgeon James Syme is one of the few operative procedures which has come down through the decades almost unchanged in technique. A landmark treatise by Harris in 1944 emphasized the value of this amputation for many conditions including trauma and certain types of peripheral vascular disease. The surgical technique as described both by Syme and Harris involves amputation at ankle joint level with removal of malleoli and a paper-thin removal of the distal articular surface of the tibia. Section of the bones must be at a right angle to the long weight-bearing axis and parallel to the floor. The calcaneus is carefully removed subperiosteally, avoiding damage to the posterior tibial artery. After the calcaneus and the rest of the tarsal and forefoot bones are removed, the flap is fashioned so as to place skin from the weight-bearing surface of the heel directly over the distal tibia with the skin incision closed anteriorly. This technique is precise. The heel skin end pad must be centered directly over the distal tibia and stabilized there. The operation can be done in one or two stages depending upon existing disease. The surgical end result is a stable, well-healed, moderately bulbous amputation at ankle level with weight-bearing heel skin over the distal tibial surface.

Earlier Syme's prostheses were unsightly, and breakage of their lateral metal stirrups was common. Women especially objected to the appearance of the prosthesis and requested reamputation to the below-knee level. Modern prostheses are not only much more cosmetic but permit an excellent gait (Fig. 24-3). Several long-term studies of well-performed

Syme's amputations indicate the excellent comfort, strength, and quality of function available. Contraindications include poor heel skin and lack of skin protective sensation.

Patients with bilateral Syme's amputations manage well, often without walking aids.

Amputations through the Leg

Below-knee amputation is statistically the commonest major amputation in the lower limb. Amputations at this level heal successfully in the majority of patients with ischemia who require major limb ablation.

Knee function is so critical to prosthetic rehabilitation that every attempt should be made to salvage the knee. Below-knee amputation is a reconstructive procedure requiring careful attention to technical detail. This level is selected on the basis of available healthy tissues including an understanding of the healing potential present at the below-knee site in the ischemic limb. The site of election is that level where enough soft tissue is available to provide a well-healed, prosthesis-tolerant stump. All length should be saved down to the junction of the middle and lower thirds of the tibia and fibula. Amputations between this site and the ankle joint are avoided because of the difficulty of obtaining appropriate soft tissue coverage. The level limit proximally is just distal to the insertion of the patellar tendon. If significant knee dysfunction is present, the very short below-knee amputation is usually contraindicated and a knee disarticulation or higher amputation is carried out.

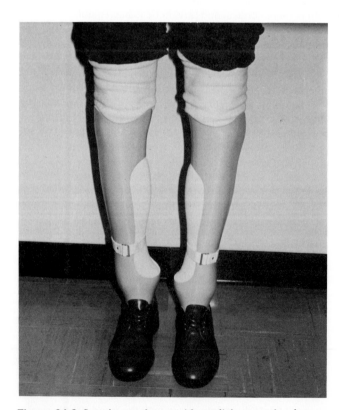

Figure 24-3 Syme's prostheses with medial cutout for donning prosthesis.

Modern technique utilizes a long posterior skin flap with an underlying myofascial flap progressively thinned to its distal end for suture to the anterior periosteum and deep fascia over the anterior tibiofibular area.[1] This myofascial stabilization permits a modest degree of distal muscle fixation to allow contractile activity. Nerves are pulled down gently and ligated high; the anterior tibia is very carefully beveled and rounded since this is the site of pressure sensitivity within the socket. The fibula is sectioned 1.5 cm higher than the tibia unless one wishes to perform a tibiofibular synostosis, in which event the bones are sectioned at the same level and the osteoperiosteal bridge developed. Routine hemostasis and drainage are used. Postsurgical management likewise must be precise and physiological. Immediate postsurgical rigid dressings have proved to be the most effective treatment system. These dressings are applied with relief pads placed under the cast for protection of pressure-sensitive areas. The immediate postsurgical rigid dressing is changed, usually 10 to 12 days after the surgery and thereafter as frequently as necessitated by loosening, while the stump matures.

Soft dressings are still used frequently following surgery. They include compression bandaging, which must be carefully monitored to prevent proximal vascular constriction and which needs to be changed frequently to maintain appropriate distal pressure control.

Much of the improvement in below-knee amputation surgery relates to muscle and skin management. The long posterior myocutaneous flap is considered standard. Other techniques are acceptable, including equal sagittal flaps and skewed flaps designed to utilize the healthiest available skin. A wide variety of reconstructive skin coverage procedures may be required to salvage the below-knee level when severe trauma including burns is encountered. These include split-skin grafts, full-thickness grafts, and, on rare occasions, composite grafts.

The surgical goal of the below-knee amputation is the formation of a cylindrical terminal motor and sensory end organ with a degree of muscle stabilization and with a nontender, nonadherent scar.

The below-knee amputation is particularly suited for immediate postsurgical rigid dressing wound management. The cast can be moderately contoured about the knee for suspension and, with the knee in extension, carried up to the upper one-third of the thigh. Knee flexion contractures are avoided; most patients can be out of bed and in a chair the day following surgery. Progressive early and rapid rehabilitation proceeds to limited weight bearing under supervision. With uneventful wound healing, light, comfortable temporary prostheses may be used to permit increasing degrees of weight bearing, generally beginning between the fourth and sixth week after surgery. Immediate weight bearing following surgery was recommended by the authors and others in the past but has now been modified. In the elderly, vertical weight loading through the temporary prosthesis and the residual limb is delayed until wound healing is sufficiently advanced that dehiscence will not occur. There is, however, still a place for immediate postsurgical prosthetic fitting and early limited ambulation for children and adults with healthier tissues than the group with peripheral vascular disease. Immediate and early weight bearing should be advised based on the surgeon's observation and experience. There are no exact time guidelines. Uncomplicated primary wound healing is the first priority.

Unhealed and infected wounds have been managed in the past by rigid dressings and limited weight bearing. This treatment was, in essence, an outgrowth of the Orr-Trueta closed-cast management of osteomyelitis. When the infection is well-localized and adequately drained and there are no sequestra or bone abscesses, the closed-cast technique including partial weight bearing may be used.

Below-knee prostheses are now of a variety of designs, lightweight, comfortable, and easy to clean (Fig. 24-4). Young, active unilateral below-knee amputees can run, jump, engage in most vigorous sports, sometimes at a high level of competition, and enjoy prolonged periods of function as in hiking, mountain climbing, playing soccer, and long-distance running. The functional potential is great and is directly dependent on the quality of surgery and prosthetic rehabilitation.

The fibula is sectioned 1 to 1.5 cm above the level of the tibial amputation. Depending on the length of the below-knee stump, there may be considerable movement between the two bones. The compressive forces of socket fit and weight bearing can irritate interosseous and contiguous structures including branches and neuromas of the peroneal nerve. Arthrodesis of the distal tibia to fibula with bone sectioned at near equal length provides a broad, stable, distal amputation with increased potential for end bearing (tibiofibular synostosis). This surgical technique was developed and popularized

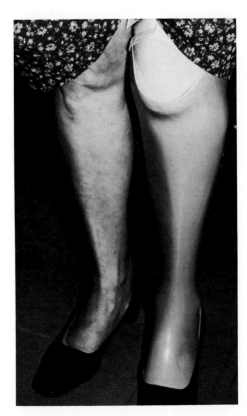

Figure 24-4 Below-knee prosthesis, exoskeletal type, patellar tendon bearing (PTB), total contact socket.

by Ertl in Germany and later by Deffer in the United States. A large World War II experience reinforced its value, but it is not indicated when ischemia is present since the additional manipulation of the distal tissues may compromise primary wound healing. The added functional benefit of tibiofibular synostosis is not so important for the elderly, less active person who can be well and comfortably fitted according to the standard below-knee technique. The procedure is justified primarily for the young, active amputee. The synostosis amputation may have to be carried out at a higher level than would otherwise be necessary in order to obtain adequate soft tissue closure. If length is critical, the operation is not indicated. The synostosis is accomplished either by interosseus bone graft using a segment of fibula or by an osteoperiosteal tube raised from the distal tibia and sutured transversely across the interosseus space to the distal fibula.

Myodesis (suture of muscle to bone) stabilizing the anterolateral muscles and calf muscles to the distal tibia has been advocated by ourselves and others. Drill holes are placed through the distal tibia to allow firm fixation of the sectioned muscles to bone. Occasional aseptic necrosis of the distal tibia may occur. This complication can be avoided by stabilizing the muscle ends to the distal soft tissues and to each other.

Through-Knee Amputation

For many years disarticulation of the knee was popular in the high-risk patient. The surgery could be performed quickly and with minimal blood loss. Surgical mortality and morbidity were considerably lower than for amputation above the knee. As elective surgery in the poor-risk patient has become less threatening, this amputation has been employed less often.

Significant advantages of the knee disarticulation included socket suspension capabilities provided by the bulbous distal femoral stump and good end-bearing capability (Fig. 24-5). In the past these advantages have been offset by prosthetic difficulties. The bulbous distal stump necessitated a bulky, unsightly prosthesis. Intrinsic knee mechanisms could not be incorporated within the limb because of asymmetrical knee joint level with the opposite intact limb. As with the Syme amputation, women often rejected this amputation for cosmetic reasons.

Modern prostheses have overcome many of these objections. They include hydraulic knee-assist mechanisms and other engineering modifications. Knee disarticulation is now a favored amputation for active persons when the alternative is an above-knee site.

Indications include neoplasms and severe distal trauma or infection where limb salvage or functional prosthetic rehabilitation cannot be obtained with a below-knee amputation. Infections involving the proximal tibia and fibula and also septic arthritis of the knee joint can be treated successfully with this procedure. The soft tissues about the knee and particularly the skin must be adequate for coverage.

Knee disarticulation for limb ischemia is no longer favored. The blood supply to the skin about the knee and in the proximal leg area is such that most patients with ischemia who were treated by knee disarticulation in the past will tolerate a short below-knee amputation using the described

posterior flap technique. Salvage of a functional knee under these circumstances can generally permit ambulation. If the knee joint cannot be preserved, in most cases the degree of skin ischemia will not allow healing. For this reason knee disarticulation in the presence of severe ischemia is confined to those individuals who are nonambulators but whose tissues will allow skin healing at the knee disarticulation level. Knee flexion contractures are thus avoided, and the long femoral lever arm may be useful in sitting and in patient transfer even though no prosthesis is used.

A sagittal incision with medial and lateral flaps is recommended.[1] The patella is retained and the patellar tendon sutured to the stump of the cruciate ligaments in the femoral intercondylar notch. The biceps femoris tendon and one or more of the medial hamstring tendons are also stabilized by intercondylar suture. A variety of techniques have been described which severely contour the bony femoral condyles. This practice is no longer routinely employed. Radical trimming of the condyles destroys the rotary stability and suspension capability which enhance the value of through-knee amputation. Only modest contouring of ridges and large, bony prominences should be carried out.

The Gritti-Stokes amputation places the patella on the distal end of the femur to accept end-weight bearing. The

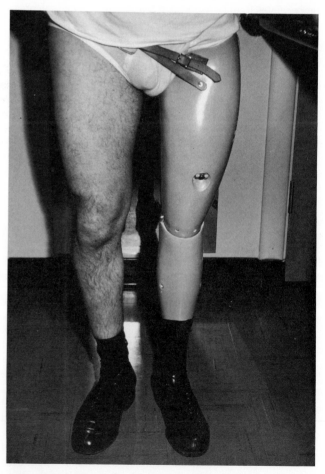

Figure 24-5 Knee disarticulation prosthesis with external knee hinges and rigid thigh socket.

TABLE 24-1 Some Commonly Described Abnormalities Requiring Correction by the Prosthetic Team

Abnormality	Definition	Common causes (not exhaustive)
A. Circumduction	Swinging of the entire prosthesis laterally in a wide arc—returning to the line of progression	a. Prosthesis too long b. Inadequate flexion of prosthetic knee c. Hip abductors weak or contracted
B. Vaulting or pelvic hike or toe stub	Rising on the toe of the sound foot to permit the prosthesis to swing through without toe stubbing	a. Prosthesis too long b. Inadequate flexion of prosthetic knee c. Excessive plantar flexion d. Toe lever arm too long
C. Medial whip	Inward movement of the prosthetic heel, outward movement of the knee, or initial flexion at the beginning of swing	a. Knee axis, normally set in 5° of external rotation to compensate for pelvic rotation, excessively rotated b. Varus knee c. Toe break not at right angle to the line of progression d. Weak muscles rotate around the femur
D. Lateral whip	Opposite to movement of medial whip: knee moves inward, heel outward	a. Knee axis *internally* rotated b. Valgus knee c. Toe break not at right angle to the line of progression d. Weak muscles rotate around the femur

Source: From Sanders, G.T.: *Lower Limb Amputations: A Guide to Rehabilitation.* Philadelphia, Davis, 1986. Modified and used with permission.

patella does not normally provide a physiological weight-bearing surface; rather, weight in the kneeling position is borne on the proximal pretibial area including the patellar tendon. This circumstance negates much of the possible value of the technique. The Gritti-Stokes amputation gives a longer limb than knee disarticulation since the patella is placed at the distal end of the femur. Prosthetists find such a stump difficult to fit. The center of axis of the prosthetic knee is well below that of the normal knee. This asymmetry is noted when the patient sits.

A number of low transcondylar techniques have been described which are designed to retain the advantages of knee disarticulation with a slightly shortened femoral lever arm thus allowing the use of intrinsic prosthetic knee units. Transcondylar amputation more often becomes in effect a very long above-knee amputation with partial loss of those very features which make knee disarticulation attractive.

Above-Knee Amputation

Indications for above-knee amputation include trauma, malignancies, congenital limb deficits, and ischemia. Classic sites of election are no longer applicable. The amputation should salvage all femoral length consistent with a painless, well-healed residual limb. Stabilization of the long thigh muscles to prevent their retraction is mandatory when surgical circumstances permit. There is no level of major amputation where muscle stabilization is more important to prosthetic

control even though the surrounding mass of muscles and fascia may prove somewhat difficult to stabilize into the relatively small distal femur. Particularly important is the stabilization under appropriate tension of the adductor muscle group and quadriceps. Weak hamstring function can be partially supplemented by an intact gluteus maximus. During weight bearing, the line of weight transfer from the pelvis through the hip joint and remaining portion of the femur shifts to the prosthetic socket. Contraction of hip abductors stabilizes the pelvic/femoral segment to prevent trunk sway. When applied to the residual femur of the above-knee amputee the abductors cause shift of the femur within its soft tissue envelope until it firmly contacts the lateral wall of the above-knee prosthetic socket. If the adductor muscles have not been attached to the distal medial femoral stump so as to oppose this displacement, a lurching Trendelenburg gait results (Table 24-1). Active, stabilized quadriceps muscles assist the hip flexors to propel the prosthesis forward and assist prosthetic toe clearance.

Loss of the knee joint by above-knee amputation significantly compounds the challenge of making the prosthesis functional. Scores of prosthetic knee mechanisms commercially available attest to this engineering challenge. While it is true that a simple peg extension can yield a stable degree of bipedal mobility, refined lower limb function using an above-knee prosthesis requires a complex bioengineering response using gravity-induced energy sources, hydraulics, pneumatics, or mechanical or electrical control systems of great ingenuity to substitute for the lost knee.

The first functional requirement for the above-knee amputee is that the prosthesis be stable in the various phases of weight bearing. Gait training is a key part of rehabilitation, much more so than at lower levels of leg loss. Properly trained, a significant number of geriatric above-knee amputees can be trained to walk well with a cane if the opposite limb is intact.

Maximum femoral length is preserved. The length of the residual lever arm is directly related to quality, suspension, alignment, and control of the prosthesis. Energy expenditure also increases as the length of the remaining limb decreases.

The skin incision is dictated by the local circumstances, including previously placed scars from vascular reconstruction or other surgery. Since the stump totally contacts the prosthetic socket, the position of skin scars is far less important than its healing. Free mobility of the skin and subcutaneous tissues, adequate blood supply, sensibility, and lack of tenderness are the important and necessary features.

Skin flaps are fashioned short using plastic technique to preserve blood supply. The flaps must be planned to avoid a tight skin closure. With the dysvascular amputee, this is the most frequently observed technical error.

The importance of muscle stabilization and means for its accomplishment have been emphasized. The technique of distal attachment of the muscles and fascia depends on the local situation. Ischemic muscles cannot be expected to heal if their blood supply is additionally disturbed by constricting sutures. When the muscle tissue is healthy and well-vascularized as with above-knee amputations for neoplasm, a careful myoplasty and/or myodesis is essential for optimum prosthetic control.

Major nerves are retracted under moderate tension and ligated before being sectioned and allowed to retract.

The bone is divided transversely, the outer cortex moderately rounded to remove sharp edges, and the periosteum purse-string sutured over the cut end of the bone. Routine hemostasis and drainage complete the operation.

Rigid immediate postoperative dressings are more difficult to apply and properly suspend at the above-knee level. Accepted practice uses soft compression dressing carried up as a spica around the pelvis for suspension. If the surgical amputee team is skilled in rigid dressing application at the above-knee level, this technique does offer the advantages previously outlined. Air splints have been used as a postoperative dressing. Lack of equipment and of experience in their use has limited the acceptance of this technique.

Hip Disarticulation

Hip disarticulation is performed infrequently. Indications include severe trauma, malignancies of the more proximal part of the lower limb, and, occasionally, ischemia. It may be necessary to perform hip disarticulation to control local infection and as a lifesaving procedure. Vascular surgical services are encountering the need for hip disarticulation more and more frequently when repeated vascular reconstructions have failed and little blood supply is present below the renal arteries. Prostheses are not generally indicated with this patient population. Adaptive mobility aids include modified wheelchairs and litters. Some of these patients can be cared for in a home setting; most are institutionalized.

Hip disarticulation for nonischemic disease and specifically trauma and malignancies is occasionally required in young people. The surgical techniques are well-standardized.

Excellent prosthetic substitution is available in the young, strong person (Fig. 24-6). Many walk without a cane or other external aid. Remarkable physical achievement with or without a prosthesis is possible. Nonetheless, the inconvenience and learning effort required for use of this heavy prosthesis discourage many individuals. The more rapid and effective the rehabilitation, the more likely that the individual will become an effective regular user of the limb. Without a prosthesis, crutches are required in order to walk or stand for any length of time. Free use of the arms is thus denied.

Hemipelvectomy and Hemicorporectomy

Hemipelvectomy and hemicorporectomy are sometimes required for elimination of malignant tumors about the pelvis, but radical local excision and reconstruction with limb salvage where possible are much preferred. Weight-bearing prostheses are rarely used after these mutilating procedures. Independent walking without crutches or walker is not achieved even when a prosthesis can be fitted.

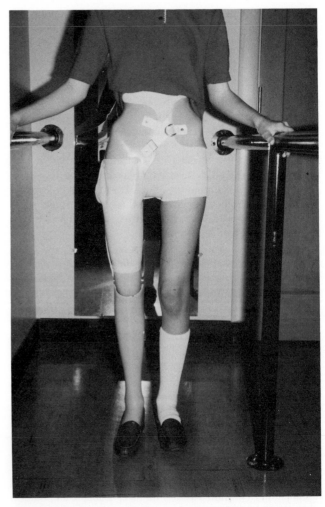

Figure 24-6 Hip disarticulation prosthesis with hydraulic knee mechanism.

Wrist Disarticulation

Preservation of both forearm bones and the distal radial ulnar articulation provides an excellent amputation result. Pronation and supination are largely preserved. Distal stump contour irregularities aid in prosthetic stability and suspension. Both body and externally powered prostheses allow significant limb rehabilitation. Wrist disarticulation amputees mostly become skilled prosthetic users and attain a remarkable degree of bimanual function. This level is widely accepted by amputees of both sexes.

Terminal devices (hand substitutes) for the wrist disarticulation amputee include those generally used for upper limb loss. In order to maintain comparable length with the intact limb when the amputation is unilateral, it may be necessary to modify the hook or hand substitute. Prosthetic modification is also required if external power sources such as electricity are used. The residual limb fills the entire socket of the unmodified prosthesis, leaving no room between the end of the amputation and the prosthetic wrist joint in which batteries and electric motor systems may be placed to activate the hook or cosmetic fingers.

Amputations through the Forearm

Amputations at the below-elbow level should conserve all length consistent with proper bone management and soft tissue coverage. Distal muscle stabilization is important, especially when myoelectric signals are to be used for externally powered electric prostheses. Individual muscle fixation is not carried out. The myoelectric signals are obtained from the mass contraction of the flexor group and the extensor group. They should be stabilized by myoplasty to or near the distal ends of both the radius and the ulna.

As the amputation level proceeds proximally from the wrist, voluntary pronation and supination are progressively more limited. The prosthetic socket further restricts rotary movement. Compensation can be partly achieved by body positioning of the limb primarily through shoulder rotation and elbow flexion/extension. It is also possible on occasion to incorporate rotary forearm prosthetic enhancement with a small planetary gear incorporated within the prosthesis.

The short below-elbow amputation is preferred over elbow disarticulation since the former preserves a useful range of active elbow movement. This implies biceps or brachialis function as well as active extension.

Below-elbow prostheses are conventionally powered by metal or plastic cables activated by body movement using a fabric loop under the opposite shoulder. A number of sources of external power, including hydraulic, pneumatic, and electric units, are also used.

Elbow Disarticulation

Amputation through the elbow joint is seldom performed. Prosthetists encounter difficulty fitting the residual limb with an acceptable substitute. This level precludes the use of intrinsic prosthetic elbow mechanisms because of their space requirements. Incorporation of the artificial elbow mechanism disproportionately lengthens the upper arm and shortens the forearm. Limb symmetry can be retained, however, by using external elbow hinges with a number of possible types of elbow control mechanisms.

In spite of these disadvantages, this amputation level does produce the advantage of a long lever arm and an irregular distal contour, making for excellent socket stability. The practice of converting the elbow disarticulation to a low above-elbow amputation is not necessary.

Through-elbow amputation is most often occasioned by trauma including burns.

Above-Elbow Amputation

There is no site of election for amputations through the upper arm. All length is saved consistent with the creation of a satisfactory residual limb. Even the very short above-elbow level, where only the head of the humerus remains, presents a more normal shoulder contour. The humeral head is not removed unless the shoulder joint is painful or its removal is necessitated by the disease.

Whenever possible, distal muscle stabilization is necessary for the above-elbow amputee to provide strength, prosthetic control, and myoelectric signals for externally powered limbs.

Both functional and purely cosmetic prostheses are available for the above-elbow amputee. Many unilateral above-elbow amputees, particularly those with amputations through the proximal half of the humerus, prefer a nonfunctional, light cosmetic limb over the heavier, more complicated functional appliance. Three types of functional prostheses are available. The terminal device can be controlled by body movement, by external electric power sources, or by a combination. As technology has improved and electric components have become miniaturized and light, more amputees are being fitted with the combination, or hybrid, prosthesis. As an example, elbow motion is controlled by myoelectric sources with terminal-device function accomplished through cables and body movement. Even though suspension of the conventional prosthesis with body-powered harnessing is somewhat uncomfortable and restrictive, both children and adults can be expected to undergo successful prosthetic rehabilitation with daily regular use of the prosthesis. The patience and assisted training necessary to develop skills is outweighed by the great advantage of bimanual function. This is particularly true in the workplace as well as in many recreational activities. Elderly above-elbow amputees are often better served by fitting them with a light, cosmetic device used primarily for dress and social occasions.

Bilateral upper limb loss whether congenital or acquired is critically disabling. Infants and children quickly learn to substitute foot function to accomplish daily living needs. Prostheses are often reserved for wear out of the home. When skillfully designed and properly fitted, however, functional prostheses can be successful. Acquired bilateral upper limb loss in adult life makes mandatory the dedicated and intense training for functional prosthetic use.

Immediate postsurgical rigid dressings with prosthetic fitting are particularly successful. The distal compression controls edema, and the immobilization minimizes postsurgical pain. Terminal devices can be fitted to the immediate postsurgical rigid dressing, often within days after surgery. Upper limb amputees rapidly acquire terminal-device control using this immediate postsurgical system. Myoelectric control electrodes can be placed in the temporary socket for early external powering. Patterns of use carry over to definitive limb use. Under this prompt progressive rehabilitation plan, very few amputees later abandon the use of the prosthesis.

Post-amputation physical therapy for all upper limb levels includes particular attention to proximal joint and muscle function. Since the terminal device is, in general, controlled by active shoulder girdle movement, it is important to prevent contractures and to maintain muscle strength.

Assuming normal mobility, the arm amputee moves freely in the environment with or without the prosthesis and is therefore less challenged than the lower leg amputee to wear the device and improve performance and skills with it. Functional goals should be set high enough to challenge the trainee yet not so great as to overwhelm and discourage prosthetic use.

Shoulder Disarticulation and Forequarter Amputation

These radical amputations usually result from malignancy. When performed on the immature skeleton, a dorsal scoliosis frequently results. In general, prosthetic substitution is aimed at cosmesis and for the fitting of clothing. Through-shoulder amputation with retention of shoulder girdle muscles results in muscle contractures and "hiking" of the scapula since the action of the scapular elevator muscles are unopposed by the weight of that portion of the arm which has been removed.

Pain Following Amputation

Complications aside from a consideration of pain have been discussed earlier. Pain can be associated with the stump itself or experienced in the phantom limb.[1,12] Occasionally both types are present. The diagnosis of these pain patterns must be carried out in a systematic manner. Early postoperative management of the amputation has a considerable influence on the degree and duration of these pain patterns. Immediate postoperative rigid dressings properly applied to control edema and provide wound stability promote a more comfortable and early healing course. Hematoma or swelling associated with a tight wound closure and wound infection produces severe, persistent pain.

As wound healing progresses, postoperative pain usually subsides and the patient then proceeds to functional rehabilitation. Pain in the phantom limb tends to subside beginning about the fifth or sixth week following amputation. Some phantom sensations including occasional pain usually persist throughout the individual's life. With most persons, it is an annoyance and does not prevent prosthetic wear, require medication, or significantly influence the pattern of daily living.

A greater challenge arises when dealing with chronic pain.[1] These sensations may be regional, phantom, or combined. A thorough history and physical and psychological examination provide a basis for diagnosis. Severe, acute, and chronic preoperative pain predisposes to a carryover of pain patterns following amputation. This is especially true when the pain has been severe and has been present for a significant time prior to surgery. Its preoperative management is also a source of important information. It should include psychosocial assessment of tolerance to previous painful experiences. The physical examination seeks areas of tenderness, particularly in relation to anatomic position of nerves, neuromas, or underlying bone irregularities. The effects of active muscle contractions on the pain should be assessed as well as the state of the soft tissues, their color, the patient's nutritional and circulatory status, and the presence or absence of edema. Local and regional nerve blockade with local anesthesia using a very small needle may be used to further explain the pain. If additional neurological information is desired, one then proceeds to regional nerve block anesthetizing the remaining limb completely. Persistence of pain indicates its central origin.

Neurocirculatory dystrophy (Sudeck's atrophy) pain is occasionally encountered. Not infrequently, pain unrelated to the amputation itself can be overlooked. Sciatica due to a herniated intervertebral disc, arthritic disease in adjacent joints, ischemia, and referred visceral pain need to be ruled out.

Following organized diagnostic screening, one can proceed to treatment. Therapy should be directed toward the diagnosed causative factors. Noninvasive methods are preferred and may include the entire spectrum of pain abatement measures: electrical, chemical, physical, and psychological. Addictive pain medication and surgical intervention are employed with *great caution.* Removal of large, tender adherent neuromas particularly in the areas of interface pressure and shear can have a moderate degree of success. Response to local anesthesia may be the major determinant in deciding upon the local removal of neuromas.

Reamputation to a higher level for pain relief is seldom indicated. Badly scarred, adherent distal tissues with difficult limb fit can benefit from appropriate revision and pain relief and improved function may follow. Revision with distal muscle stabilization is credited for occasional improvement of severe chronic stump pain. Proximal peripheral and central nervous system surgical intervention such as spinal cord tractotomy has been notoriously unsuccessful. Such intervention involving the nervous system can convert a difficult pain syndrome into a catastrophic one.

Modern amputation surgical techniques as previously described have reduced to a small number those patients who have chronic, agonizing, intractable pain. These complex problem cases are seen most often at high amputation levels, i.e., hip and shoulder disarticulations. These are best handled by experienced amputation teams cooperating with pain management specialists including psychiatrists. Fortunately the number of such cases is small.

As many as one-third of congenital amputees who have been surveyed regarding awareness of a phantom limb indicate periods of such awareness. The psychological background for this experience is poorly explained.

Diagnostic Tests for Determination of Amputation Level

Most surgeons rely on a careful history and thorough physical examination to establish the lowest effective amputation level which can be expected to heal without complication. Objective laboratory limb viability studies can assist the surgeon to select amputation levels in the presence of ischemia. Such studies do not replace clinical experience and judgment. These tests do not necessarily correspond to those used by vascular surgeons contemplating surgical reconstruction. In particular, angiography is not generally useful when determining the level of amputation in end-stage disease.

The objective information routinely used at this time by the senior author (E.M.B) includes skin temperature, Doppler segmental blood pressure with ischemic index and Doppler waveform, transcutaneous P_{O_2}, P_{CO_2}, and laser Doppler flowmetry. These are noninvasive and inexpensive and can be performed by a vascular technician. They permit "limb viability scanning" by multiple-site data accrual.

A number of other examinations used in both the research and the clinical setting are fluorescein flowmetry, skin clearance of ^{133}Xe, and nuclear magnetic resonance spectrometry.[4,5,9,10,13,15,19]

An example of the use of these tests can be demonstrated at the below-knee level. Adverse arteriographic findings and the absence of popliteal pulses are not contraindications to below-knee amputation. A segmental Doppler pressure index greater than 0.35 for the nondiabetic patient and 0.45 for the diabetic patient strongly suggests the likelihood of skin healing at that level. Skin oxygen diffusion of 25 to 30 mmHg and higher also delineates an acceptable skin healing potential.[133] Xe washout of 2.6 ml/100 g if confirmed with laser Doppler cell velocity also establishes an adequate level of skin healing.

The most reliable determinant of healing remains the appearance of the tissues at the time of surgery as judged by the experienced surgeon. This applies in particular to the observed vascularity of the skin envelope. With present preoperative diagnostic information and careful observation at surgery, uncomplicated healing rates at the below-knee level are achieved in well over 50 percent of all patients with peripheral vascular disease requiring major limb loss. Of all lower limb amputations for ischemia (which include amputations involving the foot), 75 to 90 percent should heal primarily at the below-knee level. Failure to heal requiring reamputation should not be necessary in more than 6 to 8 percent of this patient population.

PROSTHETICS

General Considerations

Historically, prostheses are as old as recorded amputations. Down through the years artificial limbs have been fabricated by a wide variety of artisans including leather workers, metalworkers, woodworkers, sculptors, medical practitioners, and, in many cases, the amputee. Prior to the development of synthetic plastics, most prostheses were constructed from organic materials and metals. Leather, linen, cotton, wool, silk, and wood were used in a variety of combinations. These materials combined with available metals completed the prosthesis.

Prostheses are now constructed primarily of composite plastics. Graphite and light metals are also in common use.[1] Today, prosthetic engineering is pursued by a small group of materials and design scientists. The demand for modern technology is stimulating increasing interest in this area of bioengineering.

The prosthesis is an artificial organ. It should replace as successfully as possible the function and appearance of the lost part. It is composed of three basic components: (1) its attachment to the body, generally by means of a socket (the human-machine interface), (2) the terminal device (replacement for the hand or foot or a portion of either organ), i.e., the physical contact with the environment, and (3) the intervening structure, or body of the prosthesis. Natural appearance is desirable when this can be obtained without compromising function. A few amputees prefer a strictly cosmetic substitute.

The prosthesis is attached to the body by straps, belts, socket contour, suction, friction, and to some degree by physiological suspension through muscle control of the stump. Comfort is an essential requisite. The energy requirement for prosthetic use particularly in the lower limb relates to the weight of the artificial limb, its components, its alignment, and the level of amputation. The higher the level of amputation, the greater the energy requirement for limb control.

The artificial limb is controlled and manipulated either by the body or by external power sources, or by a combination of both. Trunk and residual limb muscles ordinarily power lower limb prostheses. The shoulder girdle, shoulder, and residual limb activate upper limb prosthetic use. External electric power sources which are initiated by myoelectric signals arising in the muscles of the residual upper limb are used in increasing numbers as miniaturization of the engineering has developed. These myoelectric arms are available worldwide for selected users. Indications for these various types of prostheses will be described later.

FABRICATION

Most prostheses are fabricated over a plaster mold taken from the residual limb. After detailed measurements of the limb, a plaster wrap is taken and removed and a male plaster mold formed. The socket is then fabricated over the mold using thermoplastic materials. Precise socket measurements are important. It is now common practice to make a clear check socket, fit it, and then form the definitive socket after necessary modifications of the check socket. Difficult stumps may require several check sockets prior to the final fitting. Foaming techniques similar to those used in fitting ski boots can be helpful. Xeroradiography, a process of x-ray imaging, is an effective evaluation tool. This technique demonstrates both soft tissue and bone details not seen on a standard x-ray film. Computerized x-ray tomography, photogrammetry (photographic contour mapping), volume displacement measurements, and ultrasound and laser scanning are research modes being used to study and improve socket design and fabrication.

Computerized techniques for design and manufacture can rapidly and consistently fabricate, modify, and align. Shape-sensing systems can translate the physical features of the residual limb into computer-aided design and manufacturing machines. This technology is approaching practical use in prosthetics.

Necessary components for completion of the prosthesis are added following socket fabrication. A wide variety of knee, ankle/foot, wrist, and elbow joints are available. These artificial joints range from simple mechanical, single-axis hinge articulations through polycentric multiple-linkage gravity-assisted friction, hydraulic, pneumatic, and electrically controlled devices.

Structural support for the socket and the articulated components is either endoskeletal or exoskeletal. The endoskeletal units are essentially the inner frame of the prosthesis and are constructed of pylons usually of light metal graphte or composite plastics. They are covered by cosmetic synthetic foam simulating the appearance and color of the uninvolved limb. Exoskeletal units are formed in the shape of the normal limb but have no inner structural support. The strength lies in the material used.

Alignment

Prosthetic alignment is critical to proper function. This is especially true in the lower limb, where stability and gait are influenced by the alignment of the prosthesis to the socket and residual limb. The prosthetist aligns the limb after careful static and dynamic analysis. A number of alignment tools are used including jigs, plumb lines, and cinephotography. Input from the amputee is the final alignment determinant. Length, stability, control, energy consumption, and comfort can be best appreciated even in discrete variation by the amputee.

Prescription Principles

The amputee team fills its single most important role with limb prescription. The surgeon, prosthetist, and therapist are indispensable when the decision for the type of prosthetic substitute is made.[16] Input from social workers, internists, psychologists, and family may reinforce team judgment, but the three key team members can cooperatively weigh the rehabilitation potential, functional capability, and availability of the new prosthesis. A well-written prescription form avoids overlooking important but less visible needs. The practice of referring the amputee to the prosthetist with a simple request for an artificial limb is insufficient.

Specifics of limb prescription vary depending on the level of limb loss.[11] It is not intended here to outline the numerous variable entering into this process. The following short section will condense these general parameters.

Foot and Ankle Prostheses

Toe, metatarsophalangeal, and transmetatarsal amputations function well with compliant forefoot shoe fillers and shoe modifications. A stiff sole with a forward-placed rocker bar usually further improves gait and push-off.

Amputations through the midfoot up to and including the Boyd and Pirogoff levels are best fitted with a high shoe attached to an ankle, foot orthosis (AFO) to block ankle dorsiflexion, allowing gravity push-off and reducing the flatfoot gait (Fig. 24-2).

Syme's amputation requires an entire prosthetic foot rigidly attached to a patellar tendon bearing type of polymer prosthetic shell. The rigid ankle with heel cushioning and a flexible metatarsophalangeal forefoot section permit many Syme's amputees to walk with a normal gait at ordinary cadence. Walking fast or running elicits a moderately shortened gait pattern and slight limp. The distal Syme's amputation is often bulbous. A flexible insert into the rigid shin shell of the prosthesis ordinarily allows entry of the residual limb (Fig. 24-3). Some Syme's amputees need a lateral or posterior replaceable window to allow clearance for stump entry. Enlargement of the prosthesis at ankle level distorts the ankle contour. Women tend to object to this added bulk and thickness. Some are sufficiently sensitive that they request a higher level of amputation through the distal one-third of tibia and fibula to permit fitting with a more cosmetic design.

Suspension of Syme's prosthesis is accomplished by a strap above the patella attached to the sides of the prosthesis and by the contour suspension inherent in the bulbous nature of the amputation site (Fig. 24-3). Many Syme's users depend on this latter feature alone and require no additional suspension system.

Below-Knee Prostheses

The below-knee amputation is the most frequently performed major amputation. Prostheses are designed with a total-contact socket contouring around the entire residual limb up to knee level. Weight is born generally over the surface of the limb even including to a minor degree the distal end. The patellar tendon area and the proximal and medial face of the tibia are especially involved in weight bearing. Several variations in socket design are available. The medial and lateral walls can be carried up to the proximal border of the femoral condyles and the anterior section brought up over the patella (PTS). The classic total-contact patellar tendon bearing design (PTB) does not include the patella, and the trim lines of the socket superiorly lie only slightly above the knee (Fig. 24-4).

Suspension of below-knee prostheses can be accomplished by a suspension strap just above the patella and attached to the lateral and medial aspects of the socket. A variety of supracondylar wedges entrap the medial condyle so that it acts as a suspension point. An additional strap carried up the anterior thigh to a flexible pelvic belt and attached to the medial and lateral socket surfaces can further suspend the limb. When controlled muscle contraction is present in the residual limb muscles, and especially in the gastrocnemius-soleus group, it is possible to obtain some degree of suspension by muscle contraction. This is called physiological suspension and assists during the swing phase of gait to maintain socket interface stability.

The shank may be either endoskeletal and covered with a cosmetic material or exoskeletal with the leg shell supporting the weight. Ankle/feet mechanisms vary from a single-axis

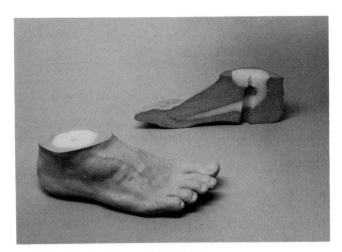

Figure 24-7 Prosthetic foot (Seattle foot) to store gravitational energy and improve physiological gait.

bolt with a fore and aft rubber bumper through a wide variety of designs including hydraulic, pneumatic, and gravity energy control. The Seattle foot is a recent development using the latter physical principles (Fig. 24-7).

For many years the below-knee prosthesis was fitted with rigid single-axis knee hinges carried from the medial and lateral proximal socket surfaces up to a thigh lacer usually encompassing about one-half to two-thirds of the thigh. The total-contact PTB and PTS designs have largely replaced this system (Fig. 24-4). The thigh lacer does provide some additional suspension and stability; however, it largely eliminates rotation of the tibia on the femur when the knee is flexed. Progressive thigh muscle atrophy under the lacer can be expected.

Prescription of this limb is now restricted to long-term users who do not wish to be converted to more physiological limbs and to people performing work and recreation that require a great deal of stability. Individuals who are up and down ladders and stairs at work, construction workers in high places, and athletes who ski, play soccer and basketball, and run will use a thigh lacer limb for these specific periods of time when extra stability and control are needed.

Function of the thigh lacer limb can be marginally improved by polycentric knee joints rather than a single-axis joint. The polycentric hinge simulates the condylar gliding motion of the knee as it flexes and extends.

Knee Disarticulation Prostheses

The knee disarticulation is to a large degree end bearing. Its bulbous nature provides excellent prosthetic suspension. Since the femur is full length, it is necessary to use side joints attached to a thigh component rather than an intrinsic knee mechanism which would require sufficient space to excessively lengthen the femoral segment and produce significant knee asymmetry when the patient sits (Fig. 24-5). Ingenious intrinsic knee mechanisms have been devised which minimize this length discrepancy. Earlier knee disarticulation prostheses used a thigh lacer of leather. Modern design consists of a semirigid thigh component with a Velcro strap support. A rigid, closed thigh section similar to that used for the above-knee prosthesis is also acceptable.

Above-Knee Prostheses

Prosthetic substitution becomes much more complicated without the knee joint. Fitting the socket to the residual limb and the proximally adjacent pelvic structures is technically more difficult than at the through-knee and below-knee levels. Since World War II, the quadrilateral socket has been standard. The brim of the socket posteriorly rests against the ischial tuberosity, and the anteroposterior dimension of the socket is narrowed to maintain the tuberosity on the posterior brim of the prosthesis during weight bearing. Unfortunately, compression in the anteroposterior plane requires a wider mediolateral dimension to accommodate the tissues, and adductor stability is compromised, accentuating the gluteus medius Trendelenburg lurch.

The present trend departs from the classic quadrilateral design and emphasizes a narrower mediolateral dimension. The ischial tuberosity slides inside the socket and is not the point of major weight bearing. The gluteal structures together with the peritrochanteric area absorb increasing load.

The femoral section of the limb itself may be endoskeletal or exoskeletal and attaches to one of more than 75 available knee mechanisms. These include mechanical, single-axis, and multiple-linkage polycentric knees; a wide variety of hydraulic mechanisms; and pneumatic, gravity friction lock, and drop-lock designs. The shin and ankle/foot units are those described in the section on the below-knee prosthesis but modified as indicated for particular alignment and individual patient needs. Proper alignment of the above-knee prosthesis following static and dynamic analysis is essential to successful stability and function. Gait abnormalities seen at differing phases of the walking cycle give important clues to help the prosthetic team improve prosthetic fitting (Table 24-1).[2]

Suspension is accomplished by suction with a suction valve at the distal end of the socket and also by socket contour. A flexible pelvic belt, a rigid hip joint to a semirigid pelvic belt, and, on rare occasions, shoulder strap suspension are worn. A combination of these suspension devices may be used. As with the below-knee residual limb, stump muscle activity enhances suspension in a physiological manner. Gait training should emphasize the advantages of muscle control of the socket.

Hip Disarticulation and Hemipelvectomy Prostheses

Removal of the hip joint increases the complexity of prosthetic fitting. Most older patients with hip disarticulation prefer not to wear a prosthesis, and use crutches, walker, and wheelchair. The younger patients can be fitted with a conforming pelvic prosthetic bucket and a hydraulic or mechanical hip joint mechanism carried down to an above-knee type of prosthesis. These prostheses are heavy even when made of the lightest available materials. Young, active amputees can use them successfully but generally require an external aid such as a cane for any prolonged walking.

Upper Limb Prosthetics

Prosthetic replacement of upper limb function is far more complicated than in the lower limb. The hand is such an exquisite motor and sensory organ, so indispensable to the human condition and so protean as a source of human sensitivity and behavior, that even the most sophisticated upper limb prostheses are but crude replicas.

Many engineers have undertaken prosthetic upper limb replacement. As they proceed, their confidence and enthusiasm is replaced by overwhelming awe at the versatility of human upper limbs. Initial disdain of the apparent crude mechanical hooks in common use also is soon overcome by an appreciation of the efficiency of these devices, largely developed by input from the amputee.

The principles of arm prostheses center about the socket, its suspension, the body of the prosthesis, and the terminal device. Like the normal hand, the prosthetic terminal device dominates upper limb function. The shoulder girdle, the shoulder, and the arm down to wrist level assist by positioning the hand or prosthetic substitute in desired positions. The forearm muscles activating hand movement are duplicated in the prosthesis either by substitute muscle groups transferring power/motion mechanically through cables or by external power sources, usually small batteries and motors housed within the prosthesis.

Wrist Disarticulation Prostheses

Modern sockets are made of semirigid composite plastics. The terminal device, hook or hand, is generally firmly fixed to the distal end of the socket without an intervening wrist joint mechanism. The socket extends to the elbow, leaving it free to move in the anteroposterior plane. When the distal radio ulnar joint is intact, a considerable degree of pronation and supination is possible. Further rotary assistance in positioning the hand and hook is accomplished by shoulder girdle and shoulder movement. For these reasons, the wrist disarticulation amputee can operate the prosthesis through a wide spatial area.

Terminal-device control is ordinarily accomplished by a contralateral axillary sling controlling a cable across the upper back down to the socket and then attached to the hook or hand. A wide variety of terminal devices are available for general and specific tasks. Excellent function can be accomplished with this prosthetic system. The artificial limb is suspended by shaping its contour to gently grasp the distal radius, ulna, and forearm.

Forearm Prostheses

Since forearm amputations should preserve all available length, the prosthesis is designed to accommodate many amputation levels. Composite plastic material forms the socket, which totally contacts the residual limb. The terminal device is attached to the socket extension designed with appropriate length for bilateral limb symmetry. The terminal device generally incorporates a mechanical wrist unit to allow prepositioning for rotation, flexion, and extension.

The hand or hook is motivated either by body powering through cables or by myoelectric-activated external energy obtained from a battery and motor housed in the socket space distal to the end of the stump. Electric signals produced by voluntary contraction of the residual forearm stump muscles are amplified to trigger battery/motor energy (Fig. 24-8). The limb is suspended by socket contouring around the remaining forearm and distal humeral condyles. When additional suspension stability is required, elbow hinges are carried from the proximal socket up to an upper arm cuff. Depending upon the length of the residual forearm, and stability requirements, a variety of elbow hinges are available including flexible, polycentric, step-up, and single-axis rigid hinges.

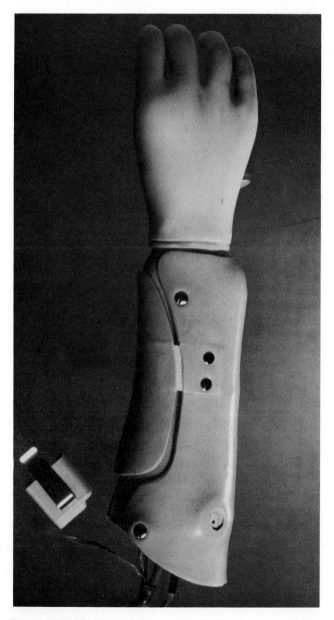

Figure 24-8 Myoelectric forearm prosthesis.

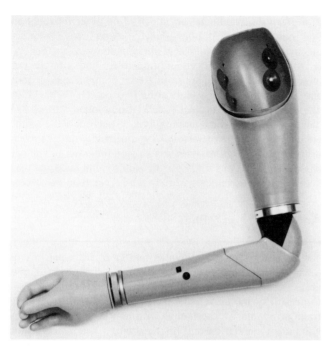

Figure 24-9 Myoelectric upper arm prosthesis (Utah arm).

Above-Elbow Prostheses

The need for elbow substitution confronts the user with a much greater challenge. The socket must be stabilized about the shoulder to prevent its rotation with prosthetic use. The substitute elbow must first be placed in a position of desired function and then locked or stabilized in this position to permit terminal-device action. The weight of the forearm and terminal device frequently tires the wearer, causing shoulder and upper back fatigue. Many individuals with amputations at this level forego function and resort to a light cosmetic replacement worn for social occasions.

Early, aggressive training following amputation develops bimanual use patterns motivating the arm amputee to become a successful wearer.

The prosthesis is composed of composite plastic material. Its socket contours the residual limb. This contact is not sufficient for suspension, so added straps are usually necessary over the shoulder to assist in prosthetic support.

A wide variety of elbow mechanisms are commercially available. The prosthetic elbow can be positioned and locked in several flexion-extension modes to stabilize the prosthesis for terminal-device use. Elbow rotation is accomplished by prepositioning the forearm through a friction mechanism using the opposite arm.

Dual-control body-powered cable systems are necessary for (1) elbow positioning and locking and (2) terminal-device function. Active shoulder and shoulder girdle motion motivates the cables.

Ingenious myoelectric prostheses are available. National pride is involved in the development of these appliances as attested by their names: the Canadian arm, the Russian arm, the Italian arm, the Boston arm, the Utah arm (Fig. 24-9), and

others. Electronics miniaturization has permitted highly sophisticated devices using a variety of initiating sources of energy including electric muscle signaling, displacement electrodes, and muscle "noise." Hybrid systems consisting of body power and external power sources are available. They are particularly useful for the upper arm prosthesis when the elbow can be controlled by electric power sources and the terminal device by body powering through cables. Bioengineering centers throughout the world are continuing research to improve these systems as well as to improve conventional materials and designs.

Conclusions

The material presented in this chapter is directed toward an understanding and working knowledge of contemporary amputation management. Since a team of disciplines is involved in amputation rehabilitation, no single monograph, treatise, or text chapter can provide complete coverage of the field. This in no way alleviates or excuses the orthopaedic surgeon from acquiring a firm working knowledge of the various services required to produce superior management.

Throughout the world, millions of amputees function at a high level of human endeavor. No one except an amputee can fully understand and appreciate what it means to be without a limb or limbs. Even the presence of a functionless, insensate limb has a different psychological impact from the empty sleeve or empty pantleg. Currently we read of amputees scaling mountains, running across continents, engaging in professional baseball and boxing, and competing in a wide array of other physical activities. Each exhibits a profile of courage and inner strength unique to the amputee. Orthopaedic surgeons involved in amputee management assume the primary responsibility for providing and directing the professional services which will allow full rehabilitation potential.

═══ **SECTION B** ═══

Amputations and Prosthetics in Children

Joan T. Gold

Advancements in the treatment of pediatric amputees are in large part due to an improved understanding of child development. The child's ability to learn permits earlier provision of and training with a prosthesis. Incorporation of a device into the child's body image results in its improved acceptance and use.[51] Newer prosthetic options and technical advancements build upon this framework.

In order to foster normal development, the emotional sequelae of these deficiencies should also be considered. A child viewed by himself or herself as defective or dependent has additional handicaps. These children require the services of an entire team including a pediatric orthopaedist, a pediatric physiatrist, a prosthetist, physical and occupational therapists, a psychologist, and a social worker in order to maximize their functional outcome.

INCIDENCE

Although the size of the amputee population under the age of 21 years is not known, it is thought to represent 10 percent of the total cases. According to Krebs's survey of 45 pediatric amputee clinics in 1980, there were 4105 children under treatment.[47] This may be an underestimation, as children with less complex deficiencies may not have been referred to these centers. Males outnumbered females 3 to 2. Eighty percent of the deficiencies were unilateral. Congenital amputees were twice as frequent as those whose deficiencies were acquired.

Incidence figures for congenital limb reductions and amputations vary. Recent studies in the United States and Sweden reveal an incidence of approximately 6.3 cases per 10,000 births.[39,45] The terminal transverse below-elbow amputation is the most common congenital deficiency, occurring in over 50 percent of the congenital cases; the left side is more commonly affected.[3,78]

Of the acquired cases, 60 percent involve the loss of a lower extremity, 30 percent involve an upper extremity, and 10 percent involve multiple extremities. Of unilateral cases, lower extremity amputations are the most likely.[47]

ETIOLOGY
Congenital Amputations and Limb Deficiencies

The causative factors of congenital amputations are mostly unknown. Embryological studies have implicated an insult to the limb buds occurring from 4 to 8 weeks of gestation.[10,86] After that time, further insults do not result in the failure of formation of parts, but rather in alterations in size. As development of upper extremities precedes that of the lower extremities, involvement of all four extremities implies a pathological process occurring over time, and not a trivial, isolated event. This is especially important in easing the guilt of a mother who has had such an infant.

The thalidomide syndrome is one of the rare exceptions in which cause could be proved. Ingestion of this drug at 34 to 50 days of gestation resulted in children with phocomelia of two to four extremities and associated facial, cardiac, and genitourinary malformations.[28] Other recognized causative factors include maternal diabetes (in association with sacral agenesis),[102] hydramnios, maternal exposure to rubella, amniotic bands, uterine cramping, and chromosomal abnormalities (trisomies 13 and 18).[39]

There may be an etiologic role for multifactorial inheritance, i.e., certain mothers being genetically more susceptible

to a given environmental agent. The role of such agents as oral contraceptives,[43] phenothiazine derivatives (such as meclizine),[38] dioxane, folic acid antagonists (such as aminopterin), anticonvulsants, endocrinopathies, and intercurrent infections has not been substantiated.[20] Smoking and alcohol use may be related to limb reduction defects.[6] The Child Amputee Prosthetic Project (CAPP) study found that of 159 patients with congenital amputations, 65 percent of the mothers had one or more of the following during their pregnancies: urinary tract infections, pneumonia, viral illnesses, or vaginal bleeding.[9] There was a 12 percent incidence of maternal diabetes. These percentages were much higher than predicted.

Acquired Amputations

Of the acquired cases, over 70 percent are trauma-related, and 90 percent of those involve one limb.[3] The majority of posttraumatic cases occur after the age of 8 years, when the child is less likely to be observed at play. Most cases occur as the result of motor vehicle accidents.[34] Other cases follow train accidents,[23,93] accidents with power tools and farm equipment,[53] electrical and chemical burns, falls, and gunshot wounds.[93] Children who are loners, have a history of behavioral disorders, and live in a low socioeconomic setting are at risk for such injuries. These factors have to be assessed in planning the rehabilitation programs of such children and have implications for prevention as well.[23,34,93]

Of the acquired cases, 30 percent result as the sequelae of disease; most are related to neoplasia, principally osteogenic sarcoma. Less commonly, infarction(s) of the limb(s) may occur in association with a disseminated intravascular coagulopathy seen with staphylococcal and streptococcal sepsis,[65] pneumococcal sepsis often in the presence of sickle cell disease,[8,83] meningococcal sepsis,[67] and varicella.[11] Other cases may represent end-stage treatment for chronic osteomyelitis or a pseudoarthrosis due to neurofibromatosis.[1]

CONGENITAL LIMB DEFICIENCIES
Classification

The Burtch revision[13] of the Frantz and O'Rahilly system[30] is the most common classification used to describe limb deficiencies; its terminology is based upon a description of the absent parts. In this system, *amelia* is defined as a complete absence of a limb, and *meromelia* as a partial deficit. Meromelias are further subdivided into those which are terminal (at the end of the limb) and those which are intercalary (in the middle of the limb). Further subgrouping denotes deficiencies which are in the preaxial (radial or tibial) or postaxial (ulnar or fibular) planes. Lastly, the missing bones or portions thereof are named.

For example, a residual hand attached to the trunk is an intercalary deficiency with absence of the humerus, radius, and ulna. An isolated absence of the fibula would be considered an intercalary deficiency; the same deficiency associated with absence of the lateral rays would be considered a terminal longitudinal postaxial deficiency. Nomenclature is made more cumbersome when several deformities coexist. A child with a proximal femoral focal deficiency has a partial intercalary transverse femoral deficiency associated with variable degrees of acetabular dysplasia and absence of the fibula.

Although applicable to many deformities, the above system does not readily describe failure of separation of parts, duplications, over- or undergrowths, amniotic band syndromes, and generalized skeletal anomalies. These exceptions are taken into account in the more complex classification system proposed by Swanson.[85] Terminal transverse congenital and acquired amputations can be described by the percentage of limb remaining. Further refinements of classification have been proposed by Kay.[46] Often, classification cannot be adequately determined at birth as ossification is incomplete.[85]

General Considerations

The infant with a congenital limb deficiency requires evaluation for associated anomalies. It is necessary to determine if there is a pattern of deformities which constitutes a recognizable syndrome, with a definable risk of recurrence in future pregnancies. Associated anomalies of other organ systems have been reported in approximately 30 percent of the population.[39,45] Malformations involving the gastrointestinal, respiratory, cardiovascular, genitourinary, and central nervous systems, or the eyes and ears, or with associated tumors have been documented.[39] An infant with multiple anomalies and high-level deficiencies may have a perinatal mortality risk as high as 20 percent.[45]

Associated congenital musculoskeletal malformations are common; long bone reductions are associated with anomalies of the hand or the foot.[45] Spinal deformities and scoliosis are prevalent, occurring in 18 percent of all upper extremity amputees. Scoliosis occurs in 100 percent of patients with bilateral upper extremity amelias. No relationship has been demonstrated between the side of the deficiency and the apex of the curve.[62]

Most terminal transverse deficiencies occur in isolation and do not have a risk of recurrence in future pregnancies. There are some exceptions such as acheiropodia (absence of the hands and feet). Also, most ulnar, tibial, and fibular deficiencies are not inherited. Amniotic bands are nongenetic anomalies but are associated with facial clefts, and eyelid and skull anomalies. The infant with the noninherited VATER syndrome, who may display vertebral anomalies, imperforate anus, tracheoesophageal fistula, and/or renal malformations (which name the syndrome), presents also with radial deficiencies.[52] However, many radial anomalies are inherited. The thrombocytopenia–absent radius (TAR) syndrome, the Fanconi syndrome, and the Holt-Oram syndrome can be associated with significant hematologic diseases (including blood dyscrasias), congenital heart disease, and renal disease, respectively. Given the degree and distribution of the deformities, a chest roentgenogram, electrocardiogram, blood count, skeletal survey, renal sonograms, and/or chromosomal analysis may be warranted.

An assessment of the infant's future functional capacities and treatment plan needs to be delineated for the family shortly after birth. According to Marquardt,[55] this requires consideration of training of potential and residual abilities, correction of dislocations and abnormal postures, provision of orthoprostheses and adaptive equipment, and consideration of surgical procedures to maintain or improve function.

Infant amputees must be handled by their parents as soon as possible and in a normal manner.[71] The defective side should not be swaddled as this could result not only in limitation in range (usually abduction) of the limb, but also in hemisensory neglect (failure to respond to stimuli presented on the affected side). Rudimentary digits should be encouraged to be used for function and to provide sensory feedback; later they can be used to activate a cable system, lock, or switch. Infants with bilateral upper extremity amelia should be engaged in activities which maximize cervical, trunk, and lower extremity range.[71] This permits them to manipulate objects with their feet and later to be independent in dressing and in performing perineal care. Infants with lower extremity amelia should be encouraged to roll, strengthen upper extremity and abdominal musculature, and improve sitting balance.

Associated deformities and contractures may need to be surgically corrected. According to Aitken, the surgical conversion rate for congenital anomalies is 8.3 percent for upper extremities and 45.4 percent for lower extremities.[3] For example, infants with amniotic bands may require serial Z-plasties. The child with a varus hip in association with a proximal femoral focal deficiency may require an osteotomy in order to attain a valgus position.[72]

Previously, provision of an upper extremity prosthesis was advised at age 4 years, just prior to school entry.[4] Current recommendations advise provision of a passive device to unilateral amputees at 3 to 6 months, when the infants are developing the propping reactions which allow them to sit when placed. The lower extremity unilateral amputee should be provided with a monolithic (unjointed) device at 6 to 12 months, when lower extremity weight bearing and pulling to standing commence.[71] Provision of more sophisticated devices, with greater degrees of freedom, occurs with advancement of developmental milestones. With this regimen, the infant learns normal patterns of movement. Up to 94 percent of lower extremity amputees and 61 percent of upper extremity amputees have been shown to use their prostheses all day at age 21 years, with the highest percentage groups having been fitted at the youngest ages.[51] With early provision of devices, atrophy, osteoporosis, and asymmetries may be avoided.

ACQUIRED LIMB DEFICIENCIES

In order to adequately evaluate the child indicated for an amputation, detailed knowledge of the underlying illness or associated injury is necessary. One should be familiar with the details of the child's medical treatment and any complications.

When the child is seen preoperatively, information concerning future medical treatment, prosthetic options, and functional outcome should be communicated to the child and the parents in order to allay the anxiety of the unknown.[64]

Preprosthetic training can be initiated in the interval between the child's initial illness or diagnostic biopsy and limb ablation. Bed rest should be discouraged as it may sabotage later rehabilitation efforts; a child at rest for 2 to 3 weeks may have up to a 50 percent reduction in muscle power.[91] Range-of-motion exercises and strengthening of selected muscle groups required for prosthetic control should be initiated.[36] For example, in a child who is to undergo an above-elbow amputation, shoulder musculature and trunk flexors should be exercised. Deep-breathing exercises should be performed, as reduction in pulmonary function is associated with higher levels of upper extremity loss.[29]

While always respecting the need for appropriate resection margins in neoplastic diseases, as much limb length as possible should be preserved at amputation, especially the epiphyses.[50] A long lever arm is able to generate larger forces with less energy expenditure, and nonstandard stump lengths can be accommodated with modern prosthetics. Preservation of the epiphyses permits additional limb growth, while avoiding spur formation.

Immediate postoperative prosthetic fitting can be considered in this group because of its advantages of decreased edema and phantom pain,[64,69] but this should be done with extreme caution. A child may not complain of discomfort, causing serious wound problems beneath the dressing to go unnoticed.[36] The child may not be able to feel pain if there is an associated neuropathy following a burn or chemotherapy. If postoperative fitting is not under consideration, the preoperative exercise program should, nevertheless, be continued; ambulation and self-care training, stump wrapping, and hygiene should be taught.[9,77]

The child with an underlying malignancy will have a more difficult course of rehabilitation. Anemia, immunosuppression, and infection may be the sequelae of chemotherapy and poor food intake. The additional energy requirements for crutch walking and prosthetic use may not be met.

Treatment protocols for osteogenic sarcoma have utilized a variety of adjuvant chemotherapeutic agents including doxorubicin, cisplatin, vincristine, methotrexate, actinomycin D, and/or cyclophosphamide.[70,101] Complications of these drugs include cardiomyopathy with failure and arrhythmias,[63,96] peripheral neuropathies, encephalopathies,[32] fractures,[59] and pulmonary fibrosis.[92] Accordingly, results of electrocardiograms and gated pool studies should be reviewed prior to prescribing an exercise program, and a maximal heart rate should be targeted. Exercises which require Valsalva maneuvers are relatively contraindicated if there is pulmonary disease present with an attendant risk of pneumothorax. Overvigorous upper extremity strengthening exercises may result in a central line's being dislodged. Splinting for a drop wrist or foot may be required in the presence of a neuropathy.[73] If deformities are left untreated, Achilles tendon lengthenings may be required. Scoliosis requiring treatment may arise secondary to the irradiation field or to a leg length discrepancy.

Medical complications result in fluctuations in the child's weight and stump size. The use of an adjustable lower extremity prosthesis permits training during the period when such fluctuations occur. Training with these devices may begin as early as 10 to 14 days postoperatively.

Vigorous rehabilitation treatment and the provision of prostheses to patients with bone tumors have been criticized as futile and not cost-effective. However, the wearing time for 50 percent of this population is over 5 years[64] and exceeds the wearing time of the elderly, dysvascular amputee by 2 to $3\frac{1}{2}$

years.[37] With survival rates as high as 60 percent at 5 years, aggressive rehabilitation should be considered for all these children.

UPPER EXTREMITY AMPUTEES AND THEIR PROSTHESES

The fabrication, components, and function of a child's upper extremity prosthesis is in many ways similar to that of an adult; unfortunately, this includes its lack of cosmesis and insufficient grasp strength. However, pediatric devices must additionally be simple to use, be light in weight, not restrict motion, and be able to accommodate for longitudinal and circumferential growth.[18,76] Both traditional exoskeletal and modular endoskeletal prostheses are available for both the upper and the lower extremities.[18,40]

For patients with distal deficiencies such as absence and/or malformation of digits, surgical alternatives may be indicated rather than provision of a prosthetic device.[57,79] Radial clubhand deformities are amenable to splinting and subsequent centralization of the hand, with possible ulnar osteotomy.[79] Other deformities, such as ulnar dysmelia, may require surgical correction, possibly elbow disarticulation, prior to attempting prosthetic fitting.[61]

A child with a partial hand deficiency may function quite well if a post for opposition attached to the wrist is provided.[76] Some posts are multipositional to accommodate holding objects of different sizes.[15] As the child gets older, a cosmetic hand may also be requested for social engagements.

A first device is supplied to the below- or above-elbow congenital amputee at 3 to 6 months. If the deficiency is unilateral, that side will be nondominant. If the child has bilateral deficiencies, the longer side will be the dominant one and is fitted first. An exoskeletal, double-walled device anchored with a figure-of-eight harness and a terminal device (TD) is the prototype. A passive mit can be supplied as the first TD, although a "hook," such as the Dorrance wafer, Dorrance 12 plastisol-coated TD or CAPP TD, with the cable system detached, is preferable. This permits toys to be placed in the TD by the adult, stimulating the infant's interest in the limb and encouraging "two-handed" activities. Normal developmental activities of rolling, sitting, crawling, pulling to standing, weight shifting, and ambulation should follow, with completion of this sequence by about 15 months.[18] The role of the therapist is to facilitate attainment of these milestones. Time without a device should also be permitted to encourage sensory feedback and stump use. The reader is referred to Blakeslee's text for further details of prosthetic training.[9]

Developmental parameters for activation of the TD include the ability to follow two-step commands, an attention span of about 10 min, and an interest in bimanual activities and toys which come apart; this usually occurs at about 18 months.[18]

Opening of the TD is achieved with flexion of the humerus. This voluntary-opening device is advantageous to the younger child as cause and effect are readily demonstrable. Once the object is grasped, continuous tension need not be maintained by the cable to hold the object in place. This permits the child to manipulate the object with the sound, contralateral extremity. Visual cues are not obscured as would be the case with a functional hand.[58] Traditionally, hands have been reserved for children of school-entry age, although they are now available in sizes as small as 24 months. CAPP TDs are being used more frequently because of their lighter weight, improved appearance, and ability to hold an object with a less precise grasp due to the larger surface area available.[15,76]

To improve prosthetic purchase around the humeral epicondyles a preflexed or Munster prosthesis may be required for the child with a short below-elbow amputation.[25] However, this option does not permit full elbow flexion. For the child with an elbow disarticulation, an outside elbow joint may be needed.[25]

An elbow-lock cable is generally added to the prosthesis of an above-elbow amputee at the developmental age of 30 to 36 months. This correlates with the child's desire to lift objects with the artificial limb, although the child cannot lift very heavy loads with it. This second system really functions to preposition the TD in the correct place. Cable locking and release are both controlled by shoulder elevation. The TD will not operate unless the elbow is locked. When the elbow lock is released, elbow flexion may be quite rapid. To prevent the child from being hit in the face with the prosthesis, a flexion stop may be required (Fig. 24-10).[75] Some children with this level of amputation may find prosthetic suspension and rotation problematic. Marquardt has suggested an angulation osteotomy of the humerus as one possible solution for this.[57]

The child with an acquired upper extremity amputation, especially when it is tumor-related, usually requires a shoulder disarticulation or a forequarter amputation. The devices which are available are the same as those available to a congenital amputee. The distal components are similar to those of the above-elbow prosthesis, and the shoulder joint is positioned passively. Occasionally, an additional shoulder or perineal strap may be required for harnessing. An older child with an underlying medical disorder may reject such a device; a shoulder cap or a passive arm prosthesis may be an acceptable cosmetic alternative. One-handed tools such as a rocker knife or a buttonhook and clothing adaptations should be offered to these patients.

The child who has bilateral deficiencies has more complex problems. When there is bilateral absence of the hands, especially when visual problems coexist, a unilateral Krukenberg procedure may be indicated. By having the forearm split into radial and ulnar portions, the child can grasp objects without a prosthetic device and with direct sensory feedback.[89] Objections to the cosmetic results of the procedure have been raised.

Patients with bilateral amelias are fitted with their first devices at 24 months. Challenor has formulated a developmental timetable for treatment of such patients.[14] These children may exhibit delays in gross motor skills such as sitting and walking, as upper extremities cannot be used to improve their balance.[71] Modular components are frequently used because of their lighter weight and ease of replacement.[15,56,76] Regardless of the components, it is essential that at least one wrist unit be positioned in flexion so that midline feeding, dressing, and perineal care activities can be performed. A va-

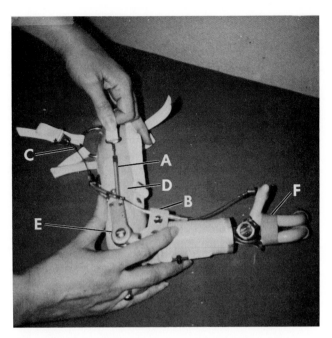

Figure 24-10 A child's standard exoskeletal above-elbow prosthesis. A = elbow lock cable, B = terminal device cable, C = figure-of-eight harness, D = double-walled socket, E = external elbow lock, F = plastisol-coated terminal device.

riety of powered prostheses are also available. Previously, carbon dioxide cartridges were used. Currently, switch-controlled or myoelectric components can be provided,[49] utilizing shoulder girdle movements for activation. Children may prefer to use their feet for activities at home but their prostheses in a social or school setting.[55] Other powered options include a prehension actuator, a motor attached to the TD to enhance grasp strength, and an electric elbow to facilitate the lifting of heavy loads.[76]

Myoelectric prostheses are generally reserved for adults with below-elbow deficiencies, with two available muscular control sites to open and close the prosthetic hand. These devices appear more natural, and a suspension harness is not needed. Recent studies have demonstrated that children as young as 16 months can use these devices effectively.[80] Their cost, their weight, and the need for refitting at 6- to 15-month intervals in addition to their frequent repairs militate against their use.[76]

Upper extremity prostheses need to be replaced about every 2 years. TDs are replaced to keep pace with the size of the contralateral hand. For the Dorrance system of TD components, a size 10P TD is provided at 2 to 3 years, 10X at 3 to 6 years, 99X at 6 to 8 years, 88 at 8 to 13 years, and 5X at 13 years or above.[9] Adjustments for growth can be made by reducing the thickness of the stump socks worn, and/or by using a triple wall socket and removing one layer when growth occurs. Newer developments permit a new customized socket to be fabricated and attached to an existing device by reheating, extending the time that a prosthesis is serviceable.[40]

LOWER EXTREMITY AMPUTEES AND THEIR PROSTHESES

For the child with a below-knee or more distal deficiency, a normal gait and absence of any functional limitations is anticipated if length and fit of the prosthesis is proper.[71] When a child is provided with a prosthesis before 12 months of age, training is a consequence of normal curiosity. Balancing on uneven surfaces, weight shifting, reaching forward to retrieve toys, and even falling down in these attempts are normal precursors to independent ambulation.[9,71] More complex tasks such as kicking a ball, hopping, and jumping should follow.[9]

The exoskeletal prosthetic components for children are similar to those supplied to the adult. A single-action, cushioned heel (SACH) foot is almost always used. Because of the lack of well-defined contours of the limb, a patellar-tendon-bearing device may be unsatisfactory for the younger child. A thigh cuff may be required to provide additional suspension, to prevent rotation while the child is climbing or engaging in sports, and to prevent genu valgum (Fig. 24-11).[27,58]

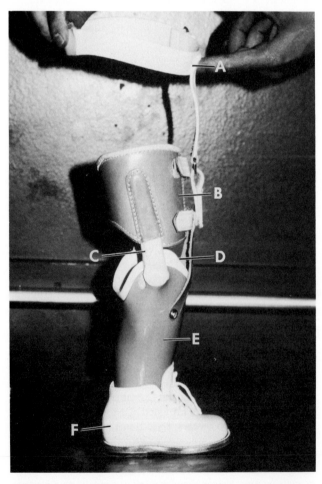

Figure 24-11 Child's standard exoskeletal below-knee prosthesis. A = pelvic belt, B = thigh corset, C = external knee joint, D = removable insert, E = double-walled socket, F = SACH foot (in shoe).

In order to allow for growth, various strategies are employed such as supplying a removable plastic liner. The prosthesis may be made intentionally too long and a lift placed on the contralateral shoe; the lift is removed when the patient has grown.[25] The shaft of the prosthesis can be lengthened just proximal to the SACH foot and relaminated. With these options, a replacement device needs to be provided every 1 to 2 years up to the age of 12 years, and then every 3 to 4 years until the age of 21 years.[51]

A standard prosthetic device can equalize the leg length discrepancy associated with congenital absence of the fibula but is suboptimal in dealing with the tibial bowing, valgus foot, talocalcaneal fusion, and ray deficiencies which may be present.[27,74,94,104] Considerations as to prosthetic fit and the need for surgical revision are made more complex by the occurrence of bilateral involvement in 25 percent and proximal femoral focal deficiency in 10 percent or more.[86] Some authors have advised soft tissue releases including Achilles tendon lengthening, posterior capsulotomy, peroneal tendon lengthening, and tibial osteotomies for the correction of such deformities.[74,94] However, the indications for such procedures have recently been brought into question. An end-weight-bearing ankle disarticulation, or Syme's amputation, is presently considered the treatment of choice for a unilateral deformity of this type;[27,100,104] this is especially true when the foot deformity is severe and a limb length inequality of over 3 in. is predicted. This procedure should be performed before the age of 2 years to lessen the psychological implications of removal of the foot. Unlike the adult who has had a Syme's procedure, the child does not have a bulbous stump with prominent malleoli. The Syme's procedure is also advantageous because the tibial epiphysis is preserved.[104] Initially, a Syme prosthesis is provided, and with growth, an end-bearing below-knee prosthesis is used. The technically more difficult Boyd procedure in which the calcaneus is fused to the tibia has also been performed when there is congenital absence of the fibula.[26]

Congenital absence of the tibia is associated with a shortened limb, a varus foot, and ray deficiencies. Instability of the ankle and knee joints and occasionally congenital hip dislocation or femoral bifurcation may be seen.[12] Classically, either a knee disarticulation and provision of an end-bearing prosthesis, or an arthroplasty to retain a below-knee stump (Brown procedure), has been advised to be performed prior to the age of 2 years.[12] If there is good quadriceps function, centralization of the fibular head in the intercondylar notch, with talectomy, and displacement of the lateral malleolus over the calcaneus have been advised to avoid amputation, but this is a much less frequently used alternative.[98](See Chap. 64, Sect. D.)

With acquired or congenital above-knee amputations, younger children are first provided with a monolithic device. At the developmental age of 36 to 48 months, when the child would normally negotiate stairs independently, a knee joint is introduced into the system.[7,58] A constant-friction knee which is light in weight but which does not adjust to changes in walking speed is most commonly used, often with an elastic anterior knee extension strap. An older child may prefer a heavier hydraulic knee which responds to changes in walking speed.[25] Suction sockets can be used in the older child in

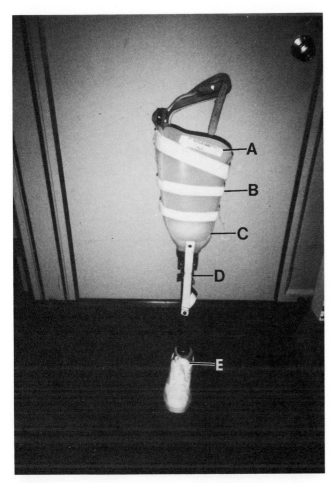

Figure 24-12 Temporary above-knee prosthesis for the adolescent. A = adjustable socket, B = Velcro straps, C = foam end pad, D = manually locking knee joint, E = SACH foot.

conjunction with a quadrilateral brim. With a short above-knee stump, extension of the prosthesis laterally to the pelvic brim may be required to provide additional stability. Pelvic suspension with a Silesian bandage or less commonly with a pelvic band with an external hip joint is also needed.

Older children with above-knee or higher acquired lesions require more training with balancing, ambulation, and stair climbing, and also conditioning and trunk-rotation exercises. Initially, prosthetic fit may be compromised by changes in stump volume and shape associated with cycles of chemotherapy.[21] Accordingly, an adjustable temporary prosthesis needs to be provided. A temporary device with an adjustable plastic socket, Velcro straps, a manually locking or safety knee, a SACH foot, and an optional cosmetic cover can be provided for use until 5 to 12 months after surgery (Fig. 24-12). As an alternative, the Icelandic–Swedish–New York University (ISNY) above-knee socket, composed of a rigid shell with a flexible interior conforming to changes in shape may be considered.[48] This has been used in several adolescent patients successfully and permits adjustments for growth.

For amputations at the thigh or above, endoskeletal components may be used because of their lighter weight. These devices are more cosmetic but more fragile, as their foam

cover may be easily torn. A CAPP endoskeletal above-knee foot with extensions at the heel, toe, and ball of the foot has recently been developed.[16,76] It is thought that these projections can better absorb the torque applied to them rather than transmitting it to the stump; this results in improved stability in the stance phase of gait, and better toe clearance. Regardless of the components used, a child with a high-level amputation can be expected to have some gait deviations such as a Trendelenburg gait or circumduction. They not infrequently require a cane or crutch on the contralateral side for ambulation.[58]

Patients with proximal femoral focal deficiency represent a special challenge. Not only is there a marked shortening of the limb, but there are associated anomalies of the femoral head and/or fibular agenesis in 50 percent of the cases.[2,72] Osteotomies to correct the neck-shaft angle or metaphyseal-epiphyseal synostosis to stabilize the joint may be required. (See Chap. 63, Sect. A.) Distally, if the fibula is lacking, a Syme's amputation with subsequent knee fusion may be indicated. If the potential growth of the patient is calculated correctly, the ankle disarticulation becomes level with the contralateral knee; a knee disarticulation prosthesis is then provided.[5,72] Alternatively, a Van Nes osteotomy with rotation of the tibia 180° can convert the deformity into a type of below-knee deficiency.[95] Prosthetic fitting may be difficult secondary to telescoping of the abnormal proximal elements. Even in the presence of a Syme's amputation distally, a modified ischial-weight-bearing flexible socket with a high lateral wall may be needed.[90] It may be difficult to convince the family to give consent for ablative surgery even if it will result in improved function; in this case, a relatively uncosmetic prosthesis with the foot held in maximal plantar flexion must be provided.

Almost one-third of patients with proximal femoral focal deficiency have bilateral involvement.[72] Amputations are usually not performed as these children can ambulate without prostheses. Such devices may be provided to lessen their significant reduction in height. For others with bilateral, symmetrical deficiencies such as phocomelia, a low to ground rocker-bottom prosthesis or "stubbies," or a swivel walker can be used by the young child to improve balance. These devices can be gradually extended upward. They are provided at about 18 months, but definitive prosthetic fitting may not occur until about 6 years (Fig. 24-13).[71] Similar treatment strategies have been advocated in patients with sacral agenesis or diastrophic dwarfism.[14]

Patients who have hip disarticulations or hemipelvectomies have much more difficulty in ambulating because of their increased energy expenditures and problems with prosthetic fit. Traditionally, a Canadian or bucket type of prosthesis is used, with the younger child requiring a shoulder harness to anchor the prosthesis (Fig. 24-14).[86]

This device is also used for patients with phocomelia; the residual foot should not be removed on such patients as it provides a good weight-bearing surface within the prosthesis. Energy for use of the Canadian type of prosthesis comes from the pelvic flexion moment. The use of an anteriorly located broad hip joint, occasionally utilizing a spring-loaded mechanism, helps to minimize energy consumption and maximize stability.[82]

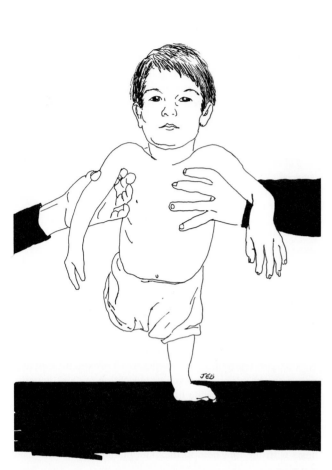 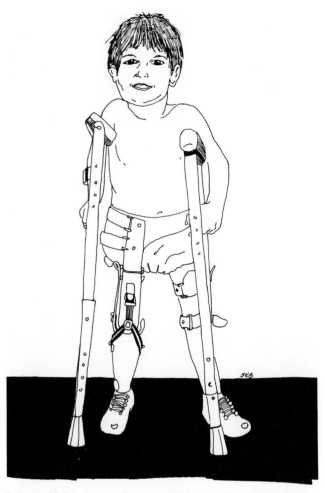

Figure 24-13 A. Patient with bilateral phocomelia. Typically one extremity is slightly longer than the other. **B.** Final prosthetic fitting, which may not be accomplished until school age (see text).

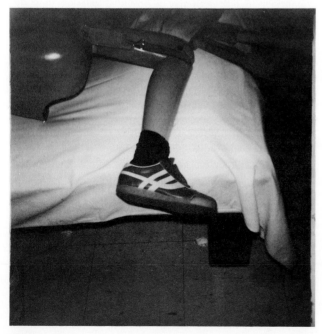 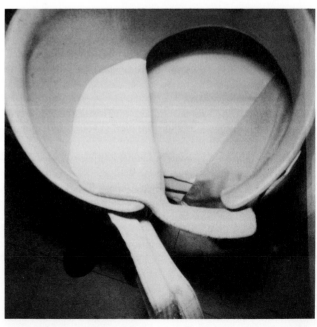

Figure 24-14 A. Typical Canadian bucket prosthesis used for patients following a hip disarticulation. **B.** The inside of the bucket must be well-padded to protect the often tender surgical site and the perineum.

Newer technical developments have included biofeedback devices[19] and computerized gait analysis[84] which facilitate prosthetic adjustments and thereby lessen gait deviations. Many sports prostheses which can hold equipment such as a baseball bat, or which can be used for swimming, have been fabricated. Amputees should be encouraged to participate in sports such as swimming, gymnastics, bicycling, soccer, and skiing with and without their prostheses.[33]

The child who is a quadruple amputee requires special considerations which cannot be dealt with in detail in this chapter.[28,56] These children may be quite fragile, being susceptible to fluctuations in body temperature because of their reduced surface area. Some children may do quite well without adaptive devices by utilizing residual limbs with or without digits, by mouthing objects, or by rolling.[28] Other children may benefit from the provision of a motorized cart which has a head or a mouth switch control.[15,105]

COMPLICATIONS

The most common physical complications seen in juvenile amputees are those associated with bone overgrowth and painful spur formation.[81] Spurs arise from appositional bone growth and occur in both the congenital and the acquired varieties. The humerus, fibula, and tibia are the bones which most commonly require surgical revision.[77] Painful bursae may develop in association with bone overgrowth, especially over the fibular head or the tibial tubercle; this is exacerbated by a poorly fitting prosthesis. The incidence of bursae formation is 8.4 percent according to Lambert.[50] Stump revisions, stump capping utilizing cartilage–cancellous bone grafting,[55,56] silastic plugs,[77,87] skin traction, and skin grafting are all methods which can be used to correct this problem.

Additional problems which may require surgery include limb length inequalities, especially when the knees are at different levels;[5] contralateral epiphysiodesis may be required. Other surgical procedures may be required for tumor recurrence or release of contractures, as treatment for skin sloughing, for excision[44] or capping of neuromas,[88] or for migration of the posterior heel pad of a Syme's amputation.[5,24]

Skin breakdown and infection may occur because of problems with prosthetic fit. The skin around an osteotomy site may be in close proximity to the pelvic band and be susceptible to breakdown. Skin lesions in a child with a neuropathy may go unreported.

Frazier states that phantom pain does not occur in congenital amputees or in those whose amputations are acquired under the age of 3 years.[31] Others state that phantom pain may occur in up to 19 percent of congenital amputees,[99] as sensory representation in the cortex still exists. If pain does exist, it is amenable to treatment with transcutaneous nerve stimulation, early prosthetic fitting, light massage, and distractions such as play.

Prolonged fabrication time and financial problems are significant obstacles which may cause emotional distress for the family.[64]

Emotional problems may arise in the parents of the amputee because of their unwarranted feelings of guilt or their mourning of their anticipated "perfect" child. Children who have acquired deficiencies and/or require surgical revision may experience depression over their loss, changes in body images, perceived social and physical inadequacies, and frequent hospitalizations. When a malignancy occurs, the concern over the side effects of chemotherapy and the fear of death compound the problem.[97]

Psychological support should be anticipatory and occur preoperatively. Intervention should not wait for the symptoms of acting out, depression, or withdrawal to occur. The child's fantasy of being provided with a "bionic" arm or leg must be gently replaced with realistic expectations. Projective play techniques, such as figure drawings or the use of specially made amputee dolls, may be helpful. For older children, prosthetic models and an amputee visitor program may be helpful.[64]

Despite the difficulties, the expectations for juvenile amputees are promising if they have had adequate social interaction and education.[51] Cognitive studies have shown them to function at or above the fiftieth percentile on the average.[17] A Danish study of 74 patients with lower extremity amputations in childhood showed that their marital status and number of children did not deviate from the norm.[44] One-third required assistance, but two-thirds were independent.

ALTERNATIVE TREATMENT TO AMPUTATION

Replantation is an accepted treatment for traumatic loss of digits but can also be performed to save limbs. Complications include limb length discrepancies in 50 to 70 percent of cases in patients aged 0 to 14 years, associated with peripheral neuropathies due to crush injuries, and the increased risk of thrombosis and septicemia.[60,68]

Limb salvage procedures offer an option to amputation for the child who has a low-grade or well-localized malignancy without involvement of the neurovascular bundle, and in whom growth is relatively complete.[66] It does not appear that these children have an increased rate of distant metastases or mortality, according to preliminary studies.[54,66]

For a malignancy of the humerus, an en bloc or Tikhoff-Lindberg resection can be performed, leaving a flail upper arm with a functional forearm.[66] For femoral involvement, an en bloc resection can be performed with surgical conversion of the foreleg and the foot, so that a below-knee type of stump can be created.

Custom-made endoprostheses, including ones which are capable of being lengthened and suitable for growing children, can be inserted after an en bloc resection.[42] Postoperative precautions are similar to those observed after total joint replacement. Continuous passive range-of-motion exercise is often indicated several days postoperatively to facilitate knee flexion. Muscle groups or the peroneal nerve may need to be sacrificed and a knee-ankle-foot orthosis required for a variable period.

Regardless of the above options, standard amputation surgery for children is still the norm rather than the exception. When the intervention strategies outlined in this chapter are followed, the pediatric amputee can be offered the appropriate treatment which can result in a functional and happy adult.

REFERENCES

Section A: Amputations and Prosthetics in Adults

1. American Academy of Orthopedic Surgeons. *Atlas of Limb Prosthetics: Surgical and Prosthetic Principles.* St. Louis, Mosby, 1981.
2. Banerjee, S.N. (ed). *Rehabilitation Management of Amputees.* Baltimore, Williams & Wilkins, 1982.
3. Burgess, E.M. Wound healing after amputation: Effect of controlled environment treatment. J Bone Joint Surg 60:245–246, 1978.
4. Burgess, E.M., and Matsen, F.A. Current concepts for determining amputation levels in peripheral vascular disease. J Bone Joint Surg 63:1493–1497, 1981.
5. Burgess, E.M., Matsen, F.A., Wyss, C.R., et al. Segmental transcutaneous measurements of PO_2 in patients requiring below-the-knee amputation for peripheral vascular insufficiency. J Bone Joint Surg 64:378–382, 1982.
6. Burgess, E.M., and Zettl, J.H. Immediate postsurgical prosthetics. Orthop Prosthet 21:105–112, 1967.
7. Finch, D.R., MacDougal, M., Tibbs, D.J., et al. Amputation for vascular disease: The experience of a peripheral vascular unit. Br J Surg 67:233, 1980.
8. Friedmann, L.W., and Thomas, C.C. (eds): *The Surgical Rehabilitation of the Amputee.* Springfield, IL, Thomas, 1978.
9. Holloway, G.A., and Burgess, E.M. Cutaneous blood flow and its relation to healing of below knee amputation. Surg Gynecol Obstet 146:750–756, 1978.
10. Holloway, G.A., and Watkins, D.W. Laser Doppler measurement of cutaneous blood flow. J Invest Dermatol 69:306–309, 1977.
11. Kegel, B. Controlled environment treatment (CET) for patients with below knee amputations. Phys Ther 56:1366–1371, 1976.
12. Kostuik, J.P. (ed): *Amputation Surgery and Rehabilitation. The Toronto Experience.* New York, Churchill Livingstone, 1981.
13. Kostuik, J.P., Wood, D., Hornby, R., et al. The measurement of skin blood flow in peripheral vascular disease by epicutaneous application of xenon 133. J Bone Joint Surg 58A:833–837, 1976.
14. Kritter, A.E. A technique for salvage of the infected diabetic gangrenous foot. Orthop Clin North Am 4:21–30, 1973.
15. Lassen, N.A., and Holstein, P. Use of radio isotopes in assessment of distal blood flow and distal blood pressure in arterial insufficiency. Surg Clin North Am 54:39–55, 1974.
16. Malone, J.M., Moore, W.S., Goldstone, J., et al. Therapeutic and economic impact of a modern amputation program. Ann Surg 189:798, 1979.
17. Malone, J.M., Moore, W.S., Leal, J.M., et al. Rehabilitation for lower extremity amputation. Arch Surg 116:93, 1981.
18. Matsen, F.A., Bach, A.W., Wyss, C.R., et al. Transcutaneous PO_2: A potential monitor of the status of replanted limb parts. Plast Reconstr Surg 65:732–737, 1980.
19. Moore, W.S. Determination of amputation level. Arch Surg 107:798, 1973.
20. Porter, J.M., Baur, G.M., and Taylor, L.M. Lower-extremity amputations for ischemia. Arch Surg 116:89, 1981.
21. Potts, J.R., Wendelken, J.R., Elkins, R.C., et al. Lower extremity amputation: Review of 110 cases. Am J Surg 138:924, 1979.
22. Slocum, D.B. (ed): *An Atlas of Amputations.* St. Louis, Mosby, 1949.
23. Stewart, R.E., and Bernstock, W.M. *Veterans Administration Prosthetic and Sensory Aids Program Since World War II.* Prosthetics and Sensory Aids Service, Department of Medicine and Surgery, U.S. Veterans Administration, Washington, D.C., 1977.
24. Syme, J. Amputation at the ankle joint. London, Month J Med Sci 2:93, 1843.

Section B: Amputations and Prosthetics in Children

1. Aitken, G.T. Amputation as a treatment for certain lower-extremity congenital abnormalities. J Bone Joint Surg 41A:1267–1285, 1959.
2. Aitken, G.T. Proximal femoral focal deficiency, in Swinyard, C.A. (ed): *Limb Development and Deformity: Problems of Evaluation and Rehabilitation.* Springfield, IL, Thomas, 1969, pp 456–476.
3. Aitken, G.T. Surgical amputations in children. J Bone Joint Surg 45A:1735–1741, 1963.
4. Aitken, G.T., and Frantz, C.H. The child amputee. J Bone Joint Surg 35A:659–664, 1953.
5. Anderson, A., Westin, G.W., and Oppenheim, W.L. Syme amputation in children: Indication, results, and long-term follow-up. J Pediatr Orthop 4:550–554, 1984.
6. Aro, T. Maternal diseases, alcohol consumption and smoking during pregnancy associated with reduction limb defects. Early Hum Dev 9:49–57, 1983.
7. Baumgartner, R.F. Above-knee amputation in children. Prosthet Orthot Int 3:26–30, 1979.
8. Bettigole, R.E. Symmetric peripheral gangrene in pneumococcal sepsis. Ann Intern Med 54:335–342, 1961.
9. Blakeslee, B. (ed): *The Limb Deficient Child* Berkeley and Los Angeles, University of California Press, 1963.
10. Blechschmidt, E. The early stages of human limb development, in Swinyard, C.A. (ed): *Limb Development and Deformity: Problems of Evaluation and Rehabilitation.* Springfield, IL, Thomas, 1969, pp 24–56.
11. Bogumill, G.B. Bilateral above-the-knee amputations: A complication of chickenpox. J Bone Joint Surg 47A:371–374, 1965.
12. Brown, F.W. Construction of a knee joint in congenital total absence of the tibia (paraxial hemimelia tibia). J Bone Joint Surg 47A:695–704, 1965.
13. Burtch, R.L. Nomenclature for congenital skeletal limb deficiencies, a revision of the Frantz and O'Rahilly classification. Artif Limbs 10:24–34, 1966.
14. Challenor, Y.B., Rangaswamy, L., and Katz, J.F. Limb deficiency in infancy and childhood, in Downey, J.A., and Low, N.L. (eds): *The Child with Disabling Illness.* New York, Raven, 1982, pp 409–447.
15. *Child Amputee Prosthetics Project: Ten Year Report 1967–1977, Research and Development Program.* U.S. Department of Health, Education and Welfare, 1977.
16. *Child Amputee Prosthetics Project: Progress Report.* U.S. Department of Health, Education, and Welfare, 1980, pp 59–61.
17. Clark, S., and French, R. Can congenital amputees achieve academically? Am Correc Ther J 32:7–11, 1978.
18. Clark, S.D., and Patton, J.G. Occupational therapy for the limb-deficient child. Clin Orthop 148:47–54, 1980.
19. Clippinger, F.W., Seaber, A.V., McElhaney, J.H., Harrelson, J.M., and Maxwell, G.M. Afferent sensory feedback for lower extremity prostheses. Clin Orthop 169:202–205, 1982.
20. Cohlan, S.Q. A review of teratogenic agents and human congenital malformations, in Swinyard, C.A. (ed): *Limb Development and Deformity: Problems of Evaluation and Rehabilitation.* Springfield, IL, Thomas, 1969, pp 161–170.
21. Cole, W.G. Prosthetic programme after above-knee amputation in children with sarcomata. J Bone Joint Surg 64B:586–589, 1982.
22. Coventry, M.B., and Johnson, E.W. Congenital absence of the fibula. J Bone Joint Surg 34A:941–955, 1952.
23. Cumming, V., and Molnar, G. Traumatic amputations in children resulting from "train-electric-burn" injuries: A social environmental syndrome? Arch Phys Med Rehabil 55:71–73, 1974.
24. Davidson, W.H., and Bohne, W.H.O. The Syme amputation in children. J Bone Joint Surg 57A:905–909, 1975.
25. Downie, G.R. Limb deficiencies and prosthetic devices. Orthop Clin North Am 7:465–473, 1976.
26. Eilert, R.E., and Jayakumar, S.S. Boyd and Syme ankle amputations in children. J Bone Joint Surg 58A:1138–1141, 1976.
27. Farmer, A.W., and Lavrin, C.A. Congenital absence of the fibula.

J Bone Joint Surg 42A:1–12, 1960.

28. Fletcher, I. Review of the treatment of thalidomide children with limb deficiency in Great Britain. Clin Orthop 148:18–25, 1980.

29. Fowler, W.M., Linde, L.M., Brooks, M.B., and Jones, M.H. Pulmonary function and physical work capacity of children who have undergone amputation of an upper extremity. Arch Phys Med Rehabil 43:409–413, 1962.

30. Frantz, C.H., and O'Rahilly, R. Congenital skeletal limb deficiencies. J Bone Joint Surg 43A:1202–1224, 1961.

31. Frazier, S.H., and Kolb, L.C. Psychiatric aspects of pain and the phantom limb. Orthop Clin North Am 1:481–495, 1970.

32. Fritsch, G., and Urban, C. Transient encephalopathy during the late course of treatment with high-dose methotrexate. Cancer 53:1849–1851, 1984.

33. Galway, H.R. Recreational activities of juvenile amputees, in Kostuik, J.P., and Gillespie, R. (eds): *Amputation Surgery and Rehabilitation: The Toronto Experience.* New York, Churchill Livingstone, 1981, pp 211–216.

34. Galway, H.R. Traumatic amputations in children, in Kostuik, J.P., and Gillespie, R. (eds): *Amputation Surgery and Rehabilitation: The Toronto Experience.* New York, Churchill Livingstone, 1981, pp 137–143.

35. Gilman, W.L., MacDougall, M.B., and Judisch, J.M. Sickle cell and disseminated intravascular coagulation. Clin Pediatr 12:600–602, 1973.

36. Griffith, E.R. Rehabilitation of children with bone and soft tissue sarcomas: A physiatrist's viewpoint. Natl Cancer Inst Monogr 56:137–143, 1981.

37. Hansson, J. Leg amputee: Clinical follow-up study. Acta Orthop Scand 69 (suppl):1–116, 1964.

38. Heinonen, O.P. Antinauseants, antihistamines, and phenothiazines, in Heinonen, O.P., et al (eds): *Birth Defects and Drugs in Pregnancy.* Littleton, MA, Publishing Sciences Group, 1977, pp 322–334.

39. Heinonen, O.P. Malformations of the musculoskeletal system, in Heinonen, O.P., et al (eds): *Birth Defects and Drugs in Pregnancy.* Littleton, MA, Publishing Sciences Group, 1977, pp 126–148.

40. Hodgins, J., Sullivan, R., and Jain, S. A modular below elbow prosthesis for children. Orthot Prosthet 36:15–21, 1982.

41. Hoy, M.G., Whiting, W.C., and Zernicke, R.F. Stride kinematics and knee joint kinetics of child amputee gait. Arch Phys Med Rehabil 63:74–82, 1982.

42. Imbriglia, J.E., Neer, C.S., and Dick, H.M. Resection of the proximal one-half of the humerus in a child for chondrosarcoma. J Bone Joint Surg 60A:262–264, 1978.

43. Janerich, D.T., Piper, J.M., and Glebatis, D.M. Congenital limb-reduction defects. N Engl J Med 291:697–700, 1974.

44. Jorring, K. Amputation in children: A follow-up of 74 children whose lower extremities were amputated. Acta Orthop Scand 42:178–186, 1971.

45. Kallen, B., Rahmani, T.M., and Winberg, J. Infants with congenital limb reduction registered in the Swedish register of congenital malformations. Teratology 29:73–85, 1984.

46. Kay, H.W., Day, H.J.B., Henkel, H.L., Kruger, L.M., Lamb, D.W., Marquardt, E., Mitchell, R., Swanson, A.B., and Willert, H.G. The proposed international terminology for the classification of congenital limb deficiencies. Dev Med Child Neurol 34:1–12, 1975.

47. Krebs, D.E., and Fishman, S. Characteristics of the child amputee population. J Pediatr Orthop 4:89–95, 1984.

48. Kristinsson, O. Flexible above knee socket made from low density polyethylene suspended by a weight transmitting frame. Orthot Prosthet 37:25–27, 1983.

49. Lamb, D.W., and Scott, H. Management of congenital and acquired amputation in children. Orthop Clin North Am 12:977–994, 1981.

50. Lambert, C.N. Amputation surgery and the child. Orthop Clin North Am 3:473–482, 1972.

51. Lambert, C.N., Hamilton, R.C., and Pellicore, R.J. The juvenile amputee program: Its social and economic value. J Bone Joint Surg 51A:1135–1138, 1969.

52. Lenz, W. Genetics and limb deficiencies. Clin Orthop 148:9–17, 1980.

53. Letts, R.M., and Gammon, W. Auger injuries in children. Can Med Assoc J 118:520–522, 1978.

54. Marcove, R.C. En bloc resection for osteogenic sarcoma. Cancer Treat Rep 62:225–231, 1978.

55. Marquardt, E.G. A holistic approach to the limb-deficient child. Arch Phys Med Rehabil 64:237–248, 1983.

56. Marquardt, E.G. The multiple limb-deficient child, in *Atlas of Limb Prosthetics: Surgical and Prosthetic Principles.* St. Louis, Mosby, American Academy of Orthopaedic Surgeons, 1981, pp 595–641.

57. Marquardt, E. The operative treatment of congenital limb malformation—part I. Prosthet Orthot Int 4:135–144, 1980.

58. Molnar, G.E., and Taft, L.T. Pediatric rehabilitation part II: Spina bifida and limb deficiencies. Curr Probl Pediatr 7:35–54, 1977.

59. Nesbit, M., Krivit, W., Heyn, R., and Sharp, H. Acute and chronic effects of methotrexate on hepatic, pulmonary, and skeletal systems. Cancer 37:1048–1054, 1976.

60. O'Brien, B., Franklin, J.D., Morrison, W.A., and MacLeod, A.M. Replantation and revascularization surgery in children. Hand 12:12–24, 1980.

61. Ogden, J.A., Watson, H.K., and Bohne, W. Ulnar dysmelia. J Bone Joint Surg 58A:467–475, 1976.

62. Powers, T.A., Haher, T.R., Devlin, V.J., Spencer, D., and Millar, E.A. Abnormalities of the spine in relation to congenital upper limb deficiencies. J Pediatr Orthop 3:471–474, 1983.

63. Pratt, C.B., Ranson, J.L., and Evans, W.E. Age-related cardiotoxicity in children. Cancer Treat Rep 62:1381–1385, 1978.

64. Pritchard, D.J. Factors that influence rehabilitation of children who undergo amputation for bone and soft tissue sarcomas: The surgeon's viewpoint. Natl Cancer Inst Monogr 56:133–135, 1981.

65. Rahal, J.J., McMahon, G.E., and Weinstein, L. Thrombocytopenia and symmetrical peripheral gangrene associated with staphylococcal and streptococcal bacteremia. Ann Intern Med 69:35–43, 1968.

66. Rao, B.N., Champion, J.E., Pratt, C.B., Carnesle, P., Dilawari, R., Flemming, I., Green, A., Austin, B., Wrenn, E., and Kumar, M. Limb salvage procedures for children with osteosarcoma: An alternative to amputation. J Pediatr Surg 18:901–908, 1983.

67. Reinstein, L., and Govindon, S. Extremity amputation: Disseminated intravascular coagulation syndrome. Arch Phys Med Rehabil 61:97–102, 1980.

68. Rich, R.H., Knight, P.J., Erickson, D.L., Broadhurst, K., and Leonard, A.S. Replantation of the upper extremity in children. J Pediatr Surg 12:1028–1032, 1977.

69. Romano, R., and Burgess, E. The immediate postsurgical prosthetic fitting technique applied to child amputees. Interclinic Info Bull 9:1–10, 1970.

70. Rosen, G., Caparros, B., Huvos, A.G., Kosloff, C., Nirenberg, A., Cacavio, A., Marcove, R.C., Lane, J.M., Mehta, B., and Urban, C. Preoperative chemotherapy for osteogenic sarcoma: Selection of postoperative adjuvant chemotherapy based on the response of the primary tumor to preoperative chemotherapy. Cancer 49:1221–1230, 1982.

71. Rosenfelder, R. Infant amputees: Early growth and care. Clin Orthop 148:41–46, 1980.

72. Rossi, T.V., and Kruger, L. Proximal femoral focal deficiency and its treatment. Orthot Prosthet 29:37–57, 1975.

73. Ryan, J.R., and Emami, A. Vincristine neurotoxicity with residual equinocavus deformity in children with acute leukemia. Cancer 51:423–425, 1983.

74. Serafin, J. A new operation for congenital absence of the fibula. J Bone Joint Surg 49B:59–65, 1967.

75. Shaperman, J. Learning patterns of young children with above-elbow prostheses. Am J Occup Ther 33:299–305, 1979.

76. Shaperman, J., and Sumida, C.T. Recent advances in research in prosthetics for children. Clin Orthop 148:26–33, 1980.

77. Shurr, D.G., Cooper, R.R., Buckwalter, J.A., and Blair, W.F. Juvenile amputees: Classification and revision rates. Orthot Prosthet 36:22–28, 1982.

78. Shurr, D.G., Cooper, R.R., Buckwalter, J.A., and Blair, W.F. Terminal transverse congenital deficiency of the forearm. Prosthet Orthot Int 35:22–25, 1981.

79. Smith, R.J., and Lipke, R.W. Treatment of congenital deformities of the hand, part I. N Engl J Med 300:344–349, 1979.

80. Sorbye, R. Myoelectric prosthetic fitting in young children. Clin Orthop 148:34–40, 1980.

81. Speer, D.P. Pathogenesis of amputation stump-overgrowth. Clin Orthop 159:294–307, 1981.

82. Stoner, E.K. Management of the lower extremity amputee, in Kottke, F.J., Stillwell, G.K., and Lehmann, J.F. (eds): *Krusen's Handbook of Physical Medicine and Rehabilitation.* Philadelphia, Saunders, 1982, p 924.

83. Stossel, T.P., and Levy, R. Intravascular coagulation associated with pneumococcal bacteremia and symmetrical peripheral gangrene. Arch Intern Med 125:876–878, 1970.

84. Sutherland, D.H. *Gait Disorders in Children and Adolescence.* Baltimore, Williams and Wilkins, 1984, pp 89–106.

85. Swanson, A.B. A classification for congenital limb malformations. J Hand Surg 1:8–22, 1976.

86. Swanson, A.B. Congenital limb defects: Classification and treatment. Clin Symp 33:3–32, 1981.

87. Swanson, A.B. Silicone-rubber implants to control the overgrowth phenomenon in the juvenile amputee. Interclinic Info Bull 11:5–8, 1972.

88. Swanson, A.B., Boeve, N.R., and Lumsden, R.M. The prevention and treatment of amputation neuromata by silicone capping. J Hand Surg 2:70–78, 1977.

89. Swanson, A.B., and Swanson, G. The Krukenberg procedure in the juvenile amputee. Clin Orthop 148:55–61, 1980.

90. Tablada, C. A technique for fitting converted proximal femoral focal deficiencies. Artif Limbs 15:27–45, 1971.

91. Taylor, H.L., Henschel, A., Brozek, J., and Key, A. Effects of bedrest on cardiovascular function and work performance. J Appl Physiol 2:223–239, 1949.

92. Tefft, M., Lattin, P.B., Jereb, B., Cham, W., Ghavimi, F., Rosen, G., Exelby, P., Marcove, R., Murphy, M.L., and D'Angio, G.J. Acute and late effects on normal tissue following combined chemo- and radio-therapy for childhood rhabdomyosarcoma and Ewing's sarcoma. Cancer 37:1201–1213, 1976.

93. Thompson, G.H., Balourdas, G.M., and Marcus, R.E. Railyard amputations in children. J Pediatr Orthop 3:443–448, 1983.

94. Thompson, T.C., Straub, L.R., and Arnold, W.D. Congenital absence of the fibula. J Bone Joint Surg 39A:1229–1237, 1957.

95. Van Nes, C.P. Rotation-plasty for congenital defects of the femur. J Bone Joint Surg 32B:12–16, 1950.

96. Von Hoff, D.D., Layard, M.W., Basa, P., Davis, H.L., Von Hoff, A.L., Rosencweig, M., and Muggia, F.M. Risk-factors for doxorubicin-induced congestive heart failure. Ann Intern Med 91:710–717, 1979.

97. Voute, P.A., Burgers, J.M.V., Van Patten, W.J., and Van Dobbenburght, O.A. Amputations in children: Clinical indications and psychological implications. Arch Chir Neerland 25:427–433, 1973.

98. Wehbe, M.A., Weinstein, S.L., and Ponseti, I.V. Tibial agenesis. J Pediatr Orthop 1:395–399, 1981.

99. Weinstein, S., and Sersen, E.A. Phantoms in case of congenital absence of limbs. Neurology 11:909–911, 1961.

100. Westin, G.W., Sakai, D.N., and Wood, W.L. Congenital longitudinal deficiency of the fibula. J Bone Joint Surg 58A:492–496, 1976.

101. Wilbur, J.R., Sutow, W.W., Sullivan, M.P., and Gottlieb, J.A. Chemotherapy of sarcomas. Cancer 36:765–769, 1975.

102. Williamson, D.A.J. A syndrome of congenital malformations possibly due to maternal diabetes. Dev Med Child Neurol 12:145–152, 1970.

103. Wolfgang, G.L. Complex congenital anomalies of the lower extremities: Femoral bifurcation, tibial hemimelia, and diastasis of the ankle. J Bone Joint Surg 66A:453–457, 1984.

104. Wood, W.L., Zlotsky, N., and Westin, G.W. Congenital absence of the fibula. J Bone Joint Surg 47A:1159–1169, 1965.

105. Zazula, J.L., and Foulds, R.A. Mobility device for a child with phocomelia. Arch Phys Med Rehabil 64:137–139, 1983.

CHAPTER 25

Radionuclide Scanning in Orthopaedics

Harold L. Atkins

GENERAL PRINCIPLES

Radiopharmaceuticals

Radiopharmaceuticals which are useful in the investigation of skeletal disease are technetium 99m, gallium 67 citrate, and indium 111–labeled white blood cells. The last two are primarily used for the evaluation of inflammatory processes.

Technetium (^{99m}Tc)

The development of a variety of technetium 99m–labeled radiopharmaceuticals beginning with technetium 99m polyphosphate has permitted the application of radionuclide bone imaging to a wide range of disorders in all age groups.[133]

The technetium phosphate complexes are adsorbed on the matrix rather rapidly, and imaging can proceed within hours following tracer administration. Methylene diphosphonate and hydroxymethylene diphosphonate are the tracers of choice because of their rapid clearance from blood, resulting in a decreased soft tissue background.[5,134]

Gallium

The precise mode of localization of gallium in neoplastic and inflammatory disease is unknown. When administered intravenously it immediately combines with transferrin in the blood and to some extent is transported as iron is but does not become incorporated into red blood cells. There is a strong affinity for lactoferrin, which is found in polymorphonuclear leukocytes, lacrimal glands, and breasts. Gallium is found to be incorporated into lysosomes. Normal sites of accumulation in the body are in liver, spleen, bone marrow, lacrimal glands, breast, and bowel. The physical characteristics of gallium 67 are far from ideal for imaging because of the multiple gamma photons, including some higher-energy photons, which are less efficiently detected by the thin crystal of the gamma camera and which require less efficient medium-energy collimators.

Indium

Indium 111–labeled leukocytes have certain advantages over gallium 67 citrate. The localization is more specific for inflammation because they are not ordinarily taken up in tumor. The usual administered activity of indium 111 leukocytes is 0.5 mCi and is limited by the rather high radiation dose to the spleen.

Techniques

Technetium 99m Bone Imaging

Approximately 20 to 25 mCi of technetium 99m methylene diphosphonate (^{99m}Tc MDP) or hydroxymethylene diphosphonate (^{99m}Tc HDP) is administered intravenously. The patient is instructed to drink substantial amounts of fluid and to empty the bladder just prior to imaging. About 50 percent of the tracer is eliminated via the urinary tract. Retained urine in the bladder at the time of imaging may obscure the bones about the pubis, the sacrum, and the hips.

Imaging is performed at 2 h or preferably 3 h following administration of the tracer. In some institutions a moving table or moving camera is used to obtain a complete skeletal image in one view, but others prefer to obtain multiple stationary images which may provide greater detail.

Normally there is good delineation of each vertebral body including pedicles and spinous processes. We obtain anterior oblique views of the ribs, which also permits clearer delineation of the sternum without overlap of the dorsal spine. Extremities usually have less uptake than the axial skeleton. A difficult area is about the shoulders, where increased activity is the norm in certain structures such as the acromioclavicular joint and the coracoid process of the scapula. More-detailed views of certain structures, such as the hips, may be necessary for aseptic necrosis. A smaller-field-of-view camera with a pinhole collimator may be used for such a purpose.

In children and adolescents the secondary growth centers accumulate a relatively greater concentration of tracer. This can create difficulties in interpretation and may obscure processes such as osteomyelitis which occur in these locations.

Gallium 67 Citrate Imaging

Gallium 67 citrate is administered intravenously at activity levels of 3 to 5 mCi for inflammatory disease and 10 mCi for detection of malignant tumors. When inflammatory lesions are being searched for, imaging may be carried out at 6 h for two reasons: (1) to be able to image prior to accumulation of activity in the large bowel and (2) to provide an earlier diagnosis. A disadvantage of early imaging is the high body background. Generally lesions retain gallium for a long time while body background activity is eliminated. When the larger administered activities are used in the search for malignancy, imaging may be carried out over many days. Usual times are 48 to 96 h.

In the detection of osteomyelitis or when other technetium 99m studies such as gated cardiac blood pool or liver imaging are to be performed, the gallium 67 study should be delayed until after completion of the technetium 99m studies. This is because the high energy of the photons from gallium 67 interfere with detection of the 140-keV gamma photons of technetium 99m.

Indium 111 Leukocyte Imaging

The use of indium 111 leukocytes for inflammatory-process imaging is no longer considered investigational. The method of labeling is complex and need not be considered here.

The tracer is administered intravenously, and imaging is performed at 4 and 24 h. The earlier imaging time is not essential. Normal accumulation is primarily in the spleen with lesser amounts in liver and bone marrow. At the earlier time some lung activity may be noted. While the photons of indium 111 are of greater energy than those of technetium 99m, much less activity is administered and there is less interference with subsequent technetium 99m imaging studies as compared to gallium. Indium 111 leukocyte imaging is more specific for inflammatory processes than gallium 67 citrate because it does not accumulate in neoplasms. Further discussion of the relative value of these two tracers is presented in the section on osteomyelitis.

TRAUMA
Fractures

Bone imaging with ^{99m}Tc MDP may be of value in the diagnosis of fractures which are not evident by radiographic examination.[130] It may also be helpful in differentiating traumatic fracture from a pathologic fracture secondary to metastatic disease in bone. Increased accumulation of the radiotracer at the fracture site may be noted within 24 h and with more certainty within 72 h.[113] The degree of uptake increases over the next several months and then decreases, with a return to normal after a year or two.[81] Uptake may persist for years in poorly united fractures or sites under abnormal stress, and especially in weight-bearing long bones.

The differentiation of traumatic from pathologic fracture requires the administration of the tracer within the first 12 to 18 h following the event. A purely traumatic fracture does not accumulate in that period, whereas a fracture secondary to metastatic disease shows avid uptake. An exception can occur if the metastasis is from a malignancy that tends not to excite new bone formation such as myeloma, thyroid cancer, and some cases of breast cancer which are purely lytic.

Radionuclide imaging of bone may be especially useful in diagnosis of child abuse.[48,132] Some controversy exists concerning relative sensitivity of radionuclide studies and radiography.[88] When injury is primarily at the ends of growing bone, abnormalities may be more readily detected by radiography, but radionuclide bone imaging may detect clinically unsuspected lesions. In the study of Sty and Starshak there were 12.3 percent false negatives with radiography and 0.8 percent with scintigraphy.[132] Merten et al found a yield of positive cases of 33 percent for radiography (161/494) and 48 percent for scintigraphy (11/23), but nonetheless they recommended radiography as the primary detection modality.[88]

In suspected cases of child abuse it is recommended that skull films be obtained because skull fractures are not readily imaged with radionuclide techniques. Radionuclide bone imaging will then pick up other areas. Further radiographic examination can then be limited to sites identified by scintigraphy for confirmation and to symptomatic sites not positive on scintigraphy.

Not infrequently scintigraphy may reveal fractures difficult to detect by radiography such as fractures of the carpal scaphoid.[98]

Stress Fractures

With the increased interest in physical fitness, more and more patients are referred for diagnosis of bone pain following such activities as running and other unaccustomed exercise. Roentgenograms are frequently negative, particularly at early times following onset of symptoms (Fig. 25-1). The technetium bone scan has a high sensitivity for detection of changes at this stage. Stress fractures are diagnosed by focal abnormalities, often in the shaft of the tibia. Stress changes may also be noted as linear cortical increases in activity at the site of muscle attachments.

The distal tibia is the most common site for stress-related injury, especially in runners. The diagnosis can be made readily in the proper clinical setting without radiographs.[117] Other common sites are the proximal femur,[26,107,153] the pubic ramus,[105] the pubic symphysis,[64] the calcaneus, and the metatarsals.[43,71]

An excellent review of scintigraphy in the diagnosis of exercise-related injuries has been published by Holder and Matthews.[53]

Avascular Necrosis

Avascular necrosis may occur as a result of extensive exercise. When this occurs in the femoral head and goes unrecognized, severe deformity and functional impairment may result. Viability of bone may also be in question following fracture of the proximal femur. In childhood and adolescence the problem is associated with idiopathic involvement of various bones (Kienböck's disease, Legg-Calvé-Perthes disease, etc.).[9,11,24,25,28,34,90,94,121,136,137] Avascular necrosis is also associated with high-dose corticosteroid therapy, slipped capital femoral epiphysis, and sickle cell disease.

In the early phase of avascular necrosis, scintigraphic images show diminished or absent uptake of the bone tracer in the affected area. Pinhole camera images may be necessary

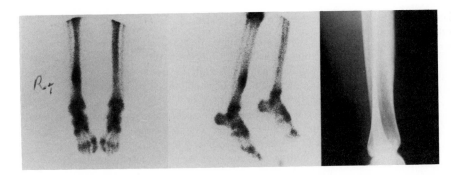

Figure 25-1 Stress fracture involving the anterior tibia. Roentgenogram (*right*) is negative. Increased activity is seen at the junction of the middle and lower third of the tibia on AP scan (*left*) and lateral view (*center*).

to visualize the abnormality adequately. In the reparative phase, which may occur 3 to 6 months later, there is increased uptake. It is useful in these cases to image all the bones, as unexpected sites of involvement may then be revealed.

Of particular interest is the question of viability of the proximal fragment following a femoral neck fracture. This question is of importance in deciding whether or not to pin the fracture or to go directly to a prosthesis. The use of technetium 99m colloid has been advocated to assess marrow perfusion at the affected site.[89,142] The colloidal particles are taken up by the phagocytes in the marrow and are an indicator of perfusion. A disadvantage of this method in older patients is normal relative inactivity and fibrosis of marrow in this location.[128] This is a particular problem in view of the age group in which these fractures frequently occur. More recently the use of technetium phosphate imaging has been in favor.[45,46,76] An alternative method is the three-phase bone study in which careful assessment is made of the dynamic phase when the tracer is in the blood pool prior to any substantial bone uptake.[3] In the later phase of the study, the use of a pinhole collimator is generally helpful.

Soft Tissue Injury

Bone-seeking tracers often localize in nonbony structures. Heterotopic bone as seen in myositis ossificans, scleroderma, and dermatomyositis is the focus of ^{99m}Tc MDP uptake.[143] Another cause of extraskeletal uptake is polymyositis.[129] In athletes extensive exercise may result in muscle necrosis which can be detected on bone scan.[82,144] Other types of injury such as direct trauma, frostbite, etc., also result in abnormal tracer distribution.[73,80,146]

OSTEOMYELITIS, TUBERCULOSIS, AND OTHER INFECTIONS

Acute Osteomyelitis

The diagnosis of acute osteomyelitis in children is difficult, particularly in the neonatal period.[1] The ^{99m}Tc MDP bone scan may appear normal, especially in the very early stages.[4,31,49] A confounding aspect is the very high uptake of bone tracer at the growing ends of bone, the usual site of osteomyelitis, which obscures any abnormality of uptake. In some instances one may observe a "cold" defect[54,93] which has been attributed to decreased perfusion secondary to an increase in pressure within the affected bone, preventing adequate blood flow, to thrombosis, or to infarction.[33,49,78]

Despite these problems the diagnosis of osteomyelitis is highly accurate and is frequently possible as early as 24 h, a time when radiographs may be normal. Howie et al obtained a sensitivity of 89 percent and a specificity of 94 percent for technetium phosphate imaging alone with an overall accuracy of 92 percent.[54] Others report results equal to or better than this.[37,38]

The three-phase technetium bone scan has been of help.[37,54] It contains (1) a flow phase, consisting of about nine sequential 5-s images which are obtained in the first minute following bolus administration of the tracer; (2) a blood-pool phase, which consists of a single static view of 500,000 to 1 million counts collected during the 5 min or so immediately following the flow phase; and (3) a conventional bone image obtained some hours following the administration of tracer. This technique enables the evaluation of hyperemia which may accompany soft tissue or bone inflammation. It is especially helpful in improving specificity by detection of soft tissue inflammation.[83]

A particularly difficult clinical problem is the evaluation of the diabetic foot. Overlying superficial soft tissue infection and postoperative changes can complicate the diagnostic process. Three-phase bone imaging has been of value.[103] The sensitivity and specificity in the study by Park et al were 83 and 75 percent, respectively, compared with the results for radiography of 62 and 69 percent.

Clinical evaluation is most important in the early diagnosis of acute osteomyelitis.[30,148] It is imperative to begin therapy despite a negative study if clinical suspicion is high.

Double-Tracer Technique

The combined use of the ^{99m}Tc MDP bone scan and gallium 67 citrate imaging is a subject of some controversy. The current belief is that gallium 67 uptake greater than the bone agent is compatible with osteomyelitis.[74,108,115] Lesser degrees of uptake may be seen in uncomplicated fractures. Gallium 67 citrate imaging has been found to have a sensitivity of 83 percent and a specificity of 96 percent for sternal osteomyelitis, a problem which can occur following many cardiac procedures.[119] However, not everyone's experience upholds this view. Osteomyelitis has been found even with low uptake of gallium. Close radiological and clinical correlation is necessary (see Chap. 22).

An alternative to gallium 67 citrate is indium 111–labeled leukocytes.[42,120] This method is most specific for acute inflammatory conditions. Its accuracy in chronic infection is not completely satisfactory. A recent study comparing gallium 67 and indium 111 showed the sensitivity of indium 111 imaging to be 100 percent in acute osteomyelitis but only 60 percent in chronic osteomyelitis.[120] While gallium 67 imaging had a high sensitivity (100 percent) overall, its specificity was rather low (25 percent).

One may conclude from the published literature and from experience that neither gallium nor indium are completely satisfactory tracers in the diagnosis of osteomyelitis. ^{99m}Tc MDP remains the best tracer so far, although its specificity is far from ideal.

Other Infections

There are several reported cases of bone imaging in miliary tuberculosis involving bone.[62,96,118] Involvement may be widespread and simulate metastatic disease in the face of normal radiographs. Following treatment the appearance of the scintigrams returns to normal in several months, although a photopenic phase may be encountered.

Bone scintigraphy in patients with mastoiditis and sinusitis may show increased uptake in these regions.[23,32,102] Such involvement may not necessarily indicate osteomyelitis but may be a reflection of hyperemia because of inflammation of the mucosal lining. However, scintigraphy may provide a clue to serious bone involvement in the appropriate clinical setting.

Bony involvement may occur in other inflammatory conditions such as sarcoidosis.[110,112,124] The exquisite sensitivity of bone scintigraphy may reveal many lesions prior to the development of symptoms or radiographic changes.

DISEASES OF THE JOINTS
Osteoarthritis

The most common abnormality noted on bone-imaging studies is osteoarthritis. In the active (but not necessarily symptomatic) phase there is increased uptake in areas of inflammatory and hypertrophic change. Common sites are cervical spine, lumbar spine, hips, and small joints of the phalanges in the hands and feet. In addition, the usual sites of marked motion such as the shoulder joint and sternoclavicular joints normally have increased uptake. Often these regions of increased tracer uptake can be confused with metastatic disease, and careful correlation with radiographs is essential. Usually the degree of concentration of tracer in hypertrophic osteoarthritis is less intense than in malignant disease, but this is not always true.

Rheumatoid Arthritis

The radionuclide bone image is usually markedly positive in rheumatoid arthritis. Differentiation from other abnormalities which can also produce intense tracer uptake in bone is aided by noting that the abnormal regions are present on both sides of the joint space. Obliteration of the joint space by advanced disease can present some problems. The increase in accumulation of tracer is in part due to increased blood flow secondary to the inflammatory process.

In the very earliest phase of inflammation, synovial imaging with ^{99m}Tc pertechnetate may be more sensitive than bone imaging. This is essentially blood-pool imaging within several minutes of tracer administration. Synovial imaging is more sensitive than radionuclide bone imaging in the small joints of the wrists, hands, knees, ankles, and feet. Pertechnetate is not especially useful for imaging of the larger joints because of the high background activity.[47] The same is true of radionuclide bone imaging.[151]

A particularly difficult area is the sacroiliac joint. Normally technetium 99m phosphate complexes show a high degree of uptake in the sacrum and adjacent ilium. Quantitative techniques have been applied with the hope of being able to differentiate the normal from the abnormal side,[38,95,126] but this has not always been successful. Gallium 67 imaging may be helpful. The use of single photon emission tomography is just becoming widespread and may prove to be a very efficacious technique.

Detection of Loosened Joint Prostheses

Following surgery for insertion of joint prostheses, there is increased uptake of technetium 99m phosphates about the surgical site as a response to the surgical trauma. This increased uptake recedes in 6 to 9 months.[21,154] After this time radionuclide bone imaging is a highly sensitive and specific means of diagnosing loosening. In the hip the diagnosis of loosening, which can be made prior to radiographic changes, is apparent when increased activity is present at the tip of the femoral component.[152] This is secondary to abnormal stress from motion of the stem against adjacent bone. Sensitivity as high as 100 percent has been found for radionuclide detection of loosening in the hip.[139,155,156]

Detection of a loosened acetabular component is more difficult.[139,152] Sensitivity may be as low as 30 percent in such cases.

Detection of infection in loosened joints utilizes the same strategy as in osteomyelitis. Gallium 67 uptake, if more extensive than in the ^{99m}Tc MDP study, is a good indication of infection, whereas gallium 67 uptake congruent with or less than the technetium 99m uptake is not indicative of infection. Williams et al reported a sensitivity of 93 percent and a specificity of 87 percent with gallium.[155]

Total knee replacements are somewhat more difficult to evaluate. Assessment of activity about the femoral component is apparently more accurate than evaluation of the tibial component. An 83 percent sensitivity and an 86 percent specificity have been reported.[59]

METABOLIC BONE DISEASE

Many metabolic conditions result in a diffuse, generalized increase in uptake of a bone tracer in the skeleton. Characteristically the images appear of superior quality with absence or near absence of renal activity. The calvarium and mandible may appear prominent, and the costochondral junctions are readily noted. The sternum may have a characteristic appearance of increased uptake along the borders and at the manubrial junction with the body of the sternum. Conditions which may give rise to this picture are renal osteomalacia, primary hyperparathyroidism, and reflex sympathetic dystrophy syndrome. There is no characteristic appearance in osteoporosis, but evidence of fracture may be seen in these patients.

Focal changes may occur in a number of metabolic disorders. Examples are progressive diaphyseal dysplasia and melorheostosis. Hypertrophic pulmonary osteoarthropathy results in increased uptake in long bone, primarily in the diaphysis. The change may be irregular, and it tapers towards the metaphysis.[20,66,114] Following treatment of the primary lesion the osteoarthropathy may resolve.[66]

PAGET DISEASE

At times Paget disease of bone may present diagnostic difficulties, although usually the diagnosis is clear-cut. Difficulties arise in differentiating monostotic Paget disease from metastasis and in differentiating metastatic prostate cancer from Paget disease. Other situations such as fibrous dysplasia, hyperparathyroidism, severe osteoarthritis, and sarcomatous degeneration must also be considered.

The uptake of bone tracer in Paget disease is usually marked. This is secondary to the hypervascularity of bone, which is the hallmark of Paget disease. Correlation with radiographs is helpful because at certain stages such as in the "burnt out" phase, uptake may be reduced but lesions may still be seen on x-ray examination.

With the development of treatment modalities for this condition, a variety of methods for assessing response have been evaluated. The bone scan is more reliable than radiography for this purpose.[67] The addition of a flow procedure to the bone scan appears to be a more sensitive method for evaluation,[8] while gallium 67 imaging may be the best way to assess response.[149] Gallium may also be useful in diagnosing sarcomatous degeneration.[161] In the latter situation, when an involved area becomes cold on bone imaging while becoming more avid for gallium, it is a good indication of sarcoma development.

PRIMARY TUMORS OF BONE
Benign Tumors

Enchondroma This is one of the more common benign bone tumors. It is cartilaginous and occurs in the medullary cavity. Uptake of bone tracers may or may not occur.[91]

Osteochondroma (Exostosis) Moderate uptake of bone tracer may occur.[36] Scintigraphy is not helpful in distinguishing a benign exostosis from an exostotic chondrosarcoma.[157]

Bone Cyst There is frequently no uptake of tracer in benign bone cysts. Uptake is seen in case of a fracture, and a slight increase in uptake may be seen around the periphery. Aneurysmal bone cysts always have increased activity, mostly around the periphery.[55]

Osteoid Osteoma and Osteoblastoma Scintigraphy with ^{99m}Tc MDP is much more sensitive than radiography for osteoblastic tumors, particularly when they occur in the spine. Sensitivity approaches 100 percent for osteoid osteoma, while radiography has a sensitivity of 55 to 93 percent.[100,125,135,159] False-negative examination with radionuclide imaging is extremely rare.[29] Differential diagnosis includes osteomyelitis, and the use of gallium 67 citrate may be useful as it is generally poorly taken up in osteoid osteoma.[75,125] The sensitivity of scintigraphy for osteoblastoma is similar to that for osteoid osteoma.[79]

Intraoperative scintigraphy has been found to be especially helpful in assessing the efficacy of removal of the tumor in osteoblastic lesions.[18,35,60,111,131,145]

Malignant Tumors

Osteosarcoma Radionuclide bone imaging is of value in the initial workup of patients with osteosarcoma. Although the yield of bone metastases at initial presentation is low,[40,85,87] the imaging procedure serves as a baseline. Subsequent bone metastasis occurs at a high rate (43 percent), and these metastases may often be asymptomatic.[87] Detection of metastatic disease is crucial to making therapeutic decisions.

Much of the time the radionuclide study provides an accurate estimate of tumor extent. However, not infrequently there is an augmented extension of increased uptake beyond the anatomic bounds of the tumor.[15,39,87,140] This may be secondary to hyperemia or abnormal stress. Rarely a lesion may display photopenia.[87,122]

At follow-up, the stump at the amputation site should have only minor increase in activity by 6 months. More than this indicates recurrence.[87] In addition to bone metastases, nonosseous uptake may be noted, especially in the lungs and lymph nodes.[50-52] In 12 patients with pulmonary metastases, there was increased bone tracer uptake in 11, and in 2 of these the radionuclide study demonstrated these prior to x-ray tomography.[51]

Chondrosarcoma In contrast to osteosarcomas, chondrosarcomas usually show no extended uptake of tracer in radionuclide imaging.[56] The anatomic extent of tumor is rather accurately portrayed by the region of increased accumulation of the imaging agent.

Multiple Myeloma Multiple myeloma does not tend to excite new bone formation and tends to be purely osteolytic in nature. Several reviews are in conformity with the idea that radiography is approximately twice as sensitive as scintigraphy in this condition.[72,77,138,147,160] In the ribs and lumbar spine the radionuclide study may be helpful and can occasionally pick up lesions missed by x-ray examination. Radiography should be the first method of survey with scintigraphy used as a supplementary procedure in symptomatic, x-ray-negative sites.

Giant Cell Tumors Extension of the region of increased uptake beyond tumor margins is a feature of giant cell tumor of bone as well as of osteosarcoma.[58,70] The appearance is that of more intense uptake about the periphery of the tumor. Computed tomography appears to be the most useful modality for estimating extent of tumor involvement, and orthotomography is helpful in determining invasion through the subchondral cortex.

Ewing Sarcoma Uptake of tracer in patients with Ewing sarcoma is secondary to reactive bone formation. The distribution of activity is more uniform than in osteogenic sarcoma and a somewhat higher percentage of patients may have osseous metastases when first diagnosed.[92] Metastases develop in 40 to 45 percent within 2 years.[41]

Soft Tissue Sarcomas Bone imaging is of value in soft tissue sarcomas in order to assess bony erosion;[14,27,63] the use of early blood-pool imaging following administration of the bone tracer and the use of gallium citrate may be particularly useful in differentiating benign from malignant lesions.[63] It is preferable to perform the radionuclide studies prior to biopsy in order to avoid misleading results.

Secondary Tumors of Bone

Bone scintigraphy is widely used for the assessment of metastatic disease because the skeleton is a frequent site of spread of malignancy. Scintigraphic survey is more accurate than radiographic survey in most forms of cancer.[84,101,123]

While most tumors metastatic to bone excite a reparative response resulting in increased bone tracer uptake, there are a few malignancies that result in no increase or even photopenic lesions. These tumors are indolent in nature or may be primarily lytic without osteoblastic response. Examples of lesions which may not elicit an increase in uptake at sites of bone metastasis are thyroid carcinoma,[10] neuroblastoma,[61] and histiocytosis X.[104]

In the past, false-negative scintigraphy has occurred secondary to extensive diffuse metastatic disease, the so-called superscan. This can be seen with carcinoma of the breast and prostate, in particular. Characteristically the kidneys and bladder may not be visualized because of the markedly avid uptake by the entire skeleton. With the improvement in instrument resolution in recent years, it is less likely that these situations would be missed because with modern gamma cameras irregularity in distribution of uptake, which would have been missed previously, can be seen.

The role of radionuclide imaging for bone metastatic disease is threefold:

1. Staging
2. Assessment of progress of disease
3. Assessment of efficacy of therapeutic intervention

Numerous articles have addressed the problem of staging using the bone scan, particularly in carcinoma of the breast.[22,65,68,84,97,157]

CONCLUSION

Radionuclide bone imaging is an important part of the clinical armamentarium and is unlikely to be replaced soon. Its high sensitivity and noninvasive character are key points in its frequent utilization. Unfortunately, the relatively low specificity requires follow-up with more definitive or complementary examinations in many instances.

Newer radiopharmaceutical developments, especially in the field of monoclonal antibodies, may provide higher specificity for scintigraphic techniques. There may also be important therapeutic implications in the development of these agents.

REFERENCES

1. Ash, J.M., and Gilday, D.L. The futility of bone scanning in neonatal osteomyelitis. J Nucl Med 21:417–420, 1980.
2. Bauer, G.C.H., Carlsson, A., and Lindquist, B. Metabolism of ^{140}Ba in man. Acta Orthop Scand 26:241–254, 1957.
3. Bauer, G., Weber, D.A., Ceder, L., et al. Dynamics of technetium-99m methylenediphosphonate imaging of the femoral head after hip fracture. Clin Orthop 152:85–92, 1980.
4. Berkowitz, I.D., and Wenzel, W. "Normal" technetium bone scans in patients with acute osteomyelitis. Am J Dis Child 134:828–830, 1980.
5. Bevan, J.A., Tofe, A.J., Francis, M.D., et al. Tc-99m hydroxymethylene diphosphonate (HMDP): A new skeletal imaging agent, in *Radiopharmaceuticals II: Proceedings 2nd International Symposium on Radiopharmaceuticals.* New York, Society of Nuclear Medicine, 1979, pp 645–654.
6. Blau, M., Nagler, W., and Bender, M.A. Fluorine-18: A new isotope for bone scanning. J Nucl Med 3:332–334, 1962.
7. Blom, J., Pauwels, E.K.J., Piso, L.N., and Taminiau, A.H.M. Misleading ^{67}Ga uptake and serial bone scintigraphy in osteoid osteoma. Diagn Imaging 52:276–279, 1983.
8. Boudreau, R.J., Lisbona, R., and Hadjipavlou, A. Observations on serial radionuclide blood-flow studies in Paget's disease: Concise communication. J Nucl Med 24:880–885, 1983.
9. Burt, R.W., and Matthews, T.J. Aseptic necrosis of the knee: Bone scintigraphy. Am J Roentgenol 138:571–573, 1982.
10. Castillo, L.A., Yeh, S.K.J., Leeper, R.D., et al. Bone scans in bone metastases from functioning thyroid carcinoma. Clin Nucl Med 5:200–209, 1980.
11. Cavailloles, F., Bok, B., and Bensahel, H. Bone scintigraphy in the diagnosis and follow up of Perthes' disease. Eur J Nucl Med 7:327–330, 1982.
12. Charkes, N.D. Some differences between bone scans made with ^{87m}Sr and ^{85}Sr. J Nucl Med 10:491–494, 1969.
13. Charkes, N.D., Young, I., and Skarloff, D.M. The pathologic basis of strontium bone scan. Studies following administration of

strontium chloride Sr 85 and strontium nitrate Sr 85. JAMA 206:2482–2488, 1968.

14. Chew, F.S., and Hudson, T.M. Radionuclide imaging of lipoma and liposarcoma. Radiology 136:741–745, 1980.

15. Chew, F.S., and Hudson, T.M. Radionuclide bone scanning of osteosarcoma: Falsely extended uptake patterns. Am J Roentgenol 139:49–54, 1982.

16. Citrin, D.L. The role of the bone scan in the investigation and treatment of breast cancer. CRC Crit Rev Diagn Imaging 13:39–55, 1980.

17. Collins, J.D., Bassett, L., Main, G.D., et al. Percutaneous biopsy following positive bone scans. Radiology 132:439–442, 1979.

18. Colton, C.L., and Hardy, J.G. Evaluation of a sterilizable radiation probe as an aid to the surgical treatment of osteoid-osteoma. J Bone Joint Surg [Am] 65:1019–1021, 1983.

19. Corcoran, R.J., Thrall, J.H., Kyle, R.W., et al. Solitary abnormalities in bone scans of patients with extraosseous malignancies. Radiology 121:663–667, 1976.

20. Costello, P., Gramm, H.F., and Lokisch, J. Detection of hypertrophic pulmonary osteoarthropathy associated with pulmonary metastatic disease. Clin Nucl Med 11:397–399, 1977.

21. Creutzig, H. Bone imaging after total replacement arthroplasty of the hip joint. Eur J Nucl Med 1:177–180, 1976.

22. Davies, C.J., Griffiths, P.A., Preston, B.J., et al. Staging breast cancer: Role of bone scanning. Br Med J 2:603–605, 1977.

23. Djupesland, G., Nakken, K.F., Muller, C., et al. Bone scintigraphy in the diagnosis of fracture and infection of the temporal bone. Acta Otolaryngol 95:670–675, 1983.

24. Dodig, D., Ugarkovic, B., and Orlic, D. Bone scintigraphy in idiopathic aseptic femoral head necrosis (IAFHN). Eur J Nucl Med 8:23–25, 1983.

25. Duong, R.B., Nishiyama, H., Mantil, J.C., et al. Kienbock's disease: Scintigraphic demonstration in correlation with clinical, radiographic, and pathologic findings. Clin Nucl Med 7:418–420, 1982.

26. El-Khoury, G.Y., Wehbe, M.A., Bonfiglio, M., et al. Stress fractures of the femoral neck: A scintigraphic sign for early diagnosis. Skeletal Radiol 6:271–273, 1981.

27. Enneking, W.F., Chew, F.S., Springfield, D.S., et al. The role of radionuclide bone-scanning in determining the resectability of soft-tissue sarcomas. J Bone Joint Surg [Am] 63:249–257, 1981.

28. Fasting, O.J., Bjerkreim, I., Langeland, N., et al. Scintigraphic evaluation of the severity of Perthes' disease in the initial stage. Acta Orthop Scand 51:655–660, 1980.

29. Fehring, T.K., and Green, N.E. Negative radionuclide scan in osteoid osteoma: A case report. Clin Orthop 185:245–249, 1984.

30. Fihn, S.D., Larson, E.B., Nelp, W.B., et al. Should single-phase radionuclide bone imaging be used in suspected osteomyelitis. J Nucl Med 25:1080–1088, 1984.

31. Fleisher, G.R., Paradise, J.E., Plotkin, S.A., and Borden, S., IV. Falsely normal radionuclide scans for osteomyelitis. Am J Dis Child 134:499–502, 1980.

32. Floyd, J.L., and Goodman, E.L. Bone scintigraphy in the diagnosis of mastoiditis. Clin Nucl Med 6:320–321, 1981.

33. Garnett, E.S., Cockshott, W.P., and Jacobs, J. Classical acute osteomyelitis with a negative bone scan. Br J Radiol 50:757–760, 1977.

34. Gelfand, M.J., Strife, J.L., Graham, E.J., and Crawford, A.H. Bone scintigraphy in slipped capital femoral epiphysis. Clin Nucl Med 8:613–615, 1983.

35. Ghelman, R., Thomson, F.M., and Arnold, W.D. Intraoperative radioactive localization of osteoid osteoma. J Bone Joint Surg [Am] 63:826–827, 1981.

36. Gilday, D.L., and Ash, J.M. Benign bone tumors. Semin Nucl Med 6:33–46, 1976.

37. Gilday, D.J., Paul, D.J., and Paterson, J. Diagnosis of osteomyelitis in children by combined blood pool and bone imaging. Radiology 117:331–335, 1975.

38. Goldberg, R.P., Genant, H.K., Shimchak, R., et al. Application and limitations of quantitative sacroiliac joint scintigraphy. Radiology 128:683–686, 1978.

39. Goldman, A.B., and Braunstein, P. Augmented radioactivity on bone scans of limbs bearing osteosarcoma. J Nucl Med 16:423–424, 1975.

40. Goldstein, H., McNeil, B.J., Zufall, E., et al. Changing indications for bone scintigraphy in patients with osteosarcoma. Radiology 135:177–180, 1980.

41. Goldstein, H., McNeil, B.J., Zufall, E., and Treves, S. Is there still a place for bone scanning in Ewing's sarcoma: Concise communication. J Nucl Med 21:10–12, 1980.

42. Goss, T.P., and Monahan, J.J. Indium-111 white blood cell scan. Orthop Rev 10:91–96, 1981.

43. Grahame, R., Saunders, A.S., and Maisey, M. The use of scintigraphy in the diagnosis and management of traumatic foot lesions in ballet dancers. Rheumatol Rehabil 18:235–238, 1979.

44. Greaney, R.B., Gerber, F.H., Laughlin, R.L., et al. Distribution and natural history of stress fractures in U.S. Marine recruits. Radiology 146:339–346, 1983.

45. Greiff, J. Determination of the vitality of the femoral head with ^{99m}Tc-Sn-pyrophosphate scintigraphy. Acta Orthop Scand 51:109–117, 1980.

46. Greiff, J., Lanng, S., Hilund-Carlsen, P.F., et al. Early detection by ^{99m}Tc-Sn-pyrophosphate scintigraphy of femoral head necrosis following medial femoral neck fractures. Acta Orthop Scand 51:119–125, 1980.

47. Greyson, N.D. Radionuclide bone and joint imaging in rheumatology. Bull Rheum Dis 30:1034–1049, 1980.

48. Haase, G.M., Ortiz, V.N., Sfakianakis, G.N., and Morse, T.S. The value of radionuclide bone scanning in the early recognition of deliberate child abuse. J Trauma 20:873–875, 1980.

49. Handmaker, H., and Leonards, R. The bone scan in inflammatory osseous disease. Semin Nucl Med 6:95–105, 1976.

50. Heyman, S. The lymphatic spread of osteosarcoma shown by Tc-99m-MDP scintigraphy. Clin Nucl Med 5:543–545, 1980.

51. Hoefnagel, C.A., Bruning, P.F., Cohen, P., et al. Detection of lung metastases from osteosarcoma by scintigraphy using ^{99m}Tc-methylene diphosphonate. Diagn Imaging 50:277–284, 1981.

52. Hoefnagel, C.A., Marcuse, H.R., and Somers, R. Pulmonary tumor-embolism from intravascular osteosarcoma demonstrated by bone scintigraphy. Clin Nucl Med 7:574–576, 1982.

53. Holder, L.E., and Matthews, L.S. The nuclear physician and sports medicine, in Freeman, L.M., and Weissmann, H.S. (eds): *Nuclear Medicine Annual 1984.* New York, Raven, 1984, pp 81–140.

54. Howie, D.W., Savage, J.P., Wilson, L.G., et al. The technetium phosphate bone scan in the diagnosis of osteomyelitis in childhood. J Bone Joint Surg [Am] 65:431–437, 1983.

55. Hudson, T.M. Scintigraphy of aneurysmal bone cysts. Am J Roentgenol 142:761–765, 1984.

56. Hudson, T.M., Chew, F.S., and Manaster, B.J. Radionuclide bone scanning of medullary chondrosarcoma. Am J Roentgenol 139:1071–1076, 1982.

57. Hudson, T.M., Chew, F.S., and Manaster, B.J. Scintigraphy of benign exostoses and exostotic chondrosarcomas. Am J Roentgenol 140:581–586, 1983.

58. Hudson, T.M., Schiebler, M., Springfield, D.S., et al. Radiology of giant cell tumors of bone: Computed tomography arthro-tomography and scintigraphy. Skeletal Radiol 11:85–95, 1984.

59. Hunter, J.C., Hattner, R.S., Murray, W.R., et al. Loosening of the total knee arthroplasty: Detection by radionuclide bone scanning. Am J Roentgenol 135:131–136, 1980.

60. Israeli, A., Zwas, S.T., Horozowski, H., and Farine, I. Use of radionuclide method in preoperative and intraoperative diagnosis of osteoid osteoma of the spine. Clin Orthop 175:194–196, 1983.

61. Kaufman, R.A., Thrall, J.H., Keyes, J.W., et al. False-negative bone scans in neuroblastoma metastatic to the ends of long bones. Am J Roentgenol 130:131–135, 1978.

62. Kimmel, D.J., and Klingensmith, W.C., III. Unusual scintigraphic appearance of osteomyelitis secondary to atypical mycobacterium. Clin Nucl Med 5:189–190, 1980.

63. Kirchner, P.T., and Simon, M.A. The clinical value of bone and gallium scintigraphy for soft-tissue sarcomas of the extremities. J Bone Joint Surg [Am] 66:319–327, 1984.

64. Koch, R.A., and Jackson, D.W. Pubic symphysitis in runners, a report of two cases. Am J Sports Med 9:62–63, 1981.

65. Komaki, R., Donegan, W., Manoli, R., et al. Prognostic value of pretreatment bone scans in breast carcinoma. Am J Roentgenol 132:877–881, 1979.

66. Kroon, H.M.J.A., and Pauwels, E.K.J. Bone scintigraphy for the detection and follow-up of hypertrophic osteoarthropathy. Diagn Imaging 51:47–55, 1982.

67. Lee, J.Y. Bone scintigraphy in evaluation of Didronel therapy for Paget's disease. Clin Nucl Med 6:356–358, 1981.

68. Lee, Y-T.N. Bone scanning in patients with early breast carcinoma: Should it be a routine staging procedure? Cancer 47:486–495, 1981.

69. Levenson, R.M., Sauerbrunn, B.J.L., Bates, H.R., et al. Comparative value of bone scintigraphy and radiography in monitoring tumor response in systemically treated prostatic carcinoma. Radiology 146:513–518, 1984.

70. Levine, E., DeSmet, A.A., Neff, J.R., and Martin, N.L. Scintigraphic evaluation of giant cell tumor of bone. Am J Roentgenol 143:343–348, 1984.

71. Levy, J.M. Stress fractures of the first metatarsal. Am J Roentgenol 130:679–681, 1978.

72. Lindstrom, E., and Lindstrom, F.D. Skeletal scintigraphy with technetium diphosphonate in multiple myeloma—A comparison with skeletal x-ray. Acta Med Scand 208:289–291, 1980.

73. Lisbona, R., and Rosenthall, L. Assessment of bone viability by scintiscanning in frostbite injuries. J Trauma 16:989–992, 1976.

74. Lisbona, R., and Rosenthall, L. Observations on the sequential use of ^{99m}Tc phosphate complex and ^{67}Ga imaging in osteomyelitis, cellulitis and septic arthritis. Radiology 123:123–129, 1977.

75. Lisbona, R., and Rosenthall, L. Role of radionuclide imaging in osteoid osteoma. Am J Roentgenol 132:77–80, 1979.

76. Lucie, R.S., Fuller, S., Burdick, D.C., and Johnston, R.M. Early prediction of avascular necrosis of the femoral head following femoral neck fractures. Clin Orthop 161:207–214, 1981.

77. Ludwig, H., Kumpan, W., and Sinzinger, H. Radiography and bone scintigraphy in multiple myeloma: A comparative analysis. Br J Radiol 55:173–181, 1982.

78. Majd, M. Radionuclide imaging in early detection of childhood osteomyelitis and its differentiation from cellulitis and bone infarction. Ann Radiol 20:9–18, 1977.

79. Martin, N.L., Preston, D.F., and Robins, R.G. Osteoblastomas of the axial skeleton shown by skeletal scanning: Case report. J Nucl Med 17:187–189, 1976.

80. Maslack, M.M., and Babyn, P.S. Methylene diphosphonate uptake in traumatized muscles. Clin Nucl Med 9:491–492, 1984.

81. Matin, P. The appearance of bone scan following fractures including intermediate and long term studies. J Nucl Med 20:1227–1231, 1979.

82. Matin, P., Lang, G., Carretta, R., and Simon, G. Scintigraphic evaluation of muscle damage following extreme exercise. J Nucl Med 24:308–311, 1983.

83. Maurer, A.H., Chen, D.C.P., Camargo, E.E., et al. Utility of three-phase skeletal scintigraphy in suspected osteomyelitis: Concise communication. J Nucl Med 22:941–949, 1981.

84. McKillop, J.H., Etcubanas, E., and Goris, M.L. The indications for and limitations of bone scintigraphy in osteogenic sarcoma. Cancer 48:1133–1338, 1981.

85. McNeil, B.J. Rationale for the use of bone scans in selected metastatic and primary bone tumors. Semin Nucl Med 8:336–345, 1978.

86. McNeil, B.J., Cassady, J.R., Geiser, C.F., et al. Fluorine-18 bone scintigraphy in children with osteosarcoma or Ewing's sarcoma. Radiology 109:627–631, 1973.

87. McNeil, B.J., and Hauley, J. Analysis of serial radionuclide bone images in osteosarcoma and breast carcinoma. Radiology 135:171–176, 1980.

88. Merten, D.F., Radkowski, M.A., and Leonidas, J.C. The abused child: A radiological reappraisal. Radiology 146:377–381, 1983.

89. Meyers, M.H., Telfer, N., and Moore, T.M. Determination of vascularity of the femoral head with 99m technetium sulphur-colloid: Diagnostic and prognostic significance. J Bone Joint Surg [Am] 59:658–664, 1977.

90. Minikel, J., Sty, J., and Simons, G. Sequential radionuclide bone imaging in avascular pediatric hip conditions. Clin Orthop 202–208, 1983.

91. Moon, N.J., Dworkin, H.J., and LaFleur, P.D. The clinical use of sodium fluoride F18 in bone photoscanning. JAMA 204:116–122, 1968.

92. Murray, I.P.C. Bone scanning in the child and young adult. Skeletal Radiol 5:1–14, 1980.

93. Murray, I.P.C. Photopenia in skeletal scintigraphy of suspected bone and joint infection. Clin Nucl Med 7:13–20, 1982.

94. Namey, T.C., and Daniel, W.W. Scintigraphic study of Osgood-Schlatter disease following delayed presentation. Clin Nucl Med 5:551–553, 1980.

95. Namey, T.C., McIntyre, J., Buse, M., et al. Nucleographic studies of axial spondylarthritides. I. Quantitative sacroiliac scintigraphy in early HLA-B27 associated sacroiliitis. Arthritis Rheum 20:1058–1064, 1977.

96. Nocera, R.M., Sayle, B., Rogers, C., and Wilkey, D. Tc-99m MDP and indium-111 chloride scintigraphy in skeletal tuberculosis. Clin Nucl Med 8:418–420, 1983.

97. Nolan, N.G., Koppikar, M.M., and Kotlyarov, E.V. Role of bone scanning in carcinoma of the breast. Ann Clin Lab Sci 10:105–110, 1980.

98. Olsen, N., Schousen, P., Dirken, H., and Christoffersen, J.K. Regional scintimetry in scaphoid fractures. Acta Orthop Scand 54:380–382, 1983.

99. O'Mara, R.E., and Subramanian, G. Experimental agents for skeletal imaging. Semin Nucl Med 2:38–49, 1972.

100. Omojola, M.F., Cockshott, W.P., and Beatty, E.G. Osteoid osteoma: An evaluation of diagnostic modalities. Clin Radiol 32:199–204, 1981.

101. Osmond, J.D., Pendergrass, H.P., and Potsaid, M.S. Accuracy of ^{99m}Tc-diphosphonate bone scans and roentgenograms in the detection of prostate, breast, and lung carcinoma metastases. Am J Roentgenol 125:972–977, 1975.

102. Ostfeld, E., Airel, A., and Pelet, D. Bone scintigraphic diagnosis in acute frontal sinusitis. Acta Otolaryngol 94:557–561, 1982.

103. Park, H-M., Wheat, L.F., Siddiqui, A.R., et al. Scintigraphic evaluation of diabetic osteomyelitis: Concise communication. J Nucl Med 23:569–573, 1982.

104. Parker, B., Pinckney, L., and Etcubanas, E. Relative efficacy of radiographic and radionuclide bone surveys in detection of skeletal lesions of histiocytosis X. Radiology 134:377–380, 1980.

105. Pavlov, H., Nelson, T.L., Warren, R.F., et al. Stress fractures of the pubic ramus. J Bone Joint Surg [Am] 64:1020–1025, 1982.

106. Pollen, J.J., Witztum, K.F., and Ashburn, W.L. The flare phenomenon on radionuclide bone scan in metastatic prostate cancer. Am J Roentgenol 142:773–776, 1984.

107. Prather, J.L., Nusynowitz, M.L., Snowdy, H.A., et al. Scintigraphic findings in stress fractures. J Bone Joint Surg [Am] 59:869–874, 1977.

108. Quinn, W.B., Graebner, J.E., and Arenson, D.G. Diagnosing osteo-

myelitis: Evaluation and significance of multiple tracer bone imaging. J Foot Surg 22:178–182, 1983.

109. Rappaport, A.H., Hoffer, P.B., and Genant, H.K. Unifocal bone findings by scintigraphy: Clinical significance in patients with known primary cancer. West J Med 129:188–192, 1978.

110. Reginato, A.J., Schiappaccasse, V., Gusman, L., and Calure, H. ^{99m}Technetium-pyrophosphate scintigraphy in bone sarcoidosis. J Rheumatol 3:426–436, 1976.

111. Rinksky, L.A., Goris, M., Bleck, E.E., et al. Intraoperative skeletal scintigraphy for localization of osteoid-osteoma in the spine: A case report. J Bone Joint Surg [Am] 62:143–144, 1980.

112. Rohatgi, P.K. Radioisotope scanning in osseous sarcoidosis. Am J Roentgenol 134:189–191, 1980.

113. Rosenthall, L., Hill, R.O., and Chuang, S. Observation on the use of ^{99m}Tc-phosphate imaging in peripheral bone trauma. Radiology 119:637–641, 1976.

114. Rosenthall, L., and Kirsh, J. Observations on radionuclide imaging in hypertrophic pulmonary osteoarthropathy. Radiology 120:359–362, 1976.

115. Rosenthall, L., Kloiber, R., Damten, B., and Al-Majid, H. Sequential use of radiophosphate and radiogallium imaging in the differential diagnosis of bone, joint and soft tissue infection: Quantitative analysis. Diagn Imaging 51:249–258, 1982.

116. Rossleigh, M.A., Lovegrove, F.T.A., Reynolds, P.M., and Byrne, M.J. Serial bone scans in the assessment of response to therapy in advanced breast carcinoma. Clin Nucl Med 7:397–402, 1982.

117. Roub, L.W., Gumerman, L.W., Hanley, E.N., et al. Bone stress: A radionuclide imaging perspective. Radiology 132:431–438, 1979.

118. Rust, R.J., Park, H.M., and Robb, J.A. Skeletal scintigraphy in military tuberculosis: Photopenia after treatment. Am J Roentgenol 137:877–879, 1981.

119. Salit, I.E., Detsky, A.S., Simor, A.E., et al. Gallium-67 scanning in the diagnosis of postoperative sternal osteomyelitis: Concise communication. J Nucl Med 24:1001–1004, 1983.

120. Schauwecker, D.S., Park, H-M., Mock, B.H., et al. Evaluation of complicating osteomyelitis with Tc-99m MDP, In-111 granulocytes, and Ga-67 citrate. J Nucl Med 25:849–853, 1984.

121. Shafa, M.H., Fernandez-Ulloa, M., Rost, R.C., and Nyquist, S.R. Diagnosis of aseptic necrosis of the talus by bone scintigraphy. Clin Nucl Med 8:50–53, 1983.

122. Siddiqui, A.R., and Ellis, J.H. "Cold spot" on bone scan at the site of primary osteosarcoma. Eur J Nucl Med 7:480–481, 1982.

123. Silberstein, E.B., Sanger, E., Tofe, A.J., et al. Imaging of bone metastases with ^{99m}Tc-Sn-EHDP (diphosphonate), F-18, and skeletal radiography. Radiology 107:551–555, 1973.

124. Silver, H.M., Shirkloda, A., and Simon, D.B. Symptomatic osseous sarcoidosis with findings on bone scan. Chest 73:238–241, 1978.

125. Smith, F.W., and Gilday, D.L. Scintigraphic appearances of osteoid osteoma. Radiology 137:191–195, 1980.

126. Spencer, D.G., Adams, F.G., Horton, P.W., et al. Scintiscanning in ankylosing spondylitis: A clinical and radiological quantitative radioisotopic study. J Rheumatol 6:426–431, 1979.

127. Spencer, R.P., Lange, R.C., and Treves, S. Use of ^{135m}Ba and ^{131}Ba as bone scanning agents. J Nucl Med 12:216–221, 1971.

128. Spencer, R.P., Lee, Y.S., Sziklas, J.J., et al. Failure of uptake of radiocolloid by the femoral heads: A diagnostic problem. J Nucl Med 24:116–118, 1983.

129. Spies, S.M., Swift, T.R., and Brown, M. Increased ^{99m}Tc-polyphosphate muscle uptake in a patient with polymyositis. Case report. J Nucl Med 16:1125–1127, 1975.

130. Starshak, R.J., Simons, G.W., and Sty, J.R. Occult fracture of the calcaneus—Another toddler's fracture. Pediatr Radiol 14:37–40, 1984.

131. Sty, J., and Simons, G. Intraoperative ^{99m}technetium bone imaging in the treatment of benign osteoblastic tumors. Clin Orthop 165:223–227, 1982.

132. Sty, J.R., and Starshak, R.J. The role of bone scintigraphy in the

evaluation of the suspected abused child. Radiology 146:369–375, 1983.

133. Subramanian, G., and McAfee, J.G. A new complex of ^{99m}Tc for skeletal imaging. Radiology 99:192–196, 1971.

134. Subramanian, G., McAfee, J.G., Blair, R.J., et al. Technetium-99m-methylene diphosphonate—A superior agent for skeletal imaging: Comparison with other technetium complexes. J Nucl Med 16:744–755, 1975.

135. Swee, R.G., McLeod, R.A., and Beabout, J.W. Osteoid osteoma: Detection, diagnosis, and localization. Radiology 130:117–123, 1979.

136. Szasz, I., Morrison, R.T., and Lyster, D.M., and Naiman, S.C. Bone scintigraphy in massive disseminated bone necrosis. Clin Nucl Med 6:97–100, 1981.

137. Tachdjian, M. 99m technetium diphosphonate bone imaging in Legg-Calve-Perthes' disease. Acta Orthop Belg 46:366–370, 1980.

138. Tamir, R., Glanz, I., Lubin, E., et al. Comparison of the sensitivity of ^{99m}Tc-methyl diphosphonate bone scan with the skeletal x-ray survey in multiple myeloma. Acta Haematol 69:236–242, 1983.

139. Tehranzadeh, J., Schneider, R., and Freiberger, R.H. Radiological evaluation of painful total hip replacement. Radiology 141:355–362, 1981.

140. Thrall, J.H., Geslien, G.E., Corcoran, R.G., and Johnson, M.O. Abnormal radionuclide deposition patterns adjacent to local skeletal lesions. Radiology 115:659–663, 1975.

141. Torg, J.S., Pavlov, H., Cooley, L.H., et al. Stress fractures of the tarsal navicular. J Bone Joint Surg [Am] 64:700–712, 1982.

142. Turner, J.H. Post-traumatic avascular necrosis of the femoral head predicted by preoperative technetium-99m antimony-colloid scan. J Bone Joint Surg [Am] 65:786–797, 1983.

143. Tyler, J.L., Derbekyan, V., and Lisbona, R. Early diagnosis of myositis ossificans with Tc-99m diphosphonate imaging. Clin Nucl Med 9:256–258, 1984.

144. Valk, P. Muscle localization of Tc-99m MDP after exertion. Clin Nucl Med 9:493–494, 1984.

145. Vigorita, V.J., and Ghelman, B. Localization of osteoid osteomas—Use of radionuclide scanning and autoimaging in identifying the nidus. Am J Clin Pathol 79:223–225, 1983.

146. Virupannavar, S., Shirazi, P.H., Khedkar, N.V., and Kaplan, E. Tc-99m PYP localization in calf muscle necrosis. Clin Nucl Med 9:286–287, 1984.

147. Wahner, H.W., Kyle, R.A., and Beabout, J.W. Scintigraphic evaluation of the skeleton in multiple myeloma. Mayo Clin Proc 55:739–746, 1980.

148. Wald, E.R., Mirro, R., and Gartner, J.C. Pitfalls in the diagnosis of acute osteomyelitis by bone scan. Clin Pediatr 19:597–600, 1980.

149. Waxman, A.D., McKee, D., Siemsen, J.K., and Singer, F.R. Gallium scanning in Paget's disease of bone: Effect of calcitonin. Am J Roentgenol 134:303–306, 1980.

150. Weingrad, T., Heyman, S., and Alavi, A. Cold lesions on bone scan in pediatric neoplasms. Clin Nucl Med 9:125–130, 1984.

151. Weissberg, D.L., Resnick, D., Taylor, A., et al. RA and its variants: Analysis of scintiphotographic, radiologic, and clinical examinations. Am J Roentgenol 131:665–673, 1978.

152. Weiss, P.E., Mall, J.C., Hoffer, P.B., et al. ^{99m}Tc-methylene diphosphonate bone imaging in the evaluation of total hip prostheses. Radiology 133:727–729, 1979.

153. Wilcox, J.R., Jr., Moniot, A.L., and Green, J.P. Bone scanning in the evaluation of exercise-related stress injuries. Radiology 123:699–703, 1977.

154. Williams, E.D., Tregonning, R.J., and Hurley, P.J. ^{99m}Tc-diphosphonate scanning as an aid to diagnosis of infection in total hip joint replacements. Br J Radiol 50:562–566, 1977.

155. Williams, F., McCall, I.W., Park, W.M., et al. Gallium-67 scanning in the painful total hip replacement. Clin Radiol 32:431–439, 1981.

156. Williamson, B.R.J., McLaughlin, R.E., Wang, G-J., et al. Radionu-

clide bone imaging as a means of differentiating loosening and infection in patients with a painful total hip prosthesis. Radiology 133:723–725, 1979.

157. Wilson, G.S., Rich, M.A., and Brennan, M.J. Evaluation of bone scan in preoperative clinical staging of breast cancer. Am J Surg 115:415–419, 1980.

158. Wilson, M.A. The effect of age on the quality of bone scans using technetium-99m pyrophosphate. Radiology 139:703–705, 1981.

159. Winter, P.F., Johnson, P.M., Hilal, S.K., and Feldman, F. Scinti-

graphic detection of osteoid osteoma. Radiology 122:177–178, 1977.

160. Woolfenden, J.M., Pitt, M.J., Durie, B.G.M., and Moon, T.E. Comparison of bone scintigraphy and radiography in multiple myeloma. Radiology 134:723–728, 1980.

161. Yeh, S.D.J., Rosen, G., and Benua, R.S. Gallium scans in Paget's sarcoma. Clin Nucl Med 7:546–551, 1982.

CHAPTER 26

Arthrography in Orthopaedics

George H. Belhobek

Arthrography is a commonly used technique. This chapter reviews the indications and modifications of the technique on a regional basis.

UPPER LIMB

Shoulder Arthrography

Both single- and double-contrast techniques have been described for shoulder arthrography. Single-contrast arthrography consists of injecting 12 to 15 ml of an equal mixture of positive contrast material (e.g., meglumine diatrizoate) and 1% lidocaine into the glenohumeral joint.[18] Care is taken not to overdistend the joint capsule so as to avoid extravasation of contrast material. X-ray views are obtained in the anteroposterior (AP), axillary, and bicipital groove projections (Fig. 26-1).

Double-Contrast Technique

The double-contrast shoulder arthrogram popularized by Goldman and Ghelman is produced by injecting 4 ml of positive contrast medium and 10 ml of room air into the shoulder joint.[32,38] A portion of the AP filming during double-contrast arthrography is carried out with the patient in the upright position to take advantage of the air-contrast interface at the inferior surface of the rotator cuff.

The double-contrast arthrogram provides more-specific information in regard to rotator cuff tears, offers better visualization of the articular cartilage and glenoid labrum, and is

more helpful in evaluating for tears or dislocations of the long head of the biceps tendon (Fig. 26-2).[38] This added information is obtained at the expense of a slightly more complicated and time-consuming filming sequence compared with the single-contrast technique. Interpretation of a double-contrast study is also considered more difficult, and Goldman and Ghelman noted that the double-contrast study might have limitations in the diagnosis of adhesive capsulitis since air tends to extravasate from the joint more easily than positive contrast material.[38]

The Normal Shoulder Arthrogram

Contrast material injected into the normal shoulder joint remains within the confines of the joint capsule except for extension into the subscapularis bursa and extension for a distance along the long head of the biceps tendon in the bicipital groove. A prominent axillary pouch is normally present. An indentation between the subscapularis recess and the axillary pouch is seen at the point of attachment of the anterior joint capsule on the glenoid labrum. Contrast material ends abruptly along the anatomic neck of the humerus and does not extend beyond the greater tuberosity (Fig. 26-1). In the axillary projection, contrast medium is identified between the glenoid cavity and the humeral head. Cartilaginous surfaces of the shoulder joint and the glenoid labrum are best visualized in this projection. Contrast material does not normally project over the surgical neck of the humerus because the joint capsule does not extend to this level. Contrast material seen overlying the surgical neck must be located within the subacromial-subdeltoid bursa and indicates a complete

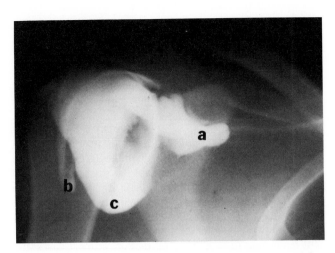

Figure 26-1 Normal shoulder arthrogram. Contrast material injected into the normal shoulder remains within the confines of the joint except for extension into the subscapular bursa *(a)*, and extension for a distance along the long head of the biceps tendon in the bicipital groove *(b)*. A prominent axillary recess *(c)* is normally present.

rotator cuff tear (see next section). The tangential view of the biceps groove should demonstrate contrast material surrounding the biceps tendon in the intertubercular groove.

The Abnormal Arthrogram

Rotator Cuff Tear The major indication for arthrography of the shoulder joint is suspected rotator cuff tear. These tears can involve the entire thickness of the cuff (complete tear) or can extend only partially through the cuff (partial thickness tear). Plain x-ray films of patients with rotator cuff tears generally do not indicate the diagnosis. Plain radiographic findings suggesting a cuff tear, such as a decrease in the humeral-acromion distance, cystic or sclerotic changes in the greater tuberosity, and a concave appearance of the acromion, have been described. These signs, however, are not diagnostic.

The diagnosis of a complete rotator cuff tear by shoulder arthrography depends on the extravasation of contrast medium through the tear into the subacromial-subdeltoid bursa (Fig. 26-3).

In the AP projection, this contrast material is seen as a collection superior and lateral to the greater tuberosity extending to the level of the anterior-inferior margin of the acromion process. This collection is separated from the articular cavity by a radiolucency of variable size which represents fragments of the torn cuff. On the axillary projection, contrast medium in the bursa will overlay the surgical neck of the humerus (saddlebag sign). The double-contrast arthrogram provides additional information about the degree of retraction of torn cuff fragments and gives an estimation of the degree of tendon degeneration present, information which may influence the surgeon's choice of an operative approach.[38]

Partial tears are seen as ulcerlike or linear collections of gas or positive contrast material extending from the articular cavity into the substance of the rotator cuff. Only tears which include the inferior surface of the cuff can be diagnosed by shoulder arthrography. Tears confined to the midsubstance or bursal side of the cuff are not visualized with contrast material injected intraarticularly.

The diagnosis of rotator cuff tears can usually be made easily on the basis of arthrographic findings (Fig. 26-4). However, several potential sources of error must be recognized. Inadequate distribution of contrast material within the joint may prevent visualization of small cuff tears. Scar formation in a small cuff tear can also lead to false-negative diagnoses (Fig. 26-5). The contrast-filled biceps tendon sheath may project slightly lateral to the greater tuberosity on a fully externally rotated AP film, simulating the filling of a small subacromial bursa and leading to a false-positive diagnosis. Inadver-

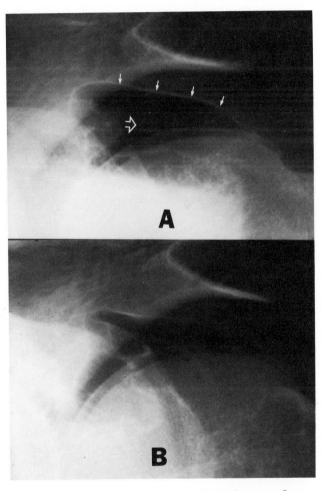

Figure 26-2 The double-contrast shoulder arthrogram. Spot films of the rotator cuff made with the patient in the upright position. **A.** External rotation. **B.** Internal rotation. This study permits a more detailed evaluation of the cuff tendons *(small arrows)*. Notice the long head of the biceps tendon *(open arrow)* as it traverses the joint from its origin on the superior glenoid labrum.

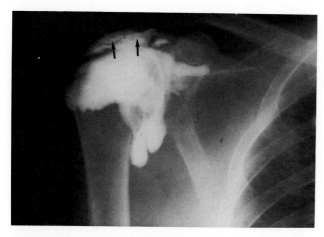

Figure 26-3 Rotator cuff tear. Single-contrast shoulder arthrogram. The intraarticular contrast material extravasates through the tear into the subacromial-subdeltoid bursa *(arrows).*

tent bursal injection may result in a false-positive diagnosis of a rotator cuff tear unless one recognizes that the articular cavity has not been opacified.[111]

There is recent evidence that ultrasonography can serve as an effective noninvasive diagnostic study for patients with suspected rotator cuff tears. Sonography images the full thickness of the rotator cuff, and it is capable of detecting partial tears of the substance or superficial surface of the cuff. These are locations where false-negative arthrograms are common. While there are disadvantages to the sonographic examination of the rotator cuff (evaluation limited to distal cuff, decreased resolution compared with arthrography, inability to differentiate between complete and incomplete tears in all cases), ultrasonography has the potential to become an effective screening examination for cuff abnormality since it appears that with a sonographic diagnosis of a normal cuff, a rotator cuff tear can be excluded with a high degree of confidence.[79,81]

Adhesive Capsulitis Adhesive capsulitis may develop following shoulder trauma. The exact pathological basis for this condition is unknown, although capsular thickening and adhesions between the capsule and the bicipital tendon or about the subacromial bursa are felt to play a part in the process.[111] Adhesive capsulitis results in a significant loss of distensibility of shoulder joint capsule and leads to a significant restriction of shoulder joint motion. In most cases, the plain shoulder x-ray views of a patient with adhesive capsulitis are normal.

The arthrographic diagnosis of adhesive capsulitis is based on the demonstration of a joint capsule of diminished size. The normal shoulder joint easily holds 10 to 15 ml of contrast medium. With adhesive capsulitis, this volume is significantly decreased (less than 10 ml), and early on during the injection of the joint, resistance is felt against the syringe plunger. There is decreased filling of the subscapular and biceps tendon recesses and narrowing of the axillary pouch. Rotator cuff tears may be associated with adhesive capsulitis.[134]

Most authors agree that single-contrast arthrography is the method of choice for demonstrating significant adhesive capsulitis.[18,111,134] Goldman and Ghelman point out that the injection of air into a joint capsule of diminished size often

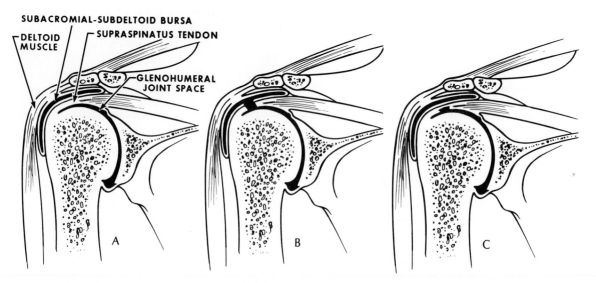

Figure 26-4 Arthrography of shoulder with different patterns of rotator cuff tear. **A.** Normal shoulder. The subacromial-subdeltoid bursa is separated from the shoulder joint capsule by the rotator cuff tendons. Contrast material introduced into the shoulder joint remains confined to this space. **B.** Shoulder with a complete tear of the rotator cuff tendons allows intraarticular contrast material to extravasate into the subacromial-subdeltoid bursa through the cuff tear. **C.** Shoulder with a partial-thickness tear involving the joint side of the cuff. Ulcerlike collections of contrast material are seen.

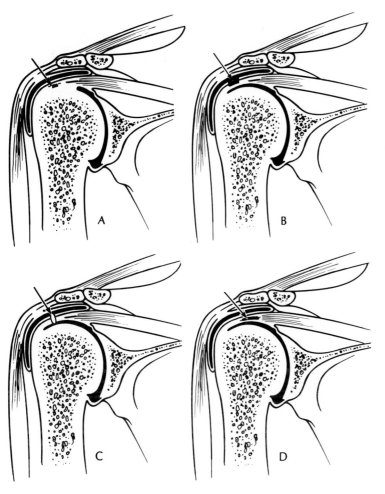

Figure 26-5 Some causes of erroneous interpretation in shoulder arthrography. Poor distribution of contrast material in the joint may cause an incomplete marginal tear to be missed **(A)**. Cuff tears confined to the midsubstance **(D)** or the subacromial bursa side of the cuff **(B)** will not be diagnosed by shoulder arthrography. Occasionally, scar formation in a cuff tear leads to a false-negative diagnosis **(C)**.

results in extravasation of the gas, thereby causing a technically poor study.[38]

Several authors have advocated distension arthrography in the treatment of adhesive capsulitis. Gilula et al reported an improved range of motion and lessening of symptoms in a small group of patients receiving diagnostic single-contrast arthrograms.[34] Loyd and Loyd treated 31 patients with adhesive capsulitis by distension of the shoulder joint capsule with a mixture of contrast medium, 1% xylocaine, and 40 mg of methylprednisolone acetate (Depo-medrol) followed by gentle manipulation of the shoulder. They described significant improvement in most of these patients following the procedure.[78] Resnick suggests that progressive enlargement of the joint capsule via a technique called *brisement* can be therapeutic in patients with adhesive capsulitis.[111]

Recurrent Dislocations Because of the inherent instability of the shoulder, this joint is dislocated more frequently than other large joints. Anterior dislocations are far more frequent than posterior dislocations. Recurrent anterior dislocations may follow the initial injury, especially in younger patients. The demonstration of a compression fracture on the posterolateral aspect of a humeral head (Hill-Sachs deformity) or a fracture of the antero-inferior margin of the glenoid labrum

on plain x-ray views allows an accurate diagnosis of a previous anterior dislocation. Documentation of such a dislocation is more difficult when the humeral head has relocated and there are no accompanying bony abnormalities. Shoulder arthrography can demonstrate soft tissue abnormality which confirms previous shoulder dislocations.

Enlargement of the joint capsule (balloon capsule) and disruption of the glenoid labrum are arthrographic findings seen with shoulder dislocations. Tomograms made in the axial projection following double-contrast arthrography (arthrotomography) have been shown to significantly increase the accuracy of diagnosis of glenoid labrum abnormalities.[28,67] Computed tomography (CT) scans following double-contrast arthrography (computed arthrotomography) have been advocated as a more comprehensive and more easily obtainable method than conventional arthrotomography in this regard.[24,125] Deutsch et al published data from a study comparing computed and conventional arthrotomography in the diagnosis of glenoid labrum abnormalities. They found both techniques to be sensitive methods of assessing the labrum. However, CT showed a slightly higher accuracy (96 to 86 percent) and required less technical expertise and radiation exposure.[24] Computed arthrotomography of the shoulder has the added advantage of being able to detect Hill-Sachs deformities and to delineate the tendon of the long head of the biceps within the biceps groove, and has the potential to assess disorders of osseous development of the glenoid fossa and humerus which are thought to predispose to glenohumeral joint instability.[24,117,125]

Abnormalities of the Tendon of the Long Head of the Biceps Abnormalities of the bicipital tendon and sheath can be diagnosed by arthrography. These include complete and partial tendon ruptures, tendon dislocations and subluxations, and tenosynovitis. Interpretation of the studies is complicated by the many normal variations of the tendon sheath.[111] Contrast filling of the biceps tendon sheath in the intertubercular groove is not constant, and, therefore, nonvisualization of the tendon in the groove is not a reliable sign of tendon rupture. Similarly, leakage of contrast medium from the sheath can be due to overdistension of the joint and is not diagnostic of tendon abnormality. The arthrographic diagnosis of a complete tear of the biceps tendon is made when the radiolucent filling defect of the normal tendon is not seen in the contrast-filled tendon sheath or when the sheath is grossly distorted. Incomplete tears of the tendon may result in an increase in the width of the tendon shadow. Medial dislocation of the tendon is suggested when the position of the structure does not change on the internal and external rotation AP views of the shoulder or when the tendon is visualized medial to the groove on the biceps groove projection.[18,111] Computed arthrotomography can be helpful in evaluating biceps tendon abnormalities.[24]

Articular Abnormalities As in the knee joint, arthrography can be helpful in the investigation of patients with various articular disorders of the shoulder joint. Synovial thickening, synovial nodularity, and synovial masses are demonstrated by arthrography. Contrast filling of paraarticular lymphatics may be seen with inflammatory arthropathies. Loose bodies are best evaluated with single-contrast studies using air alone as contrast medium.

Shoulder Impingement Syndrome Plain radiographs of the shoulder may show subacromial spurs at the insertion of the ligamentous coracoacromial arch and corresponding bony proliferation and cystic changes on the greater tuberosity. A fluoroscopic examination of the shoulder during manipulation of the humerus is considered positive for impingement when a patient's symptoms are reproduced at the point of contact between the greater tuberosity and the undersurface of the acromion or subacromial spur.[14] Shoulder arthrography in these patients may demonstrate complete or partial rotator cuff tears at the point of impingement.

Subacromial bursography has been advocated by a few as a means of documenting impingement of an intact rotator cuff against the coracoacromial arch. The bursogram is obtained by injecting 3 to 4 ml of water-soluble contrast material into the subacromial-subdeltoid bursa under fluoroscopic control. Abnormal distribution of contrast material during abduction of the shoulder suggests impingement.[73] Irregularity of the outline of the bursa would suggest adhesions or synovial proliferations. Theoretically, partial tears of the outer surface of the rotator cuff should be diagnosable by

subacromial bursography. Practically speaking, however, these are difficult to identify due to overlapping of structures. Subacromial bursography is performed only as an adjunctive study usually following shoulder arthrography.[73,130]

Elbow Arthrography

Elbow arthrography can be carried out using either single- or double-contrast techniques.

With single-contrast arthrography, standard radiographs in the AP, lateral, and both oblique planes are obtained after the injection of contrast material. Fluoroscopy of the joint is noted to be helpful by several authors.[6,55] Similar projections are obtained for the double-contrast technique. Pavlov et al feel that with the double-contrast technique, additional filming to include radiographs with the elbow in positions to vary the dependent portions of the joint can be helpful in evaluation of intraarticular loose bodies.[102]

The application of tomography to elbow arthrography is felt by many authors to be the best method of evaluating elbow joint abnormality.[29,55,85] The complex anatomy of the elbow makes it difficult to demonstrate all of the articular cartilage in profile on standard radiographic projections. Loose bodies are often multiple and quite small and may be difficult to visualize on the plain radiographs made during arthrography. Arthrotomography improves the ability to localize articular cartilage defects and to demonstrate small loose bodies. Tomography is particularly effective when coupled with the double-contrast arthrographic technique. Scout tomograms at 3-mm intervals in the AP and lateral projections should precede the arthrogram. Identical sections are then made after the injection of contrast medium. A fluoroscopic examination following arthrotomography can add additional diagnostic information.

The Normal Elbow Arthrogram

There are a number of important features of the anatomy of the elbow joint. A fibrous capsule encloses the articular surfaces of the elbow. A synovial membrane lines the fibrous capsule and is attached to the articular margins of the humerus, radius, and ulna. It is reflected under the annular ligament to line the pararadial recess about the neck of the radius. Three joint recesses can be identified: (1) the coronoid recess (anterior), (2) the olecranon recess (posterior), and (3) the pararadial recess (annular). They form potential reservoirs for loose bodies. The articulating cartilages of the elbow joint are smooth and uniform in thickness except for a portion of the ulna in the trochlear notch where the cartilage is normally deficient and the bone roughened. The articular cartilage of the capitellum is limited to its anterior and inferior surfaces. Cartilage is present on the trochlea anteriorly, inferiorly, and posteriorly.[29,55]

Certain features of normal anatomy must not be confused with abnormality. The anterior border of the coronoid recess often appears wrinkled during elbow flexion, and the border adjacent to the medial collateral ligament is typically irregular. This irregularity resolves with the elbow in extension. A small, concentric projection of normal synovium ex-

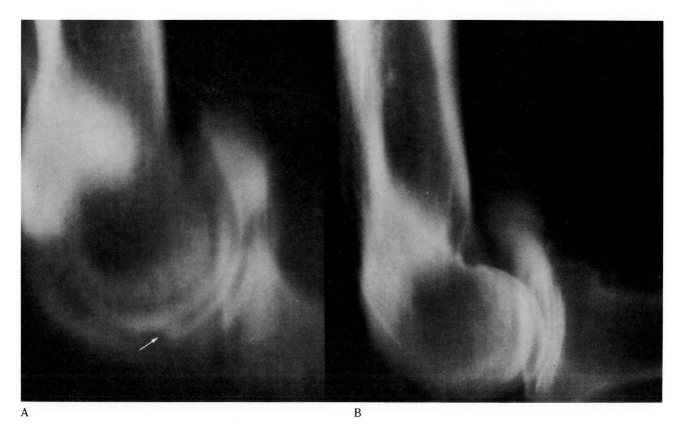

A   B

Figure 26-6 Double-contrast elbow arthrotomogram demonstrates the normal appearance of the articular surfaces of the ulnar-trochlear joint (**A**) and the radial-capitellar joint (**B.**) The small cartilaginous defect normally present within the trochlear notch *(arrow)* should not be confused with an osteochondral defect.

tends from the lateral capsule into the radiocapitellar joint. The small cartilaginous defect normally present deep within the trochlear notch should not be confused with an osteochondral defect (Fig. 26-6).[55]

The Abnormal Elbow Arthrogram

Articular Cartilage Abnormalities and Loose Body Formation Elbow arthrography is most commonly employed for the evaluation of articular cartilage abnormalities and for the detection and localization of loose bodies. Arthrography can determine which paraarticular calcific densities seen on plain radiographs lie within the joint cavity and which are embedded in the soft tissues. Double-contrast arthrotomography has the potential to demonstrate loose bodies which are not readily apparent on plain x-ray views or in plain arthrographic studies. Occasionally, arthrotomography demonstrates a cartilaginous loose body which has not been suspected on plain radiographs. Arthrotomograms must be compared with prearthrography scout tomograms so that small ossified bodies are not overlooked because of masking by positive contrast material. Double-contrast arthrotomography also has the greatest potential to demonstrate articular cartilage abnormalities.

Intraarticular loose bodies are diagnosed when they are shown to be completely surrounded by contrast material and are shown to move freely within the joint. Postarthrography fluoroscopy can be helpful in demonstrating this. Calcifications that are fixed in the periarticular tissues may move, but less freely than loose bodies; they do not roll over and they do not fall into dependent portions of the joint.[55] Joint impingement by thickened synovium or bony prominences resulting in decreased joint motion can also be documented during arthrotomography and fluoroscopy.

Arthrography may be used to assess the condition of the articular cartilage involved with osteochondritis dissecans. Because fissures in the cartilage may be thin and difficult to see, it is desirable to evaluate the articular surfaces with arthrotomography. Deformity or irregularity of the articular surfaces may also be demonstrated (Fig. 26-7).[55]

Trauma Acute and chronic osteochondral fractures may be documented by double-contrast arthrotomography in much the same fashion as osteochondritis dissecans. The location and extent of condylar fractures in the immature skeleton and deformities resulting from remote trauma can also be evaluated with this procedure. Single-contrast techniques have been suggested for this purpose.[6] Mink et al have used single-contrast arthrotomography to evaluate recurrent dislocations of the elbow.[85]

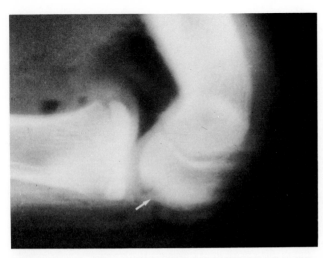

Figure 26-7 This arthrotomogram section through the radial-capitellar portion of the elbow joint of a 12-year-old baseball pitcher demonstrates an osteochondral fracture *(arrow)* of the articular surface of the capitellum. This fracture was not apparent on plain x-ray examination of the elbow.

Wrist Arthrography

Wrist arthrography is a well-established technique which can be useful in the evaluation of patients with chronic wrist pain. Early investigators stressed the application of this procedure to patients with rheumatoid arthritis.[51,108] Subsequent publications point out the usefulness of this procedure in studying various rheumatologic diseases,[112] paraarticular masses,[3] and abnormality induced by trauma.[72,93]

The Normal Wrist Arthrogram

Most arthrographers recommend primary injection of the radiocarpal joint for wrist arthrography.[19,51,68,72,108,112] Contrast material injected into the radiocarpal joint should remain within this compartment except for filling of the pisiform-triquetrum joint, which has been noted to fill in as many as 69 percent of patients.[72] The high percentage of pisiform-triquetrum joint filling has prompted the feeling that this communication represents a normal human variant or degenerative phenomenon.[72,93]

Small recesses or excrescences are seen beneath the volar aspect of the distal radius.[19,112] Medial indentation of the compartment produces a proximal pouch called the *prestyloid recess* and a distal pouch which is proximal to the ulnar aspect of the triquetrum.

Communication between the radiocarpal compartment and either the midcarpal or the distal radioulnar compartments is considered abnormal.[72] Tendon sheaths and lymphatics are not normally opacified.

The Abnormal Wrist Arthrogram

Evaluation of Arthritides Arthrography in patients with inflammatory arthritis may demonstrate synovial, soft tissue, or cartilaginous abnormalities which are not visualized on routine roentgenograms.[51,108,112] Multiple authors have described synovial irregularities and a corrugated appearance of the joint capsule as common findings in rheumatoid arthritis. Communications between the midcarpal and distal radioulnar joints and filling of the flexor and extensor tendon sheaths are frequent findings in the rheumatoid wrist. Contrast filling of paraarticular lymphatics is also seen frequently. Lymphatic filling is a phenomenon common to the inflammatory arthritides, the result of synovial inflammation and hypertrophy.[112] Arthrographic findings identical to those seen in rheumatoid arthritis may be seen in other inflammatory conditions such as infectious arthritis and ankylosing spondylitis.

The arthrographic pattern of abnormality in wrists with posttraumatic arthritis includes compartment communications, tendon sheath opacification, mild synovial irregularity, and articular cartilage destruction.[112] Lymphatic filling can occasionally be seen with this process.[72]

Arthrography of the Posttraumatic Wrist Arthrography may be useful in the evaluation of patients with chronic posttraumatic wrist pain. Routine radiographs may be normal or equivocal in patients with disruptions of carpal ligaments. Motion series or fluoroscopic examinations of the wrist are helpful in demonstrating wrist deformities which relate to carpal ligament injuries. These procedures, however, can have false-negative results. Wrist arthrography can be used to document these ligamentous tears. Wrist arthrography is performed if the routine and special x-ray studies have revealed no explanation for the wrist pain and ligamentous disruption is strongly suspected clinically.[93]

Contrast material injected into the radiocarpal joint normally remains within this joint compartment with the exception of the previously noted communication between the radiocarpal compartment and the pisiform-triquetrum joint. Communication between the radiocarpal and midcarpal joints would indicate a disruption of either the scapholunate or the lunotriquetral ligament. Fluoroscopic monitoring during contrast injection allows identification of the site of leakage. Tirman et al have recently suggested that contrast injection of the midcarpal joint is a more effective method for evaluating scapholunate and lunotriquetral ligament tears.[135] Care must be taken to correlate clinical, plain radiographic, motion series, and fluoroscopic findings with the arthrographic findings since isolated communication between the radiocarpal and midcarpal joints has been shown to occur in 13 to 47 percent of asymptomatic individuals.[19] The number of asymptomatic communications has been shown to increase with patient age, which suggests that these communications can be the result of a degenerative process.[19,93,112] In a young individual who has sustained trauma to the wrist, however, opacification of the midcarpal compartment after the introduction of contrast material into the radiocarpal joint or opacification of the radiocarpal joint after injection of the midcarpal joint strongly suggests acute disruption of the scapholunate or the lunotriquetral ligament.[113]

The triangular fibrocartilage normally separates the radiocarpal joint from the distal radioulnar joint. Tears of this structure allow communication between the radiocarpal and distal radioulnar joints. Tears in the triangular fibrocartilage can result in clinical symptoms. However, it has been re-

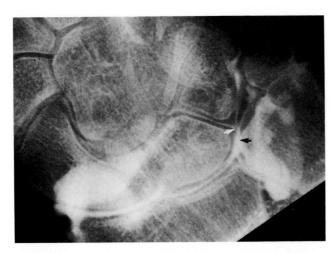

Figure 26-8 Abnormal wrist arthrogram. Contrast material injected into the radiocarpal joint normally remains within this compartment. Extravasation of contrast material into the midcarpal joint indicates a tear of either the scapholunate or lunotriquetral ligaments. Here the white arrow indicates the tear of the lunotriquetral ligament. Contrast material in the inferior radioulnar joint is diagnostic of a triangular fibrocartilage perforation *(black arrow)*.

ported that communication between these two compartments occurs in between 7 and 40 percent of cadavers and asymptomatic individuals, indicating that not all triangular fibrocartilage tears can be indicted as the cause of a patient's symptoms. The incidence of this compartment communication increases with age and is felt to be the result of cartilage degeneration, a traumatic tear, or disruption of the fibrocartilage by an inflammatory process. Palmer et al feel that a perforated triangular cartilage in a wrist with a negative ulnar variance is more likely to be a true traumatic tear than a perforation in a wrist with a positive ulnar variance.[93] The arthrographic demonstration of this compartment communication must be correlated with clinical findings before symptoms are attributed to this abnormality (Fig. 26-8).[68]

Wrist arthrography in conjunction with tomography may help to differentiate fibrous unions from nonunions of scaphoid bone fractures.[19]

LOWER LIMB

Hip Arthrography

The specific indications for hip arthrography vary with the age of the patient.

In infants and children, an important indication for contrast arthrography is the suspicion of a septic hip. Significant damage to the hip joint can occur with bacterial infections if treatment is delayed for even a short time. Plain x-ray findings are generally negative early in the course of the infection. The hip arthrogram is carried out primarily to obtain culture material and secondarily to assess joint damage. A second indi-

cation for arthrography in infants and children is the evaluation of congenital hip dysplasias (congenital hip dislocation, proximal focal femoral deficiency, multiple epiphyseal dysplasia, and congenital coxa vara). While the diagnosis of hip dysplasia is usually established on the basis of a clinical examination and plain x-ray findings, contrast arthrography is useful in demonstrating the severity of the deformity and the degree of joint incongruity. A third indication for hip arthrography in children is the evaluation of Legg-Calvé-Perthes disease. As with the congenital conditions, arthrography is not usually necessary to establish the diagnosis but is useful in determining the severity of the deformity and in diagnosing complications.

In the adolescent and adult, the most frequent indication for contrast studies of the hip joint is the evaluation of primary arthritides. In arthritides such as rheumatoid arthritis and degenerative joint disease, arthrography is performed to evaluate the severity of cartilage destruction and to demonstrate the presence of loose bodies. In diseases such as pigmented villonodular synovitis, synovial osteochondromatosis, and septic arthritis, the plain x-ray examination remains relatively normal for a long period of time. Contrast studies of the joint may be the earliest means of suggesting the diagnosis. Arthrography can also be helpful in the diagnosis of osteochondral fractures and acute chondrolysis.

In adults with hip prostheses, indications for arthrography are related to complications of the procedure. These include loosening of prosthesis components, infection, pseudoarthrosis of a trochanteric osteotomy, and persistent dislocations due to foreign matter within the acetabular component.

Hip Arthrography in Infants and Children

Injection Technique Preliminary AP and frog lateral scout films are made prior to arthrography. It is recommended that children over 6 months of age be sedated with a combination of meperidine hydrochloride (Demerol), diazepam (Valium), and promethazine hydrochloride (Phenergan). Children younger than 6 months of age are restrained during the procedure and generally require no anesthesia.[40] Arthrocentesis is carried out under fluoroscopic control using a 22-gauge 1.5-in. or spinal needle as necessary to reach the joint. The medial aspect of the femoral neck is selected as the preferential site of injection because the normal redundancy of the medial joint capsule gives the arthrographer greater leeway for positioning the needle in an intraarticular position. Anteromedial, anterolateral, and inferomedial approaches to the joint have been described. Strife et al prefer the inferomedial approach because any extravasation of contrast material occurring medially will not obscure the important details of the intracapsular structures.[129] After positioning of the needle, aspiration of the joint is attempted. If fluid is obtained, the material should be sent for culture and sensitivity studies. If no fluid is withdrawn, 5 ml of sterile, nonbacteriostatic saline is injected and reaspirated. Contrast material is not injected prior to joint aspiration since this substance may be bactericidal. The intracapsular position of the needle is checked with a few drops of contrast medium. Confirmation of an intraar-

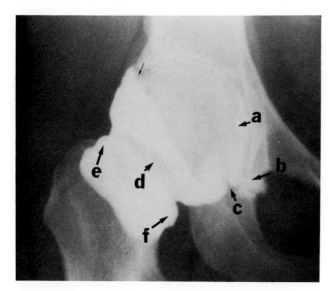

Figure 26-9 Normal hip arthrogram. This AP view obtained during a single-contrast hip arthrogram examination demonstrates a thin, uniform line of contrast material between the femoral head and the acetabulum. The articular cartilage at the superior lateral aspect of the acetabulum is referred to as the limbus *(arrow)*. It is triangular, has a pointed tip, and is outlined both medially and laterally by contrast material. The thin line of contrast material lateral to the limbus is referred to as the limbus thorn. Additional anatomic landmarks are fovea centralis femoris *(a)*, the fossa acetabuli *(b)*, indentation from the ligamentum transversum *(c)*, zona orbicularis *(d)*, superior recess coli *(e)*, and inferior recess coli *(f)*.

ticular position is made when the contrast material is seen to flow away from the end of the needle. Then 2 to 4 ml of a 30% solution of positive contrast material (e.g., Renografin) is injected into the joint. Too great a volume or too dense a concentration of contrast material can obscure normal cartilaginous structures. Routine films include AP, frog lateral, and maximal abduction views.[40]

Normal Arthrographic Anatomy (Fig. 26-9)

The articular cartilage of the acetabulum appears as a radiolucent shadow that is outlined by a thin line of contrast material. Its superolateral aspect, the limbus, has a sharp pointed tip and extends lateral to the osseous acetabulum.[64,123] Both the medial and the lateral side of the limbus are outlined by contrast material. The contrast material that extends lateral to the margin of the limbus is called the limbus "thorn."[123,124] If the femoral head is well-seated in the acetabulum, the tip of the limbus thorn should be no more than 2 to 3 mm above the triradiate cartilage.[124] On all views, the height of the femoral head should measure one-half of its width.[59] The ossific nucleus, if present, should be in the center of the cartilaginous head, and the entire cartilaginous head is normally covered by the acetabulum.[53] On the arthrogram, contrast material normally pools in the two areas of capsular redundancy: the coli recesses and the fossa acetabuli. There is a band of radiolucency across the femoral neck relating to the thick fibers of the orbicular ligament (zona orbicularis).[53,59,64,123,124]

The Septic Hip

The primary role of contrast arthrography in the diagnosis of septic hip is to confirm the intraarticular location of the needle during aspiration. Hip arthrography also may be useful in evaluating late abnormalities of treated septic hips. These include coxa vara deformities, incongruity, and subluxation and pseudosubluxation (the asymmetrical position of the ossific nucleus in the cartilaginous head which gives a false impression of lateral displacement on a plain film).

Congenital Hip Dislocation

The diagnosis of congenital hip dislocation is usually established early in life on the basis of a clinical examination.[39,40] The arthrogram is useful, however, in evaluating those patients who fail to respond to conservative therapy or who are not diagnosed at birth.

The contrast study is helpful in differentiating between complete dislocation and subluxation. The arthrographic criteria for subluxation and dislocation are based on a classification described by Leveuf.[69,70] In the cases of subluxation, the cartilaginous acetabulum incompletely covers the femoral head (less than 50 percent). The limbus thorn becomes elongated since the displaced femoral head rests directly beneath it.[53,124] In complete dislocation, the femoral head is completely uncovered by the cartilaginous acetabulum and is displaced superiorly and laterally. The flexible limbus flips inward to rest between the femoral head and the acetabulum. The joint capsule of the dislocated hip has a characteristic hourglass shape because it is compressed between the limbus and the ligamentum teres.[53,124] Causes of failed hip reduction such as a thickened ligamentum teres; an infolded, blunted limbus; or atrophy and deformity of the acetabulum or femoral head are also demonstrated on the arthrographic study. In older children, the arthrogram is useful in demonstrating femoral acetabular incongruity and can help in the selection of candidates for femoral or innominate osteotomies.[40]

Other Dysplasias

Arthrography can provide useful information concerning the severity of deformity, the presence of incongruity, and the efficacy of therapy in other congenital growth disturbances such as proximal focal femoral deficiency, multiple epiphyseal dysplasias, and congenital coxa vara.[39,40]

Legg-Calvé-Perthes Disease

The diagnosis of Legg-Calvé-Perthes disease is made on the basis of the clinical examination, radionuclide bone scan findings, and plain x-ray abnormalities. Arthrography, however, is useful in demonstrating the two major complications of this disease: incongruity and a persistently detached fragment. The early demonstration of femoral acetabular incongruity is essential in determining the prognosis of avascular necrosis of the femoral head. Plain x-ray films are of little help in obtaining this information. In the first months of the disease, the arthrogram is always normal since in the early stages of Perthes disease, the abnormalities are limited to the

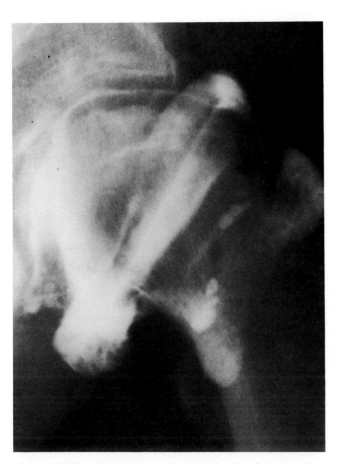

Figure 26-10 Arthrography can be useful when demonstrating the two major complications of Legg-Perthes disease: incongruity and a persistently detached fragment. This arthrogram of a patient with Legg-Perthes disease demonstrates several of the criteria indicative of joint incongruity, including an abnormal shape and irregular contour of the cartilaginous femoral head, incomplete coverage of the femoral head by the acetabulum, and the inferiomedial pooling of contrast material.

ossific nucleus. In the later stages of fragmentation and repair, the cartilaginous structures become involved and the arthrogram becomes useful in demonstrating incongruity.[59,60]

The arthrographic criteria indicative of incongruity and therefore a poor prognosis include (1) an abnormal shape of the cartilaginous femoral head with a decrease in the ratio of the height to one-half the width, (2) an irregular contour of the cartilaginous femoral head, (3) irregularity of the superolateral aspect of the acetabular cartilage, with or without blunting of the limbus, (4) incomplete coverage of the femoral head by the acetabulum, and (5) inferior medial pooling of contrast material (Fig. 26-10).[59,60]

An unusual, late complication of Legg-Calvé-Perthes disease is a persistent, nonunited fragment of the femoral head. Information concerning the integrity of the articular cartilage over this fragment is important in determining the need for surgical treatment. Arthrography, particularly with the addition of tomography (arthrotomography), is an excellent means of evaluating the condition of the articular cartilage overlying a fragment and in determining the potential for a fragment to become a loose body.[53]

Chondrolysis

Chondrolysis or acute cartilaginous necrosis is a serious complication of slipped femoral capital epiphysis. It is thought to be the result of an autoimmune synovitis in genetically susceptible individuals.[41] Routine roentgenograms may demonstrate only juxtaarticular osteoporosis, or osteoporosis plus joint space narrowing. The primary role of arthrography is to obtain aspiration material to rule out infection. High levels of IgM antibodies relating to autolysis of the articular cartilage may be found in the joint aspirate.[41] The contrast study can also demonstrate cartilaginous erosions which may not be apparent on plain x-ray films.

Hip Arthrography in Adolescents and Adults

Normal Hip Arthrogram The criteria for a normal hip arthrogram in the adolescent or the adult are essentially the same as for a child. The principal difference in the arthrographic anatomy is the absence of a cartilaginous component to the femur and acetabulum.[59]

Evaluation of Arthritis There are several ways in which aspiration arthrography can be helpful in the evaluation of arthritides. Analysis of the aspirated joint fluid may establish the diagnosis of septic arthritis (bacterial growth), pigmented villonodular synovitis (bloody fluid), or chondrolysis (high levels of immunoglobulins).[41] The contrast study may demonstrate synovial proliferation characteristic of certain arthritides such as pigmented villonodular synovitis, synovial osteochondromatosis, and tuberculosis. The arthrogram can also demonstrate the severity of cartilage destruction.

In all types of inflammatory arthritides, the outline of the contrast-coated capsule becomes corrugated and irregular. Lymphatic drainage of contrast material can be identified. Abnormal communication with the iliopsoas bursa or greater trochanteric bursa is also seen. Communication between the joint capsule and other cavities suggests abscess formation and septic arthritis.[39]

Long-standing inflammatory arthritis may result in contraction of the joint capsule with loss of normal recesses and retraction of the normal insertions of the joint capsule. The demonstration of a small, thick joint capsule (less than 8 ml capacity) in the absence of chronic infection should suggest the diagnosis of adhesive capsulitis.[42]

Osteochondral Injuries Hip arthrography can demonstrate small avulsion fractures, particularly those arising from the posterior aspect of the femoral head. Klein et al suggest that the application of CT scanning to the arthrographic study enhances the ability to visualize cartilaginous fragments and capsular defects.[66]

Hip arthrography can be helpful in demonstrating the size and number of loose bodies within the joint. Pneumoarthrography or double-contrast arthrography may be more useful in this regard, particularly if tomograms are to be included with the study.

Arthrography of Total Hip Replacements This is discussed in Chap. 71, Sect. A.

Knee Arthrography

Arthrography versus Arthroscopy

The relation of arthrography and arthroscopy in the diagnosis of knee joint abnormality has been a subject of debate for several years. The issue is whether there is a need for arthrography in a setting which includes adequate arthroscopy. There are numerous reports in the literature indicating that both procedures are important adjuncts to the clinical diagnosis of knee joint abnormality.[12,15,20,56,105,128] Neither one of these procedures should ever be substituted for a careful history and physical examination, however.

Knee arthrography is a safe, minimally invasive procedure which is useful as an initial screening study in patients suspected of having knee joint abnormality. A good-quality arthrogram delineates the entire medial meniscus and the anterior two-thirds of the lateral meniscus and demonstrates the integrity of the joint capsule. A high degree of confidence can be attached to a positive arthrographic diagnosis of meniscus abnormality.[9] While the accuracy of knee arthrography in the diagnosis of cruciate ligament abnormality is generally less than that of an arthroscopic examination, arthrography can be a useful screening procedure in those patients with an equivocal clinical examination or when clinical symptoms hinder the ability of the examiner to make a diagnosis. Arthroscopy complements arthrography by demonstrating portions of the knee joint which are not well seen arthrographically: the apex and the posterior horn of the lateral meniscus, the articular surfaces of the patellofemoral and knee joints, and the cruciate ligaments. Arthrography complements arthroscopy by its ability to readily visualize the periphery and under surfaces of the menisci, areas which are not easily visualized by arthroscopy.[12,15,20] Even a nondiagnostic arthrogram may be helpful by pointing out questionable areas of abnormality which can be further evaluated arthroscopically. The role of MRI scan in this regard is discussed in Chap. 27.

Abnormalities of the Meniscus

Modern knee arthrography is performed using either single- or double-contrast techniques.[10,31,43,57,62,131] Numerous authors have shown that a high degree of accuracy can be obtained when arthrography is used to diagnose meniscus tears.[9,10,61,71,88,131] Brown and Allman studied 295 arthrograms and showed that a positive diagnosis of a meniscus tear was correct 96 percent of the time while 93 percent of all meniscus lesions were demonstrated arthrographically.[9] Tegtmeyer et al, using single-contrast arthrography, obtained accuracies of 96 percent for the diagnosis of medial meniscus injury and 95 percent for lateral meniscus tears. With double-contrast arthrography, figures of 95 percent for medial meniscus tears and 90 percent for lateral meniscus tears were obtained.[131]

Interpretation of Meniscus Abnormalities Contrast material in the knee joint defines a triangular cross section of meniscus on arthrographic images. The presence of contrast material within the confines of the triangular cross section indicates a meniscus tear. Deformity of the contour of the meniscus indicates that a portion of the structure has been

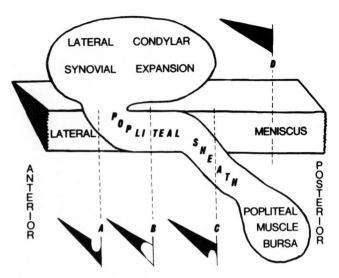

Figure 26-11 This diagrammatic representation of the posterior horn of the lateral meniscus demonstrates the arthrographic appearance of the meniscus as it relates to the popliteus tendon sheath. Interruption of the coronary ligament attachments (level C) and the connective tissue supports (level A) of the meniscus allow passage of the popliteus tendon through the meniscus. These attachments are intact at the midportion of the sheath (level B). The lateral meniscus is firmly attached to the joint capsule posterior to the tendon sheath (level D). *(From Jelasco, D.V., Radiology 114:335–339, 1975. Reproduced with permission.)*

torn and a fragment displaced or that significant meniscus degenerative changes have taken place.

Since the medial meniscus is completely attached to the joint capsule at its periphery, any contrast material within the outline of this meniscus indicates a tear or peripheral separation. The normal lateral meniscus has a complete peripheral attachment of its anterior two-thirds. Posteriorly it is more loosely bound because of the popliteus tendon's crossing the periphery of the meniscus in this region (Fig. 26-11). This results in greater mobility of the lateral meniscus and makes the structure more difficult to project in profile. Gas and contrast material accumulated in the popliteus tendon sheath overlap the posterior horn of the lateral meniscus, making it more difficult to identify tears. Additionally, the posterior one-fifth of the lateral meniscus curves anteriorly to insert in a position just posterior to the tibial attachment of the anterior cruciate ligament, a point that is difficult to demonstrate arthrographically. The posterior one-fifth is a segment of lateral meniscus which, according to Clancy, is commonly damaged in association with anterior cruciate ligament injuries.[12] These features of the lateral meniscus account for the decreased accuracy of arthrographic diagnosis of tears of this structure compared with the medial meniscus.

Each type of meniscus tear has a characteristic arthrographic appearance, although in some cases it is impossible to accurately characterize a tear because of the complex nature of the lesion. Generally speaking, tears in both the medial and the lateral meniscus have similar appearances.

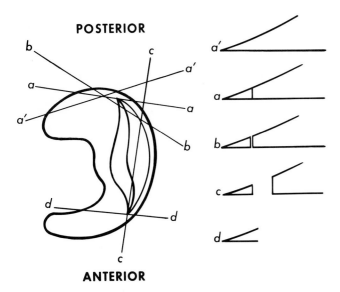

POSTERIOR

ANTERIOR

Figure 26-12 The vertical concentric ("longitudinal") tear diagrammed here is the most common meniscus tear seen in younger patients. Lines *a* through *d* represent a series of x-ray beam projections made during the spot film examination of a meniscus. Images *a* through *d* represent the fluoroscopic spot film images that correspond to the various portions of the tear. A complete examination of the meniscus requires that the entire meniscus be visualized and filmed.

With a displaced longitudinal or bucket handle tear, the peripheral fragment is seen as a shortened, irregular structure with the central fragment projecting near or in the intercondylar notch (Fig. 26-12). Occasionally, the peripheral fragment of such a tear has a shortened but symmetrical appearance which could be confused with a developmentally small meniscus. In these cases the diagnosis of meniscus tear is confirmed when the displaced central fragment is displayed on the examination.[47] The addition of a tunnel projection to the arthrography filming routine can be useful in demonstrating these displaced fragments.

Vertical radial (i.e., "transverse") tears begin at the apex of the meniscus and extend into the body, partially splitting the meniscus into anterior and posterior fragments. These tears are less common than the vertical concentric variety.[61] On arthrography, a vertical radial tear is seen as a localized opacification of the apex of the meniscus. The so-called parrot beak tear which extends diagonally into the meniscus from its apex has a similar arthrographic appearance (Fig. 26-13).

Horizontal tears extend into the meniscus from its apex or from its superior or inferior surfaces, separating the structure into upper and lower fragments. Arthrography demonstrates these tears as linear collections of contrast material (Fig. 26-14*A* and *B*). Horizontal tears are more common in patients with degenerating menisci. Cystic degeneration of the meniscus is occasionally demonstrated in association with horizontal meniscus tears. The cysts are seen as collections of contrast material at the periphery of the tear. They are more common in the lateral than in the medial meniscus.[122]

Combinations of the basic tear configurations result in a meniscus that arthrographically appears deformed with multiple collections of contrast material within it. These are referred to as complex tears.

Degenerative changes can be diagnosed by arthrography. The earliest arthrographic sign of meniscus degeneration is decreased resiliency of the structure, a finding that can be appreciated during the fluoroscopic examination of the joint. More-extensive degeneration is seen as focal surface irregularities and excessive absorption of positive contrast medium into the substance of the meniscus. These findings are most frequently seen along the inferior surface of the posterior medial meniscus.[44]

Discoid Meniscus The discoid lateral meniscus is well shown by arthrography. Hall reported an incidence of 2.7 percent in a series of 985 consecutive arthrograms.[49] The increased size of these menisci causes them to be injury-prone, sometimes tearing with insignificant trauma (Fig. 26-15). Symptoms of a torn meniscus in a child should raise suspicion of a torn discoid lateral meniscus. Discoid medial menisci have been reported but are extremely uncommon to encounter.[110]

Ligamentous Injuries

The integrity of the cruciate ligaments can be evaluated during knee arthrography. The cruciate ligaments, while they are intraarticular, are extrasynovial structures. Intraarticular contrast material, therefore, only outlines their synovial reflections (Fig. 26-16). This indirect visualization of the cruciate ligaments leads to inherent problems with the arthro-

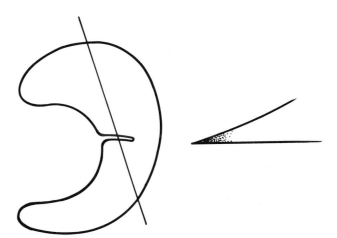

Figure 26-13 Vertical radial (transverse) tear. The vertical radial tear begins at the apex of the meniscus and extends into the body, partially splitting the meniscus into anterior and posterior fragments. The line crossing the tear indicates the direction of the x-ray beam. Intraarticular contrast material collected in this tear is projected as a localized opacification of the apex of the meniscus.

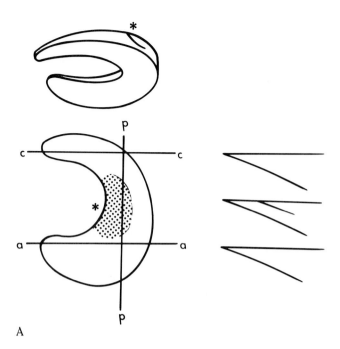

A

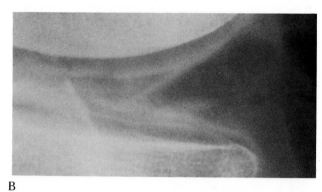

B

Figure 26-14 Horizontal tear. **A.** The horizontal tear extends into the meniscus from its apex or its superior or inferior surfaces, separating the structure into upper and lower fragments. Sections at the right show the image obtained in regions *a-a, c-c,* and through the middle of the tear when the x-ray beam is directed along *b-b.* **B.** In a arthrogram tears are seen as linear collections of contrast material.

graphic evaluation of these structures. In patients who have intact synovial reflections surrounding torn or attenuated cruciate ligaments, false-negative diagnosis can result. Synovitis, synovial scarring, synovial clot formation, and an infrapatellar plica can all hinder contrast coating of these investing membranes and can lead to inaccurate diagnoses. In spite of these drawbacks, many authors have demonstrated that the accuracy of arthrography in the diagnosis of anterior cruciate ligament injuries reaches a level where the procedure can be considered a useful diagnostic tool, particularly in the patient with a difficult clinical examination.[1,8,96,97,109,138] Inaccuracies can be held to a minimum when careful attention is paid to filming techniques and when there is strict adherence to diagnostic criteria.

Contrast material within extracapsular structures is the hallmark of acute collateral ligament or capsular disruptions.

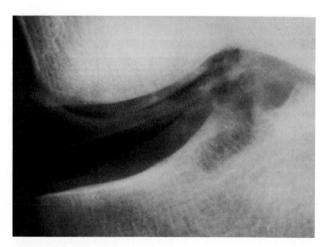

Figure 26-15 Discoid lateral meniscus. Notice that the meniscus extends through the entire lateral joint compartment, and that an internal edge to the structure is not well-defined.

However, examinations obtained more than 48 h postinjury may give false-negative results because of sealing of the synovial tears. Acute third-degree tears of the medial collateral ligament are seen as a feathery pattern of contrast medium in the medial soft tissues. Disruptions involving only the deep layer of the medial collateral ligament are seen as sharply defined collections of contrast material outlined by the intact superficial layer of ligament. Tears of the middle portion of the lateral capsular ligament have an arthrographic appearance similar to that of medial collateral ligament tears. Chronic collateral ligament tears can be diagnosed if extreme widening of the joint is noted during the meniscus examination.[101]

Abnormalities of Articular Cartilage

A portion of the articular cartilage of the medial and lateral joint compartments is visualized during knee arthrography. The cartilage that is demonstrated is only that which can be made tangent to the x-ray beam. Early changes of degenerative joint disease include cartilage surface irregularities and cartilage thinning. Advanced degenerative disease is manifested as deep cartilaginous erosions and denuded subchondral bone. Chondral fractures are seen as localized avulsions of articular surface. The patellar cartilage is best seen on lateral spot films made with the knee extended. An axial view of the patella is also helpful in this evaluation. In its early stages, chondromalacia patella is generally not diagnosed by arthrography. In the later stages of this disease, arthrography demonstrates articular cartilage surface irregularities, fissures, and imbibed contrast material in denuded cartilaginous surfaces. Large articular cartilage erosions are seen in advanced cases of chondromalacia patella.

The articular surface involved with osteochondritis dissecans can also be evaluated arthrographically. If positive contrast material or gas surrounds the osteochondral fragment, the articular surface is disrupted and the fragment has

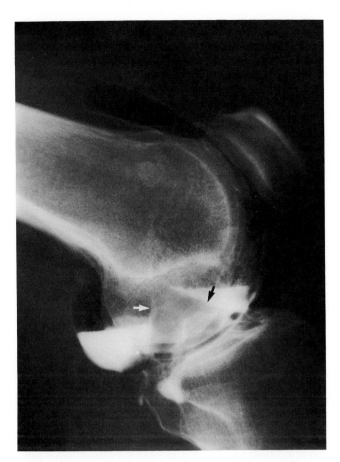

Figure 26-16 A properly projected horizontal beam radiograph demonstrates the cruciate ligaments as a well-defined triangle with the anterior limb representing the anterior cruciate ligament anatomy *(black arrow)* and the posterior limb the posterior cruciate ligament anatomy *(white arrow)*. It is important to remember that intraarticular contrast material outlines the synovial membrane surrounding the ligaments and not the ligaments themselves.

a high potential to become a loose body. If the articular surface over the fragment is shown to be intact, loose body formation is less likely to occur. Arthrotomography can often provide better detail of these lesions.

Loose Bodies

In patients in whom loose bodies are suspected, arthrography can be helpful in (1) detecting the presence of cartilaginous bodies that are not seen on plain radiographs, (2) determining whether paraarticular osseous densities seen on plain x-ray films are intraarticular or extraarticular, and (3) determining whether small osseous densities seen on plain x-ray films have large cartilaginous components.[101] When arthrography is performed specifically for the evaluation of loose bodies, it is recommended that the procedure be carried out as a pneumoarthrogram (gas only) so that small bodies are not obscured by positive contrast material, and air bubbles in positive contrast material are not confused as abnormality.

Synovial Abnormality

The normal synovial joint lining appears smooth and sharply outlined with contrast material during arthrography. Various inflammatory and neoplastic conditions of the synovium such as the inflammatory arthritides, pigmented villonodular synovitis, lipoma arborescens, and synovial hemangioma can cause generalized synovial proliferation or localized synovial masses.[30,36,77,106,116,139,140] Synovial proliferation and thickening are seen as an enlarged and irregular capsule on the arthrogram. The arthrographic appearance of these conditions may resemble each other, and a specific diagnosis is usually not possible. Evaluation of the joint aspirate may be helpful in limiting the differential diagnosis.

Popliteal cysts represent a distended gastrocnemio-semimembranosus bursa which communicates with the posterior aspect of the knee joint. On arthrography, a popliteal cyst appears as a contrast-containing sac posterior and medial to the knee joint. Extravasation of contrast material into the soft tissue surrounding a popliteal cyst would suggest dissection of the cyst, a condition which causes painful swelling of the calf. The clinical presentation of a dissecting popliteal cyst can mimic thrombophlebitis, and a positive Homans' sign can often be elicited. Arthrography is usually diagnostic and prevents unnecessary anticoagulation therapy.[101]

The suprapatellar plica is seen as a band of tissue crossing the suprapatellar bursa from anterior to posterior on lateral arthrogram films of the knee. The medial patellar plica is the most common plica causing clinical symptoms, and it is also the most difficult to visualize at arthrography. Several methods of demonstrating the medial patellar plica during arthrography have been described, including horizontal beam lateral views in varying degrees of flexion,[4] axial views of the patella-femoral joint,[25] and CT scanning of the knee joint.[7]

Ankle Arthrography

Ankle arthrography was first described by Hansson in 1940.[50] Ankle arthrography is useful in the evaluation of both acute and chronic injuries of the ankle joint. In cases of acute trauma, it can be used to document ligamentous injuries. In the case of a chronically unstable ankle, it is useful in detecting intraarticular loose bodies, articular cartilage defects, and synovial abnormalities.[62,91,92,103,121,127]

For the patient with suspected articular cartilage abnormality or loose bodies, double-contrast arthrotomography is the procedure of choice. Plain tomograms of the ankle joint in the mortise and lateral projections should be obtained at 3-mm intervals prior to the contrast study. Similar tomographic projections are then obtained postarthrography.[103] Postarthrography fluoroscopy can also be helpful in patients with articular cartilage damage and loose body formation.

The Normal Ankle Arthrogram

Both single- and double-contrast techniques of ankle arthrography have been described.[91,92,103] In the normal ankle, no extraarticular leakage of contrast material occurs except for filling of the tendon sheaths of the flexor hallucis longus and the flexor digitorum longus in 20 percent of patients.[92,103] In addition, contrast medium has been noted to fill the posterior aspect of the talocalcaneal joint in 10 percent of normal ankles.[62,92,103]

There are three recesses in the normal ankle: the anterior recess, the posterior recess, and the interosseous recess which extends proximally for approximately 1 to 2.5 cm between the distal tibia and fibula.

The Abnormal Ankle Arthrogram

Acute Injuries Ankle arthrography has been shown to be helpful in assessing acute ligamentous injuries of the ankle joint. Although acceptance of this procedure has grown considerably in recent years, it is still not in widespread use.[92]

Inversion, eversion, and anterior drawer stress x-ray views are the traditional noninvasive method of evaluating the integrity of the ankle joint ligaments. Recently, however, the literature has emphasized the lack of reliability of stress x-ray views in diagnosing these injuries.[92,121,127,137] Many authors feel that arthrographic studies are more definitive than stress x-ray studies in diagnosing ankle ligament injuries, especially if performed within 72 h of the trauma.[62,92,121,137] False-negative studies can be decreased if the procedure is performed within 24 to 36 h postinjury, before capsular tears have the opportunity to be sealed by organizing clot or adhesions.[103]

The rationale for using arthrography to diagnose ligament tears is based on the fact that the major ankle ligaments are intimately associated with the joint capsule such that posttraumatic ruptures of these ligaments cause associated tears of the joint capsule. The pattern of leakage of contrast material from the joint is determined by the specific ligament that is injured.[63,91,92,103,127] Single, positive contrast arthrography is the technique of choice for evaluating acute ligamentous injuries.

Rupture of the anterior talofibular ligament is the most common of all ligamentous tears at the ankle. With this injury, contrast material leaks from the joint into the soft tissues around the tip of the distal fibula, especially anteriorly and laterally. On the laterally projected x-ray view, a space may be visualized between the extravasated contrast material and the anterior tibiofibular ligament.[91,92] This finding helps to differentiate tears of the anterior talofibular ligament from tears of the anterior tibiofibular ligament where the clear space is absent.

Ruptures of the calcaneofibular ligament invariably have an associated tear of the anterior talofibular ligament.[92] Therefore, arthrographic signs of rupture of both ligaments are seen together. Rupture of the calcaneofibular ligament results in simultaneous tearing of both the joint capsule and the inner aspect of the peroneal tendon sheath. This allows intraarticular contrast material to leak into the sheath (Fig. 26-17).[122,125,128] Spiegel has reported that the calcaneofibular ligament can be torn without leakage of contrast material into the peroneal tendon sheath.[127] Olson feels that this is the result of insufficient intraarticular contrast pressure secondary to decompression of the joint through the associated anterior talofibular ligament tear.[92] Direct injection of the peroneal

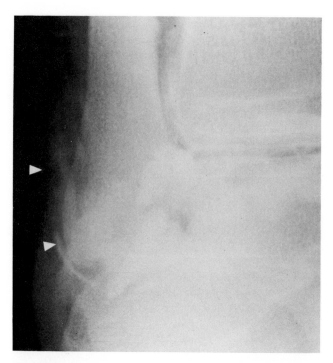

Figure 26-17 Use of ankle arthrography for ligament injury. The pattern of contrast leakage through capsular tears is characteristic for the specific ligament injury. Here the positive contrast material seen in the peroneal tendon sheath *(arrowheads)* indicates a tear of the calcaneofibular ligament. Single-contrast arthrography is more suitable for the evaluation of ligament ruptures than the double-contrast technique.

tendon sheath (peroneal tenography) is an alternative method of demonstrating ruptures of the calcaneofibular ligament. Eichelberger et al feel that peroneal tenography is now the method of choice for demonstrating calcaneofibular ligament tears because it has a lower false-negative rate than ankle arthrography.[27]

Tears of the posterior talofibular ligament do not occur as isolated injuries, and contrast material extravasated through this tear is obscured by the extravasated contrast material from the other lateral ligament tears.[92]

Isolated tears of the deltoid ligament are unusual but can occur, resulting in extravasation of intraarticular contrast medium around the tip of the medial malleolus. These tears usually occur in conjunction with tears of the distal tibiofibular syndesmosis. This disruption results in the leakage of contrast material both anterior and superior to the syndesmosis.[92,103]

Isolated ruptures of the anterior tibiofibular ligament are rare. When they do occur, contrast material is extravasated anterior to the ligament and is seen immediately adjacent to the tibia on lateral x-ray views. Ruptures of the anterior tibiofibular ligament are usually accompanied by ruptures of the syndesmosis.[92]

Chronic Injuries Osseous and osteocartilaginous abnormalities causing chronic ankle symptoms are often evident on routine x-ray films. Lesions of the articular cartilage and sy-

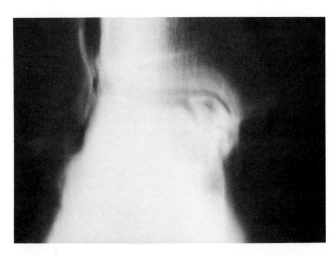

Figure 26-18 Double-contrast arthrotomography of the ankle joint is the technique of choice for the evaluation of articular cartilage abnormalities. This AP arthrotomogram demonstrates a linear collection of positive contrast material in a chondral fracture of the medial aspect of the talar dome.

novium, and nonopaque loose bodies, however, cannot be diagnosed without an arthrographic procedure.

The integrity of the articular cartilage is best demonstrated with double-contrast arthrotomography. Small loose bodies located in the corners of the ankle joint are also best seen with this technique (Fig. 26-18). Tehranzadeh and Gabrielle have suggested that CT scanning following double-contrast arthrography is useful in locating intraarticular loose bodies, especially when conventional arthrotomography is inconclusive.[133] Postarthrography fluoroscopy can be helpful in diagnosing loose bodies located in the major ankle joint recesses.

Proliferative and edematous changes of the synovium, as in other joints, are seen as a lobulated contour of the joint capsule. Posttraumatic adhesive capsulitis is diagnosed by the demonstration of a decrease in the size of the joint capsule, obliteration of the normal anterior and posterior recesses, and extravasation of contrast material along the needle tract.[103]

REFERENCES

1. Aglietti, P., Pimpinelli, G.P., and Burini, M. Is double contrast arthrography of any value in lesions of the anterior cruciate ligament? Ital J Orthop Traumatol 6:135–145, 1980.
2. Anderson, L.S., and Staple, T.C. Arthrography of total hip replacement using subtraction technique. Radiology 109:470–472, 1973.
3. Andren, L., and Eiken, O. Arthrographic studies of wrist ganglions. J Bone Joint Surg 53A:299–302, 1971.
4. Aprin, H., Shapiro, J., and Gershwind, M. Arthrography (plica views): A non-invasive method for diagnosis and prognosis of plica syndrome. Clin Orthop 183:90–95, 1984.
5. Bircher, E., and Oberholzer, J. Die Kniegelenkkapsel in Pneumoradiographie-Bilde. Acta Radiol 15:452–466, 1934.
6. Blane, C.E., Kling, T.F., Andrews, J.C., Dipietro, M.A., Hensinger, R.N. Arthrography in the post-traumatic elbow in children. Am J Radiol 143:17–21, 1984.
7. Boven, F., DeBoeck, M., and Potvliege, R. Synovial plicae of the knee on computed tomography. Radiology 147:805–809, 1983.
8. Braunstein, E.M. Anterior cruciate ligament injuries: A comparison of arthrographic and physical diagnosis. Am J Radiol 138:423–425, 1982.
9. Brown, D.W., Allman, F.L., and Eaton, S.B. Knee arthrography: A comparison of radiographic and surgical findings in 295 cases. Am J Sports Med 6:165–172, 1978.
10. Butt, W.P., and McIntyre, J.L. Double contrast arthrography of the knee. Radiology 91:487–499, 1969.
11. Casperi, R.B. Shoulder arthroscopy: A review of the present state of the art. Contemp Orthop 4:523–530, 1982.
12. Clancy, W.G. The role of arthrography and arthroscopy in the acutely injured knee. Medi Times 109:22–27, 1981.
13. Codman E.A. *The Shoulder: Rupture of the Subacromal Bursa.* Boston, Mass. T. Todd Company Printers, 1934.
14. Cone, R.O., Resnick, D., and Danzig, L. Shoulder impingement syndrome: Radiographic evaluation. Radiology 150:29–33, 1984.
15. Curran, W.P., and Woodward, E.P. Arthroscopy: Its role in diagnosis and treatment of athletic knee injuries. Am J Sports Med 8:415–418, 1980.
16. Dalinka, M.K., Gohel, V.K., and Rancier, L. Tomography in the evaluation of the anterior cruciate ligament. Radiology 108:31–33, 1973.
17. Dalinka, M.K., and Garofola, J. The infrapatellar synovial fold: A cause for confusion in the evaluation of the anterior cruciate ligament. Am J Radiol 127:589–591, 1976.
18. Dalinka, M.K., Osterman, A.L., Albert, A.S., Harty, M. Arthrography of the wrist and shoulder. Orthop Clin North Am 14:193–215, 1983.
19. Dalinka, M.K., Turner, M.L., Osterman, A.L., Batra, P. Wrist arthrography. Radiol Clin North Am 19:217–226, 1981.
20. DeHaven, K.E., and Collins, H.R. Diagnosis of internal derangements of the knee: The role of arthroscopy. J Bone Joint Surg 57A:802–810, 1975.
21. DelBuono, M.S., and Solarino, G.B. Arthrography of the elbow with double contrast media. Ital Clin Orthop 14:223–232, 1962.
22. DeSmet, A.A., and Neff, J.R. Knee arthrography for the preoperative evaluation of juxta-articular masses. Radiology 143:663–666, 1982.
23. Deutsch, A.L., Resnick, D., Dalinka, M.K., Gilula, L., Danzig, L., Guerra, J. Jr., Dunn, F.H. Synovial plicae of the knee. Radiology 141:627–634, 1981.
24. Deutsch, A.L., Resnick, D., and Mink, J.H. Computed and conventional arthrotomography of the glenohumeral joint: Normal anatomy and clinical experience. Radiology 153:603–609, 1984.
25. Dory, M.A. Arthrographic recognition of the mediopatellar plica. Letter to the editor. Radiology 150:608, 1984.
26. Dussalt, R.G., Goldman, A.B., and Ghelman, B. Roentgenographic diagnosis of loosening and/or infection in hip prostheses. Correlation between roentgen and surgical findings. J Can Assoc Radiol 28:119–123, 1977.
27. Eichelberger, R.P., Lichtenstein, P., and Brogdon, B.G. Peroneal tenography. JAMA 247:2587–2591, 1982.
28. El-Khoury, G.Y., Albright, J.P., Abu-Yousef, M.M., Montgomery, W.J., Tuck, S.L. Arthrotomography of the glenoid labrum. Radiology 131:333–337, 1979.
29. Eto, R.T., Anderson, P.W., and Harley, J.D. Elbow arthrography with the application of tomography. Radiology 115:283–288, 1975.
30. Forrest, J., and Staple, T.W. Synovial hemangioma of the knee.

Demonstration by arthrography and arteriography. Am J Radiol 112:512–516, 1971.

31. Freiberger, R.H., Killoran, P.J., and Cardona, G. Arthrography of the knee by double contrast method. AJR 97:736–747, 1966.

32. Ghelman, G., and Goldman, A.B. The double contrast arthrogram: Evaluation of rotary cuff tears. Radiology 124:251–254, 1977.

33. Ghelman, B., and Freiberger, R.H. The adult hip, in Freiberger, R.H., and Kay, J.J. (eds): *Arthrography.* New York, Appleton-Century-Crofts, 1979, pp 192–194.

34. Gilula, L.A., Schoenecker, P.L., and Murphy, W.A. Shoulder arthrography as a treatment modality. Am J Radiol 131:1047–1048, 1978.

35. Glassburg, G.B., and Ozonoff, M.B. Arthrographic findings in septic arthritis of the hip in infants. Radiology 128:151–155, 1978.

36. Goergen, T.G., Resnick, D., and Niwayama, G. Localized nodular synovitis of the knee: A report of two cases with abnormal arthrograms. Am J Radiol 126:647–650, 1976.

37. Goldberg, R.P., Hall, F.M., and Wyshak, G. Pain in knee arthrography: Comparison of air versus CO_2 and reaspiration versus no reaspiration. Am J Radiol 136:377–379, 1981.

38. Goldman, A.B., and Ghelman, B. The double contrast shoulder arthrogram. Radiology 127:655–663, 1978.

39. Goldman, A.B. Arthrography of the hip joint. CRC Crit Rev Diagn Imaging 13:111–171, 1980.

40. Goldman, A.B. Hip arthrography. Radiol Clin North Am 19:329–348, 1981.

41. Goldman, A.B., Schneider, R., and Martel, W. Acute chondrolysis complicating slipped capital femoral epiphysis: Roentgen diagnosis and differential diagnosis. Am J Radiol 130:945–950, 1978.

42. Griffiths, H.J., Utz, R., Burke, J., Bonfiglio, T. Adhesive capsulitis of the hip and ankle. Am J Radiol 101–105, 1985.

43. Hall, F.M. Methodology in knee arthrography. Radiol Clin North Am 19:269–275, 1981.

44. Hall, F.M. Double and single arthrography of the knee. Letter to the editor. Radiology 134:796, 1980.

45. Hall, F.M. Epinephrine enhanced knee arthrography. Radiology 111:215–217, 1974.

46. Hall, F.M. Pitfalls in knee arthrography. Radiology 118:55–62, 1976.

47. Hall, F.M. Further pitfalls in knee arthrography. J Can Assoc Radiol 29:179–184, 1978.

48. Hall, F.M. Pitfalls in the assessment of the menisci by knee arthrography. Radiol Clin North Am 19:305–328, 1981.

49. Hall, F.M. Arthrography of the discoid lateral meniscus. Am J Radiol 128:993–1002, 1977.

50. Hansson, C.J. Arthrographic studies of the ankle joint. Acta Radiol 22:281–287, 1941.

51. Harrison, M.O., Freiberger, R.H., and Ranawat, C.S. Arthrography of the rheumatoid wrist joint. Am J Radiol 112:480–486, 1971.

52. Hendrix, R.W., and Anderson, T.M. Arthrographic and radiologic evaluation of prosthetic joints. Radiol Clin North Am 19:349–363, 1981.

53. Heublein, G.W., Greene, G.S., and Conforti, V.P. Hip joint arthrography. Am J Radiol 68:736–748, 1952.

54. Hudson, T.M., Schiebler, M., Springfield, D.S., Enneking, W.F., Hawkins, I.F. Jr., Spanier, S.S. The radiology of giant cell tumors of bone: Computed tomography, arthrotomography, scintigraphy. Skeletal Radiol 11:85–95, 1984.

55. Hudson, T.M. Elbow arthrography. Radiol Clin North Am 19:227–241, 1981.

56. Ireland, J., Trickey, E.L., and Stoker, D.J. Arthroscopy and arthrography of the knee: A critical review. J Bone Joint Surg 628:3–6, 1980.

57. Jelasco, D.V. Positive contrast arthrography of the knee. Am J Radiol 103:669–673, 1968.

58. Jelasco, D.V. The fascicles of the lateral meniscus: An anatomic-arthrographic correlation. Radiology 114:335–339, 1975.

59. Jonsater, S. Coxa plana: A histopathologic and arthrographic study. Acta Orthop Scand 12(suppl):5–98, 1953.

60. Katz, J.F. Arthrography and Legg-Calve-Perthes disease. J Bone Joint Surg 50A:467–472, 1968.

61. Kaye, J.J., and Nance, E.P. Meniscal abnormalities in knee arthrography. Radiol Clin North Am 19:277–286, 1981.

62. Kaye, J.J. The ankle, in Freiberger, R.H., and Kaye, J.J. (eds): *Arthrography.* New York, Appleton-Century-Crofts, 1979 pp 237–256.

63. Kaye, J.J., and Bohne, W.H. A radiographic study of the ligamentous anatomy of the ankle. Radiology 125:659–667, 1977.

64. Kenin, A., and Levine, J. A technic for arthrography of the hip. Am J Radiol 68:107–111, 1952.

65. Killoran, P.J., Marcove, R.C., and Freiberger, R.H. Shoulder arthrography. Am J Radiol 103:658–668, 1968.

66. Klein, A., Sumner, T.E., Volberg, F.M., Orbon, R.J. Combined CT-arthrography in recurrent traumatic hip dislocation. Am J Radiol 138:963–964, 1982.

67. Kleinman, P.K., Kanzaria, P.K., and Goss, T.P. Axillary arthrotomography of the glenoid labrum. Am J Radiol 141:993–999, 1984.

68. Kricun, M.E. Wrist arthrography. Clin Orthop 187:65–71, 1984.

69. Leveuf, J. Primary congenital subluxation of the hip. J Bone Joint Surg 29:149–162, 1947.

70. Leveuf, J. Results of open reduction of true congenital luxation of the hip. J Bone Joint Surg 30A:875–882, 1948.

71. Levinsohn, E.M., and Baker, B.E. Prearthrotomy diagnostic evaluation of the knee: Review of 100 cases diagnosed by arthrography and arthroscopy. Am J Radiol 134:107–111, 1980.

72. Levinsohn, E.M., and Palmer, A.K. Arthrography of the traumatized wrist. Radiology 146:647–651, 1983.

73. Lie, S., and Mast, W.A. Subacromial bursography. Radiology 144:626–630, 1982.

74. Lindblom, K. Arthrography of the knee: A roentgenographic and anatomical study. Acta Radiologica 74(suppl):1–112, 1948.

75. Lindblom, K. Arthrography and roentgenography in ruptures of tendons of the shoulder joint. Acta Radiol 20:548–562, 1939.

76. Lindblom, K. Arthrography. J Fac Radiol 3:151–163, 1952.

77. Lowenstein, M.B., Smith, J.R., and Cole, S. Infrapatellar pigmented villonodular synovitis: Arthrographic detection. Am J Radiol 135:279–282, 1980.

78. Loyd, J.A., and Loyd, H.M. Adhesive capsulitis of the shoulder: Arthrographic diagnosis and treatment. South Med J 76:879–883, 1983.

79. Mack, L.A., Matsen, F.A., Kilcoyne, R.F., Davies, P.K., Sickler, M.E. US evaluation of the rotator cuff. Radiology 157:205–209, 1985.

80. McIntyre, J.L. Arthrography of the lateral meniscus. Radiology 105:531–536, 1972.

81. Middleton, W.D., Edelstein, G., Reinus, W.R., Melson, G.L., Tatty, W.G., Murphy, W.A. Sonographic detection of rotator cuff tears. Am J Radiol 144:349–353, 1985.

82. Mink, J.H., and Dickerson, R. Air or CO_2 for knee arthrography. Am J Radiol 134:991–993, 1980.

83. Mink, J.H., Richardson, A., and Grant, T.T. Evaluation of glenoid labrum by double contrast shoulder arthrography. Am J Radiol 133:883–887, 1979.

84. Mink, J.H., Harris, E., and Rappaport, M. Rotator cuff tears: Evaluation using double-contrast shoulder arthrography. Radiology 157:621–623, 1985.

85. Mink, J.H., Eckardt, J.J., and Grant, T.T. Arthrography in recurrent dislocation of the elbow. Am J Radiol 136:1242–1244, 1981.

86. Mittler, S., Freiberger, R.H., and Harrison-Stubbs, M. A method of improving cruciate ligament visualization in double contrast arthrography. Radiology 102:441–442, 1972.

87. Neviaser, T.J. Arthrography of the shoulder. Orthop Clin North Am 11:205–217, 1980.

88. Nicholas, J.A., Freiberger, R.H., and Killoran, P.J. Double contrast arthrography of the knee. J Bone Joint Surg 52A:203–220, 1970.

89. Oberholzer, J. Die arthropneumoradiographie bei habitueller schulterluxation. Rontgenpraxis 5:589–590, 1933.

90. Olson, R.W. Knee arthrography. Am J Radiol 101:897–914, 1967.

91. Olson, R.W. Arthrography of the ankle: Its use in the evaluation of ankle sprains. Radiology 92:1439–1446, 1969.

92. Olson, R.W. Ankle arthrography. Radiol Clin North Am 19:255–268, 1981.

93. Palmer, A.K., Levinsohn, E.M., and Kuzma, G.R. Arthrography of the wrist. J Hand Surg 8:15–23, 1983.

94. Pastershank, S.P., Resnick, D., Niwayama, G., Danzig, L., Haghighi, P. The effect of water-soluble contrast media on the synovial membrane. Radiology 143:331–334, 1982.

95. Patel, D. Arthroscopy of the plicae—synovial folds and their significance. Am J Sports Med 6:217–225, 1978.

96. Pavlov, H., and Torg, J.S. Double contrast arthrographic evaluation of the anterior cruciate ligament. Radiology 126:661–665, 1978.

97. Pavlov, H., Warren, R.F., Sherman, M.F., Cayea, P.D. The accuracy of double contrast evaluation of the anterior cruciate ligament. J Bone Joint Surg 65A:175–183, 1983.

98. Pavlov, H., and Freiberger, R.H. An easy method to demonstrate the cruciate ligaments by double contrast arthrography. Radiology 126:817–818, 1978.

99. Pavlov, H., Hirschy, J.C., and Torg, J.S. Computed tomography of the cruciate ligaments. Radiology 132:389–393, 1979.

100. Pavlov, H., and Goldman, A.B. The popliteus bursa: An indicator of subtle pathology. Am J Radiol 134:313–321, 1980.

101. Pavlov, H., and Schneider, R. Extrameniscal abnormalities as diagnosed by knee arthrography. Radiol Clin North Am 19:287–304, 1981.

102. Pavlov, H., Ghelman, B., and Warren, R.F. Double contrast arthrography of the elbow. Radiology 130:87–95, 1979.

103. Pavlov, H. Ankle and subtalor arthrography. Clin Sports Med 1:47–69, 1982.

104. Phillips, W.C., and Kattapuram, S.V. Prosthetic hip replacements: Plain films and arthrography for component loosening. Am J Radiol 138:677–682, 1982.

105. Poehling, G.G., Bassett, F.H., and Goldner, J.L. Arthroscopy: Its role in treating non-traumatic and traumatic lesions of the knee. South Med J 70:466–469, 1977.

106. Prager, R.J., and Mall, J.C. Arthrographic diagnosis of synovial chondromatosis. Am J Radiol 127:344–346, 1976.

107. Preston, B.J., and Jackson, J.P. Investigations of shoulder disability by arthrography. Clin Radiol 28:259–266, 1977.

108. Ranawat, C.S., Freiberger, R.H., Jordan, L.R., Straub, L.R. Arthrography in the rheumatoid wrist joint. J Bone Joint Surg 51A:1269–1281, 1969.

109. Reider, B., Clancy, W., and Langer, L.O. Diagnosis of cruciate ligament injury using single contrast arthrography. Am J Sports Med 12:451–454, 1984.

110. Resnick, D., Goergen, P.G., Kaye, J.J., Ghelman, B., Woody, P.R. Discoid medial meniscus. Radiology 121:575–576, 1976.

111. Resnick, D. Shoulder arthrography. Radiol Clin North Am 19:243–253, 1981.

112. Resnick, D. Arthrography in the evaluation of arthritic disorders of the wrist. Radiology 113:331–340, 1974.

113. Resnick, D., Andre, M., Kerr, R., Pineda, C., Guerra, J. Jr., Atkinson, D. Digital arthrography of the wrist: A new radiographic-pathologic investigation. Am J Radiol 142:1187–1190, 1984.

114. Roebuck, E.J. Double contrast knee arthrography; some new points of technique including the use of dimer X. Clin Radiol 28:247–257, 1977.

115. Rokous, J.R. Modified axillary roentgenogram: A useful adjunct in the diagnosis of recurrent instability of the shoulder. Clin Orthop 82:84, 1972.

116. Rosenthal, D.I. Medicine or meddling? Use of arthrography in rheumatology. Clin Rheum Dis 9:453–471, 1983.

117. Saha, A.K. Anterior recurrent dislocation of the shoulder. Acta Orthop Scand 38:479–493, 1967.

118. Salvati, E.A., Freiberger, R.H., and Wilson, P.D., Jr. Arthrography for complications of total hip replacement. J Bone Joint Surg 53A:701–709, 1971.

119. Salvati, E.A., Im, V.C., Aglietti, P., Wilson, P.D., Jr. Radiology of total hip replacements. Clin Orthop 121:74–82, 1976.

120. Samilson, R.L., Raphael, R.L., Noonan, C., Siris, E., Raney, F.L., Jr. Shoulder arthrography. JAMA 175:773–778, 1961.

121. Sauser, D.D., Nelson, R.C., Lavine, M.H., Wu, C.W. Acute injuries of the lateral ligaments of the ankle: Comparison of stress radiography and arthrography. Radiology 148:653–657, 1983.

122. Schuldt, D.R., and Wolfe, R.D. Clinical and arthrographic findings in meniscal cysts. Radiology 134:49–52, 1980.

123. Severin, E. Arthrograms of the hips of children. Surg Gynecol Obstet 72:601–604, 1941.

124. Severin, E. Arthrography in congenital dislocation of the hip. J Bone Joint Surg 21:304–313, 1939.

125. Shuman, W.P., Kilcoyne, R.F., and Matsen, F.A. Double contrast computed tomography of the glenoid labrum. Am J Radiol 141:581–584, 1983.

126. Spataro, R.F., Katzberg, R.W., Burgener, F.A., Fischer, H.W. Epinephrine enhanced knee arthrography. Invest Radiol 13:286, 1978.

127. Spiegel, P.K., and Staples, O.S. Arthrography of the ankle joint: Problems in diagnosis in acute lateral ligament injuries. Radiology 114:587–590, 1975.

128. St. Pierre, R.K., Sones, P.J., and Fleming, L.L. Arthroscopy and arthrography of the knee: A comparative study. South Med J 74:1322–1328, 1981.

129. Strife, J.L., Towbin, R., and Crawford, A. Hip arthrography in infants and children: The inferomedial approach. Radiology 152:536, 1984.

130. Strizak, A.M., Danzig, L., Jackson, D.W., Resnick, D., Staple, T. Subacromial bursography. J Bone Joint Surg 64A:196–201, 1982.

131. Tegtmeyer, C.J., McCue, F.C., Higgins, S.M. Arthrography of the knee: A comparative study of the accuracy of single and double contrast techniques. Radiology 132:37–41, 1979.

132. Tehranzadeh, J., Schneider, R., and Freiberger, R.H. Radiological evaluation of the painful hip replacement. Radiology 141:355–362, 1981.

133. Tehranzadeh, J., and Gabrielle, O.F. Intra-articular calcified bodies: Detection by computed tomography. South Med J 77:703–709, 1984.

134. Tirman, R.M., Nelson, C.L., and Tirman, W.S. Arthrography of the shoulder: State of the art. CRC Crit Rev Diagn Imaging 17:19–76, 1981.

135. Tirman, R.M., Weber, E.R., Snyder, L.L., Koonce, T.W. Midcarpal wrist arthrography for detection of tears of the scapholunate and lunotriquetral ligaments. Am J Radiol 144:107–108, 1985.

136. Turner, A.F., and Budin, E. Arthrography of the knee. Radiology 97:505–508, 1970.

137. Van den Hoogenband, C.R., VanMoppes, F.I., Stapert, J.W., Greep, J.M. Clinical diagnosis, arthrography, stress examination and surgical findings after inversion trauma of the ankle. Arch Orthop Trauma Surg 103:115–119, 1984.

138. Wang, J., and Marshall, J. Acute ligamentous injuries of the knee: Single contrast arthrography—a diagnostic aid. J Trauma 15:40–43, 1975.

139. Weitzman, G. Lipoma arborescens of the knee. J Bone Joint Surg 47A:1030–1033, 1965.

140. Wolfe, R.D., and Giuliano, V.J. Double contrast arthrography in the diagnosis of pigmented villonodular synovitis of the knee. Am J Radiol 110:793–799, 1970.

CHAPTER 27

Orthopaedic Applications of Magnetic Resonance Imaging

William J. Montgomery and Georges Y. El-Khoury

Magnetic resonance imaging (MRI) is dramatically changing the way we approach diagnostic problems in the musculoskeletal system.[21,31,35] Because of enhanced tissue contrast, spatial resolution, and the possibility of tissue characterization, MRI has had a tremendous impact on musculoskeletal imaging.[7] Since MRI exams are initiated by the treating physician, some understanding of the basic principles and the potentials and limitations of this technique is appropriate. Some advantages and disadvantages of MRI are summarized in Table 27-1.

PHYSICAL PRINCIPLES

Magnetic resonance is very different from any other imaging modality. It uses no ionizing radiation but obtains image contrast information by the reaction of particular tissue when stimulated by a radiofrequency (RF) pulse while in a strong magnetic field. The axial images may seem similar to computed tomographic (CT) images, but in reality they are very different. An RF antenna (coil) is used to broadcast a pulsed signal directed at a body part and the same or another coil receives the response from the stimulated nuclei. How the image signal characteristics appear and whether the image of

a particular tissue appears bright or dark is basically a function of the RF pulse strength and timing, the "listening" or receiving time intervals, and the types of tissue imaged. This enables the examiner to look at tissue with different pulse sequences and so learn about its nature and whether it is normal or abnormal.

Another way in which MRI differs from CT is that, with the exception of reconstructed images, most CT images are usually obtained and displayed in the axial plane. MRI can directly acquire and display images in virtually any plane without loss of resolution. Therefore studying MRI sections requires a thorough grasp of sectional anatomy.

The basic principle[18,27] underlying magnetic resonance imaging is that nuclei with an odd number of protons or neutrons exhibit spin. As they spin they precess, at a particular frequency, about an axis somewhat like a spinning top or gyroscope (Fig. 27-1). Because spinning nuclei are charged they

TABLE 27-1 Advantages and Disadvantages of MRI

Advantages:
   High soft-tissue contrast (greater than CT)
   No beam hardening artifact from cortical bone
    as exists with CT
   Multiple pulse sequences available
   Increased tissue specificity
   No known biological hazard

Disadvantages:
   Does not demonstrate calcific densities well
   Cortical bone usually less well imaged than with CT
   Longer scan time (relative to CT) for most studies
   Claustrophobic reactions by some patients
   High cost
   Limited clinical availability of contrast agents

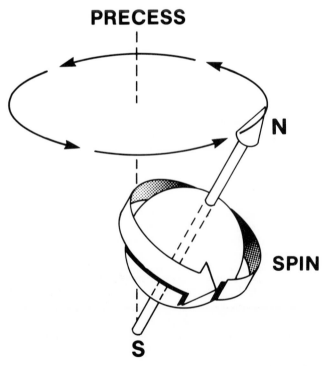

Figure 27-1 Diagram distinguishing the inherent nuclear spin from the precession.

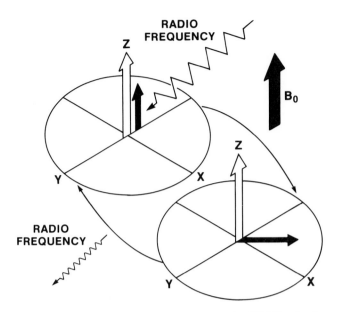

Figure 27-2 The sequence of events when the 90° RF pulse is applied. B_0 is the external magnetic field. The X-Y plane is perpendicular to the external magnetic field (B_0). Z denotes the axis of precession when the hydrogen atoms are in the thermal equilibrium state.

behave like small magnets. The nucleus which is most commonly used for medical imaging is hydrogen, since it is abundant in tissues and has favorable magnetic characteristics. When hydrogen nuclei are placed in a strong magnetic field the randomly oriented nuclei precess at a frequency determined by the magnetic field and align themselves parallel to the external magnetic field. If a specific RF pulse, resonant with (equal to) the precessing frequency, is applied to these nuclei, it causes deflection of the nuclear magnetic moment proportional to the strength of the RF pulse (Fig. 27-2). If, for example, the pulse strength is chosen to cause a 90° deflection of the nuclear magnetic moments, the nuclei rotate and continue to precess perpendicular to the external magnetic field. Magnetic moments perpendicular to the external field are capable of producing alternating current in receiver coils placed around the patient. When the RF pulse stops, the nuclei return to their original positions, or thermal equilibrium state, in alignment with the external field, and in so doing their ability to induce a current in the receiver coils decreases.

Some commonly used terms when discussing MR imaging are resonance, T1, T2, TR, TE, spin echo, and pulse sequence. A brief explanation of these terms will follow.

Definitions

Resonance

Resonance is the synchronizing of the RF emitted by the transmitter with the precessing frequency of the hydrogen nuclei in the tissue being studied. When this synchrony is

achieved energy can be transmitted to the nuclei efficiently and selectively, causing the axis of precession to deflect (Fig. 27-2). This is a fundamental principle governing all magnetic resonance imaging. The frequency at which a particular nucleus precesses depends on the strength of the external magnetic field and on an inherent property characteristic of each nucleus, called the *gyro-magnetic ratio.*

Pulse Sequence

A *pulse sequence* is a schedule of radiofrequency stimulation used to obtain images reflecting relaxation properties of the tissue or, in other words, characterizing the return of hydrogen nuclei to the thermal equilibrium state after being stimulated by the RF pulse.

The pulse sequences most commonly used are the spin echo, inversion recovery, chemical shift, and small flip angle. For the purposes of this discussion, only spin echo sequences will be considered since currently these are the most commonly used sequences for imaging the musculoskeletal system. Chemical shift and small flip angle techniques have promise in evaluation of the musculoskeletal system but are still in the development phase. In *spin echo* sequence, a 90° pulse is followed by a 180° pulse. The 90° pulse deflects the collective magnetic moments of hydrogen nuclei in the stimulated tissue into the transverse plane. The magnetic moments of hydrogen start to dephase or move away from each other as they precess because of local influence by neighboring atoms and molecules. A 180° pulse rephases them, and, as they come together, a current is produced in the receiver coil which is translated into a signal.

TE, or *echo time,* is the time between the 90° pulse and the *peak signal,* or *echo,* emitted from the excited tissue. *TR,* or *repetition time,* is the time between the 90° pulses. Spin echo sequences with relatively short TE and short TR are said to be *T1-weighted,* and sequences with long TE and TR are called *T2-weighted.*

Transverse and Longitudinal Relaxation Times

T1 and T2 are tissue-related characteristic time constants. T1 is known as the *longitudinal relaxation time* (also as the *spin-lattice relaxation time*). This is a tissue-specific time constant related to the time required to realign the magnetic moment of the nuclei with the external magnetic field after it has been deflected by a 90° RF pulse. T2 is the *transverse relaxation time,* also known as the *spin-spin relaxation time.* After the magnetic moment of the nuclei is deflected to 90° by an RF pulse, all of the nuclei are in phase with one another, i.e., all the nuclei precess as one unit. However, in a short time (a matter of milliseconds) they slip out of phase because of interactions between neighboring nuclei. As a result, transverse magnetization ceases and the signal from the scanned tissue is lost. The maximum value of this transverse magnetization is achieved immediately after the 90° RF pulse and then decreases by the tissue-specific time constant T2. For most soft tissues, the range of T1 with clinical MR units (0.15–1.5 tesla) is 220–3000 ms. T2 varies from 55 to 200 ms. In general, T1-

weighted images show anatomy best and T2-weighted images show pathology best.[14]

On T1-weighted sequences:

Tissues with short T1 have high signal intensity (bright).
Tissues with a long T1 have low signal intensity (dark).

On T2-weighted sequences:

Tissues with short T2 have low signal intensity (dark).
Tissues with a long T2 have high signal intensity (bright).

Although a detailed explanation of what influences relaxation times in healthy and diseased tissues is beyond the scope of this chapter, some basic facts are worth keeping in mind (Table 27-2). Inflamed tissue appears darker on T1-weighted images and brighter on T2-weighted images because the T1 and T2 are increased relative to normal tissue. The edema, or free water component, is probably responsible. Neoplastic tissues usually have increased relaxation times relative to the host tissue; thus the images are darker or isointense on T1- and brighter on T2-weighted images. This is also thought to be due to an increase in the free water content. Fibrous tissue has a long T1 and therefore appears dark on T1-weighted sequences. The T2 relaxation time is also reduced and therefore the signal intensity is darker than that of the host tissue. Hematoma demonstrates several changes and the signal intensities are a function of the composition of the hematoma based on its age and chemical degradation products.[17] Generally there is an increase in the T1 and T2 relaxation times, again probably because of the increased edema and inflammatory changes.[12,37]

In addition to the T1 and T2 relaxation times, signals emitted from excited tissue also depend on the proton density or availability of free hydrogen in the tissue. Flow also has

an effect on the signal intensity. For example, a glass of water would appear bright on a T2-weighted sequence; on the other hand, if the water is changed into ice, the hydrogen, now bound in the ice crystals, appears dark. With regard to flow, blood in arteries shows dark signals on both T1- and T2-weighted images. This is explained to be due to the migration of the excited cylinder of blood from the scanning field and replacement by unexcited blood before the receiver coil is turned on to detect the echo.

Finally, the selection of the proper pulse sequences for a particular examination involves careful clinical judgment coupled with firm understanding of the technology. Keeping open a two-way channel of communication between the orthopaedist and radiologist is essential when ordering these studies. An understanding of the exact question to be answered significantly affects the design of the MRI examination.

Technical Aspects

No significant health risks have been demonstrated for MRI of normal individuals. It has been noted that for some pacemakers magnetic resonance may alter the function from demand to permanent mode. Also, paramagnetic material residing within the body may undergo torque and become displaced, thus injuring the surrounding tissue. Examples of this would be some types of cerebral artery aneurysm clips and metallic foreign bodies lodged within the eye. In general, metallic orthopaedic appliances are not magnetic enough to produce heat or motion, but they do create a significant local artifact which precludes scanning for information in their immediate vicinity. This artifact is less widely disseminated in MR images than with CT.

TABLE 27-2 Relative Relaxation Times of Practical Value in the Musculoskeletal System

Normal tissue	T1	T2
Water	Long (dark)	Long (bright)
Cerebrospinal fluid	Long (dark)	Long (bright)
Fat	Short (bright)	Medium (gray, bright)
Fibrous connective tissue	Long (dark)	Very short (dark)
Tendons and ligaments	Very long (dark)	Very short (dark)
Bone	Very long (dark)	Very short (dark)
Muscle	Medium (gray)	Medium (gray)
Cartilage		
Hyaline cartilage	Intermediate (gray)	Intermediate (gray)
Fibrocartilage	Long (dark)	Very short (dark)
Abnormal process	**T1**	**T2**
Infection/inflammation	Long (dark)	Long (bright)
Neoplasm	Long (dark) or medium (isointense)	Long (bright)
Fibrosis	Long (dark)	Very short (dark)
Fatty infiltration	Short (bright)	Intermediate (bright)
Hemorrhage (acute)	Long (dark)	Long (bright)

Source: Ehman, R.L.[14] and Mitchell, D.G., et al.[21]

There are three types of magnets used in magnetic resonance: resistive, permanent, and superconductive. By far the most widely used magnet in the clinical MR setting is the superconductive magnet.

The superconductive magnet can achieve high field strengths necessary for both imaging and spectroscopy. It operates at close to $0°$ kelvin, at which current flows without resistance. To keep the magnet cooled, liquid helium and liquid nitrogen are used, which adds to the expense of operating the system. It requires more space than the other systems and has an increased shielding requirement because of higher magnetic fields. As research leads to higher-temperature superconductivity capabilities, some of the cumbersome features of a superconductive system will probably be eliminated.

CLINICAL APPLICATIONS

Avascular Necrosis

There is mounting evidence that MRI may be the most sensitive method for early detection of avascular necrosis.[16,22,24] MRI is usually not necessary when the plain film or plain tomographic findings are diagnostic; however, occasionally MRI is performed for the purpose of mapping a known involved segment[20] prior to a rotational osteotomy designed to reposition the necrotic portion of the head away from the weight-bearing area.

Bone marrow in the peripheral skeleton in adults is fatty and therefore appears bright on T1-weighted images. Avascular necrosis reveals well-defined areas with irregular margins

of low signal intensity on T1-weighted images adjacent to bright normal marrow signal (Fig. 27-3). The peripheral sclerotic margin of the necrotic segment observed on plain films or plain tomography exhibits a thin black line (low signal intensity) on magnetic resonance images. T2-weighted images show variable signal intensities in the involved areas; however, with this sequence it is easy to detect a joint effusion which is present in most patients.[23] It is possible that the T2-weighted images may have some role in staging this process, but, as this time, the correlation with other staging schemes has not been consistent or useful. It is still uncertain as to how rapidly changes of avascular necrosis will be reflected in magnetic resonance imaging after a traumatic incident (e.g., in the hip following fracture and/or dislocation). Therefore, currently we cannot recommend this technique to predict prognosis following such injuries.

Imaging in the coronal plane is usually sufficient. If volume and spatial relationships of the necrotic segment are desired then axial sections can be obtained. Both of these projections allow examination of the contralateral side for comparison. T1-weighted images are usually adequate to detect the abnormality.

Differentiating between infarction and infection in patients with sickle cell anemia is not yet possible. Both acute infarcts and infection would show decreased signal intensity on T1-weighted images and high signals on T2-weighted images. This area is currently being investigated.

In Legg-Perthes disease, involved areas in the femoral capital epiphysis show diminished or absent signal intensity.[8,38] Magnetic resonance is at least as sensitive as a radionuclide scan, but because of better spatial resolution with magnetic resonance, the extent of the lesion is accurately de-

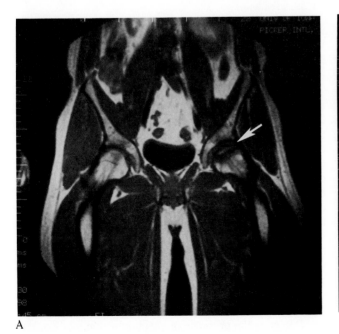

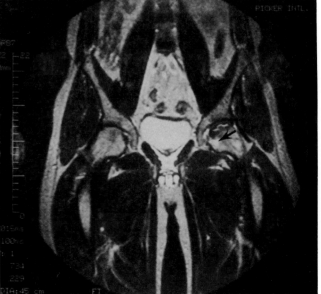

A

B

Figure 27-3 Avascular necrosis of the femoral head. **A.** Relatively T1-weighted coronal image through the femoral heads demonstrates necrotic segment (arrow) of the left femoral head. **B.** Relatively T2-weighted image again demonstrates the segment of necrosis but also a region of focally increased signal from within the femoral head and neck (arrow). Effusion in the left hip is also noted (bright areas).

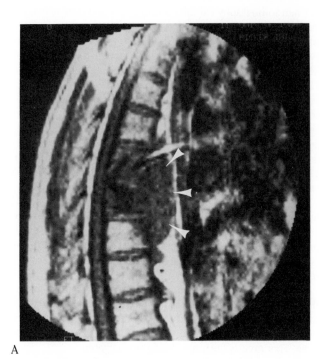

A

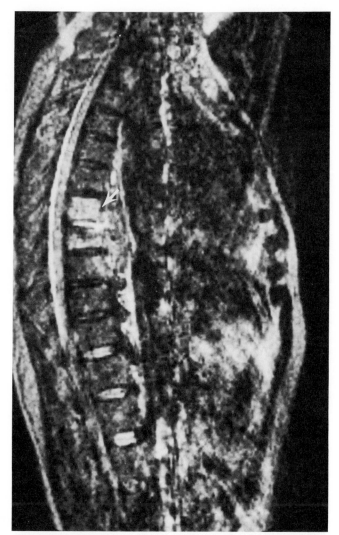

B

Figure 27-4 Imaging of vertebral osteomyelitis. **A.** A T1-weighted image demonstrating regions of low signal intensity from contiguous vertebral body marrow spaces, and a large soft-tissue low signal intensity mass confluent with these (arrowheads). The linear high signal region anterior to the vertebral bodies is an artifact. **B.** A relatively T2-weighted image demonstrates a region of high signal intensity (arrow) which involves the same vertebral bodies and is contiguous with the soft-tissue mass. This image also demonstrates the absence of significant extension into the spinal canal.

lineated, and this imaging technique may have an impact on the treatment.

Magnetic resonance has been successfully used in studying avascular necrosis of the lunate,[26] talus,[36] and knee.[32]

Infection

Because of its excellent sensitivity to an increase in free water, magnetic resonance promises to be very helpful in the diagnosis of musculoskeletal infections. Recent reports[2,4,5] compared MRI with other modalities used to diagnose osteomyelitis, septic arthritis, and abscess formation. The overall conclusion is that MRI is superior to radionuclide scan, tomography, CT, and plain films for establishing the early presence and extent of infectious processes.

Because of the increase in edema associated with an inflammatory response, there is increased signal intensity on T2-weighted images, usually accompanied by diminished marrow signal intensity in T1-weighted images (Fig. 27-4). This higher signal intensity is readily seen even in small

amounts or in small body parts, and is easily distinguished from the surrounding lower signal intensity regions of normal tissue. Since the bright signal seen on T2-weighted images in tissues with infection is caused by the increasing amounts of free water, it is also, therefore, less specific. The current MRI diagnostic criterion employed by most investigators for osteomyelitis is the presence of either diffuse or localized increase in marrow signal in T2-weighted images.[4] In the soft tissues if the signal is increased in a diffuse pattern, and there is no associated low signal band peripherally, this is most consistent with cellulitis and/or edema. With a focally increased signal pattern surrounded by a thin peripheral band with low signals, an abscess must be considered.[2] The abscess on T1-weighted images usually has a corresponding low signal intensity.

Detecting the presence of infection within joints or tendon sheaths is more difficult. When there is intracapsular or synovial fluid there should be marked increased signal intensity on T2-weighted images and decreased signal intensity on the T1-weighted images. Pyarthrosis or infected tenosynovial fluid is suggested if, in addition to the above criteria for the presence of fluid, there is also evidence of increased signal intensity in the soft-tissue structures, indicating inflammation or infection.[2]

Trauma

Acute muscle hematomas and muscle tears or avulsions are nicely demonstrated by MRI.[15] We had the opportunity to study a few patients with suspected avulsion of the hamstring group from the ischial tuberosity (Fig. 27-5). With the help of MRI the certainty of this diagnosis is greatly enhanced. Acute hematomas show low signal intensity on T1-weighted and high signal intensity on T2-weighted images. This pattern, however, changes as the hematoma becomes subacute or chronic.

The role of MRI in evaluation of spinal fractures is becoming better defined.[34] Magnetic resonance permits direct visualization of the spinal canal and cord in the sagittal plane. Magnetic resonance can frequently differentiate cord hematoma from cord edema, and may permit us to predict a better prognosis for patients with edema.[28] Retropulsed bone fragments and hematomas impinging on the thecal sac and cord can be well seen.

Soft-tissue injuries in and about the knee have received a good deal of attention in recent literature.[11] MRI, in contradistinction to arthrography and arthroscopy, is capable of demonstrating intra- and extracapsular abnormalities.[6] The posterior cruciate ligament is consistently and reliably visualized on magnetic resonance exams in the sagittal plane and is seen as a thick low signal band on both T1- and T2-weighted

images. The anterior cruciate is more difficult to show with consistency because of its smaller size and oblique course, and because it has slightly more internal signals than the posterior cruciate and therefore appears grayish black, instead of black, on the T1-weighted images (Fig. 27-6).

Menisci are well demonstrated by MRI; however, because its images reflect both structure and biochemical composition, minor chemical changes in the substance of the menisci could be misinterpreted as tears. Most investigators are still on the learning curve; however, certain criteria for diagnosing the presence or absence of tears are slowly emerging.[11] The majority of mistakes and false-positive interpretations are made in the posterior horns.[35] Tears are diagnosed with more certainty when abnormal signals clearly reach the surface of the meniscus and if they are associated with abnormalities in the contour of the meniscus.

The muscles, tendons, and collateral ligaments around the knee are also demonstrated by MRI (Fig. 27-7).

Neoplasm

Skeletal

MRI is sensitive in the early detection of primary and metastatic bone tumors.[9,30] The technique is especially helpful to the surgeon in staging primary malignant bone tumors by demonstrating medullary and soft-tissue extension.[33] The ability to image in any plane, including direct coronal and sagittal, has helped in surgical planning. With some exceptions, magnetic resonance images lack bony tissue specificity. Therefore, for making a specific diagnosis and assessing bio-

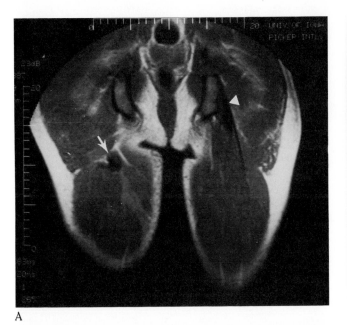

A

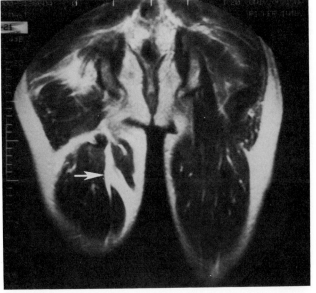

B

Figure 27-5 Tendinous avulsion of the hamstrings at their origin on the right. **A.** A T1-weighted image in the coronal plane at the level of the origin of the hamstring complex from the ischial ramus demonstrates inferior displacement of the large tendinous portion of the right hamstring (straight arrow). Neither plain films nor MRI suggested bony avulsion. The normal tendinous origin of the left hamstring is seen for comparison (arrowhead). **B.** A coronal T2-weighted image at the same level shows the extensive hemorrhage and edema within the fascial compartments and the retracted hamstring muscle (arrow).

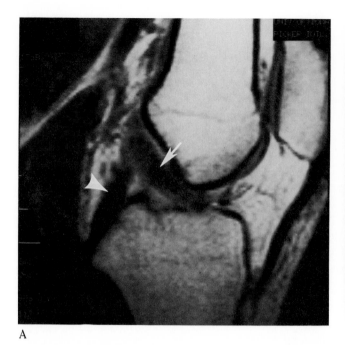

A

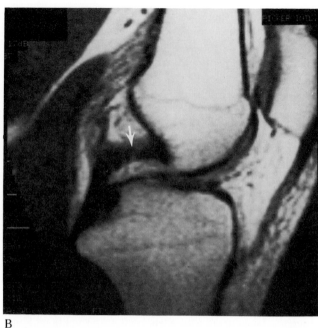

B

Figure 27-6 Magnetic resonance images of normal cruciate ligaments. **A.** A T1-weighted image demonstrates the normal course and appearance of the anterior cruciate ligament (straight arrow). The most posteroinferior portion of the posterior cruciate ligament is also imaged (arrowhead). **B.** The remainder of the

posterior cruciate ligament (arrow) is seen as it curves to attach at the medial aspect of the femoral condyles. The posterior cruciate ligament normally demonstrates lower signal intensity than the anterior cruciate ligament.

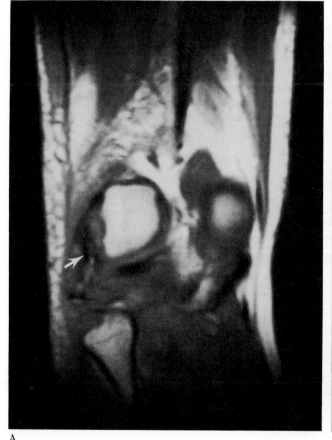

A

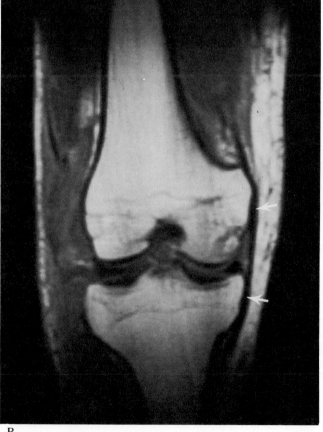

B

Figure 27-7 T1-weighted images demonstrating lateral collateral ligament disruption about the knee. **A.** A coronal image through the posterior portion of the knee demonstrates disrup-

tion of the fibular collateral ligament (arrow). **B.** More anterior coronal imaging demonstrates a normal appearing medial collateral ligament (arrows).

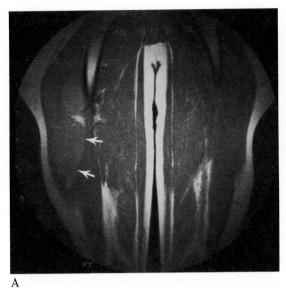

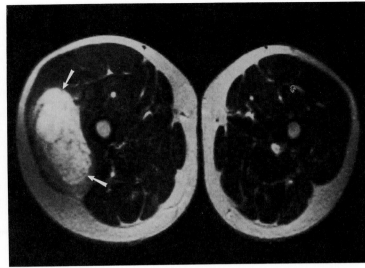

A

B

Figure 27-8 Malignant soft tissue tumor in the right vastus lateralis. **A.** This relatively T1-weighted, coronal image demonstrates a large mass in the right vastus lateralis with signal intensity slightly greater than muscle (arrows). **B.** Axial T2-weighted images demonstrate nearly complete replacement of the vastus lat-

eralis on the right by very high signal intensity neoplastic tissue (arrows), which proved to be a rhabdomyosarcoma. The extent of the tumor is particularly well visualized on T2-weighted images.

logical activity of a bone lesion one has to rely on plain radiographs and CT. Soft-tissue calcifications, cortical destruction, and periosteal reaction are not well detected by MRI.[1]

Both T1 and T2 relaxation times usually increase relative to the surrounding normal tissue and therefore tumors appear as areas of decreased signal intensity on T1-weighted images and show increased signal intensity on T2-weighted images.[3]

In searching for metastatic foci in the bone, radionuclide scanning remains the examination of choice. Minor areas of bone destruction may not be clearly detected by MRI. However MRI has had a great impact in studying spinal metastasis and is the preferred investigation when canal invasion and cord compression are suspected. MRI in most institutions has replaced myelography for evaluation of the patient with suspected metastatic disease of the spine accompanied by

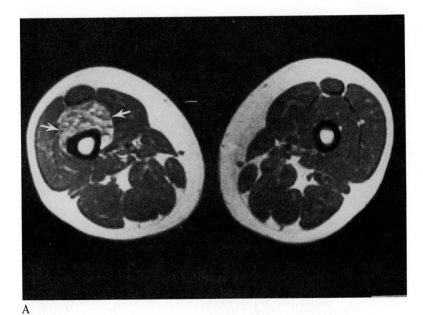

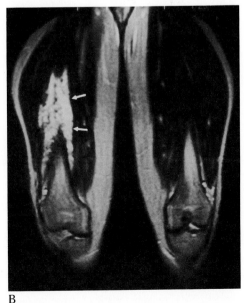

A

B

Figure 27-9 Benign hemangiolipoma involving the vastus intermedius muscle. **A.** Axial, relatively T1-weighted images through the distal thigh demonstrate a moderately high signal intensity mass (arrows) nearly completely replacing the vastus intermedius muscle. The high signal is thought to be caused by the blood

and/or fat component of the mass. **B.** Coronal T2-weighted images just anterior to the femurs demonstrate very high signal intensity regions (arrows) on the right caused by the large hemangiomatous component of this mass.

lower-extremity weakness or paralysis. For these patients, it is more expedient and less invasive to perform MRI. Use of a T2-weighted sequence and the appropriate surface coils yields exquisite images of thecal sac and surrounding bone and soft-tissue structures. These images are always obtained in conjunction with T1-weighted images, which tend to delineate the anatomy better than T2-weighted images.

Soft Tissue

MRI is by far the best available diagnostic modality for a suspected soft-tissue tumor.[30] In patients with known soft-tissue tumors, MRI can demonstrate the size and extent of the lesion as well as the neurovascular invasion (Fig. 27-8). It is not always possible to tell benign from malignant soft-tissue tumors. The tumors that can be characterized by MRI are lipoma, which appears bright (increased signal intensity) on both T1- and T2-weighted images; hemangioma, which is very bright (hyperintense) on T2-weighted images (Fig. 27-9); and desmoplastic fibroma or aggressive fibromatosis, which appears as black areas (decreased signal intensity) on both T1- and usually T2-weighted images (Fig. 27-10).

MRI is also helpful in the follow-up of patients who had resection of a soft-tissue tumor. It is also conceivable that in the near future paramagnetic contrast agents such as gadolinium (Gd-DTPA), which shortens both T1 and T2 relaxation time of tumors, will be available for clinical use. Such contrast agents carry the promise that they may be capable of differentiating postsurgical change and fibrosis from tumor recurrence.

Synovial Disease

In patients with severe rheumatoid arthritis (RA) and cervical spine involvement, most centers now perform MRI to study cord compromise or impingement on the brain stem. Anterior atlantoaxial subluxation and cranial settling are serious complications of craniovertebral junction involvement with RA. These patients were previously studied with myelography followed by plain tomography or CT. With MRI, abnormal signals from the cord substance and brain stem have been detected in symptomatic patients, which is an advantage over myelography. Massive pannus with destruction of the odontoid process also can be shown (Fig. 27-11). Images of the cervical spine acquired with cardiac gating are superior to images acquired without gating; however, they require more time to perform.

A

Figure 27-10 Recurrent desmoplastic fibroma in the region of the previously resected left hamstring complex. **A.** Axial T1-weighted images in the upper thigh demonstrate a homogeneous low signal intensity mass (arrow) occupying the region of the left hamstring muscles, which have been previously resected, and lying adjacent to the anteromedial sciatic nerve (arrowhead). **B.** Sagittal T2-weighted images also demonstrate the homogeneous lack of signal from within this mass (lower arrows). This is characteristic of dense desmoid tumors. The infiltrative nature of the lesion can be seen at the superior margin of the tumor in the low signal mass infiltrating fibers of the gluteus maximus muscle (upper arrows). The absence of the hamstring muscle complex inferior to the mass is readily apparent.

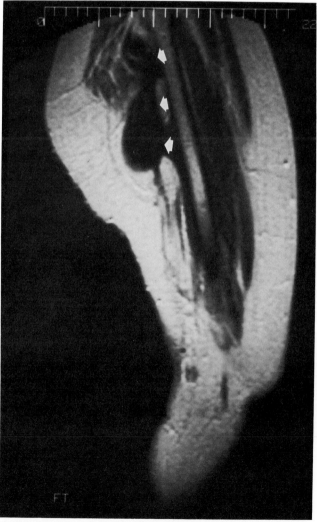

B

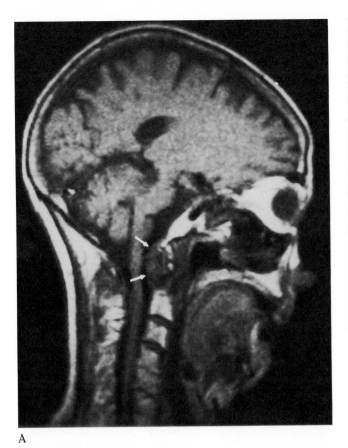

A

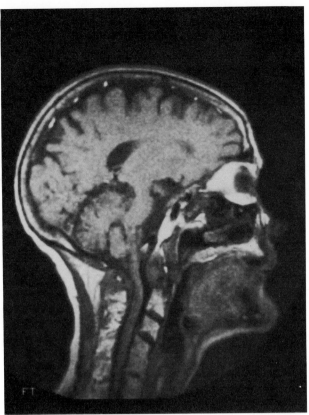

B

Figure 27-11 Rheumatoid pannus from the occiput to the C2 region. **A.** T1-weighted images in the midline sagittal position demonstrate a large intermediate signal intensity mass extending from the anterior portion of the foramen magnum down to the mid-body of C2 (arrows). The patient has rheumatoid arthritis, and this represents inflammatory pannus. This view is in flexion. **B.** A similar T1-weighted image obtained at the same level but in extension demonstrates motion at the junction of the inflammatory mass of pannus and the mid-body of C2 with posterior displacement of the upper cervical cord and brain stem.

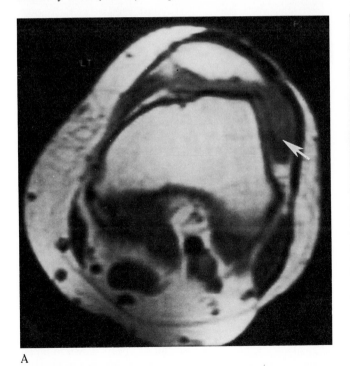

A

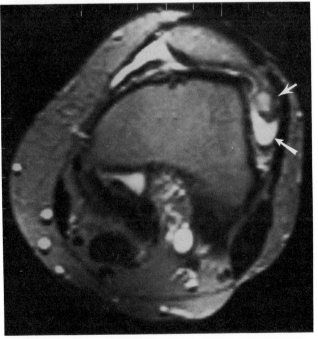

B

Figure 27-12 Magnetic resonance images of focal pigmented villonodular synovitis of the left knee. **A.** A relatively T1-weighted axial image through the right femur at the level of the patella demonstrates a mass with inhomogeneous signal intensity (arrow) in the lateral portion of the intraarticular space. **B.** A T2-weighted image at the same level demonstrates a focal pedunculated mass (short arrow). This was surgically proved to be focal pigmented villonodular synovitis. Surrounding synovial fluid is seen as a homogeneous, high signal intensity (long arrow) region.

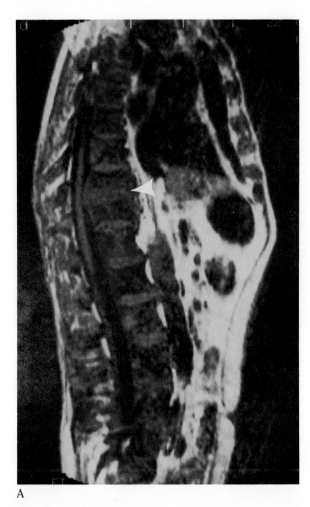

A

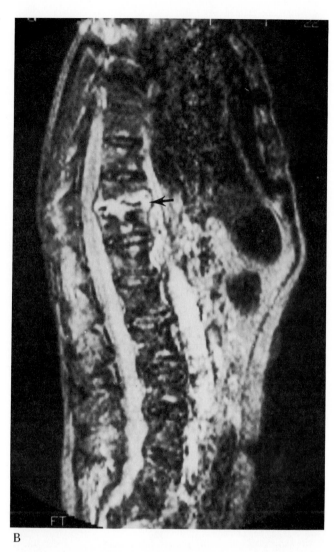

B

Figure 27-13 Diffuse metastatic carcinoma of the prostate involving nearly the entire vertebral column. **A.** A T1-weighted, nearly midline, sagittal image demonstrates a diffuse, inhomogeneous appearance of the entire spine with a central mass (arrow head) pushing the midthoracic cord posteriorly. The marrow of the vertebral bodies has been inhomogeneously replaced by tumor deposits. **B.** A T2-weighted image at the same level demonstrates more specifically that the focal mass in the midthoracic spine is indeed part of a pathological fracture complex with hematoma (arrow) and posterior longitudinal ligament impinging on the anterior portion of the thecal sac, displacing the cord posteriorly.

In other joints with RA synovial hypertrophy, cartilage thinning and erosions, cysts, and joint and tendon sheath effusions are easily demonstrated by MRI.

MRI is an ideal way to study patients with pigmented villonodular synovitis[19] (Fig. 27-12) and synovial osteochrondromatosis.

Marrow Packing Disorders

Marrow packing diseases such as Hodgkin's disease, lymphomas, leukemias, multiple myeloma, and Gaucher's disease are primarily medical diseases. The orthopaedic surgeon gets involved when fractures occur in weakened bone or when avascular necrosis and infection develop as a complication of the treatment. As has been shown in the section on metastasis, MRI is a sensitive method of detecting tumor deposits in bone marrow (Fig. 27-13).[10,35] These deposits appear as areas of decreased signal intensity on T1-weighted images (Fig. 27-14). Diffuse marrow involvement with any of the marrow packing diseases results in a generalized decrease in signal intensity of the bone marrow. MRI has been shown to be effective in following the results of treatment and in locating optimal sites for biopsy. Chemical shift imaging and the technique known as "STIR" (short T1 inversion recovery sequence) have been preferred by some investigators in evaluating these diseases over the spin-echo sequences.[35]

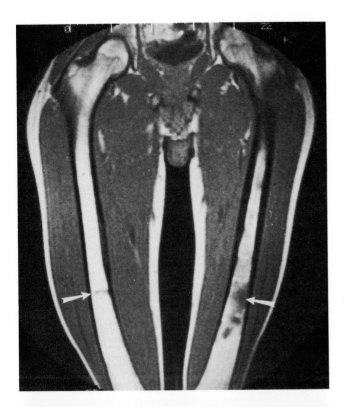

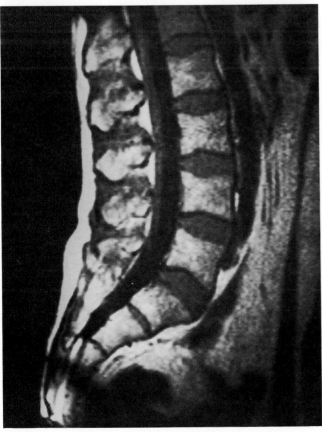

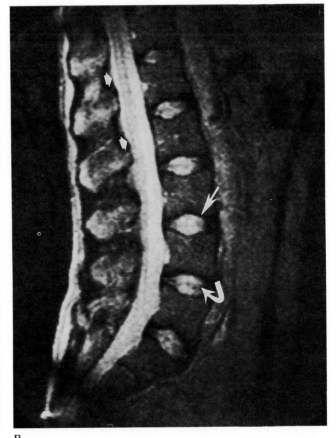

Figure 27-14 Lymphoma. Coronal T1-weighted image through the shaft of the femurs demonstrates patchy replacement of bone marrow (arrows) by lymphoma with apparent preservation of cortical margins. The replacement is very extensive on the left and only spotty on the right.

Disc Disease

MRI has capabilities which combine the advantages of CT, myelography, and discography without being invasive. Because magnetic resonance is sensitive to free hydrogen in tissues it shows early disc dehydration and degeneration.[25,29,35] Healthy discs appear bright on T2-weighted images (Fig. 27-15B), whereas degenerated discs lose their brightness. In general, most herniated discs are also degenerated, but not all (Fig. 27-16).

T2-weighted sequences yield what is known as the *myelographic effect,* showing the thecal sac as bright and resembling a myelogram very closely.

In all disc studies appropriate surface coils are used to improve the signal-to-noise ratio of the images.[13] As mentioned before, cardiac gating may add to the clarity of the images.

A

B

Figure 27-15 Midline sagittal images of a normal lumbar spine. **A.** A T1-weighted image shows normal appearance of lumbar vertebrae and intervertebral discs using a surface coil. **B.** A T2-weighted image at the same level shows the high signal from the cerebral spinal fluid (short arrows), known as the "myelographic effect," and bright signals from the intervertebral disc nuclear material (large arrow). The intranuclear cleft (curved arrow), with lower signal, is also demonstrated at the L4–5 level.

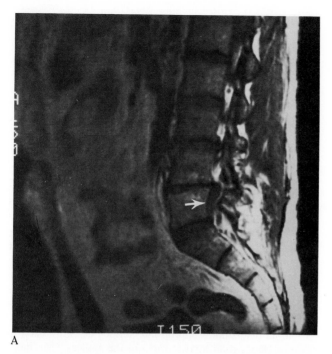

A

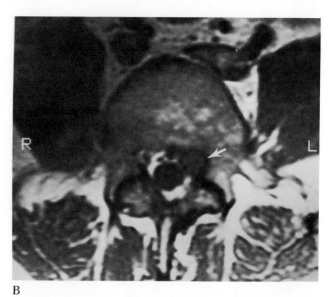

B

Figure 27-16 Extruded disc at L4–5 with migration posterior to the L5 vertebral body. **A.** A sagittal T1-weighted image to the left side of the spinal canal shows a low signal intensity mass (arrow) behind the body of L5 and a narrowed L4–L5 intervertebral disc space. **B.** An axial T1-weighted image through the body of L5

demonstrates that the lateral recess is filled with a low signal intensity mass (arrow). **C.** An axial T1-weighted image through the L5, S1 disc shows a normal appearance for comparison with the disc above and demonstrates normal-appearing nerve roots (arrow), surrounded by fat.

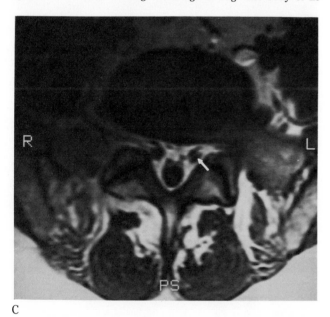

C

MRI is slowly becoming the primary study for evaluation of disc disease. There are also indications that, by using Gd-DTPA, it may be effective in differentiating scar tissue from recurrent disc herniation following surgery.[35] MRI is also being used to screen patients for the presence of spinal dysraphism and also for scoliosis patients prior to surgery (Fig. 27-17).

REFERENCES

1. Aisen, A.M., Martel, W., Braunstein, E.M., McMillin, K.I., Phillips, W.A., and Kling, T.F. MRI and CT evaluation of primary bone and soft tissue tumors. AJR 146:749–756, 1986.
2. Beltran, J., Noto, A.M., McGhee, R.B., Freedy, R.M., and McCalla, M. Infections of the musculoskeletal system: High-field strength MR imaging. Radiology 164:449–454, 1987.
3. Berquist, T.H. Bone and soft tissue tumors, in Berquist, T.H., et al (eds): *Magnetic Resonance of the Musculoskeletal System.* New York, Raven, 1987, chap 4, pp 85–108.
4. Berquist, T.H. Musculoskeletal infection, in Berquist, T.H., et al (eds): *Magnetic Resonance of the Musculoskeletal System.* New York, Raven, 1987, chap 5, pp 109–126.
5. Berquist, T.H., Brown, M.L., Fitzgerald, R.H., and May, G.R. Magnetic resonance imaging: Application in musculoskeletal infection. Magnet Reson Imag 3:219–230, 1985.
6. Berquist, T.H., Ehman, R.L., Rand, J.A., and Scott, S. Musculoskeletal trauma, in Berquist, T.H., et al (eds): *Magnetic Resonance of the Musculoskeletal System.* New York, Raven, 1987, chap 6, pp 127–163.
7. Berquist, T.H., Ehman, R.L., and Richardson, M.L. (eds): *Magnetic Resonance of the Musculoskeletal System.* New York, Raven, 1987.
8. Blueman, R.G., Falke, T.H.M., Ziedes des Plantes, B.G., Jr., and Steiner, R.M. Early Legg-Perthes disease (ischemic necrosis of the femoral head) demonstrated by magnetic resonance imaging. Skeletal Radiol 14:95–98, 1985.
9. Bohndorf, K., Reiser, M., Lochner, B., deLacroix, W.F., and Steinbrich, W. Magnetic resonance imaging of primary tumors and tumor-like lesions of bone. Skeletal Radiol 15:511–517, 1986.
10. Cohen, M.D., Klatte, E.C., Baehner, R., et al. Magnetic resonance imaging of bone marrow disease in children. Radiology 151:715–718, 1984.

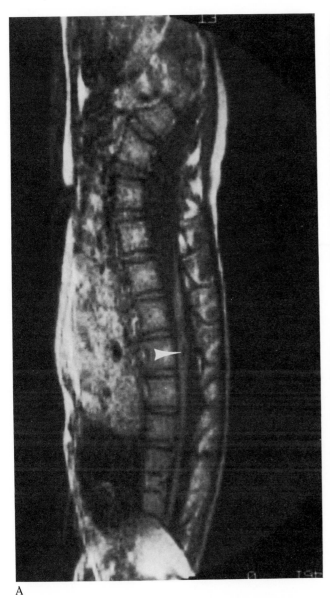

A

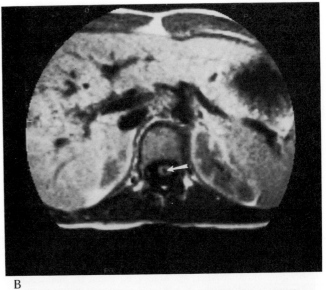

B

C

Figure 27-17 Images of the spinal cord of an 11-year-old female made for evaluation of very mild scoliosis associated with neurological deficit. **A.** A sagittal image near mid-line with relative T1-weighting demonstrates central widening of the cord with a low signal intensity region (arrowhead) suggestive of at least a focal portion of hydromyelia. **B.** A T1-weighted axial image through this level of low signal intensity confirms the lesion's central location (arrow). **C.** An axial T1-weighted image slightly lower than *B* shows diastematomyelia (arrow) not readily appreciated from the sagittal imaging.

11. Crues, J.V., III, Mink, J., Levy, T.L., Lotysch, M., and Stoller, D.W. Meniscal tears of the knee: Accuracy of MR imaging. Radiology 164:445–448, 1987.

12. Dooms, G.C., Fisher, M.R., Hricak, H., and Higgins, C.B. MR imaging of intramuscular hemorrhage. J Comput Assist Tomogr 9:908–913, 1985.

13. Edelman, R.R., Shoulimas, G.M., Stark, D.D., et al. High resolution surface-coil imaging of lumbar disk disease. Am J Radiol 144:1123–1129, 1985.

14. Ehman, R.L. Interpretation of magnetic resonance images, in Berquist, T.H., et al (eds): *Magnetic Resonance of the Musculoskeletal System.* New York, Raven, 1987, chap 2, pp 23–64.

15. Ehman, R.L., and Berquist, T.H. Magnetic resonance imaging of musculoskeletal trauma. Radiol Clin North Am 24:291–319, 1986.

16. Gillespy, T., III, Gerrant, H.K., and Helms, C.A. Magnetic resonance imaging of osteonecrosis. Radiol Clin North Am 24:193–208, 1986.

17. Gomori, F.M., Grossman, R.I., Goldberg, H.I., Zimmerman, R.A., and Bilaniuk, L.T. Intracranial hematomas: Imaging by high field MR. Radiology 157:87–93, 1985.

18. Harms, S.E., Morgan, T.J., Yamanaski, W.S., Harli, T.S., and Dodd, G.D. Principles of nuclear magnetic resonance imaging. Radiographics 4:26–43, 1984.

19. Hartzman, S., Reicher, M.A., Bassett, L.W., Duckwiler, G., Mandelbaum, B., and Gold, R.H. MR imaging of the knee. Part II. Chronic disorders. Radiology 162:553–557, 1987.

20. Markisz, J.A., Knowles, R.J.R., Altchek, D.W., Schneider, R., Whalen,

J.P., and Cahill, P.T. Segmental patterns of avascular necrosis of the femoral heads: Early detection with MR imaging. Radiology 162:717–720, 1987.

21. Mitchell, D.G., Burk, D.L., Jr., Vinitski, S., and Rifkin, M.D. The biophysical basis of tissue contrast in extracranial MR imaging. Am J Radiol 149:831–837, 1987.

22. Mitchell, M.D., Kundel, H.L., Steinberg, M.E., Kressel, H.Y., Alavi, A., and Axel, L. Avascular necrosis of the hip: Comparison of MR, CT and scintigraphy. Am J Radiol 147:67–71, 1986.

23. Mitchell, D.G., Rao, V., Dalinka, M., Spritzer, C.E., Geftel, W.B., Axel, L., Steinberg, M., and Kressel, H.Y. MRI of joint fluid in the normal and ischemic hip. Am J Radiol 146:1215–1218, 1986.

24. Mitchell, D.G., Rao, V.M., Dalinka, M.K., Spritzer, C.E., Alavi, A., Steinberg, M.E., Fallon, M., and Kressel, H.Y. Femoral head avascular necrosis: Correlation of MR imaging, radiographic staging, radionuclide imaging, and clinical findings. Radiology 162:709–715, 1987.

25. Modic, M.T., Pavlicek, W., Weinstein, M.A., Boumphrey, F., Ngo, F., Hardy, R., and Duchesneau, P.M. Magnetic resonance imaging of intervertebral disk disease. Radiology 152:103–111, 1984.

26. Naegele, M., Kuglstatter, W., Krauss, B., Hahn, D., Markl, A.A., Lissner, J., and Wilhelm, K. Ischemic necrosis of the lunati: Correlative study of MR imaging, bone scintigraphy, conventional radiography, and surgical perspectives. Radiology 161(P): 24, 1986.

27. Nixon, J.R. Basic principles and terminology, in Berquist, T.H., et al (eds): *Magnetic Resonance of the Musculoskeletal System.* New York, Raven, 1987, chap 1, pp 1–21.

28. Paushter, D.M., and Modic, M.T. Magnetic resonance imaging of the spine. Appl Radiol 13:61–68, 1984.

29. Pech, P., and Haughton, V.M. Lumbar intervertebral disk: Correlative MR and anatomic study. Radiology 156:699–701, 1985.

30. Petterson, H., Gillespy, T., III, Hamlin, D.J., Enneking, W.F., Springfield, D.S., Andrew, E.R., Spainer, S., and Slone, R. Primary musculoskeletal tumors: Examination with MR imaging compared with conventional modalities. Radiology 164:237–241, 1987.

31. Petterson, H., Hamlin, D.J., Mancuso, A., and Scott, K.N. Magnetic resonance imaging of the musculoskeletal system. Acta Radiol 26:225–235, 1985.

32. Pollack, M.S., Dalinka, M.K., Kressel, H.Y., Lotki, P.A., and Spritzer, C.E. Magnetic resonance imaging in the evaluation of suspected osteonecrosis of the knee. Skeletal Radiol 16:121–127, 1987.

33. Richardson, M.L., Kilcoyne, R.F., Gillespy, T., III, Helms, C.A., and Genant, H.K. Magnetic resonance imaging of musculoskeletal neoplasms. Radiol Clin North Am 24:259–267, 1986.

34. Richardson, M.R. Magnetic resonance imaging of the spine, in Berquist, T.H., et al (eds): *Magnetic Resonance of the Musculoskeletal System.* New York, Raven, 1987, chap 7, pp 165–184.

35. Sartoris, D.J., and Resnick, D. MR imaging of the musculoskeletal system: Current and future status. Am J Radiol 149:457–467, 1987.

36. Sierra, A., Potchen, E.J., Moore, J., and Smith, H.G. High-field magnetic resonance imaging of aseptic necrosis of the talus. J Bone Joint Surg [Am] 68A:927–928, 1986.

37. Swenson, S.J., Keller, P.L., Berquist, T.H., McLeod, R.A., and Stephens, D.H. Magnetic resonance imaging of hemorrhage. Am J Radiol 145:921–927, 1985.

38. Toby, E.B., Koman, L.A., and Bechtold, R.E. Magnetic resonance imaging of pediatric hip disease. J Pediatr Orthop 5:665–671, 1985.

PART IV

General Considerations in Pediatric Orthopaedics

CHAPTER 28

Orthopaedic Management of Cerebral Palsy

Mark Hoffer

CLASSIFICATION

The cerebral palsies are a group of diseases whose common etiology is brain damage, either intrauterine or soon after birth. Excluded from the strict definition of cerebral palsy are those congenital problems that are familial, those problems that are progressive, and those problems that are acquired in childhood as a result of head injuries. So far as the orthopaedic surgeon is concerned, however, as long as the brain damage is static, the treatment is essentially the same. In the acquired brain damage patient it takes at least 2 years to reach such a static state. Brain-damaged children can be roughly classified into groups depending on the type of involvement the patient has and the geographic distribution of the involvement on the body (Table 28-1). In general, there are three types of cerebral palsy: spastic, motion disorder, and mixed. The child with spasticity has hyperactive reflexes, tends to develop contractures, and may be amenable to orthotic and surgical therapeutic approaches. A child with motion disorder (athetosis, chorea, tremor, etc.) has major problems with control of limb position and limb balance. These patients rarely are amenable to orthopaedic and orthotic measures; however, therapists have a major impact on their lives in terms of self-care and occupational programs. Many children have a mixed picture of spasticity and motion disorder. It is important to identify these children because the extent to which the patient is disabled by a motion disorder affects the prognosis of many surgical procedures.

The geographic distribution of the disability in the cerebral-palsied or head-injured individual has a profound effect on function and the need for orthopaedic care. The *hemiplegic* patient has involvement predominantly on one side. It is not infrequent to see the opposite lower limb slightly involved in the hemiplegic patient. The hemiplegic patient tends to have more involvement distally, that is, in the hands and feet, than proximally. Nearly all hemiplegic cerebral palsy patients eventually walk and talk. This is not necessarily true of those with acquired hemiplegia. The most common deformities in the spastic hemiplegic child are equinovarus and the pronated flexed forearm, wrist, and finger combination.

The *spastic diplegic* patient has involvement predominantly of the lower extremities, although there is practically always some involvement in the upper extremities and there may in fact be strabismus associated with this spastic diple-

gia. These patients have more problems with their hips than their feet. They may be ambulatory if they develop balance reactions by 3 years of age. This means that they will have lost the perinatal reflexes prior to that time, usually in a gradual fashion. Thus, the examination for asymmetrical tonic neck reflex (perinatal reflex) versus parachute reaction (early balance reaction) is a key factor in estimating a prognosis for eventual balance and ambulation (see Table 28-2). These are the patients who frequently decrease their ambulation as they get larger in late adolescence. Persistent contractures and dislocated hips also tend to decrease the ambulatory ability in this group of patients.

TABLE 28-1 Classification of Cerebral Palsy

A. Type:
   Spastic
   Motion disorder
   Athetoid ataxia, etc.

B. Geographic distribution:
   Quadriplegia
   Diplegia
   Hemiplegia

C. Reflex level:
   Brainstem: Symmetrical tonic neck reflexes
   Midbrain: Parachute reaction
   　　　　　Upright balance

D. Motor testing:
   Contractures, joint or myotendon
   Myotendinous tone, spasticity
   Pattern posture
   Selective control

E. Sensory testing:
   Object identification
   Two-point discrimination

F. Intelligence

G. Communication:
   Verbal
   Nonverbal

TABLE 28-2 Reflex Testing

A. Brainstem reflex level: Present normally to 6 months of age; when obligatory thereafter, diagnostic of cerebral palsy. If persists past 3 years, walking doubtful. If persists past 6 years, independent sitting doubtful.
  1. Asymmetrical tonic neck reflex: occiput side extremities flex; face side extremities extend.
  2. Symmetrical tonic neck reflex: upper extremities flex, lower extremities extend with neck flexed; upper extremities extend, lower extremities flex with neck extended.

B. Midbrain reflex level: Present normally at 4 to 6 months and throughout life.
  Signs of balance reaction:
  1. Parachute. Arms and legs abduct and extend when prone child is lowered a few inches.
  2. Upright balance. Arms and trunk balance with sideward challenge.

The *totally involved* patient (called *spastic quadriplegic* by some; we would rather reserve the term *quadriplegia* for a spinal palsy) has involvement in all four extremities but in addition has significant problems in balance, swallowing, and communication. They rarely ambulate and most of them have great problems with activities of daily living (ADL) skills. These patients have a higher incidence of scoliosis and dislocating hips.

GENERAL ORTHOPAEDIC APPROACH AND MANAGEMENT

Types of Deformities

Deformities that the orthopaedic surgeon is asked to deal with in these spastic patients may be of three varieties. First, there is the dynamic deformity which accompanies abnormal muscle tone. The degree of tone is difficult to estimate unless the patient is totally asleep, and then one may also see how much fixed deformity there is. Second, many deformities that are initially dynamic eventually develop fixed contractures of the musculotendinous structures. Third, fixed joint contractures may develop, and the joints may eventually dislocate.[41,42]

In the totally involved cerebral palsy patient and in the spastic diplegic patient who has not developed balance, hip and knee deformities may become a problem in sitting and ability to transfer.[30] Surgical procedures are usually not performed on deformed feet in nonambulatory patients because of the unpredictability of such procedures.

Deformities and Ambulation Potential

Dynamic deformities in potentially ambulatory children rarely prevent ambulation, although they may make gait less efficient. Thus, these dynamic deformities should be addressed after the patient begins ambulating and when therapist and surgeon perceive that a plateau has been reached which cannot be overcome by therapy and orthotic devices.[16] On the other hand, fixed deformities can interfere with the onset of ambulation in individuals with balance problems and either spastic diplegia or spastic hemiplegia. This is especially true of hip flexion contractures in excess of 45°, adduction contractures prohibiting 30° of abduction, and knee flexion contractures that are greater than 20°. Fixed deformities of the foot rarely interfere with the onset of ambulation, although they may affect the efficiency of gait. To estimate where the knee and foot deformities have an effect on ambulatory ability, one should see if the patient can ambulate by knee walking.

Pelvic Obliquity and Hip Stability

The child with scoliosis and pelvic obliquity has instability of the high side hip.[23,24,25] It is debatable whether the scoliosis causes this instability or the unstable hip causes the scoliosis.[26,31,37] Most now believe that the two cannot be separated in a cause-and-effect relation. In terms of treatment, however, the pelvic obliquity must be eliminated before the hip is dealt with. Thus, a spine fusion is necessary when there is fixed pelvic obliquity, and a release of the abducted opposite side is necessary if there is dynamic pelvic obliquity.

Release of Hip Deformities

Adduction contractures prohibiting abduction of 30° and hip flexion contractures of 45° or greater should be released, especially when they are increasing in younger children. This is advised even when x-ray views of the hip are normal. This is not necessary, however, in older adolescents with normal-appearing hips.

Adductor Release

Indications In ambulatory patients, overactivity of the adductors tends to decrease the width of the gait.[32,36,39,46] Overactive adductors may cause hip dislocations, especially in the nonambulatory patient. Releases of the adductor longus and the gracilis are the easiest and most proven procedures to decrease this width of gait when tone alone is the problem. When there is a fixed contracture prohibiting 30° of abduction, lengthening of the brevis should be carried out in addition. If there is concern about subluxation, obturator neurectomy should be added.[2,53] Overzealous adductor lengthenings and obturator neurectomies can result in an abducted hip. This penalizes gait and even makes it difficult for patients to sit. Furthermore, it may force the opposite hip to adopt an adducted position when sitting.

Surgical Technique The adductors are approached through a transverse incision 1 cm beneath the groin crease. The length of the incision should be 3 to 5 cm, and care should be taken to avoid the femoral triangle laterally. The adductor longus can be easily located because it is tendinous and is released in its entirety. The gracilis is a thick band just medial to the adductor longus, and it is also released in its entirety. The brevis lies beneath these two muscles, and on the surface of the brevis one can see the anterior branch of the obturator nerve. If an obturator neurectomy is to be carried out, it should be performed upon this branch alone. The brevis is released to the extent of allowing abduction to 50°. The wound is closed with interrupted sutures and a drain. This is necessary because the incidence of hematomas and infections is high in this procedure. Abduction is maintained utilizing two long leg plasters and a bar with the thighs adducted 45° from each other. In the hip that is stable, this is all that is necessary and is utilized for only 3 weeks, after which it is utilized as a night splint for another 3 to 4 weeks.

Flexor Release

Indications Flexed hip postures in the ambulatory patient may cause a lumbar lordosis and a compensatory knee flexion posture. Overactivated hip flexors may cause hip dislocations, especially in the nonambulatory patient. There is some discussion in the literature about whether the psoas or all the other flexors cause this problem.[6,7,20,33] The only definite way to find which is the offending muscle is an ambulatory electromyogram.[28] In general we have found that the psoas tends to be the main problem in this posture. Lengthening of the psoas is advised especially when there is an increased sacral femoral angle seen on a standing lateral view and there is a fixed contracture of the hip exceeding 45°. Overzealous psoas lengthenings may be a problem, especially in patients with "extensor thrust" (tendency to a spastic extensor posture of knees and hips). In these patients an extension contracture of the hips may result, and this makes sitting even more difficult.[8] Finally, a rare complication of the extensor posture of the hip may be an anterior dislocation. Therefore, these hip flexor lengthenings should only be performed on patients with fixed contractures who have defined flexed hip postures documented by lateral sacral femoral views.

Surgical Technique Psoas lengthening is best performed through an anterolateral hip approach and not through the groin. This is because the groin approach releases the psoas from its insertion but the degree of lengthening is difficult to ascertain. Through the anterolateral approach using either the traditional Smith-Petersen or a more transverse "bikini" incision, the sartorius is located and released. Beneath the sartorius the first muscle encountered is the psoas. Care should be taken not to damage the femoral nerve which lies within the psoas sheath itself. We generally perform a partial myotomy of the psoas, although a formal psoas recession as described by Bleck may also be performed. The patient is managed postoperatively with a prone program, and no plas-

ter is necessary. The patient is permitted to ambulate whenever comfortable enough.

Hamstring Release

Indications The internally rotated thighs may be a problem in gait in the ambulatory patient.[4] The stride angle is decreased and patients may trip. There are many causes for dynamic internally rotated thigh when there is adequate passive external range. The gait electromyogram can help differentiate the muscle imbalance.[10,52] Generally hamstring overactivity is the cause for this dynamic posture.[49] When such exists, especially when there is a fixed knee flexion contracture, tenomyotomy of the hamstrings is advised. If there is a dynamic internally rotated gait with adequate external rotation of the hip in the absence of a knee flexion contracture, transfer of the medial hamstring laterally may improve the gait. In that case the semitendinosus alone is transferred. This prevents a recurvatum from occurring as a consequence of decreasing the overall hamstring tone. Another approach to this problem is the anteromedial transfer of the greater trochanter, thus allowing the abductors of the hip to act as external rotators.[44] Tenomyotomy of the hamstrings is the commonest of these procedures and will be described in the next section.

The knee-flexed position in the ambulatory patient may be due to a postural problem involving either the hip or the ankle. When there is no fixed contracture, attention should be given to these other joints before dealing with the knee itself. If this precaution is not taken and hamstring lengthenings are carried out, recurvatum may be the result. Proximal hamstring lengthenings have been advocated in the past for this problem, but they may give patients profound weakness in hip extension. Proximal hamstring lengthening should not be performed except in the rare patient with extensor thrust and hip extension posture.[3,9,40] Extensor thrust is that pattern of tone involving hip and knee extensors in uncontrolled overactivity. In ambulatory or nonambulatory patients with knee flexion contractures of greater than 20°, hamstring lengthenings are a safe and appropriate procedure. In addition, hamstring procedures may be necessary to balance an internally rotated gait as noted above. In both cases, the identical approach is taken.

Surgical Technique The patient is placed prone, and a sterile tourniquet is used. A longitudinal incision is made across the middle third and distal third of the thigh. This incision should avoid the popliteal space. The hamstrings and sciatic nerve are located and the sciatic nerve protected. The semitendinosus may be transferred through the lateral hamstring incision in the case of the internally rotated gait. In the case of a fixed contracture, tenomyotomies may be carried out to allow the knee to fully extend. In general it is wise to keep at least one hamstring intact during this procedure unless there is a fixed contracture of all. Long leg plaster is placed and utilized for at least 3 weeks. Care is taken in the extension of the knee prior to closure of the wound to ensure that the sciatic nerve is not unduly stretched so that peroneal palsy will be avoided.

Femoral Osteotomy

Indications

When there is a fixed internal rotation of the thigh, it is usually due either to contracted muscles as noted above or to anteversion. This is evaluated clinically by examining the patient in the prone position and internally rotating the hip until the greater trochanter lies parallel to the table. The radiological examination by anteroposterior and horizontal lateral views or by CT scan may also be utilized. The involved contracted muscles should then be released, and derotation osteotomy should be carried out. If this is an ambulatory child, such a set of procedures is appropriate and may improve the stride angle and gait. In nonambulatory patients, such procedures are necessary only when the hip is subluxed. Thus, there are two separate situations when proximal femoral derotation osteotomy is required: (1) anteversion with a dislocated hip in an ambulatory patient; (2) anteversion with a subluxed hip in an ambulatory or nonambulatory patient. When a combination of valgus and anteversion is associated with a subluxed hip, a proximal varus derotation osteotomy should be performed.[11,51,52]

Distal Derotation Femoral Osteotomy[18]

Surgical Technique Through a lateral incision in the distal thigh using a sterile tourniquet, the bone is approached subperiosteally, and an osteotomy is performed with guide pins in place to note the amount of rotation. Usually, 30° to 45° of derotation is carried out. Then parallel pins are placed and the patient is placed in long leg plaster. Of necessity these pins lie close to the wound. Therefore, a modification of this procedure has been carried out by Rosenfeld. He advises a medial approach, placing the pins through both cortices in the uncorrected position. Then after the osteotomy the pins lie parallel to one another and are driven through the lateral cortex and out the skin. The medial wound is closed, and the pins are incorporated in the plaster.

Proximal Varus Derotation Osteotomy

Surgical Technique A routine lateral hip incision is carried out. The incision is carried down to the subperiosteum. A transverse osteotomy is carried out between the greater and lesser trochanters. The hip is carried into external rotation of 30° and a varus position of approximately 110°. This is done by use of an opening wedge and cross pinning in children from 3 to 8 years of age. In children over age 8, a closing wedge with excision of the medial wedge gives better stability than either smooth pins across the osteotomy site or a nail plate combination. The problem with nail plate combinations, especially in younger children, is that there is not a great deal of freedom to allow for both the varus and derotation neces-

sary in this procedure. It is more easily used in the older adolescent.

Pelvic Osteotomy

Indications When there is lateral displacement of the head associated with valgus and/or anteversion, a varus derotation osteotomy as described above is necessary to hold the hip in the acetabulum. However, if there is inadequate acetabular coverage, cartilage-sparing pelvic osteotomies (Pemberton) double innominate,[47] triple innominate,[45] or buttress support osteotomies (Shelf osteotomy,[54] Chiari osteotomy) may be carried out. Salter osteotomy gives better coverage anterolaterally, and the problem tends to be posterior; thus the Salter osteotomy is not recommended for these hips. The cartilage-sparing osteotomies and the Shelf procedure may be effective in the relatively mildly subluxed hip that can be well-contained. In the problem hip, however, the Chiari osteotomy is the most effective procedure.

Surgical Procedure: Chiari Osteotomy The Chiari osteotomy is carried out through an anterolateral (Smith-Petersen) approach, the incision being carried farther back posteriorly than usual, exposing the anterior half of the iliac crest. Dissection proceeds subperiosteally to the hip capsule and the sciatic notch. X-ray films are taken with a pin just above the hip joint in the direction of 15° posterosuperiorly. This verification is needed because too high an osteotomy gives a poor buttress. A curved hemostat is placed in the sciatic notch to protect the structures therein. A motor saw is utilized to get the proper angle all along the interval between the pin below the anteroinferior iliac spine and to approximately 1 in. above the sciatic notch. Then a Gigli saw is placed in the notch and an osteotomy performed from the notch to the original saw cut. The hip is abducted, and this should allow displacement of about half the iliac crest. A pin is then placed to fix the osteotomy and x-ray films taken to verify its position.

On rare occasions, in the younger child with a high dislocation, an open reduction of the hip and shortening varus osteotomy are helpful. However, it is not wise to perform this procedure in children over 8 years of age or when there is cartilage irregularity. Then one should avoid surgery until the patient has pain.[29] If pain becomes a problem, especially limiting sitting, a head and neck resection of femur can be carried out. This is not always a benign procedure, and postoperatively many of these children have residual discomfort and develop heterotopic bone.[22]

Treatment of the Extended Knee Deformity

The extended knee posture results in recurvatum of the knee during gait in the ambulatory patient and also presents difficulty in sitting in the nonambulatory patient. It is difficult for the hip to flex when the knee is not flexed. The stiff extended knee in the cerebral palsy patient is due to either overactivity of the quadriceps mechanism, overlengthening of the hamstrings, or overactivity of the triceps surae mechanism. In the ambulatory patient it is important to control the ankle equinus deformity or tip the tibia forward with an ankle brace or a heel raise to overcome the straight knee position. If the triceps surae mechanism does not prove to be the basic problem, a rectus femoris lengthening may be required.[48] It is advisable to obtain a preoperative gait electromyogram to verify that the other quadriceps muscles are active in stance so that the rectus femoris may be lengthened without causing a flexed knee posture. The rectus femoris lengthening is also helpful in the stiff knee posture of a sitting patient to help flex the knee and allow the hip thus to flex.

Rectus Femoris Lengthening

Surgical Technique A longitudinal transverse incision is made over the distal third of the thigh. The transverse incision is better cosmetically, but in patients with fixed extension contractures, skin closure may be difficult with a transverse incision; thus judgment must be utilized in selecting the approach. The rectus femoris is located and lengthened just above its insertion in the patella. The patient is placed in a flexed knee plaster at 90°, and this is kept for 2 to 3 weeks, after which the patient is allowed to walk or sit and range-of-motion exercises carried out.

Treatment of Foot and Ankle Deformities

Talipes Equinus Deformity

Indications for Surgery The foot in cerebral palsy is most commonly involved in the spastic hemiplegic patient. Of the various deformities, equinus is seen most often. In general, equinus deformities, even when fixed, should not be operated upon unless it can be demonstrated that they interfere with the patient's gait. Stretching exercises and even sequential plasters should be tried first. Then triceps surae–lengthening procedures should be performed.[3] The two-joint muscle tests to differentiate between gastrocnemius and soleus spasticity are probably not a valid differential. A gait electromyogram is necessary to note precisely which of the two muscles is hyperactive. In most cases it is the soleus, and therefore a heel cord lengthening is required.[27,50] Overzealous lengthening of the Achilles tendon can result in calcaneus deformities.[9,38] Thus, care in lengthening and postoperative management is advised.

Surgical Technique: Heel Cord Lengthening A small percutaneous tenotomy with a no. 11 blade is carried out at the Achilles tendon insertion, incising the medial half of the tendon; another incision at the musculotendinous junction severs the middle half of the tendon; a third tenotomy incision between the two incises the lateral half of the Achilles tendon. Then the foot is dorsiflexed, gaps are palpated in the regions of the three tenotomies, and plaster is placed with the ankle in slight equinus. The patient is permitted to walk whenever comfortable. The cast is kept on for 6 weeks followed by a

brace for 6 months, and then the orthosis may be continued as necessary.

Talipes Varus Deformity

Indications for Surgery Varus foot deformities are also frequent, especially in hemiplegics.[5,34] When these deformities are fixed, they interfere with bracing and ambulation and become rapidly progressive. When this varus deformity is fixed, a posterior tibial tendon lengthening is necessary.[12,35] The dynamic deformity is more complex to analyze and can be evaluated by gait analysis. Either the posterior tibial or the anterior tibial muscles may be the deforming force.[13,17] If it is felt that the posterior tibial muscle is the deforming force, the inferior half of its tendon may be split, and one of the split portions transferred laterally into the peroneus brevis tendon.[14,21] On the other hand, if it is felt that the anterior tibial muscle is the deforming force, its tendon may be split and transferred laterally.[19]

Surgical Technique: Posterior Tibial Tendon Lengthening A longitudinal incision is made above the medial malleolus at the musculotendinous junction of the posterior tibial tendon, and the tendon is lengthened within its musculotendinous sheath.

Surgical Technique: Split Anterior Tibial Tendon Transfer Three incisions are made: one over the insertion of the anterior tibial tendon, another in the distal third of the tibia over the anterior tibial tendon, and a third over the dorsum of the cuboid. All three incisions are longitudinal. In the first incision the anterior tibial tendon is located and split. An umbilical tape is placed in the split, and the tape is passed up into the second incision. The lateral half of the tendon is released and carried into the second wound. The tendon is then passed subcutaneously into the third wound, and a drill hole is placed in the cuboid in tunnel fashion. The tendon is driven through the drill hole and sutured to itself. A short leg plaster is placed and the patient allowed to walk whenever comfortable. The cast is used for 6 weeks. A brace is utilized thereafter for at least 6 months.

Talipes Valgus Deformity of the Foot

Indications for Surgery Valgus deformities are common in ambulatory spastic diplegic patients. Here tendon transfers fail to control the deformity, and eventually the deformity may become fixed and painful. In addition, the forefoot may develop a painful hallux valgus. On the other hand, many of these valgus feet are asymptomatic. When the deformity is progressing, it is wise to utilize a polypropylene ankle, foot orthosis (AFO) to hold the foot and hindfoot in neutral as much as possible. When this becomes difficult a hindfoot stabilization is advised.[15,43] If a fixed deformity is permitted to occur, the only remedy is to wait until the child is 12 or 13 years of age and perform a triple arthrodesis.

Surgical Technique: Alban-Grice Hindfoot Stabilization[1] An oblique incision is made over the dorsolateral aspect of the foot halfway between the lateral malleolus and the fifth metatarsal base and in line with skin folds. The extensor tendons and the peroneal tendons are located and protected. The incision is carried down to the sinus tarsi, which is debrided. Another portion of the incision distal to the peroneal tendons is developed over the lateral aspect of the heel. A Cloward drill, usually size 12, is placed in the sinus tarsi. This drill cleans out the perichondral tissues while the foot is held in a corrected position. A larger Cloward dowel cutter, usually size 14, is placed in the heel, and a block is removed from the calcaneus. The size 14 dowel of bone is then transferred into the size 12 gap created in the sinus tarsi. A staple is placed across the gap, which also holds the foot in position. The postoperative management is by plaster immobilization for 8 weeks and weight bearing in a polypropylene AFO for at least 6 months thereafter. At the same time, if there is a developing bunion deformity, a release of the adductor hallucis should be carried out and a smooth pin placed across the great toe to be removed at 4 to 6 weeks.

GAIT ANALYSIS IN CEREBRAL PALSY

Motion systems, force plate studies, and dynamic electromyography are the three modalities of gait analysis that have been utilized to evaluate cerebral palsy ambulatory patients. The motion system analysis documents trunk, thigh, leg, and foot segments throughout the gait cycle, so that one can compute the various joint positions and more accurately assess the inappropriate postures throughout the gait cycle. Force plate studies generate information about the reaction of the foot on the ground in the cerebral palsy patient and thus can estimate the efficiency of gait. Dynamic electromyography usually utilizes fine wire electrodes in muscles whose activity is in question. The patient is then allowed to ambulate, and one can see which muscles are working in an appropriate phase of the gait cycle. A number of complex postures have been analyzed by gait analysis, and answers are found to be unique for the individual tested. In the hip-flexed posture, gait analysis can separate overactivity of the rectus from that of the iliopsoas. In the internally rotated hip posture, the medial hamstrings can be separated from the other internal rotators. In the adducted posture, the gracilis and adductor longus can be separated from the less commonly overactive adductors. In the patient with a flexed knee posture, active hamstrings can be separated from postural reaction to tip or ankle position. Patients with varus ankle and hindfoot in gait can be separated into those patients who have posterior tibial inappropriate activity and those with hyperactivity of the anterior tibial muscle. Patients with equinus ankle and gait can be separated into the group with overactivity of the gastrocnemius, of the soleus, or of both.

REFERENCES

1. Alban, S., and Alban, H. Subtalar extra-articular arthrodesis with calcaneal bone in children with cerebral palsy. *Proceedings, American Academy of Cerebral Palsy,* 1975.

2. Banks, H., and Green, W.T. Adductor myotomy and obturation neurectomy for correction of adduction contracture of the hip in cerebral palsy. J Bone Joint Surg 42A:111–126, 1960.
3. Banks, H.H., and Green, W.T. Correction of equinus deformity in cerebral palsy. J Bone Joint Surg 40A:1359–1370, 1958.
4. Basset, F.H. Deformities of the foot in cerebral palsy. Instr Course Lect 20:35–40, 1971.
5. Bisslar, R.S., and Lewis, H.L. Transfer of the tibialis posterior tendon in cerebral palsy. J Bone Joint Surg 52A:137–141, 1975.
6. Bleck, E.E. The hip in cerebral palsy. Orthop Clin North Am 11:79–104, 1980.
7. Bleck, E.E. Postural and gait abnormalities caused by hip-flexion deformity in spastic cerebral palsy. Treatment by iliopsoas recession. J Bone Joint Surg 53A:1468–1488, 1971.
8. Bowen, J.R., MacEwen, G.D., and Mathews, P.A. Treatment of extension contracture of the hip in cerebral palsy. Dev Med Child Neurol 23:23–29, 1981.
9. Bradley, G., and Coleman, S. Treatment of the calcaneo cavus foot deformity. J Bone Joint Surg 63A:1159–1166, 1981.
10. Chong, K.C., Vojnic, C.D., and Quanbury, A.O. The assessment of the internal rotation gait in cerebral palsy: An electromyographic gait analysis. Clin Orthop 132:145–150, 1978.
11. Eilert, R.E., and MacEwen, G.D. Varus derotational osteotomy of the femur in cerebral palsy. Clin Orthop 125:168–172, 1977.
12. Frost, H.M., and Ruda, R. Cerebral palsy spastic varus treated by intramuscular posterior tibial tendon lengthening. Clin Orthop 79:61–70, 1971.
13. Gitzka, T.L., Staheli, L.T., and Duncan, W.L. Posterior tibial transfers through the interosseous membrane to correct equinovarus deformity in cerebral palsy. Clin Orthop 89:201–206, 1972.
14. Green, N.E., Griffin, P.P., and Shiavi, R. Splint posterior tibial tendon transfers in spastic cerebral palsy. J Bone Joint Surg 65A:748–754, 1983.
15. Grice, D.S. Extra-articular arthrodesis of the subastragalar joint with paralytic flat foot of children. J Bone Joint Surg 9:927–940, 1952.
16. Hoffer, M.M., and Koffman, M. Cerebral palsy: The first three years. Clin Orthop 151:222–227, 1980.
17. Hoffer, M.M., and Perry, J. Pathodynamics of gait alterations in cerebral palsy. Foot Ankle 4:128–134, 1983.
18. Hoffer, M.M., Prietto, C., and Koffman, M. Supracondylar derotation osteotomy of the femur for internal rotation of the thigh in cerebral palsied children. J Bone Joint Surg 63A:389–393, 1981.
19. Hoffer, M., Rieswig, J., Garret, A.A., and Perry, J. Split anterior tibial tendon transfer in the treatment of spastic varus hindfoot of childhood. Orthop Clin North Am 5:31–37, 1974.
20. Kalen, V., and Bleck, E.E. Prevention of spastic paralytic dislocation of the hip. Dev Med Child Neurol 27:17–24, 1985.
21. Kling, T., and Hensinger, R. Results of split posterior tibial tendon transfer in children with cerebral palsy. Orthop Trans 7:100–107, 1983.
22. Koffman, M. Proximal femoral resection or total hip replacement in severely disabled cerebral-spastic patients. Orthop Clin North Am 12:91–100, 1981.
23. Letts, M., Shapiro, L., Mulder, K., and Klassen, O. The windblown hip syndrome in total body cerebral palsy. J Pediatr Orthop 4:55–62, 1984.
24. Mackenzie, I.G. Abnormalities of the hip in cerebral palsy. Dev Med Child Neurol 17:797–799, 1975.
25. Madigan, R.R., and Wallace, S.L. Scoliosis in the institutionalized cerebral palsy population. Spine 6:583–590, 1981.
26. Moreau, M., Drummond, D.S., Rogala, E., Ashworth, A., and Porter, T. Natural history of the dislocated hip in spastic cerebral palsy. Dev Med Child Neurol 21:749–753, 1979.
27. Perry, J., Hoffer, M., Antonelli, D., Giovan, P., and Greenberg, R. Electromyography of the triceps surae in cerebral palsy. J Bone

Joint Surg 56A:511–514, 1974.

28. Perry, J., Hoffer, M., Antonelli, D., Plut, J., Lewis, G., and Greenberg, R. Electromyography before and after surgery for hip deformity in children with cerebral palsy. A comparison of clinical and electromyographic findings. J Bone Joint Surg 58A:201–208, 1976.

29. Pritchett, J.W. The untreated unstable hip in severe cerebral palsy. Clin Orthop 184:169–172, 1983.

30. Rang, M., Douglas, G., Bennet, G.C., and Koreska, J. Seating for children with cerebral palsy. J Pediatr Orthop 1:279–287, 1981.

31. Reimers, J. The stability of the hip in children. A radiological study of the results of muscle surgery in cerebral palsy. Acta Orthop Scand 184 (suppl):1–100, 1980.

32. Reimers, J., and Poulsen, S. Adductor transfer versus tenotomy for stability of the hip in spastic cerebral palsy. J Pediatr Orthop 1:52–54, 1984.

33. Roosth, H.P. Flexion deformity of the hip and knee in spastic cerebral palsy: Treatment by early release of spastic hip-flexor muscles. J Bone Joint Surg 53A:1489–1510, 1971.

34. Root, L. Transfer of posterior tibial tendon in cerebral palsy. *Proceedings, American Academy of Cerebral Palsy,* 1971.

35. Root, R., and Frost, H.M. Spastic varus treated by inner muscular posterior tibial tendon lengthening. Clin Orthop 79:61–70, 1971.

36. Root, L., and Spero, C.R. Hip adductor transfer compared with adductor tenotomy in cerebral palsy. J Bone Joint Surg 63A:767–772, 1981.

37. Samilson, R.L. Orthopedic surgery of the hips and spine in retarded cerebral palsy patients. Orthop Clin North Am 12:83–90, 1981.

38. Schneider, M., and Balon, K. Deformity of the foot following anterior transfer of the posterior tibial tendon and lengthening of the Achilles tendon for spastic equinovarus. Clin Orthop 125:113–118, 1977.

39. Schultz, R.S., Chamberlain, S.E., and Stevens, P.M. Radiographic comparison of adductor procedures in cerebral palsied hips. J Pediatr Orthop 4:741–744, 1984.

40. Sharps, C.H., Clancy, C., and Steel, H.H. A long-term retrospective study of proximal hamstring release for hamstring contracture in cerebral palsy. J Pediatr Orthop 4:443–447, 1984.

41. Sharrard, W.J., Allen, J.M., and Heaney, S.H. Surgical prophylaxis of subluxation and dislocation of the hip in cerebral palsy. J Bone Joint Surg 57B:160–166, 1975.

42. Sherk, H.H., Pasquariello, P.D., and Doherty, J. Hip dislocation in cerebral palsy: Selection for treatment. Dev Med Child Neurol 25:738–746, 1983.

43. Silver, C.M., Simon, S.D., Spindell, E., Litchman, H.M., and Scala, M. Calcaneal osteotomy for valgus and varus deformities of the foot in cerebral palsy; a preliminary report on twenty-seven operations. J Bone Joint Surg 49A:232–236, 1967.

44. Steel, H.H. Gluteus medius and minimus insertion advancement for correction of internal rotation gait in spastic cerebral palsy. J Bone Joint Surg 62A:919–927, 1980.

45. Steel, H.H. Triple osteotomy of the innominate bone. A procedure to accomplish coverage of the dislocated or subluxated femoral head in the older patient. Clin Orthop 122:116–127, 1977.

46. Stevenson, T., and Donovan, M.M. Transfer of the hip adductor origin to the ischium in spastic cerebral palsy. Dev Med Child Neurol 13:247–258, 1971.

47. Sutherland, D.A., and Greenfield, K. Double innominate osteotomy. J Bone Joint Surg 59A:1082–1091, 1977.

48. Sutherland, D.H., Larsen, L.J., and Mann, R. Rectus femoris release in selected patients with cerebral palsy: A preliminary report. Dev Med Child Neurol 17:26–34, 1975.

49. Sutherland, D.H., Schottstaedt, E.R., Larsen, L.J., Ashley, R.K., Callander, J.N., and James, P.M. Clinical and electromyographic study of seven spastic children with internal rotation gait. J Bone Joint Surg 51A:1070–1082, 1969.

50. Tohen, A., Carmona, J., and Barrera, J. The utilization of abnormal reflexes in the treatment of spastic foot deformities. Clin Orthop 47:77–82, 1966.

51. Tylkowski, C.M., Rosenthal, R.K., and Simon, S.R. Proximal femoral osteotomy in cerebral palsy. Clin Orthop 151:183–192, 1980.

52. Tylkowski, C.M., Simon, S.R., and Mansour, J.M. Internal rotation gait in spastic cerebral palsy. The Frank Stinchfield Award Paper. Hip 1:89–125, 1982.

53. Wheeler, M.E., and Weinstein, S.L. Adductor tenotomy-obturator neurectomy. J Pediatr Orthop 4:48–51, 1984.

54. Zuckerman, J.D., Staheli, L.T., and McLaughlin, J.F. Acetabular augmentation for progressive hip subluxation in cerebral palsy. J Pediatr Orthop 4:436–442, 1984.

CHAPTER 29

Orthopaedic Management of Myelomeningocele

Earl Feiwell and Samuel Rosenfeld

DEFINITIONS

Spinal dysraphism is the term often used to categorize congenital defects of the neural tube. The term *myelodysplasia* is used to broadly categorize associated congenital defects of the neural elements. Following are specific definitions of the abnormality which may be found.

Spina bifida occulta is a localized defect in the arch of one or more vertebrae with the spinal cord and meninges remaining confined within the canal.

Meningocele is a defect of the vertebral arch with protrusion of the meninges from the canal. The skin remains intact over the protrusion. Some neural tissue abnormality may be present. *Myelomeningocele* is used when the meningocele has associated neural elements within it which are usually not covered by epithelium. *Lipomeningocele* is meningocele which also includes a lipomatous growth.

Lumbosacral dysgenesis and *diastematomyelia* are dealt with in the chapter on congenital anomalies of the spine (Chap. 52).

GENERAL CONSIDERATIONS

A child may be born with a combination of these lesions and other associated congenital anomalies. The incidence of these abnormalities varies with location, race, maternal age, and socioeconomic status. The overall incidence in the United States is 1 or 2 cases per 1000 live births. However, it is low as 0.3 cases per 1000 in Japan and over 4 cases per 1000 in parts of Britain. Both inherited and environmental factors affect the etiology, but the exact interrelation is ill-understood.

Developmental Pathology

Although there are multiple theories, the Gardner hydrodynamic theory explains most of the associated abnormality.[33] It is postulated that the opening of the fourth ventricle does not occur at its normal time in the sixth to seventh week of intrauterine life and, consequently, hydrostatic pressure rises in the neural tube. This pressure causes bulging caudally and cranially. Different deformities are created depending upon the amount of deformation and its timing. Ordinarily the central canal closes and disappears as soon as the fourth ventricle opens, but in myelomeningocele patients the canal remains patent.

Normal cord advancement to birth level L2–3 frequently does not occur, and some degree of tethering is present. Additionally, scarring from any attempted surgical closure procedures contributes to tethering during subsequent growth.

Hydrocephalus is frequently associated with myelomeningocele (72 percent) most frequently with higher lesions (83 percent thoracic and upper lumbar) and less so with lower-level lesions (60 percent). The Arnold Chiari malformation is usually present with the hydrocephalus.[55] There is a downward elongation of the cerebellar tonsils and vermis into the spinal canal along with similar displacement of the brainstem. This abnormality explains the often-observed motor coordination problems causing spasticity when the lesion is at higher neurological levels. Other complications occur during growth as a result of tethering-associated hydrocephalus or expansion of the central canal (hydromyelia). Diastematomyelia may occur and be an additional cause of tethering.

Lumbosacral dysgenesis differs from myelomeningocele in that there is rarely involvement of the central nervous system, other than in the area directly involved with the deformity. Associated deformities such as meningocele or diastematomyelia occur. Partial sacral agenesis is associated with unilateral neurological involvement. When lumbar vertebral absence extends to L2, ambulatory potential is poor and transarticular knee amputation or subtrochanteric amputation is likely.

Etiology of Deformity

Deformities result from muscle imbalance, uterine positioning, positional contractures, spasticity, and factors related to growth.[56] Consequences of muscle imbalance are seen about the hips (subluxation and dislocation), knees (hyperextension deformity when no flexors are present at birth), and feet (dorsiflexion causing calcaneal gait and contractures). Uterine positioning problems are seen with windswept deformities of the feet at birth when no muscle function is present, i.e., vertical talus on one foot and forefoot adductus or equinovarus on the other. Talipes equinovarus is frequently seen in infants born with only hip flexors and adductors and knee extensors. Postural contractures such as knee and hip flexion contractures occur with wheelchair usage without appropriate intermittent extension positioning.[57] Spasticity brings on rapid deformity and limits overall usage of the extremity. Spasticity may result from the primary neurological problem of hydrocephalus and Arnold Chiari malformation, or from other acquired factors such as injury from shunt placement, infection, recurrent hydrocephalus, hydromyelia, or tethering of the cord.[41,62] Loss of functional capacity results from spasticity in upper and/or lower extremities.[53]

Progressive deformities occur during growth associated with asymmetry of soft tissue forces.[76] Spinal deformity increases during rapid growth periods. Tethering of the spinal cord increases scoliosis and/or lordosis during growth.[41] Deformities most commonly treated by the orthopaedist are below the level of the lesion. The spine, pelvis, hips, knees, ankle, and foot are primarily involved. The upper extremities must not be forgotten in the evaluation as loss of function interferes with activities of daily living (ADL).[89] Upper extremity function may progressively deteriorate secondary to neurological impairment associated with hydromyelia or hydrocephalus. The extent of any motor weakness and neurological impairment should be routinely and regularly recorded.

Functional Evaluation

Treatment is based upon the prognosis for future function. Patients who will be primarily "wheelchair ambulatory" require straight spines, level pelvis with mobile hips with 90° of flexion, no abduction or adduction contractures, 90° of flexion of the knees, and shoeable feet. Ambulatory patients will require straight spines, level pelvis, extended hips and knees, and plantigrade feet.[3]

Ambulation potential is primarily related to anatomic level of the lesion.[37] Multiple other factors modify this potential, most specifically any spasticity. Few patients will ambulate if spasticity is present in both upper and lower extremities.[53] A gradual onset of spasticity indicates progressive neurological abnormality. Early treatment of the neurological problem may preempt the need for orthopaedic treatment. Intelligence level does not affect ambulation unless IQ is less than 50.[24] Fractures impair ambulation potential because of adjacent joint stiffness and deformity.[3,21,37] The period of immobilization may also be a factor. Obesity seems to be more important in contributing to cessation of ambulation rather than delaying or preventing its initiation.[3,37]

Anatomic Levels of the Lesion

Anatomic levels determine not only the potential for ambulatory activities but also the orthotic requirements (see Table 29-1).[28]

A lesion at T12 or above results in no functioning muscles beyond the pelvis. Ambulation in childhood occurs with a maximal orthosis, i.e., a hip, knee, ankle, foot orthosis (HKAFO) or parapodium-type device. Patients who are beyond adolescence rarely are able to walk, and the wheelchair is used for mobility.

An L1 lesion preserves some function by the iliopsoas,

enabling hip flexion. However, significant hip flexion does not occur above the L2 level, where both the iliopsoas and sartorius flex the hip. If the lesion is within the L1 segment the patients function primarily at the thoracic level. These patients require at least an HKAFO, but their trunk support is good. However, as the teenage period approaches, they cease ambulation.

Preservation of function at the L2 level provides strong hip flexion with weak hip adduction. These patients also require HKAFOs by adolescence. Most of these patients are nonambulatory.

With function at L3 the quadriceps are grade 3 to grade 4 and hip adductors are strong. However, no abduction is present, and there is no active knee flexion. These patients require knee, ankle, foot orthoses, KAFOs, although some may require an HKAFO in early childhood. The majority are wheelchair ambulators as adults or at best household ambulators (see definitions in the following section). This is related to the high energy requirement for use of KAFOs.[91] It is at this level that other physical factors are the most influential in affecting potential ambulatory status. These factors include scoliosis, pelvic obliquity, and, most notably, flexion contractures.[3,85]

With function preserved at the L4 segment level, there is activity of the tibialis anterior. There is also a minimal amount of hip abduction. Medial hamstring function occurs primarily from the semimembranosus and some from the semitendinosus. Medial hamstrings provide knee flexion as well as some hip extension. Ankle, foot orthosis (AFO) is now sufficient because of increased knee stability.

With function preserved at the L5 level, strong dorsiflexion results from a normally functioning tibialis anterior muscle and some toe extensors. The tibialis posterior also functions to assist the foot and ankle. Community ambulation (see next section) is anticipated with an AFO.

Paralysis below the S1 segment involves primarily the foot intrinsics, eliminating the need for anything other than a shoe orthosis. With lesions in the upper sacral levels, all forms of muscle imbalance about the foot are seen. Multiple foot operations may be necessary throughout the period of growth to achieve a plantigrade foot.

Functional Levels

It is important to remember that each segment is named after the nerve root that leaves the neuroforamen. The anterior horn cells contributing to each spinal nerve root occupy a segment of the spinal cord. The cells innervating any individual muscle or muscle group may occupy several segments. Consequently, the precise pattern of muscle weakness is variable depending on the level and extent of neuronal dysgenesis.

For this reason we classify patients into functional levels based upon the voluntary muscles that move the joints. Thoracic-level patients have no function in voluntary muscles crossing the hip joint. High lumbar–level patients have hip flexors and/or adductors and/or knee extensors. Low lumbar patients have functioning voluntary muscles that flex the knee, dorsiflex the ankle, and/or abduct the hip. Sacral-level patients have gluteus maximus and/or ankle and foot plantar flexors.

TABLE 29-1 Functional Classification of Patients and Their Ambulation Potential

Level	Anatomical (neurosegmental) level of lesion	Significant motor function at level	Common major deformity related to muscle imbalance	Childhood (1) requirements (2) mobility	Adult (1) requirements (2) mobility
Thoracic	T12 or above, L1 (some patients)	(No significant function in lower limbs)	Scoliosis and pelvic obliquity	(1) Standing brace and wheelchair; (2) exercise (nonfunctional) ambulators only	(1) and (2) wheelchair only
High lumbar	L1	Hip flexion	Hip flexion contracture or dislocation*	(1) Crutches and long braces with hip support; (2) household ambulators or community wheelchair	(1) Long braces (KAFO) with crutches; (2) 75% of patients wheelchair only; remainder will be household ambulators
	L2	Hip adduction			
	L3, L4 (some patients)	Knee extension			
Low lumbar	L4	Knee flexion (medial hamstrings)			(1) Will require short braces (AFO); crutches may also be needed; (2) 75% of patients will be community ambulators
	L5	Ankle extension, hip abduction	Calcaneus deformity of ankle; foot ulceration†	(1) Short braces, crutches for long distances; (2) community ambulator	
	S1 (some patients)	Knee flexion (lateral hamstrings)			
Sacral	S1	Ankle flexion, inversion, and eversion	Claw toes, high arch foot	(1) Supports in shoes; (2) community ambulator	(1) May require shoe supports; (2) 100% will be community ambulators for a limited distance (but for up to 90% of their requirements)
	S2	(Foot intrinsics are nonfunctional)			
	S3, S4	(Motor function essentially intact)	Minimal or no deformity		

*Some patients with lesions at this level will also have scoliosis and pelvic obliquity.
†Some patients with lesions at this level will also have hip flexion contracture or dislocation.

Using this classification, we find that the majority of the thoracic-level patients function only in wheelchairs. The upper-lumbar patients, for the most part, require KAFOs and HKAFOs in early childhood and wheelchairs in adolescence and adulthood. Low lumbar–level patients usually ambulate with AFOs, and the majority are community ambulators in adulthood. Sacral-level patients are anticipated to be community ambulators with or without foot orthosis (see Table 29-1 for summary).

Ambulation categories are as defined by Hoffer et al:[37]

1. *The community ambulator.* These patients walk indoors and outdoors for most of their activities and may need crutches or braces in both. They use a wheelchair only for long trips out of the community or for greater speed of ambulation.

2. *Household ambulator.* These patients walk only indoors and with apparatus. They are able to get in and out of the chair and bed with little if any assistance. They may use a wheelchair for some indoor activities at home and school, and for all activities in the community.

3. *Nonfunctional ambulators.* Walking for these patients is a therapy session at home, school, or the hospital. Afterward they use their wheelchairs to get from place to place and satisfy all their needs for transportation.

4. *Nonambulators.* These patients are wheelchair-bound but usually can transfer from chair to bed.

Treatment

The goal of treatment is maximum habilitation taking into account the anatomic level of involvement as well as any secondary factors which may be limiting the patient (Table 29-1). Patients are best treated by the team approach. The therapeutic team should include physician specialists such as neurosurgeon, urologist, pediatrician, and orthopaedist together with a physical therapist, orthotist, occupational therapist, psychologist, and social worker. All are required in evaluating and staging treatment. Accurate documentation is essential to detect changes secondary to progressive neurological lesions.[41,62]

The orthopaedic surgeon must be familiar with the abnormality involved. Starting from the prognosis made on the basis of neurosegmental level and other associated factors, realistic goals should be set and surgical, orthotic, and physical therapy treatment planned accordingly. Any deviation from the prognosis for achievement must be evaluated, bearing in mind the possibility of progressive complications occurring within the central nervous system. If such neurological changes are not responsible, other causes must be sought and corrected if possible. Early orthotic and physical therapy management should be related to helping the child achieve normal milestones of development. Surgical planning, on the other hand, should be related to anticipated adult needs.

Treatment is tempered by the maturational needs of the infant and child. Close bonding is necessary for infant security. Children must have the ability to explore, handle, and manipulate objects as well as devices. Trial-and-error experience is self-motivating. Progressive upright experience is necessary. In early childhood, standing and ambulatory attempts may be gratifying to the child as well as the parent. However, for older children, life becomes a more painful experience. The children find themselves being left behind by more agile playmates, unable to participate in many activities because their hands are occupied with crutches or a walker, and unable to expend the energy required in rapid transport from one classroom to another in junior high and high school years. In addition, short lower extremities result in short stature. The wheelchair, during these years, becomes far more socially acceptable and useful for the thoracic and high-lumbar patients.

It is up to the orthopaedist to provide the aids and the therapy to help the child meet the milestones of development required for appropriate maturation. More severely involved patients require more orthotics and devices in infancy to allow head support, sitting, and accomplishment in the crawling stage.[13] The lower-level patients achieve these goals without additional devices unless they are markedly hampered by frequent surgeries and casting.

Orthotic Treatment

The basic principle of orthotic treatment consists of using lightweight devices to supply stability to the joints that do not have adequate control. In later childhood, cosmesis too becomes an important factor. Improvement of mobility is paramount. Devices such as the caster cart should be provided when needed to aid crawling or other forms of exploration close to the floor.[13]

When a child is ready to stand but requires full support (thoracic- or upper lumbar–level patients), a standing orthosis may be utilized.[16] Generally the child is between 12 and 18 months of age. Standing devices should be simple and lightweight and allow for growth to age 2 years. Polypropylene formed orthoses may be used to maintain correct foot positioning after surgery or cast correction, even before attempts at standing and walking.

Orthotics for mobility should be provided when the child demonstrates a desire for ambulation or after 18 months in high-level lesions when it is believed the child is capable. Trunk stabilization is required for thoracic patients without pelvic control. Hip stabilization should be provided for those with adequate trunk control but no knee control (high lumbar level).

The parapodium,[13,16] Shrewsbury,[70] or reciprocating brace,[94] or standard HKAFO with locked hip, knee, and ankle, can be used in these patients. The parapodium provides a flat base which allows mobility by pivoting the body from side to side, thereby advancing the patient. Swing gait can be used. The Shrewsbury brace uses the same principle but is spring-loaded so that shifting weight from side to side unloads one side and automatically shifts the brace forward. The reciprocating brace allows alternating hip motion. It functions best with active hip flexors, although low thoracic–level patients can utilize it if they are free of flexion contracture.

Improved balance associated with increasing age, practice, and strength allows use of the KAFOs in high lumbar–level patients. Low lumbar–level patients require ankle stabilization but generally have adequate knee stabilizers. Polypropylene orthoses vacuformed for close fit around the calf, ankle, and foot provide stability, are lightweight, and are cosmetically desirable. Their disadvantage is that there is no accommodation for growth. Prior to age 3 years, we prefer a single upright metal brace with growth adjustment and double-adjustable ankle joint in order to reduce expense.

Patients with borderline knee extension strength benefit from the posterior entry type of orthosis (Glancy or floor reaction brace).[45] Polypropylene AFOs are used in nonambulatory patients for foot and ankle positioning. Sacral-level patients may require shoe orthotics because of foot deformities.

Surgical Treatment

Surgical treatment should be planned to interrelate with the child's other surgical specialty needs. Menelaus has summarized the principles of orthopaedic surgery as follows:[54,55]

1. Surgery should be selected with regard to the anticipated adult needs.
2. Minimum orthopaedic surgery which will completely and permanently correct the deformities is required. A single surgical procedure is preferred to multiple partial procedures repeated over a long period of time.
3. As much surgery as possible is performed under one anesthetic with as little immobilization as possible. Early weight bearing should be carried out with the patient in plaster.
4. Muscle imbalance should be corrected in all circumstances.

REGIONAL CONSIDERATIONS

Pelvic Obliquity

Obliquity of the pelvis is a seriously disabling problem for the myelodysplastic patient. Pelvic obliquity causes difficulty in the sitting patient by creating poor balance and predisposing to the development of pressure sores on the downside ischial prominence. The walking patient exhibits leg length inequality, and dislocation of the hip on the elevated side may occur.

Scoliosis is the primary cause of significant pelvic obliquity in the myelodysplastic patient. However, hip contractures may also be a cause. In a fixed abduction contracture caused by a tight iliotibial band, the pelvis becomes tilted when the legs are brought together parallel with the body axis. Since the patient cannot ambulate with one leg fully abducted and also tends to lie supine with the legs parallel, the tilted pelvis is the position routinely adopted. The pelvic tilt causes the contralateral hip to adopt an increasingly adducted position. If there is a fixed adduction contracture, there is elevation of the affected side of the pelvis and the contralateral hip takes up an abducted position. Only when the pelvis is leveled by placing the two anterior superior iliac spines in the horizontal plane is the appropriate hip deformity revealed.

Correction of the hip contractures brings about correction of the pelvic obliquity. If the contractures are left long enough, however, fixed secondary contracture develops in the lumbar spine.[39]

If the pelvic obliquity is caused by scoliosis, rotation of the pelvis occurs in conformity with the lumbar curve. Pelvic obliquity in this situation is fixed and unaffected by the position of the legs. However, the hip joint on the elevated side of the pelvis adopts a secondary position of adduction. If there is associated weakness of the adductor musculature in the same hip and if the obliquity occurs sufficiently early in childhood, hip dislocation will occur.

Methods of evaluating pelvic obliquity have not been well-defined. Lindseth described a method relating the transverse axis of the pelvis to the end plate of the uppermost vertebra of the lumbar curve.[44] We have not found this entirely satisfactory and instead use a measurement on a complete spine x-ray film that includes the pelvis. The "weight-bearing line of the spine" is estimated to be from the midpoint of the T1 vertebra to the midpoint of S2. Patients in the sitting position tend to bring this line into a vertical position, thereby creating a functional type of pelvic obliquity (Fig. 29-1). Sitting x-ray views show a similar result, but accurate balance is difficult for these patients. Many times patients need their arms for balance and are therefore constantly changing the overall weight-bearing line. A good transverse pelvic axis is also difficult to obtain on a sitting film since the pelvis is frequently obscured.

If there has been an extensive spine fusion, there will be no significant differences if the measurements are taken on sitting or supine films, and therefore the latter x-ray views are taken and these measurements used. In a patient who has not had a spine fusion, we find it is satisfactory to take both the supine and the sitting view for comparison. In practice there is usually little difference in the two measurements. The transverse axis of the pelvis is determined by a line connect-

ing two comparable landmarks on each side. The angle this line makes with the vertical weight-bearing line measures the degree of pelvic obliquity.

Treatment of pelvic obliquity associated with spinal deformity is by the use of a body jacket (TLSO) to reduce progression. In our pelvic obliquity clinic, a polyurethane cushion with appropriate cutouts has been most successful in reducing the incidence of pressure sores.

Surgical treatment consists of early spine correction when it is apparent that the spinal deformity is becoming fixed. The spinal fusion should be performed to obtain a balanced spine and eliminate the pelvic obliquity. If the obliquity remains after spinal fusion, additional surgery may be required. Osteotomy of the spine which some authors recommend has a high complication rate, and correction is often inadequate.[31,61] Lindseth recommends bilateral posterior osteotomy where there is fixed pelvic obliquity due to uncorrectable lumbosacral scoliosis. A wedge of bone is removed from the posterior ilium on the low side of the obliquity and inserted on the opposite side to maintain the correction (Fig. 29-2).[43] A 41 percent correction of pelvic obliquity and 69 percent correction of trunk list from the midline has been reported with an acceptable complication rate.[43] Indications for surgery are the occurrence of frequent pressure sores and demonstrated imbalance during sitting requiring at least one

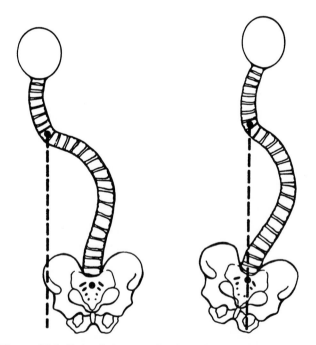

Figure 29-1 Sitting balance and pelvic obliquity. *Left:* Schematic depiction of person with severe scoliosis placing the pelvis level on a surface. The weight-bearing line would be far to the right, and the person would fall or be required to push with the right arm in order to keep from falling over to the right. *Right:* How the same person would sit by directing the weight-bearing line centrally over the S2 area. Balance would be maintained on one ischium. Unless a sitting x-ray was taken or the entire spine was x-rayed with the pelvis, functional pelvic obliquity would be difficult to determine.

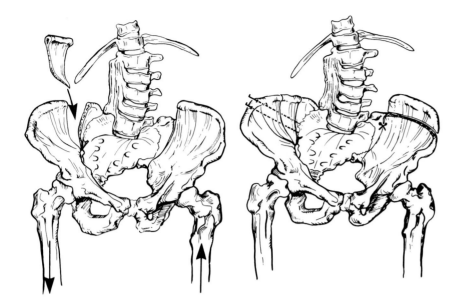

Figure 29-2 Posterior iliac osteotomy for fixed pelvic obliquity. *Left:* After bilateral osteotomy and removal of the wedge of predetermined size from the low side of the obliquity, the pelvis is rotated from the sacrum in the frontal plane by pulling down on the limb on the high side and pushing up on the limb on the low side. This maneuver closes one osteotomy site, where the bone was removed, and opens the one on the opposite side to receive the bone graft. *Right:* The transferred iliac wedge is fixed with two Kirshner wires. While the closed wedge osteotomy is held with nonabsorbable sutures through drill holes, enough of the upward projecting iliac wing is removed to permit two halves of the previously split iliac epiphysis to be approximated back to the top of the iliac wing during closure. (From Lindseth, R.R., J Bone Joint Surg 60A:17, 1978. Reproduced with permission.)

hand to stabilize the individual in the upright position and prevent falling over.

The Hip

Contractures

All patients who have muscle imbalance tend to develop contractures unless they have been prevented by appropriate stretching or muscle release. Flexion and adduction contractures which predispose to hip instability are common.

Release of contractures about the hip is necessary for successful ambulation. In nonambulatory patients, hip flexion contractures are not of too much concern, but unilateral abduction or adduction contractures which will create pelvic obliquity are important. A level pelvis is necessary for appropriate sitting. In addition, adequate hip flexion beyond 90° is necessary.

Patients with external rotation contractures are treated by extensive posterior release dividing the short lateral rotators and posterior hip capsule. At the same time, any associated contractures are dealt with.[55,56]

Abduction contractures may result iatrogenically from prolonged abduction splinting or postsurgical contractures. If they are the result of tight iliotibial band, an Ober-Yount procedure provides adequate release for contracted iliotibial band. In those older patients who have intraarticular or pericapsular scarring, osteotomy of the proximal femur is appropriate.[89] Similarly in patients with flexion contractures of greater than 40°, it is necessary to carry out an extension osteotomy along with appropriate soft tissue releases anteriorly. Patients who are confined to wheelchairs are usually not appropriate candidates for flexion contracture releases as the contractures will readily recur. Only in cases of severe flexion contracture such as greater than 50° should consideration be given to undertaking releases. Pure rotational deformities occurring about the hip in older patients may be best treated by osteotomies either proximally or distally on the femur.

Hip Dysplasia

Hip dysplasia occurs as a result of an imbalance of muscle forces in which the flexors and abductors are strong and the adductors and extensors are weak or absent. The result may be a hip at risk for dislocation or one that is already dislocated at birth. The activity in the abductor muscles is the most important factor. Evaluation of patients with poliomyelitis has demonstrated that dislocation does not occur if the abductor muscle power is better than poor-grade.[59] If the opposite hip is in relative abduction, there is an increasing tendency for the adducted hip to dislocate. The individual with no hip muscle imbalance but with a paralyzed (flail) hip joint develops dislocation gradually over a period of time if other factors are present which tend to place the hip at risk in an adducted position. In a low lumbar–level patient the problem may be a slow subluxation without frank dislocation. The importance of pelvic obliquity due to uncorrected lumbar

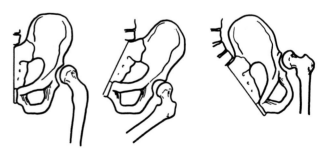

Figure 29-3 Relation between hip stability and femoral neck shaft angle, hip deformity, and pelvic obliquity. *Left:* The neck is in valgus, and the weight-bearing pressures are on the outer aspect of the acetabulum. *Center:* The neck is in normal or even varus position, but the adduction contracture places the weight-bearing pressure on the outer aspect of the acetabulum. *Right:* The femoral angle is normal; however, because of pelvic obliquity the weight-bearing pressure is again on the outer aspect of the acetabulum.

scoliosis or hip contractures has already been discussed. If such obliquity is present the adducted upside hip is at particular risk, especially if there is associated acetabular dysplasia and weak abductors. To emphasize the role of the adducted position promoting instability in the circumstances, Somerville stated that "the nearer the angle between the neck of the femur and the horizontal of the pelvis approaches $90°$ the more unstable the hip will become" (Fig. 29-3).[82]

In the newborn the iliopsoas muscle produces a flexed and external position of the limb.[51] Its contracture is believed to be the predominant cause of the flexion contracture which may be seen in the midlumbar myelomeningocele hip.[7] Under these circumstances it exerts a bowstring effect on the femoral head, displacing it posteriorly and laterally. The deforming force increases with attempts to relieve the hip flexion contracture by passive hip extension. Breed and Healey point out that under these circumstances it often grooves the femoral head and produces dysplasia of the posterior acetabulum.[7]

The increased valgus of the femoral neck is believed to be due to alteration of bone shape secondary to iliopsoas predominance during the intrauterine and postnatal growth period.[8] In the newborn child the neck shaft angle at birth approximates $160°$, ordinarily, diminishing to $120°$ in adolescence. In the myelomeningocele child, however, the valgus may increase. Additional factors involved include a lack of stimulation to the activity of the lateral aspect of the growth plate, and the trochanteric apophysis associated with weak or absent abductor muscles. In addition, lack of weight bearing in the early years may selectively inhibit physeal growth.

The inequality of muscle action may promote torsional deformities. This was shown on decalcified femurs by Brookes and Wardle.[8] They observed that imbalance in flexor over extensor force tends to increase anteversion. The role of the iliopsoas muscle may be more important in the etiology of valgus deformity in the high lumbar–level patient (L2–3 range), where the adductors are still quite weak but the iliopsoas is at full strength. The presence of a valgus femoral neck with increased anteversion in a joint maintained in an adducted position promotes anterior and lateral acetabular dysplasia, since those portions of the femoral head tend to remain uncovered. The final consequence is hip instability.

Surgical Indications

It is the authors' opinion that the ability to ambulate is more dependent upon the neurological level than upon hip reduction.[28,37] Contractures of the knees, spine, and pelvic area seem to be more important than whether the hip is dislocated as a prognosticator for ambulation in lower-level patients. Ascher and Olson demonstrated that patients in the L3-level category are the only ones adversely affected by lack of hip reduction.[3] Lee and Carroll have concluded that hip stability definitely improves ambulatory status.[42] They reviewed their statistics over 10 years and reported excellent results for hip reduction and ambulation compared with their earlier patients, in whom a lower percentage of hip stability had been accompanied by correspondingly poorer ambulation statistics. There may, however, have been some bias in the study associated with the improvement in overall care over the years.

Menelaus has indicated that patients with lesions above L3 level are primarily benefited by elimination of contractures about the hip and by achieving an extended position.[55,56] However, he believes that hip stability is a reasonable goal when it can be obtained. Contractures are more readily eliminated in ambulatory patients with reduced hips. It is doubtful whether extensive multiple procedures should be carried out in an upper lumbar patient. In such patients the likelihood of ambulation is poor, and if they do ambulate they will use crutches and a KAFO. In these circumstances simply correcting the contractures is sufficient.

Unilateral dislocations in low lumbar patients should be treated. However, if the muscular deficit is symmetrical, bilateral transfers should be performed as the opposite hip will undoubtedly sublux and subsequently dislocate. Bilateral subluxations in low lumbar patients should also be treated. High bilateral dislocations are best left alone. Displacement in sacral-level patients should definitely be treated since these may in reality be congenital rather than paralytic dislocations. Also, if a specific muscle group such as the abductors is paralyzed while all others are functional, appropriate transfer in these patients results in more stable ambulation.

Treatment

Treatment of hip dysplasia requires that concentric reduction be obtained and maintained and the muscle forces be balanced. Various muscle-balancing procedures have been described. Because of the risks which may accompany surgery on a newborn baby, many authors believe that even if a patient is identified as an appropriate candidate for hip stabilization, no treatment should be carried out until the child is between 12 and 20 months of age. McKibbin recommends abduction extension splinting of the hip in infants up to 24 months of age who have functional muscles crossing the hip joint to promote good acetabular development.[51] Raycroft also recommends early reduction of the hip by performing adductor (and possibly also iliopsoas) release and then splinting in a similar position until definitive lateral muscle transfers can be performed at a later date.[70] He describes better long-term hip stability with prompt rather than delayed treatment.

Breed and Healey point out that by 1 year of age, virtually all the hips of lumbar-level patients are unstable either with subluxation or dislocation.[7] They recommend the early performance of iliopsoas recession. They believe that this procedure is better than splintage alone and must be done early, consistent with their view of the importance of the iliopsoas tendon in maintaining and promoting hip stability and reducing acetabular dysplasia.[7]

The use of a Palvik harness may improve hip positioning and maintain reduction of the hips during the early months, but its prolonged use will bring about iliopsoas contracture and create difficulty in achieving extension; also prolonged splinting of the child in abduction deters maturation and limits the child's abilities to achieve normal developmental milestones. Its use can be modified, however, splinting only at night and at nap time, allowing the child free movement during the rest of the day.

As a step toward balancing adductor-abductor forces, it has been recommended that the origins of the adductors longus brevis and gracilis be detached from the pelvis and then transferred posteriorly to the ischial tuberosity. In some cases this procedure is combined with a lateral transfer of the iliopsoas from the lesser to the greater trochanter when the abductors have been severely weakened.[46,59] Any transfer to increase abductor muscle force only works provided there is a satisfactory fulcrum represented by a stable concentric hip joint. Any instability significantly affects success of such a transfer.

Mustard[58] reported transferring the iliopsoas through a notch in the anterior portion of the ilium to the greater trochanter in paralytic poliomyelitis, and Sharrard[77] then modified the operation by transferring the muscle posteriorly through a foramen made in the ilium. The modification was designed to make up for the lack of extensor muscles as well as the abductor muscles in myelomeningocele and was reported to provide improved extensor strength and a more upright posture in addition to benefiting abduction. Electromyographic studies, however, do not support this contention, and the iliopsoas continues to function with the flexor musculature.[9]

There is a definite place for posterolateral iliopsoas transfer to the greater trochanter in the myelodysplastic patient. In addition to providing lateral muscle power, there is diminution of the force, producing femoral neck valgus.[8] There also seems to be improved hip extension from better hamstring function.[7] Patient selection is critical if good results are to be achieved. Jackson et al noted that factors which predispose to failure are the presence of a dysplastic acetabulum (acetabular index more than 30°), prior hip surgery, limb length inequality, and a patient over 5 years of age.[40] The presence of strong secondary hip flexors is critical (rectus femoris and sartorius). Otherwise the patient may lose vital hip flexor function.[83] With good selection and if performed early, excellent results have been reported.[42,63,64]

The procedure described by Sharrard[76] may be altered by leaving the iliacus partially attached within the pelvis. The hole in the iliac wing should be large enough to allow passage of tendon and muscle and may be made somewhat lateral to the position recommended by this author. The aperture in the ilium characteristically enlarges if the transfer is functioning successfully. We find that an important technical factor is to avoid creating a tunnel in the proximal femur which may fracture with avulsion of the transfer. Instead we prefer to create a perichondral or periosteal flap, anchoring the tendon by drill hole and suture.

The external oblique is a muscle which does not have the bulk of the iliopsoas but does have a more advantageous position of origin, being further lateral on the trunk and extending straight down to the greater trochanter after transfer.[35] Its transfer may reduce body sway or Trendelenburg lurch during ambulation, but it will not completely eliminate it.[35] This transfer also spares the iliopsoas and allows its use as a flexor. As discussed, sectioning the psoas may be an advantage or disadvantage depending on the individual patient. The external oblique transfer is performed by developing a flap a few centimeters wide parallel with the fibers of the aponeurosis in the groin. The distal end of the flap is then divided in the region of the pubic tubercle, tubed, and passed subcutaneously to be inserted into the greater trochanter. This operation was first described by Thompson, Thomas, and Straub.[86] It is important to make a long enough muscle flap by completing the proximal dissection of the external oblique muscle posterior and anteriorly to the rib cage and rotating it sufficiently so that after transfer of the tubed structure, tension is placed on all aspects of the muscle.

Varus Osteotomy

If the child is over 2 years of age and has a significant valgus deformity, varus osteotomy is an additional procedure which may help stabilize the hip. The procedure gives additional coverage to the femoral head and may be combined with muscle-balancing procedures to resist recurrence of the valgus. A closing wedge osteotomy is the most stable. Parallel threaded pins inserted across the osteotomy are sufficient to maintain position.[26] A wide variety of internal fixation devices have been described and may be used. The iliopsoas tendon can be easily reached when the wedge of bone is taken and dealt with appropriately.

Acetabuloplasty

Acetabular procedures are performed when the acetabulum is deficient in patients over the age of 2 years. The Salter osteotomy is not recommended as the posterior aspect of the acetabulum may become defective and posterior dislocation occur.[72] In such cases posterior shelf operations such as the Pemberton have been performed.[66] This osteotomy has been effective in that it decreases the volume of the enlarged acetabulum and brings normal cartilage down over the femoral head.

A combination of the Pemberton and Salter procedures has been recommended by Perlik et al (Fig. 29-4).[67] The osteotomy commences a centimeter or so above the anterior inferior iliac spine and follows the attachment of the joint capsule paralleling the acetabular dome. It extends posteriorly through the ilioischial limb of the triradiate cartilage deep

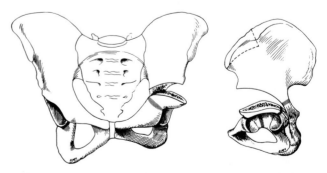

Figure 29-4 A combination pelvic osteotomy for acetabular dysplasia combines the key aspects of the Pemberton and the Salter osteotomy. *Left:* Anteroposterior view. *Right:* Lateral view. For explanation see text. (From Perlik, P.C., Westin, G., and Marafiot, R.L., J Bone Joint Surg 67A:843, 1985. Reproduced with permission.)

into the body of the ischium. Opening up this osteotomy creates a greenstick fracture to the remaining portion of the body of the ischium and enables the acetabulum to be displaced forward and downward. Capsulorrhaphy may be an additional procedure performed with acetabuloplasty.[14,42,56] If it is decided to perform an acetabular procedure for dysplasia, it should be carried out at the same time as the iliopsoas transplant since the exposure is similar.

Good results in stabilizing the hip have been reported with the Chiari osteotomy.[12] Other authors, however, report poor results when Chiari procedures have been combined with iliopsoas transfers.[40] It seems that poor results occur when the iliopsoas transfer acts as a tenodesis, tending to displace the femoral head out of the acetabulum. The Colonna arthroplasty is a procedure that is mentioned only for condemnation. The procedure can stabilize the hip, but postoperatively movement is often significantly limited. Madigan and Worrall observed that over 80 percent of flexion-extension range of motion is lost after this procedure.[47] The most favorable results were in those patients whose lesion level was above T12.

Combined Procedures

A combination of procedures to eliminate muscle imbalance and correct skeletal dysplasia is logical. Sharrard used such a combination of procedures and noted that some of his failures were the result of failure to either appropriately balance muscles or obtain good congruent relations between the femoral head and the acetabulum at the time of transfer.[14] Both Carroll and Menelaus strongly recommended capsulorrhaphy for the lax capsule after reduction.[42,56]

Nichols et al recommended multiple procedures for the paralytic hip; these included posterior transfer of the abductor muscles, femoral osteotomy, and iliopsoas transfer accompanied by Pemberton osteotomy, when indicated, in a mixed population of patients, including those with myelodysplasia. London and Nichols used a similar combination with posterior lateral iliopsoas transfer and considered their most successful patients were those who had adductor muscle posterior transfer.[46] McKay described using a similar group of procedures to stabilize the hip and used the external oblique muscle as an abductor.[50] Bunch and Hakala had excellent success in lower lumbar patients when varus osteotomy was combined with posterior lateral iliopsoas transfer.[10] It should be noted, however, that if, some time after a transfer, a varus osteotomy is performed, it may create apparent lengthening of the transferred muscle and considerably weaken its action. Consequently, the transfer must be tightened at the time of osteotomy.

Complications of Surgical Reduction of the Hip

All the usual surgical complications occur and are to be considered, such as anesthetic complications and neurological or vascular complications and infection. Failure to stabilize the hip can follow even if all the appropriate measures have been taken.[8,14,40,63] Additionally, postoperative stiffness or contracture with intra- and extraarticular fibrosis can occur.[14,28] Heterotopic bone formation[14,63] or fracture[22,28,63] can compro-

mise the result. Dislocation of the opposite hip may also occur secondary to the treatment of the affected side, and one should be aware of this possibility.

Knee Deformities and Rotational Deformities of the Lower Extremities

Isolating the knee deformities in the patient with myelomeningocele is difficult as deformities about the hips and ankles influence the knees. Also any deformity about the knee can accentuate other deformities in the lower extremities. In myelomeningocele lower extremities often present a complex pattern of deformities involving all the lower extremity joints.

These deformities may be conveniently discussed as flexion contractures, extension contractures, and varus and valgus deformities. Rotational deformities in the lower extremities will be discussed separately. They are directly related to the anatomic level of the patient's lesion and often can be predicted after the neurological examination. Many knee contractures are secondary to postural contractures and not muscle imbalance. These problems are difficult to deal with and also produce significant functional limitations for these patients.

Orthotics

The role of orthotics in the management of knee deformities is straightforward. When there is quadriceps weakness, the orthosis must provide extension support for the knee during weight-bearing activities. In the patient with flexion contractures, orthotics can be used as an adjunct for guided gradual extension of the knee using appropriately placed hinges in the mechanical axis of the extremity. Care to prevent posterior subluxation of the tibia is essential. Varus and valgus deformities of small degrees can be maintained with double upright metal knee hinges. For hip joint rotational problems, twister cables are used to maintain the neutral position in gait; they have limited use with bony deformity to enhance gait while awaiting surgical correction. We use lightweight cables attached to a pelvic band and polypropylene AFO, or heavier cables attached to KAFOs.

Knee Deformities

Flail knee is present in the patient with thoracic-level myelomeningocele. These patients usually are not ambulatory, and the flail knee is not a clinical problem. These knees can be managed with simple orthoses for positioning. The flail knee frequently develops contractures based on prolonged or repeated flexed position, i.e., full wheelchair usage.[19] When any quadriceps activity is present, extension contractures often result. Management of specific contractures will be dealt with in the subsequent section.

Flexion Contractures Flexion contractures about the knee in the spina bifida patient can be due to intrauterine positioning, positional contractures in the older child, muscle imbalance, and muscle paralysis. Flexion contractures present at birth are secondary to intrauterine positioning and often not

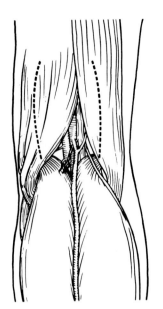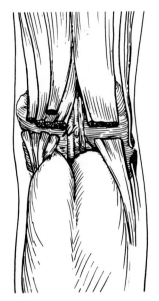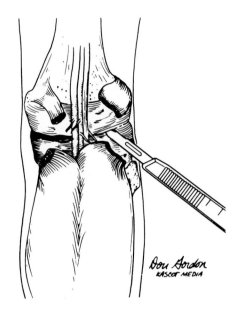

Figure 29-5 Posterior release of knee contracture in myelomeningocele. *Left:* Medial and lateral longitudinal incisions. *Center:* All flexor tendons have been divided and part of the tendons excised. *Right:* The gastrocnemius has been elevated from the femoral condyles. An extensive posterior capsulectomy has been done. The posterior cruciate, medial, and lateral collateral ligaments may be divided when full extension is not obtained after the capsulectomy. (From Dias, L.S., J Pediatr Orthop 21:129, 1985. Reproduced with permission.)

related to muscle imbalance. These contractures demonstrate spontaneous correction within the first 6 months of life and an appropriate exercise program. Positional knee flexion contractures are usually secondary to hip flexion contractures with resultant external rotation of the extremity. These patients are often supine for long periods of time. The hips are flexed and abducted. The lower extremity is subsequently externally rotated, and the knees are flexed.

Knee flexion contractures due to muscle imbalance are usually due to increased spasticity in hamstring tone. Hamstring spasticity can be seen in the upper or lower lumbar patients. Contractures about the knee greater than 15° significantly increase the workload of a possibly weakened quadriceps, and this may lead to progressive contracture.[68]

Treatment of knee flexion contractures is based upon the degree of contracture and the functional level of the patient. In the nonambulatory patients who are not weight bearing for transfers, knee flexion contractures are rarely a problem. For ambulatory patients with knee flexion contractures of less than 20°, physiotherapy programs for stretching and orthotic management are appropriate.[1,80] In the ambulatory patient with knee flexion contractures above 20°, surgical management is indicated.[19] Depending on the degree of contracture, surgical management commences with specific tendon lengthening. If this does not bring the knee out to less than 20°, posterior capsulotomy carefully protecting the neurovascular structures is the next step (Fig. 29-5).

With flexion contractures not amenable to tendon lengthening or posterior capsulotomy, a distal femoral extension osteotomy should be considered.[74] Osteotomy in the presence of persistent muscle imbalance should not be performed; however, remodeling is rapid and recurrence of the flexion deformity is frequent.[1] Long-term orthotic management postoperatively is indicated. Hamstring transfer to the patellar tendon has been suggested by Abraham,[1] but we have no experience with this procedure in our spina bifida population. Sharrard states that surgical management of knee flexion contractures exceeding 30° must precede surgical management of hip flexion contractures.[1] Sharrard also states that IQs of less than 65 combined with arm weakness are a contraindication for operative management of knee flexion contractures.[1]

Extension Contracture of the Knee Extension contracture of the knee is frequently associated with ipsilateral hip dislocation. These dislocations are often teratologic, the children being born with extension contractures of the knee. Patients with knee extension contractures often have external rotation deformities at the hip, internal tibial torsional deformities of the legs, and talipes equinovarus deformities of the hindfoot. The hip dislocation is not reducible until the knee extension contracture is treated. The cause of knee extension contractures is muscle imbalance. This is usually seen in the patient with a high lumbar lesion. Unopposed quadriceps activity is present. This leads to quadriceps contracture and resultant fibrosis. Often there is a lateral dislocation of the patella. With progressive extension contracture, knee recurvatum is present. Often this is followed by anterior subluxation of the hamstrings. These abnormal positions of the knee lead to internal derangement of the knee.[74]

Treatment of knee extension contractures have received attention in recent literature.[2,19] Attempts at nonoperative management of extension contractures are appropriate prior to any surgical intervention. In the ambulatory patient, knee extension contractures are often helpful in decreasing the amount of orthotic assistance the patient needs for weight-bearing activities. In the nonambulatory patient, extension contractures pose a problem in wheelchair activities. During sitting, the leg is exposed to gravitational forces, and this often helps in the treatment of the contracture. Vigorous physiotherapy should be initiated early on and may preclude surgical management. In the nonambulatory patient with residual extension contracture, simple surgical release of the quadriceps through a transverse incision is appropriate.[2] In the patient with some quadriceps activity, some quadriceps function can be maintained with some type of quadricepsplasty (Fig. 29-6).[2,19] Prolonged postoperative splinting is recommended to prevent recurrent extension contracture.[19] We have little experience in elaborate quadriceps release in our spina bifida population.

Angular Deformities about the Knee

Varus and valgus deformities about the knee are common in the myelomeningocele patient. The valgus deformity is usually secondary to an iliotibial band contracture.[74] The valgus deformity can also be seen in the rare patient with isolated biceps femoris spasticity. This is commonly seen in association with external tibial torsion and ankle valgus deformities. Valgus deformity about the knee is also common secondary to malunited supracondylar femur fractures. Another group of spina bifida patients that develop progressive valgus deformity of the knee are those ambulatory patients with weak quadriceps that have been weight bearing with no orthotic protection about the knee. These patients often externally rotate the lower extremity and present the medial aspect of the knee forward, allowing their medial collateral ligament to act as their knee stabilizer. With time this leads to medial collateral ligament instability and secondary valgus deformity.

Varus deformities about the knee are less common than other knee deformities in this patient population. Varus deformity is usually secondary to malunited supracondylar femur fractures. The patient with poor quadriceps strength who is ambulating with no orthotic protection may also collapse into a varus knee deformity.

Management of angular deformities about the knee usually is nonsurgical. Appropriate orthotic management as previously discussed provides knee stability and prevents future deformity. In the patient with an iliotibial band contracture, a Yount procedure is appropriate and usually successful.[74] Osteotomies about the knee are also successful in correcting the angular deformities. Meticulous preoperative planning is essential for satisfactory results. Care must be taken to protect the distal femoral and proximal tibial epiphyseal plates in the skeletally immature patient.

Angular deformities following fracture about the knee have been addressed above. Residual knee stiffness with limitation of motion is common following fractures about the knee.[21] The limitation of motion is usually established by 6 months after the fracture, and Drabu and Walker found that the majority of contractures that are secondary to fractures resolve by 3 years after the fracture. No surgery is usually indicated in these patients to regain range of motion.[21] We commonly take advantage of a fracture about the knee to correct any preexisting deformity by manipulation and immobilization.

Torsional Deformities in the Lower Extremities

Torsional deformities in the lower extremities are often difficult to evaluate in view of the multiple deformities present. It is very important to fully evaluate the patient clinically. The foot progression angle should be observed. Orthotic systems may be malaligned because of torsional deformity. The entire mechanical axis of the extremity must be evaluated to check relation of hip to knee to ankle in a weight-bearing position.

External Torsional Deformities External rotation of the lower extremity may be secondary to femoral or tibial abnormality. Femoral torsional deformities are most commonly postural in the thoracic-level patient. Muscle imbalance can be responsible for the production of torsional deformities about the femur. This is most commonly due to contracture of the iliotibial band. Femoral retroversion is also common in these patients. External rotation of the femur is often asso-

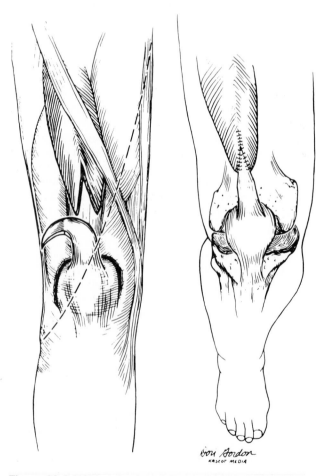

Figure 29-6 V-Y lengthening of the quadriceps mechanism for knee extension contracture in myelomeningocele. *Left:* Medial and lateral release of the knee capsule is performed proximally. *Right:* The quadriceps is sutured with the knee in 45° of flexion. (From Dias, L.S., J Pediatr Orthop 2:130, 1985. Reproduced with permission.)

ciated with ankle and foot deformities. These are most commonly calcaneus, calcaneovalgus, calcaneovarus, and abductovarus deformities of the foot.[56]

Treatment of external femoral rotation can be temporarily managed with twister cable. Operative management is primarily bony, but occasionally by soft tissue surgical procedures. These have not been successful in our hands. Femoral osteotomy is successful in treatment of femoral torsional deformities. We prefer distal supracondylar femoral osteotomies.[38] We reserve proximal derotational osteotomies for those patients who need simultaneous hip angular osteotomies.

External rotation deformities about the tibia are also usually secondary to iliotibial band contractures. These patients often have shortening of the fibula.[47] This leads to ankle valgus and external tibial torsion. Commonly medial malleolar pressure sores are seen in these patients secondary to orthotic use. Management for external tibial torsion is with orthotically tempered twister cables. Patients with residual external tibial torsion require a tibial osteotomy. A distal osteotomy is preferable to a proximal one.[20] It can often be combined with an angular osteotomy for ankle abnormality.

Internal Torsional Deformities Internal torsional deformities about the femur are usually due to excessive femoral anteversion. These are frequently associated with hip dislocation and hip adductor spasticity. These patients often have associated talipes varus, equinovarus, equinus, and cavovarus deformities.[55]

Internal torsional deformities about the tibia are usually secondary to muscle imbalance with spasticity of the medial hamstring. They can also occur secondary to muscle imbalance at the ankle associated with activity of the tibialis posterior muscle. Physiological internal tibial torsion may also play a role in the younger child.

Treatment of internal torsional deformities in the lower extremities can be with orthotic management. Twister cables have been successful in the young patient who is beginning to ambulate.

In the older child, surgical management is indicated. We prefer distal femoral as well as distal tibial osteotomies unless otherwise indicated.[38] Menelaus has described lateral hamstring transfers.[56] Dias was successful performing distal tibial osteotomies with transfers of the semitendinosus to the biceps tendon.[20]

In the patient with asymmetric neurological levels, windswept deformities are common. These deformities must be dealt with individually and obviously provide a considerable management challenge.

The Foot

The goal of treatment depends on the functional ability of the patient. Patients who are not ambulatory or whose prognosis is a nonambulatory status require a shoeable foot but do not require full mobility or a perfectly plantigrade foot. Patients who will be wearing orthotics (KAFOs, AFOs) do not require full normal mobility of their joints but sufficient amount of mobility that they can accommodate the slight changes of

position with pressures. Ambulatory patients must be provided with plantigrade feet that do not result in excessive pressure on any portion of the plantar surface during stance.

Basic Foot Deformities

The primary types of deformities seen in myelomeningocele feet are talipes equinus; talipes equinovarus or equinovalgus; calcaneus with valgus or varus; valgus foot; convex pes valgus (vertical talus); cavus foot; and toe deformities.

Talipes Equinus Talipes equinus is seen primarily in completely paralyzed legs and is an early deformity. It apparently develops as a contracture of the gastrocsoleus despite the muscle's lack of function. At times isolated function is present within the gastrocsoleus, and this leads to contracture.

Treatment varies with the age group as well as with function. In the nonfunctioning gastrocsoleus, tendon lengthening can be done by subcutaneous tenotomy at a very early age. Frequently there is no sensation in the area and the procedure may be carried out (as done by Menelaus in 1976) without anesthesia in infants during the first few weeks of life.[54]

Subcutaneous tenotomy is performed in our clinic by cutting the medial half of the tendon just at the heel level, the lateral half about $\frac{3}{4}$ in. above that, and the medial half for a second time about $\frac{3}{4}$ in. above the lateral cut.

In older patients with rigid ankle joints, who would not be improved by tendon and posterior capsule releases, anterior-based wedge osteotomies of the distal tibia have been successful in providing a plantigrade foot. Extreme deformities have been overcome with this method. In children with growing distal tibial epiphyses and fixed equinus, Sharrard and Grosfeld described posterior soft tissue release followed by anterior tibiofibular ligament release permitting widening of the mortise and enabling the talus to be brought back up into neutral from its plantarflexed position.[78]

Talipes Equinovarus Talipes equinovarus appears to occur more frequently in paralysis above the L4 level. Treatment schedules are variable. Other than early release of the Achilles tendon through subcutaneous tenotomies, cast corrections are utilized during the early months of life, and surgical correction is delayed until at least 6 months of age. Most patients require complete posterior medial, plantar, and lateral releases of the foot. Postoperative pinning in the corrected position is necessary. Insensitive feet must be carefully protected against excessive or localized cast pressure. For this reason, casting should be used only to protect the foot from outside deforming forces after full correction has been achieved surgically.[25] Cast immobilization for 12 to 16 weeks, followed by brace immobilization in the corrected position, is required.

Recurrent deformities undergo repeat releases. In patients who have been neglected or are seen late, and in patients who have had repeated corrections with gross deformity of the talus, talectomy is carried out at the same time as soft tissue releases.[56] In recurrent deformities in which the lateral column of the foot is longer than the medial column, lateral column shortening is necessary. Evans resection and fusion of calcaneocuboid joint[23] and Lichtblau distal calcaneal resection[43] are examples.

Adduction and supination deformities in the 5- to 10-year-old age group can be benefited by cuneiform-cuboid wedge osteotomy[25] through two vertical incisions over the dorsum of the foot, one over the first cuneiform–second cuneiform area and the other one at the third cuneiform–cuboid junction. A lateral-based wedge can be removed, and this allows derotation of the forefoot as well as correction of the adduction angulation. The advantage of this is that it preserves the joints proximal and distal to the cuneiforms and allows for maximum growth of the foot.

Triple arthrodesis is used in more mature feet, those over the age of 12 years or its equivalent bony age. Residual deformities in teenagers and young adults that cause ulceration over the proximal portion of the fifth metatarsal are best treated by triple arthrodesis.

Calcaneus deformity of the myelodysplastic foot is generally related to excessive dorsiflexion of the ankle. The deformity is benefited by bracing which prevents excessive dorsiflexion. However, gradually the contracture becomes greater and plantigrade stability is lost. Severe deformities defy the wearing of shoes because of lack of posterior heel prominence. Stance is affected as there is no posterior stability. Knee stability is decreased because a knee-flexed position is required to maintain a plantigrade position of the foot. The deformity is secondary to a poor to absent gastrocsoleus and a strong dorsiflexor of the foot. The tibialis anterior is innervated by the highest nerve roots of the muscles crossing the ankle, beginning at about the L4 level, and is the strongest of the L5-level muscles at the ankle. A full-strength tibialis anterior may be present and no gastrocsoleus strength exist. The peroneus tertius is also frequently functional with lesions at this level. Treatment consists of removing the deforming force, namely the tibialis anterior, and passing the muscle through the interosseous membrane to the os calcis (Peabody procedure).[36,65,89] The peroneus tertius, if functional, should also be transplanted. Treatment is best carried out between 6 and 24 months of age. Banta et al demonstrated improved gait with a combined procedure of anterior tibial transplantation and Achilles tenodesis.[5]

Calcaneovarus deformity may be present initially or may occur after transfer if the tibialis posterior was unrecognized as being functional.[56] This muscle should be transferred to the os calcis or may be sectioned if it is relatively weak. Calcaneovalgus is treated in the same manner with transfers, along with the tibialis anterior, through the peronei to the heel.

Talipes Valgus Talipes valgus causes instability in weight bearing, since weight is transferred to the medial side of the ankle. Pressure occurs over a medial malleolus, and in an insensitive foot, ulcerations occur. Talipes valgus is difficult to control and is usually seen with excessive dorsiflexion of the ankle. Problems appear to become more significant as the child reaches the age of 7 to 10 years and becomes heavier. The earliest and most severe deformities occur from muscle imbalance, secondary to strong active lateral muscles such as the peronei with absent medial muscles such as the posterior tibialis. The tibialis posterior muscle ordinarily is innervated by higher levels than the peronei. Spastic peronei may create the problem. Talipes valgus occurs in flaccid feet secondary to dorsiflexion and eversion. It is necessary, in all these cases, to have an absent soleus muscle.[17] The fibula is short compared with a normal fibula, and containment of the talus on the lateral aspect is poor.[48] This allows excessive valgus of the joint with wedging of the distal tibial epiphysis.[27] As the weight-bearing center passes more medial, the subtalar joint responds by also going into valgus. The external rotation of the lower extremities further accentuates the problems of pushing the foot into valgus.

Treatment of apparent muscle imbalance is necessary with section of the spastic tendons as well as transfers required. Weight-bearing anterior and posterior radiographs of the ankle joint demonstrate the valgus position of the talus. A CT scan of the tibiotalar joint and subtalar joint as suggested by Smith and Staples[81] is helpful in defining whether the subtalar joint is also involved. With the valgus ankle, treatment of the subtalar joint alone is doomed to failure. Treatment of the ankle valgus is carried out in several ways. Patients with no gastrocsoleus function and excessive dorsiflexion can have a tenodesis of the distal portion of the Achilles tendon into the fibula.[92] This provides a blockage of dorsiflexion past neutral. In addition, it applies stress to the fibula with each step, pulling the fibula distalward as the patient rolls forward off the foot. It has been noted that the fibula is stimulated and does pull down to the talus, and the distal tibial epiphysis loses its wedging.[27] Patients with significant eversion of the subtalar joint may require a subtalar fusion. Patients who have ankle problems above the age of 10 years, with remaining growth potentials in their distal tibia, undergo medial epiphyseal stapling to allow growth on the lateral side, thereby straightening out the valgus ankle.[11]

Supramalleolar osteotomy has been used in patients who are approaching or have already achieved closure of their distal tibial epiphysis.[80] In these patients, definitive corrective treatment is achieved. The wedge of bone that is removed can be utilized for subtalar fusion if that is desired. Achilles tenodesis can be utilized along with any of the other procedures mentioned for excessive dorsiflexion prevention. Patients with eversion of the subtalar joint and abduction of the midfoot require the stabilization of a triple arthrodesis as described by Williams and Menelaus.[94] Distal tibial rotational and wedge osteotomies can be performed at the same time.[60]

Paralytic Vertical Talus This deformity consists of a dislocation of the foot around the talus bringing the foot in valgus. The os calcis is in equinus. The navicular sits on the neck of the talus, and there is a convexity at the plantar surface of the calcaneal-cuboid joint. There is marked rockering at the weight-bearing surface, placing pressure around the head of the talus and at the calcaneal-cuboid joint. The muscular imbalance is associated with strong dorsiflexors and evertors along with weakness of balancing toe flexors, tibialis posterior, and intrinsics. A tight Achilles tendon is present but is not necessarily functioning. Uterine position as well as muscle imbalance may be a cause of the development of this type of foot deformity.[56] Treatment is surgical and requires placing the tibialis anterior into the neck of the talus after reduction.[75] Dias[18] has demonstrated that patients over the age of

4 years require subtalar fusion, and Menelaus recommends subtalar fusion in patients without a functioning anterior tibial muscle.[56]

Talipes Cavus Cavus foot is primarily seen in sacral-level patients and is due to the lack of intrinsics with all the other muscles being present. The toes are also clawed. Early treatment consists of sectioning the plantar fascia, and lengthening the tibialis posterior tendon to provide relief for the high arch. In older children and adults, a metatarsal osteotomy may be performed. Clawing of the toes has been adequately treated in our patients by the performance of the Taylor-Girdlestone[86] transfer, placing the long toe flexors into the extensor hood. The extensor tendon is lengthened or resected and a dorsal capsulotomy performed. The long toe extensors may be placed into the necks of the metatarsals if forefoot equinus is present. Sharrard recommended a flexor tenodesis of the first toe.[79]

Spastic intrinsic muscles create a cavus foot with extended toes. In patients with no foot sensation, sectioning of the posterior tibial nerve and release of the plantar ligament cure the problem. In patients who have sensation about the bottom of the foot, selected sectioning of the motor branches in the plantar surface of the foot is appropriate.[32]

Ulcerations Plantar pressure sores are usually the result of residual deformity causing prominences on the plantar surface of the foot. Occasionally ulcerations occur in an insensitive foot secondary to the patient's walking barefooted. The use of a protective cast brings about rapid closure of the ulceration.[6] However, if it is due to bony prominence, the prominence itself must be treated. Determination must be made whether it is a localized prominence or whether the entire foot deformity must be corrected. If there is infection around the metatarsal head, causing persistent drainage and ulceration, it is necessary to resect the head before healing occurs. A rocker-bottom shoe helps prevent additional ulcerations. Wheelchair patients may suffer ulcerations secondary to not wearing shoes. Severe foot deformity may prevent the donning of shoes. In those cases, surgical correction is required.

REFERENCES

1. Abraham, E., Verinder, D.G.R., and Sharrard, W.J.W. The treatment of flexion contracture of the knee in myelomeningocele. J Bone Joint Surg 59B:433–438, 1977.
2. Aprin, H., and Kilfoyle, R.M. Extension contracture of the knees in patients with myelomeningocele. Clin Orthop 144:260–263, 1979.
3. Ascher, M., and Olson, J. Factors affecting the ambulatory status of patients with spina bifida cystica. J Bone Joint Surg 350–356, 1983.
4. Baker, L.D., Dodelin, R., and Bassett, F.H. Pathological changes in the hip in cerebral palsy. J Bone Joint Surg 44A:1331–1342, 1962.
5. Banta, J., Sutherland, D.H., and Wyatt, M. Anterior tibialis transfer to os calcis with Achilles tenodesis for calcaneal deformity in myelomeningocele. J Pediatr Orthop 1:125–130, 1981.
6. Brand, P.W. The insensitive foot, in Jahss, M.H. (ed): *Disorders of the Foot,* Philadelphia, Saunders, 1982.
7. Breed, A.L., and Healey, P.M. The mid lumbar myelomeningocele

8. hip. Mechanics of dislocation and treatment. Pediatr Orthop 2(1):15–23, 1982.
8. Brookes, M., and Wardle, E.N. Muscle action and the shape of the femur. J Bone Joint Surg 44B:398–411, 1962.
9. Buisson, J.S., and Hamblen, D.L. Electromyographic assessment of the transplanted iliopsoas muscle in spina bifida cystica. Dev Med Child Neurol 14:29–33,1972.
10. Bunch, W.H., and Hakala, M.W. Iliopsoas transfers in children with myelomeningocele. J Bone Joint Surg 66A:224–227, 1984.
11. Burkus, J.K., Moore, D.W., and Raycroft, M.D. Valgus deformity of the ankle in myelodysplastic patients. J Bone Joint Surg 65A:1157–1162, 1983.
12. Canale, S.T., Hammond, N.L., Cotler, J.M., and Snedden, H.E. Pelvic displacement osteotomy for chronic hip dislocation in myelodysplasia. J Bone Joint Surg 57A:177–182, 1975.
13. Carroll, N. The orthotic management of the spina bifida child. Clin Orthop 102:108–115, 1974.
14. Carroll, N.C., and Sharrard, W.J.W. Long-term follow-up of posterior iliopsoas transplantation for paralytic dislocation of the hip. J Bone Joint Surg 54A:551–560, 1972.
15. Compere, E.L., Garrison, M., and Fahey, J.J. Deformities of the femur resulting from arrestment of growth of the capital and greater trochanteric epiphyses. J Bone Joint Surg 22:909–914, 1940.
16. DeSouza, L.J., and Carroll, N. Ambulation of the braced myelomeningocele patient. J Bone Joint Surg 58A:1112–1118, 1974.
17. Dias, L.S. Ankle valgus in children with myelomeningocele. Dev Med Child Neurol 20:627–633, 1978.
18. Dias, L.S. Vertical talus. *Foot and Ankle Society Annual Meeting.* Las Vegas, 1984.
19. Dias, L.S. Surgical management of knee contractures in myelomeningocele. J Pediatr Orthop 2:127–131, 1982.
20. Dias, L.S., Jasty, M.J., and Collins, P. Rotational deformities of the lower limb in myelomeningocele, evaluation and treatment. J Bone Joint Surg 66A:215–223, 1984.
21. Drabu, K.J., and Walker, G. Stiffness after fractures around the knee in spina bifida. J Bone Joint Surg 67B:266–267, 1985.
22. Drummond, D.S., Moreau, M., and Cruess, R.L. Post-operative neuropathic fractures in patients with myelomeningocele. Dev Med Child Neurol 23:147–150, 1981.
23. Evans, D. Relapsed club foot. J Bone Joint Surg 43B:722–733, 1961.
24. Feiwell, E. Selection of appropriate treatment for patients with myelomeningocele. Orthop Clin North Am 12:101–106, 1981.
25. Feiwell, E. The foot in myelodysplasia, in Mann, R.A. (ed): *Surgery of the Foot.* St. Louis, 5th ed. Mosby, 1985.
26. Feiwell, E. The unstable hip: Infra-acetabular osteotomy, in McLaurin, R. (ed): *Myelomeningocele.* New York, Grune & Stratton, 1977.
27. Feiwell, E., and Miller, G. Valgus of the foot in myelodysplasia. *American Orthopaedic Foot Society, 13th Annual Meeting,* Anaheim, CA 1983.
28. Feiwell, E., Sakai, D., and Blatt, T. The effect of hip reduction of function in patients with myelomeningocele. J Bone Joint Surg 60A:169–173, 1978.
29. Ferguson, A.B., Jr. Primary open reduction of congenital dislocation of the hip using a median adductor approach. J Bone Joint Surg 55A:671–689, 1973.
30. Fleming, J.L. Iliopsoas transplant and femoral osteotomy for paralytic dislocation. J Bone Joint Surg 39A:697, 1957.
31. Floman, Y., Penny, J.N., Micheli, L.J., Riseborough, E.J., and Hall, J.E. Osteotomy of the fusion mass in scoliosis. J Bone Joint Surg 64A:1307–1316, 1982.
32. Garceau, G.J., and Brahms, M.A. A preliminary study of selective plantar-muscle denervation for pes cavus. J Bone Joint Surg 38A:553–562, 1956.
33. Gardner, W.J. Hydrodynamic mechanism of syringomyelia: Its re-

lationship to myelocele. J Neurol Neurosurg Psychiatry 28:247–259, 1965.

34. Hall, P.V., Lindseth, R.E., Campbell, R.L., and Kalsbeck, J.E. Myelodysplasia and developmental scoliosis—A manifestation of syringomyelia. Spine 1: 48–56, 1976.

35. Hammesfohr, R., Topple, S., Yoo, K., Whitesides, T., and Paulin, A.M. Abductor paralysis and the role of the external oblique transfer. Orthopedics 6:315–321, 1983.

36. Hayes, J.T., Gross, H.P., and Dow, S. Survey for paralytic defects in myelomeningocele. J Bone Joint Surg 46A:1577–1597, 1964.

37. Hoffer, M.M., Feiwell, E., Perry, R., Perry, J., and Bonnett, C. Functional ambulation in patients with myelomeningocele. J Bone Joint Surg 55A:137–148, 1973.

38. Hoffer, M.M., Prietto, C., and Koffman, M. Supracondylar derotational osteotomy of the femur for internal rotation of the thigh in the cerebral palsied child. J Bone Joint Surg 63A:389–393, 1981.

39. Irwin, C.E. The iliotibial band. Its role in producing deformity in poliomyelitis. J Bone Joint Surg 31A:141–146, 1949.

40. Jackson, R.D., Padgett, T.S., and Donovan, M.M. Posterior iliopsoas muscle transfer in myelodysplasia. J Bone Joint Surg 61A:40–45, 1979.

41. Jackson, R., and Feiwell, E. Functional decline due to occult neurological changes in older children with myelomeningocele. *Presented at the Western Orthopedics Meeting,* October 1985.

42. Lee, E.H., and Carroll, N.C. Hip stability and ambulatory status in myelomeningocele. J Pediatr Orthop 5:522–527, 1985.

43. Lichtblau, S.A. A medial and lateral release operation of club foot. J Bone Joint Surg 55A:1377–1384, 1973.

44. Lindseth, R.R. Posterior iliac osteotomy for fixed pelvic obliquity. J Bone Joint Surg 60A:17–22, 1978.

45. Lindseth, R., and Glancy, J. Polypropylene lower extremity braces for paraplegia due to myelomeningocele. J Bone Joint Surg 56B:556–563, 1974.

46. London, J.T., and Nichols, O. Paralytic dislocation of the hip in myelodysplasia. J Bone Joint Surg 57A:501–506, 1975.

47. Madigan, R.R., and Worrall, V.T. Paralytic instability of the hip in myelomeningoceles. Clin Orthop 125:57–64, 1977.

48. Makin, M. Tibio-fibular relationship in paralized limbs. J Bone Joint Surg 47B:500–506, 1965.

49. McCall, R., Douglas, R., and Richtor, N. *Surgical Treatment in Patients with Myelodysplasia Before Using the LSU Reciprocation-Gait System.* Orthopedics 6:843–848, 1983.

50. McKay, D.W. McKay hip stabilization in meningo-myelocele. Presented at the AAOS Meeting, 1977.

51. McKibbin, B. The action of the iliopsoas muscle in the newborn. J Bone Joint Surg 50B:161–165, 1968.

52. McKibbin, B. The use of splintage in the management of paralytic dislocation of the hip in spina bifida cystica. J Bone Joint Surg 56B:163–172, 1973.

53. Mazur, J.M., Stillwell, A., Menelaus, M. The significance of spasticity in the upper and lower limbs in myelomeningocele. J Bone Joint Surg 68B:213–218, 1986.

54. Menelaus, M.B. Orthopaedic management of children with myelomeningocele: A plea for realistic goals. Dev Med Child Neurol 18(suppl 37):3–11, 1976.

55. Menelaus, M.B. The hip in myelomeningocele. J Bone Joint Surg 58B:448–452, 1976.

56. Menelaus, M.B. *The Orthopaedic Management of Spina Bifida Cystica.* Livingstone, Edinburgh, 1980.

57. Mooney, V., et al. Comparison of pressure distribution qualities in seat cushions. *Bulletin of Prosthetic Research.* Spring 1971.

58. Mustard, W.T. Iliopsoas transfer for weakness of the hip abductors. J Bone Joint Surg 34A:647, 1952.

59. Nickel, V., Perry, J., Garrett, A., and Feiwell, E. Paralytic dislocation of the hip. *Proceedings of the AAOS* 48A:1021, 1966.

60. Nicol, R.O., and Menelaus, M.B. Correction of the combined tibial torsion and valgus deformity of the foot. J Bone Joint Surg 65B(5):641–645, 1983.

61. O'Brien, J.P., Dwyer, A.P., and Hodgson, A.R. Paralytic pelvic obliquity. J Bone Joint Surg 57A:626–631, 1975.

62. Park, T.S., et al. Progressive spasticity and scoliosis in children with myelomeningocele. J Neurosurg 62:367–375, 1985.

63. Parker, B., and Walkers, G. Posterior psoas transfer and hip instability in lumbar myelomeningocele. J Bone Joint Surg 57B:53–58, 1975.

64. Parsch, K., and Goessens, H. Surgical treatment of spinal column and hip deformities in spina bifida. Acta Orthop Belg 37 (3):230–239, 1971.

65. Peabody, C. Tendon transplantation in the lower extremity. Instr Course Lect 6:178–188, 1949.

66. Pemberton, P.A. Pericapsular osteotomy of the ilium for treatment of congenital subluxation and dislocation of the hip. J Bone Joint Surg 47A:65–86, 1965.

67. Perlik, P.C., Westin, G., and Marafioti, R.L. A combination pelvic osteotomy for acetabular dysplasia in children. J Bone Joint Surg 67A:842–850, 1985.

68. Perry, J., Antonelli, D., and Ford, W. Analysis of knee joint forces during flexed knee stance. J Bone Joint Surg 57A:961–967, 1975.

69. Peterson, M., and Adkins, H. Measurements and redistribution of excessive pressures during wheelchair sitting. J Am Phys Ther Assoc 62(7):990–994, 1982.

70. Raycroft, F. Abduction splinting of the hips of infants with myelodysplasia. *Second Symposium on Spina Bifida—A Multidisciplinary Approach.* Cincinnati, November 1984.

71. Rose, G.K., Sankarankutty, M., and Stallard, J. A clinical review of the orthotic treatment of myelomeningocele patients. J Bone Joint Surg 65B:242–246, 1983.

72. Rose, G.K., Henshaw, J.T. A swivel walker for paraplegics: Medical and technical considerations. Bio-Med Eng 7(9):420–425, October 1972.

73. Salter, R.B. Innominate osteotomy in the treatment of congenital dislocation and subluxation of the hip. J Bone Joint Surg 43B:426–444, 1964.

74. Schafer, M.F., and Dias, L.S., *Myelomeningocele, Orthopaedic Treatment.* Baltimore, Williams & Wilkins, 1983.

75. Sharrard, W.J.W. Paralytic convex pes valgus, in McLauren, R. (ed): *Myelomeningocele.* New York, Grune & Stratton, 1977.

76. Sharrard, W.J.W. Paralytic deformities in the lower limb. J Bone Joint Surg 49B:731–747, 1967.

77. Sharrard, W.J.W. Posterior iliopsoas transplantation in the treatment of paralytic dislocation of the hip. J Bone Joint Surg 46B:426–444, 1964.

78. Sharrard, W.J.W., and Grosfeld, I. Management of foot deformities in myelomeningocele. J Bone Joint Surg 50B:456–465, 1968.

79. Sharrard, W.J.W., and Smith, T.W.D. Tenodesis of flexor hallucis longus for paralytic clawing of the hallux in childhood. J Bone Joint Surg 58B:224–226, 1976.

80. Sharrard, W.J.W., and Webb, J. Supramalleolar wedge osteotomy of the tibia in children with myelomeningocele. J Bone Joint Surg 56:458–461, 1974.

81. Smith, R.W., and Staple, T.W. Computerized tomography (CT) scanning technique for the hindfoot. Clin Orthop 177:34–38, 1983.

82. Somerville, E.W. Paralytic dislocation of the hip. J Bone Joint Surg 41B:279–288, 1959.

83. Stevens, P.M., and Coleman, S.S. Coxa breva: Its pathogenesis and a rationale for its management. J Pediatr Orthop 5:515–521, 1985.

84. Stillwell, A., and Menelaus, M.B. Walking ability after transplantation of the iliopsoas. J Bone Joint Surg 66B:656–659, 1984.

85. Stillwell, A., and Menelaus, M.B. Walking ability in mature patients with spina bifida. J Pediatr 3(2):184–190, 1983.

86. Taylor, R.G. Treatment of claw toes by multiple transfer flexors to extensor tendon. J Bone Joint Surg 33B:539–542, 1951.

87. Thomas, L.I., Thompson, T.C., and Straub, L. Transplantation of the external oblique muscle for abductor paralysis. J Bone Joint Surg 32A:207–217, 1950.

88. Trumble, T., Banta, J.V., Raycroft, J.F., and Curtis, B.H. Talectomy for equinovarus deformity in myelodysplasia. J Bone Joint Surg 67A:1:21–29, 1985.

89. Turner, A. Hand function in children with myelomeningocele. J Bone Joint Surg 67B:268–272, 1985.

90. Turner, J., and Cooper, R. Posterior transposition of tibialis anterior through the interosseus member. Clin Orthop 79:71–74, 1971.

91. Waters, R.L., and Lunsford, R.P.T. Energy cost in paraplegic loco-

motion. J Bone Joint Surg 67A:1245–1249, 1985.

92. Weissman, S.L., Torok, G., and Khermosh, O.J. Intertrochanteric osteotomy in fixed paralytic obliquity of the pelvis. J Bone Joint Surg 43A:1135–1154, 1961.

93. Westin, G.W. Achilles tenodesis to fibular. Personal communication, 1975.

94. Williams, P.F., and Menelaus, M.B. Triple arthrodesis by inlay graft—A method suitable for underformed or valgus foot. J Bone Joint Surg 59B(3):333–336, 1977.

95. Yngve, D.A., Douglas, D., and Roberts, J.M. The reciprocation gait orthosis in myelomeningocele. J Pediatr Orthop 4:304–310, 1984.

CHAPTER 30

Miscellaneous Neuromuscular Disorders of Orthopaedic Interest

Roger Dee

THE MUSCULAR DYSTROPHIES

Duchenne's Muscular Dystrophy

This X-linked-recessive myopathy generally affects only males.[37] Estimates of its incidence range from 13 to 33 per 100,000 males, of which one-third arise from new mutations.[103]

Clinical Features

Affected males may show mild delay in their early motor milestones or may toe walk but usually are diagnosed between the age of 3 to 5 years when they begin to lose skills that they have already acquired. Lumbar lordosis is universally present at this stage, and the classic pseudohypertrophy of the calf muscles is common. The muscle weakness is steadily progressive, with the proximal musculature being more affected than the distal.[159] It is because of this proximal weakness that these boys exhibit a positive Gowers' sign (using the hands to "climb" up the legs) on arising from the floor (Fig. 30-1).[55,56]

Patients with Duchenne's dystrophy have an average loss of 15 IQ points when compared with their siblings.[1,105] Nevertheless, education is stressed because of their physical limitations.

Recurrent respiratory infections, including pneumonia, become more common as the child gets older and respiratory function deteriorates.[83] Cardiomyopathy also becomes prominent. Death usually ensues before the end of the second dec-

ade. Approximately three-quarters are pulmonary deaths, and approximately one-quarter are cardiac deaths.

Genetic counseling is necessary for the families of these patients to identify carrier females. Usually carriers are asymptomatic, but occasionally they may show evidence of a mild myopathy—the so-called manifesting carrier.[41]

Etiology

In this condition changes have been seen in the distribution and density of intramembrane particles in the muscle fiber plasmalemma together with abnormal anastomoses between the sarcoplasmic reticulum and the T system.[106] Both the muscle biopsy and the electromyogram (EMG) are consistent with the view that there may be some form of defective excitation-contraction coupling.[106] This is consistent with the observed increase in the isometric contraction and relaxation time.[106]

Diagnosis

Laboratory Tests There is a very high level of serum creatine phosphokinase (CPK), particularly in the first year of life before the disease manifests itself. If this test is normal at this age, it is strong evidence against the possibility of the disease.[9]

A high CPK level identifies a female as a carrier and is a useful screening test, but even three negative tests do not entirely rule out the carrier state.[26,127]

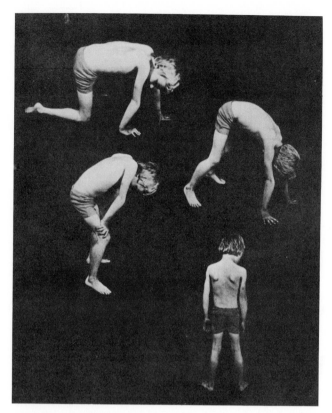

Figure 30-1 Duchenne's muscular dystrophy in a 6-year-old boy. Gowers' sign is present (see text). There is enlargement of the calf muscles and atrophy of the shoulder muscles with scapular winging. *(From McComas, A.J.: Neuromuscular Function and Disorders, Butterworth, London, 1977. Reproduced with permission.)*

Orthopaedic Management

During the stage of independent ambulation, patients with Duchenne's muscular dystrophy usually have little scoliosis but require active physical therapy for stretching of the hips, iliotibial bands, hamstrings, and heelcords. Night splints are also frequently used to minimize contractures. In the ambulatory stage, internal fixation is indicated for fractures of the hip or femur that otherwise require prolonged recumbency.

Children with this disorder may ambulate independently until the end of their first decade. Some children are more severely affected than others, but the diagnosis of any child still ambulating independently after the age of 12 years should be reevaluated. As the child ceases to ambulate independently, many centers advocate releasing existing contractures and bracing with long-leg braces to allow the child to ambulate or stand for an additional $2\frac{1}{2}$ to 3 years.[20,144] The surgery frequently consists of hip flexor releases, iliotibial band releases, Achilles tendon lengthening, and tibialis posterior lengthening or transfer.[111,141,143,160,167] Surgery must be done immediately if the patient is to remain ambulatory. In the long-leg braces, the patients actually "sit" on the posterior portions of the thigh cuffs when standing and use trunk sway to help themselves ambulate. In the later part of the bracing phase, scoliosis may begin to develop. If a total contact brace is used, this may significantly affect trunk shift and convert the patient from a braced walker to a braced stander. If the child is only standing, total contact bracing does not seem to affect motor ability. Nevertheless, most patients take longer to adjust to their braces, and pulmonary function studies in and out of braces should be considered to rule out respiratory compromise.

Eventually, however, because of progressive muscle weakness, patients become wheelchair-bound. Approxi-

Muscle Biopsy The muscle biopsy is fairly typical in this disease. It shows foci of necrosis with phagocytosis and interstitial infiltration by connective tissue (Fig. 30-2). Between the muscle fibers there is an increase in the amount of connective tissue which has been identified as type III collagen.[106] An increased number of undifferentiated large type IIC fibers are present.[11] Such abnormalities as multisegmented hypertrophied fibers, lateral sarcoplasmic masses, and ringlike structures known as annulets are also seen on light microscopy (Fig. 30-3). These latter changes, however, are characteristic of various forms of muscular dystrophy and are not specific for Duchenne's.[47]

EMG Changes On electromyography, one occasionally sees small-amplitude polyphasic potentials, with fibrillation, which is associated with necrosis.[11,112]

ECG Recording Abnormal changes in the ECG, associated with cardiomyopathy, are seen in 70 percent of cases. Abnormalities are also seen in the carrier state but are not helpful as a screening test.[11]

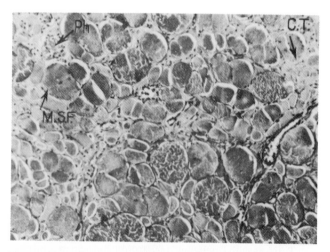

Figure 30-2 Muscular dystrophy (H&E). There is irregularity in the size of the muscle fibers and some abnormally large and multisegmented fibers *(MSF)*; loci of necrosis with phagocytosis *(Ph)*; and interstitial infiltration by connective tissue *(CT)*. *(From Escourelle, R., and Poirier, J.: Manual of Basic Neuropathology. Philadelphia, Saunders, 1978. Reproduced with permission.)*

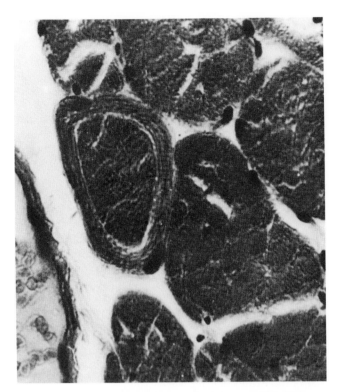

Figure 30-3 Striated annulet (ring fiber) in muscular dystrophy (H&E). *(From Escourelle, R., and Poirier, J: A Manual of Basic Neuropathology. Philadelphia, Saunders, 1978. Reproduced with permission.)*

mately 75 percent do not develop significant, progressive scoliosis.[140] With the advent of the Luque instrumentation for posterior spinal fusion, surgery in these patients has become more feasible.[99] Progressive curves over 30° are now considered for fusion if the patient's respiratory status allows. There is evidence that curves associated with a flexed spine are more likely than those with a hyperextended spine to progress and require fusion.[165] Fusions should be done early because respiratory insufficiency worsens with time and increases the surgical morbidity and mortality.

In this late wheelchair-bound stage, hip and knee flexion contractures continue to develop.[2] If the patient has previously had heelcord and tibialis posterior procedures, the feet remain in good alignment and are shoeable. If not, severe acquired talipes equinovarus is frequently seen, with recurrent lateral ankle sprains and inability to wear shoes. Sometimes, tendon releases, triple arthrodesis, or tarsal curettage may be necessary to alleviate pain and ameliorate the deformities.

Also, in the wheelchair stage, self-feeding may become more of a problem. Upper extremity contractures are frequently present, and the child no longer has the muscle power to lift his hand to his mouth. Most patients bend forward, but if they are being braced or have had a posterior spinal fusion, this may be difficult.

Becker's Muscular Dystrophy

Becker's muscular dystrophy[8] is a severe X-linked myopathy which shows close linkage to red-green color blindness.[42,43] The genes for both Becker's and Duchenne's dystrophy may be on the short arm of the X chromosome.[70,90] Precise diagnosis is again important for appropriate genetic counseling. An affected male will have no sons with the disorder, but all his daughters will be carriers. A female carrier will have a 50 percent chance that any son has the disorder and a 50 percent chance that any daughter is a carrier.

Clinical Features

Patients with Becker's dystrophy typically have evidence of proximal weakness either at the end of the first decade or during the second. Most patients are fully ambulatory until after skeletal maturity, and that in part may explain why few show significant scoliosis. Equinus foot deformities are not infrequent as the disorder progresses. Hip and knee flexion contractures may be seen in the wheelchair-bound patient. Drennan gives the average age for loss of ambulatory status as 30, and average age of death as 36.[31] There is significant interfamilial variability, however. Intelligence is not diminished in this disorder, and many patients lead productive lives.

Differential Diagnosis

It is important to distinguish this disease from limb girdle dystrophy. A very high CPK level and degenerative changes on the muscle biopsy together with the presence of pseudohypertrophy point to Becker's dystrophy as the correct diagnosis, however.[70]

Limb Girdle Dystrophy

Limb girdle dystrophy is an autosomal recessive disorder; therefore, males and females are equally affected. Although siblings usually show the same age of onset and degree of progression, there is considerable interfamilial variability. Onset may be in the first decade or as late as the fourth. Proximal musculature is more affected than distal.[35] Those patients who ambulate until after skeletal maturity do not generally develop significant scoliosis or contractures. However, some severely affected patients may show these deformities. Inappropriate genetic counseling may be given if a patient with this condition is confused with a patient who is instead a manifesting carrier for Duchenne's dystrophy.[70]

Facioscapulohumeral Dystrophy

Facioscapulohumeral dystrophy is an autosomal dominantly inherited myopathy which is quite variable in its presentation. Some patients are very minimally affected, whereas in some children the disorder may be more marked. In this disorder it is particularly necessary to exclude those patients

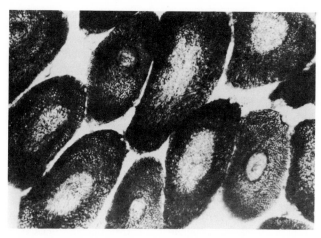

Figure 30-4 Central core disease. The central portion of each muscle fiber contains a zone of absent oxidative activity (succinic dehydrogenase) $\times 450$. *(From Banker, B.Q., Clin Orthop 194:30-43, 1985. Reproduced with permission.)*

with presentation similar to that of true facioscapulohumeral dystrophy but who have rather one of the congenital myopathies or other progressive neuromuscular disorders.[11]

The earliest presentation is usually facial weakness causing difficulty in closing the eyelids tightly or in pursing the lips or puffing out the cheeks. Scapular weakness, however, is frequently the most disabling component of the disorder, causing difficulty in abducting the arms and inability to adequately stabilize the scapula against the thoracic cavity so that work can be carried out. Copeland has described a thoracoscapular fusion to stabilize the scapula in this disorder.[19]

Other orthopaedic problems include scoliosis and hyperlordosis, which occasionally may be disabling. Some patients may have ambulatory difficulties and benefit from lower extremity bracing.

OTHER CONGENITAL MYOPATHIES

Central Core Disease

Central core disease is an autosomal dominant congenital myopathy. Its hallmark is an axon with amorphous central zone devoid of enzymatic activity and therefore not stained using histochemical methods (Fig. 30-4).[11,35,53] The fibers affected are predominantly type I.[47] Also, a predominance of type I fibers is seen in the biopsy. The muscle weakness is usually nonfocal in these patients and may vary from mild to severe. Motor milestones are commonly delayed. Progressive scoliosis, foot deformity, and congenital dislocation of the hips are all orthopaedic problems commonly seen with this disorder.[3,44,118] Malignant hyperthermia (discussed later on in this chapter) is the most feared complication of central core disorder.[23-25,44] Dantrolene sodium is the treatment of choice for malignant hyperthermia.[91]

Congenital Fiber-Type Disproportion

Fiber-type disproportion is characterized by relative disproportion of the size and number of type I to type II muscle fiber, with type I fibers being smaller and more common.[35] Generalized hypotonia is the hallmark of the disorder and is sometimes noted to be progressive in early life. Progressive scoliosis, torticollis, congenital dislocation of the hips, and multiple joint contractures of the hands and feet are the most common orthopaedic problems seen. There is frequently a familial pattern.

Mitochondrial Myopathies

The mitochondrial myopathies are a group of neuromuscular disorders characterized by "ragged-red" fibers, which are disrupted red-staining fibers seen with Gomori trichrome staining.[11,35] On electron microscopy, the mitochondria typically have bizarre, giant forms. Frequently there are inclusions within the mitochondria. Abnormal mitochondria have been recognized in many disorders including some of the cardiomyopathies, lipid storage disorders such as carnitine deficiency, and the oculocraniosomatic syndrome, in which a varied pattern of systemic muscle weakness accompanies that of the extraocular muscles.[89,113]

Myotubular Myopathy

Myotubular myopathy, or centronuclear myopathy, is characterized by an appearance in the muscle fibers superficially resembling the myotubules seen in the developing fetus.[35,145]

With the histochemical ATPase reaction a central pale area resembling a doughnut is seen on muscle fiber biopsy.[11] Patients with this disorder show generalized weakness which is either nonprogressive or slowly progressive. More than one disorder may be characterized by this histological appearance, as differing patterns of inheritance have been reported.

Nemaline Myopathy

Nemaline myopathy is usually an autosomal dominant myopathy characterized by a mild, usually nonprogressive weakness.[35,54,139] Muscle biopsy may show changes in fiber-type distribution compared with normal muscle. There may be diminution or increase in the number of type I fibers. The rods, which may only be seen in a small percentage of fibers, are best seen with Gomori trichrome stain.[47] Progressive scoliosis, chest wall deformity, and foot deformities are frequently seen.

Congenital Dystrophy

Congenital dystrophy is an autosomal-recessive myopathy which is characterized by severe hypotonia in the newborn. Type II fibers are completely absent in the muscle biopsy.[11] Little progression in the disorder occurs after the first few

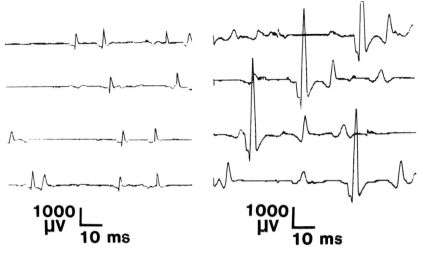

Figure 30-5 The motor unit potential (MUP) in patients with denervation and myopathy. *Left panel:* Small short MUP in myopathy. *Right panel:* Long high-amplitude MUP in the denervation process. *(From Oh, S.J.: Clinical Electromyography. Baltimore, University Park Press, 1984. Reproduced with permission.)*

years of life. Congenital dystrophy is one cause of multiple congenital contractures, and scoliosis, congenital dislocation of the hips, and talipes equinovarus may all be seen by the orthopaedist.[35]

Electrodiagnostic Tests in Myopathy

When recorded with a concentric needle electrode, the normal motor unit potential (MUP) has a duration of 3 to 15 ms with a peak amplitude of 300 V to 3 mV.[112] In myopathy the number of functioning cells is reduced and the MUP is characteristically small in amplitude and of short duration. By contrast, in denervation disorders the MUP is usually increased, a development associated with collateral sprouting from residual intact axons (Fig. 30-5).

Recently the technique of single-fiber EMG (SFEMG) recording has been made available; it uses a small electrode which is less than the diameter of a single muscle fiber.[112] By using the action potential recorded from one muscle fiber to generate the sweep, action potentials in phase with that single muscle fiber (and therefore with others of the same motor unit), can be identified and counted and an average fiber density (FD) within that motor unit calculated. In primary myopathies, SFEMG typically shows increased FD.[146] SFEMG can also measure the variability in the time interval between two potentials from two single muscle fibers belonging to the same motor unit. This variability of the interpotential interval difference is called *jitter* and is abnormal in a number of diseases but in only less than a third of cases of Duchenne's dystrophy.

MYOTONIA

In this group of diseases the muscle fiber membrane is hyperexcitable. Changes in the resting membrane potential have been detected which render the membrane more easily depolarized.[106] Needle EMG shows waxing and waning in fre-

quency and amplitude (Fig. 30-6). When a loudspeaker is used to monitor the activity, the sound is like that of a dive-bomber or a motorcycle revving up.[11,112]

Steinert's Myotonic Dystrophy

Steinert's myotonic dystrophy[149] is a progressive systemic illness characterized by progressive distal weakness, frontal baldness, heart disease, mental deficiency, cataracts, and in-

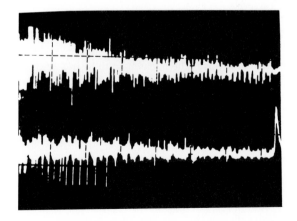

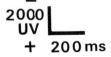

Figure 30-6 Myotonic potentials. The waxing and waning in frequency and the amplitude of potentials are characteristic of myotonic potentials. *(From Oh, S.J.: Clinical Electromyography. Baltimore, University Park Press, 1984. Reproduced with permission.)*

fertility.[7,69] It is inherited as an autosomal dominant but is unusual in that patients whose mothers were also affected by the disorder have more severe illness, manifesting itself in early childhood, than those who inherit the disorder from their father.[71] Patients with maternally inherited disease may indeed present in the newborn nursery with failure to thrive, respiratory distress, and marked hypotonia.[158] Although they may initially appear to improve, the steadily downhill course of myotonic dystrophy becomes all too apparent.

Fifty percent of patients with the congenital form of Steinert's myotonic dystrophy have talipes equinovarus. Although these foot deformities may initially appear to correct well with serial casting, they invariably recur. Soft tissue transfers appear to offer little hope of balancing the foot, and usually triple arthrodesis is required in early adolescence. Commonly there are associated hallucal deformities which may also require surgical intervention.[119,125]

Patients with the congenital form of Steinert's myotonic dystrophy may also be more prone to congenital dislocation of the hips as well as scoliosis than patients with the so-called adult form of the disorder. Mental deficiency is also much more common in those with the congenital form of the problem.[13] It should be noted that in infants with the congenital form of Steinert's myotonic dystrophy, myotonia is not a presenting problem but hypotonia is. It is only in the late first or early second decade that the myotonia begins to appear in these patients.

As the disorder progresses in both the congenital and the adult forms, foot-drop gait appears. Plastic AFOs may be used to ameliorate this, but some patients ultimately require a wheelchair. In addition, heart disease is common, and patients must have serial ECGs. Additionally, ophthalmologic screens are necessary to detect cataracts.

Diagnosis

The creatine phosphokinase level is usually only mildly elevated.[103] The EMG changes are characteristic for myotonia.[112]

The Muscle Biopsy The nuclei tend to lie in a central position, and there is increased connective tissue and variation of fiber size.[103] The type I fibers are selectively involved in about half the cases, particularly during the early stages of the disease (Fig. 30-7).[11,103]

Myotonia Congenita (Thomsen's Disease)

In spite of the similarity of terms, myotonia congenita, or Thomsen's disease,[78,156] is a condition distinct from the congenital form of myotonic dystrophy. Thomsen's disease is an autosomal-dominant condition in which myotonia is most marked on an initial movement and decreases with repetition. The disorder usually appears in childhood but is compatible with normal life span. Frequently there is hypertrophy of the musculature. There are no associated systemic abnormalities.[75] The defect in this condition seems to be abnormal calcium permeability in the muscle fiber membrane.[106] The EMG

is useful in diagnosis. Muscle biopsy reveals an absence of type IIB fibers.[11]

Paramyotonia Congenita (Eulenburg's Disease)

Paramyotonia congenita, or Eulenburg's disease,[48] is an autosomal dominant condition characterized by episodes of myotonic paralysis precipitated by exposure to cold. The disorder particularly affects the hands and face. Frequently, there is a hypertrophy of the muscles in these patients.

MALIGNANT HYPERTHERMIA

Certain susceptible patients exposed to succinylcholine, halothane, and various other anesthetic agents may experience tachycardia, contracture of muscles, and a considerable rise in body temperature. Unless appropriate treatment is undertaken immediately, death is likely. Treatment consists of immediate cessation of anesthesia, changing all anesthetic tubing still contaminated by anesthetic agents, administration of sodium bicarbonate (1 mg/kg) and dantrolene sodium (2.5 mg/kg), icing of the patient, and immediate closure of incisions. Dantrolene lowers the sarcoplasmic calcium levels and is thought to act on the coupling between the sarcoplasmic reticulum and the T system in the muscle.[106]

Malignant hypothermia may be found in families, inherited as an autosomal dominant. CPK screening has been found to be of little benefit in screening potential carriers, and the diagnostic test of choice is the caffeine-tested muscle biopsy.

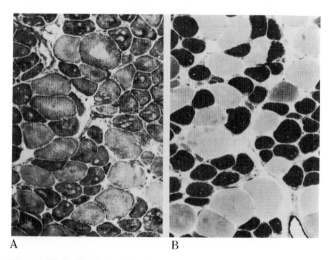

A   B

Figure 30-7 Myotonic dystrophy: **A.** NADH tetrazolium reductase preparation. Numerous atrophied fibers with changes in their sarcoplasm. **B.** ATPase preparation at pH 4.35. × 80. All atrophied fibers are of type I; most type II fibers are hypertrophied. *(From Escourelle, R., and Poirier, J.: A Manual of Basic Neuropathology. Philadelphia, Saunders, 1978. Reproduced with permission.)*

MYASTHENIA GRAVIS

This is an uncommon disease with no particular pattern of inheritance and with several separate presentations.[10,102,108] It is estimated that 1 person in 5000 contract it during the course of their lives. In young adult cases, females predominate by a ratio of 3:1, whereas at an older age fewer female cases occur and males predominate.[4] Transient neonatal myasthenia occurs in 15 percent of children born to myasthenic mothers, and this is thought to be due to passive transfer of anti-acetylcholine receptor IgG from mother to fetus. This condition generally spontaneously improves after 2 to 4 weeks and does not recur, but neostigmine treatment may be required.

Clinical Features

The increased fatigability of the muscle characteristic of this disease is common in the ocular muscles or the muscles involved in speaking and swallowing. Approximately 1 in 5 patients has generalized weakness of the limbs.[11]

Juvenile Myasthenia Gravis

Juvenile myasthenia gravis generally develops after the age of 10 years and initially involves the ocular muscles. Weakness may be restricted to the facial muscles, in which case spontaneous remission may occur. Alternatively the disease may extend to the extremities, when the myasthenia is then usually most marked in the proximal upper extremities.

Congenital or Infantile Myasthenia

Congenital or infantile myasthenia is probably an autosomal recessive condition characterized by ptosis, ophthalmoplegia, and sometimes generalized muscle weakness. There may sometimes be episodes of respiratory distress.

Diagnostic Tests

It is considered that this disease is due to a humorally mediated autoimmune condition which blocks the acetylcholine (Ach) receptors of the neuromuscular junction. Although in these patients one finds antibodies that bind to the Ach receptors (and although in animals such antibodies are capable of producing systemic manifestations when passively transferred), their titer correlates poorly with the severity of the disease. There is often a correlation with other autoimmune diseases, and 10 percent of patients have a thymoma.[4,16]

The response to neostigmine or edrophonium (both of which drugs relieve the symptoms) is a useful diagnostic test.

The muscle biopsy is not as helpful as the EMG but does show some type II fiber atrophy. The easy fatigability of the muscle is demonstrated electromyographically by the repetitive nerve stimulation test (Jolly test).[112] At low rates of repetitive stimulation, a decremental response is seen in involved muscle. Raising the rate of stimulation often abolishes the response. When SFEMGs are used, an increase in jitter is also shown in these patients[112] (Fig. 30-8).

Treatment

Thymectomy is valuable in selected candidates and can give long-term relief. Curiously enough, the results are not so good if the patient has a thymic tumor. Emergency treatment may require the administration of neostigmine. Pyridostigmine, which has a longer duration of action, has been used in maintenance therapy. Plasmapheresis as well as steroids and immunosuppressive drugs such as azathioprine have also been used.[16]

DISEASES OF THE MOTOR NEURONS
Spinal Muscular Atrophy

Classification

Spinal muscular atrophy is a collection of disorders characterized by degeneration of the anterior horn cells and in some cases of the bulbar motor nuclei. The more severe infantile form, usually characterized by poor head control, inability to obtain sitting balance, and early death, is usually known by the term *Werdnig-Hoffmann disease*.[75-77,79,163,164] The other well-known form, characterized by later onset usually in the late first or early second decade and with slower progression, is known by the eponym *Kugelberg-Welander disease* (juve-

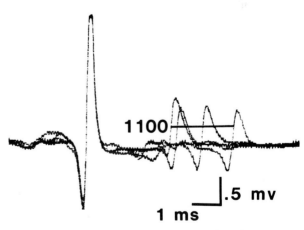

Figure 30-8 Abnormal jitter during single-fiber electromyography in myasthenia gravis. The horizontal line and number indicate the range between the shortest and longest interpotential interval. The mean value of the consecutive interpotential interval difference *(MCD)* is 1100 ms. The normal MCD is 55 ms. *(From Oh, S.J.: Clinical Electromyography. Baltimore, University Park Press, 1984. Reproduced with permission.)*

nile spinal muscular atrophy).[92,162] Both these disorders appear to be autosomal recessive conditions, but there are other spinal muscular atrophies which appear to be dominantly inherited. Subclassification is frequently difficult and based more on clinical criteria than on specific neurochemical classification. Dubowitz suggests the following classification of the childhood spinal muscular atrophies: (1) Severe, unable to sit unsupported; (2) intermediate, able to sit unsupported but unable to stand or walk unaided; (3) mild, able to stand and walk.[35]

In the severe spinal muscular atrophy group, or Werdnig-Hoffmann disease, children either may be affected from birth or may show weakness within the first few months of life. There are frequently decreased tendon reflexes, and tongue fasciculations are common. Generalized hypotonia, poor head control, swallowing difficulties, and recurrent upper respiratory infections are common. Survival past 1 year of life is rare.

In the intermediate group, children commonly develop normally for the first few months of life and frequently achieve the ability to sit unaided. Nevertheless, in this group the children commonly are unable to crawl or walk, and they begin to show progressive motor weakness. The tendon reflexes are decreased, and tongue fasciculations may be seen. These patients may survive into their teenage years or early adulthood and commonly show severe progressive scoliosis.[49,72,80,136]

In the mild group, or the group with Kugelberg-Welander disease, the children commonly achieve the early milestones but beginning in the late first decade and early second decade have difficulty keeping up with their peers. They frequently use a Gowers' maneuver to get up from the floor. Some may have normal reflexes, but commonly, most reflexes are depressed. Many of these patients are in wheelchairs by their mid-thirties.[31]

Diagnosis

In Werdnig-Hoffmann disease the muscle biopsy shows hypertrophy of type I fibers in a uniform manner which is fairly characteristic of this disease when evaluated with the histochemical ATPase reaction (Fig. 30-9). In this condition, however, CPK levels may be normal, and the EMG is often difficult to interpret, although fibrillation potentials are common.[11,103]

In Kugelberg-Welander disease the biopsy shows the fiber-type grouping characteristic of neurogenic atrophy. Instead of the usual mosaic distribution of motor units, there is a tendency for muscle fibers of the same type to group themselves together; type II fibers predominate. CPK levels may be mildly elevated. The EMG changes are consistent with the muscle biopsy and show a mixed pattern of denervation and reinnervation.[11]

Motor Neuron Disease (Amyotrophic Lateral Sclerosis)

Clinical Features

This condition presents most commonly in the fifth to seventh decade, in men twice as frequently as in women. There is

progressive degeneration involving the anterior horn cells and the nuclei of the cranial nerves (predominantly 10,11, and 12) combined with demyelination and gliosis of the anterior and lateral columns of the spinal cord.[103] This progressive disorder may confine the patient to a wheelchair within a year or two, and the patient may end up bedridden and unable to move, talk, or swallow.[11] In the early stages, the disorder may be mistaken for many orthopaedic conditions, particularly the myopathy of cervical disc disease and cervical stenosis. The etiology of the condition is unknown but may be a viral agent, since there is a resemblance to poliomyelitis.

Laboratory Test

Concentric needle EMG typically shows fibrillation potentials and sharp waves in most muscles. These are evidence of denervation. The motor unit potentials are long and often of increased amplitude, indicating reinnervation with an increased number of fibers near the electrode. Fasciculations are prominent. A very abnormal degree of jitter seen on SFEMG indicates rapid clinical progression.[146]

POLIOMYELITIS

Clinical Features

Poliomyelitis is an infectious disease caused by a neurotropic virus. It produces a degenerative lesion with massive neuronal loss and gliosis in the anterior horns and degeneration of the ventral nerve roots.[47] It gains access by the gut or res-

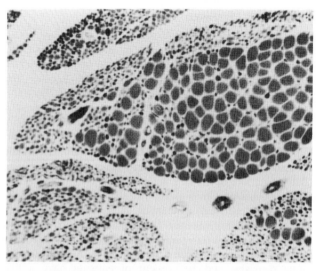

Figure 30-9 The muscle biopsy findings in infantile spinal muscular atrophy show characteristics of "denervation"-type muscle biopsies. There are large numbers of round atrophic fibers. Fiber-type groupings are seen here as clumps of hypertrophic type 1 fibers. This uniform histochemical type is well shown (ATPase reaction, pH 9.4). *(From Brooke, M.A.: A Clinician's View of Neuromuscular Disease. Baltimore, Williams & Wilkins, 1977. Reproduced with permission.)*

piratory tract and spreads to the central nervous system via the blood. It has an incubation period of 6 to 20 days. The acute phase generally lasts 7 to 10 days before the temperature returns to normal. If paralysis occurs it usually appears on the third or fourth day.[57] There is a period of convalescence following the acute disease when some recovery in muscle power may occur. This period, which may last 18 months, is characterized by an early period of weeks or months when the muscles are tender and painful and a later period when although no longer sensitive, they still may be recovering.[152]

Since the development of the Sabin[132] and Salk[133] vaccines, acute poliomyelitis has been almost eradicated in the developed world but is still occasionally seen in unvaccinated groups.

The *chronic phase* of the disease lasts for the rest of the patient's life, and there may be some deterioration later on in life presumably related to either the activity of slow virus in the anterior horn cells or attrition of anterior horn cells occurring from some other cause. This deterioration later on in life can be very distressing to patients who have managed to function despite the level of disability and had been accustomed to the apparently static nature of their disease.

Management

During the acute phase, bulbar involvement may lead to respiratory difficulties, which are outside the scope of this volume. For the orthopaedist, the usual policy of preventing the development of contracture and maintaining joint mobility should not commence until the acute period has been over for at least 48 h. During the convalescence the full range of physical reeducation of muscles and muscle strengthening of recovering muscles should be employed. Careful charting of all muscle groups at regular intervals is essential throughout the disease and should be performed by personnel skilled in accurate testing of individual muscles. Appropriate orthotics and night splints are utilized. Such measures prevent paralyzed muscles from being overstretched. Bracing may restore ambulatory status, which is important for the patient's morale.

Later on it may be necessary to restore by muscle and tendon transfers an essential joint motor or stabilizer which has been permanently lost. Fixed deformity may require correction by soft tissue releases, osteotomies, or wedge incisions. A major goal is to stabilize flail joints in this condition. This may require reducing dislocations or performing extra- or intraarticular fusions, sometimes combined with tendon transfers across the stabilized joint.

Hip Joint

Operations for Muscle Paralysis The aponeurosis of the external oblique muscle may be transferred to the greater trochanter to substitute for a paralyzed abductor.[82] The erector spinae or tensor fasciae latae muscles can be transferred to compensate for lost gluteus medius and maximus function. Transferring the origin of the tensor fasciae latae posteriorly changes its line of action so that it may function as an abduc-

tor.[27,96] Ober transferred the lateral two-thirds of the erector spinae and sutured it to a strip of fasciae latae reflected upward from the thigh to obtain the necessary length and reconstruct abductor function.[110] Paralysis of the abductors in the presence of good adductor and flexor function in the hip joint predisposes to dislocation of the hip. For this reason Mustard devised an operation transferring the psoas anteriorly to the tip of the greater trochanter to restore abductor function and restore muscle balance.[109] It seems, however, that this transfer and its modification by Sharrard[138] function primarily as a tenodesis, as do most of these major muscle transfers around the hip in all probability. In Sharrard's modification the psoas and iliacus are passed through a hole made in the ilium and approach the greater trochanter, to which they are reattached by passing posterior to the hip joint.

Correction of Deformity Flexion abduction contracture of the hip is common in poliomyelitis despite good preventive treatment. It is due primarily to contractures of the iliotibial band and may be corrected by fasciotomy at the hip and knee. Transfer of the crest of the ilium may be necessary to release the abduction contracture.[82]

Flexion contracture of the hip occasionally responds to conservative treatments such as prone nursing and traction. Occasionally, however, the Soutter procedure is required. In this procedure, via an anterior Smith-Petersen approach, the tensor fasciae latae and sartorius are freed from the iliac crest and the rectus femoris and anterior joint capsule detached from the ilium, enabling the flexion contracture to be overcome.[142]

Occasionally femoral osteotomy may be required for long-standing flexion abduction contractures. This is particularly indicated when one hip has a fixed abduction contracture and the opposite hip has a fixed adduction contracture and the pelvic obliquity is not fixed.

Stabilization Prevention of hip dislocation is most important. This may be achieved by muscle balancing and appropriate tenodesis procedures such as the iliopsoas transplant. Varus osteotomy of the femur may also be necessary to maintain stability and correct the valgus deformity of the neck commonly seen as an adaptive change. Acetabular osteotomy may be required if the center-edge (CE) angle is diminished. The procedure described by Salter has been recommended.[134]

A flail hip may be treated by hip arthrodesis, if the patient has good spinal and abdominal musculature. In such cases, extension of the knee despite paralyzed quadriceps is then rendered possible as the patient advances the pelvifemoral skeletal unit by using the trunk muscles. It is possible for the patient to flick the knee into extension. This is often helped by the presence of some residual equinus in the foot and ankle.

The Knee Joint

Muscle Balance Transference of the hamstrings (the biceps femoris and semitendinosus) or the iliotibial tract to the patella has been used for quadriceps paralysis. EMG studies have shown that phasic conversion during gait can occur in these muscles after transference in this region. These patients should probably have an intact triceps surae before this transfer is performed; otherwise they risk developing a recurvatum deformity.

Correction of Deformities Wedging casts with polycentric hinges may be used, but one should be ever alert for the problem of the subluxing tibia. Release of the iliotibial band is usually required, and additional soft tissues such as the posterior capsule and the hamstrings may also require lengthening. Once again one should beware lest one produce a recurvatum deformity; also one should be cautious of the effect of any release of the triceps surae muscles at the knee on the balanced foot.

Recurvatum deformity is common, and several procedures have been described to prevent it by performing posterior tenodesis at the knee joint.[74,117] Tibial osteotomy has also been used to correct recurvatum deformity and also valgus or torsional deformities which occur because of the pull of the contracted iliotibial band.

Stabilization Stabilization is usually performed by tenodesis procedures when the posterior structures are paralyzed and deficient as described above. Occasionally arthrodesis is necessary for the painful completely flail joint but is an uncommon procedure in poliomyelitis.

Foot and Ankle

Muscle Balancing The principles of tendon transfers will be briefly recapitulated. It is important that the motor to be used has adequate strength for its designed purpose since it will certainly lose one power during the transfer. The joint across which the tendon is to act must not be stiff or contracted. The tendon should run straight to its point of attachment without changes in direction and must be transferred under sufficient tension. When it has been transferred it should have a similar range of excursion to the paralyzed muscle it is replacing. Care must be taken also not to damage the neurovascular supply to the muscle during the transfer.

The principal tendon transfers used in poliomyelitis have been well summarized by Tachdjian (Table 30-1). Note that when the long toe extensors are used to substitute for paralyzed ankle dorsiflexors (Table 30-1), clawing of the toes occurs. This can also occur when long toe flexors substitute for a weak triceps surae group during pushoff.[82] Paralysis of the intrinsic muscles, which also contributes to these toe deformities, can be helped by performing a Girdlestone flexor-to-extensor tendon transfer.[153] For clawing of the great toe, the classic Robert Jones operation of fusion of the interphalangeal joint and transference of the extensor hallucis longus tendon into the neck of the first metatarsal is still useful.[87] Clawing of the great toe may be caused by inadequate pushoff associated with weak plantar flexors of the ankle. In this case, after the interphalangeal joint is fused, the extensor hallucis longus tendon may be transferred to the flexor hallucis longus tendon to reinforce its action, relying upon the extensor hallucis brevis alone to dorsiflex the hallux.[28] When the ankle dorsiflexors are weak and the tendo Achillis is contracted, the Jones operation is preferred since the first metatarsal is depressed.

In dorsal bunion the first metatarsal is elevated and there is plantar flexion of the great toe at the metatarsophalangeal joint. This is caused by weakness of the plantar flexor of the first metatarsal (the peroneus longus muscle). In this case it is possible to promote flexion of the first metatarsal by transferring the flexor hallucis longus tendon into its head.[152] Alternatively, the flexor hallucis brevis together with the abductor and adductor hallucis can be transferred into the neck of the first metatarsal to depress it.[100] In addition to transferring motors to depress the first metatarsal, one may have to release the tibialis anterior, which is the dorsiflexor of the first metatarsal, and transfer its insertion posteriorly. This is the Lapidus procedure for dorsal bunion.[95]

Cavus deformity may be treated at any early stage by Steindler soft tissue stripping of the plantar fascia and the muscles from the os calcis.[148] Occasionally, if the deformity is fixed, wedge tarsectomy is required.

Stabilizing Procedures Equinovarus and equinovalgus deformity in the skeletally mature foot may require tendo Achillis lengthening and triple arthrodesis followed some 6 weeks later by the appropriate tendon transfers.[82] It is important not to perform triple arthrodesis, however, if there is any instability of the ankle joint. Otherwise, anterior subluxation of the ankle will occur. Careful clinical and radiological examination of the ankle joint is therefore required preoperatively. Pantalar arthrodesis may then be required if the ankle is unstable.

With a calcaneal deformity, stabilization is always required, but soft tissue surgery may, in the skeletally immature foot, minimize the severity of the deformity.[82] After puberty, triple arthrodesis is the operation of choice. For this condition rather more of the talar head is resected so that the foot may be posteriorly displaced to increase the length of the lever arm posteriorly and diminish the amount of muscle power required to lift the heel.[60] When triple arthrodesis for equinus deformities is performed, this displacement is not required. However, the arthrodesis position is such that when the foot is in a plantigrade position, the talus is fully plantarflexed in the ankle joint. When the cast is removed the equinus position is thus permanently corrected in the presence of paralyzed dorsiflexors.

Stabilization fusions performed in the skeletally immature should avoid restricting growth of the foot. Such a procedure is the Grice procedure which is an extraarticular bone block operation for correction of the valgus heel.[60] In this operation a rigid corticocancellous or fibular bone graft is inserted into the sinus tarsi by way of prepared slots on the inferior surface of the talus and the os calcis. This procedure restores lateral height to the longitudinal axis of the foot.

In the rare event that ankle fusion is required before skeletal maturity, the Chuinard procedure is useful. The surgeon carefully resects the articular surfaces via an anterior approach without disturbing the growth plate, and inserts a corticocancellous bone block under compression after distracting the opposing bone surfaces.[15] The treatment of leg length inequality which may occur in poliomyelitis and also the treatment of the neuromuscular problems in the upper limb and spine are dealt with in separate chapters elsewhere in this book.

TABLE 30-1 Tendon Transfers for Paralytic Deformities of the Foot and Ankle

Dynamic Imbalance				
Paralyzed or weak	Normal or strong	Deformity of foot	Tendon transfer	Remarks
Peroneus longus Peroneus brevis	Anterior tibial Extensor hallucis longus Extensor digit. communis Posterior tibial Gastrocnemius-soleus Flexor hallucis longus Flexor digit. longus	Varus Dorsal bunion (first metatarsal dorsiflexed because of unopposed action of anterior tibial)	Lateral transfer of anterior tibial to base of second metatarsal	Perform transfer before fixed deformity develops Lateral stability will be retained Do not transfer more lateral than second metatarsal in presence of strong extensor digit. communis (will cause pes valgus)
Peroneus longus Peroneus brevis Extensor digit. communis Extensor hallucis longus	Anterior tibial Posterior tibial Gastrocnemius-soleus Flexor hallucis longus Flexor digit. longus	Varus, some equinus	Lateral transfer of anterior tibial to base of third metatarsal	Do not transfer more lateral than base of third metatarsal (will cause pes valgus)
Peroneus longus Peroneus brevis Extensor digit. communis Extensor hallucis longus Anterior tibial	Posterior tibial Gastrocnemius-soleus Flexor hallucis longus Flexor digit. longus	Equinovarus	Anterior transfer of posterior tibial tendon through interosseous space to base of third metatarsal	Preoperatively, equinovarus deformity should be fully corrected by stretching cast or soft tissue surgery May consider reinforcing posterior tibial transfer by adding flexor hallucis longus or flexor digit. longus to anterior transfer through interosseous space; anterior tenodesis to prevent dropping down of foot is another choice Postoperatively, support transfer by dorsiflexion assist below-knee orthosis
Anterior tibial	Peroneus longus Peroneus brevis Extensor hallucis longus Extensor digit. communis Gastrocnemius-soleus Posterior tibial Flexor hallucis longus Flexor digit. longus	Equinovalgus Cockup deformity of toes (overactivity of toe extensors displaces proximal phalanges of toes into hyperextension and depresses metatarsal heads) Occasionally cavovarus deformity of foot results (unopposed peroneus longus acts as depressor of first metatarsal)	Anterior transfer of peroneus longus to base of second metatarsal (suture peroneus brevis to distal stump of peroneus longus)	Do not attach peroneus longus to first metatarsal (will displace it upward and cause dorsal bunion) Transfer long toe extensors to heads of metatarsals if cockup deformity of toes is present If both peroneals are transferred, lateral instability of foot will develop, necessitating stabilization of subtalar extraarticular or triple arthrodesis

(Continued on next page)

TABLE 30-1   *(Continued)*

Dynamic Imbalance				
Paralyzed or weak	**Normal or strong**	**Deformity of foot**	**Tendon transfer**	**Remarks**
Gastrocnemius-soleus (motor strength zero or trace)	Peroneus longus Peroneus brevis Flexor hallucis longus Posterior tibial Flexor digit. longus Anterior tibial Extensor hallucis longus Extensor digit. communis	Calcaneus or Calcaneocavus	Posterior transfer (to os calcis) of both peroneals, posterior tibial, and flexor hallucis longus	*Caution*—Prevent development of dorsal bunion by lateral transfer of anterior tibial to base of second metatarsal within a year In adolescent patient with fixed calcaneus deformity, before tendon transfers, perform triple arthrodesis with posterior shift of os calcis to correct bony deformity In young child, calcaneus deformity will correct with subsequent growth; however, subtalar extraarticular arthrodesis may be required for lateral stability
Gastrocnemius-soleus (motor strength poor)	As already described	Calcaneus or Calcaneocavus	Posterior transfer (to os calcis) of posterior tibial and peroneus longus	Suture distal stump of peroneus longus to peroneus brevis Watch closely for possible development of dorsal bunion; lateral transfer of anterior tibial to base of second metatarsal may be indicated
Gastrocnemius-soleus Posterior tibial Peroneus longus Peroneus brevis	Anterior tibial Flexor hallucis longus Extensor hallucis longus Extensor digit. communis Flexor digit. longus	Calcaneovarus	Posterior transfer (to os calcis) of anterior tibial and flexor hallucis longus	Suture distal stump of flexor hallucis longus to flexor hallucis brevis Interphalangeal joint fusion of great toe may be necessary
Anterior tibial Gastrocnemius-soleus	Peroneus longus Peroneus brevis Posterior tibial Flexor hallucis longus Flexor digit. longus Extensor hallucis longus Extensor digit. longus	Calcaneovarus	Posterior transfer (to os calcis) of both peroneals and posterior tibial	Perform triple arthrodesis in adolescence to provide lateral stability to hindfoot.
Gastrocnemius-soleus Posterior tibial Peroneus longus Peroneus brevis Flexor hallucis longus Flexor digit. longus	Anterior tibial Extensor hallucis longus Extensor digit. communis	Calcaneovarus	Posterior transfer (to os calcis) of anterior tibial	Protect transfer with plantar flexion assist orthosis until skeletal maturity Consider tendo Achillis tenodesis In adolescence, if adequate function exists in transferred anterior tibial, foot is stabilized by triple arthrodesis If anterior tibial function is inadequate, Chuinard-type ankle fusion is performed (will provide stability, and gait will improve considerably)

TABLE 30-1 *(Continued)*

	Dynamic Imbalance			
Paralyzed or weak	Normal or strong	Deformity of foot	Tendon transfer	Remarks
Gastrocnemius-soleus Posterior tibial Peroneus longus Peroneus brevis Flexor hallucis longus Flexor digit. longus Anterior tibial	Extensor hallucis longus Extensor digit. communis	Calcaneovalgus (minimal)	Ankle fusion (Chuinard type)	Stability and muscle control of knee should be adequate Full knee extension and functioning hamstrings are prerequisite
Flail ankle and foot (all muscles paralyzed)	None except short toe flexors and intrinsic muscles of foot	Flexion of toes and metatarsus varus Hindfoot neutral or valgus (may be in inversion due to contracture of plantar fascia)	Pantalar arthrodesis Resect motor branches of plantar nerves	As above
Anterior tibial Extensor hallucis longus Extensor digit. communis Peroneus longus Peroneus brevis Posterior tibial	Gastrocnemius-soleus Flexor digit. longus Flexor hallucis longus	Equinus	Anterior transfer of flexor digit. longus and flexor hallucis through interosseous space Anterior tenodesis	Do not lengthen tendo Achillis (will produce calcaneus deformity) Disability is little (patient must lift leg to clear toes) Stretch triceps surae; use night support to prevent fixed equinus deformity

Anterior tibial = tibialis anterior muscle. Posterior tibial = tibialis posterior muscle.
Source: Tachdjian, M.O.: *The Child's Foot.* Philadelphia, Saunders, 1985. Used with permission.

ARTHROGRYPOSIS

In 1841 Otto first described arthrogryposis multiplex congenita as a condition of multiple deformities associated with severe contracture of the muscles.[114,115] It is now recognized that there are many causes of multiple congenital contractures and that "arthrogryposis" is not a single disease entity but a large number of specific entities having a similar clinical picture.[64] Hall points out that there are over 150 specific known causes of multiple congenital contractures (Table 30-2). Of her 186 cases, 28 percent had a known recognizable genetic disorder of single-gene, chromosome, or multifactorial cause; in 6 percent of cases a recognized environmental insult or teratogen exposure was responsible for the syndrome. There were 70 patients undiagnosed (20 percent). This is important information with regard to genetic counseling. In Hall's series, 46 percent of cases had a known syndrome that was determined to have no recurrence risk for arthrogryposis within the family. Of the 28 percent of cases which followed Mendelian patterns, one-half were inherited as autosomal dominant and one-quarter as autosomal recessive disorders.[64]

If a specific diagnosis is made, it is possible for the physician to assess the risk of another child in that family being affected as anywhere from zero to 50 percent. Hall has also calculated and made available the risks in those patients in whom a specific diagnosis is not able to be made.[64]

In the classic presentation of arthrogryposis multiplex congenita, which is currently believed to be secondary to an in utero viral infection,[12,21,166] the child suffers multiple congenital contractures in all four limbs (Fig. 30-10). The wrists and hands are typically in flexion and the shoulders internally rotated with extended elbows. The lower limbs typically exhibit knee flexion contractures and talipes equinovarus bilat-

TABLE 30-2 Differential Diagnosis of Multiple Congenital Contractures

Amyoplasia
Beals syndrome
Cerebral palsy
Congenital muscular dystrophy
Craniocarpotarsal (whistling face) syndrome
Fetal alcohol syndrome
Fetal hydantoin syndrome
Intrauterine postural malformations
Larsen syndrome
Mietens syndrome
Möbius syndrome
Pierre Robin syndrome
Poland syndrome
Potter syndrome
Sacral agenesis
Schwartz syndrome
Skeletal dysplasia
   Metatrophic dwarfism
   Diastrophic dwarfism
Spina bifida
Spinal dysraphism
Turner syndrome
Zellweger syndrome

Source: Thompson, G.H., Bilenker, R.M., Clin Orthop 194:6–14, 1985. Reproduced with permission.

erally.[32,34,51,98] There may be unilateral or bilateral hip dislocations, but in general the more proximal joints tend to be less involved, and the trunk is often spared. However, scoliosis can be present.[12,33,73] The skin over the affected joints is typically featureless and lacks the flexion creases. There are no sensory abnormalities.[155]

This classic picture of arthrogryposis multiplex congenita has been called amyoplasia by Hall because of the fibrotic replacement of muscle. However, this term has been criticized since it implies absence of limb muscles and their replacement by fatty and fibrous tissue. It has been pointed out that since joint spaces (present in these patients) do not develop in the absence of fetal movements, which require functioning muscle, the concept of primary amyoplasia may be untenable.[151]

In the other forms of arthrogryposis, the primary disorder may be neurogenic, myopathic, environmental, or associated with skeletal dysplasia. Each seems to bring about the clinical effects by producing severe weakness early in fetal life, which immobilizes the joints at various stages in their development (Table 30-3).[155] Multiple congenital contractures have been produced experimentally in laboratory animals by the use of curare.[29,30] A child with these deformities born to a mother treated by paralytic agents for tetanus occurring during the pregnancy has also been reported.[85]

The neurogenic or myopathic disorders affect some component of the motor unit.[155] The etiologic categories are shown in Table 30-3, and an abbreviated differential diagnosis is shown in Table 30-2.

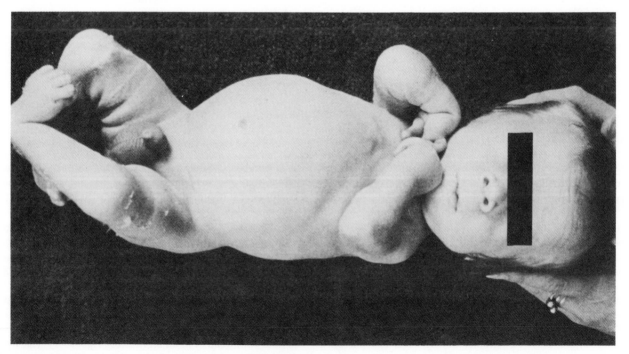

Figure 30-10 Appearance of an infant with arthrogryposis. *(From Palmer, P.M., et al, Clin Orthop 194:54-59, 1985. Reproduced with permission.)*

TABLE 30-3   A Schematic View of Etiologic Categories and Agents and the Sequence of Events Leading to Joint Contracture

Etiologic category	Primary agent	Secondary effect	Reciprocal response	Final result
Mutagenic agent	Gene defect	Muscle fiber loss	Collagenic	Joint contracture
Mitotic pressure	Chromosomal defect	Muscle fiber hypodevelopment	Collagenic	Joint contracture
Viral or bacterial infection		Upper or lower motor neuron loss	Collagenic	Joint contracture
Chemical or drug agents		Upper or lower motor neuron loss	Collagenic	Joint contracture
Environmental and pregnancy factors	Hyperthermia, polyhydramnios, plural births	Upper or lower motor neuron loss, immobilization	Collagenic	Joint contracture

Source: Swinyard, C.A., Bleck, E.E., Clin Orthop 194:15–27, 1985. Reproduced with permission.

Diagnosis

The orthopaedist, neurologist, geneticist, and pediatrician must participate in diagnosing and managing these conditions.[155] Risk factors which may be elicited in the history include an increased familial incidence of talipes equinovarus, vaginal bleeding in the first trimester, diminution of fetal movements during the third trimester, and an abnormal lie of the fetus. Other risk factors include oligohydramnios and a history of maternal illness, treatment with such drugs as phenytoin or insulin, or addiction to ethanol or other chemicals.[155]

Careful neurological evaluation together with assessment of muscle enzymes (determination of CPK levels may be helpful in a myopathy) should identify specific neuromuscular diseases. Chromosome analysis is indicated in infants and children with multisystem defects or central nervous system involvement. Chromosomal abnormalities such as trisomy 18 and trisomy 8 mosaicism can present at birth with congenital contractures.

Muscle biopsy may be recommended in some patients to accurately differentiate between neurogenic and myopathic processes.[6] In the former there is loss of mosaicism and fiber type grouping associated with reinnervation. In the latter the two fiber types are affected unevenly depending on the disease process.[47] The biopsy must be taken between muscle clamps to retain resting length, and it is better if an area of muscle is chosen where a small portion of peripheral nerve and associated motor end plates are also within the specimen.[155]

In Banker's series of 74 children with congenital contractures, there was only one patient with central core disease, one patient with nemaline myopathy, and only a handful of children with congenital muscular dystrophy. Seven percent of children had Arnold-Chiari syndrome, and 1 percent had lumbosacral agenesis; 23 percent, however, had some form of dysgenesis of the central nervous system. Biopsies occasionally may be indicated and characteristically show that adipose tissue fills in areas that should contain fasciculi of muscle fibers (Fig. 30-11).[5]

There may be many congenital anomalies associated with the congenital contractures (Table 30-4).[46,51,88,135] Radiographic assessment is required for these multiple skeletal abnormalities, and spinal CT may be helpful in assessing the central nervous system.[155]

Management

In the past, regimes often included long-term casting, but it is now realized that this may lead to further atrophy of muscle. In most forms of congenital contractures, modern management stresses an aggressive passive motion therapy program consisting of daily stretching of all involved joints with orthotic treatment to maintain joint mobility.

The Knee

The treatment of upper limb deformities and also of scoliosis is dealt with elsewhere in this book. In the lower limb in most of these disorders, it is important to correct the flexed knee before treating the flexed hip.[34] This is particularly so if a congenital dislocation of the hip is present since if it is reduced first, attempting to straighten the knee may thereafter cause the hip position to be lost.[116] An increased range of motion of 60 percent can be achieved by the stretching program and maintained with lightweight orthotics. When soft tissue surgery is required, it should include the posterior capsule since hamstring release without capsulotomy is less effective.[154] Osteotomy has a role in patients who cannot otherwise be braced. This operation must be performed after the age of 12 years if it is not to be followed by recurrence of the deformity.[34,154] Partial epiphysiodesis of the distal femur to correct deformity is not recommended.[154]

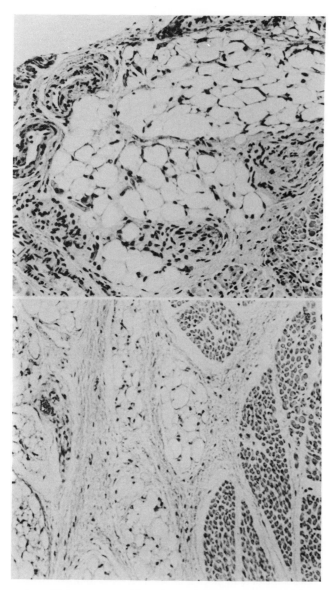

Figure 30-11 In a newborn infant with dysgenesis of motor nuclei of the spinal cord, the muscle fibers are small. Adipose tissue fills in the area that should contain fasciculi of muscle fibers (H&E; ×180). This is seen in 7 percent of cases of arthrogryposis. *(From Banker, B.Q., Clin Orthop 194:30-43, 1985. Reproduced with permission.)*

The Hip

Knee contractures occur in 60 percent of these patients, but 80 percent have some kind of hip involvement. The unilateral dislocation should be treated aggressively.[81,116] If it is not, persistent dislocation will cause pelvic obliquity and subsequent scoliosis which cannot then be corrected by reducing the hip.[81] Open reduction is always necessary[81] and may require femoral shortening.[116]

Hip contracture without dislocation should be treated by gentle manipulation early on, avoiding forceful extension, which has a high risk of causing fracture or anterior dislocation. Conservative treatment is usually successful and pre-

ferred to surgical correction. Traction using long leg casts has been recommended.[81,98] Occasionally anterior soft tissue release including capsulotomy may be required. Some authors believe the hip flexion contractures are more disabling than dislocations and point out that when the flexed knee is treated first, conservative treatment of the flexed hip is frequently successful.[34] Femoral osteotomy at the end of the growth period is also a successful treatment for the flexed hip. Varus derotation has been recommended combined with femoral shortening as a one-stage procedure during open reduction of the hip for all unilateral hip dislocations.[147] This procedure is also recommended for those patients with bilateral hip dislocations with less severe generalized involvement.[147] However, other authors disagree and suggest that bilateral hip dislocations are best left unreduced unless there is a flexion contracture of more than 35°, when some type of intervention is necessary.[81]

The Foot

In the foot, where talipes equinovarus is the commonest deformity, talectomy has been recommended as a corrective procedure.[62] This procedure can be accompanied by tenotomy of the Achilles tendon if required to enable the calcaneus to be placed under the tibia and held there by K wire for 3 weeks. Immobilization in plaster is required for 3 months.[34]

TABLE 30-4 Congenital Anomalies Associated with Arthrogryposis

Head and neck	Craniosynostosis
	Abnormal brains
	Mandibulofacial dysostosis
	Hypoplasia of the mandible (Pierre Robin syndrome)
	Congenital facial diplegia (Möbius' syndrome)
	Microphthalmia
	Klippel-Feil syndrome
Shoulder girdle	Sprengel's deformity
Spine	Kyphoscoliosis
	Segmentation disorders
	Spina bifida
	Agenesis of sacrum
Cardiovascular system	Congenital heart disease
Genitourinary system	Renal anomalies
	Ureteral anomalies
	Cryptorchidism
	Scrotal defects
Respiratory system	Pneumonia
	Tracheoesophageal fistula
Abdomen	Inguinal hernia
Extremities	Absence of patellas
	Syndactylism
	Constriction bands
	Synostosis

Source: Drummond, D.S., et al, Instr Course Lect 23:82, 1974. Reproduced with permission.

The Verebelyi-Ogston procedure has been recommended by Gross for the rigid myelodysplastic or arthrogrypotic foot.[61] In this procedure, through windows in the cartilaginous shells of the talus and cuboid, cancellous bone is removed from the ossific nucleus, allowing collapse and correction of these shells as the foot is manipulated into a corrected position. Prolonged orthotic support is necessary to prevent recurrence.[61]

Surgery for congenital convex pes valgus, which is the second most common deformity, seems to be unsuccessful, and a specialized AFO incorporating the Gillette modification of the University of California at Berkeley's type of foot control has been recommended.[62]

It seems that mild to moderate deformity in the growing child may be managed by posteromedial release,[34] but these procedures have been found by others to be unsuccessful and associated with a high complication rate,[62] so that some type of bony procedure is usually required. In the older child triple arthrodesis is recommended.[34]

POLYNEUROPATHY

Guillain-Barré Syndrome

According to McComas,[103] this condition is characterized by four features: (1) paralysis involving the legs and spreading upward to involve the upper limbs and sometimes the respiratory muscles and cranial nerves, (2) sensory loss with a generalized feeling of pins and needles, (3) a history of viral infection, usually respiratory, 2 to 4 weeks before the onset of these neurological symptoms, and (4) a rise in protein content of the cerebrospinal fluid with little increase in white cells (cytoalbuminological dissociation). Recovery usually commences a few weeks after the onset of neurological symp-

toms and may be incomplete. The EMG shows F-wave latency, which may be the sole abnormality in this peripheral neuropathy when other nerve conductions are all normal.[112]

It is thought that Guillain-Barré syndrome is probably an immunologic response to infection. The pathology has been shown to be demyelination affecting the nerve roots and to a lesser extent the peripheral nerve trunks.[47]

Hereditary Motor and Sensory Neuropathies

The hereditary motor and sensory neuropathies are a group of disorders classified together by Dyck et al and having the following characteristics: they are inherited, they are slowly progressive, and they are characterized by predominantly peripheral motor neuron involvement with lesser involvement of peripheral sensory and autonomic neurons.[38,40] The disorders are symmetrical, nonfocal, and characterized by axonal atrophy and degeneration. The electrodiagnostic abnormalities seen in these conditions are summarized in Table 30-5.

Hereditary Motor and Sensory Neuropathy Type I

Hereditary motor and sensory neuropathy type I includes the peroneal type of progressive muscular atrophy, or Charcot-Marie-Tooth disorder,[14] and Roussy-Lévy syndrome.[128,130] The hallmarks of the disorder are autosomal dominant inheritance, progressive foot-drop gait, cavovarus foot deformity, scoliosis, and progressive involvement starting peripherally and evolving centrally.[17,18,84,86,93,97,125,131,137,148] Recently there have been reports of hip dysplasia and dislocation in patients with this type of neuropathy.[120] The peripheral nerves are commonly enlarged and palpable. In some patients an essential tremor is seen, but in the same kindred affected individu-

TABLE 30-5   Nerve Conduction Abnormalities in Hereditary Motor and Sensory Neuropathies

Neuropathy	Clinical findings	Electrophysiological findings*
Type I: Hypertrophic type of the Charcot-Marie-Tooth disease (CMT) including Roussy-Lévy syndrome	Distinction between type I and II is not always possible. Earlier onset, weakness of intrinsic hand and neck flexor muscles, sensory impairment of hands, and kyphosis are common in type I. Roussy-Lévy syndrome has the combination of type I and essential tremor.	Marked slowing in motor NCV (below 20 m/s) and sensory NCV. Frequent absence of CNAP. Dispersion phenomenon and marked diminution of the amplitude of CNAP.
Type II: Neuronal type of CMT		Normal or near normal (NCVs are no more than 40% below normal).
Type III: Hypertrophic neuropathy of infancy (Déjerine-Sottas disease)	Hypertrophic neuropathy from infancy. No pes cavus. Thickened nerves and high CSF protein.	Very marked slowing in motor NCV (2–10 m/s). Frequent absence of CNAP.
Type IV: Refsum's disease	CMT-like findings, retinitis pigmentosa, neuronal hearing loss, ataxia, ichthyosis.	Very marked slowing of motor NCV (below 10 m/s). Absence of CNAP.
Type V: Familial spastic paraplegia with neuronal type of CMT	Combination of spastic paraplegia with CMT.	Normal motor NCV; low amplitude or absence of CNAP.

*CNAP = compound nerve action potential. NCV = Nerve conduction velocity.
Source: Oh, S.J.: *Clinical Electromyography,* Baltimore, University Park Press, 1984.

als may have only the peroneal muscular atrophy. Bird et al have recently shown that the type I disorder is linked to the Duffy locus on the long arm of chromosome 1.[9] However, Dyck et al have shown that one of their large kindreds does not show a similar linkage.[39] Therefore it can be surmised that patients with similar clinical presentations may have dissimilar disorders.

Hereditary Motor and Sensory Neuropathy Type II

Hereditary motor and sensory neuropathy type II is also known as the neuronal type of peroneal muscular atrophy. These patients differ from those of type I in having later onset of symptoms, no enlargement of peripheral nerves, and less severe weakness of hand musculature but greater weakness of plantar flexor musculature. Cavovarus foot deformities, scoliosis, and hip dysplasia may all be seen in this disorder.

Hereditary Motor and Sensory Neuropathy Type III

Hereditary motor and sensory neuropathy type III is also known as Déjerine-Sottas disorder,[22] or hypertrophic neuropathy of infancy. It is an autosomal recessive disorder characterized by severe onset in childhood and with multiple orthopaedic manifestations including talipes equinovarus, scoliosis, and severe incoordination.

Hereditary Motor Sensory Neuropathy Type IV

Hereditary motor sensory neuropathy type IV, or Refsum's disorder, is a rare autosomal recessive disorder characterized by an accumulation of phytanic acid.[121,122] The onset is usually insidious either in the first, second, or third decades, but it is occasionally precipitated by infection. It is characterized by marked exacerbations and remissions. Night blindness or pigmentary retinal degeneration is present in all cases. There is also a symmetrical neuropathy which chiefly affects the distal portion of the lower limbs, but which gradually becomes more widespread, involving the trunk musculature. Ataxia and other cerebellar signs may also be present, and occasionally such patients are diagnosed as having Friedreich's ataxia. Cardiomyopathy, ichthyosis, pes cavus, claw toes, epiphyseal dysplasia, irregular length of the metatarsals, and psychosis have also been reported.

Hereditary Motor Sensory Neuropathy Type V

Hereditary motor sensory neuropathy type V is an autosomal dominant disorder characterized by spastic paraplegia. The onset of the disorder is usually in the second or latter decades, and difficulty in walking or running is usually the earliest symptom. Tightness of the adductors, hamstring contractures, and contractures of the tendo Achillis may ensue, leading to progressive gait disturbance. Sensory examination is usually normal.

Hereditary Motor Sensory Neuropathy Type VI

Hereditary motor sensory neuropathy type VI is a rare disorder characterized by optic atrophy in association with peroneal muscular atrophy. The genetic pattern of this disorder is not fully elucidated.

Hereditary Motor Sensory Neuropathy Type VII

Hereditary motor sensory neuropathy type VII has an association with retinitis pigmentosa in addition to the peroneal muscular atrophy. It is probably an autosomal recessive disorder.

SPINOCEREBELLAR DEGENERATION

The spinocerebellar degeneration disorders are characterized by neuronal degeneration in the cerebellum as well as the peripheral nervous system. Friedreich's ataxia is the most commonly seen spinocerebellar degeneration.[52] There are both autosomal recessive and autosomal dominant forms of Friedreich's ataxia, with the autosomal recessive form being the most common. In these patients, progressive unsteadiness of the gait is usually the first sign. Ataxia, positive Romberg's sign, and depressed or absent lower extremity reflexes are also common. Orthopaedically progressive cavovarus foot deformities as well as scoliosis frequently require attention.[104,137] Patients are commonly wheelchair-bound by the late second or third decade.

Ataxia-telangiectasia is an autosomal recessive disorder characterized by progressive ataxia, telangiectasias of both the eyes and the skin, and immunodeficiency. Onset is usually in early childhood.

Marinesco-Sjögren syndrome is an autosomal recessive disorder characterized by ataxia, moderate to severe mental deficiency, and cataracts. These patients may present to the orthopaedist with scoliosis.

CONGENITAL INSENSITIVITY TO PAIN

There are several separate entities which result in congenital insensitivity to pain. These include congenital indifference to pain, which appears to be of sporadic occurrence and which is characterized by indifference to noxious stimuli even though the threshold for perception of these stimuli is normal. Congenital sensory neuropathy, however, is generally inherited as an autosomal dominant and is characterized by self-mutilation as well as decreased sensation, temperature perception, and touch perception. The distal portions of the extremities are frequently more involved than the proximal portions. In the Riley-Day syndrome, or familial dysautonomia,[123,124] there is abnormal temperature control and difficulty controlling the autonomic reflexes. There are no fungiform papillae on the tongue, and there is absence of the normal axonal reflex response to histamine. Sudden death during anesthesia is not uncommon in the Riley-Day syndrome.

The orthopaedic complications of these disorders include the development of Charcot joints secondary to repeated trauma in the absence of protective sensation. Additionally because of the decrease in perception of pain, fractures and/or osteomyelitis may go undetected if not actively pursued. Scoliosis may also develop, particularly in the Riley-Day syndrome.[101,107,123,124]

NEURALGIC AMYOTROPHY

This unusual condition can cause confusion if one is not aware of its existence. The patient may present with wasting of the deltoid or winging of the scapula due to the paralysis of the serratus anterior muscle, but other muscles may be involved including the supraspinatus, infraspinatus, and trapezius.[11] Occasionally the only abnormality is winging of the scapula due to involvement of the nerve supply to the serratus anterior muscle. A history is elicited of a period of acute pain in the shoulder for a variable period preceding the paralysis (usually several weeks but often forgotten). The usual pattern is recovery by 4 weeks, but it sometimes takes up to 2 years. There is a suggestion that the disease is an autosomal dominant.[11] The pathology is currently unknown.

REFERENCES

1. Allen, J.E., and Rodgin, D.W. Mental retardation in association with progressive muscular dystrophy. Am J Dis Child 100:208, 1960.
2. Archibald, K.C., and Vignos, P.J. A study of contractures in muscular dystrophy. Arch Phys Med Rehabil 40:150–157, 1959.
3. Armstrong, R.M., Koenigsberger, R., Mellinger, J., and Lovelace, R.E. Central core disease with congenital hip dislocation: Study of two families. Neurology 21:369, 1971.
4. Arnasen, B.G.W. Immunology and neurological disease, in Swash, M., and Kennard, C. (eds): *Scientific Basis of Clinical Neurology.* Edinburgh, Churchill Livingstone, 1985, pp 603–618.
5. Banker, B.Q. Neuropathologic aspects of arthrogryposis multiplex congenita. Clin Orthop 194:30–43, 1985.
6. Banker, B.Q., Victor, M., and Adams, R.D. Arthrogryposis multiplex due to congenital muscular dystrophy. Brain 80:319, 1957.
7. Batten, F.E., and Gibb, H.P. Myotonia atrophica. Brain 32:187–205, 1909.
8. Becker, P.E. Two new families of benign sex-linked recessive muscular dystrophy. Rev Can Biol 21:551, 1962.
9. Bird, T.D., Ott, J., and Giblett, E.R. Linkage of Charcot-Marie-Tooth neuropathy to the Duffy locus on chromosome 1. Am J Hum Genet 34:388, 1982.
10. Bowman, J.R. Myasthenia gravis in young children. Pediatrics, 1:472, 1948.
11. Brooke, M.H. *A Clinician's View of Neuromuscular Disease.* Baltimore, Williams & Wilkins, 1977.
12. Brown, L.M., Robson, M.J., and Sharrard, W.J.W. The pathophysiology of arthrogryposis multiplex congenita neurologica. J Bone Joint Surg 62B:291–296, 1980.
13. Calderon, R. Myotonic dystrophy: A neglected cause of mental retardation. J Pediatr 68:423, 1966.
14. Charcot, J.M., and Marie, P. Sur une forme particuliere d'atrophie musculaire progressive, souvent familiale, debutant par les pieds et les jambes et atteignant plus tard les mains. Rev Med (Paris) 6:97–138, 1886.
15. Chuinard, E.G., and Peterson, R.F. Distraction compression bone graft arthrodesis of the ankle, a method especially applicable for children. J Bone Joint Surg 45A:481–490, 1963.
16. Chujid, J.G. The nervous system, in *Current Medical Diagnosis and Treatment.* Los Altos, CA, Lange, 1984, pp 581–621.
17. Cole, W.H. The treatment of clawfoot. J Bone Joint Surg 22:895–908, 1940.
18. Coleman, S.S., and Chestnut, J. A simple test for hindfoot flexibility in the cavovarus foot. Clin Orthop 123:60–62, 1977.
19. Copeland, S.A., and Howard, R.C. Thoracoscapular fusion for facioscapulohumeral dystrophy. J Bone Joint Surg 60B:547–551, 1978.
20. Curtis, B.H. Orthopaedic management of muscular dystrophy and related disorders. Instr Course Lect 19:78, 1970.
21. Davidson, J., and Beighton, P. Whence the arthrogrypotics? J Bone Joint Surg 58B:492–495, 1976.
22. Dejerine, J., and Sottas, J. Sur la neurite interstitielle hypertrophique et progressive de l'enfance. C R Soc Biol (Paris) 45:63–96, 1893.
23. Denborough, M.A., Dennett, X., and Anderson, R. McD. Central-core disease and malignant hyperplexia. Br Med J 2:272, 1973.
24. Denborough, M.A., Ebeling, P., King, J.O., and Zapt, P. Myopathy and malignant hyperpyrexia. Lancet 2:1138, 1970.
25. Denborough, M.A., and Lovell, R.R.H. Anaesthetic deaths in a family. Lancet 2:45, 1960.
26. Dennis, N.R., Evans, K., Clayton, B., and Carter, C.O. Use of creatine kinase for detecting severe X-linked muscular dystrophy carriers. Br Med J 2:577–579, 1976.
27. Dickson, F.D. An operation for stabilizing paralytic hips: A preliminary report. J Bone Joint Surg 9:1–7, 1927.
28. Dickson, F.D., and Diveley, R.L. Operation in correction of mild clawfoot, the result of infantile paralysis. JAMA 87:1275, 1926.
29. Drachman, D.B., and Coulombre, A. Experimental club foot and arthrogryposis multiplex congenita. Lancet 2:523, 1962.
30. Drachman, D.B., and Sokoloff, L. The role of movement in embryonic joint development. Dev Biol 14:401, 1966.
31. Drennan, J.C. *Orthopaedic Management of Neuromuscular Disorders.* Philadelphia, Lippincott, 1983.
32. Drummond, D.S., and Cruess, R.L. The management of the foot and ankle in arthrogryposis multiplex congenita. J Bone Joint Surg 60B: 96–99, 1978.
33. Drummond, D.S., and MacKenzie, D.A. Scoliosis in arthrogryposis multiplex congenita. Spine 3:146–151, 1978.
34. Drummond, D.S., Siller, T.M., and Cruess, R.L. Management of arthrogryposis multiplex congenita. Instr Course Lect 23:79–95, 1974.
35. Dubowitz, V. *Muscle Disorders in Childhood.* Philadelphia, Saunders, 1978.
36. Dubowitz, V., and Brooke, M.H. *Muscle Biopsy: A Modern Approach.* London, Saunders, 1973.
37. Duchenne, G.B. Recherches sur le paralysie musculaire pseudo-hypertrophique ou paralysie myosclerosique. Arch Gen Med 11:5, 179, 305, 421, 552, 1868.
38. Dyck, P.J., and Lambert, E.H. Lower motor and primary sensory neuron diseases with peroneal muscular atrophy. Part I. Neurologic, genetic and electrophysiologic findings in hereditary polyneuropathies. Arch Neurol 18:603–618, 1968; Part II. Neurologic, genetic, and electrophysiologic findings in various neuronal degenerations. Arch Neurol 18:619–625, 1968.
39. Dyck, P.J., Ott, J., Moore, S.B., Swanson, C.J., and Lambert, E.H. Linkage evidence for genetic heterogeneity among kinships with hereditary motor and sensory neuropathy type I. Mayo Clin Proc (submitted for publication)
40. Dyck, P.J., Thomas, P.K., Lambert, E.H., and Bunge, R. (eds): *Peripheral Neuropathy.* Philadelphia, Saunders, 1984.
41. Emery, A.E.H. Clinical manifestations in two carriers of Du-

chenne muscular dystrophy. Lancet 1:1126, 1963.

42. Emery, A.E.H., and Skinner, R. Clinical studies in benign (Becker type) X-linked muscular dystrophy. Clin Genet 10:189–201, 1976.

43. Emery, A.E.H., Smith, C.A.B., and Sanger, R. The linkage relations of the loci for benign (Becker type) X-borne muscular dystrophy, colour blindness and the Xg blood groups. Ann Hum Genet, 32:261–269, 1969.

44. Eng, G.D., Epstein, B.S., Engel, W.K., McKay, D.W., and McKay, R. Malignant hyperthermia and central core disease in a child with congenital dislocating hips. Arch Neurol 35(4):189, 1978.

45. Erb, W. *Die Thomsen'sche Krankheit (Myotonia Congenita).* Leipzig, 1886.

46. Escobar, V., Bixler, D., Gleiser, S., Weaver, D.D., and Gibbs, T. Multiple pterygium syndrome. Am J Dis Child 132:609–611, 1978.

47. Escourelle, R., and Poirier, J. *Manual of Basic Neuropathology.* Philadelphia, Saunders, 1978.

48. Eulenburg, A., von. Ueber eine familiare, durch 6 generationen verfolgbare Form congenitaler Paramytonic. Neurol Zentralbl 5:265, 1886.

49. Fisk, J.R., and Bunch, W.H. Scoliosis in neuromuscular disease. Orthop Clin North Am 10(4):863, 1979.

50. Freeman, E.A., and Sheldon, J.H. Cranio-carpo-tarsal dystrophy. Arch Dis Child 13:277–283, 1938.

51. Friedlander, H.L., Westin, G.W., and Wood, W.L. Arthrogryposis multiplex congenita. J Bone Joint Surg 50A:89–112, 1968.

52. Friedreich, N. Eigene beobachtungen, in *Ueber Progressive Muskelatrophie.* Berlin Hirschwald, 1873, p 11.

53. Gonatas, N.K., Perez, M.C., Shy, G.M., and Evangelista, I. Central core disease of skeletal muscle. Ultrastructural and cytochemical observations in two cases. Am J Pathol 47:503–524, 1965.

54. Gonatas, N.K., Shy, G.M., and Godfrey, E.H. Nemaline myopathy. The origin of nemaline structures. N Engl J Med 274:535–539, 1966.

55. Gowers, W.R. *Pseudohypertrophic Muscular Paralysis.* London, Churchill, 1879.

56. Gowers, W.R. A lecture on myopathy of a distal form. Br Med J 2:89, 1902.

57. Green, W.T., and Grice, D.S. The treatment of poliomyelitis: Acute and convalescent stages. Instr Course Lect 8:261, 1951.

58. Green, W.T., and Grice, D.S. The management of chronic poliomyelitis. Instr Course Lect 9:85, 1952.

59. Green, W.T., and Grice, D.S. The surgical correction of the paralytic foot. Instr Course Lect 10:343, 1953.

60. Grice, D.S. An extraarticular or subastragalar arthrodesis joint for correction of paralytic flat feet in children. J Bone Joint Surg 34A:927–940, 1952.

61. Gross, R.H. The role of the Verebelyi-Ogston procedure in the management of the arthrogrypotic foot. Clin Orthop 194:99–103, 1985.

62. Guidera, K.J., and Drennan, J.C. Foot and ankle deformities in arthrogryposis multiplex congenita. Clin Orthop 194:93–98, 1985.

63. Hall, J.G. An approach to congenital contractures (arthrogryposis). Pediatr Ann 10:15, 1981.

64. Hall, J.G. Genetic aspects of arthrogryposis. Clin Orthop 194:44–53, 1985.

65. Hall, J.G., Reed, S.D., and Driscoll, E.P. Part I. Amyoplasia. A common sporadic condition with congenital contractures. Am J Med Genet 15(4):571, 1983.

66. Hall, J.G., Reed, S.D., and Greene, G. The distal arthrogryposes: Delineation of new entities—Review and nosologic discussion. Am J Med Genet 11:185, 1982.

67. Hall, J.G., Reed, S.D., McGilivray, B.D., Herrman, J., Partington, M.W., Schinzel, A., Shapiro, J., and Weaver, D.D. Part II. Amyoplasia. A specific type of arthrogryposis with an apparent excess of discordantly affected identical twins. Am J Med Genet 15(4):591, 1983.

68. Hall, J.G., Reed, S.D., Scott, C.I., Rogers, J.G., Jones, K.L., and Camarano, A. Three distinct types of X-linked arthrogryposis seen in six families. Clin Genet 21:81–97, 1982.

69. Harper, P.S. *Myotonic Dystrophy.* Philadelphia, Saunders, 1979.

70. Harper, P.S. Genetics of neurological disease, in Swash, M., and Kennard C. (eds): *Scientific Basis of Clinical Neurology.* Edinburgh, Churchill Livingstone, 1985, pp 680–693.

71. Harper, P.S., and Dyken, P.R. Early onset dystrophia myotonica, evidence supporting a maternal environment factor. Lancet 2:53–55, 1972.

72. Hensinger, R.N., and MacEwen, G.D. Spinal deformity associated with heritable neurological conditions: Spinal muscular dystrophy, Friedreich's ataxia, familial dysautonomia, and Charcot-Marie-Tooth disease. J Bone Joint Surg 58A:13, 1976.

73. Herron, L.D., Westin, G.W., and Dawson, E.G. Scoliosis in arthrogrypsosis multiplex congenita. J Bone Joint Surg 60A:293–299, 1978.

74. Heyman, C.H. A method for the correction of paralytic femur (?) recurvatum: Report of a bilateral case. J Bone Joint Surg 6:689, 1924.

75. Hoffmann, J. Uber chronische spinale Muskelatrophie im Kindesalter auf familiarer Basis. Dtsch Z Nervenheilk 3:427–470, 1893.

76. Hoffmann, J. Weitere Beitgräge zur Lehrevon der hereditaren progressiven spinalen Muskelatrophie im Kindesalter. Dtsch Z Nervenheilk 10:292, 1897.

77. Hoffmann, J. Ueber die hereditare progressive spinale Muskelatrophic im Kindesalter. Munch Med Wochen 47:1649–1651, 1900.

78. Hoffmann, J. Zur Lehre von der Thomsen'schen Krankheit mit besonderer Berucksichtigung des dabei vorkommenden Muskelschwundes. Dtsch Z Nervenheilk 18:198, 1900.

79. Hoffmann, J. Dritter Beitrag zur Lehre von der hereditaren progressiven spinalen Muskelatrophic im Kindesalter. Dtsch Z Nervenheilk 18:217–224, 1900.

80. Hsu, J.D., Groolman, T.B., Hoffer, M.N. et al. The orthopaedic management of spinal muscular atrophy. J Bone Joint Surg 55B:663, 1973.

81. Huurman, W.W., and Jacobsen, S.T. The hip in arthrogryposis multiplex congenita. Clin Orthop 194:81–86, 1985.

82. Ingram, A.J. Anterior poliomyelitis, in Munsor, A.S., and Crenshaw, A.H. (eds): *Campbell's Operative Orthopaedics,* 6th ed. St. Louis, Mosby, 1969.

83. Inkley, S.R., Oldenburg, F.C., and Vignos, P.J. Pulmonary function in Duchenne muscular dystrophy related to stage of disease. Am J Med 56:297–306, 1974.

84. Jacobs, J.E., and Carr, C.R. Progressive muscular atrophy of the peroneal type (Charcot-Marie-Tooth disease), orthopaedic management and end-result study. J Bone Joint Surg 32A:27, 1950.

85. Jago, R.H. Arthrogryposis following treatment of maternal tetanus with muscle relaxants. Arch Dis Child 45:277, 1970.

86. Japas, L.M. Surgical treatment of pes cavus by tarsal V-osteotomy. J Bone Joint Surg 58A:927, 1968.

87. Jones, R. The soldier's foot and the treatment of common deformities of the foot. Part II: Clawfoot. Br Med J 1:749, 1916.

88. Kasai, T., Oki, T., Osuga, T., and Nogami, H. Familial arthrogryposis with distal involvement of the limbs. Clin Orthop 166:182–184, 1982.

89. Kearns, T.P., and Sayre, G.P. Retinitis pigmentosa, external ophthalmoplegia and complete heart block. Arch Ophthalmol (Chicago) 60:280, 1958.

90. Kingston, H.M. et al. Genetic linkage between Becker's muscular dystrophy and a cloned DNA sequence of the short arm of the X chromosome. J Med Genet 20:255–258, 1983.

91. Kolb, M., Horn, M.L., and Martz, R. Dantrolene in human malignant hyperthermia, multi-center review. Anesthesiology 56:254, 1982.

92. Kugelberg, E., and Welander, L. Heredofamilial juvenile muscular atrophy simulating muscular dystrophy. Arch Neurol Psychiatry 75:500–509, 1956.

93. Lambrinudi, C. New operation on dropfoot. Br J Surg 15:193, 1927.

94. Landouzy, L., and Dejerine, J. De la myopathie atrophique progressive (myopathie hereditaire), debutant, dans l'enfance, par le face, sans alteration du systeme nerveux. C R Acad Sci Paris 98:53, 1884.

95. Lapidus, P.W. Dorsal bunion, its mechanics and operative correction. J Bone Joint Surg 22:621, 1940.

96. Legg, A.T. Transplantation of tensor fasciae femoris in cases of weakened gluteus medius. N Engl J Med 209:61, 1933.

97. Levitt, R.L., Canale, S.T., Cooke, A.J., Jr., and Gartland, J.J. The role of foot surgery in progressive neuromuscular disorders in children. J Bone Joint Surg 55A:1396, 1973.

98. Lloyd-Roberts, G.C., and Lettin, A.W.F. Arthrogryposis multiplex congenita. J Bone Joint Surg 52B:494–508, 1970.

99. Luque, E.D., and Cardoso, A. Sequential correction of scoliosis with rigid internal fixation. Orthop Trans 1:136, 1977.

100. McKay, D.W. A new technique for correction of dorsal bunion. Referred to as a personal communication by Tachdjin, M.O., in *The Child's Foot.* Philadelphia, Saunders, 1985.

101. MacEwen, G.D., and Floyd, G.C. Congenital insensitivity to pain and its orthopaedic implications. Clin Orthop 68:100, 1970.

102. Macrae, D. Myasthenia gravis in early childhood. Pediatrics 13:511, 1954.

103. McComas, A.J. *Neuromuscular Function and Disorders.* London, Butterworth, 1977.

104. Makin, M. The surgical treatment of Friedreich's ataxia. J Bone Joint Surg 35A:425–436, 1953.

105. Marsh, G.G., and Munsat, T.L. Evidence of early impairment of verbal intelligence in Duchenne muscular dystrophy. Arch Dis Child 49:118, 1974.

106. Mastaglia, F.L. Structure and function of skeletal muscle, in Swash, M., and Kennard, C. (eds): *Scientific Basis of Clinical Neurology.* Edinburgh, Churchill Livingstone, 1985, pp 410–435.

107. Mazar, A., Herold, H.Z., and Vardy, P.A. Congenital sensory neuropathy with anhidrosis. Orthopaedic complication and management. Clin Orthop 118:184–187, 1976.

108. Millichap, J.G., and Dodge, P.R. Diagnosis and treatment of myasthenia gravis in infancy, childhood and adolescence. Neurology 10:1007–1014, 1960.

109. Mustard, W.T. A follow-up study of iliopsoas. Transfer for hip instability. J Bone Joint Surg 41B:289–298, 1969.

110. Ober, F.R. An operation for relief of paralysis of the gluteus maximus muscle. JAMA 88:1063, 1927.

111. Ober, F.R. The role of the iliotibial band and fascia lata as a factor in the causation of low back disabilities and sciatica. J Bone Joint Surg 18:105, 1936.

112. Oh, S.J. *Clinical Electromyography.* Baltimore, University Park Press, 1984.

113. Olson, W., Engel, W.K., Walsh, G.O., and Einaugler, R. Oculocraniosomatic neuromuscular disease with "ragged-red" fibers. Arch Neurol 26:193–211, 1972.

114. Otto, A.G. Monstrorum sexcentorum descripto anatomica, in *Museum Anatomico Pathologicum Vratislaviense.* 1841, p 323.

115. Otto, A.G. A human monster with inwardly curved extremities. Trans by Dr. L.S. Peltier from the Latin. Clin Orthop 194:4–5, 1985.

116. Palmer, P.P., MacEwan, G.D., Gowen, J.R., and Matthews, P.A. Passive motion therapy for infants with arthrogryposis. Clin Orthop 194:54–59, 1985.

117. Perry, J., et al. Triple tenodesis of the knee: A soft tissue operation for the correction of paralytic genu recurvatum. J Bone Joint Surg 58A:978–985, 1976.

118. Ramsey, P.L., and Hensinger, R.N. Congenital dislocation of the hip associated with central core disease. J Bone Joint Surg 57A:648–651, 1975.

119. Ray, S., Bowen, J.R., and Marks, H.G. Foot deformity in myotonic dystrophy. Foot Ankle 5:125–130, 1984.

120. Ray, S., Bowen, J.R., and Marks, H.G. Congenital dislocation of the hip and hip dysplasia in Charcot-Marie-Tooth disease. Contemp Orthop 11:19–23, 1985.

121. Refsum, S. Heredopathia atactica polyneuritiformis: A familial syndrome not hitherto described. Acta Psychiatr Neurol (Suppl 38):1–303, 1946.

122. Refsum, S., Salmonsen, L., and Skatvedt, M. Heredopathia atactica polyneuritiformis in children. J Pediatr 35:335, 1949.

123. Riley, C.M., Day, R.L., Greeley, D.M., and Langford, W.S. Central autonomic dysfunction with defective lacrimation. Pediatrics 3:468, 1949.

124. Riley, C.M., and Moore, R.H. Familial dysautonomia differentiated from related disorders. Pediatrics 37:435, 1966.

125. Rochelle, J., Bowen, J.R., and Ray, S. Pediatric foot deformities in progressive neuromuscular disease. Contemp Orthop 8:41–50, 1984.

126. Rose, G.K. Arthropathy of the ankle in congenital indifference to pain. J Bone Joint Surg 35B:408–410, 1953.

127. Roses, A.D., Roses, M.J., Miller, S.E., Hull, K.L., and Appel, S.H. Carrier detection in Duchenne muscular dystrophy. N Engl J Med 294:193, 1976.

128. Roussy, G., and Levy, G. Sept cas d'une maladie familiale particuliare. Rev Neurol (Paris) 54:427–450, 1926.

129. Roussy, G., and Levy, G. La dystasie areflexique hereditaire. Presse Med 2:1733, 1932.

130. Roussy, G., and Levy, G. A propos de la dystasie areflexique hereditaire. Rev Neurol (Paris) 62:763, 1934.

131. Ryerson, E.W. Arthrodesis operations of the foot. J Bone Joint Surg 5:453, 1923.

132. Sabin, A.B. Oral poliovirus vaccine. History of its development and prospects. Eradication of poliomyelitis. JAMA 194:872, 1965.

133. Salk, J.E. Studies in human subjects on active immunization against poliomyelitis. JAMA 151:1081, 1953.

134. Salter, R.B. Pelvic osteotomy in the treatment of congenital dislocation and subluxation of the hip. J Bone Joint Surg 43B:518–539, 1961.

135. Schwartz, O., and Jampel, R.S. Congenital blepharophimosis associated with a unique generalized myopathy. Arch Ophthalmol 68:52, 1962.

136. Schwentker, E.P., and Gibson, D.A. The orthopaedic aspects of spinal muscular atrophy. J Bone Joint Surg 58A:32–38, 1976.

137. Shapiro, F., and Brennan, M.J. Orthopaedic management of childhood neuromuscular disease. Part II: Peripheral neuropathies, Friedreich's ataxia and arthrogryposis multiplex congenita. J Bone Joint Surg 64A:949–953, 1982.

138. Sharrard, W.J. Posterior iliopsoas transplantation in the treatment of paralytic dislocation of the hip. J Bone Joint Surg 46B:426, 1964.

139. Shy, G.M., Engel, W.K., Somers, J.E., and Wanko, T. Nemaline myopathy. A new congenital myopathy. Brain 86:793, 1963.

140. Siegel, I.M. Scoliosis in muscular dystrophy. Clin Orthop 93:235–238, 1973.

141. Siegel, I.M. The management of muscular dystrophy. A clinical review. Muscle Nerve 1:453, 1978.

142. Soutter, R. A new operation for hip contractures in poliomyelitis. Med Surg J 170:380, 1914.

143. Spencer, G.E. Orthopaedic care of progressive muscular dystrophy. J Bone Joint Surg 49A:1201–1204, 1967.

144. Spencer, G.E., and Vignos, P.J. Bracing for ambulation in childhood progressive muscular dystrophy. J Bone Joint Surg 44A:234–242, 1962.

145. Spiro, A.J., Shy, G.M., and Gonatas, N.K. Myotubular myopathy. Persistence of fetal muscle in an adolescent boy. Arch Neurol

14:1–14, 1966.

146. Stalberg, E. The motor unit: Electromyography, in Swash, M., and Kennard, C. (eds): *Scientific Basis of Clinical Neurology.* New York, Churchill Livingstone, 1985, pp 448–462.

147. St. Clair, H.S., and Zimbler, S. A plan of management and treatment results in the arthrogrypotic hip. Clin Orthop 194:74–86, 1985.

148. Steindler, A. The stripping of the os calcis. J Orthop Surg 2:8, 1920.

149. Steinert, H. Myopathologische Beitrage 1. Uber das klinische und anatomische Bild des Muskelschwunds der Myotoniker. Dtsch Z Nervenheilk 37:58–104, 1909.

150. Sutherland, D.M., Bost, F.C., and Schottstaedt, E.R. Electromyographic study of transplanted muscles about the knee in poliomyelitis patients. J Bone Joint Surg 42A:919–939, 1960.

151. Swinyard, C.A., and Bleck, E.E. The etiology of arthrogryposis (multiple congenital contracture). Clin Orthop 194:15–29, 1985.

152. Tachdjian, M.O. *The Child's Foot.* Philadelphia, Saunders, 1985.

153. Taylor, R.G. The treatment of clawtoes by multiple transfers of flexor into extensor tendons. J Bone Joint Surg 33B:539–542, 1981.

154. Thomas, B., Schopler, S., Wood, W., and Oppenheim, W.L. The knee and arthrogryposis. Clin Orthop 194:87–92, 1985.

155. Thomsen, G.H., and Bilenker, R.M. Comprehensive management of arthrogryposis multiplex congenita. Clin Orthop 194:6–14, 1985.

156. Thomsen, J. Tonische Krampfe in willkurlich beweglichen Muskeln infolge von erebter psychischer Disposition (Ataxia muscularis). Arch Psychiatr Nervenkr 6:702–718, 1876.

157. Tooth, H.H. *The Peroneal Type of Progressive Muscular Atrophy.* London, Lewis, 1886.

158. Vanier, T.M. Dystrophia myotonia in childhood. Br Med J 2:1284–1288, 1960.

159. Vignos, P.J. Diagnosis of progressive muscular dystrophy. J Bone Joint Surg 49A:1212, 1967.

160. Vignos, P.J., Spencer, G.E., and Archibald, K.C. Management of progressive muscular dystrophy in childhood. JAMA 184:89, 1963.

161. Weissman, S.L., Torok, G., and Khermosh, O. Intertrochanteric osteotomy for fixed paralytic obliquity of the hips. J Bone Joint Surg 43A:1135–1154, 1961.

162. Welander, L. Myopathia distalis tarda hereditaria. Acta Med Scand 265(suppl):1, 1951.

163. Werdnig, G. Zwei fruhinfantile hereditare Falle von progressiver Muskelatrophie unter dem Bilde der Dystrophie, aber auf neurotischer Grundlage. Arch Psychiatr Nervenkr 22:437–481, 1891.

164. Werdnig, G. Die fruhinfantile progressive spinale Amyotrophie. Arch Psychiatr Nervenkr 26:706–744, 1894.

165. Wilkins, K.E., and Gibson, D.A. The patterns of spinal deformity in Duchenne muscular dystrophy. J Bone Joint Surg 58A:24–32, 1976.

166. Wynne-Davies, R., Williams, P.F., and O'Connor, J.C.B. The 1960's epidemic of arthrogryposis multiplex congenita. J Bone Joint Surg 63B:76–82, 1981.

167. Yount, C.C. The role of the tensor fasciae femoris in certain deformities of the lower extremities. J Bone Joint Surg 8:171–193, 1926.

CHAPTER 31

Bone Dysplasias

Suzanne Ray

In 1977, an attempt was made to standardize the terms used for different bone dysplasias and dysostoses. As a result, the International Nomenclature of Constitutional Diseases of Bone was drawn up, and was later revised in 1983 (see Table 31-1). This nomenclature lists only those bone dysplasias and dysostoses which are considered well-defined entities. More newly recognized disorders or those which may represent so-called private syndromes are not included.

Since it is beyond the scope of this chapter to deal exhaustively with each of the bone dysplasias or dysostoses, only those likely to be seen by the orthopaedist are discussed in detail. For further reading, References 10, 48, 54, 60, 64, 68, 85, 95, and 98 are suggested.

OSTEOCHONDRODYSPLASIAS

Chondrodysplasia Punctata

Chondrodysplasia punctata is seen in at least two distinct forms,[99] an autosomal recessive form which is almost invariably lethal and a dominant form which is compatible with life. Characteristically, stippled epiphyses are seen in both disorders. The autosomal recessive form has marked rhizomelic shortening together with cataracts and multiple joint contractures. The stippling is most noted in the femora and humeri. The autosomal dominant form, also known as the Conradi-Hunermann type,[20,41,84] frequently results in severe spinal abnormalities including kyphoscoliosis and limb

TABLE 31-1 Disorders of Bone

Osteochondrodysplasias—Abnormalities of cartilage and/or bone growth and development

I. Defects of growth of tubular bones and/or spine identifiable at birth
   A. Usually lethal before or shortly after birth
      1. Achondrogenesis type I (Parenti-Fraccaro)
      2. Achondrogenesis type II (Langer-Saldino)
      3. Hypochondrogenesis
      4. Fibrochondrogenesis
      5. Thanatophoric dysplasia
      6. Thanatophoric dysplasia with cloverleaf skull
      7. Ateloosteogenesis
      8. Short rib syndrome (with or without polydactyly)
         a. Type I (Saldino-Noonan)
         b. Type II (Majewski)
         c. Type III (lethal thoracic dysplasia)
   B. Usually nonlethal dysplasia
      1. Chondrodysplasia punctata
         a. Rhizomelic form autosomal recessive
         b. Dominant X-linked form
         c. Common mild form (Sheffield)
      Exclude: symptomatic stippling (warfarin, chromosomal aberration)
      2. Campomelic dysplasia
      3. Kyphomelic dysplasia
      4. Achondroplasia
      5. Diastrophic dysplasia
      6. Metatrophic dysplasia (several forms)
      7. Chondroectodermal dysplasia (Ellis–van Creveld)
      8. Asphyxiating thoracic dysplasia (Jeune)
      9. Spondyloepiphyseal dysplasia congenita
         a. Autosomal dominant form
         b. Autosomal recessive form
      10. Kniest dysplasia
      11. Dyssegmental dysplasia
      12. Mesomelic dysplasia
         a. Type Nievergelt
         b. Type Langer (probable homozygous dyschondrosteosis)
         c. Type Robinow
         d. Type Rheinardt
         e. Others
      13. Acromesomelic dysplasia
      14. Cleidocranial dysplasia
      15. Otopalatodigital syndrome
         a. Type I (Langer)
         b. Type II (André)
      16. Larsen syndrome
      17. Other multiple dislocation syndromes (Desbuquois)
II. Defects of growth identifiable in later life
      1. Hypochondroplasia
      2. Dyschondrosteosis
      3. Metaphyseal chondrodysplasia: type Jansen
      4. Metaphyseal chondrodysplasia: type Schmid
      5. Metaphyseal chondrodysplasia: type McKusick
      6. Metaphyseal chondrodysplasia with exocrine pancreatic insufficiency and cyclic neutropenia
      7. Spondylometaphyseal dysplasia
         a. Type Kozlowski
         b. Other forms
      8. Multiple epiphyseal dysplasia
         a. Type Fairbank

(Continued on next page)

TABLE 31-1 *(Continued)*

Osteochondrodysplasias—Abnormalities of cartilage and/or bone growth and development

    b. Other forms
  9. Multiple epiphyseal dysplasia with early diabetes (Wolcott-Rallisson)
 10. Arthroophthalmopathy (Stickler)
 11. Pseudoachondroplasia
    a. Dominant
    b. Recessive
 12. Spondyloepiphyseal dysplasia tarda (X-linked recessive)
 13. Progressive pseudo-rheumatoid chondrodysplasia
 14. Spondyloepiphyseal dysplasia, other forms
 15. Brachyolmia
    a. Autosomal recessive
    b. Autosomal dominant
 16. Dyggve-Melchior-Clausen dysplasia
 17. Spondyloepimetaphyseal dysplasia (several forms)
 18. Spondyloepimetaphyseal dysplasia with joint laxity
 19. Otospondylomegaepiphyseal dysplasia (OSMED)
 20. Myotonic chondrodysplasia (Catel-Schwartz-Jampel)
 21. Parastremmatic dysplasia
 22. Trichorhinophalangeal dysplasia
 23. Acrodysplasia with retinitis pigmentosa and nephropathy (Saldino-Mainzer)
III. Disorganized development of cartilage and fibrous components of skeleton
  1. Dysplasia epiphyseal hemimelia
  2. Multiple cartilaginous exostoses
  3. Acrodysplasia with exotoses (Giedion-Langer)
  4. Enchondromatosis (Ollier)
  5. Enchondromatosis with hemangioma (Maffucci)
  6. Metachondromatosis
  7. Spondyloenchondroplasia
  8. Osteoglophonic dysplasia
  9. Fibrous dysplasia (Jaffe-Lichtenstein)
 10. Fibrous dysplasia with skin pigmentation and precocious puberty (McCune-Albright)
 11. Cherubism (familial fibrous dysplasia of the jaws)
IV. Abnormalities of density of cortical diaphyseal structure and/or metaphyseal modeling
  1. Osteogenesis imperfecta (several forms)
  2. Juvenile idiopathic osteoporosis
  3. Osteoporosis with pseudoglioma
  4. Osteopetrosis
    a. Autosomal recessive lethal
    b. Intermediate recessive
    c. Autosomal dominant
    d. Recessive with tubular acidosis
  5. Pyknodysostosis
  6. Dominant osteosclerosis type Stanescu
  7. Osteomesopyknosis
  8. Osteopoikilosis
  9. Osteopathia striata
 10. Osteopathia striata with cranial sclerosis
 11. Melorheostosis
 12. Diaphyseal dysplasia (Camurati-Engelmann)
 13. Craniodiaphyseal dysplasia
 14. Endostealhyperostosis
    a. Autosomal dominant (Worth)
    b. Autosomal recessive (Van Buchem)
    c. Autosomal recessive (sclerosteosis)
 15. Tubular stenosis (Kenny-Caffey)

(Continued on next page)

TABLE 31-1 *(Continued)*

Osteochondrodysplasias—Abnormalities of cartilage and/or bone growth and development

16. Pachydermoperiostosis
17. Osteodysplasty (Melnick-Needles)
18. Frontometaphyseal dysplasia
19. Craniometaphyseal dysplasia (several forms)
20. Metaphyseal dysplasia (Pyle)
21. Dysosteosclerosis
22. Osteoectasia with hyperphosphatasia
23. Oculodentoosseous dysplasia
    a. Mild type
    b. Severe type
24. Infantile cortical hyperostosis (Caffey disease, familial type)

Dysostoses—Malformation of individual bones, singly or in combination

A. Dysostoses with cranial and facial involvement
    1. Craniosynostosis (several forms)
    2. Craniofacial dysostosis (Crouzon)
    3. Acrocephalosyndactyly
        a. Type Apert
        b. Type Chotzen
        c. Type Pfeiffer
        d. Other types
    4. Acrocephalopolysyndactyly (Carpenter and others)
    5. Cephalopolysyndactyly (Greig)
    6. First and second branchial arch syndromes
        a. Mandibulofacial dysostosis (Treacher-Collins, Franceschetti)
        b. Acrofacial dysostosis (Nager)
        c. Oculoauriculovertebral dysostosis (Goldenhar)
        d. Hemifacial microsomia
        e. Others (probably parts of a large spectrum)
    7. Oculomandibulofacial syndrome (Hallermann-Streiff-Francois)
B. Dysostoses with predominant axial involvement
    1. Vertebral segmentation defects (including Klippel-Feil)
    2. Cervicooculoacoustic syndrome (Wildervanck)
    3. Sprengel anomaly
    4. Spondylocostal dysostosis
        a. Dominant form
        b. Recessive form
    5. Oculovertebral syndrome (Weyers)
    6. Osteoonychodysostosis
    7. Cerebrocostomandibular syndrome
C. Dysostoses with predominant involvement of extremities
    1. Acheiria
    2. Apodia
    3. Teraphocomelia syndrome (Roberts) (SC pseudothalidomide syndrome)
    4. Ectrodactyly
        a. Isolated
        b. Ectrodactylyectodermal dysplasia, cleft palate syndrome
        c. Ectrodactyly with scalp defects
    5. Oroacral syndrome (aglossia syndrome, Hanhart syndrome)
    6. Familial radioulnar synostosis
    7. Brachydactyly, types A, B, C, D, E (Bell's classification)
    8. Symphalangism
    9. Polydactyly (several forms)
    10. Syndactyly (several forms)
    11. Polysyndactyly (several forms)
    12. Camptodactyly

(Continued on next page)

TABLE 31-1 (*Continued*)

Dysostoses—Malformation of individual bones, singly or in combination

13. Manzke syndrome
14. Poland syndrome
15. Rubinstein-Taybi syndrome
16. Coffin-Siris syndrome
17. Pancytopenia-dysmelia syndrome (Fanconi)
18. Blackfan-Diamond anemia with thumb anomalies (Aase syndrome)
19. Thrombocytopenia-radial-aplasia syndrome
20. Orodigitofacial syndrome
    a. Type Papillon-Leage
    b. Type Mohr
21. Cardiomelic syndromes (Holt-Oram and others)
22. Femoral focal deficiency (with or without facial anomalies)
23. Multiple synostoses (includes some forms of symphalangism)
24. Scapuloiliac dysostosis (Kosenow-Sinios)
25. Hand-foot-genital syndrome
26. Focal dermal dypoplasia (Goltz)

D. Idiopathic osteolyses
1. Phalangeal (several forms)
2. Tarsocarpal
    a. Including François form and others
    b. With nephropathy
3. Multicentric
    a. Hajdu-Cheney form
    b. Winchester form
    c. Torg form
    d. Other forms

Miscellaneous Disorders with Osseous Involvement

1. Early acceleration of skeletal maturation
   a. Marshall-Smith syndrome
   b. Weaver syndrome
   c. Other types
2. Marfan syndrome
3. Congenital contractural arachnodactyly
4. Cerebrohepatorenal syndrome (Zellweger)
5. Coffin-Lowry syndrome
6. Cockayne syndrome
7. Fibrodysplasia ossificans congenita
8. Epidermal nevus syndrome (Solomon)
9. Nevoid basal cell carcinoma syndrome
10. Multiple hereditary fibromatosis
11. Neurofibromatosis

Chromosomal Aberrations: Primary Metabolic Abnormalities

A. Calcium and/or phosphorus
1. Hypophosphatemic rickets
2. Vitamin D dependency or pseudo-deficiency rickets
    a. Type I with probable deficiency in 25-hydroxy vitamin D 1 α hydroxy-lase
    b. Type II with target-organ resistancy
3. Late rickets (McCance)
4. Idiopathic hypercalciuria
5. Hypophosphatasia (several forms)
6. Pseudohypoparathyroidism (normo- and hypocalcemic forms, including acrodysostosis)

(*Continued on next page*)

TABLE 31-1 *(Continued)*

Chromosomal Aberrations: Primary Metabolic Abnormalities

B. Complex carbohydrates
   1. Mucopolysaccharidosis type I (α_1 iduronidase deficiency)
     a. Hurler form
     b. Scheie form
     c. Other forms
   2. Mucopolysaccharidosis type II—Hunter (sulfoiduronate sulfatase deficiency)
   3. Mucopolysaccharidosis type III—Sanfilippo
     a. Type IIIA (heparan sulfamidase deficiency)
     b. Type IIIB (N-acetyl-α-glucosaminidase deficiency)
     c. Type IIIC (α-glucosaminide-N-acetyl transferase deficiency)
     d. Type IIID (N-acetyl-glucosamine-6-sulfate sulfatase deficiency)
   4. Mucopolysaccharidosis type IV
     a. Type IVA (Morquio (N-acetyl-galactosamine-6-sulfate sulfatase deficiency)
     b. Type IVB (β-galactosidase deficiency)
   5. Mucopolysaccharidosis type VI—Maroteaux-Lamy (arylsulfatase β deficiency)
   6. Mucopolysaccharidosis type VII (β-glucosaminidase deficiency)
   7. Aspartylglucosaminuria (aspartylglucosaminidase deficiency)
   8. Mannosidosis (α-mannosidase deficiency)
   9. Fucosidosis (α-fucosidase deficiency)
  10. G_{M1}-Gangliosidosis (β-galactosidase deficiency)
  11. Multiple sulfatases deficiency (Austin-Thieffry)
  12. Isolated neuraminidase deficiency—several forms including:
     a. Mucolipidosis I
     b. Nephrosialidosis
     c. Cherry red spot myoclonia syndrome
  13. Phosphotransferase deficiency—several forms including:
     a. Mucolipidosis II (I cell disease)
     b. Mucolipidosis III (pseudopolydystrophy)
  14. Combined neuraminidase-galactosidase deficiency
  15. Salla disease
C. Lipids
   1. Niemann-Pick disease (sphingomyelinase deficiency) (several forms)
   2. Gaucher disease (β-glucosidase deficiency) (several types)
   3. Farber disease lipogranulomatosis (ceraminidase deficiency)
D. Nucleic acids
   1. Adenosine-deaminase deficiency and others
E. Amino acids
   1. Homocystinuria and others
F. Metals
   1. Menkes syndrome (kinky hair syndrome and others)

Source: Courtesy of Dr. P. Maroteaux.

length discrepancy. In these latter patients, the stippling is primarily seen in the spine and epiphyses. It is necessary to differentiate patients with either of these disorders from other causes of stippled epiphysis including chromosomal abnormalities.

Campomelic Dysplasia

The term *campomelic dysplasia* is used to describe at least three different conditions: (1) the long-limbed type, (2) the short-limbed craniosynostotic type, and (3) the short-limbed normocephalic type.[51] The classic, long-limbed form of campomelic dysplasia is usually identified by symmetrical bowing in the long bones, particularly the tibia, fibula, and femur, although spinal anomalies are also common[67,81] (Fig. 31-1). Congenital dislocation of the hips is frequently present, and the ossification centers of the distal femur, proximal tibia, and talus are usually not present at birth. The feet are usually described as "clubfeet," but there are complex anomalies of both the feet and ankles.[81] Cleft palate, tracheomalacia, as

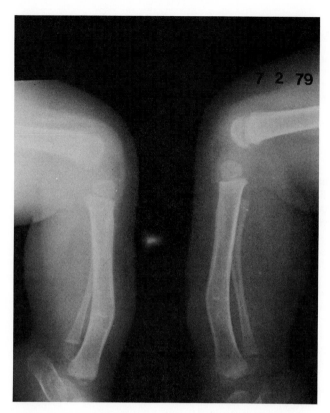

Figure 31-1 Bowing of the tibias in campomelic dysplasia. (*Courtesy of J. Richard Bowen and the Medical Photography Department, Alfred I. Dupont Institute. Reproduced with permission.*)

well as cardiac, renal, and central nervous system anomalies, are all common findings. Patients frequently do not survive past 1 year of age. The syndrome is autosomal recessive, but all phenotypic females require a karyotype since many are XY.

Achondroplasia

Achondroplasia is undoubtedly the most common cause of dwarfism.[39] Although it is an autosomal dominant condition, the rate of spontaneous mutation is high. Heterozygous achondroplasia is usually consistent with long-term survival. Homozygous or double-dominant achondroplasts are occasionally seen in the newborn period, but do not survive.[34]

Patients with achondroplasia can be recognized in the newborn nursery by the rhizomelic shortening of the long bones, characteristic frontal bossing with depressed nasal bridge (Fig. 31-2) and characteristic radiographic changes. The tubular bones are shortened and thickened with widened metaphyses. The epiphyses frequently indent the central areas of the metaphyses. One of the hallmarks of achondroplasia is the progressive narrowing of the interpedicular distances in the lumbar spine when proceeding in a caudal di-

rection. Additionally, the acetabular roof is horizontal, and the pelvic outlet is said to have a "champagne glass" configuration. The trident hand, although another hallmark of achondroplasia, does not usually lead to functional disability.[5]

Many infants are hypotonic and may have a thoracolumbar gibbus when sitting. If this increases, spinal fusion may be necessary to prevent cord compression. Foramen magnum stenosis should not be overlooked in the patient with either delayed motor development[106] or progressive neurological signs. As achondroplastic patients get older, they develop marked lumbar lordosis and have a high incidence of spinal stenosis even in the late teens or early twenties.

Diastrophic Dysplasia

Diastrophic dysplasia is an autosomal recessive bony dysplasia that, prior to Lamy and Maroteaux in 1960, was considered a variant of achondroplasia.[56] These patients have marked short stature, unusually rigid talipes equinovarus (Fig. 31-3), hitchhiker's thumbs, cartilaginous calcification of the ear pinnae, progressive kyphoscoliosis, and frequently cleft palate. Multiple joint dislocations including those of the elbow, knees, and hips are often present, and symphalangism of the proximal interphalangeal joints of the hands may be seen. Careful evaluation of the cervical spine is necessary as cervical kyphospondylosis and spina bifida occulta may all contribute to instability in this region. Scoliosis may rapidly progress with weight bearing and may be unrelenting in spite of early bracing.[11,36,52] Both the hitchhiker's thumb deformity and a similar deformity of the great toe helps in the ready identification of these patients. The so-called diastrophic variant is now considered to be a milder version of the same disorder and not a separate entity.[55] The recent work of Stanescu et al suggests that it is type II collagen which is defective in this disorder.[101]

Metatrophic Dysplasia

Metatrophic dysplasia is an autosomal recessive dysplasia which presents at birth with short extremities and a relatively long trunk, but with growth and progressive kyphoscoliosis it gradually becomes characterized by relatively long extremities when compared with the shortened trunk. In the sacral region, there is frequently a small "tail" which helps in the identification of these patients.[45,83] Orthopaedically, kyphoscoliosis and atlantoaxial instability frequently present the greatest problems.

Chondroectodermal Dysplasia

Chondroectodermal dysplasia, or Ellis–van Creveld syndrome,[28,29] is an autosomal recessive dwarfism characterized by postaxial polydactyly, cardiac defects, and anomalies of teeth and nails. Cone-shaped epiphyses may be seen in the hands and feet. This disorder is not uncommon among the Amish.[61]

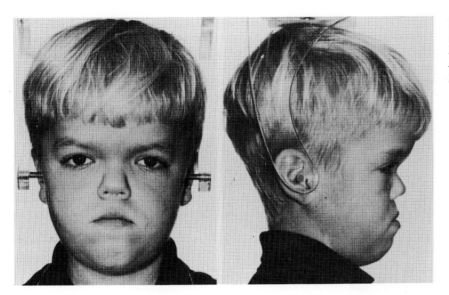

Figure 31-2 Characteristic facies of achondroplasia. (*From Cohen, M.J., Jr., in Hall, B., ed: Cartilage, vol. 3. New York, Academic Press, 1983. Reproduced with permission.*)

Asphyxiating Thoracic Dysplasia (Jeune)

Asphyxiating thoracic dysplasia is usually considered to be autosomal recessive. It is characterized by a narrow thorax with short ribs and frequent respiratory distress during the newborn period. At one time it was thought that most of these children died in the newborn period, but survivors do exist. As the children get older, the pulmonary problems appear to diminish, but renal failure may develop.[35]

Spondyloepiphyseal Dysplasia Congenita

The autosomal dominant form of spondyloepiphyseal dysplasia congenita is undoubtedly one of the more common bone disorders. It is characterized by short trunk dwarfism with marked vertebra plana (Fig. 31-4). Progressive spinal deformities are common. Atlantoaxial instability secondary to odontoid hypoplasia may lead to severe complications if not recognized. Coxa vara and genu valgum are seen secondary to the epiphyseal changes.[97,98,100] In adulthood, the epiphyseal irregularities may also predispose toward degenerative arthritis. Fifty percent of patients may have myopia and/or retinal detachment. It is important to distinguish spondyloepiphyseal dysplasia from the spondylometaepiphyseal dysplasias and also from the spondyloepimetaphyseal dysplasias, which are heterogeneous groups of disorders classified according to whether epiphyseal or metaphyseal changes predominate.

Kniest Syndrome

Kniest syndrome is an autosomal dominant, short trunk and short-limbed dwarfism, characterized by severe progressive kyphoscoliosis. Multiple joint contractures are frequently present as are sometimes visual and hearing difficulties.[83]

Mesomelic Dysplasia

The *mesomelic dysplasias* are heterogeneous groups of bone dysplasias characterized by shortening of the middle sections of the extremities.[47] The Nievergelt type of mesomelic dysplasia is an autosomal dominant trait with multiple tarsal and carpal synostoses and severe shortening in the tibia and fibula.[25,76] The Langer type, however, represents the homozygous condition of dyschondrosteosis. In other words, both

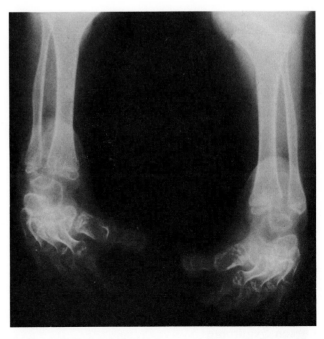

Figure 31-3 Rigid bilateral talipes equinovarus in diastrophic dysplasia. (*From Ray S., and Cowell, H., Contemporary Orthopaedics 9:51–58, 1984. Reproduced with permission.*)

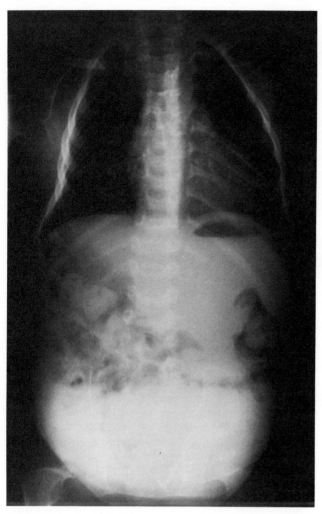

Figure 31-4 Spondyloepiphyseal dysplasia congenita. There is a short trunk dwarfism with vertebra plana.

parents of a patient with a Langer type of mesomelic dwarfism would have dyschondrosteosis, which usually is characterized only by a mild shortness of stature and Madelung's deformity.[57]

Cleidocranial Dysplasia

Cleidocranial dysplasia is an autosomal dominant disorder characterized by severe hypoplasia or absence of the clavicles with resultant hypermobility of the shoulders (Fig. 31-5). The pubic symphysis is frequently widened and should not be confused with a traumatic separation. The anterior fontanelle is frequently open even in adulthood, and multiple wormian bones are seen on lateral skull radiographs.[54,64] Occasionally, scoliosis is seen.

Larsen Syndrome

Larsen syndrome is a heterogeneous group of disorders, of which one is probably an autosomal recessive condition and

another, an autosomal dominant. In both, the face is commonly flattened and there are usually multiple joint dislocations including elbows, hips, and knees.[58] Spinal anomalies are common and may lead to progressive deformities in both the cervicothoracic and lumbar regions.[12] Two centers of ossification in the calcaneus may be seen.

Hypochondroplasia

Hypochondroplasia is an autosomal dominant disorder with an essentially normal facies and milder shortening of the extremities than in achondroplasia.[90] There may sometimes be some mild narrowing of the intrapedicular distances in the lumbar region.[110]

Metaphyseal Chondrodysplasia

The *metaphyseal chondrodysplasias* are a heterogeneous group of disorders characterized by significant involvement of the metaphyseal regions of the long bones but with relative sparing of the epiphyseal regions.[53] Both the Jansen and Schmidt types are autosomal dominants.[88] The McKusick type, also known as cartilage hair hypoplasia, is common among the Amish. Patients may have fine hair as well as immunodeficiency in addition to their skeletal involvement.[62] The disorder is autosomal recessive, as is the Schwachman syndrome, which is characterized by immunodeficiency and pancreatic insufficiency.[89]

Spondylometaphyseal Dysplasia

The *spondylometaphyseal dysplasias* are, again, a heterogeneous group of disorders with both autosomal recessive and

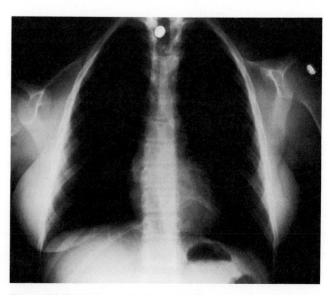

Figure 31-5 Cleidocranial dysplasia. The clavicles are absent bilaterally.

autosomal dominant patterns possible. They are characterized by involvement of the spine as well as the metaphyseal changes seen in the previous group of disorders.[53] Stanescu et al suggests that the Kozlowski type may be a lysosomal disorder.[101]

Multiple Epiphyseal Dysplasia

Both autosomal dominant and autosomal recessive forms of *multiple epiphyseal dysplasia* are possible, although the autosomal dominant form is the more common. Both show mild shortening of stature with irregular, sometimes fragmented, epiphyses. Degenerative arthritis later in life is not uncommon, and reconstructive surgery, especially about the hips, may be necessary.[102] In addition, patients with multiple epiphyseal dysplasia may be misdiagnosed as having bilateral Legg-Calvé-Perthes disease since the clinical symptoms and radiographs may be quite similar. Obtaining shoulder radiographs in children with such pathological hip conditions should help to differentiate the two conditions.

Arthroophthalmopathy

Arthroophthalmopathy, or the Stickler syndrome, may occasionally be confused with Marfan syndrome. It, too, is an autosomal dominant disorder, and the patients have a marfanoid appearance. However, cleft palate as well as progressive osteoarthropathy help to distinguish it.[103,104]

Pseudoachondroplasia

Pseudoachondroplasia is found in both autosomal dominant and autosomal recessive forms. Stanescu et al believe that the disorder is secondary to an abnormal proteoglycan core protein not being transported properly from the rough endoplasmic reticulum to the golgi apparatus.[101] The facial appearance appears normal, but there is a micromelic shortening of the extremities. In some patients progressive spinal disorders are seen.[83]

Spondyloepiphyseal Dysplasia Tarda

Spondyloepiphyseal dysplasia tarda may be either an X-linked recessive or an autosomal recessive disorder. Patients with this disorder are usually not diagnosed until mid-childhood. Progressive spinal disorders as well as progressive arthropathy involving the major joints may be seen.[10,54]

Myotonic Chondrodysplasia

Myotonic chondrodysplasia, or the Schwartz-Jampel syndrome, is an autosomal recessive bone dysplasia with myotonia present from birth. The skeletal changes are severe and similar to spondyloepiphyseal dysplasia congenita. Blepharophimosis as well as relative lack of facial expression also help to distinguish the syndrome.[10,54]

Trichorhinophalangeal Dysplasia

Trichorhinophalangeal dysplasia is an autosomal dominant disorder characterized by fine hair, bulbous nose, and cone-shaped epiphyses.[54,64]

Dysplasia Epiphysealis Hemimelica

Dysplasia epiphysealis hemimelica is a sporadic condition in which there is asymmetrical overgrowth of a tarsal bone or of a portion of an epiphysis. It is most common about the lower extremity and is always unilateral.[31]

Multiple Cartilaginous Exostosis

Multiple cartilaginous exostosis (multiple hereditary exostosis, diaphyseal aclasis) is a common autosomal dominant condition characterized by multiple cartilaginous exostoses about the ends of the long bones, particularly the knees. These exostoses commonly grow away from the joint and are much larger than they appear radiographically because of large cartilaginous caps. They can cause deformity of the long bone, impinge on nerves and vessels, and may undergo malignant transformation. Concern exists when a lesion grows rapidly, causes pain, and/or historically, grows after skeletal maturity. Removal, when necessary, must be extraperiosteal to minimize the likelihood of recurrence. Osteotomy for correction of the bony deformities, especially of the ulna and fibula, may also be necessary in this condition.[44]

Multiple Enchondromatosis (Ollier)

Multiple enchondromatosis, or Ollier disease,[77] is a sporadic disorder characterized by irregular radiolucencies in the metaphysis and diaphysis of the long bones (Fig. 31-6). Frequently one side of the body may be more affected than the other resulting in significant limb length inequality. Fractures and osteotomies through the enchondromatous lesions heal well. However, just as in multiple hereditary exostosis, malignant degeneration may not be uncommon. When the disorder is seen in conjunction with multiple hemangiomas, it is known as Maffucci syndrome.[63]

Metachondromatosis

Metachondromatosis is an autosomal dominant condition which combines features of both multiple hereditary exostosis and enchondromatosis. Cartilaginous exostoses, particularly about the hands and feet, are common. These have sometimes been reported to regress or to disappear completely. In addition, multiple enchondromatoses, particularly about the pelvis, are seen. Finally, this disorder may show soft tissue calcifications in the juxtaarticular area.[10,54] Treatment is symptomatic when the exostoses interfere with function or are otherwise disabling.

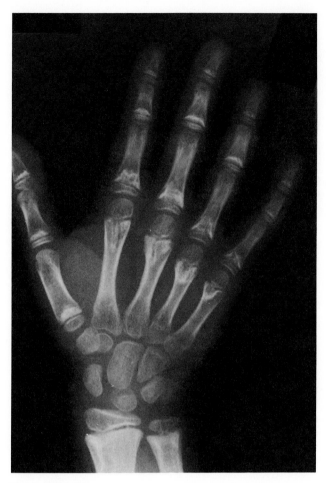

Figure 31-6 The hand of a patient with enchondromatosis (Ollier disease).

Fibrous Displasia

Fibrous dysplasia is usually of sporadic occurrence. Typically, the bone has a ground-glass appearance. The diaphysis may be expanded, and the modeling pattern of the bone is distorted. Frequent fractures, microfractures, and bowing are common. The shepherd's crook deformity of the femur may be seen as a result of these multiple fractures. Both monostotic and polyostotic cases are seen. Irregular café au lait ("coast of Maine") spots are common. When polyostotic fibrous dysplasia is associated with precocious puberty, it is frequently known as the McCune-Albright syndrome.[1]

Osteogenesis Imperfecta

Osteogenesis imperfecta is a very heterogeneous category of disorders, characterized by extreme bone fragility and multiple fractures. Initially, the disorder was characterized into congenita and tarda forms, depending on the onset of fractures. This proved inadequate, and subsequently Sillence developed a four-category classification of the disorder.[92] Unfortunately, even this classification does not adequately take into account the multiplicity of conditions known as osteogenesis imperfecta.

The patients most severely affected by osteogenesis imperfecta may have in utero fractures leading to a "crumpled bone" appearance. These patients usually do not survive.

Other patients may have long slender bones with multiple fractures in the postnatal period. These fractures commonly lead to severe skeletal deformities if untreated. It is in this group of patients that multiple surgical procedures are frequently necessary to help minimize deformity and improve the quality of life. Multiple osteotomies of the long bones, especially in the lower extremities, together with rods of either the expandable or nonexpandable type have been used to reduce the number of fractures, ameliorate the deformities, and improve ambulation.[6,96] Progressive scoliosis, particularly in adolescence, becomes an increasing problem and is resistant to brace therapy. Early fusion may be indicated. Otherwise, progressive scoliosis becomes a leading cause of death in the older patient. In addition, the cervical spine must be carefully evaluated for an evidence of atlantoaxial subluxation due to odontoid hypoplasia.

Finally, some patients may be seen who only begin to sustain fractures in mid- to late childhood (the old "tarda"

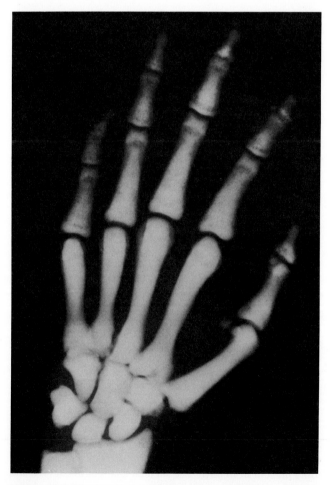

Figure 31-7 The hand of a patient with osteopetrosis. (*From Ray, S., and Daniels, K., Contemporary Orthopaedics 11:59–61, 1985. Reproduced with permission.*)

form of the disorder). These patients may be managed symptomatically.

Osteopetrosis

Osteopetrosis refers to any of several bone disorders leading to increased sclerosis of the bones (Fig. 31-7). The most severe autosomal recessive form leads to obliteration of the narrow space in the long bones, widened metaphyses, "bone within a bone" appearance, hepatosplenomegaly, and anemia. There is progressive narrowing of the foramina within the skull leading to neurological deficits, blindness, and deafness. The condition was generally lethal in early childhood until the advent of bone marrow transplantation. Adequate engraftment of donor osteoclasts appears to lead to regression of the disorder.[19,46,91]

The autosomal dominant form, which is frequently termed *Albers-Schonberg disease,* usually shows generalized osteosclerosis, most noted in the skull. Symptoms may include fractures or osteomyelitis, but are frequently so minimal that the disorder may be discovered while examining radiograph studies taken for other reasons. There do appear to be intermediate forms of osteopetrosis, and, in addition, there is an autosomal recessive form associated with renal tubular acidosis and cerebral calcification (carbonic anhydrase II deficiency).[93]

Pycnodysostosis

Pycnodysostosis is an autosomal recessive disorder characterized by general osteosclerosis. However, in contrast to osteopetrosis there is relatively normal bone modeling in this disorder. Stature is usually short and the fontanelles are generally open even into adulthood. Fractures with malunion or nonunion may be the presenting problem in this disorder.[65,66] Stanescu et al report that abnormal inclusions in the growth plate chondrocytes contain lipid in this disorder.[101]

Osteopoikilosis

Osteopoikilosis is an autosomal dominant disorder which is characterized by numerous, symmetrical round areas of increased density in the long bones, pelvis, and scapula. The spine is usually not involved.[54] These areas are usually asymptomatic.

Osteopathia Striata

Osteopathia striata is an autosomal dominant disorder in which striations are seen in the long bones and pelvis. These may be seen in association with cranial sclerosis.[54]

Melorheostosis

Melorheostosis is a sporadic condition in which linear areas of dense bone are seen to be running down an extremity. The radiographic changes are frequently likened to candle drippings. Melorheostosis may be asymptomatic or may be seen in an area with increasing pain and soft tissue sclerosis.[15,59,72]

Diaphyseal Dysplasia

Diaphyseal dysplasia (Camurati-Engelmann)[16,30] is an autosomal dominant condition in which there is sclerosis and fusiform enlargement of the diaphyses of the long bones as well as occasional sclerosis of the skull. It may be asymptomatic, but in some patients it is associated with muscular pain and weakness.[7,18,40]

Craniodiaphyseal Dysplasia

Craniodiaphyseal dysplasia may be heterogeneous, although an autosomal recessive form has certainly been reported. It is distinguished from diaphyseal dysplasia by the greater amount of cranial involvement leading to facial changes (leontiasis ossea), cranial nerve palsies, and, sometimes, retardation.[7]

Metaphyseal Dysplasia

Metaphyseal dysplasia (Pyle disease)[80] is an autosomal recessive disorder in which expansion of the metaphyses of the long bones, particularly about the knee, is seen. There may sometimes be sclerosis in the skull. In general these patients are asymptomatic, although occasionally they may have minor skeletal problems such as mild genu valgum or pes planus. It is important to distinguish this disorder from the more severe craniometaphyseal dysplasia and frontometaphyseal dysplasia.[7]

Infantile Cortical Hyperostosis

Infantile cortical hyperostosis (Caffey disease) may be a sporadic disorder, although some believe that it may be an autosomal dominant condition with incomplete penetrance. Adults are clinically asymptomatic and may be radiographically normal.[54] However, in infancy, affected patients develop periosteal elevation of multiple bones, particularly the mandible, together with inflammation and fever. These symptoms may last for several weeks but invariably resolve spontaneously. It is important to differentiate this condition from more serious disorders associated with periosteal elevation including congenital syphilis, disseminated osteomyelitis, and tumor.[54,64]

DYSOSTOSES

Acrocephalosyndactyly

The acrocephalosyndactylies are generally considered to be a heterogeneous class of disorders characterized by craniosyn-

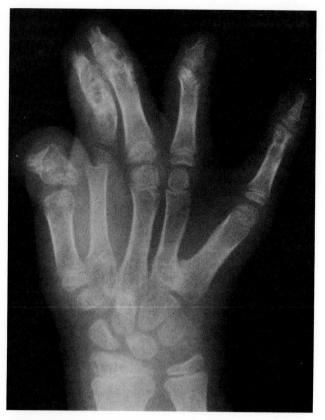

Figure 31-8 The "mitten" hand of a patient with Apert syndrome (acrocephalosyndactyly).

ostosis as well as complex syndactylies of the hands and feet. The most well-known acrocephalosyndactyly is Apert syndrome.[2,8] The hands are affected by severe complex syndactyly, often called "mitten hands" (Fig. 31-8). The reconstructive procedures can be extremely challenging to even the most skilled surgeon.[33,38] The feet are similarly affected and may require osteotomies as well as special shoes to enable the child to walk comfortably.[23,70] The base of the skull and upper cervical spine should be carefully evaluated for any possible anomalies. Acrocephalopolysyndactyly or Carpenter syndrome may be distinguished by its autosomal recessive pattern of inheritance as well as its preaxial polydactyly.[17]

Osteoonychodysostosis

Osteoonychodysostosis, or nail-patella syndrome, is an autosomal dominant condition in which the nails and patellae may range from hypoplastic to absent. The abnormal patellae may lead to recurrent knee problems, including instability. The iliac horns, although pathognomonic for the nail-patella syndrome, are of no functional significance. Similarly, the hypoplasia seen in the elbows of these patients does not usually lead to functional problems.[10,95]

Ectrodactyly

Ectrodactyly, or lobster claw deformity, may be seen as an isolated phenomenon or may be seen in conjunction with other disorders particularly the EEC syndrome (ectrodactyly, ectrodermal dysplasia, and cleft palate). In these latter patients the condition is inherited as an autosomal dominant with variability in expressivity.[10,95]

Brachydactyly

Brachydactyly refers to a heterogeneous group of disorders which are generally inherited as autosomal dominant conditions and which are characterized by shortened hands and feet. They may be subclassified according to the complexity of the brachydactyly.[105]

Symphalangism

Symphalangism is an autosomal dominant condition which is generally characterized by fusion of the proximal interphalangeal joints of the fingers. It may also be associated with carpal and tarsal coalitions.[105]

Rubinstein-Taybi Syndrome

Rubinstein-Taybi syndrome is a sporadically occurring syndrome characterized by mental and growth retardation. The facies is broadened with a beaklike nose. The thumbs and great toes are also broadened.[10,95]

Thrombocytopenia-Radial-Aplasia Syndrome

Thrombocytopenia-radial-aplasia syndrome is an autosomal recessive condition in which the radii have varying degrees of hypoplasia and the patients may have thrombocytopenia, as well as other hematologic abnormalities, including granulocytosis and eosinophilia. The degree of thrombocytopenia does not correlate with the radial hypoplasia.[10,95]

Cardiomelic Syndrome

The *Holt-Oram syndrome* is the most well known of the cardiomelic syndromes. In this autosomal dominant disorder, abnormalities of the heart including atrial septal defects and ventricular septal defects are found together with upper extremity abnormalities ranging from triphalangeal thumbs to radial hypoplasia to phocomelia.[37,49,78]

Focal Dermal Hypoplasia

Focal dermal hypoplasia syndrome (Goltz syndrome) is a mesoectodermal disorder characterized by linear areas of hypoplasia. There are frequently congenital amputations, spina bifida, linear striations in the bone, nail and dental abnormalities, syndactylies, and multiple other nonspecific abnormalities present in patients with this syndrome. It is believed to be an X-linked dominant that is lethal in males.[54]

Idiopathic Osteolysis

There are many different syndromes in which osteolysis of the phalanges and the carpal and tarsal bones are common. They may be either autosomal recessive or autosomal dominant syndromes, except for Gorham osteolysis which may involve any bone and is believed to be of sporadic occurrence.[32,107]

Marfan Syndrome

Marfan syndrome is an autosomal dominant condition, well known for its skeletal and cardiac problems. In general, patients with this syndrome are relatively tall and endomorphic. Arachnodactyly and hyperextensibility are common. Progressive scoliosis not infrequently requires surgery, and may be associated with other chest wall anomalies including pectus carinatum and pectus excavatum. Myopia and lens subluxation are common. In general, the lens subluxes superiorly in Marfan syndrome because of a defect in the suspensory ligament. Dilation of the aorta and dissecting aneurysm are the most common cardiovascular problems.[60]

Congenital Contractural Arachnodactyly

Congenital contractural arachnodactyly is an autosomal dominant condition which is not infrequently confused with Marfan syndrome. Unlike Marfan syndrome, however, there are multiple, symmetrical contractures of the large joints including hips, knees, ankles, and elbows. Arachnodactyly may be present as may increasing scoliosis. Cardiac anomalies are less common than in Marfan syndrome.[60]

Cerebrohepatorenal Syndrome

Cerebrohepatorenal (Zellweger) *syndrome* is an autosomal recessive syndrome with hypotonia, hepatomegaly, characteristic facies, and mental retardation. Punctate calcifications similar to those of chondrodysplasia punctata may be seen. The condition is fatal in early life.[79]

Fibrodysplasia Ossificans Congenita

Fibrodysplasia ossificans congenita, or myositis ossificans progressiva, is an autosomal dominant with high mutation rate. In this condition, there is progressive ossification of the connective tissues leading eventually to immobility of the extremities and usually early demise. The symptoms initially appear on the trunk, but subsequently spread. One of the earliest features is shortening of the first ray of both the foot and hand, with the hallux usually in valgus position. This finding is usually present from the time of birth and antecedes the development of the fibrodysplasia.[95]

Neurofibromatosis

Neurofibromatosis, or Von Recklinghausen disorder,[109] is an autosomal dominant disorder with variable expressivity. Crowe et al[22] suggest that two or more characteristic features of neurofibromatosis are necessary in order to make a definite diagnosis. These features include six or more café au lait spots, a positive tissue biopsy, a positive family history, or characteristic skeletal features such as pseudarthrosis of the tibia, limb hypertrophy, or sharply angulated spinal curvature. Skeletal manifestations of neurofibromatosis may also include periosteal dysplasia, and those secondary to metabolic disturbances. Although the rate of malignancy in neurofibromatosis is high, primary bone tumors are rare.[26]

The cervical spine should be examined radiographically in all patients with neurofibromatosis, especially those with scoliosis, as there may be an up to 44 percent incidence of abnormality.[112] Scoliosis, kyphoscoliosis, congenital scoliosis, spondylolisthesis, and meningomyelocele are frequently seen in the thoracic or lumbar spine. It is important to distinguish the dystrophic curve because of its poor results with bracing. Wedging of the vertebral body, marked rotation of an apical vertebra, scalloping, foraminal enlargement, and spindling of the transverse processes and ribs may all signal dystrophic curves.[111]

Although pseudarthrosis of the tibia is seen in 5 to 10 percent of patients with neurofibromatosis, 50 percent of patients with congenital pseudarthrosis of the tibia will have neurofibromatosis. Also in neurofibromatosis, pseudarthrosis of other long bones is occasionally seen. Surgical treatment for congenital pseudarthrosis have included prophylactic grafting prior to fracture, Boyd dual-onlay graft, Farmer composite cross-leg pedicle graft, McFarland bypass bone graft, free vascularized bone graft, dual rod internal fixation, electromagnetic coil stimulation, and amputation.[13,21,74,75,82,108] Attempts to correlate the radiographic findings at the time of presentation with ultimate outcome have been mixed.[21,73,75,82]

Down Syndrome

The most common genetic abnormality in *Down syndrome* is nondisjunction of a G chromosome (trisomy 21). Ninety-four percent of patients with Down syndrome will have this abnormality. However, translocation of a G chromosome to a D chromosome or to another G chromosome occurs in 3.3 percent of cases, and mosaicism occurs in 2.4 percent of cases.[95]

Down syndrome is common relative to the other conditions discussed and is readily recognized by the characteristic facies, Brushfield spots, simian creases, mental retardation, and hypotonia. Orthopaedic problems are common in this disorder and include atlantoaxial subluxation (either secondary to a hypoplastic odontoid process or to hyperextensibility of the transverse ligament), scoliosis, slipped capital femoral epiphysis, subluxed or dislocated hips, subluxed or dislocated patellae, and metatarsus primus varus with resultant hallux valgus or hallux varus.[24] Early intervention in the young child with Down syndrome with dislocated or subluxed hips may be indicated. Nevertheless, in the older child, surgical intervention produces the same results as nonintervention.[9] The patellae, if symptomatic, may be treated conservatively with exercises, and rarely require surgery. Comfortable shoes with wide toe boxes are important in order to minimize foot deformity.

Nonorthopaedic abnormalities include congenital heart disorder, such as atrioventricular canal, and thyroid abnormalities.

Trisomy 18 Syndrome

Trisomy 18, or Edward syndrome,[27] is the second most common chromosomal malformation syndrome, with an incidence of approximately 0.3 per 1000 newborns.[95] The patients have severe mental and growth retardation, and only 10 percent survive the first year.[95] Orthopaedically, the hands are clenched with overlapping fingers. Multiple contractures of other joints are common, but the distal ones tend to be more significant than the proximal ones. Congenital dislocation of the hips has been reported. Vertical tali are also common but are usually not treated surgically because the overall prognosis for these individuals is poor.

Mucopolysaccharidosis Type I

Mucopolysaccharidosis type I, also known as α-L-iduronidase deficiency, is an autosomal recessive condition characterized by coarsening of the facies, restricted motion of the joints, progressive mental deficiency, and clouding of the corneas. The syndrome was initially described by Hurler in 1919.[43] The majority of the patients with this disorder show symptoms beginning in early childhood, usually within the first two years of life, and die before the age of 10. Orthopaedically, patients have restriction of multiple joints, particularly the elbow. There is a characteristic broadening of the phalanges and metacarpals, as well as broadening and irregularity of the metaphyses.[50] Anterior wedging is commonly seen in the vertebrae, and there is frequently a gibbus at the thoracolumbar junction. Odontoid hypoplasia is not uncommon, and all patients require cervical films to rule out atlantoaxial subluxation.

Initially an allelic form of Hurler disease was categorized as mucopolysaccharidosis type 5, or Scheie syndrome.[87] However, with further research, these were found to be patients with the same lysosomal enzyme anomaly, although with different clinical presentations.[4] Patients with this allelic form commonly live into mid- to late adulthood with corneal clouding and joint stiffness being the predominant features.

Mucopolysaccharidosis Type II

Mucopolysaccharidosis type II, or *Hunter syndrome,*[2] is an X-linked recessive condition characterized by deficiency of

sulfoiduronate sulfatase.[3] It was initially described in two brothers by Hunter in 1917. Typically the onset is slightly later than Hurler syndrome, but coarsening of the facies and mental and neurological deterioration progress just as in the other mucopolysaccharidoses. Orthopaedically there are restrictions about many joints, as well as the typical changes of dysostosis multiplex seen in the mucopolysaccharidoses. Once again atlantoaxial subluxation may be present, secondary to odontoid hypoplasia. In contrast to Hurler syndrome, patients with Hunter syndrome have neither clouding of the cornea nor a thoracolumbar gibbus.

Mucopolysaccharidosis Type III

Mucopolysaccharidosis type III, or *Sanfilippo syndrome,*[86] describes a group of autosomal recessive conditions. At this point in time, at least four different enzymatic deficiencies have been described causing this syndrome. These are now termed type 3A (heparan sulfamidase deficiency), type 3B (N-acetyl-α-glycosaminidase deficiency), type 3C (α-glucosaminide-N-acetyl transferase deficiency), and type 3D (N-acetyl-glucosamine-6-sulfate sulfatase deficiency). These patients are characterized by severe mental deterioration, although, in general, the physical and bony changes are not as marked as in the other mucopolysaccharidoses. Most patients die by the end of the second decade.

Mucopolysaccharidosis Type IV

Mucopolysaccharidosis type IV has now been discovered to be two different disorders, both of which are autosomal recessive. The first, type 4A, is the classic Morquio-Brailsford disorder[14,71] which is now known to be caused by N-acetyl-galactosamine-6-sulfate sulfatase deficiency. The other disorder, type 4B, is caused by β-galactosidase deficiency. These patients are usually mentally normal but have the most severe bone and growth disturbances of all the mucopolysaccharidoses. The changes of dysostosis multiplex are the most marked in these patients, who show marked platyspondyly of the vertebral bodies, shortened long bones with widened metaphyses, coxa vara, genu valgum, as well as short stubby hands. Although there may be some evidence of joint laxity among the hand and wrist bones, there is frequently joint restriction at the larger joints, particularly the hips. Corneal clouding is present. The life span is variably shortened.

Mucopolysaccharidosis Type VI

Mucopolysaccharidosis type VI, or the *Maroteaux-Lamy syndrome,* is an autosomal recessive, caused by aryl sulfatase B deficiency. These patients have somewhat milder courses than patients with Hurler syndrome.[64] Nevertheless, they show coarsening of the facies, progressive growth retardation, stiffness of the joints, dysostosis multiplex, and early demise, usually by the end of the second decade. In contrast to Hurler syndrome, mental deterioration is not common.

Mucopolysaccharidosis Type VII

Mucopolysaccharidosis type VII, also known as *β-glucuronidase deficiency,* is an autosomal recessive disorder of complex carbohydrate metabolism. Most patients become symptomatic either within the first year of life with coarsening of the facies, corneal clouding and dysostosis multiplex. Nevertheless, other patients with milder symptoms in the second decade have also been reported.[94]

Homocystinuria

The most common form of *homocystinuria* is an autosomal recessive condition resulting from a block in cystathionine synthetase. Clinically, many patients resemble those with Marfan syndrome: a tall, thin habitus; chest wall deformity; and scoliosis. Dislocation of the lenses is common, with the lenses typically dislocated inferiorly. Mental retardation is also common.[60]

Menkes Syndrome

Menkes syndrome, or the so-called kinky hair syndrome, is an autosomal recessive condition characterized by severe mental retardation, hypertonicity, and seizures. Osteoporosis at a few months of age is common, as is cortical hyperostosis. The disorder appears to be secondary to abnormal copper metabolism.[69]

REFERENCES

1. Albright, F., Butler, A.M., Hampton, A.O., and Smith, P.A. Syndrome characterized by osteitis fibrosa disseminata. N Engl J Med 216:727–746, 1937.
2. Apert, E. De l'acrocephalosyndactylie. Bull Soc Med Hop Paris 23:1310–1330, 1906.
3. Bach, G., Eisenberg, F., Cantz, M., and Neufeld, E.F. The defect in the Hunter syndrome. Deficiency of sulfoiduronate sulfatase. Proc Natl Acad Sci 70:2134–2138, 1973.
4. Bach, G., Friedman, R., Weissman, B., and Neufeld, E.F. The defect in the Hurler and Scheie syndromes: Deficiency of α-L-iduronidase. Proc Natl Acad Sci 69:2048–2051, 1972.
5. Bailey, J.A. Orthopaedic aspects of achondroplasia. J Bone Joint Surg 52A:1285–1301, 1970.
6. Bailey, R.W., and Dubow, H.I. Experimental and clinical studies of longitudinal bone growth utilizing a new method of internal fixation crossing the epiphyseal plate. J Bone Joint Surg 47A:1669, 1965.
7. Beighton, P., and Cremin, B.J. *Sclerosing Bone Dysplasias.* Springer Verlag, Berlin, 1980.
8. Beligere, N., Harris, V., and Pruzansky, S. Progressive bony dysplasia in Apert's syndrome. Radiology 139:593–597, 1981.
9. Bennet, G.C., Rang, M., Roye, D.P., and Aprin, H. Dislocation of the hip in trisomy 21. J Bone Joint Surg 64B:289–294, 1982.
10. Bergsma, D. *Birth Defects Compendium,* 2d ed. New York, Liss, 1979.
11. Bethem, D., Winter, R.B., and Lutter, L. Disorders of the spine and diastrophic dwarfism. J Bone Joint Surg 62A:529–536, 1980.
12. Bowen, J.R., Ortega, K., Ray, S., and MacEwen, G.D. Spinal deformities in Larsen's syndrome. Clin Orthop 197:159–163, 1985.
13. Boyd, H.B. Pathology and natural history of congenital pseudarthroses of the tibia. Clin Orthop 166:5–13, 1982.
14. Brailsford, J.F. Chondro-osteodystrophy. Am J Surg 7:404–410, 1929.
15. Campbell, C.J., Papademetriou, T., and Bonfiglio, M. Melorheostosis. A report of the clinical, roentgenographic and pathologic findings in fourteen cases. J Bone Joint Surg 50A:1281–1304, 1968.
16. Camurati, M. Di un raro caso di osteite simmetrica ereditaria degli arti inferiori. Chir Organi Mov 6:622–665, 1922.
17. Carpenter, G. Case of acrocephaly with other congenital malformations. Proc R Soc Med 2:45–53, 1909.
18. Clawson, D.K., and Loop, J.W. Progressive diaphyseal dysplasia (Engelmann's disease). J Bone Joint Surg 46A:143–150, 1964.
19. Coccia, P.F., Krivit, W., Cervenka, J., et al. Successful bone marrow transplantation for infantile malignant osteopetroses. N Engl J Med 302:701–708, 1980.
20. Conradi, E. Vorzeitiges Auftreten von Knochen und eigenartigen Verkalkungskernen bei Chondrodystrophia foetalis hypoplastica. Z Kinderheilk 80:86–97, 1914.
21. Crawford, A.H. Neurofibromatosis in childhood. Instr Course Lect 30:56–74, 1981.
22. Crowe, F.W., Schull, W.J., and Neel, J.V. *A Clinical, Pathological and Genetic Study of Multiple Neurofibromatosis.* Springfield, MA, Thomas, 1956.
23. Dell, P.C., and Sheppard, J.E. Deformities of the great toe in Apert's syndrome. Clin Orthop 157:113–118, 1981.
24. Diamond, L.S., Lynne, D., and Sigman, B. Orthopaedic disorders in patients with Down's syndrome. Orthop Clin North Am 12:57–71, 1981.
25. Dubois, H.J. Nievergelt-Pearlman syndrome. Synostosis in feet and hands with dysplasia of elbows. Report of a case. J Bone Joint Surg. 52B:325–329, 1970.
26. Ducatman, B.S., Scheithauer, B.W., and Dahlin, D.C. Malignant bone tumors associated with neurofibromatosis. Mayo Clin Proc 58:578–582, 1983.
27. Edwards, J.H., Harnden, D.G., Cameron, A.H., Crosse, V.M., and Wolff, O.H. A new trisomic syndrome. Lancet 1:787–789, 1960.
28. Ellis, R.W.B., and Andrew, J.D. Chondro-ectodermal dysplasia. J Bone Joint Surg 44B:626–636, 1962.
29. Ellis, R.W.B., and Van Creveld, S. A syndrome characterized by ectodermal dysplasia, polydactyly, chondrodysplasia and congenital morbus cordis. Arch Dis Child 15:65–84, 1940.
30. Engelmann, G. Ein Fall von Osteopathia hyperostotica (Sclerosis) multiplex infantilis. Fortschr Rontgenstr 39:1101–1106, 1929.
31. Fairbank, T.J. Dysplasia epiphysialis hemimelica. J Bone Joint Surg 38B:237–242, 1956.
32. Gorham, L.W. Disappearing bones. J Bone Joint Surg 37A:985–1004, 1955.
33. Green, S.M. Pathological anatomy of the hands in Apert's syndrome. J Hand Surg 7(5):450–453, 1982.
34. Hall, J.G., Dorst, J.P., Taybi, H., Scott, C.I., Langer, L.O., and McKusick, V.A. Two probable cases of homozygotes for the achondroplasia gene. Birth Defects 5(4):29–34, 1969.
35. Herdman, R.C., and Langer, L.O. The thoracic asphyxiant dystrophy and renal disease. Am J Dis Child 116:192–201, 1968.
36. Herring, J.A. The spinal disorders in diastrophic dwarfism. J Bone Joint Surg 60A:177–182, 1978.
37. Holt, M., and Oram, S. Familial heart disease with skeletal malformations. Br Heart J 22:236–242, 1960.
38. Hoover, G.H., Flatt, A.E., and Weiss, M.W. The hand and Apert's syndrome. J Bone Joint Surg 52A:878–895, 1970.
39. Horton, W.A., Rotter, J.I., Rimoin, D.L., Scott, C.I., and Hall, J.G.

Standard growth curves for achondroplasia. J Pediatr 93:435–438, 1978.

40. Hundley, J.D., and Wilson, F.C. Progressive diaphyseal dysplasia. Review of the literature and report of seven cases in one family. J Bone Joint Surg 55A:461–474, 1973.

41. Hunermann, C. Chondrodystrophia calcificans congenita als abortive Form der Chondrodystrophie. Z Kinderheilk 51:1–19, 1931.

42. Hunter, C. A rare disease in two brothers. Proc R Soc Med 10:104–116, 1917.

43. Hurler, G. Ueber einem Typ multipler Abartungen vorwiegend am Skelettsystem. Z Kinderheilk 24:220–234, 1919.

44. Jaffe, H.L. Hereditary multiple exostosis. Arch Pathol 36:335–357, 1943.

45. Jenkins, P., Smith, M.B., and McKinnell, J.S. Metatropic dwarfism. Br J Radiol 43:561–565, 1920.

46. Kadota, R.P., and Smithson, W.A. Bone marrow transplantation for disease of childhood. Mayo Clin Proc 59:171–184, 1984.

47. Kaitila, I.I., Leisti, J.T., and Rimoin, D.L. Mesomelic skeletal dysplasias. Clin Orthop 114:94–106, 1976.

48. Kaufman, H.J. Classification of the skeletal dysplasias and the radiologic approach to their differentiation. Clin Orthop 114:12–17, 1976.

49. Kaufman, R.L., Rimoin, D.L., McAlister, W.H., and Hartman, A.F. Variable expression of the Holt-Oram syndrome. Am J Dis Child 127:21–25, 1974.

50. Kelly, T.E. The mucopolysaccharidoses and mucolipidoses. Clin Orthop 114:116–136, 1976.

51. Khajavi, A., Lachman, R., Rimoin, D., Schimke, R.N., Dorst, J., Handmaker, S., Ebbin, A., and Ferreault: Hererogeneity in the campomelic syndrome. Radiology 120:641–647, 1976.

52. Kopits, S.E. Orthopaedic complications of dwarfism. Clin Orthop 114:153–179, 1976.

53. Kozlowski, K. Metaphyseal and spondylometaphyseal chondrodysplasias. Clin Orthop 114:83–93, 1976.

54. Kozlowski, K., and Beighton, P. *Gamut Index of Skeletal Dysplasias.* Berlin, Springer-Verlag, 1984.

55. Lachman, R.S., Sillence, D., Rimoin D., Horton, W., Hall, J., Scott, C., Spranger, J., and Langer, L. Diastrophic dysplasia. The death of a variant. Radiology 140:79–86, 1981.

56. Lamy, M., and Maroteaux, P. Le namisme diastrophique. Presse Med 68:1977–1980, 1960.

57. Langer, L.O. Mesomelic dwarfism of the hypoplastic ulna fibula mandible type. Radiology 89:654–660, 1967.

58. Larsen, L.J., Schottstaedt, E.R., and Bost, R.C. Multiple congenital dislocations associated with characteristic facial abnormality. J Pediatr 37:574–581, 1950.

59. Leri, A., and Lievre, J.A. La melorheostose, l'hyperostose d'un membre "en coulee." Presse Med 36:801–805, 1928.

60. McKusick, V.A. *Heritable Disorders of Connective Tissue,* 4th ed. St. Louis, Mosby, 1972.

61. McKusick, V.A., Egeland, J.A., Eldridge, R., and Kusen, D.E. Dwarfism in the Amish. I. The Ellis-Van Creveld syndrome. Bull Johns Hopkins Hosp 115:306–336, 1964.

62. McKusick, V.A., Eldridge, R., Hostetler, J.A., Ruangwit, V., and Egeland, J.A. Dwarfism in the Amish. II. Cartilage-hair hypoplasia. Bull Johns Hopkins Hosp 115:306–336, 1964.

63. Maffucci, A. Di un caso di encondroma e d'angioma multiplo. Movem Med Chir Napoli 25:399–412, 1881.

64. Maroteaux, P. *Bone Diseases of Children.* Philadelphia, Lippincott, 1979.

65. Maroteaux, P., and Lamy, M. La pycnodysostose. Presse Med 70:999–1002, 1962.

66. Maroteaux, P., and Lamy, M. The malady of Toulouse-Lautrec. JAMA 191:715–717, 1965.

67. Maroteaux, P., Spranger, J., Opitz, J.M., Kucera, J., Lowry, R.B.,

Schimke, R.N., and Kagan, S.M. Le syndrome campomelique. Presse Med 79:1157–1162, 1971.

68. Maroteaux, P., Stanescu, V., and Stanescu, R. The lethal chondrodysplasias. Clin Orthop 114:31–45, 1976.

69. Menkes, J.H., Alter, M., Steigler, G.K., Weakley, D.R., and Snug, J.H. A sex-linked recessive disorder with retardation of growth, peculiar hair, and focal cerebral and cerebellar degeneration. Pediatrics 29:764–779, 1962.

70. Meyer, J.L. Apert's syndrome: Acrocephalosyndactylism. J Foot Surg 20:210–213, 1981.

71. Morquio, L. Sur une forme de dystrophie osseuse familiale. Bull Soc Pediatr 27:145–152, 1929.

72. Morris, J.M., Samilson, R.L., and Corley, C.L. Melorheostosis. J Bone Joint Surg 45A:1191–1206, 1963.

73. Morrissy, R.T. Congenital pseudarthrosis of the tibia: Factors that affect results. Clin Orthop 166:21–27, 1982.

74. Morrissy, R.T., Riseborough, E.J., and Hall, J.E. Congenital pseudarthrosis of the tibia. J Bone Joint Surg 63B:367–375, 1981.

75. Murray, H.H., and Lovell, W.W. Congenital pseudarthrosis of the tibia: A long-term follow-up study. Clin Orthop 166:14–20, 1982.

76. Nievergelt, K. Positiver Vaterschaftsnachweis auf Grund erblicher Missbildungen der Extremitaten. Arch Klaus-Stift Vererb-Forsch 19:157–194, 1944.

77. Ollier, M. De la dyschondroplasie. Bull Soc Chir (Lyon) 3:22–27, 1899.

78. Poznanski, A.K., Gall, J.C., and Stern, A.M. Skeletal manifestations of the Holt-Oram syndrome. Radiology 94:45–53, 1970.

79. Poznanski, A.K., Nosanchuk, J.S., Baublis, J., and Holt, J.F. The cerebro-hepato-renal syndrome (CHRS) (Zellweger's syndrome). Am J Roentgenol 109:313–322, 1970.

80. Pyle, E.C. A case of unusual bone development. J Bone Joint Surg 13:874–876, 1931.

81. Ray, S., and Bowen, J.R. Orthopaedic problems associated with survival in campomelic dysplasia. Clin Orthop 185:77–82, 1984.

82. Ray, S., Goral, A.B., and Bowen, J.R. Syndrome identification in orthopaedics: Neurofibromatosis. Contemp Orthop 11:43–46, 1985.

83. Rimoin, D.L., Siggers, D.C., Lachman, R.S., and Silberberg, R. Metatropic dwarfism, the Kniest syndrome and the pseudoachondroplastic dysplasias. Clin Orthop 114:70–82, 1976.

84. Rimoin, D.L., Silberberg, R., and Hollister, D.W. Chondro-osseous pathology in the chondrodystrophies. Clin Orthop 114:137–152, 1976.

85. Rubin, P. *Dynamic Classification of Bone Dysplasias.* Chicago, Year Book, 1964.

86. Sanfilippo, S.J., Podosin, R., Langer, L., and Good, R.A. Mental retardation associated with acid mucopolysacchariduria (haparan sulfate type). J Pediatr 63:837–838, 1963.

87. Scheie, H.G., Hambrick, G.W., and Barness, L.A. A newly recognized forme fruste of Hurler's disease (gargoylism). Am J Ophthalmol 53:753–769, 1962.

88. Schmidt, B.J., Becak, W., Becak, M.L., Soibelman, I., Queiroz, A.S., Lorga, A.P., Secaf, F., Antonio, C.F., and Carvalho, A.A. Metaphyseal dysostosis. J Pediatr 63:106–112, 1963.

89. Schwachman, H., Diamond, L.K., Oski, F.A., and Khaw, K.T. The syndrome of pancreatic insufficiency and bone marrow dysfunction. J Pediatr 65:645–663, 1964.

90. Scott, C.I. Achondroplastic and hypochondroplastic dwarfism. Clin Orthop 114:18–30, 1976.

91. Sieff, C.A., Chessells, J.M., Levinsky, R.J., Pritchard, J., Rogers, D.W., Casey, A., Muller, K., and Hall, C.M. Allogenic bone-marrow transplantation in infantile malignant osteopetrosis. Lancet 1:437–441, 1983.

92. Sillence, D. Osteogenesis imperfecta: An expanding panorama of variants. Clin Orthop 159:11–25, 1981.

93. Sly, W.S., Hewett-Emmett, D., Whyte, M.P., Yu, Y.L., and Tashian,

R.E. Carbonic anhydrase II deficiency identified as the primary defect in the autosomal recessive syndrome of osteopetrosis with renal tubular acidosis and cerebral calcification. Proc Natl Acad Sci 80:2752–2756, 1983.

94. Sly, W.S., Quinton, B.A., McAllister, W.H., and Rimoin, D.L. Beta glucuronidase deficiency: Report of clinical, radiologic and biochemical features of a new mucopolysaccaridosis. J Pediatr 82:249–257, 1973.

95. Smith, D.W. *Recognizable Patterns of Human Malformation,* 3d ed. Philadelphia, Saunders, 1982.

96. Sofield, H.A., and Miller, E.A. Fragmentation realignment and intramedullary rod fixation of deformities of the long bones in children. J Bone Joint Surg 41A:1371–1391, 1959.

97. Spranger, J.W., and Langer, L.O. Spondyloepiphyseal dysplasia congenita. Radiology 94:313–322, 1970.

98. Spranger, J.W., Langer, L.O., and Wiedemann, H.R. *Bone Dysplasias.* Philadelphia, Saunders, 1974.

99. Spranger, J.W., Opitz, J.M., and Bidder, U. Heterogeneity of chondrodysplasia punctata. Hum Genet 11:190–212, 1971.

100. Spranger, J.W., and Wiedemann, H.R. Dysplasia spondyloepiphysaria congenita. Helv Pediatr Acta 21:598–611, 1966.

101. Stanescu, V., Stanescu, R., and Maroteaux, P. Pathogenic mechanisms in osteochondrodysplasias. J Bone Joint Surg 66A:817–836, 1984.

102. Stanescu, V., Stanescu, R., and Maroteaux, P. Articular degeneration as a sequela of osteochondrodysplasias. Clin Rheum Dis 11:239–270, 1985.

103. Stickler, G.B., Belau, P.G., Farrell, F.J., Jones, J.D., Pugh, D.G., Steinberg, A.G., and Ward, L.E. Hereditary progressive arthroophthalmopathy. Mayo Clin Proc 40:433–455, 1965.

104. Stickler, G.B., and Pugh, D.G. Hereditary progressive arthroophthalmopathy. Mayo Clin Proc 42:495–500, 1967.

105. Temtamy, S.A., and McKusick, V.A. The genetics of hand malformations. Birth Defects 14(3):328–350, 413–426, 1978.

106. Todorov, A.B., Scott, C.I., Warren, A.E., and Leeper, J.D. Developmental screening tests in achondroplastic children. Am J Med Genet 9:19–23, 1981.

107. Torg, J.S., and Steel, H.H. Sequential roentgenographic changes occurring in massive osteolysis. J Bone Joint Surg 51A:1649–1655, 1969.

108. Umber, J.S., Moss, S.W., and Coleman, S.S. Surgical treatment of congenital pseudarthrosis of the tibia. Clin Orthop 166:28–33, 1982.

109. Von Recklinghausen, F. *Uber die multiplen Fibrome der Haut und ihre Beziehung zu den multiplen Neuromen.* Berlin, August Hirschwald, 1882.

110. Walker, B.A., Murdoch, J.L., McKusick, V.A., Langer, L.O., and Beals, R.K. Hypochondroplasia. Am J Dis Child 122:95–104, 1971.

111. Winter, R.B., Moe, J.H., Bradford, D.S., Lonstein, J.E., Pedras, C.V., and Weber, A.H. Spine deformity in neurofibromatosis. J Bone Joint Surg 61A:677–694, 1979.

112. Yong-Hing, K., Kalamchi, A., and MacEwen, G.D. Cervical spine abnormalities in neurofibromatosis. J Bone Joint Surg 61A:695–699, 1979.

PART V

The Upper Extremity

CHAPTER 32

Surgical Anatomy of the Upper Extremity

Roger Dee, Steven Sampson, and David Chiu

SECTION A

The Shoulder and Arm

Roger Dee

THE SHOULDER JOINT

Since the glenoid is relatively shallow, it is the fibrous capsule and its ligamentous thickenings together with the overlying subscapular muscle which are primarily responsible for anterior stability (Fig. 32-1). Between the important superior glenohumeral ligament and the less strong middle glenohumeral

ligament, there is often a foraminal defect recognized by the arthroscopist as the subscapularis recess. The thick inferior glenohumeral ligament seems to be responsible for maintaining shoulder stability at 90 degrees of abduction in external rotation. At 45 degrees there is some contribution from the subscapularis muscle and also the middle glenohumeral ligament.[2] Severance of all the posterior capsule will not render the shoulder joint unstable unless the superior glenohumeral ligament is also severed anteriorly.[3]

Surgical Relationships of the Shoulder Joint

Access to the structures around the shoulder anteriorly (Fig. 32-2) is between the pectoralis major and the deltoid muscles. The cephalic vein marks the deltopectoral groove. Abduction of the arm may avoid the need to detach the clavicu-

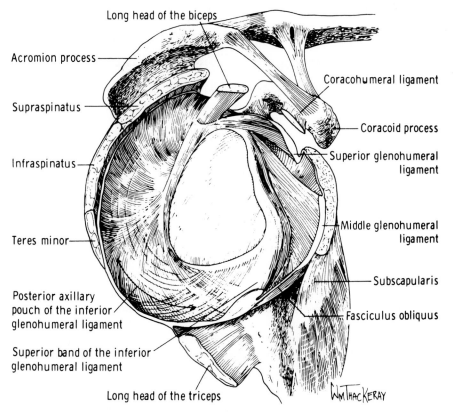

Figure 32-1 The anatomy of the glenohumeral ligaments and other stabilizers of the shoulder joint. (*From Turkel, S. J., et al, J Bone Joint Surg 63A:1209, 1981. Reproduced with permission.*)

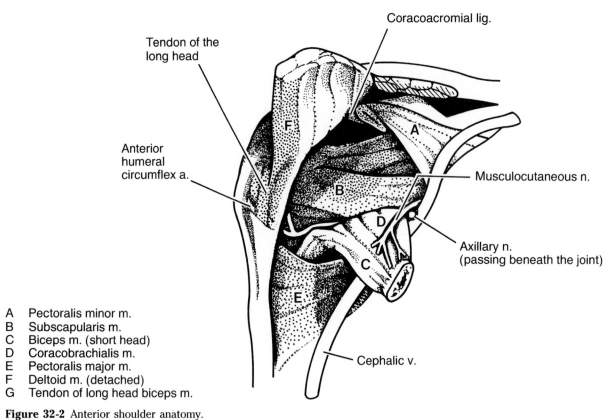

A Pectoralis minor m.
B Subscapularis m.
C Biceps m. (short head)
D Coracobrachialis m.
E Pectoralis major m.
F Deltoid m. (detached)
G Tendon of long head biceps m.

Figure 32-2 Anterior shoulder anatomy.

lar fibers of deltoid. The coracobrachialis and the short head of the biceps muscles are both retracted aside or reflected inferiorly after detachment of the coracoid tip. Other important structures attached to the coracoid include the conoid and trapezoid ligaments, which are responsible for the integrity of the acromioclavicular joint, and the fan-shaped coracoacromial ligament, which passes over the long head of the biceps in its groove and may be a factor in impingement syndromes. The subclavian vessels lie just beneath the coracoid.

The key muscle then exposed is the subscapularis. At its lower border are the circumflex scapular arteries and some large veins. Crossing it more medially is the neurovascular bundle entering the arm. The axillary nerve passes posteriorly beneath its lower border to reach a position inferior to the joint capsule before entering the quadrilateral space. Division of this muscle is difficult since it may be adherent to its immediate posterior relationship, the shoulder joint capsule, which may thus be entered inadvertently. After dividing the subscapularis, there is good access to the joint and to the glenoid labrum for major reconstructive shoulder joint surgery including joint replacement.

An alternative approach is to perform a limited split between the anterior and middle third of the deltoid muscle fibers (limited to 5 cm so that there will not be damage to axillary nerve branches to the anterior fibers). Such a split downward from the tip of the acromion will give limited access to the rotator cuff. To gain access to the supraspinous fossa, for example, to do a supraspinatus muscle slide for an old rotator cuff injury, the acromioclavicular joint must be excised.[1]

To gain access to the supraclavicular region for major brachial plexus or vascular work, it is occasionally necessary to remove all or part of the clavicle.

Posterior Relationships of the Shoulder Joint

The cape of the deltoid covers the shoulder joint posteriorly (Fig. 32-3). Its fibers may be detached from the spine of the scapula and the posterior acromial margin and retracted inferiorly to allow access to the next layer of muscles. The infraspinatus muscle may be divided to give direct access to the posterior shoulder joint capsule. Preserving all of or a portion of the teres minor muscles protects the axillary nerve and its important deltoid branch as it emerges from the quadrilateral space. Medially, the circumflex scapular vessels pass through the triangular space. The blending of the lateral and the long heads of the triceps forms the important seam of Henry. "Splitting the seam" gives access to the posterior aspect of the proximal humeral shaft and displays the ulnar and radial nerves as they diverge, the former eventually to reach the position behind the medial epicondyle and the latter to pass into the spiral groove to reach the anterior compartment on the lateral side.

Important relationships of the nerves originating from a brachial plexus to the artery and vein in the upper arm are shown in Fig. 32-4.

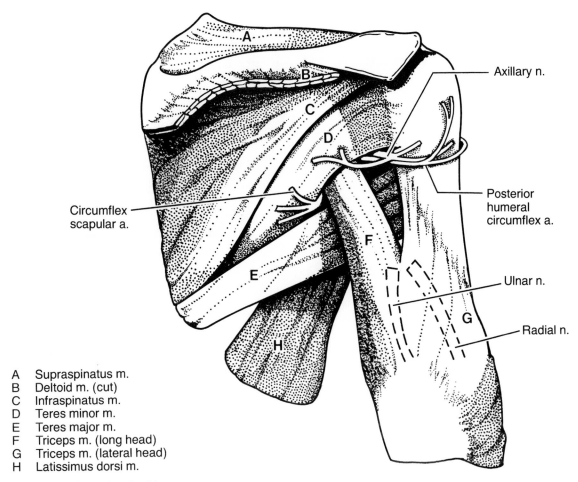

A   Supraspinatus m.
B   Deltoid m. (cut)
C   Infraspinatus m.
D   Teres minor m.
E   Teres major m.
F   Triceps m. (long head)
G   Triceps m. (lateral head)
H   Latissimus dorsi m.

Figure 32-3 Posterior shoulder anatomy.

Figure 32-4 Transverse section of upper arm at lower border of subscapularis muscle.

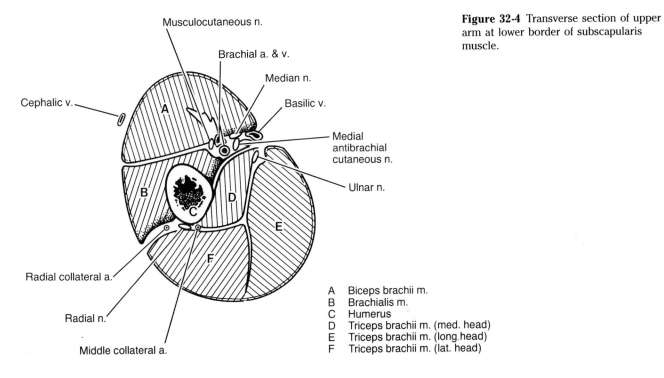

A   Biceps brachii m.
B   Brachialis m.
C   Humerus
D   Triceps brachii m. (med. head)
E   Triceps brachii m. (long head)
F   Triceps brachii m. (lat. head)

SECTION B

Surgical Anatomy of the Elbow

Roger Dee

The medial and lateral ligaments of the elbow are surgically significant. The *medial ligament* (Fig. 32-5) is composed of anterior and posterior oblique components and a small transverse nonfunctioning part in between.[3] The anterior oblique ligament runs from the under surface of the medial epicondyle to a small bony prominence on the medial aspect of the ulna just below the coronoid process. The posterior oblique ligament arises slightly posteriorly to its anterior component but inserts in a fan-shaped fashion across the entire length of the olecranon process. The anterior oblique fibers are more significant in maintaining stability than the posterior fibers. The anterior oblique ligament is essential for the stability of the elbow throughout its entire range of motion. If its integrity is maintained, the joint is stable even after removal of a large portion of the olecranon. The *lateral ligament complex* fans out from its origin from the lateral epicondyle to be inserted primarily into the annular ligament. It consequently has an indirect insertion into the ulna via the annular ligament but in addition there may also be some posterior marginal fibers passing directly from the lateral epicondyle into the ulna and comprising the lateral ulnar collateral ligament.[2] The anconeus muscle may function as an accessory lateral ligament.[1]

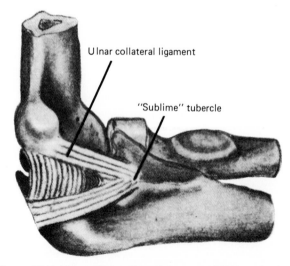

Figure 32-5 The medial collateral ligament (MCL) is divided into anterior and posterior bands and attached to a definite bony prominence on the ulna which also gives rise to some fibers of flexor digitorum superficialis (formerly called *sublimis* hence the term *sublime tubercle*). (*From Last, R. J., ed: Anatomy, Regional and Applied, 7th ed. New York, Churchill Livingstone. Reproduced with permission.*)

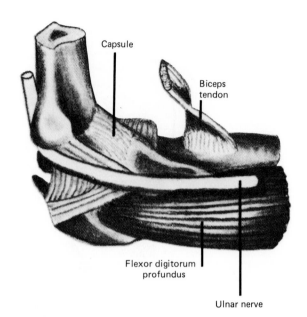

Figure 32-6 The relationship of the ulna nerve to the MCL and the bone. (*From Last, R. J., ed: Anatomy, Regional and Applied, 7th ed. New York, Churchill Livingstone. Reproduced with permission.*)

RELATIONS AND APPROACHES TO THE ELBOW JOINT

The proximity of the ulnar nerve to the medial elbow joint capsule deters routine medial approach to the elbow joint. This nerve, after passing behind the medial epicondyle and between the two heads of the flexor carpi ulnaris lies in immediate relationship to the ulna at its *sublime tubercle*. This tubercle gives part origin to the flexor digitorum superficialis muscle (Fig. 32-6). In this location it is particularly vulnerable during arthroplasty. However, if the nerve is identified and anteriorly displaced from its groove, access to both the posterior and anterior aspects of the elbow joint is available. This approach has been used for such procedures as medial joint synovectomy.

The most common surgical approaches to the elbow are the posterior approach, the lateral approach, or some combination thereof. In the posterior approach it is possible to split or flap the triceps tendon to obtain direct access to the elbow joint capsule. Palpation during pronation and supination will identify the posterolateral portion of the superior radial ulnar joint. Here between the anconeus muscle and the main extensor origin is a useful lateral portal of entry into the elbow (Kocher approach). It divides no muscles and there are no major neurovascular structures to be avoided except distally where the posterior interosseous nerve passes around the neck of the radius to reach the posterior compartment (Fig. 32-7). This incision is easily extended proximally by detaching the muscles from the lateral supracondylar ridge and freeing the triceps posteriorly. If the lateral ligament is detached from its lateral epicondylar origin, the whole joint can be opened for major reconstructive joint surgery including prosthetic arthroplasty while maintaining the integrity of the me-

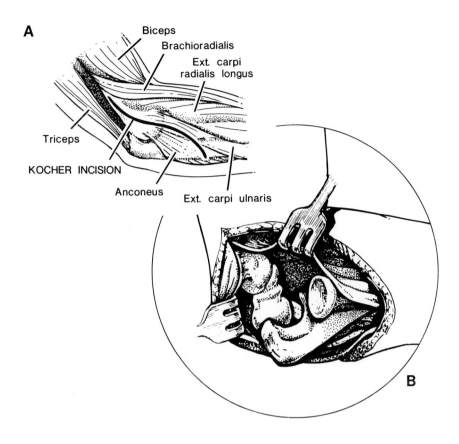

A

Biceps

Brachioradialis

Ext. carpi radialis longus

Triceps

KOCHER INCISION

Anconeus

Ext. carpi ulnaris

B

Figure 32-7 The lateral Kocher approach to the elbow. **A.** The skin incision. **B.** The view obtained after dislocation. It is necessary to fully supinate and flex the elbow if adequate exposure of the trochlear notch is required, e.g., in order to insert an ulnar component during total elbow arthroplasty. (*Modified from Crenshaw, A. H., ed: Campbell's Operative Orthopaedics, 6th ed. St. Louis, Mosby, 1980. Reproduced with permission.*)

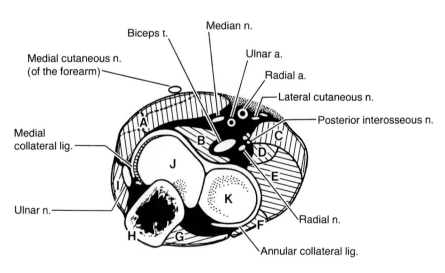

Biceps t.

Median n.

Medial cutaneous n. (of the forearm)

Ulnar a.

Radial a.

Lateral cutaneous n.

Posterior interosseous n.

Medial collateral lig.

Radial n.

Ulnar n.

Annular collateral lig.

Figure 32-8 Transverse section of right forearm at the level of the superior radio-ulnar joint. Note how a surgical approach between the brachialis and brachoradialis muscles will give access to important structures (anterior Henry approach).

A Superficial flexor muscles
B Brachialis m.
C Brachioradialis m.
D Extensor carpi radialis brevis m.
E Extensor carpi radialis longus m.
F Common extensor tendon
G Anconeus m.
H Olecranon process (cut)
I Flexor carpi ulnaris m.
J Trochlear notch
K Head of radius

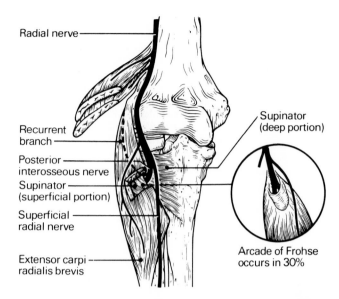

Figure 32-9 Diagram showing where the posterior interosseous nerve may be compressed either by the edge of the extensor carpi radialis brevis during pronation or where it passes between the deep and superficial layers of the supinator muscle. In 30 percent of adults there is a fibrous arch in the supinator termed the arcade of Frohse (see inset). (*From Wadsworth, T. G., ed: The Elbow, New York, Churchill Livingstone, 1982. Reproduced with permission.*)

dial collateral ligament. At the end of the procedure, the lateral ligament is carefully reattached to its origin.

A more anterior approach on the lateral side is between the extensor digitorum communis arising from the lateral epicondyle and those muscles arising from the lateral supracondylar ridge (the brachioradialis and extensors carpi radialis longus and brevis). This route usually has little advantage over the more posterolateral approach, and it is possible to lose the plane between these muscles. Moving more anteriorly, the Henry approach to the structures of the antecubital fossa and the proximal one-third of the radius is via the interval between the brachioradialis and the brachialis. This approach exposes the radial nerve and its posterior interosseous branch (Fig. 32-8). This branch and the radial recurrent artery pass beneath the arcade of Frohse in the superficial head of the supinator muscle. The supinator muscle is a key muscle in this area, and an understanding of its anatomy aids greatly in comprehension not only of the mode of displacement of proximal radial fractures but also the mode of entrapment of the posterior interosseous nerve (Fig. 32-9). The supinator consists of two separate bands of muscle. Deep fibers arise from the supinator crest of the ulna, wrap around the proximal radius, and insert into the radius between the anterior and posterior oblique lines in such a direction that they can axially rotate the bone into supination. Superficial fibers sweep downward and anteriorly from a separate origin at the humerus and insert similarly into the radius. The proximal medial margin of these superficial fibers is tendinous and forms the arcade of Frohse. The posterior interosseous nerve passes beneath the arcade and comes to lie superficial to the

deeper supinator fibers of the ulnar origin. The posterior interosseous nerve supplies this muscle only after it passes through it between the superficial and deep layers of fibers. Consequently, abnormal electromyographic changes may be detected in the muscle if the nerve is constricted beneath the arcade or within its intramuscular path.

Anteromedially, the brachial artery, accompanied by the median nerve, passes beneath a strong medial prolongation of the bicipital aponeurosis called the *lacertus fibrosus.* The brachial artery is close to bone in the supracondylar region and easily damaged by a fracture.

SECTION C

The Hand, Wrist, and Forearm: Anatomy of Surgical Exposures

Steven Sampson and David Chiu

SURGICAL EXPOSURE OF THE DIGITS

In the hand, anatomical considerations are paramount in planning the surgical approach. Optimal exposure can be attained by following four axioms of surgical exposures:[25] (1) Incisions must be designed so that the resultant scar does not cause restraint of joint motion. (2) The incision should not transgress flexion creases. An incision perpendicular to a flexion crease is certain to cause some restriction to extension but longitudinal midline incisions are permissible dorsally.[19] (3) The design of the incision should be tailored to avoid invasion of diamond contact zones and should border functional units[9,41] (Fig. 32-10). (4) Incisions must be topographically accurate. Littler and Chase have shown that any incision planned around intersecting diamond contact zones will allow excellent exposure and will minimize restriction of joint motion secondary to scar contracture.[1–4,9,14,19,24–26,29,33,41]

Surgical exposure of the digit is additionally guided by three basic interaxial digital lines:[9,23–25,41] (1) longitudinal, (2) transverse, and (3) oblique (see Figs. 32-12 to 32-14). Surgical incisions carried out in these planes undergo minimal change in length during active flexion and extension of the digit.

Distal Phalanx and Distal Interphalangeal Joint

Volarly, the DIP flexion crease lies 1 to 2 mm proximal to the joint space of the DIP joint.[22,23] The center of the dermal

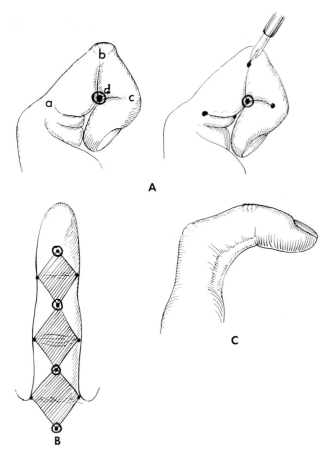

Figure 32-10 A. Preoperative planning of skin incisions may be carried out by flexing the interphalangeal joints maximally and by placing a mark (black dot) at the dorsal extent of each digital flexion crease (a, b, c). **B.** With digital extension, the polar contact points (circled dot) become evident as midvolar apices of the three basic diamond contact zones of the digit. **C.** Scar contracture is inevitable when incisions longitudinally transgress a diamond contact zone. (*From Chase, R. A.: Atlas of Hand Surgery, vol I. Philadelphia, Saunders, 1973. Reproduced with permission.*)

ridges of the whirl pattern of each terminal unit correspond to the region of the flexor digitorum profundus insertion as well as the center of the sterile matrix of the nail. Therefore, surgical exposure of the terminal flexor tendon insertion need not be extended beyond this central landmark. Also, a K-wire traction pin placed perpendicular to the axis of the distal phalanx through this landmark will not injure the germinal matrix.[2]

At the apex of the volar interaxial approach to the DIP joint, the neurovascular bundles are extremely superficial and vulnerable to injury. In addition, at this level, the neurovascular bundles tend to ramify into small branches to the nail fold, the terminal fingertip, and the pulp.[44,45] The drastic decrease in artery diameter as it ramifies makes this a critical level in consideration of the feasibility of replantation of the fingertip.

The longitudinal midaxial or dorsolateral exposure to the terminal zone of the digit is useful for gaining exposure to the

articular surfaces of the distal interphalangeal joint, the terminal extensor tendon, and the proximal portion of the distal phalanx. On approaching the base of the distal phalanx, it is important to maintain a plane dorsal to the insertion of the lateral intraosseous ligaments on either ungual spine and lateral tubercle of the distal phalanx. Such an incision will not compromise the vascular supply of the pulp of that region, which passes through a fibroosseous hiatus called the rima ungualum[35,36] (Fig. 32-11).

The dorsal exposure of the distal interphalangeal joint and the terminal tendon insertion can be carried out by combining modifications of the longitudinal midaxial and transverse axial incisions in the so-called H incision (line A on Fig. 32-12). In developing the distal extent of the H incision, care must be taken to avoid injury to the germinal matrix by preserving the distal 4 mm of the eponychium.

Middle Phalanx, Proximal Interphalangeal Joint, and Proximal Phalanx

This phalangeal segment includes the important PIP joint and its surrounding complex anatomy which must be preserved. In this zone, the extensor mechanism embraces the proximal and middle phalanges along its dorsal and lateral borders. Any surgical exposure dorsal to the longitudinal midaxial plane must also preserve the primary venous and lymphatic drainage of the digit.[12,21,27,31] These vessels are located in the subareolar tissue plane above the aponeurosis or the exten-

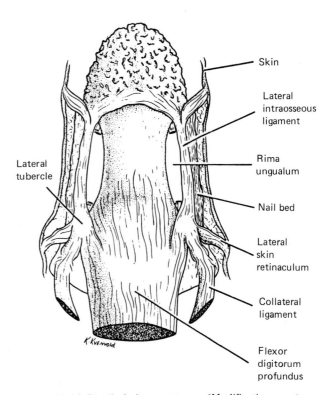

Figure 32-11 Distal phalanx anatomy. (*Modification courtesy of Marvin Shrewsbury; from Shrewsbury, M. M., and Johnson, R. K., J Bone Joint Surg 57A:785, 1975.*)

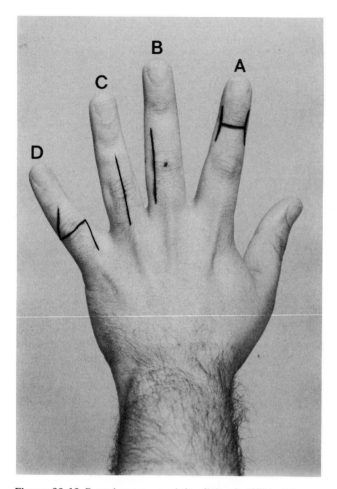

Figure 32-12 Dorsal exposure of the digits. **A.** "H" incision—greater extensile articular exposure may require division of a collateral ligament. **B.** Dorsolateral approach. **C.** Middorsal approach. **D.** Bayonette incision.

sor mechanism. The dorsal veins are readily visible when the hand is placed in a dependent position prior to exsanguination. Careful preoperative planning of the skin incision ensures preservation of these vessels. By following a middorsal longitudinal incision (line C on Fig. 32-12) throughout this segment, large skin flaps of skin exposure can be raised in the subareolar plane, providing good access to deeper structures. Through a dorsolateral approach[16] (line B on Fig. 32-12) to the base of the middle phalanx, the head of the proximal phalanx as well as the shaft of the proximal phalanx can be exposed by entering a plane between the central tendon and the lateral band. This exposure is aided by a flexion maneuver of the PIP joint, thereby causing the migration of the lateral bands volarly. Pratt[32] has advised a central tendon splitting exposure at the level of the shaft of the proximal phalanx. However, a gently curved incision through the skin would be recommended to avoid the greater likelihood of scar adherence if this were carried out in one single line of exposure from skin to bone. A bayonette incision (line D on Fig. 32-12) with the central limb crossing the PIP joint may also be selected. However, with this approach, a greater opportunity

exists to injure the contralateral dorsal venous drainage of the digit.

The lateral approach to this middle phalangeal segment can be accomplished by two routes:[4,25,26] (1) a midlateral Bunnell approach and (2) a midaxial longitudinal approach (Fig. 32-13). The classic midlateral or true lateral exposure is initiated within the volar skin containing papillary ridges and passes in a plane just volar to the neurovascular bundle. A midaxial longitudinal exposure of the digit passes in a plane that lies dorsal to the neurovascular bundle.

The topographical surgical landmarks of the midaxial approach are guided by three anatomical considerations.[25] Firstly, the volar proximal interphalangeal joint flexion crease coincides with the corresponding joint space which is unique among the other small joints of the hand.[33] Secondly, the line of exposure through the skin passes through the line connecting the lateral apices of the volar diamond pattern, i.e., the edges of these flexion creases (Fig. 32-13). Finally, this plane coincidentally passes longitudinally through a plane on the skin surface that can be identified by a change in skin texture between the relatively smooth dorsal skin versus the volar skin with its distinct papillary ridges.

One major advantage of the longitudinal midaxial incision is that it allows early postoperative motion to begin because little tension is generated on flexion and extension in this axis. Likewise, it is important to realize that this axis will tend to migrate dorsally in the swollen edematous state and that it may also do so in a child whose subcutaneous fat may distort the normal landmarks present in the adult.[23-26]

Utilizing these lateral approaches, one may gain entry to the dorsolateral and volar-lateral portions of the middle phalangeal segment, i.e., the proximal interphalangeal joint. These lateral approaches may be combined with volar oblique transaxial incisions (Fig. 32-14) which will enable one to gain access to both sides of the flexor tendon sheath and the accompanying neurovascular bundles. An important anatomical consideration in this combined approach is the relationship of the neurovascular bundle to the lateral retaining skin ligaments of the digits.[1,10,15,18,25,28,29,38] These retaining or retinacular ligaments attain their greatest fiber diameter and functional significance in this middle phalangeal segment. These ligaments act as a sling with the more dorsal ligaments called Cleland's and the more volar ones called Grayson's (Fig. 32-15). Upon entering through the midaxial skin plane, deeper dissection may be made dorsal to this sling in order to obtain adequate exposure to the PIP joint and its collateral ligaments, or it may be made volar to the sling with retraction of the neurovascular bundle dorsally, in order to expose the flexor tendon sheath (Fig. 32-13). Thus, these ligaments are important for locating and protecting the neurovascular bundle.

The volar approach to this phalangeal zone is primarily for zone 2 flexor tendon injuries. In general, strategic extension of any laceration along an interaxial skin incision will minimize dissection and provide adequate exposure of the zone of injury. Such a concept must be incorporated in the overall design of the skin incision in order to minimize the primary injury. Therefore, it is often necessary to combine a longitudinal midaxial incision with a volar oblique interaxial incision to gain adequate exposure of the tendon sheath. These incisions are easily extended into the palm (Fig. 32-14).

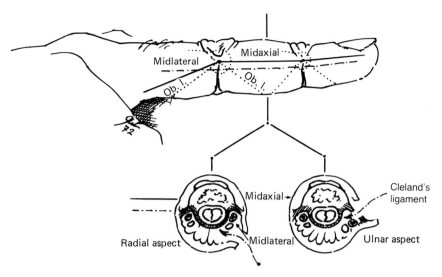

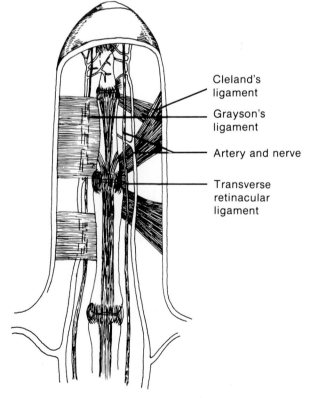

Figure 32-13 Lateral approaches of the digit: (1) midlateral (Bunnell); (2) midaxial; (3) oblique. Release of retinacular (Cleland's) ligaments allows the volar skin flap to be mobilized while the neurovascular bundle remains in place. (*From Littler, J. W., in Littler, J. W., et al, eds: Symposium on Reconstructive Hand Surgery. St. Louis, Mosby, 1974. Reproduced with permission.*)

Technically, the skin incisions are planned to optimize exposure of the sheath as well as to provide healthy flap coverage in an attempt to minimize scar adherence postoperatively.

In summary, the volar approach to the digit is by way of the oblique interaxial line.[24] In 1967, Bruner described the zigzag volar incision for flexor tendon surgery.[5,6] The major difference between these two volar zigzag approaches is that Littler has emphasized that digital exposure should extend to the midaxial line in order to minimize secondary scar contracture at the level of the flexion crease. His concept is of utmost importance in the region of the PIP joint in that this joint contributes 80 percent of motion to the extrinsic arc.[23]

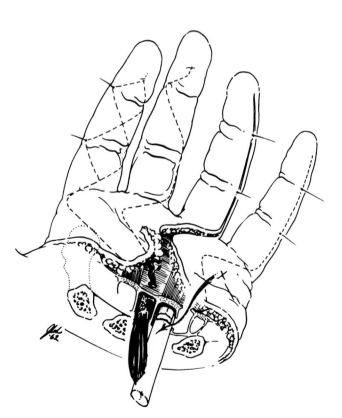

Figure 32-14 Volar oblique transaxial zigzag approach (1962). This approach has been outlined on the long finger, whereas a midaxial approach has been incised on the ring finger. (*From Littler, J. W., in Converse, J. M., ed: Reconstructive Plastic Surgery, Philadelphia, Saunders, 1977. Reproduced with permission.*)

Figure 32-15 Retinacular ligaments of the digit (volar exposure): (1) Grayson's ligament lies more volar than the neurovascular bundle. (2) On the right, Grayson's ligament has been removed. The neurovascular bundle is seen lying on the more dorsal Cleland's ligament. (*From Milford, L. W.: Retaining Ligaments of the Digits of the Hand. Philadelphia, Saunders, 1968. Reproduced with permission.*)

Proximal Phalanx, Metacarpophalangeal Joint, and Metacarpal

The topographical landmarks of this zone are primarily located on the palmar surface of the hand. In the extended hand, the distal palmar crease lies approximately 1 to 2 mm proximal to the metacarpophalangeal joint of the long ring and little fingers.[33] Likewise, the proximal palmar crease lies in similar proximity to the MP joint space of the index finger. The digital palmar flexion creases at the level of the web space correspond approximately to the midproximal phalanx level. Thus, incisions crossing this plane do not cause scar contracture as much as incisions crossing the plane of the joint. However, incisions crossing the commissure of the web spaces often cause significant skin contracture. Therefore, surgical exposure of the web space is always carried out by avoiding incisions that traverse the commissure perpendicularly. For extensile exposure to one or two of the four ulnar metacarpal bones or their respective joints a dorsolateral approach is favored with gently curved proximal or distal extensions. These longitudinal skin exposures also tend to parallel the extensive venous and lymphatic drainage of the hand. For the specific purpose of elective reconstructive surgery of the MP joints of the ulnar for digits, a transverse inci-

sion at the level of the MP joints is favored.[39] However, care must be taken to preserve the venous drainage of the digits and the dorsal sensory nerves. Deeper dissection requires longitudinal exposure either through an extensor tendon splitting incision or a dorsolateral exposure through the sagittal band and then entry into the metacarpophalangeal joint itself. More proximally, access to the metacarpals may be obtained by middorsal exposure with retraction of the extensor tendons.

The exposure of the palmar structures of the hand can be carried out in an individualized manner or by using an extensile total palmar exposure approach.[25] When individualized digital palmar exposures require proximal extension toward the wrist crease, incisions should parallel the thenar crease in an intereminential plane. Distal to the distal palmar crease, the neurovascular structures are more easily injured. Just distal to the superficial transverse metacarpal ligament, the neurovascular bundles lie much more volar and superficial.[18,38] When a more proximal extensile exposure is required, an incision paralleling the distal palmar crease is carried out with an oblique extension toward the intereminential point of the wrist crease. This oblique extension should coincide with the radial border of the ring fin-

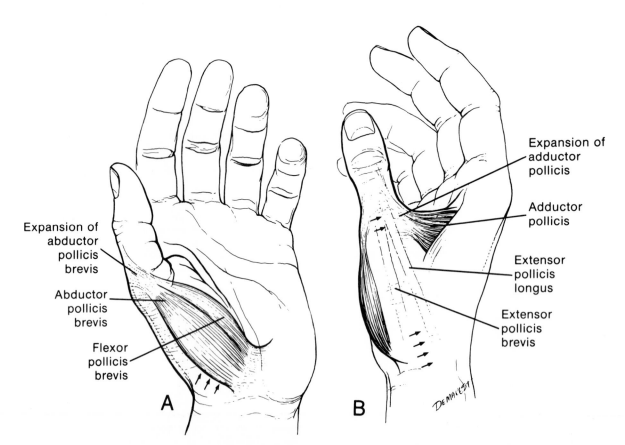

Figure 32-16 Exposure of thumb. **A.** Carpometacarpal joint of the thumb. The dorsoradial exposure interval lies between the extensor pollicis brevis and the abductor pollicis brevis (arrows). **B.** Metacarpophalangeal joint of the thumb. The dorsal exposure interval lies between the long and short extensors (arrows). (*Modified from Kaplan, E. B., and Riordan, D. C., in Spinner, M., ed: Kaplan's Functional and Surgical Anatomy of the Hand, 3d ed. Philadelphia, Lippincott, 1984. Reproduced with permission.*)

ger so as to correspond to the deeper ulnar border of the transverse flexor retinaculum, i.e., the ulnar border of the carpal tunnel.[7,8,40]

SURGICAL EXPOSURE OF THE THUMB

Interphalangeal Joint

The basic surgical anatomy for exposure of the IP joint of the thumb closely corresponds to that which has already been described for the DIP joint of the digits.

Metacarpophalangeal Joint

Metacarpophalangeal joint exposure closely corresponds to that described for exposure of the digital middle phalangeal segment and proximal interphalangeal joint. An exception to this generalized statement is that once the dorsum of the MP joint is approached through the skin, the deeper exposure is usually aided by splitting the interval between the extensor pollicis brevis and the extensor pollicis longus[20,38] (Fig. 32-16B). The remainder of the dorsal approach closely parallels the middle phalangeal zone, carefully avoiding injury to the dorsal venous supply of the thumb and the sensory branches of the radial nerve. A midaxial incision along the radial aspect of the thumb provides excellent exposure for the volar aspect of the digit (Fig. 32-16A). When exposure is required proximal to the MP flexion crease, incisions should be placed parallel to the dorsoradial aspect of the thumb metacarpal along the periphery of the functional cutaneous zone of the thenar eminence.[41]

Carpometacarpal Joint

There are two basic surgical approaches to the basal joint of the thumb: Firstly, a dorsoradial approach[18,39] begins with a longitudinal incision over the radialmost edge of the first metacarpal extending proximally with a gentle curve. The incision is carried down through the interval between the abductor pollicis longus and the extensor pollicis brevis with care to protect the branches of the radial nerve and the dorsoradial branches of the radial artery from injury. A more extensile approach to this region is a radiopalmar (Wagner)[13,43] approach that begins distally in the midaxial line of the first metacarpal along its radial axis. This axis is again noted similar to that found in the digit where a change in skin texture aids in its localization. As the incision passes proximally along the axis of the first metacarpal, it is gently curved into the line of the wrist flexion crease. Deeper extraperiosteal elevation of the abductor pollicis brevis will enable excellent exposure of the basal joint (Fig. 32-16A).[11]

SURGICAL EXPOSURE OF THE WRIST

Dorsal Exposure

Major surgical reconstructions of the wrist can be safely performed through a straight or gently angled dorsal incision.[1,18–20,30,39] Various S-shaped incisions have also been used for major reconstructive procedures of the wrist, but such incisions often place the distalmost corner of the skin flap in jeopardy in susceptible patients. Otherwise, where limited surgical dissection is required, a dorsal transverse wrist crease incision is perhaps more cosmetic. Limited exposure of the distal ulna can be accomplished by a gently curved dorsoulnar longitudinal incision in the region just distal to the ulnar styloid. Care must be taken to avoid injury to the dorsal sensory branch of the ulnar nerve. Likewise, a dorsoradial approach may be used in order to expose the scaphoid. This approach may be carried out with a zigzag skin incision with the central limb of the Z within the lines of Langer in the dorsoradial wrist flexion crease. The deeper interval of dissection is carried between the extensor pollicis brevis and the extensor pollicis longus, with the former being retracted volarly along with the sensory branch of the radial nerve. Care is taken to avoid injury to the radial artery which passes dorsally between the first and third extensor compartments.[18]

Volar Approach

The most important volar approach to the wrist and surrounding region is one that is a continuation of the carpal tunnel approach previously described. Continuing proximally from the intereminential point at the wrist crease, the incision is carried obliquely and ulnarward toward the radial border of the flexor carpi ulnaris tendon in the distal forearm. This is carried out in order to avoid injury to the palmar cutaneous branch of the median nerve.[7,8] Upon deeper dissection, the antebrachial fascia is traversed longitudinally, the median nerve with its sensory branch and radial artery are retracted radially, and the flexor tendons are then retracted ulnarly. Exposure of the volar distal radius may be obtained by elevating the pronator quadratus from the distal radius. Exposure to the volar-carpal region is carried out by T'ing the volar capsule in such a way as to be able to resuture the flaps once dissected. This incision can be extended both proximally and distally as described below.[16,18]

A more direct and limited exposure of the scaphoid may be carried out by the Russe approach.[18,34] This is carried out through a longitudinal incision in the region of the flexor carpi radialis tendon and extended distally a short distance in a gently curved manner toward the midaxis of the radial border of the first metacarpal. The incision is then carried deeper following retraction of the radial artery radially and the flexor carpi radialis ulnarly. The floor of the flexor carpi radialis tendon sheath is incised and the capsule of the wrist is also incised and T'd so as to allow adequate exposure of the operative site.

SURGICAL EXPOSURE OF THE MID- AND DISTAL FOREARM

Knowledge of the internervous planes of the forearm[17,37] is critically important for surgical exposure in that region. Utilizing these planes between muscle groups innervated by dif-

TABLE 32-1 Internervous Planes of the Forearm

Exposure	Muscle group interval	Neural interval	Anatomical region	Figure
Dorsal	FCU-ECU	Ulnar-radial	Ulnar shaft	13
Dorsoradial	Anconeus-ECU	Radial-PIN	Radial head	14
Dorsoradial (Thompson)	EDC-ECRB	PIN-radial	Dorsal radius	15
Volar-radial (Henry)	BR/flexor-pronator	Radial-median	Volar radius	16
Volar-ulnar	FDS-FCU	Medial-ulnar	Ulnar nerve and artery	17

Key:
FCU: Flexor carpi ulnaris
ECU: Extensor carpi ulnaris
EDC: Extensor digitorum communis
ECRB: Extensor carpi radialis brevis
BR: Brachioradialis
FDS: Flexor digitorum superficialis
PIN: Posterior interosseous nerve

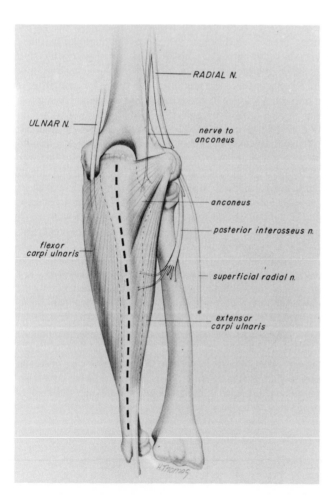

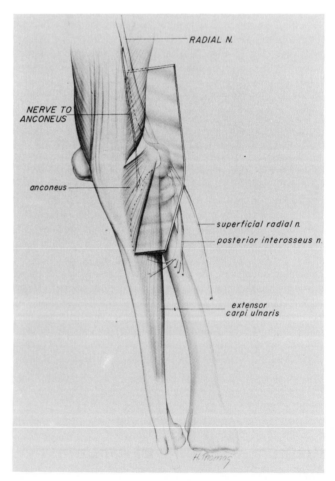

Figure 32-17 Dorsal exposure of ulnar shaft. (See also Table 32-1.) (*From Spinner, M.: Injuries to the Major Branches of Peripheral Nerves of the Forearm, 2d ed. Philadelphia, Saunders, 1978. Reproduced with permission.*)

Figure 32-18 Plane for proximal dorsoradial exposure in the region of radial head. (See Table 32-1.) (*From Spinner, M.: Injuries to the Major Branches of Peripheral Nerves of the Forearm, 2d ed. Philadelphia, Saunders, 1978. Reproduced with permission.*)

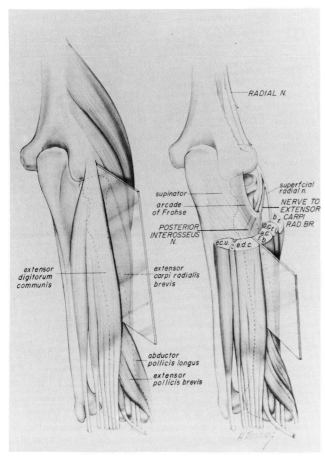

Figure 32-19 Plane for dorsoradial exposure to radial shaft (Thompson). (See also Table 32-1.) (*From Spinner, M.: Injuries to the Major Branches of Peripheral Nerves of the Forearm, 2d ed. Philadelphia, Saunders, 1978. Reproduced with permission.*)

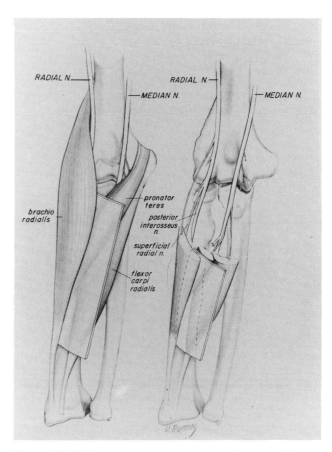

Figure 32-20 Plane for volar approach to radial shaft (Henry). (See also Table 32-1.) (*From Spinner, M.: Injuries to the Major Branches of Peripheral Nerves of the Forearm, 2d ed. Philadelphia, Saunders, 1978. Reproduced with permission.*)

ferent peripheral nerves, one will not only accurately expose the required structures but minimize postoperative complications such as nerve injury and fibrosis of the forearm. Spinner has superbly illustrated the required internervous planes of exposure and this can be seen in Table 32-1 as well as in Fig. 32-17 to 32-21.

Finally, the surgical plan of forearm exposure should not only incorporate accurate localization of the deeper structures by way of internervous planes; it should also take into consideration the required flap coverage for any future surgical reconstruction which may be necessary.[25]

REFERENCES

Section A: The Shoulder and Arm

1. Haleri, G.B., and Wiley, A.M. Advancement of the supraspinatus muscle in the repair of the rotator cuff. J Bone Joint Surg 63A:232–238, 1981.
2. Turkel, S.J., et al. Stabilising mechanisms preventing anterior dislo-

cation of the gleno-humeral joint. J Bone Joint Surg 63A:1208–1217, 1981.
3. Warren R.F. Subluxation of the shoulder in athletes. Clin Sports Med 2:339–354, 1983.

Section B: Surgical Anatomy of the Elbow

1. Basmajian, J.V., and Griffin, W.R. Function of Anconeus muscle. J Bone Joint Surg 54A:1712–1714, 1972.
2. Morrey, B.F., and An, K. Functional anatomy of the ligaments of the elbow. Clin Orthop 201:84–90, 1985.
3. Schwabe, G.H., Bennett, J.B., Woods, G.W., and Tullos, H.S. The role of the medial collateral ligament. Clin Orthop 146:42–52, 1980.

Section C: The Hand, Wrist, and Forearm

1. Adamson, J.E., and Fleury, A.F. Incisions in the hand and wrist, in Green, D.P. (ed): *Operative Hand Surgery.* New York, Churchill Livingstone, 1982, pp 1263–1281.
2. Beasley, R.W. *Hand Injuries,* Philadelphia, Saunders, 1981 pp 79, 138.
3. Borges, A.F. *Elective Incisions and Scar Revision.* Boston, Little, Brown, 1973, pp 1–14.

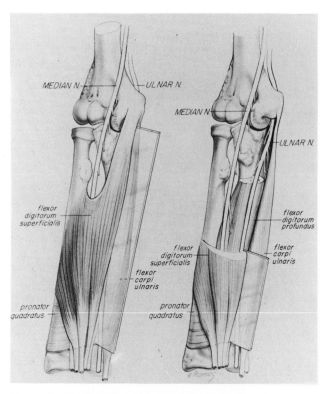

Figure 32-21 Plane for volar exposure to ulnar neurovascular structures. (See also Table 32-1.) (*From Spinner, M.: Injuries to the Major Bnches of Peripheral Nerves of the Forearm, 2d ed. Philadelphia, Saunders, 1978. Reproduced with permission.*)

4. Boyes, J.H. *Bunnel's Surgery of the Hand,* 5th ed. Philadelphia, Lippincott, 1970.
5. Bruner, J.M. The zig-zag volar-digital incision for flexor tendon surgery. Plast Reconstr Surg 40:571–574, 1967.
6. Bruner, J.M. Surgical exposure of flexor tendons in the hand. Ann R Coll Surg Engl 53:84–94, 1973.
7. Burton, R., and Littler, J.W. Non-traumatic soft tissue afflictions of the hand, in *Current Problems in Surgery.* Chicago, Year Book, 1975, pp 1–56.
8. Carroll, R.E., and Green, D.P. The significance of the palmer cutaneous nerve at the wrist. Clin Orthop 83:24–28, 1972.
9. Chase, R.A. Atlas of Hand Surgery, Philadelphia, Saunders, 1973, pp 35–39.
10. Cleland, F. The cutaneous ligaments of the phalanges. J Anat Physiol 12:526, 1878.
11. Eaton, R.G. *Joint Injuries of the Hand.* Springfield, Thomas, 1971, pp 69–72.
12. Eaton, R.G. The digital neurovascular bundle—A microanatomic study of its contents. Clin Orthop 61:176–185, 1968.
13. Eaton, R.G., and Littler, J.W. Ligament reconstruction for the painful thumb carpometacarpal joint. J Bone Joint Surg 55A:1655, 1973.
14. Graham, W.P. Incisions, amputations and skin grafting in the hand. Orthop Clin North Am 1:213–218, 1970.
15. Grayson, J. The cutaneous ligaments of the digits. J Anat 75:164, 1941.
16. Heim, U., and Pfeiffer, K.M. *Small Fragment Set Manual.* Berlin, Springer-Verlag, 1982, pp 129–194.
17. Henry, A.K. *Extensile Exposure,* 2d ed. Baltimore, Williams & Wilkins, 1970, pp 100–106.
18. Hoppenfeld, S., and deBoer, P. *Surgical Exposures in Orthopaedics.* Philadelphia, Lippincott, 1984, pp 141–208.
19. Howard, F.M., and McFarlane, R.M. Lacerations, incisions and scars, in Sandzen, S.C. (ed): *The Hand and Wrist.* Baltimore, Williams & Wilkins, 1985, pp 99–106.
20. Kaplan, E.B. *Surgical Approaches to the Neck, Cervical Spine and Upper Extremity.* Philadelphia, Saunders, 1966, pp 135–227.
21. Lampe, E.W. Surgical anatomy of the hand. Ciba Found Symp 3(8): 66–109, 1951.
22. Lister, G. *The Hand: Diagnosis and Indications.* Edinburgh, Churchill Livingstone, 1984.
23. Littler, J.W. The severed flexor tendon. Surg Clin North Am 39:435, 1959.
24. Littler, J.W. The hand, in Cooper, P. (ed): *The Craft of Surgery.* Boston, Little, Brown, 1964, pp 1287–1313.
25. Littler, J.W. Hand, wrist and forearm incisions, in Littler J.W., et al (eds): *Symposium on Reconstructive Surgery.* St. Louis, Mosby, vol 9, 1974, pp 89–97.
26. Littler, J.W. Principles of reconstructive surgery of the hand, in Converse, J.M. (ed): *Reconstructive Plastic Surgery.* Philadelphia, Saunders, 1977, pp 3102–3153.
27. Lucas, G. The pattern of venous drainage of the digits. J Hand Surg 9A:448–450, 1984.
28. Milford, L. *Retaining Ligaments of the Digits of the Hand.* Philadelphia, Saunders, 1968, p 39.
29. Milford, L. The hand, in Crenshaw, A.H. (ed): *Campbell's Operative Orthopaedics,* 6th ed. St. Louis, Mosby, 1987, pp 111–149.
30. Millender, L.H., and Nalebuff, E.A. Arthrodesis of the rheumatoid wrist; an evaluation of sixty patients and description of a different surgical technique. J Bone Joint Surg 55A:1026–1034, 1973.
31. Moss, S.H., Schwartz, K.A., von-Drasek-Ascher, G., Ogden, L.L., Wheeler, C.S., and Lister, G.D. Digital venous anatomy. J Hand Surg 10A:473–482, 1985.
32. Pratt, D.R. Exposing fractures of the proximal phalanx of the finger longitudinally through the dorsal extensor apparatus. Clin Orthop 15:22–26, 1959.
33. Rank, B.K., Wakefield, A.R., and Hueston, J.T. *Surgery of Repair as Applied to Hand Injuries,* 4th ed. Edinburgh, Churchill Livingstone, 1973, pp 15–59.
34. Russe, O. Fracture of the carpal navicular. J Bone Joint Surg 42A: 759–768, 1960.
35. Shrewsbury, M.M., and Johnson, R.K. The fascia of the distal phalanx. J Bone Joint Surg 57A:784–788, 1975.
36. Shrewsbury, M.M., and Johnson, R.K. Form, function and evolution of the distal phalanx. J Hand Surg 8:475–479, 1983.
37. Spinner, M. *Injuries to the Major Branches of Peripheral Nerves of the Forearm,* 2d ed. Philadelphia, Saunders, 1978, pp 67–77.
38. Spinner, M. *Kaplan's Functional and Surgical Anatomy of the Hand,* 3d ed. Philadelphia, Lippincott, 1984, pp 361–397.
39. Swanson, A.B. Reconstructive surgery in the arthritic hand and foot. Ciba Found Symp 31(6): pp 8, 20, 25, 26, 1979.
40. Taleisnik, J. The palmar cutaneous branch of the median nerve and the approach to the carpal tunnel. J Bone Joint Surg 55:1212–1217, 1973.
41. Tubiana, R. Surgical exposure and skin coverage, in Tubiana, R. (ed): *The Hand,* vol II, chap 33. Philadelphia, Saunders, 1985, pp 226–241.
42. Tubiana, R. Methods of skin closure, in Tubiana, R. (ed): *The Hand,* vol II, chap 33, Philadelphia, Saunders, 1985, p 245.
43. Wagner, C.J. Method of treatment of Bennett's fracture dislocation. Am J Surg 80:230–231, 1950.
44. Zook, E., Van Beel, A.L., Russel, R.C., and Beatty, M.C. Anatomy and physiology of the perionychium: A review of the literature and anatomical study. J Hand Surg 5:528–536, 1980.
45. Zook, E. The perionychium. Clin Plast Surg 8:21–31, 1981.

CHAPTER 33

Biomechanics of the Upper Extremity

Michael D. Ries, Lawrence C. Hurst, and Roger Dee

SECTION A

Biomechanics of the Shoulder

Michael D. Ries

The upper limb is suspended from the axial skeleton primarily by muscle and ligament attachments. The suspension system is provided by the scapulothoracic articulation and by three synovial joints: the glenohumeral, acromioclavicular, and sternoclavicular. Motion at these joints permits the upper limb and hand to be positioned in space, and the system provides a fulcrum for load-bearing activities of the upper extremity.

KINEMATICS

Either abduction from zero to 180 degrees or forward flexion from zero to 180 degrees will place the arm at the same overhead position. In this position, the medial epicondyle points forward and medially.[13]

Abduction to 180 degrees in the coronal plane requires external rotation of the humerus to prevent impingement of the greater tuberosity on the coracoacromial arch.[4] The greater tuberosity rotates posteriorly with external rotation and slides underneath the arch so that the arm can be fully abducted. With the arm in 60 degrees of internal rotation, abduction is blocked beyond 120 degrees, and patients with internal rotation contractures will have limited abduction because of this anatomical relationship.[20]

The plane of the scapula, rather than the coronal plane, has been recommended as the reference plane for consideration of shoulder motion.[7,9,19] The scapular plane is oriented 30 degrees anterior to the coronal plane (Fig. 33-1).[31] In the scapular plane, the inferior portion of the capsule is not twisted, the supraspinatus and deltoid are optimally aligned for elevation of the arm,[19] and no rotation of the humerus is required for full abduction.[9]

The full range of abduction involves approximately 120 degrees of glenohumeral and 60 degrees of scapulothoracic

motion (Fig. 33-2).[31] The ratio of glenohumeral to scapulothoracic motion is termed *scapulohumeral rhythm*. This ratio is dependent upon the reference plane used. For abduction in the coronal plane between 30 and 170 degrees, Inman, Saunders, and Abbott found a constant glenohumeral to scapulothoracic ratio of 2:1.[8] For each 15 degrees of abduction, 10 degrees occurred at the glenohumeral joint and 5 degrees occurred at the scapulothoracic articulation. Abduction from zero to 30 degrees involves primarily glenohumeral motion. For abduction in the scapular plane, Freedman and Monro determined a ratio of 1.35:1.[7] Poppen and Walker found a similar ratio of 1.25:1 for abduction beyond 30 degrees in the scapular plane and abnormal scapulohumeral rhythm was associated with significant shoulder disease.[19]

Scapulothoracic movement during abduction involves the sum of motion at the sternoclavicular and acromioclavicular joints. The clavicle elevates 4 degrees at the sternoclavicular joint for each 10 degrees of abduction.[8] Beyond 90 degrees of abduction, further elevation of the clavicle is negligible. Approximately 20 degrees of motion occurs at the acromioclavicular joint. This occurs during the early phase of abduction, between zero and 30 degrees, and beyond 135 degrees.[8] Between 30 and 135 degrees of abduction, acromioclavicular motion is negligible.

Motion between the scapula and clavicle at the acromioclavicular joint is possible due to rotation of the clavicle around its long axis. Without this rotation the coracoclavicular ligament would prevent acromioclavicular motion during abduction. The curve of the clavicle acts as a crankshaft allowing a relative elongation of the coracoclavicular ligament.

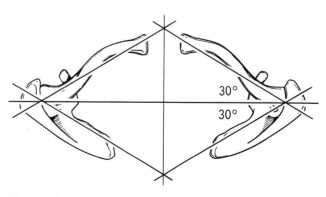

Figure 33-1 Relation of scapular plane to coronal and sagittal planes.

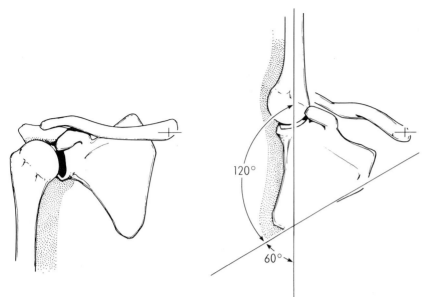

Figure 33-2 Glenohumeral and scapulothoracic motion during abduction. From 0 degrees to 180 degrees of abduction it involves approximately 60 degrees of scapulothoracic and 120 degrees of glenohumeral motion.

Approximately 50 degrees of clavicular rotation occurs during abduction. If this rotation is prevented, abduction is limited to 110 degrees.[8]

MUSCLES CONTROLLING GLENOHUMERAL MOTION

The main abductors of the glenohumeral joint are the deltoid and supraspinatus.[5] The long head of the biceps is active during abduction when the forearm is supinated.[2] The infraspinatus, subscapularis, and teres minor act to depress the humeral head during abduction.

Since the relatively shallow glenoid does not provide a stable fulcrum during elevation of the arm, the deltoid tends to displace the humeral head out of the glenoid.[3] With the arm by the side, the deltoid acts to pull the humerus up, subluxing the head superiorly. On further abduction, the deltoid pulls the humeral head into the glenoid. When the arm is overhead the deltoid tends to sublux the humeral head inferiorly. The rotater cuff prevents this subluxation by pressing the humeral head into the glenoid. The deltoid and rotator cuff are considered a *force couple.* A force couple consists of two opposing forces acting on an object and separated by some distance so that rotation of the object results. In this case the deltoid and rotator cuff provide the two forces necessary to cause rotation, i.e., abduction of the humerus (Fig. 33-3). The rotator cuff alone is capable of abducting the arm, but with about 50 percent of normal power.[30] Full abduction is also possible with loss of the supraspinatus alone, although the endurance and force of abduction are diminished.[34] Rupture of the rotator cuff is associated with pain and limited ability to abduct the arm.[16]

Saha has described a "zero position" of the glenohumeral joint where the humeroscapular aligned axis coincides with the axes of muscles crossing the shoulder.[27,28] This position is approximately 165 degrees of abduction in the plane of the

scapula. The deforming muscle forces are minimized, and Milch has recommended the position for reduction of dislocations and fracture dislocations of the shoulder.[14]

The effectiveness of the deltoid is enhanced by its multipennate fiber arrangement. With the fibers arranged in this angular manner, the overall change in length of the deltoid required for a given contraction force is less than that for a muscle with a parallel arrangement of fibers such as the biceps. The deltoid is thus designed for powerful activity, whereas the biceps is designed for rapid activity.[6] In addition, as the scapula rotates during abduction, the acromium moves away from the deltoid insertion which maintains the deltoid nearer to its resting length.[12] This explains the powerful shoulder strength possible with the arm overhead.

The muscles involved in adduction of the humerus are the latissimus dorsi, clavicular and sternal heads of the pectoralis major, and teres major.[6,31]

Forward flexion is controlled by the clavicular portion of the pectoralis major and the anterior fibers of the deltoid.

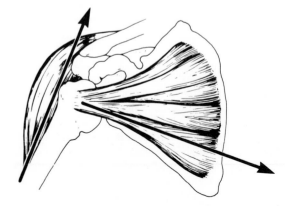

Figure 33-3 Muscle force vectors showing the force couple created by the deltoid and the rotator cuff. *(From Perry, J., Phys Ther 58:265–278, 1978. Reprinted with permission.)*

Both heads of the biceps are also active during flexion.[22] The pectoralis major and anterior deltoid tend to rotate the humerus internally, but such rotation is resisted by the teres minor and infraspinatus.[6] The trapezius and subclavius stabilize the scapula.[20]

Extension of the humerus is controlled primarily by the latissimus dorsi. The activity of the sternal portion of the pectoralis major decreases as extension progresses.[20] The posterior fibers of the deltoid resist the tendency of the latissimus dorsi and pectoralis major to internally rotate the humerus. Backward extension is controlled primarily by the posterior fibers of the deltoid, latissimus dorsi, and teres major.[20]

Internal rotation is controlled by the subscapularis and teres major. This motion is assisted by the latissimus dorsi, anterior deltoid, and pectoralis major.

External rotation is controlled by the infraspinatus, teres minor, and posterior deltoid. The supraspinatus also participates when the arm is abducted.[6]

MUSCLES CONTROLLING SCAPULAR MOTION

The upper trapezius, levator scapulae, and upper digitations of the serratus anterior elevate and passively support the scapula during abduction.[8] This muscle group forms the upper component of a force couple which rotates the scapula during abduction of the arm. The lower trapezius and lower digitations of the serratus anterior form the lower portion of the force couple. In this manner the upper trapezius elevates the acromium and the lower trapezius depresses the base of the scapular spine to rotate the scapula[17] (Fig. 33-4). The mid-

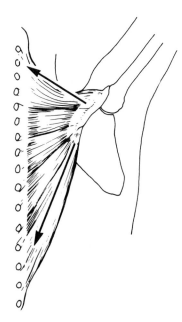

Figure 33-4 Muscle force vectors showing the force couple created by the upper and lower portions of the trapezius to rotate the scapula during abduction. *(From Perry, J., Phys Ther 58:265–278, 1978. Reprinted with permission.)*

dle portion of the trapezius and rhomboids fix the scapula in its plane of motion during abduction of the arm and relax during flexion to permit the scapula to rotate around the thorax.

The scapula adducts through the action of the trapezius and rhomboids. Abduction of the scapula is achieved by the serratus anterior and pectoralis minor.

The pectoralis major abducts the scapula as it adducts the arm across the chest. The latissimus dorsi adducts the scapula as it extends the humerus.

FORCES AT THE GLENOHUMERAL JOINT

An approximation of glenohumeral joint forces can be obtained from free body force analysis.[18] The muscle force necessary to hold the arm at 90 degrees of abduction may be assumed to be the deltoid, ignoring the rotator cuff (Fig. 33-5A). For an arm weighing 0.052 times body weight acting at a center of mass 318 mm from the center of glenohumeral rotation and a deltoid force D acting at a moment arm, or perpendicular distance from the muscle to the center of glenohumeral rotation of 30 mm, the sum of the moments about the center of glenohumeral rotation gives

$$D \times (30\,mm) = (0.052\ \text{body weight}) \times (318\,mm)$$
$$D = 0.551\ \text{body weight}^{18}$$

In this simplified analysis, the deltoid force which roughly approximates the joint force is about 10 times the weight of the arm or one-half body weight.

In a more detailed analysis, Poppen and Walker[18] determined the forces at the glenohumeral joint for abduction in the scapular plane based on the EMG analysis of the muscles participating at various angles of abduction. Each muscle force was assumed to be proportional to its cross-sectional area multiplied by the integrated EMG signal. The force vectors or line of muscle pull and moment arm, or perpendicular distance from the muscle to the center of glenohumeral rotation, was determined from an analysis of anatomical and radiographic findings. Glenohumeral forces were then resolved into shearing and compressive components relative to the face of the glenoid (Fig. 33-5B). The maximum glenohumeral force was 0.89 times body weight at 90 degrees of abduction and the maximum shearing force was 0.42 times body weight at 60 degrees of abduction. At 0 degrees of abduction, the resultant glenohumeral force indicated a slight downward sag of the humeral head. From 30 to 60 degrees the humeral head tended to sublux upward. Beyond 60 degrees the humeral head was compressed against the center of the glenoid.

GLENOHUMERAL STABILITY

The glenoid is slightly concave and much smaller than the articular surface of the humeral head. The average vertical dimension of the humeral articular surface is 48 mm with a transverse diameter of 45 mm. The glenoid has an average

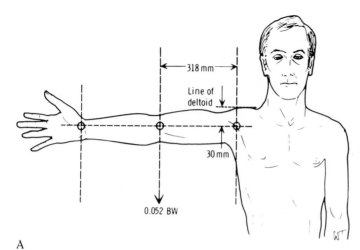

A

Figure 33-5 A. Arm held at 90 degrees of abduction. Weight of the arm is 0.052 times body weight at a center of mass 318 mm from the center of the humeral head. Deltoid force at 30 mm from the center of the humeral head gives a joint force of approximately 10 times the weight of the arm of one-half body weight (see calculation in the text). **B.** Resultant glenohumeral joint force vectors at varying degrees of abduction with the arm in neutral (N), internal rotation (I), and external rotation (X). *(From Poppen, N.K., and Walker, P.S., Clin Orthop 135:165–170, 1978. Reprinted with permission.)*

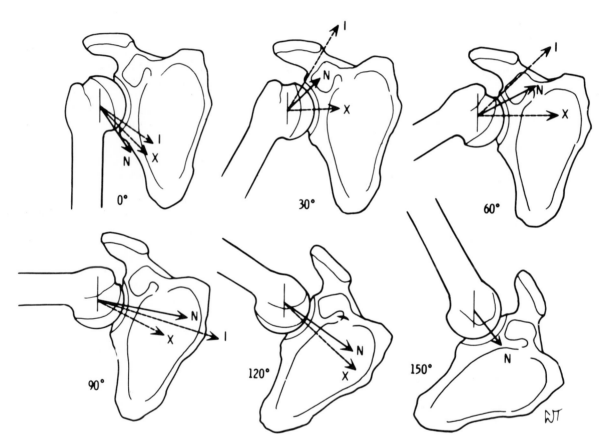

B

vertical height of 35 mm and a transverse diameter of 25 mm.[29] Although this lack of articular congruity permits a wide range of glenohumeral motion, it provides little stability and the shoulder is the most commonly dislocated joint in the body.[11]

The humeral head is inclined at an angle of 120 to 135 degrees to the axis of the shaft and retroverted 20 to 30 degrees in normal individuals.[26,31] The glenoid usually has a slight retrotilt relative to the scapula, but may be neutral or tilted slightly anteriorly.[25] Excessive anterior tilt of the glenoid may predispose to anterior dislocation.[24]

The glenoid labrum, which is predominantly fibrous, does not substantially increase the depth of the concave surface. Developmentally, the labrum appears as a separate structure from the glenoid.[32]

The capsule and ligaments provide static stability to the shoulder. The volume of the shoulder capsule is approximately two times the size of the humeral head to permit shoulder mobility.[23] The capsule is thickened anteriorly into superior, middle, and inferior glenohumeral ligaments which enhance stability to anterior dislocation (see Chap. 32, Sect. A).

The superior glenohumeral ligament appears to function to prevent downward subluxation of the arm in the dependent position and does not contribute substantially to resistance to anterior dislocation.[33] At the midrange of abduction the subscapularis covers the humeral head anteriorly and stability to anterior dislocation is provided by the subscapularis, middle, and inferior glenohumeral ligaments. However, beyond 90 degrees of abduction, the tendon does not cover the inferior portions of the humeral head anteriorly. Stability at this position is provided primarily by the inferior glenohumeral ligament and axillary pouch.[33]

Mechanical testing studies indicate that the strength of the shoulder capsule decreases with age.[10] In the young the weakest point occurs at the glenoid labrum attachment, but ruptures in the capsule and subscapularis tendon more commonly occur in the older age groups.[21] This correlates with the increased frequency of dislocations in the young in which there are intracapsular disruptions with the labrum or capsule avulsed in continuity with the periosteum.[21] Capsular and rotator cuff ruptures occur more commonly in the elderly.

SECTION B

Biomechanics of the Elbow

Michael D. Ries, Lawrence C. Hurst, and Roger Dee

The elbow functions to position the hand in the sagittal plane by flexion-extension and provides pronation-supination which positions the hand in the transverse plane. Three articulations consisting of the humeroulnar, radioulnar, and radiocapitellar joints permit this motion. The elbow also acts as a fulcrum, thus functioning as a load-bearing joint in actions such as lifting, overhead throwing, and pushing.

KINEMATICS

The elbow is a trochoginglymus joint which permits flexion-extension and axial rotation or pronation-supination. The normal range of flexion-extension is from 0 to 146 degrees.[7] Most activities of daily living may be accomplished with a functional arc of 100 degrees from 30 to 130 degrees.[23] Mall[19] found the axis of rotation for elbow flexion at the center of the trochlea. This conclusion was supported in three-dimen-

sional analyses done by Morrey and Chao[24] and by Youm et al[39] using independent coordinate systems for the humerus and ulna on cadaver specimens. This evidence supports the concept that elbow flexion is represented as a uniaxial hinge. In contrast, Ewald[10] and Ishizaki[14] found a changing center of rotation with flexion. London[18] found the axis of rotation passed through concentric arcs formed by the trochlear sulcus and capitellum. However, at the extremes of flexion and extension, the axis of rotation changed so that joint motion became a rolling instead of a sliding movement. In addition,

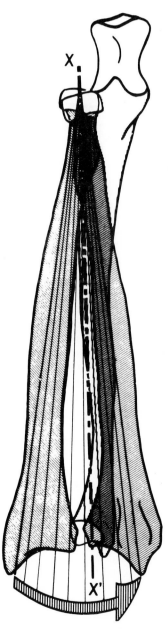

Figure 33-6 Arrow shows the arc formed by the distal radius about a line $X X'$ through the heads of the radius and ulna during pronation-supination. *(From Kapandji, I.A.: The Physiology of the Joints, vol 1. New York, Churchill Livingstone, 1982. Reproduced with permission.)*

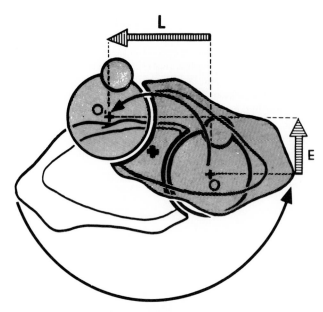

Figure 33-7 The right radius and ulna viewed from distal aspect. Ulna moves in the arc shown during supination but does not rotate on its own axis. Motion consists of a lateral component, L, and an extension component, E. The complementary motion of the radius is also shown, but this bone also rotates as shown in Fig. 33-6. Radius moves in a larger arc. Center of rotation for pronation-supination passes through the point around which both bones move (marked with cross). *(From Kapandji, I.A.: The Physiology of the Joints, vol 1. New York, Churchill Livingstone, 1982. Reproduced with permission.)*

Morrey and Chao[24] found slight internal axial rotation of the ulna occurred during early flexion and slight external axial rotation during terminal flexion. Dempster[9] noted humeral rotation relative to the ulna with joint flexion. Thus it appears that the elbow may not be represented by a uniaxial hinge throughout the flexion-extension range. The changing center of rotation and the sliding movement at the extremes of joint movement may be related to the high incidence of loosening seen with constrained hinge-type total elbow replacements.

The average normal range of pronation-supination is from 71 degrees of pronation to 81 degrees of supination.[7] Most activities of daily living may be accomplished in 100 degrees of forearm rotation from 50 degrees of pronation to 50 degrees of supination.[23]

The axis of forearm rotation is usually considered to pass through the capitellum and head of the radius extending to the distal ulna.[8,31] The rotation axis is oblique to the anatomical axis of the radius and ulna so that pronation-supination outlines a cone. The head of the radius rotates within the annular ligament, and the distal radius rotates around the ulna in an arc (Fig. 33-6). Ray et al[28] found slight motion of the distal ulna during pronation and supination about an axis passing through the index finger. The motion of the ulna was opposite to that of the radius in the latéral plane so that the ulna was abducted during pronation and adducted during supination. Youm et al[39] found slight distal ulnar motion to be a combination of flexion-extension and abduction-adduction.

This motion was noted to be greatest when the axis of pronation-supination was more radial. However, proximal ulnar motion was found to be negligible. Kapandji[16] suggests that the distal ulna is displaced on a small arc consisting of a lateral component and an extension component, whereas the distal radius rotates on a larger arc (Fig. 33-7). The center of both arcs is the point through which the axis of pronation-supination passes.

The axis of the radial head is displaced laterally approximately 2 mm in pronation; this is due to the ovoid shape of the radial head. This lateral displacement permits room for the radial tuberosity to move medially in pronation[16] (Fig. 33-8).

CARRYING ANGLE

The *carrying angle* is the angle formed by the long axis of the humerus and the long axis of the ulna. Potter[27] first quantitated the carrying angle. He reported an angle of 6.83 degrees in males and 12.65 degrees in females. Others have noted sim-

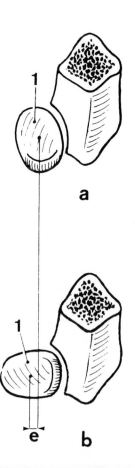

Figure 33-8 Radial head in contact with radial notch of ulna. Due to the ovoid shape of the radial head (1), the axis of the radial head is shifted laterally from **a,** the pronated position, to **b,** the supinated position, by the distance *e. (From Kapanji, I.A.: The Physiology of the Joints, vol 1. New York, Churchill Livingstone, 1982. Reproduced with permission.)*

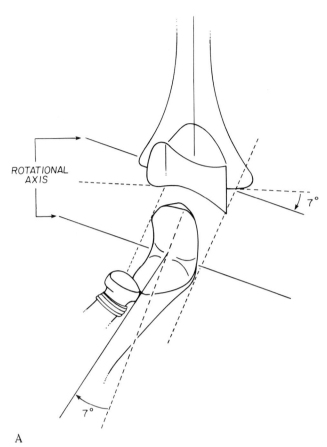

A

B

Figure 33-9 A. A perpendicular to the axis of the humeral diaphysis forms an oblique angle (of about 7 degrees) to the axis of joint rotation. A similar oblique angle exists between a perpendicular to the axis of the ulnar diaphysis and the axis of rotation.

B. Carrying angle formed by long axis of humerus H and long axis of ulna U. Oblique angle of humerus is equal to oblique angle of ulna so that the carrying angle disappears with flexion as the ulna superimposes on the humerus at U_1.

ilar differences in the carrying angle between males and females.[5,11,19,26,31]

The carrying angle changes as the elbow joint is flexed. Thompson[32] described the disappearance of the carrying angle during flexion, although the forearm did not cross the axis of the humerus. Dempster[9] found an oscillatory pattern of change. Amis et al[1] described a decrease in carrying angle similar to a sinusoidal curve with flexion. Youm et al[39] found a variation in pattern for different specimens with either a sinusoidal or linear change in carrying angle to 90 degrees of flexion and a constant angle beyond 90 degrees. Morrey and Chao[24] described a change in the carrying angle from valgus in extension to slight varus in extreme flexion. In contrast, London[18] found the carrying angle to be constant through the flexion range.

If the oblique angle of the humerus, formed by the long axis of the humerus and the axis of joint rotation, is equal to the oblique angle of the ulna, formed by the long axis of the ulna and the axis of rotation, the carrying angle will disappear with joint flexion (Fig. 33-9A and B). Recently, An et al[4] defined the carrying angle in terms of three variables which are the angle of joint flexion and the oblique angles of the humerus and ulna. If the carrying angle is defined as the angle

between the long axis of the humerus and the projection of the long axis of the ulna on a plane containing the humerus, or if it is defined as the angle between the long axis of the ulna and the projection of the long axis of the humerus on a plane containing the ulna, the carrying angle changes minimally with joint flexion. If, however, the carrying angle is defined as the abduction-adduction angle of the ulna relative to the humerus using Eularian angles to define the position of the humerus and ulna, the carrying angle decreases with joint flexion. Depending on the values of the oblique angles of the humerus and ulna, the carrying angle may change from valgus in extension to slight varus in flexion.[5]

ELBOW JOINT FORCES

The magnitude and direction of forces acting at the elbow joint may be determined from free body force analysis (Fig. 33-10).

Since the flexor muscles act through a relatively short moment arm, a large muscle force is needed to hold a weight in the hand at a greater distance from the center of elbow

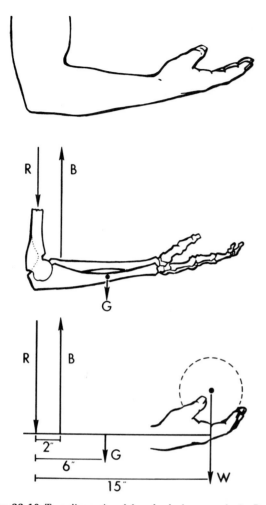

Figure 33-10 Two-dimensional free body force analysis: $B =$ flexor muscle force, $G =$ weight of forearm, $W =$ weight at hand, and $R =$ joint reaction force. Conditions of equilibrium are satisfied by the following equation for the sum of the moments about the center of the elbow joint. $(G \times 6'') + (W \times 15'') - (B \times 2'') = 0$. For a weight W of 20 lb and a forearm weight of 5 lb, $(5 \text{ lb} \times 6'') + (20 \text{ lb} \times 15'') - (B \times 2'') = 0$, or $B = 165$ lb; the sum of forces in the vertical direction must also equal zero. Thus: $R + 5 + 20 - 165 = 0$, or $R = 140$ lb. *(From Williams and Lissner in LeVeau, B., ed: Biomechanics of Human Movement. Philadelphia, Saunders, 1977. Reprinted with permission.)*

flexion. A large joint reaction force is created as a consequence of the large muscle force which may predispose the joint to degenerative arthritis. The short moment arm of the muscle force is mechanically inefficient. However, a short excursion or length of muscle contraction is necessary to achieve a larger arc of motion at the hand. This is the mechanism of the pulley system in the hand which maintains the tendon forces at short moment arms to the center of joint rotation.

Rapid distal motion of the limb is possible by short excursions of proximal muscles lying close to the axis of joint rotation to permit actions such as throwing.[35] However, because of the large joint reaction forces that occur during these activities, the elbow joint should not be considered as a "non-weight-bearing" joint.

Flexor muscles exert joint compressive as well as flexion forces which may be separated by vector addition[37] (Fig. 33-11). The magnitude of these forces will depend upon the angle of joint flexion as the length of the flexor moment arm changes with elbow flexion. Since the flexor moment arm is shortest at full extension, a large muscle force is necessary to cause a flexion component and the joint compressive load at this position is relatively large.[2]

Strenuous forearm adduction against resistance with the elbow flexed at 90 degrees can generate substantial torque across the elbow. This torque is resisted by tension in the medial collateral ligament of up to 1.28 kilonewtons (kN) and a radiocapitellar compressive force of up to 1.84 kN.[2] After total elbow replacement, these torques are transmitted to the stem and cement mantle. Such forces have been considered an additional cause of loosening after total elbow replacement.[3,13] Current nonconstrained designs rely more on the ligaments to transmit this torque.

STABILITY

The articular congruity of the elbow joint as well as soft tissue constraints contribute to its stability. However, dislocation is not uncommon.[17] The medial aspect of the elbow is supported by an anterior oblique portion of the medial collateral ligament and a weaker posterior oblique portion. The posterior oblique is absent in many primates.[29] The anterior oblique ligament is taut throughout the flexion-extension range, whereas the posterior oblique ligament is taut only during flexion.[29,34] The lateral ligament originates at the lateral epicondyle of the humerus and inserts on the annular ligament, although a bundle of posterior fibers attach to the supinator crest[20] and some anterior fibers insert on the coronoid.[12] The anconeus muscle crosses the lateral side of the elbow and may act as a joint stabilizer.[6]

The medial collateral ligament is the primary stabilizer to valgus stress. The anterior oblique portion of the medial ligament appears to bear the major component of the resistance to valgus stress. In cadaver specimens, the stability is maintained when the posterior oblique is sectioned and the anterior oblique is left intact.[34] However, the elbow is unstable when the anterior oblique is sectioned and the posterior oblique is left intact. Morey and An[22] found that the medial collateral ligament is the primary stabilizer at 90 degrees of flexion, contributing 54 percent of the resistance to valgus stress. The remainder was provided by the shape of the articular surfaces and the anterior capsule. In extension, the olecranon becomes locked in its fossa. An equal contribution from the medial collateral ligament, shape of joint surfaces, and anterior capsule were equally important to resisting valgus stress in extension.[22] Valgus stress encountered during

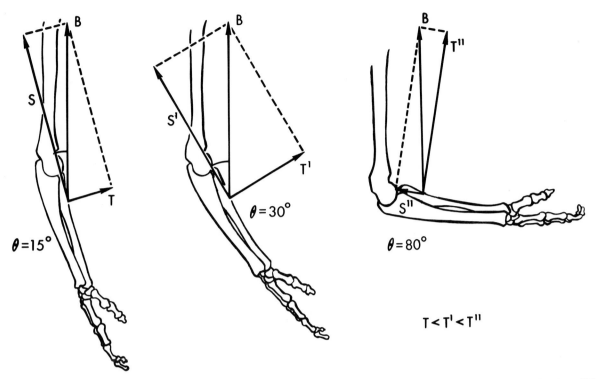

$T < T' < T''$

Figure 33-11 Flexor muscle force (B) may be separated into vector components. These are T (elbow flexion) and S (joint compression). Flexion component increases and compressive component decreases as joint flexion angle (ϕ) increases. *(From Williams and Lissner, in LeVeau, B., ed: Biomechanics of Human Movement. Philadelphia, Saunders, 1977. Reprinted with permission.)*

overhead throwing activities is associated with medial collateral ligament rupture.[33,36] Valgus deformity occurs in 30 percent of professional baseball players.[34] Compression at the radiocapitellar joint provides a secondary stabilizer to valgus stress when the medial collateral ligament becomes attenuated.

On the lateral side of the elbow, the capsule and joint surfaces principally contribute to resistance to varus stress. The lateral ligament contributes only 9 percent of the restraint to varus stress at 90 degrees of flexion.[22] Approximately 78 percent is provided by joint articulation and 13 percent by the capsule. In extension, the lateral ligament contributes 14 percent of this restraint with 54 percent provided by joint articulation and 32 percent from the capsule.[22]

Hyperextension has been postulated as a mechanism of posterior elbow dislocations. The olecranon is levered into the olecranon fossa causing a tear of the medial collateral ligament. Josefsson et al[15] found complete rupture of both the medial and lateral ligaments in every dislocation regardless of the type. These injuries are usually stable after reduction if the radiocapitellar joint, which is the secondary stabilizer, remains intact.[34]

SECTION C

Biomechanics of the Hand and Wrist

Michael D. Ries and Lawrence Hurst

The skeletal components of the hand are arranged in series of arches. The concave side of these arches faces the palm. There are two transverse arches. The proximal ridge arch passes through the carpus, and the more mobile distal arch passes through the metacarpal heads. Each of five longitudinal arches is formed by the five finger rays. The shape of the longitudinal arches and distal transverse arch are controlled by a balance of muscle forces and ligamentous constraints. Since the extrinsic extensors and flexors are not equal antagonists, the additional force needed for their balance is pro-

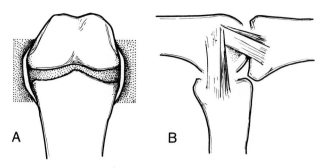

Figure 33-12 Collateral ligaments at the metacarpophalangeal joints. **A.** Viewed from its distal aspect, the metacarpal head resembles a trapezoid. **B.** Viewed laterally, the origin of the collateral ligament on the metacarpal head is slightly dorsal to the midline. The ligament is tightened with flexion since it crosses a greater distance. *(From Eaton, R.G.: Joint Injuries of the Hand. Springfield, Ill., Charles C Thomas, 1971. Modified and reprinted with permission.)*

vided by the intrinsics. Loss of the intrinsic muscles results in a disruption of the mobile arches.[17]

THE INTERPHALANGEAL JOINTS

The structure of the proximal (PIP) and distal (DIP) interphalangeal joints is similar: They are simple diarthrodial hinge joints. The average range of motion at the PIP joint is 110 degrees and 80 degrees at the DIP joint.[22] The interphalangeal joints have a tongue-and-groove contour. This joint congruity contributes to their resistance to rotatory, lateral, and shearing stresses.[13] The collateral ligaments are important in maintaining stability. They are proportionally larger than they might appear, and the ligament-to-articular-surface-area ratio is greater than that of any other joint in the body.[14] The volar plate, a fibrocartilaginous structure, blends with the collateral ligaments at the distal lateral margins. The central distal portion of the plate is poorly attached to the base of the middle phalanx.[5] Sectioning the central 80 percent of the volar plate at the PIP joint permits only 5 degrees of hyperextension.

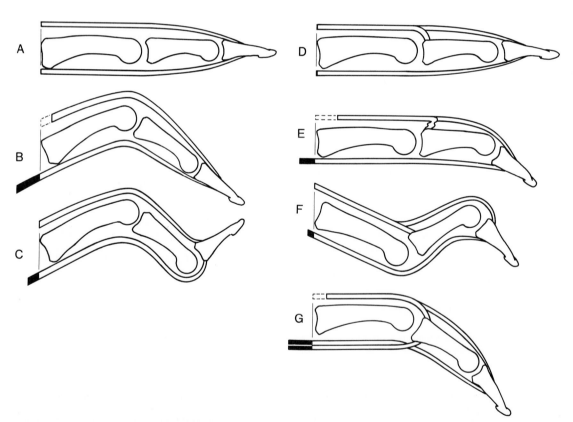

Figure 33-13 A. Landsmeer's model of intercalated bones considers the situation if only two tendons (flexor and extensor) are fixed proximally and act on three articulating phalanges. **B** and **C.** Pulling on the flexor tendons (*B*) will cause flexion of the PIP joint. The extensor tendon is functionally shortened and will provoke hyperextension of the DIP joint (*C*). **D–F.** Adding a central slip to the model (*D*) changes the behavior of the system. Pulling on the flexor tendon will again functionally shorten the extensor tendon, but since the extensor tendon is tethered by the central slip, the functional shortening occurs proximal to this slip (*E*). This causes the PIP joint to become hyperextended (*F*). **G.** To prevent this deformity, it is necessary to add to the model a flexor of the PIP joint (flexor superficialis).

However, when the distal lateral portions are cut the joint is unstable, permitting hyperextension to 35 degrees.[5]

METACARPOPHALANGEAL JOINTS

Metacarpophalangeal (MP) joints are condyloid joints. The condyloid shape allows for rotation and lateral movement as well as flexion and extension. An MP joint permits a flexion arc of 100 degrees and an abduction-adduction arc of 60 degrees.[3] The lateral movement is possible due to the ovoid shape of the metacarpal head. Viewed directly from its distal aspect the metacarpal head resembles a trapezoid with the narrow portion dorsal (Fig. 33-12A). This allows the collateral ligaments to be relaxed in extension when they lie beside the narrow portion of the head, permitting abduction-adduction and rotation. When the joint is flexed, the ligaments tighten around the wide portion of the metacarpal head and lateral motion is restricted. In addition, the origin of the collateral ligaments on the metacarpal head is slightly dorsal to the midline. This enhances their relative laxity in extension (Fig. 33-12B). The distance between origin and insertion is different for the separate parts of the collateral ligament at different points in the flexion arc. The distance from the dorsal origin to the insertion lengthens 3 or 4 mm and the volar portion shortens 1 or 2 mm during this arc. With the MP joint in hyperextension, the dorsal portion of the ligament shortens 2 or 3 mm and the volar portion lengthens slightly.[34] Thus, the dorsal portion of the collateral ligament supplies joint constraint in flexion, and the volar plate and volar portion of the collateral ligament constrains the joint in extension. The MP joints are also constrained by the deep transverse intermetacarpal ligaments which go between the volar plates.

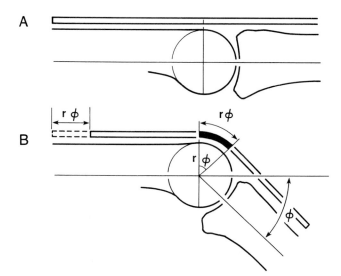

Figure 33-14 Extensor tendon excursion. **A.** The metacarpal or phalangeal head is represented by a semicircle with radius **B.** When the joint is flexed at angle ϕ, expressed in radians, extensor tendon excursion is equal to $r\phi$. *(From Landsmeer, J.F.M., Acta Morphol Neerl Scand 3:287–321, 1961. Modified and reprinted with permission.)*

FINGER POSITION AND TENDON EXCURSION
Equilibrium of Muscle Forces

Landsmeer[29] described a simple model of the finger to explain the muscle balance necessary to maintain the functional position (Fig. 33-13). The model consists of a linked chain of bone segments which responds passively to the muscle forces acting upon it and is controlled by two terminal antagonistic muscles inserting on the distal phalanx.

Tendon Excursion

The amount of tendon lengthening or shortening at a specific finger joint may be calculated based on the anatomical dimensions of the joint and the arc of joint motion. This gives the *tendon excursion* required to turn a joint through its range of motion (Fig. 33-14).

Landsmeer[29] has proposed geometric models to determine tendon excursion for various types of tendons. He calculated the extensor tendon excursions during joint motion from the radius of curvature or the metacarpal or phalangeal head and the degree of joint motion. He assumed that the joint surface has a constant radius of curvature and may be represented by a semicircle. Similar calculations for the flexor tendon assume it to be contained in a rigid sheath which holds it in a constant position against the volar shaft of the phalanx or metacarpal, but which permits it to curve smoothly within the angle of the joint. This means the distance from the tendon to the center of the joint will increase as the joint flexes (Fig. 33-15). This distance is a function of the anatomy of the pulley system. If it is also assumed that the curve of the tendon at the volar side of the joint forms part of a circle, an equation can be used to determine flexor tendon excursion.[29]

More recently a three-dimensional mathematical model, based on measurements in cadaver specimens, has been used to determine flexor profundus excursion at the PIP joint.[1] Results of this method and Landsmeer's flexor tendon model are remarkably consistent.

Flexor tendon excursion is dependent on the length of tendon not contained in the rigid part of the sheath and upon the distance from the tendon to the center of the joint. This length is controlled by the pulley system which holds the tendon near the center of the joint. If the pulley system is defective and bowstringing is permitted, the length of the tendon not contained in the rigid part of the sheath as well as tendon excursion is increased.

The pulley mechanism at the level of the MP joint may be ineffective due to disease, trauma, or surgery. The effect of this is to increase the excursion required at the MP joint with inadequate tendon excursion at the interphalangeal joints. Release of the A1 pulley is commonly used in the treatment of trigger finger. This slightly increases the excursion required for flexion. In the otherwise normal hand, this will not interfere with function.[50] However, incising the A1 and A2 pulleys at the MP joint region to a level of 1 mm distal to the finger web, leaving a 5 mm distal band of the A2 pulley, produces loss of finger flexion power equivalent to that incurred by 40

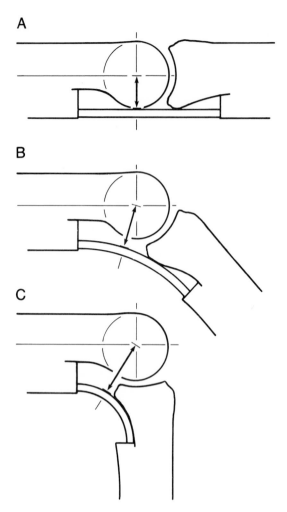

Figure 33-15 Flexor tendon held in a rigid sheath against the volar shaft of the metacarpal or phalanx, but curving smoothly in the joint angle. As the joint flexes (**A** through **C**) the distance from the tendon to the center of the joint, represented by arrows, increases.

degrees of wrist volar flexion.[6] Preservation of the A2 and A4 pulleys is necessary to maintain normal finger flexion.[22]

If a tendon is permitted to bowstring, the moment arm or distance from the tendon to the joint center is increased. The moment of a tendon is the tension in the tendon multiplied by its moment arm. If bowstringing occurs, the moment or power required to turn the joint is decreased but at the expense of increasing the excursion required to turn the joint.

PINCH AND GRASP

The functional positions of the hand may be separated into two types which are pinch and power grasp.[37] Precision handling is dynamic manipulation or movement of an object from the static pinch position.[28]

As shown in Fig. 33-16, pinch can further be divided into tip (A), palmar (B), lateral (C), and three-point pinch (D). In

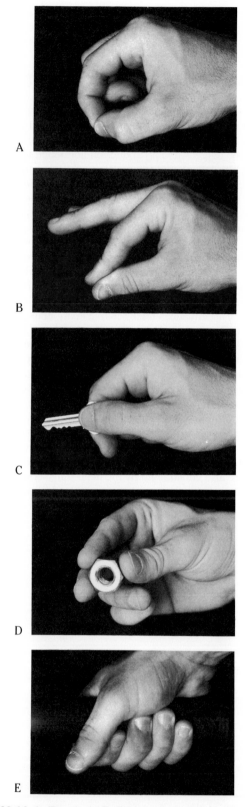

Figure 33-16 A. Tip pinch. **B.** Palmar pinch. **C.** Lateral or key pinch. **D.** Three-point, or chuck, pinch. **E.** Power grasp.

power grasp (E), the fingers are flexed to grip an object with the thumb as a stabilizer. The long finger provides most of the gripping force. The ring and little fingers supinate toward the midline.[21]

There are wide variations in the force of pinch and grasp in different individuals. Handedness, state of nutrition, pain, fatigue, age, and sex will influence hand strength. Average grasp strengths of 47.6 kg for males and 24.6 kg for females have been reported based on measurements with a hydraulic dynamometer.[55] Average strengths of 7.9 kg for males and 5.2 kg for females were measured during three-point pinch. With lateral pinch, similar strengths were found with 7.5 kg for males and 4.9 kg for females. Most simple activities of daily living can be achieved with a grasp strength of 4 kg and a pinch strength of 1 kg.[55] During pinch, the compressive force is provided primarily by the extrinsics.[33] In a two-dimensional analysis, Smith et al[51,52] determined that a flexor tendon force of 6 times the fingertip compressive force is necessary for pinch. This results in a volar dislocation force of three times the fingertip force at the level of the MP joint. This tendency of the tendon to bowstring in a volar-ulnar direction has been proposed as a factor in the development of ulnar drift in rheumatoid arthritis.

Power grasp generates larger tendon tension than pinch. However, the DIP and PIP joint compressive loads are less than those in pinch.[8] This suggests that the hand is better constructed to perform powerful grasp since less joint compressive load is required to maintain stability at the distal joints.

Although the joint loads during pinch increase from the DIP joint proximally to the MP joint and contact areas also increase, the contact pressures do not remain constant. The contact pressure is equal to the joint load divided by contact area. This difference in pressures occurs because the increase in area and the increase in load from the distal joints to the proximal joints are not equal. The highest contact pressures occur at the DIP joint and decrease toward the MP joint during pinch because of the extremely small contact area at the DIP joint.[36] This may be related to the high incidence of degenerative disease and presence of Heberden's nodes that occur at the distal interphalangeal joint.

The contact pressures during pinch are higher than those during grasp. During grasp, the contact pressures increase from the DIP joint to the MP joint.[36] This pattern of contact pressures is consistent with the clinically observed pattern of degenerative joint disease. The distal joints of the index and long finger are more frequently involved with degenerative joint disease in occupations which involve primarily pinching activities compared to a relative sparing of these joints in occupations which involve primarily grasping activities.[18,44]

For a pinch force of 1 kg, compressive loads at the thumb have been determined of 3.0 kg at the interphalangeal joint, 5.4 kg at the MP joint, and 12.0 kg at the trapeziometacarpal joint.[10] During pinch, the trapeziometacarpal joint is in a position of adduction. Adduction is not a stable position of this joint. This instability may contribute to subluxation and the development of degenerative disease at the trapeziometacarpal joint.[11]

The Extensor Mechanism

The extensor tendon at the finger divides into the central slip and two lateral bands at the level of the proximal interphalangeal joint (Fig. 33-17). The central slip inserts on the proximal border of the middle phalanx, and the two lateral bands combine to form the terminal extensor tendon. This tendon inserts on the dorsum of the distal phalanx. The lateral bands are a conjoint tendon formed by the tendons of the lumbricals and interossei. Extension of the finger is accomplished by tension in the central slip and lateral bands.

Since the condylar radius of the middle phalanx is larger than that of the proximal phalanx, extensor excursion required at the DIP joint is about one-third less than that at the PIP joint.[62] Thus, for DIP and PIP extension to occur together, the lateral bands must compensate for the added excursion required at the PIP joint. This is accomplished with volar and lateral shifts of 3 or 4 mm of the lateral bands during PIP joint flexion.[20] When the PIP joint is in the flexed position, more tension occurs in the central slip. In the extended position, more tension occurs in the lateral bands. In midflexion, tension is balanced in both the central slip and lateral bands.[35,47]

Function of the Oblique Retinacular Ligament

The oblique retinacular ligament, described by Weitbrecht,[59] extends from the flexor tendon sheath at the level of the proximal phalanx to the terminal extensor tendon but is an inconsistent finding.[49] Landsmeer[27,30] postulated that during DIP joint flexion the oblique retinacular ligament is tightened and causes PIP joint flexion. In addition, when the PIP joint is brought into extension, the oblique retinacular ligament is again tightened and now causes DIP joint extension.

However, Harris and Rutledge[20] found that the oblique retinacular ligament was relaxed from 0 to 70 degrees of DIP joint flexion with the PIP joint at full extension. The ligament may only contribute to DIP joint extension from 90 to 70 degrees.

When the oblique retinacular ligament is not present, an osteocapsular ligament is found in the position of the proximal segment of the oblique retinacular ligament. After excision of the oblique retinacular ligament, coordinated motion of the interphalangeal joint is unaltered.[20,49]

The lateral bands are held dorsally by the triangular ligament between the lateral bands and volarly by the transverse retinacular ligaments.[53] The transverse retinacular ligaments merge with the lateral bands and insert on the lateral portions of the volar plate. A disruption of balance at the lateral bands may result in either swan neck or boutonniere deformity.

Swan Neck Deformity

A swan neck deformity (hyperextension of the PIP joint and flexion of the DIP joint) occurs when the transverse retinacular ligaments are lax in some individuals. This allows hyperextension of the PIP joint by "bowstringing" the lateral bands dorsally. Voluntary flexion at the DIP joint with the flexor pro-

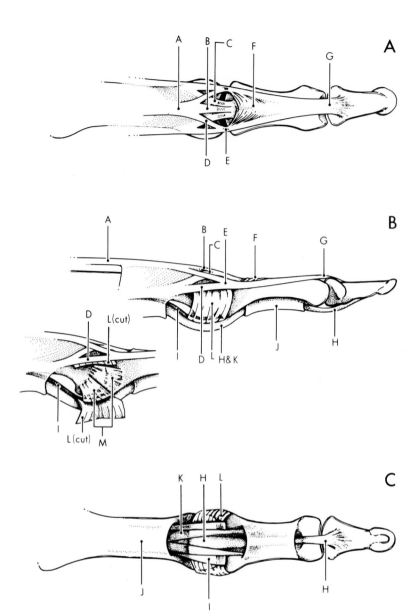

Figure 33-17 A. Dorsal view of normal PIP joint anatomy. **B.** Lateral view of normal PIP joint anatomy with inset figure showing anatomy after cutting and reflecting of the transverse retinaculum. **C.** Volar view of normal PIP joint anatomy. Abbreviations: (A) extensor digitorum communis tendon, (B) central slip, (C) medial band of oblique intrinsic expansion, (D) lateral slip, (E) conjoint lateral band, (F) triangular ligament, (G) terminal extensor tendon, (H) flexor digitorum profundus, (I) volar plate, (J) flexor tendon sheath, (K) flexor digitorum superficialis, (L) transverse retinaculum, (M) collateral ligament (proper and accessory). *(From Smith, R.J., Clin Orthop 104:92–111, 1974. Modified and reproduced with permission.)*

fundus is still possible. Excessive tension on the extensor mechanism, such as intrinsic muscle contracture in rheumatoid arthritis, may also result in a swan neck deformity. Furthermore, volar subluxation of the proximal phalanx in rheumatoid arthritis may add increased tension to the extensor mechanism through the sagittal bands at the MP joint, thus pulling the PIP joint into more hyperextension.[53]

Boutonniere Deformity

A *boutonniere deformity* is the opposite of a swan neck deformity: The PIP joint is in a position of flexion, and the DIP joint is in a position of hyperextension. This occurs after the central slip ruptures during acute PIP joint flexion with the lateral bands pulled laterally, tearing the triangular ligament.[16] The excursion of the extensor mechanism is transmitted to the DIP joint through the lateral bands and results in

DIP joint hyperextension. The flexor superficialis, without an adequate antagonist, flexes the PIP joint. The retinacular ligaments further shorten with pull from the flexor tendon, and a boutonniere deformity follows.[53]

Function of Sagittal Bands

Extension at the MP joint is achieved through a sagittal band of fibers which connect the extensor tendon to the volar plate (Fig. 33-18). Although there is sometimes a fibrous insertion from the extensor tendon to the base of the proximal phalanx,[30] this is tight only in hyperextension. If this insertion were responsible for MP joint extension, it would create laxity at the extensor expansion distal to it and thus limit interphalangeal extension. With the normal range of finger extension, this insertion is never tight.[19] In hyperextension, the extensor tendon distal to the MP joint is lax and the interphalangeal joints fall into flexion. In this position of forced hyperextension, the interphalangeal joints can be extended only with the intrinsics.

THE THUMB

The skeletal constituents of the thumb are the proximal and distal phalanges, the metacarpal, and the trapezius, which comprise the interphalangeal, metacarpophalangeal, and trapeziometacarpal joints. The three joints permit 5 degrees of freedom.[11] One degree of freedom (flexion-extension) is provided at the interphalangeal joint; 2 degrees at the MP joint (flexion-extension and abduction-adduction); and 2 degrees at the trapeziometacarpal joint (flexion-extension and abduction-adduction). A small degree of axial rotation is also possible at both the MP[17] and trapeziometacarpal[26] joints.

The interphalangeal joint of the thumb is structurally and functionally similar to the finger interphalangeal joints. This has been modeled as a hinge joint. It provides a flexion range of 0 to 90 degrees.[24]

The MP joint differs from the finger MP joints in that lateral motion is more limited. An average abduction range of 0 to 20 degrees and a variable degree of flexion-extension ranging from 0 to 90 degrees has been reported in a study of 1000 thumbs.[12,23] In addition to the static stability afforded by the collateral ligaments and volar plate, the thenar intrinsics, which insert on the two sesamoids, and the extensor mechanism also provide dynamic restraints to hyperextension and excessive abduction and adduction. The trapeziometacarpal joint is a saddle joint with a ridge on the surface of the trapezium, concave in one plane and convex in another. This geometry permits flexion-extension, abduction-adduction, and

during distraction, axial rotation.[11] The metacarpophalangeal and trapeziometacarpal joints have been modeled as universal joints.[10]

The trapeziometacarpal joint is supported by the capsule and ligaments on the volar, dorsal, and ulnar aspects. The dorsal radial facet provides the main resistance to dorsal subluxation and becomes eroded early in degenerative arthritis of this joint.[14]

Cooney et al[11] determined an average total motion for the trapeziometacarpal joint of 53 degrees of flexion-extension, 42 degrees of abduction-adduction, and 17 degrees of axial rotation, using an in vivo study based on a constant relationship between the trapezium and third metacarpal.

Opposition of the thumb consists of abduction and rotation of the thumb as a unit involving the interphalangeal, metacarpophalangeal, and trapeziometacarpal joints. Kaplan[25] noted that rotation is provided primarily by the trapeziometacarpal joint, and this motion is enhanced by abduction at the metacarpophalangeal joint. Cooney et al[11] also found that axial rotation occurs at both the trapeziometacarpal and MP joints. However, MP arthrodesis does not functionally limit opposition as much as trapeziometacarpal arthrodesis.[25] After trapeziometacarpal arthrodesis, a compensatory increase in metacarpophalangeal and carpal motion results in useful thumb function.[15]

THE WRIST

The wrist functions to position the hand. The motions of the wrist are flexion, extension, radial deviation, and ulnar deviation. Rotation is provided by pronation and supination of the

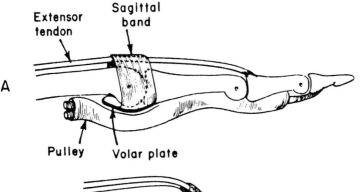

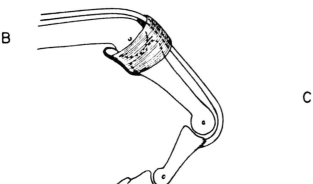

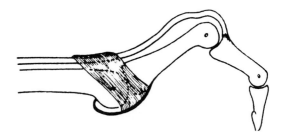

Figure 33-18 Diagrammatic representation of the sagittal bands. The sagittal bands are attached dorsally to the extensor tendon and volarly to the volar plate.
A. In extension, the bands overlie the MP joint.
B. With flexion, the bands migrate distally. In this position the extensor tendon can extend the PIP joint.
C. In hyperextension, the extensor tendon distal to the MP joint is lax and the PIP joint falls into flexion.
(From Smith, R.J., Clin Orthop 104:92–111, 1974. Reproduced with permission.)

forearm, although a small amount of rotation can occur within the carpus.[43] The average combined range of radial and ulnar deviation is 50 degrees, with 15 degrees of radial deviation and 35 degrees of ulnar deviation.[58] During ulnar deviation the proximal row moves radially and the distal row moves ulnarly. With radial deviation this motion is reversed,[58] although the motion of the proximal row is negligible,[60,61] with radial deviation at only 20 degrees. Thus, ulnar deviation involves both intercarpal and radiocarpal motion, while radial deviation involves intercarpal motion.

The carpus may also be considered in terms of three functional columns.[56] The flexion-extension or central column is formed by the distal carpal row and the lunate. This functions as a longitudinal link attached to the radius and is dependent upon the integrity of the carpal ligaments since the muscles which produce wrist motion attach distal to the central column. The scaphoid forms the second mobile column. The triquetrum is the rotation column. A small degree of carpal rotation appears to take place around the triquetrum as a pivot point independent of forearm pronation-supination.[56]

The amount of flexion-extension is variable with a range of 84 to 169 degrees and an average of 121 degrees reported based on a radiographic study of 55 normal wrists.[48] The average range of flexion is 66 degrees and of extension 55 degrees. This motion involves both radiocarpal and intercarpal motion. The radiocarpal joint contributes 66 percent of total wrist extension with 34 percent at the intercarpal joint. During flexion the intercarpal joint contributes 60 percent, with 40 percent at the radiocarpal joint.[48] For most activities of daily living, the wrist functions from 10 degrees of flexion to 35 degrees of extension.[7]

The center of rotation for both flexion-extension and radioulnar motion is located in the head of the capitate.[2,57,60,61] The center of rotation for flexion-extension is slightly more proximal than the center of rotation for radial-ulnar deviation. Thus, a universal joint has been used to model the wrist with the axes of both hinge joints passing through the respective centers of rotations in the head of the capitate.[2]

With trauma or disease, such as rheumatoid arthritis, loss of carpal height and ulnar translation of the carpus may occur. The loss of cartilage and bony compression in rheumatoid arthritis leading to loss of carpal height results in ligament laxity and ulnar translation of the carpus.[32] This increases the moment arm of the tendons acting on the radial side and decreases the moment arm of the tendons acting on the ulnar side. A zigzag collapse of the carpus results, demonstrating that the wrist as well as the hand follows Landsmeer's intercalated bone model.[32,60] The degree of carpal collapse may be assessed radiographically based on the ratio of carpal height to the length of the third metacarpal (Fig. 33-19A). In normal subjects this ratio is remarkably constant at 0.54.[61] In a similar manner the degree of ulnar translation can be determined. Since the center of rotation in the radial-ulnar direction lies at a fixed point in the head of the capitate, the carpoulnar distance can be measured from the center of rotation in the capitate to a projection of the long axis of the ulna. Dividing this distance by the length of the third metacarpal gives a ratio of 0.30 in the normal wrist (Fig. 33-19B).[61]

Ulnar Variance

Ulnar variance is the term used to define the relative lengths of the radius and ulna. The ulnar variance is zero when the lengths of the radius and ulna are equal. A positive ulnar variance is present when the ulna is longer than the radius, and a

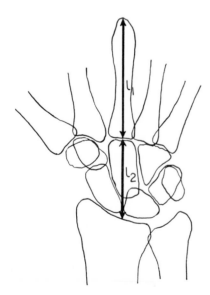

A

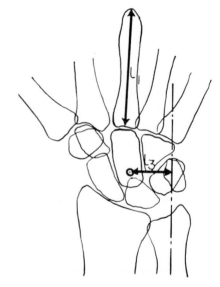

B

Figure 33-19 A. Carpal height ratio used to assess carpal collapse. Length of third metacarpal divided by carpal height: L2/L1. In normal wrists, this ratio is 0.54. **B.** Carpoulnar distance ratio used to assess ulnar translation. Distance from center of radioulnar deviation at head of capitate to longitudinal axis of ulna divided by length of third metacarpal: L3/L1. In normal wrists, this ratio is 0.3. *(From Youm, Y., et al, J Bone Joint Surg 60A:423–431, 1978. Reproduced with permission.)*

negative ulnar variance is present when the ulna is shorter than the radius.[4] Forearm rotation of up to 150 degrees occurs at the distal radioulnar joint.[38,40,46] The position of the distal ulna relative to the position of the distal radius, or apparent ulnar variance, will depend upon forearm position (see Sect. B). A standard position of 90 degrees of elbow flexion with the forearm in neutral pronation-supination is recommended for radiographic measurement of ulnar variance.[40]

Loads are distributed across the carpus to the distal radius, and to the distal ulna through the triangular fibrocartilage complex, between the distal ulna and ulnar carpus. Palmer et al[42] have shown that the distal radius bears 82 percent of load transmitted across the wrist to the forearm, with 18 percent carried by the distal ulna. Ulnar lengthening or shortening significantly affects the distribution of this load. Ulnar lengthening of 25 mm increases the ulnar load to 42 percent, and ulnar shortening of 2.5 mm reduces the load to 4 percent. A positive ulnar variance is associated with a thinner triangular fibrocartilage complex and with perforations of the triangular fibrocartilage complex.[39] The beneficial effect of this shift in load distribution with differing ulnar variance at the level of the distal radioulnar joint is demonstrated with ulnar lengthening used in the treatment of Kienbock disease[54] and with ulnar shortening in the treatment of degenerative perforations of the triangular fibrocartilage complex.[41]

REFERENCES

Section A: Biomechanics of the Shoulder

1. Basmajian, J.V., and Bazant, F.J. Factors preventing downward dislocation of the adducted shoulder joint. J Bone Joint Surg 41A:1182–1186, 1959.
2. Basmajian, J.V., and Latif, A. Integrated actions and functions of the chief flexors of the elbow. J Bone Joint Surg 39A:1106–1118, 1957.
3. Bechtol, C.O. Biomechanics of the shoulder. Clin Orthop 146:37–41, 1980.
4. Codman, E.A. *The Shoulder.* Brooklyn, NY, Miller, 1934.
5. DeDuca, C.J., and Forrest, W.J. Force analysis of individual muscles acting simultaneously on the shoulder joint during isometric abduction. J Biomech 6:385–393, 1973.
6. DePalma, A.F. *Surgery of the Shoulder.* Philadelphia, Lippincott, 1983.
7. Freedman, L., and Munro, R.R. Abduction of the arm in the scapular plane: Scapular and glenohumeral movements. J Bone Joint Surg 48A:1503–1510, 1966.
8. Inman, V.T., Saunders, M., and Abbott, L.C. Observation on the function of the shoulder joint. J Bone Joint Surg 26:1–30, 1944.
9. Johnston, T.B. The movements of the shoulder-joint. A plea for the use of the plane of the scapula as the plane of reference for movements occurring at the humero-scapular joint. Br J Surg 25:252–260, 1937.
10. Kaltsas, D.S. Comparative study of the properties of the shoulder joint capsule with those of other joint capsules. Clin Orthop 173:20–26, 1983.
11. Linscheid, R.L., and Wheeler, D.K. Elbow dislocations. JAMA 194:1171–1176, 1965.
12. Lucas, D.B. Biomechanics of the shoulder joint. Arch Surg 107:425–432, 1973.
13. Martin, C.P. A note on the movements of the shoulder joint. Br J Surg 20:61–66, 1932.
14. Milch, H. The treatment of recent dislocations and fracture dislocations of the shoulder. J Bone Joint Surg 31A:173–180, 1949.
15. Moseley, H.F., and Overgaard, B. The anterior capsular mechanism in recurrent anterior dislocation of the shoulder. J Bone Joint Surg 44B:913–927, 1962.
16. Nixon, J.E., and DiStefano, V. Ruptures of the rotator cuff. Orthop Clin North Am 6:423–447, 1975.
17. Perry, J. Normal upper extremity kinesiology. Phys Ther 58:265–278, 1978.
18. Poppen, N.K., and Walker, P.S. Forces at the glenohumeral joint in abduction. Clin Orthop 135:165–170, 1978.
19. Poppen, N.K., and Walker, P.S. Normal and abnormal motion of the shoulder. J Bone Joint Surg 58A:195–201, 1976.
20. Radin, E.L. Biomechanics and functional anatomy, in Post, M. (ed): *The Shoulder, Surgical and Nonsurgical Management.* Philadelphia, Lea and Febiger, 1978.
21. Reeves, B. Experiments on the tensile strength of the anterior capsular structures of the shoulder in man. J Bone Joint Surg 50B:858–865, 1968.
22. Rothman, R.H., Marvel, J.P., and Heppenstall, R.B. Anatomic considerations in the glenohumeral joint. Orthop Clin North Am 6:341–352, 1975.
23. Rothman, R.H., Marvel, J.P., and Heppenstall, R.B. Recurrent anterior dislocation of the shoulder. Orthop Clin North Am 6:415–422, 1975.
24. Saha, A.K. Anterior recurrent dislocation of shoulder. Acta Orthop Scand 68:479–493, 1967.
25. Saha, A.K. Dynamic stability of the glenohumeral joint. Acta Orthop Scand 42:491–505, 1971.
26. Saha, A.K. Mechanics of elevation of glenohumeral joint. Acta Orthop Scand 44:668–678, 1973.
27. Saha, A.K. Mechanism of shoulder movements and a plea for the recognition of "zero position" of glenohumeral joint. Indian J Surg 12:153–165, 1950.
28. Saha, A.K. Mechanism of shoulder movements and a plea for the recognition of "zero position" of glenohumeral joint. Clin Orthop 173:3–10, 1983.
29. Sarrafian, S.K. Gross and functional anatomy of the shoulder. Clin Orthop 173:11–19, 1983.
30. Staples, O.S., and Watkins, A.L. Full active abduction in traumatic paralysis of the deltoid. J Bone Joint Surg 25:85–89, 1943.
31. Steindler, A. *Kinesiology of the Human Body.* Springfield, IL, Thomas, 1955.
32. Tullos, H.S., Bennett, J.B., and Braly, W.G. Acute shoulder dislocations: Factors influencing diagnosis and treatment. Instr Course Lect 33:364–385, 1984.
33. Turkel, S.J., Panio, M.W., Marshall, J.L., and Girgis, F.G. Stabilizing mechanisms preventing anterior dislocation of the glenohumeral joint. J Bone Joint Surg 63A:1208–1217, 1981.
34. Van Linge, B., and Mulder, J.D. Function of the supraspinatus muscle and its relation to the supraspinatus syndrome. J Bone Joint Surg 45B:750–754, 1963.

Section B: Biomechanics of the Elbow

1. Amis, A.A., Dowson, D., Unsworth, A., Miller, J.H., and Wright, V. An examination of the elbow articulation with particular reference to variation of the carrying angle. Eng Med 6:76–80, 1977.
2. Amis, A.A., Dowson, D., and Wright, V. Elbow joint force predictions for some strenuous isometric actions. J Biomech 13:765–775, 1980.
3. Amis, A.A., Dowson, D., Wright, V., and Miller, J.H. The derivation of elbow joint forces and their relation to prosthesis design. J Med Eng Tech 3:229–234, 1979.

4. An, K.N., Morrey, B.F., and Chao, E.Y.S. Carrying angle of the human elbow joint. J Orthop Res 1:369–378, 1984.

5. Atkinson, W.B., and Elftman, H. The carrying angle of the human arm as a secondary sex character. Anat Rec 91:49–52, 1945.

6. Basmajian, J.V., and Griffin Jr., W.R. Function of anconeus muscle. J Bone Joint Surg 54A:1712–1714, 1972.

7. Boone, D.C., and Azen, S.P. Normal range of motion of joints in male subjects. J Bone Joint Surg 61A:756–759, 1979.

8. Burman, M. Induced pseudarthrosis of the radius in congenital radioulnar synostosis. Geometric analysis of the consequent mechanical situation. Bull Hosp Joint Dis 13:269–321, 1952.

9. Dempster, W.T. Space requirements of the seated operator. *Wright Air Development Center Technical Report,* 1955, pp 55–159.

10. Ewald, F.C. Total elbow replacement. Orthop Clin North Am 6:685–696, 1975.

11. Fick, R. *Handbuch der Anatomie und Mechanik der Gelenke.* Gustav Fischer, Jena, 1911, pp 304–312.

12. Frazer, J.E. *The Anatomy of the Human Skeleton.* Philadelphia, Blakiston's, 1920.

13. Gurtowski, J., Stern, L., Manley, M.T., Dubrow, E., and Dee, R. Loosening of semi-constrained total elbow prostheses. Trans Orthop Res Soc 8:102, 1983.

14. Ishizuki, M. Functional anatomy of the elbow joint and three-dimensional quantitative motion analysis of the elbow joint. J Jap Orthop Assoc 53:989–996, 1979.

15. Josefsson, P.O., Johnell, O., and Gentz, C.F. Long term sequelae of simple dislocation of the elbow. J Bone Joint Surg 66A:927–930, 1984.

16. Kapandji, I.A. *The Physiology of the Joints,* vol 1. Edinburgh, Churchill Livingstone, 1982.

17. Linscheid, R.L., and Wheeler, D.K. Elbow dislocations. JAMA 194:1171–1176, 1965.

18. London, J.T. Kinematics of the elbow. J Bone Joint Surg 63A:529–535, 1981.

19. Mall, F.P. On the angle of the elbow. Am J Anat 4:391–404, 1905.

20. Martin, B.F. The annular ligament of the superior radioulnar joint. J Anat 92:473–481, 1958.

21. Mikic, Z.D., and Vukadinovic, S.M. Late results in fractures of the radial head treated by excision. Clin Orthop 181:220–228, 1983.

22. Morrey, B.F., and An, K.N. Articular and ligamentous contributions to the stability of the elbow joint. Am J Sports Med 11:315–319, 1983.

23. Morrey, B.F., Askew, L.J., An, K.N., and Chao, E.Y. A biomechanical study of normal functional elbow motion. J Bone Joint Surg 63A:872–877, 1981.

24. Morrey, B.F., and Chao, E.Y. Passive motion of the elbow joint. J Bone Joint Surg 58A:501–508, 1976.

25. Morrey, B.F., Chao, E.Y., and Hui, F.C. Biomechanical study of the elbow following excision of the radial head. J Bone Joint Surg 61A:63–68, 1979.

26. Nagel, K. Untersuchungen uber den Armwinkel des Menschen. Morphol Anthropol 10:317–352, 1907.

27. Potter, H.P. The obliquity of the arm of the female in extension. The relation of the forearm with the upper arm in flexion. J Anat Physiol 29:488–491, 1895.

28. Ray, R.D., Johnson, R.J., and Jameson, R.M. Rotation of the forearm. An experimental study of pronation and supination. J Bone Joint Surg 33A:993–996, 1951.

29. Schwab, G.H., Bennett, J.B., Woods, G.W., and Tullos, H.S. Biomechanics of elbow instability: The role of the medial collateral ligament. Clin Orthop 146:42–52, 1980.

30. Steel, F.L.D., and Tomlinson, J.D.W. The "carrying angle" in man. J Anat 92:315–317, 1958.

31. Steindler, A. *Kinesiology of the Human Body.* Springfield, Ill, Thomas, 1955, pp 499–507.

32. Thompson, A.R. Some features of the elbow joint. J Anat 58:368–373, 1924.

33. Tullos, H.S., Erwin, W., Woods, G.W., Wukasch, D.C., Cooley, D.A., and King, J.W. Unusual lesions of the pitching arm. Clin Orthop 88:169–182, 1972.

34. Tullos, H.S., Schwab, G., Bennet, J.B., and Woods, G.W. Factors influencing elbow instability. Instr Course Lect 30:185–199, 1981.

35. Wadsworth, T.G. *The Elbow.* Edinburgh, Churchill Livingstone, 1982.

36. Waris, W. Elbow injuries of javelin-throwers. Acta Chir Scand 93:563–575, 1946.

37. Williams and Lissner, B., in LeVeau, B. (ed): *Biomechanics of Human Movement.* Philadelphia, Saunders, 1977.

38. Wilson, F.D., Andrews, J.R., Blackburn, T.A., and McCluskey, G. Valgus extension overload in the pitching elbow. Am J Sports Med 11:83–88, 1983.

39. Youm, Y., Dryer, R.F., Thambyrajah, K., Flatt, A.E., and Sprague, B.L. Biomechanical analysis of forearm pronation-supination and elbow flexion-extension. J Biomech 12:245–255, 1979.

Section C: Biomechanics of the Hand and Wrist

1. An, K.N., Chao, E.Y., Cooney, W.P., and Linscheid, R.L. Normative model of human hand for biomechanical analysis. J Biomech 12:775–788, 1979.

2. Andrews, J.G., and Youm, Y. A biomechanical investigation of wrist kinematics. J Biomech 12:83–93, 1979.

3. Berme, N., Paul, J.P., and Purves, W.K. A biomechanical analysis of the metacarpophalangeal joint. J Biomech 10:409–412, 1977.

4. Bowers, W.H. Distal radioulnar joint, in Green, D.P. (ed): *Operative Hand Surgery.* Edinburgh, Churchill Livingstone, 1982.

5. Bowers, W.H., Wolf, J.W., Nehil, J.L., and Bittinger, S. The proximal interphalangeal joint volar plate. An anatomical and biomechanical study. J Hand Surg 5:79–88, 1980.

6. Brand, P.W., Cranor, K.C., and Ellis, J.C. Tendon and pulleys at the metacarpophalangeal joint of a finger. J Bone Joint Surg 57A:779–784, 1975.

7. Brumfield, R.H., and Champoux, J.A. A biomechanical study of normal wrist motion. Clin Orthop 187:23–25, 1984.

8. Chao, E.Y., and Cooney, W.P. Internal forces in normal hands, in Walker, P.S. (ed): *Human Joints and Their Artificial Replacements.* Springfield, IL, Thomas, 1977.

9. Chao, E.Y., Opgrande, J.D., and Axmear, F.E. Three-dimensional force analysis of finger joints in selected isometric hand functions. J Biomech 9:387–396, 1976.

10. Cooney, W.P., and Chao, E.Y.S. Biomechanical analysis of static forces in the thumb during hand function. J Bone Joint Surg 59A:27–36, 1977.

11. Cooney, W.P., Lucca, M.J., Chao, E.Y.S., and Linscheid, R.L. The kinesiology of the thumb trapeziometacarpal joint. J Bone Joint Surg 63A:1371–1381, 1981.

12. Coonrad, R.W., and Goldner, J.L. A study of the pathological findings and treatment in soft-tissue injury of the thumb metacarpophalangeal joint. J Bone Joint Surg 50A:439–451, 1968.

13. Eaton, R.G. *Joint Injuries of the Hand.* Springfield, IL, Thomas, 1971.

14. Eaton, R.G. Joints and their ligaments. *Symposium on Reconstructive Hand Surgery,* vol 9, 1972, pp 13–19.

15. Eaton, R.G., and Littler, J.W. A study of the basal joint of the thumb. J Bone Joint Surg 51A:661–668, 1969.

16. Elliot, R.A. Injuries to the extensor mechanism of the hand. Orthop Clin North Am 1:335–354, 1970.

17. Flatt, A.F. Kinesiology of the Hand. Instr Course Lect 18:266–281, 1961.

18. Hadler, N.M., Gillings, D.B., Imbus, H.R., Levitin, P.M., Makuc, D., Utsinger, P.D., Yount, W.J., Slusser, D., and Moskovitz, N. Hand

structure and function in an industrial setting. Arthritis Rheum 21:210–220, 1978.

19. Haines, R.W. The extensor apparatus of the finger. J Anat 85:251–259, 1951.

20. Harris, C., and Rutledge, G.L. The functional anatomy of the extensor mechanism of the finger. J Bone Joint Surg 54A:713–726, 1972.

21. Harrison, S.H. The functional relationship of the thumb to the fingers, in Tubiana, R. (ed): *The Hand,* vol 1. Philadelphia, Saunders, 1981.

22. Idler, R.S. Anatomy and biomechanics of the digital flexor tendons. Hand Clin 1:3–11, 1985.

23. Joseph, J. Further studies of the metacarpo-phalangeal and interphalangeal joints of the thumb. J Anat 85:221–229, 1951.

24. Kapandji, I.A. Biomechanics of the interphalangeal joint of the thumb, in Tubiana, R. (ed): *The Hand,* vol 1. Philadelphia, Saunders, 1981.

25. Kaplan, E.B. The participation of the metacarpophalangeal joint of the thumb in the act of opposition. Bull Hosp Joint Dis 27:39–45, 1966.

26. Kuczynski, K. Carpometacarpal joint of the human thumb. J Anat 118:119–126, 1974.

27. Landsmeer, J.M.F. Anatomical and functional investigations on the articulation of the human fingers. Acta Anat 24(Suppl):5–69, 1955.

28. Landsmeer, J.M.F. Power grip and precision handling. Ann Rheum Dis 21:164–170, 1962.

29. Landsmeer, J.M.F. Studies in the anatomy of articulation. Acta Morphol Neerl Scand 3:287–321, 1961.

30. Landsmeer, J.M.F. The anatomy of the dorsal aponeurosis of the human finger and its functional significance. Anat Rec 104:31–44, 1949.

31. Landsmeer, J.M.F. The coordination of finger-joint motions. J Bone Joint Surg 45A:1654–1662, 1963.

32. Linscheid, R.L., and Dobyns, J.H. Rheumatoid arthritis of the wrist. Orthop Clin North Am 2:649–665, 1971.

33. Long, C., Conrad, P.W., Hall, E.A., and Furler, S.L. Intrinsic-extrinsic muscle control of the hand in power grip and precision handling. J Bone Joint Surg 52A:853–867, 1970.

34. Minami, A., An, K-N, Cooney, W.P., Linscheid, R.L., and Chao, E.Y.S. Ligamentous structures of the metacarpophalangeal joint: A quantitative anatomic study. Orthop Res 1:361–368, 1984.

35. Micks, J.E., and Reswick, J.B. Confirmation of differential loading of the lateral and central fibers of the extensor tendon. J Hand Surg 6:462–467, 1981.

36. Moran, J.M., Hemann, J.H., and Greenwald, A.S. Finger joint contact areas and pressures. J Orthop Res 3:49–55, 1985.

37. Napier, J.R. The prehensile movements of the human hand. J Bone Joint Surg 38B:902–913, 1956.

38. Palmer, A.K. The distal radioulnar joint. Orthop Clin North Am 15:321–335, 1984.

39. Palmer, A.K., Glisson, R.R., and Werner, F.W. Relationship between ulnar variance and triangular fibrocartilage complex thickness. J Hand Surg 9A:681–683, 1984.

40. Palmer, A.K., Glisson, R.R., and Werner, F.W. Ulnar variance determination. J Hand Surg 7:376–379, 1982.

41. Palmer, A.K., and Nevaiser, R.J. Triangular fibrocartilage complex abnormalities—Results of surgical treatment. Orthop Trans 7:506, 1983.

42. Palmer, A., and Werner, F.W. Biomechanics of the distal radioulnar joint. Clin Orthop 187:26–35, 1984.

43. Palmer, A.K., Werner, F.W., Murphy, D., and Glisson, R. Functional wrist motion: A biomechanical study. J Hand Surg 10A:39–46, 1985.

44. Radin, E.L., Parker, H.G., and Paul, I.L. Pattern of degenerative arthritis. Preferential involvement of distal finger joints. Lancet 1:377–379, 1971.

45. Ratliff, A.H. Deformities of the thumb in rheumatoid arthritis. Hand 3:138–143, 1971.

46. Ray, R.D., Johnson, R.J., and Jameson, R.M. Rotation of the forearm. An experimental study of pronation and supination. J Bone Joint Surg 33A:993–996, 1951.

47. Sarrafian, S.K., Kazarian, L.E., Topouzian, L.K., Sarrafian, V.K., and Siegelman, A. Strain variation in the components of the extensor apparatus of the finger during flexion and extension. A biomechanical study. J Bone Joint Surg 52A:980–990, 1970.

48. Sarrafian, S.K., Melamed, J.L., and Goshgarian, G.M. Study of wrist motion in flexion and extension. Clin Orthop 126:153–159, 1977.

49. Shrewsbury, M.M., and Johnson, R.K. A systematic study of the oblique retinacular ligament of the human finger: Its structure and function. J Hand Surg 2:194–199, 1977.

50. Simmons, B.P., and de la Caffiniere, J.Y. Physiology of flexion of the fingers, in Tubiana, R. (ed): *The Hand,* vol 1. Philadelphia, Saunders, 1981.

51. Smith, E.M., Juvinall, R.C., Bender, L.F., and Pearson, J.R. Flexor forces and rheumatoid metacarpophalangeal deformity. JAMA 198:130–134, 1966.

52. Smith, E.M., Juvinall, R.C., Bender, L.F., and Pearson, J.R. Role of the finger flexors in rheumatoid deformities at the metacarpophalangeal joints of the fingers. Arthritis Rheum 7:467–480, 1964.

53. Smith, R.J. Balance and kinetics of the fingers under normal and pathological conditions. Clin Orthop 104:92–111, 1974.

54. Sundberg, S.B., and Linscheid, R.L. Kienbock's disease: Results of treatment with ulnar lengthening. Clin Orthop 187:43–51, 1984.

55. Swanson, A.B., Hagert, C.G., and Swanson, G. Evaluation of impairment of hand function. J Hand Surg 8:709–723, 1983.

56. Taleisnik, J. Wrist: Anatomy, function, and injury. Instr Course Lect 27:61–87, 1978.

57. Voltz, R.G. The development of a total wrist arthroplasty. Clin Orthop 116:209–214, 1976.

58. Voltz, R.G., Lieb, M., and Benjamin, J. Biomechanics of the wrist. Clin Orthop 149:112–117, 1980.

59. Weitbrecht, J. *Syndesmology. A description of the Ligaments of the Human Body.* Kaplan, E.B. (translator). Philadelphia, Saunders, 1969.

60. Youm, Y., and Flatt, A.E. Kinematics of the wrist. Clin Orthop 149:21–32, 1980.

61. Youm Y., McMurtry, R.Y., Flatt, A.E., and Gillespie, T.E. Kinematics of the wrist. J Bone Joint Surg 60A:423–431, 1978.

62. Zancolli, E. *Structural and Dynamic Bases of Hand Surgery.* Philadelphia, Lippincott, 1968.

CHAPTER 34

Congenital Anomalies of the Hand and Upper Extremity

Melvin Rosenwasser

The incidence of congenital hand deformities is difficult to ascertain because of the heterogeneity of the population subgroups. Recent figures from the Centers for Disease Control in Atlanta, Georgia,[10] reveal that approximately 1 out of every 1000 live births, demonstrate a congenital deformity. Relative incidence as studied by Flatt[9] in a series from Iowa showed syndactyly, polydactyly, camptodactyly, clinodactyly, and radial agenesis to be the five most frequent diagnoses, which accounted for 50 percent of the total.

In order to study this diverse group of conditions, the International Federation of Hand Societies adopted a classification of limb anomalies based on anatomical and embryological defect. The classification was outlined by Swanson in the first issue of the *Journal of Hand Surgery,*[17] citing seven major groups: (I) failure of formation of parts, (II) failure of separation of parts, (III) duplication, (IV) overgrowth (gigantism), (V) undergrowth (hypoplasia), (VI) congenital constriction bands, and (VII) generalized skeletal abnormalities.

The cause is unknown in more than 50 percent of congenital limb deformities, with the remaining half divided among environmental factors, genetic factors, or a combination of both. The evidence that thalidomide, coumadin, and dilantin cause limb deformities is conclusive.[10]

Chromosomal defects including trisomy 21 (Down syndrome), trisomy 18, trisomy 13 are associated with syndactyly, polydactyly, clinodactyly, and camptodactyly.

Brachydactyly, syndactyly, and camptodactyly can also be transmitted as single-gene autosomal defects either dominant, recessive, or sex-linked. The risk of recurrence varies with the mode of transmission. A partial list of the five most common defects with their known inheritance is in Table 34-1.

An example of autosomal dominant transmission is Aperts syndrome, or acrocephalosyndactyly.[10] An autosomal recessive transmission would be thrombocytopenia-absent-radius syndrome (TAR), which presents as a radial clubhand. An example of X-linked transmission would be whistling face syndrome.[1,3,7,8,9,13] The reason that the surgeon must be cognizant of some of the associated conditions is that a thorough organ system review with pediatric consultation is necessary prior to any reconstructive surgery.

It is necessary to understand the neuromuscular development of the upper extremity so that proper staging for reconstruction will be integrated into the overall maturation of skills. Most child behaviorists and hand surgeons believe that the hand functions of grasp and release and pinch are well integrated by 1 year and that further refinement, coordination, and control continue to age 3 or 4. Surgical reconstruction must be timed to allow for normal cortical development.

Thumb reconstructions, therefore, are performed at 1 year of age, or when the child is large enough to safely un-

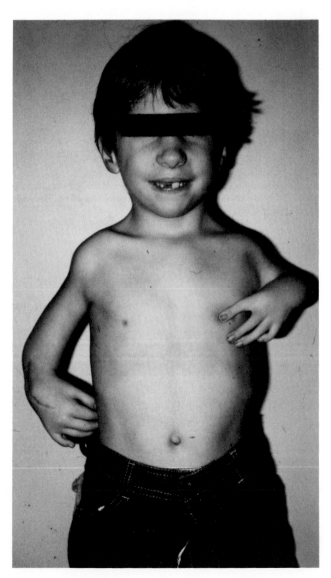

Figure 34-1 Phocomelia; absence of left humerus.

TABLE 34-1 The Five Most Common Congenital Deformities

Diagnosis	Incidence/inheritance	Characteristics
Syndactyly	1 in 2000 live births 20 percent genetic, all types	Simple: skin only Complex: conjoined bone, tendon, nerve, or blood vessel Complete: skin bridge to tip Incomplete: not to tip Most common: 3rd–4th interspace; next: 4th–5th interspace
Radial agenesis	1 in 100,000 live births Sporadic; autosomal dominant, drug effect (thalidomide)	May involve loss of all or any part of thumb, radial carpus, radius, extensor muscles
Clinodactyly: bent finger, radial or ulnar, in coronal plane	Normal adults: 1%–19.5% Patients with Down syndrome: 35%–79% Sporadic; autosomal dominant with variable penetrance	Greater than 10 degrees angulation of joint Usually DIP Caused by maldevelopment of middle phalanx (delta phalanx)
Camptodactyly: Infancy: onset 84% Adolescence: onset 16%	1 in 1000 live births; sporadic; few cases with autosomal dominant	Two-thirds are bilateral; flexion contracture of PIP joint with compensatory hyperextension of MP Progression in 80% of cases during growth spurt Tight or deficient skin of absent or deficient intrinsic extensors
Polydactyly: Preaxial: duplicate thumbs	0.08 in 1000 live births; mostly sporadic; no firm genetic passage	Wassal classification types I–VII (50% are type IV: duplication of distal and proximal phalanges)
Central: duplicate index, long, or ring fingers	Unknown; autosomal dominant	Complex duplication Mostly type II duplicate distal and middle phalanx
Postaxial: duplicate little finger Type A: well-formed with articulation Type B: rudimentary skin tag	*Blacks:* 1 in 300 live births *Whites:* 1 in 3000 live births Autosomal dominant with complete and incomplete penetrance	Often bilateral Most are type B with skin tag only

dergo general anesthesia. Priorities must be set for the staged procedures in cases such as thumb-index syndactyly when tethering structures would increase deformity during longitudinal growth.

ARM ABNORMALITIES

The shoulder may be involved in congenital defects such as congenital amputation, phocomelia, and arthrogryposis. Upper limb amputations are extremely rare, with a frequency of 1 in 270,000 live births.[1,3,7,8,9,13] When amputation is complete, prosthetic rehabilitation is the sole indication in most cases.

Longitudinal deficiencies such as phocomelia yield an extremely short limb, which again does not lend itself to lengthening or other reconstructive procedures (Fig. 34-1). Phocomelia is seen in 0.8 percent of congenital anomalies but is related to the mother's ingestion of thalidomide. Prosthetic rehabilitation can be performed successfully even in the young child and should not be delayed. Late introduction of such devices past ages 3 to 5 years will not allow integration for bimanual activities, and the child will reject the prosthesis.

Congenital synostosis of the elbow is a rare but disabling condition when complete, especially so when bilateral, which is frequently the case. There is no genetic inheritance pattern for this defect. Many synostoses are associated with other generalized skeletal anomalies such as congenital hip dislocation and clubfoot.[1,3,7,8,9,13]

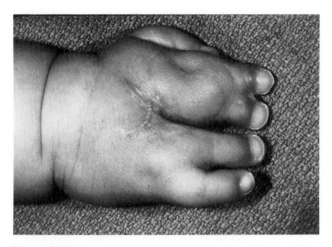

Figure 34-2 Complete and incomplete syndactyly.

Humeroradioulnar synostosis fixes the elbow in marked flexion, and surgical attempts to provide motion have not been successful. Radioulnar synostosis, when complete, can also greatly limit function when a marked pronation deformity is present and especially when it is bilateral. Derotational osteotomy has been successful in repositioning the forearm in mild pronation. If the condition is bilateral, one forearm may be positioned into mild supination to aid perineal care.

Radial head dislocation can be associated with radioulnar synostosis. The dislocation can be anterior, posterior, or lateral. Two-thirds are posterior, with the remainder equally divided between anterior and lateral. Differentiation from the more common posttraumatic condition is enhanced by the presence of relative ulnar shortening or radial lengthening, a dome-shaped radial head with a long narrow neck, bilaterality, certain other anomalies, and a family history.[1,3,7,8,9,13]

Genetic inheritance is high, 60 to 100 percent having an autosomal dominant or recessive pattern. Many associated conditions that demonstrate a short ulna may predispose to radial head dislocation. Ulnar deficiency, multiple exostosis, and multiple enchondromatosis are only a few conditions that may present with a dislocated radial head.

Radial head dislocation leads to a mild to moderate loss of motion at the elbow, with most loss seen in rotation. Surgery is indicated for pain, limited mobility, and cosmesis. Radial head excision may be performed at skeletal maturity.

HAND ABNORMALITIES

Syndactyly

Syndactyly is one of the most common congenital hand deformities. It is classified as *complete* if the skin bridge is present to the distal tip, and as *complex* (rather than *simple*) if other structures such as nail, bone, tendon, nerve, or blood vessel are conjoined[1,3,7,8,9,13] (Fig. 34-2).

The most common site is the interspace of the long and ring fingers, followed by the interspace of the ring and little fingers, and then that of the index and long fingers. The thumb-index interspace is rarely involved in the isolated cases of syndactyly, but is involved with associated anomalies such as Apert syndrome (Fig. 34-3).

Treatment of this condition depends upon the complexity and site. Division of border digits is done early to prevent progressive angular deformity. Dorsal and volar flaps are raised to resurface the commissures and reestablish the proper web depth and slope. The anatomical constraint to the amount of deepening is the bifurcation of the proper digital arteries. The lateral sides of the separated fingers can only be partially surfaced with the flaps because of the increased surface area of the separated digits, which always require a thick split skin graft.

There is an unknown but definite incidence of recurrence of web contracture secondary to longitudinal growth and the contraction of the skin graft. In division of simple syndactyles, a normal cosmetic and functional result is to be expected.

Polydactyly

Polydactyly is a very common entity with an increased incidence in the black race, especially in the postaxial or ulnar duplication presentation.[1,3,7,8,9,13] There is a genetic transmission of polydactyly in both spontaneous cases and associated syndromes. Polydactyly is classified into preaxial (thumb), central (index, long, and ring), and postaxial (little finger) categories (Fig. 34-4). Within these types there is further classification based on the extent to which the extra digit is fully formed. For thumb duplication the classification proposed by Wassel is used, outlining types I to VII.[18] Fifty percent of thumb duplications are type IV, which is a duplication of both phalanges and a common metacarpal.

In general, it is best to ablate the most radial thumb, but a careful preoperative evaluation should always be done because there are occasions when preservation of the radial thumb is indicated because it has the most intact composite parts. If the duplication is a triphalangeal thumb, it is most frequently ablated with maximal utilization of bone, skin, and nail matrix to reconstruct the adjacent thumb. It is important to recognize that the remaining thumb must be rebalanced following ablation of the supernumerary digit. The tendon

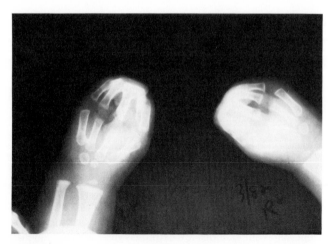

Figure 34-3 Complex syndactyly. Rosebud hand of Apert's syndrome.

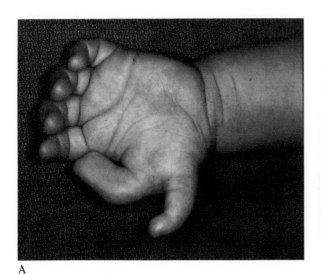

A

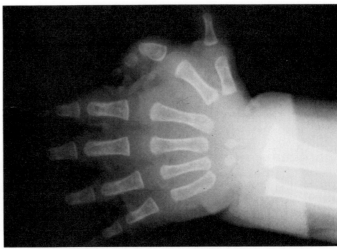

B

Figure 34-4 A. Thumb duplication. Type VI. **B.** Radiograph of same hand.

insertions, collateral ligaments, and capsule must be restored or a late collapsing zig-zag deformity will result. The Bilhaut-Cloquet procedure divided the type II duplicate thumb (Fig. 34-5), excised the middle one-half, and then rejoined the remainder.[2] This procedure requires division of the epiphyseal plate and germinal nail matrix, leading to nail and growth deformities. Therefore authors have not favored the Bilhaut-Cloquet procedure for type II deformity because of increased interphalangeal joint stiffness and nail deformities. Postaxial duplication is usually easier to treat, and simple ablation for the skin tag or more formal tissue rearrangement for complete duplication should be performed in the operating suite when the child is around 1 year old.

Camptodactyly

Camptodactyly, or bent finger, is frequently seen involving the proximal interphalangeal joint of the fifth finger (Fig. 34-6). The deformity has a bimodal distribution, that is to say: infancy and adolescence. It is usually progressive, and can be functionally limiting when it approaches 90 degrees of flexion.[1,3,7,8,9,13]

The cause is unknown, but a rudimentary or absent intrinsic extensor mechanism has been implicated. This condition must be differentiated from trauma or juvenile aponeurotic fibromatosis. Trauma could injure the dorsal extensor mechanism, causing a boutonniere deformity, and juvenile aponeurotic fibromatosis can involve palmar fascia and skin, creating a flexion deformity.

Treatment of camptodactyly is reserved for severe progressive deformities and includes Z-plasty of skin, joint capsule, and collateral ligament–volar plate releases, and transfer of the flexor sublimis to the extensor hood. In skeletally mature individuals with fixed deformities, a dorsal closing wedge osteotomy is preferred. Excessive straightening may cause vascular injury and must be avoided.

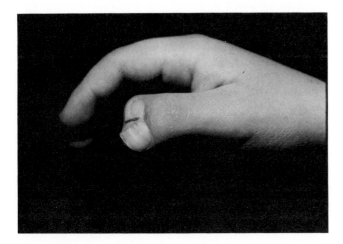

Figure 34-5 Thumb duplication. Type II.

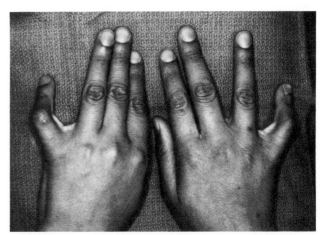

Figure 34-6 Camptodactyly.

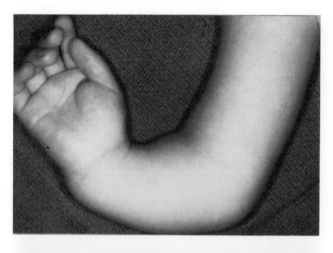

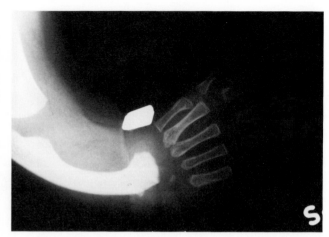

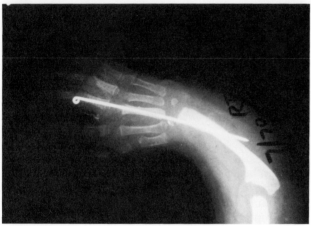

Figure 34-7 **A.** Radial agenesis. **B.** Radiograph of same limb. **C.** Centralization of carpus over ulna.

Clinodactyly

Clinodactyly is a bending or curvature in the radioulnar plane usually seen with the fingertip curved toward the midline.[1,3,7,8,9,13] Clinodactyly occurs in otherwise normal children in a 1 to 20 percent frequency. Rarely this curvature is caused by a delta phalanx involving malalignment of the epiphyseal plate of the middle phalanx with progressive angular deformity. This entity rarely requires treatment, but if a delta phalanx is present, an epiphyseodesis and wedge osteotomy will correct and prevent further deformity. Excision of the delta phalanx may be performed but will lead to excessive shortening of the digit.

Radial Clubhand

Radial clubhand is a manifestation of radial agenesis with a longitudinal deficiency which may be total or partial[1,3,7,8,9,13] (Fig. 34-7A and B). It may involve all or part of the extensor muscle mass, radial carpus, or thumb ray. It may be associated with cardiac and hematologic disorders such as the Holt-Oram, TAR, or Vater syndromes.[11,12,15] The treatment is based on the child's functional needs. Indeed the European literature advocates no specific treatment for bilateral cases especially if a rudimentary thumb is present. Most American authors have advocated early splinting of the radial and palmar flexed hand and subsequent centralization of the carpus over the ulna with secondary thumb reconstruction[1,3,7,8,9,13] (Fig. 34-7C). This reconstruction may be a distraction lengthening and stabilization if adequate thumb components are present, or more likely will be an index pollicization, which involves a local vascularized transposition with a restoration of thenar intrinsic function.[6] This reconstruction works very well if the index to be pollicized is itself not too hypoplastic. New microsurgical procedures, for example, transplantation of toe to thumb, have provided additional ways of allowing active prehension.[4,5] Elbow mobility is a prerequisite for centralization procedures for radial clubhand to ensure that hand-to-mouth feeding activities are possible. Centralization

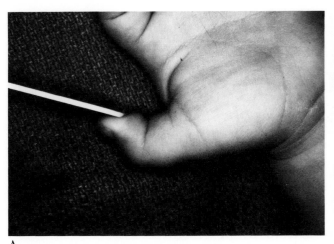

A

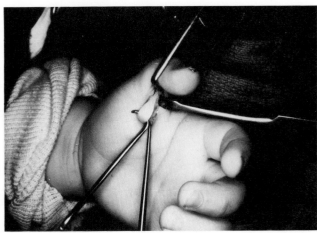

B

Figure 34-8 A. Congenital trigger thumb, preoperative view. **B.** Release of proximal pulley. Note proximal thickening of tendon.

will not always prevent a recurrence. Recurrence often necessitates a wrist arthrodesis at skeletal maturity.

Less Common Congenital Deformities

The above five diagnoses account for one-half of the patients in Flatt's series. The remaining half are represented by less common diagnoses but require the same thoughtful evaluation of functional requirements before contemplating any surgical exercise. Congenital trigger thumb is easily diagnosed, and treatment can yield a normal hand (Fig. 34-8A and B). Many of the hypoplastic syndromes, including annular congenital bands, require digital lengthenings via transposition or distraction.[14] It is clear that joint mobility, sensibility, and bilaterality are important determinants of whether the patient will be able to use the reconstructed limb. Each patient is unique, and no algorithm can be fashioned to treat all children with the same diagnosis. Photographs of the end results will often prepare parents and child for what can be realistically expected from reconstruction.

One day we may be able to predict the potential for and prevent these upper limb anomalies, thus obviating oftimes imperfect reconstruction.[16]

REFERENCES

1. Barsky, A.J. *Congenital Anomalies of the Hand and Their Surgical Treatment.* Springfield, IL, Thomas, 1958.
2. Bilhaut, M. Guerison d'un pouce bifide par un nouveau procede operatoire. Congr Fr Chir 4:576, 1890.
3. Boyes, J.H. (ed.): *Bunnell's Surgery of the Hand,* 5th ed. Philadelphia, Lippincott, 1970.
4. Buncke, H.J. Toe digital transfer. Clin Plast Surg 3(1):49–57, 1976.
5. Buncke, H.J., McLean, D.H., George, P.T., Breevator, J.C., Chater, N.L., and Commons, G.W. Thumb replacement. Great toe transplantation by microvascular anastomosis. Br J Plast Surg 26:194–201, 1973.
6. Carroll, R.E. Pollicization, in Green, D.P. (ed): *Operative Hand Surgery.* New York, Churchill Livingstone, 1982, pp 1619–1634.
7. Dobyns, J.H., Wood, V.E., Bayne, L.G., and Frykman, G.K. Congenital hand deformities, in Green, D.P. (ed): *Operative Hand Surgery.* New York, Churchill Livingstone, 1988, pp 255–536.
8. Entin, M.A. Congenital anomalies, in Flynn, J.E. (ed): *Hand Surgery,* 3d ed. Baltimore, Williams & Wilkins, 1982, pp 45-73.
9. Flatt, A.E. *The Care of Congenital Hand Anomalies.* St. Louis, Mosby, 1977.
10. Goldberg, M.J., and Bartoshesky, L.E. Congenital hand anomaly. Etiology and associated malformations. Hand Clin 1(3):405–415, 1985.
11. Hays, R.M., Bartoshesky, L.E., and Feingold, M. New features of thrombocytopenia and absent radius syndrome. Birth Defects 18(3B):115–121.
12. Holt, M., and Oram, S. Familial heart disease with skeletal malformations. Br Heart J 22:336–342, 1960.
13. Kelikian, H. *Congenital Deformities of the Hand and Forearm.* Philadelphia, Saunders, 1974.
14. Matev, I.B. Thumb reconstruction in children through metacarpal lengthening. Plast Reconstr Surg 64:665–669, 1979.
15. Quan, L., and Smith, D.W. The VATER association; vertebral defects, anal atresia, T-E fistula with esophageal atresia. Radial and renal dysplasia. A spectrum of associated defects. J Pediatr 82:104–107, 1973.
16. Smith, R.J. Preventive surgery for congenital deformities of the hand. Hand Clin 1(3):373–382, 1985.
17. Swanson, A.B. A classification for congenital limb malformations. J Hand Surg 1:8–22, 1976.
18. Wassel, H.D. The results of surgery for polydactyly of the thumb. A review. Clin Orthop 64:175–193, 1969.

CHAPTER 35

Traumatic Injury to the Upper Extremity

Steven Sampson, Edward Akelman, Robert J. Garroway,
Frank C. McCue III, Roger Dee, Enrico Mango, Craig Ordway,
Louis U. Bigliani, and David S. Morrison

SECTION A

Fractures and Dislocations of the Hand, Wrist, and Forearm

Steven Sampson and Edward Akelman

The estimated cumulative average incidence rate of fractures of the hand, wrist, and forearm per thousand population is 9.1 percent.[69] These injuries often affect people during their wage-earning years and cause significant disabilities and, particularly, loss of useful motion.

PHALANGEAL BONES

Fractures of the Distal Phalanx

Fractures of the distal phalanx are the most common fractures found in the hand and are frequently complicated by soft tissue loss, severe pulp compartmental crush, and nail bed lacerations.[170] The majority are comminuted but nondisplaced, and may be dorsally splinted to immobilize the distal joint. Associated nail bed lacerations must have thorough irrigation, debridement, and careful repair of the nail bed. Associated subungual hematomas should be drained, permitting the nail to remain intact.[220]

Displaced transverse fractures of the base of the distal phalanx are usually reducible by closed means with the aid of a metacarpal or wrist block. In order to obtain and maintain reduction, flexion of the distal fragment and dorsal splintage of the distal interphalangeal (DIP) joint in slight flexion are often necessary so as to overcome the flexor profundus pull on the proximal fragment (Fig. 35-1).[146] Displaced fractures

may require longitudinal K-wire fixation in order to maintain reduction. Fractures associated with a gap of greater than 2 mm may require open reduction so as to extricate the nail matrix driven into the fracture site.

Distal Interphalangeal Joint Dislocations

These dislocations are extremely rare.[16,40,139,150,169,191] They are usually dorsal and sometimes open, associated with an innocent-appearing laceration in the region of the distal interphalangeal joint flexion crease.[219] Following irrigation and debridement of the skin edges, the joint is easily reduced by gentle traction preceded by flexing the wrist and metacarpophalangeal joints. A dorsal splint is applied with the DIP joint in slight flexion for approximately 3 weeks with active proximal interphalangeal (PIP) motion initiated from the onset.

Fractures of the Middle and Proximal Phalanges

Fractures within this phalangeal zone of injury are called "no man's land" fractures.[20,189,190] Overall skeletal stability of the middle and proximal phalanx is essential for normal PIP func-

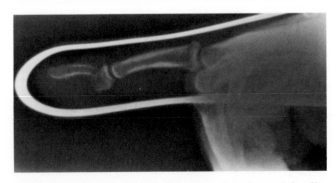

Figure 35-1 Dorsally displaced fracture of the base of the distal phalanx.

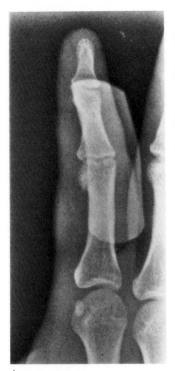
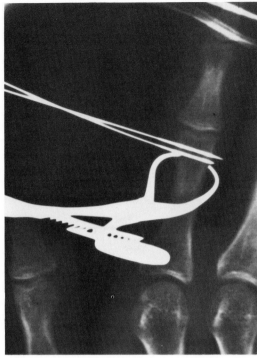

A   B

Figure 35-2 **A.** Condylar fracture of the proximal phalanx with an articular stepoff. **B.** Anatomical closed reduction held with percutaneous K-wire pins.

tion. In this region, fractures will usually displace because of the deforming muscle forces acting on the fracture fragments.[15]

Intracondylar Fractures

Intracondylar fractures of the middle and proximal phalanges are often displaced. These fractures should have an attempted closed reduction utilizing a fracture clamp and percutaneous K-wire fixation (Fig. 35-2).[11,75,146] However, more typically, these fractures require an open reduction because of malrotation of the condylar fragment.[185] When these fragments are large enough, 1.5-mm miniscrew fixation may be utilized.[31,32,84,93,178,182] Otherwise, transverse K-wire fixation may be adequate with motion of the involved segment delayed for approximately 3 to 4 weeks. Because of the intraarticular nature of these fractures, protected early motion is helpful if fracture stability can be obtained.

Middle Phalanx Fractures

Extraarticular fractures of the middle phalanx are relatively less common than proximal phalangeal fractures. The displacement of middle phalangeal fractures is usually determined by the relationship of the fracture to the flexor digitorum superficialis insertion.[75,186] Extraarticular fractures of the base of the middle phalanx usually collapse and angulate dorsally. Fractures of the neck, distal to the superficialis insertion, collapse and angulate volarly. Fractures located in the midshaft region between these two extremes may angulate in either direction.

Stable fractures of the middle phalanx may be treated with dorsal splintage allowing active PIP motion when possible. Because of the increased cortical content of this phalanx, x-ray manifestation of fracture healing will lag significantly behind clinical healing.[10] When these fractures are malrotated, displaced, or angulated greater than 20 degrees, a closed reduction should be carried out. The hand and wrist should than be placed in a short arm cast incorporating the

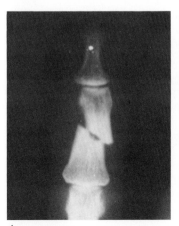
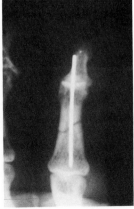

A   B

Figure 35-3 **A.** AP x-ray view showing angulated fracture of the middle phalanx that failed attempted closed reduction. **B.** Anatomical reduction with K-wire fixation.

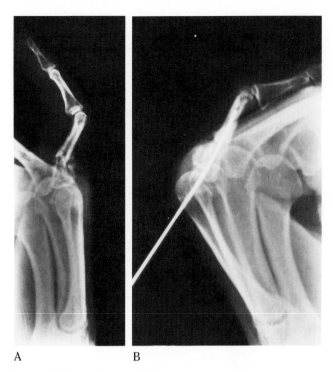

A   B

Figure 35-4 A. Zigzag collapse of fracture of the proximal third of proximal phalanx presenting 12 days after injury. **B.** Anatomical reduction held with K-wire fixation.

immediately adjacent digit or digits in such a way as to restore the longitudinal and transverse arches of the hand and wrist. This restoration may be accomplished by placing the hand in an "intrinsic plus" position with the wrist resting in 20 degrees of dorsiflexion, the metacarpophalangeal (MP) joints flexed 60 to 70 degrees, and the interphalangeal (IP) joints flexed minimally.[95]

Unstable middle phalangeal fractures may be longitudinally stabilized avoiding PIP joint fixation (Fig. 35-3).[15,20] A K-wire passed in line with the midaxial skin landmarks will accurately guide pin placement along the midaxis of the bone. Following stabilization, carefully supervised exercises of the PIP joint may be performed during the 4-week splinting period.

Proximal Phalanx Fractures

Transverse fractures in the proximal third to midshaft regions of the proximal phalanx collapse with a volar angulatory deformity (Fig. 35-4A). An adequate closed reduction can usually be obtained by traction applied to the middle phalanx while flexing the metacarpophalangeal joint to 90 degrees. This reduction maneuver uses the intact dorsal periosteal sleeve of the proximal phalanx as a hinge. In addition, by flexing the proximal fragment 90 degrees, the deforming forces of the intrinsic musculature will be overcome.

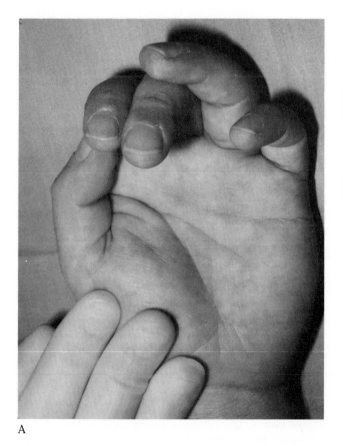

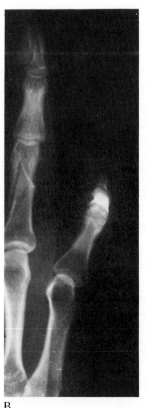

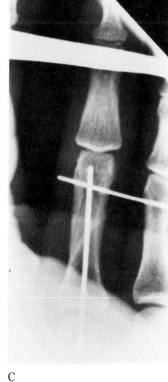

A   B   C

Figure 35-5 A. Malrotation secondary to a spiral oblique fracture of the proximal phalanx. **B.** Shortened spiral oblique fracture of proximal phalanx. **C.** Near anatomical reduction obtained utilizing both longitudinal and transverse K-wires.

Spiral and oblique proximal phalangeal fractures may be unstable and are usually associated with shortening and malrotation (Fig. 35-5*A* and *B*).[20] These fractures are usually easy to reduce, but tend to redisplace in the direction of their prior deformity. Malrotation must be carefully checked by finger flexion and comparison with the opposite hand.

Fractures at the base of the proximal phalanx frequently occur in osteopenic metaphyseal bone and usually deform with the apex volar. These fractures can usually be reduced by similar traction and flexion maneuver,[118] but are usually associated with dorsal comminution and consequently commonly redisplace.

Unstable transverse and short oblique proximal phalangeal fractures can usually be stabilized with a K-wire following anatomical closed reduction (Fig. 35-4). The wire is passed into the proximal phalanx in an antegrade fashion with the MP joint flexed at 60 to 70 degrees and advanced across the fracture to the phalangeal metaphysis but not into the PIP joint.[11] The K-wire acts as "an internal suture" allowing provisional stabilization and early PIP joint motion. Incorporation of adjacent digits in plaster helps maintain rotational stability. The K-wire is maintained for approximately 3 weeks, and the pin is then removed. Complications of this technique are avoided by expeditious removal of the K-wire.[53,189,190]

Unstable oblique proximal phalangeal fractures with greater than 45 degrees of angulation may be reduced with a fracture clamp (Fig. 35-5*C*).[11,20] This clamp also serves as a x-ray marker for the placement of pins as far apart as possible in the midaxis of the phalanx.[6,165] These fractures are usually maintained with the adjacent digit incorporated. Postoperatively, extension block splinting should be begun in the early postoperative period in order to allow active PIP flexion. If anatomical closed reduction cannot be obtained, open reduction with K-wires or 2.0-mm screw fixation may be considered.[31,32,49,84,93,127,178,182] Motion of the digit should be initiated within 48 h of stable operative fixation.

Proximal Interphalangeal Dislocations and Fracture Dislocations

PIP joint dislocations are common. Dorsal dislocations with resultant hyperextension injuries to the volar plate are by far the most common type of dislocation.[17] Following metacarpal or wrist block anesthesia, these dislocations are usually easy to reduce. Treatment includes dorsal PIP joint splintage in approximately 30 degrees of flexion for approximately 1 week, followed by "buddy" tape splinting to the adjacent digit for the next 6 weeks. Following reduction, all dislocations should be tested for stability with an "active motion test" and a collateral ligament stress test while the patient is under anesthesia.[40,42] These tests will determine those dislocations which are stable and able to be moved early as opposed to those which will require extension block splinting for more prolonged periods of time.

Frequently, intraarticular fractures at the base of the middle phalanx are associated with dorsal dislocation and/or subluxation of the PIP joint. These volar plate fractures are usually stable if less than one-third of the articular surface is involved on examination of a true lateral x-ray view.[140] Frac-

tures with greater than one-third of the articular surface involved are usually unstable because the displaced volar middle phalangeal fragment also contains the distal attachment of the collateral ligament, thereby allowing dorsal displacement (Fig. 35-6).[3,40,42,43,121,185,215,217] In the acute state, reduction of these subluxations can usually be carried out with flexion of the PIP joint between 60 and 80 degrees. If a closed reduction can be obtained, an extension block splinting program with active PIP joint flexion is carried out.[122] Alternatively, loss of reduction is associated with joint incongruity necessitating open reduction accompanied by collateral ligament excision, debridement of comminuted volar fragments, and advancement of the volar plate.[43,151]

Volar dislocations of the proximal interphalangeal joint are rare injuries.[156,157,183,201] These injuries may be treated conservatively when congruent reduction is obtained with less than a 30-degree extension lag actively at the PIP joint. However, these injuries are sometimes irreducible, and they may reveal evidence of joint incongruity due to interposition of the central slip[61,158] or herniation of the proximal phalangeal condyle through the extensor mechanism with associated rupture of the volar plate and the collateral ligament.[40] These irreducible complex dislocations require open reduction and K-wire pinning of the PIP joint in extension for approximately 4 weeks; they are treated like acute boutonniere tendon injuries during the postoperative period. As opposed to dorsal dislocations, volar dislocations of the PIP joint are frequently associated with significant loss of motion.[156]

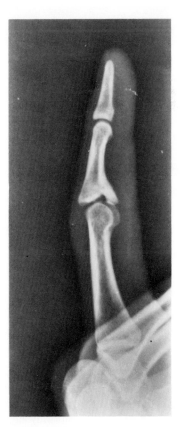

Figure 35-6 True lateral x-ray view reveals volar plate fracture subluxation with impaction of the middle phalanx and joint incongruity.

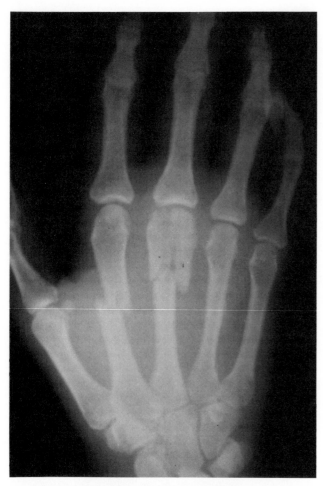

Figure 35-7 A dune buggy rolled over this hand causing severe soft tissue swelling as well as an oblique shortened midshaft fracture of the index metacarpal with an adjacent comminuted intraarticular fracture of the long metacarpal head, neck-shaft region.

METACARPAL BONES

Fractures of the Metacarpal

Biomechanically, the index and long metacarpals act as the stabilizing central *fixed* unit of the hand and wrist. The ring, little, and thumb metacarpals are portions of the *mobile* unit of the hand. Fracture displacement, angulation, and shortening occurring within the central fixed unit of the hand have dramatically more functional impact than those same injuries sustained in the mobile unit of the hand. Anatomically, the carpometacarpal (CMC) joints of the index and long fingers have stable joint configurations and strong ligamentous attachments, whereas the CMC joints of the ring and little fingers allow flexion, extension, and supination.[79]

The intrinsic muscles are the primary deforming force of fractures occurring within the longitudinal arch of the hand. Instead of flexion occurring at the metacarpophalangeal (MP) joint, the intrinsic muscles act to dorsally angulate fractures in this region. Generally, unstable *fixed-unit* metacarpal fractures are evident by compensatory MP joint hyperextension, whereas metacarpal *mobile-unit* fractures tend to compensate primarily at their mobile CMC joints and then secondarily at the MP joint.

Intraarticular Metacarpal Fractures

Intraarticular metacarpal head fractures are relatively rare injuries.[107,123] These fractures are most commonly seen involving the border digits, with the index and little fingers most commonly involved. They may be associated with open osteochondral fractures, and joint sepsis is a key concern. Most fractures in this region are comminuted and are associated with significant soft tissue trauma including adjacent metacarpal and phalangeal fractures (Fig. 35-7). Large articular fragments should be considered for open reduction and internal fixation, whereas severely comminuted fractures should have controlled early motion initiated, with MP joint arthroplasty as a salvage alternative. Transverse fractures of the metacarpal head have been associated with a avascular necrosis as a late complication.

Intraarticular fractures of the base of the metacarpals are most common in the thumb and little fingers. The most significant clinical problem associated with these injuries is subluxation of the CMC joint. In a *Bennett's fracture;* the strong volar ligament remains attached to the volar-ulnar tubercle of the thumb metacarpal (Fig. 35-8A).[63,70,208,212] Due to the continued pull of the abductor pollicis longus, the thumb metacarpal subluxes dorsoradially and the adductor pulls the shaft toward the second metacarpal.[15] Articular congruity must be reestablished with a closed reduction and percutaneous pinning (Fig. 35-8B). Closed reduction may be obtained by traction of the thumb metacarpal followed by radial abduction and finally by a pronation rotatory torque, placing the thumb metacarpal in the palmar abduction in opposition to the second metacarpal.[80]

Comminuted intraarticular fractures associated with the thumb metacarpal are also known as *Rolando's fractures* (Fig. 35-8C).[70] These fractures may be initially stabilized in a thumb spica cast with the thumb metacarpal placed in palmar abduction in apposition to the index finger. Early mobilization in 10 to 14 days should be considered, depending upon individual circumstances. Rolando's fractures associated with large intraarticular fragments should be considered for open reduction and internal fixation with either 2.0- or 2.7-mm screws or K-wire stabilization.[31,32,84,93,127,178,182]

Fractures of the little metacarpal base simulate Bennett's fracture subluxation of the thumb.[13] Articular congruity must be obtained by a reduction that overcomes the pull of the extensor carpi ulnaris on the metacarpal base and also that of the hypothenar intrinsic musculature. Reduction must be carried out by traction and ulnar abduction of the little finger metacarpal followed by a slight supination torque. Percutaneous pinning is then carried out, pinning the little to the ring metacarpal and to the hamate. The best x-ray picture taken to visualize reduction of this joint is shot with the forearm pronated 30 degrees from the routine anteroposterior position. Late sequelae of unreduced subluxation dislocations include posttraumatic arthrosis sometimes requiring ligament interposition arthroplasty, prosthetic arthroplasty, or arthrodesis.[192]

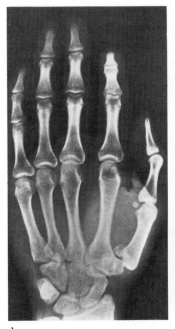 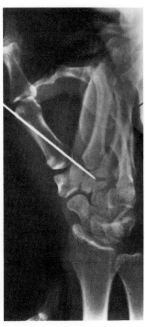

A   B

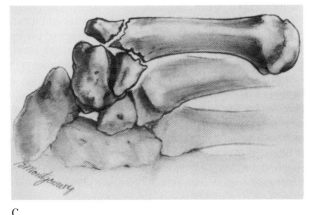

C

Figure 35-8 A. Bennett's fracture with subluxation of first metacarpal and loss of joint congruity. **B.** Closed anatomical reduction maintained with an axial K-wire. **C.** Rolando's fracture. *(From Green, D.P. and O'Brien, E.T., South Med J 65:807, 1972. Reproduced with permission.)*

Extraarticular Metacarpal Fractures

Fractures of the *metacarpal neck* are generally unstable injuries because of the concomitant comminution of the volar cortex (Fig. 35-9A). Within this region, there is a relatively dramatic transition from thin corticocancellous metaphyseal bone to thickened diaphyseal cortex.[10,109] Anatomically, the dorsal cortices of the metacarpals are relatively straight in contour, whereas the volar cortices have a concavity corresponding to the contour of the palm. Radiographically, a true lateral of the average metacarpal will reveal a 10- to 15-degree neck-shaft angulation.[1]

When metacarpal neck fractures are associated with significant dorsal soft tissue swelling following a clenched fist mechanism of injury, the possibility of a human bite infection must be meticulously excluded.

Controversy exists as to how much dorsal angulation in the ring and little metacarpal neck fracture is acceptable.[68,77,90,170,182] Because of compensatory carpometacarpal motion, up to 30 or 40 degrees of dorsal angulation may be acceptable for these mobile-unit neck fractures. This is in contrast to the fixed-unit (index and long) metacarpal neck fractures in which minimal angulation (10 to 15 degrees) is acceptable.

Closed reduction of metacarpal neck fractures is carried out by traction, disimpaction followed by the Jahss reduction maneuver. This entails 90 degrees of MP and PIP flexion, thereby controlling the distal metacarpal fragment by the relative tautness of the MP collateral ligaments. Counterpressure is then applied to the dorsum of the proximal fragment at the fracture site. Typically, reduction is easy to obtain but difficult to maintain.[50] A short arm cast is applied incorporating the adjacent digit to the level just proximal to the PIP joint. The wrist is held in 20 degrees of extension, the MP joints are held in 60 to 70 degrees of flexion, and the PIP joints are left free. Molding the cast in the 90-90 degree reduction position is contraindicated because of the resultant stiffness and potential skin or tendon slough over the dorsum of the MP joint.[94]

Rowland and Green have described a simple clinical test to identify those patients who may be treated by closed reduction and cast immobilization. Following wrist block anesthesia, those patients who are able to fully extend the fractured finger without concomitant MP joint hyperextension and flexion at the PIP joint may be treated conservatively.[75] If "clawing" or zigzag collapse becomes apparent on this clinical test (Fig. 35-9A), then percutaneous pin fixation is recommended to maintain the reduction (Fig. 35-9B).

Technically, various methods of percutaneous pin fixation of these metacarpal neck fractures have been described.[19,45,77,146,170,212] An anatomical reduction is essential prior to K-wire stabilization paralleling the straight dorsal cortex of the involved metacarpal.[109] In the majority of cases, stabilization of the fracture has occurred by the end of 3 weeks, and the K-wire is then removed. Removal of the K-wire at this time avoids the feared complication of MP joint arthrofibrosis and sepsis. Following K-wire removal, the involved digits are splinted with buddy tape. Additional indications for closed-reduction internal fixation of metacarpal neck fractures is any fracture associated with malrotation or complete displacement.

Fractures occurring in the region of the *metacarpal shaft* may result in similar dorsal angulatory deformities related to the intrinsic muscular forces. Less than 10 degrees of dorsal angulation is acceptable in the index and long metacarpals. Twenty degrees is acceptable in the ring and little fingers. The closer a fracture is to the midshaft level, the greater the probability that such a fracture will cause a claw deformity on extension of the digit. Oblique fractures of the metacarpal shaft tend to be unstable and tend to shorten according to the initial deforming force and to the degree of obliquity at the fracture site. The intervolar plate (deep transverse metacar-

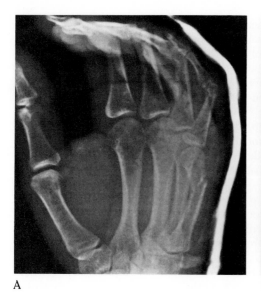
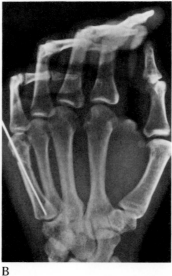

Figure 35-9 A. Clawing is evident with MP hyperextension and PIP flexion in this metacarpal neck-shaft fracture. X-ray films reveal 40 degrees of dorsal angulation. **B.** Anatomical closed reduction held with percutaneous K-wire.

A   B

pal) ligament will usually prevent significant central metacarpal (i.e., long and ring fingers) shortening.[40] However, greater than 3 or 4 mm of shortening is more likely to occur in the border metacarpals (i.e., index and little fingers and thumb).

Unstable metacarpal shaft fractures are treated initially by attempted closed reduction and application of a short arm cast incorporating the adjacent digits to the level just proximal to the PIP joint. Reduction can usually be accomplished by longitudinal traction, extension of the wrist with fixation of the CMC joints followed by MP flexion, and, finally, "third-point" molding dorsally over the fracture site. If a closed reduction cannot be maintained as swelling subsides, percutaneous K-wire fixation is carried out.

When two adjacent unstable oblique metacarpal fractures occur, a single longitudinal intramedullary K-wire is usually inadequate to control angulation, rotation, and shortening. Therefore, besides a longitudinal pin to control dorsal angulation, a distal transmetacarpal pin may be utilized to prevent shortening. This type of treatment may be complicated by delayed union due to overdistraction at the fracture site. Alternatively, unstable oblique fractures of the metacarpal shaft may be treated by open reduction and internal fixation with 2.0- or 2.7-mm screws. Plate fixation may be indicated when the obliquity of the fracture is less than 45 to 60 degrees from the axis of the metacarpal shaft. In general, rigid internal fixation should be reserved for situations in which immediate skeletal stability is required to mobilize joints within the first 48 h (Fig. 35-7).[31,32,84,93,97,127,178]

Metacarpophalangeal Joint Dislocations

MP joint dislocations of the ulnar four digits are relatively rare injuries.[40] The history is of a significant hyperextension injury of either the index or little metacarpal with resultant rupture of the volar plate. Anatomically, the MP joints are structurally the most unstable phalangeal joints and are dependent on ligamentocapsular restraint to check increased motion. The MP joints allow abduction, adduction, and some rotation as these joints progress from a flexed to an extended posture.[40] Thus, when forces are applied in the hyperextended position, the collateral ligaments are lax and tension is borne by the volar plate. The central MP joints of the long and ring fingers are relatively more stabilized by their bordering digits and their respective intervolar plate ligaments.[40,42]

Simple MP joint dislocations should undergo an attempted closed reduction under wrist block anesthesia.[22,40] While flexing the wrist, the head of the proximal phalanx is gently grasped. In order to secure reduction, the dorsally displaced proximal phalanx base is gently pushed distally, while the fingers grasping the proximal phalanx are initially hyperextending and then flexing its base. Any overt traction maneuver may convert the simple reducible dislocation into a complex or irreducible one.

The pathognomonic sign of a complex MP dislocation is the presence of an associated skin puckering in the region of the distal palmar crease of the hand.[72,91,98,129,217] The most common anatomical structure preventing closed reduction is the interposition of the volar plate which ruptures proximally. This differs from the dorsal dislocations of the PIP joint in which the volar plate most commonly ruptures distally.[17,40,42] Reduction is carried out after incision of the flexor tendon sheath in the region of the Al pulley. Care must be taken when using a volar approach because the radial neurovascular bundle may be displaced volarly under tension. Following reduction, the joint is placed in 45 degrees of flexion and a short arm cast is applied incorporating the adjacent digit for approximately 3 weeks allowing PIP flexion. During the fourth postoperative week, a program of MP joint extension block splinting is begun.[40,42]

Dislocations of the MP joint of the thumb are much more common than those seen in the ulnar four digits. They may be simple or complex, and they may be dorsally, volarly, or laterally displaced. The reduction maneuver recommended is as previously described for other MP joints.[22,129] Complex dislocations have been attributed to the volar plate, sesamoids, and flexor pollicis longus. Following reduction, a short-arm thumb spica cast is applied with the MP joint in approximately 20 degrees of flexion with the IP joint left free. Few patients develop late collateral ligamentous instability following dorsal and volar dislocations; however, ulnar instability must be carefully checked especially after lateral dislocations.[40,42]

Carpometacarpal Joint Dislocations

Dislocations of the carpometacarpal joints of the ulnar four metacarpals are among the most commonly overlooked dislocations in the hand.[79,82,87,104,113,190] These injuries are usually associated with extensive soft tissue swelling which obscures the true reason for the flattening of the proximal transverse metacarpal arch contour. Dislocations in this region may be dorsal or volar, but most are dorsal with involvement of the fourth and fifth metacarpal bases (Fig. 35-10A). As with other ulnar-sided metacarpal injuries, a true lateral radi-

ograph will commonly be difficult to interpret because of the multiple overlapping shadows of the adjacent four metacarpals.[99] Much more information may be derived from lateral x-ray films taken with the forearm pronated 30 degrees from the routine lateral position.[13]

Dislocations of the ulnar four carpometacarpal joints are generally easy to reduce by gentle traction.[79] However, the maintenance of these reductions often requires percutaneous K-wire fixation. When more than one carpometacarpal joint is dislocated, these wires are passed longitudinally following reduction and restoration of the proximal transverse carpal arch (Fig. 35-10B). Reductions that are held with transverse K-wires at the base tend to flatten this arch, thereby possibly preventing congruous reduction of the CMC joints. A short arm cast is applied with the CMC joints in extension. The involved and the adjacent digits are incorporated with the MP joints flexed approximately 60 degrees. The pins are removed at 4 weeks, and immobilization is then continued an additional 2 to 3 weeks. Chronic dislocations in this region are associated with pain and loss of grip strength.[92] Either inter-

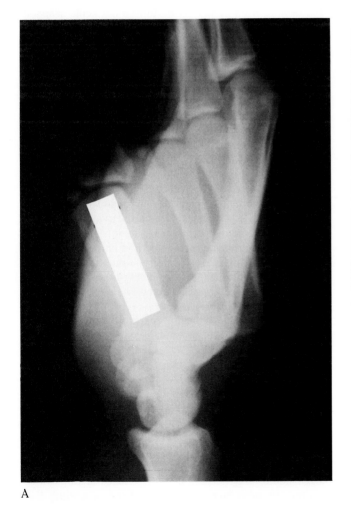

A

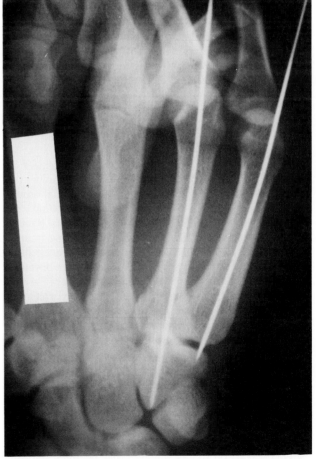

B

Figure 35-10 A. Dislocation of the carpometacarpal joints of the ring and little finger. Lateral x-ray view reveals loss of the normal joint congruity between the ring and little metacarpal bases with the hamate. **B.** Anatomical closed reduction obtained with longitudinal percutaneous K-wire fixation.

position arthroplasty or arthrodesis have been the recommended treatments for this condition.

Carpometacarpal dislocations of the thumb are rare.[40] Again, these dislocations are generally dorsoradial. Generally, reduction is easy to obtain, but difficult to maintain. A pin placed longitudinally in a retrograde fashion from the region of the MP joint across the CMC joint can be used to overcome this difficulty. A short-arm thumb spica cast is applied allowing IP motion for approximately 3 to 4 weeks. The pin is then removed and a thumb stabilizer splint is applied for an additional 3 weeks. Chronic CMC dislocations of the thumb usually present with pain, deformity, and weakness of pinch. Treatment is dependent upon the chronicity of the dislocation and the degree of arthrosis found in the basal joint. Treatment options include volar ligament reconstruction, tendon interposition arthroplasty, trapezium arthroplasty, or arthrodesis.[40,41,42]

CARPAL BONES

Greater than 90 percent of carpal bone fractures occur within the proximal carpal row.[203] Because it is a vulnerable link between the proximal and distal carpal rows, the scaphoid is the most common carpal bone to be fractured, but such injuries are only one-tenth as common as distal radius fractures.[125] Carpal bone fractures usually occur in a relatively young population group and are frequently complicated by severe soft tissue swelling, ligamentous disruption, and/or neurovascular compromise.[58,195,196]

Scaphoid Fractures

Considerable controversy exists regarding the treatment of scaphoid fractures.[86,116,124,125,149,166,190,195,196,203] A thorough understanding of scaphoid anatomy and its blood supply are important in determining the prognosis for fracture union.[64,65,196] Anatomically, this small boat-shaped carpal bone is almost completely covered with hyaline cartilage. There are two extremely important areas that are devoid of hyaline cartilage.[196] One area is the volar insertion of the radioscaphoid-capitate ligament or "sling" ligament which obliquely crosses the waist of the scaphoid. Dorsally, a second area void of hyaline cartilage lies along the spiral groove also coincident with the waist region of the scaphoid. The main intraosseous blood supply to the proximal two-thirds of the scaphoid enters through this dorsal ridge region. Vascular injection studies of the scaphoid have revealed that approximately 13 percent of the specimens would have lost the retrograde blood supplied to the proximal pole following a waist fracture.[64,65,145,193,196] Vascular variation from individual to individual contributes to the difficulty in predicting which patients will go on to develop avascular necrosis following similar fractures of the scaphoid.

Weber and Chao[209,210] have demonstrated the mechanism of scaphoid fractures in vitro by loading the radial side of the palm thereby dorsiflexing the wrist beyond its physio-logical range (greater than 95 degrees). The wrist then also assumes a posture of radial deviation. This loading position produces a bending moment in the region of the waist of the foreshortened and volar flexed scaphoid, and fracture occurs.

A general guiding principle in the acute management of wrist trauma is that following a fall on the "outstretched" hand and wrist, the presence of any snuffbox tenderness even in the absence of radiographic evidence of a fractured scaphoid should be considered a fracture until proved otherwise. Leslie and Dixon[110] reviewed a series of 222 consecutive patients with acute scaphoid fractures. They included four standard radiographic positions in the wrist trauma series: a posterior-anterior view, a lateral view, a posterior-anterior view with the wrist pronated 45 degrees, and a similar view supinated 45 degrees. The initial PA and semipronated views enabled these authors to diagnose a clear fracture 98 percent of the time. According to the authors, the remaining 2 percent of fractures became radiographically evident over the ensuing weeks of treatment. These false-negative fractures were incomplete and were located on the compression (concave) side of the scaphoid. The initial lateral radiograph is essential for the diagnosis of concomitant carpal instability.

It is noteworthy that myriad radiographic positions[196] have been devised in an attempt to rule out acute scaphoid fracture. Terry and Ramin[199] have emphasized the adjacent soft tissue planes to the scaphoid, which they call the *navicular* (scaphoid) *fat stripe.* Obliteration or displacement of this soft tissue plane would dictate treatment as an acute fracture.[214] In rare instances, nondiagnostic plain films may be supplemented by bone scan and/or by tomography.[60,143,162,188] In order to avoid falsely negative bone scans, imaging should be delayed at least 48 h following wrist trauma.

Weber[210] and Cooney[27,28] have developed a radiographic classification that is based on the degree of initial fracture displacement, i.e., fracture stability. Those scaphoid fractures which are nondisplaced and which have a fracture gap of less than 1 mm have an intact periosteal hinge and are considered stable fractures.[44] Acute stable fractures, treated in a thumb spica short-arm cast with the wrist positioned in slight flexion and radial deviation, had a near-perfect union rate with an immobilization time of 9 or 10 weeks. Exceptions to the rule of fracture stability were those patients whose treatment was delayed, those patients with concomitant Colles' fracture, and those patients noted to have a late carpal collapse deformity.[114,153] The authors have emphasized that the above immobilization position of the wrist may be critical in avoiding late carpal collapse.[27,28]

A displaced scaphoid fracture with greater than 1 mm of stepoff on any radiographic view, with or without evidence of carpal instability, is considered an unstable fracture.[27,44,86,125] Although Cooney's series was small, approximately 50 percent of such displaced fractures went on to nonunion despite attempt at closed reduction and casting. The average healing time to union was approximately 4 months in those fractures which healed. Thus, a general recommendation for these displaced fractures is one of attempted closed anatomical reduction with percutaneous K-wire fixation and casting. If an anatomical reduction cannot be obtained, open reduction is recommended with emphasis on correction of any carpal instability at the time of open reduction.

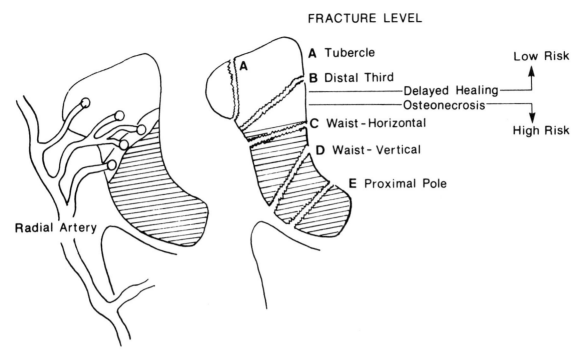

FRACTURE LEVEL

A Tubercle — Low Risk

B Distal Third — Delayed Healing

Osteonecrosis

C Waist - Horizontal — High Risk

D Waist - Vertical

E Proximal Pole

Radial Artery

Figure 35-11 Vascular and regional factors affecting prognosis in scaphoid fractures. Fractures within the proximal two-thirds are at high risk for the development of osteonecrosis. *(From Melone, C.P., Clin Plast Surg 8:86, 1981. Reproduced with permission.)*

The prognosis for the management of acute scaphoid fractures is thus based on two important factors: (1) anatomical location of the fracture and (2) fracture stability.[125] Fractures of the proximal and middle thirds of the scaphoid are at high risk for delayed union and avascular necrosis (Fig. 35-11). Since approximately 70 percent of fractures occur in the middle third or waist region and 20 percent occur within the proximal third region, it is not surprising that healing time is prolonged.[125,166,203] In contrast, fractures of the distal third region of the scaphoid (approximately 10 percent of scaphoid fractures) go on to uneventful union in approximately 6 weeks. Displaced or unstable fractures are also at high risk for delayed union, malunion, or nonunion. Any fracture offset greater than 1 mm is usually associated with malrotation and thus poor fragment apposition.

High-risk scaphoid fractures should be treated with long-arm casting incorporating the thumb to the interphalangeal joint level for 6 weeks, followed by short-arm casting with supracondylar extension to limit forearm rotation for 6 more weeks, and finally with a short-arm thumb spica cast. The patient is x-rayed in plaster at weekly intervals for 2 weeks from the onset of immobilization and then x-rayed out of plaster at the above-prescribed intervals. Fracture healing is determined clinically by the disappearance of snuffbox tenderness and the bridging trabeculae radiographically. Overall, the literature is controversial as to the position of the wrist and thumb during the immobilization period as well as the extension of the cast at or above the elbow level.[27,28,48,56,125,149] Those patients who present acutely and adhere to an immobilization protocol will generally go on to

uneventful union. Those patients who are noncompliant,[100] present late,[44] and have sporadic cast immobilization, will have a higher rate of nonunion.

The distinction between delayed union and nonunion is at times extremely arbitrary. A roentgenographic definition of scaphoid nonunion[14] is a fracture that fails to show a progression of fracture healing on three separate monthly examinations after a treatment period of 6 months. The natural history of scaphoid nonunion has recently been reviewed.[119,164] Clearly, the pattern of posttraumatic osteoarthritis that extends into the radiocarpal joint over a 20-year period places those individuals with displaced or unstable fractures at high risk. Those displaced scaphoid nonunions should be reduced and bone grafted prior to the onset of panscaphoid arthrosis. It remains unclear whether panscaphoid arthrosis is inevitable in those patients who have stable nonunions without carpal instability. The treatment of symptomatic scaphoid nonunion has been well-studied.[52,78,86,102,166,218] Lichtman and Alexander[112] have succinctly summarized a treatment algorithm for decision making in scaphoid nonunion (Fig. 35-12). In light of the complications associated with the use of unaugmented Silastic scaphoid prosthesis, salvage procedures such as augmented prosthesis with limited carpal arthrodesis, fascial interposition arthroplasty, proximal row carpectomy, and wrist arthrodesis should be considered.

Other Carpal Fractures

Simple fractures are the more common and are characterized by ligamentous avulsion fracture patterns.[19,147] The *tri-*

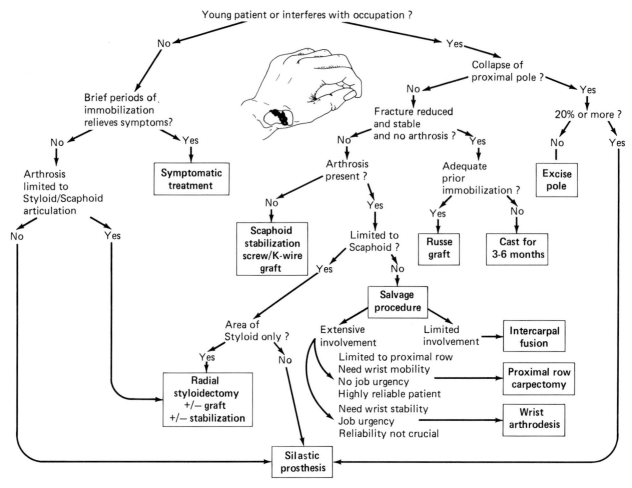

Figure 35-12 Algorithm for treatment of scaphoid nonunions. *(From Lichtman, D.M., and Alexander, C.E., Orthop Rev 11:66, 1982. Reproduced with permission.)*

quetrum avulsion fracture is primarily associated with a dorsal fleck of bone with concomitant severe soft tissue swelling over the dorsum of the wrist. Posteroanterior and lateral x-ray films may be nondiagnostic and must be supplemented by 30-degree semipronated oblique films. The treatment of choice is short-arm casting for approximately 4 to 6 weeks' duration. Fractures of the hook of the hamate[21,186] are associated with a history of athletic injury, especially during racket sporting events. Patients complain of pain radiating to the dorsum of the ulnar side of the wrist associated with hypothenar swelling. On physical exam, point tenderness is located directly over the hook of the hamate palmarly. Once again, standard positioning for x-ray filming is inadequate to reveal the fracture.[144] Acutely, patients may not permit carpal tunnel view positioning due to pain (Fig. 35-13). Lateral tomography of the hamate will then be diagnostic. Treatment of choice acutely is short-arm casting for approximately 4 to 6 weeks' duration. When seen chronically, symptomatic nonunion of hook of the hamate is usually treated by excision of the ununited fragment.[8,21]

Complex carpal bone fractures are rare but extremely disabling injuries.[19,147] The mechanism of injury usually results from high-energy loading associated with compression and shear. Complex injuries are typified by their concomitant injury to an adjacent joint which is usually subluxed or dislocated. The extent of osteochondral injury is usually unrecognized and may be associated with late carpal arthrosis. The remainder of the carpal bones have been implicated in this complex pattern of injury. Beginning with the distal carpal row, fractures of the trapezium[54,96,152] are often associated with dorsal dislocation of the first metacarpal. Alternatively, compressive loading of the first metacarpal may split the trapezium, requiring open reduction in order to restore the articular congruity of the basal joint. Fractures of the trapezoid are extremely rare and are often associated with fixed-unit disruption of the carpometacarpal joints of the index and long fingers. These trapezoid fractures are usually ligamentous avulsion injuries and require careful reduction of the injured carpometacarpal joints. Fractures of the body of the hamate[148] are usually intraarticular in nature and can be associ-

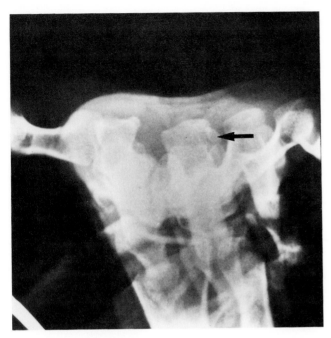

Figure 35-13 Atrophic hook (see arrow) of the hamate secondary to nonunion.

ated with carpometacarpal dislocations of the ring and little fingers. Closed or, possibly, open reduction may be the required treatment in order to restore articular congruity. Fractures of the pisiform are extremely rare injuries.[81,206] A positive grind test may be elicited by gently compressing the pisotriquetral joint surfaces together. Late pisotriquetral arthrosis may be treated by excision of the pisiform.[74] Lunate fractures have been implicated in the pathophysiology of Kienböck disease. These injuries much more commonly present as a cause of chronic wrist pain. Finally, the most common capitate fracture[2,159] is associated with fracture of the middle third of the scaphoid. The so-called scaphocapitate fracture syndrome[204] involves fracture at the level of the neck of the capitate and malrotation of the body. These injuries may be associated with avascular necrosis of the head of the capitate nonunion[55] and late carpal collapse.[114,153] Acutely displaced fractures are treated by open reduction and K-wire fixation.

Radiocarpal Dislocation

Radiocarpal dislocations[12,39,136,213] are extremely rare and are usually associated with multiple trauma. They are classified according to extent of injury. Type I dislocations are usually associated with dorsal or volar rim distal radial articular fractures. These dislocations are primarily dorsal and are associated with palmar radiocarpal ligament ruptures. Closed reduction followed by immobilization in plaster has been occasionally successful in the management of these injuries. When the closed reduction cannot be maintained or obtained, open reduction is indicated. Type II radiocarpal dislocations are associated with carpal fractures and dislocations. These

fractures have uniformly required open reduction and ligament reconstruction. Overall, type I radiocarpal dislocations have a much better prognosis. Posttraumatic arthrosis of the wrist frequently requires arthrodesis.

RADIUS

Fractures of the Distal Radius

Classification

Fractures of the distal radius are commonly classified by numerous eponyms such as Colles',[24] Smith's,[46] Barton's, and reverse Barton's.[35,202] Confusion in the usage of these eponyms has led to the development of various classification systems.[29,57,62] These systems, however, fail to differentiate intraarticular from extraarticular fractures adequately and, as a result, are severely limited in their prognostic value.

The author's modification of Frykman's classification[57] descriptively names each distal radius fracture subtype (Table 35-1 and 35-2). There are two significant prognostic risk factors: the extent of apparent articular involvement and the presence or absence of fracture stability. Any distal radius fracture may be stable or unstable, dorsally or volarly displaced, and extra- or intraarticular.

Stable fractures are those fractures in which clinically acceptable alignment and joint congruity can be maintained by plaster immobilization with or without a closed reduction. The inherent stability of any closed reduction is primarily dependent upon the presence of fracture comminution and related factors such as the patient's age and the degree of osteopenia, of energy applied, and of soft tissue injury. Thus, all unstable distal radius fractures are at high risk for increased morbidity, i.e., loss of motion, strength, and posttraumatic arthritis.[23–26,29,36,51,57,62,68,73,106,126,157,161,172,179,195,205,211]

Radiographic Analysis

Van der Linden and Ericson have shown that anatomical displacement of distal radius fractures may reliably be described by two radiographic measurements.[205,214] A lateral x-ray view of the distal radius shows loss of the normal radial tilt of 11 degrees (dorsal angulation), and the anteroposterior x-ray view shows the presence of a radial shift, an increase in the distance from the long axis of the radius to the most radial part of the styloid process. The presence of any radial shift is usually indicative of a displaced intraarticular fracture. Both the degree of dorsal angulation and radial shift correlate directly with the degree of radial shortening. However, conversely, large radial shifts may be present independent of the degree of dorsal angulation. Thus, both parameters are necessary in order to adequately define and interpret the guidelines and the results of treatment.

Treatment

Dorsally Displaced Extraarticular Fractures (Table 35-1) Stable extraarticular fractures that require no reduction may initially be placed in a sugar tong splint and converted once the initial swelling has subsided to a short arm cast. If

TABLE 35-1 Dorsally Displaced Fractures: Distal Radius

Joint involvement	Eponym/description	Position of reduction	
		Wrist	Forearm
Extraarticular*			
None	Colles'	V/F†	Pronation
Intraarticular*			
Radiocarpal (R/C) alone	Dorsal Barton's Dorsal marginal rim Fracture/subluxation	D/F‡	Pronation
Radioulnar (R/U) alone	Colles' type	V/F†	Pronation
Both R/C and R/U	Dorsomedial lunate "Die-punch" fracture	V/F†	Pronation

*All fractures may be stable or unstable.
†V/F = volar flexion.
‡D/F = dorsiflexion.

there is any suspicion of latent clinical instability, the patient should be x-rayed again at weekly intervals for the first two weeks. From the onset, elevation and full active range of motion of the interphalangeal and metacarpophalangeal joints is emphasized in order to avoid reflex sympathetic dystrophy and arthrofibrosis of the fingers with associated intrinsic contracture.[57,73,75]

Fractures Requiring Reduction Since Colles' first clinical description (1814) of this foreshortened fracture, treatment has been focused on the restoration of radial length.[14,73,175] Fracture displacement occurs both in the flexion-extension axis of the radiocarpal joint as well as the rotational axis of the forearm through the head of the ulna. These axial displacements must be taken into consideration when any closed reduction is required.

The authors believe that those fractures which present with greater than 0 degrees of dorsal angulation and a resulting loss of radial length require an attempted closed reduction. Under anesthesia, the fracture is disimpacted by applying 10 to 15 lb of longitudinal fingertip traction for approximately 15 min. While traction is maintained, dorsal and rotational displacement may be corrected by pronating the distal radial fragment, thereby "locking" the reduction.[24] In order to correct the dorsal angulation, the final reduction maneuver includes volar flexion and mild ulnar deviation of the wrist as the traction is released. Postreduction x-ray films are obtained following the application and three-point molding of the sugar tong splint.

Minimal acceptable reduction criteria for extraarticular dorsally displaced fractures are not clearly defined in the literature. Most authors agree that the better the anatomical reduction, the better the functional outcome. The possible

exception is the elderly, osteopenic, low-demand patient whose functional requirements may be meager in comparison to the young adult. Fernandez has analyzed the results of treatment in this latter population following malunited extraarticular fractures of the distal radius.[51] Those patients who presented with a dorsal angulation greater than 25 degrees associated with a loss of radial length greater than 6 mm, apparently lost greater than 50 percent of their palmar flexion arc of motion as well as 50 percent of their grip strength. Additionally, a dynamic midcarpal stability has been observed to a rise from even smaller magnitudes of dorsal angulation (loss of palmar tilt), i.e., malunion.[194]

The authors' prerequisites for an acceptable closed reduction are based upon Cooney's criteria for an unstable extraarticular fracture.[29] These included the inability to maintain fracture reduction without loss of dorsal angulation of more than 5 degrees or with 5 mm of radial shortening.

In order to maintain reduction of these unstable extraarticular fractures, most authors recommend a distraction technique (external fixator or pins-in-plaster).[23,25,26,29,34,68,73] Internal fixation techniques are rarely indicated except for the treatment of malunions.

Dorsally Displaced Intraarticular Fractures (Table 35-1)
The closed treatment of dorsally displaced intraarticular fractures of the distal radius is not significantly different from that given to extraarticular fractures. However, additionally, the critical prerequisite for an acceptable closed reduction is articular congruity. Knirk and Jupiter found that those fractures which had 2 mm or more of articular depession had a 100 percent incidence of radiographic stigmata of posttraumatic arthritis,[106] whereas those fractures which healed with articular congruity had an incidence of arthritis of only 11 percent.

Fractures Requiring Reduction Intraarticular fractures of the dorsal rim of the distal radius associated with dorsal subluxation of the carpus are usually inherently unstable fractures.[35,46,75,101,149,202] Unlike other dorsally displaced fractures, attempted closed reduction requires dorsiflexion of the wrist in order to reduce the lunate on a stable volar radiocarpal buttress. When reduction cannot be maintained, dorsal rim fractures are usually too comminuted to allow individual fragment fixation. Instead, distraction fixation or dorsal buttress plate fixation may be required.

Dorsally displaced intraarticular fractures may involve the radioulnar joint alone. Unstable displaced fractures may be treated by closed reduction and percutaneous pin fixation with or without a fixed distraction apparatus. Late complications of these fractures usually involve pain with a limitation of forearm rotation that may be treated by a partial distal ulna excision.[37,83]

Fractures involving both the radiocarpal and radioulnar joints are usually unstable due to the impacted dorsomedial articular fragment—the "die-punch" fracture (Fig. 35-14).[106,126] If articular congruity cannot be obtained by closed means, open reduction may be required with elevation of the articular depression and bone grafting for the subchondral defect. Again, reduction may be maintained by pin or screw fixation if the fragment is large enough. Otherwise, distraction fixation or buttress plating may be required.[134]

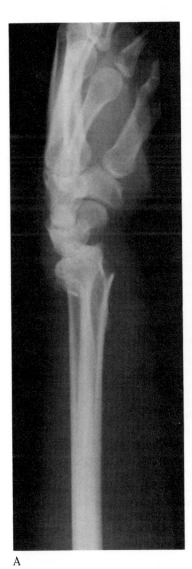
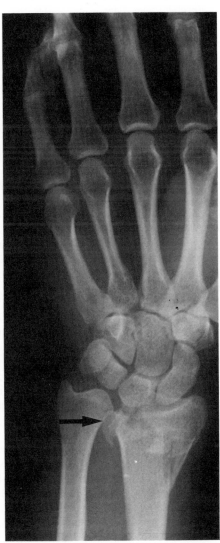
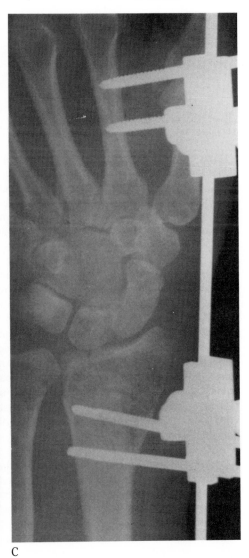

A   B   C

Figure 35-14 A. A 30-year-old woman, a homemaker, sustained this unstable, dorsally displaced intraarticular fracture of the distal radius with involvement of both the radiocarpal and radioulnar joints. Lateral x-ray film reveals 35 degrees of dorsal angulation and mild shortening. **B.** AP x-ray film reveals the impacted dorsomedial "die-punch" fracture (see arrow) with minimal radial shift of the distal radial fragment. **C.** AP x-ray film reveals near anatomical reduction and joint congruity following the application of an external fixator.

TABLE 35-2 Volar Displaced Fractures: Distal Radius

Joint involvement	Eponym/description	Position of reduction	
		Wrist	Forearm
Extraarticular*			
None	Smith's type I Reverse colles' type	D/F†	Supination
Intraarticular*			
Radiocarpal (R/C) alone	Volar Barton's Smith's type II Volar marginal rim Fracture subluxation	V/F‡	Supination
Radioulnar (R/U) alone	Reverse Colles' type Smith's type III	D/F†	Supination
Both R/C and R/U	Reverse Colles' type	D/F†	Supination

*All fractures may be stable or unstable.
†D/F = dorsiflexion
‡V/F = volar flexion.

Volarly Displaced Extraarticular Fractures (Table 35-2)
When someone falls on an outstretched, fixed, and pronated palm, the extraarticular proximal radial fracture fragment supinates around its rotational axis, i.e., the ulnar head.[46,182,200] Ultimately, the distal radius fragment is driven volarward relative to a clinically prominent ulnar head.

Fractures Requiring Reduction Under anesthesia, closed reduction may be carried out by disimpaction and supination of the distal radial fragment. By dorsiflexing the wrist, the volar carpal ligaments become taut, thereby "locking" the reduction. Postreduction x-ray films are obtained following the application and three-point molding of a sugar tong splint.

Like dorsally displaced extraarticular fractures, reduction criteria for volarly displaced fractures are not clearly defined. As previously mentioned, Fernandez also studied malunions within this fracture displacement subtype.[51] He concluded that those fractures with at least 25 degrees of volar angulation and greater than 6 mm of radial shortening presented with at least a 50 percent loss of dorsiflexion and grip strength.

The authors consider those volarly displaced fractures that cannot be maintained in a neutral or near-anatomical position as clinically unstable. Following reduction, these unstable fractures may be maintained with the aid of an external fixator or pins-in-plaster treatment. This treatment may be augmented by percutaneously pinning a relatively large distal radial fracture fragment with associated volar cortical comminution.

Volarly Displaced Intraarticular Fractures (Table 35-2)
Intraarticular fractures involving the radiocarpal joint are characterized by their instability.[35,46,101,149,202] Anatomically, the volar carpal ligaments are probably avulsed from the comminuted volar articular rim of the radius. Because this articular rim is insufficient to buttress against the volar shear forces, the wrist subluxes volarly.

Fractures Requiring Reduction Attempted closed reduction of the volar rim fracture subluxation should include longitudinal traction followed by supination and slight volar flexion of the wrist. As opposed to the closed reduction maneuver required for other volarly displaced fractures, the volar carpal ligament tether that occurs by dorsiflexing the wrist will have little effect on the avulsed volar rim fracture fragments in this subgroup. Instead, slight volar flexion of the wrist may tend to reduce the volar shear force, thereby preventing redisplacement. Unstable fractures may require open reduction with buttress plating or at times, an attempt at distraction fixation with an external fixator or pins-in-plaster treatment.

Volarly displaced intraarticular fractures may involve the radioulnar joint alone. These fractures are extremely rare, but are more stable than the volar rim fracture subtypes. Closed reduction should be carried out in a similar fashion as described for other volarly displaced extraarticular fractures. Following reduction, unstable fractures may be pinned in order to avoid pain and limitation of forearm rotation.

Fractures involving both the radiocarpal and radioulnar joints clinically have their volar counterpart. In a similar fashion, articular congruity must be restored. Impacted articular fragments depressed greater than 2 mm must be elevated and bone-grafted. Volar buttress plating will help maintain this reduction.

Complications

Complications of distal radius fractures are frequent.[29,51,195] They include loss of reduction and malunion,[51,106,126] radioulnar joint symptoms,[37,128] extensor pollicis longus rupture, degenerative arthrosis,[106,126] reflex sympathetic dystrophy and shoulder-hand syndrome,[57,108,133] compressive neuropathy,[29,57,117] compartment syndrome, and intrinsic contracture.

Radial Styloid Fractures (Table 35-3)

These fractures, originally described as having been caused by sudden reversal of the starter crank were called chauffeur's fractures.[149] Most of these injuries now are caused by forced radial deviation during falls or during motor vehicle accidents. An anteroposterior x-ray shows the fracture line best. The line usually runs from the scaphoid fossa radially toward the lateral radial cortex. It is, therefore, an intraarticular fracture. Depending on the position of the wrist when the injury occurs, there may be associated radiocarpal ligamentous injuries.

Nondisplaced fractures may be treated by short arm casting for 4 to 6 weeks. If significant displacement is noted, distraction and reduction in an ulnar direction facilitates reduction. Reduction can be maintained by placing the wrist in slight ulnar deviation. Plaster immobilization for 6 weeks is usually sufficient for healing to occur. If the reduction cannot be maintained, open reduction and fixation with either two Kirschner wires or a lag screw, should be done.

Middle to Distal Third Diaphyseal Fracture of the Radius with Dorsal Dislocation of the Radioulnar Joint (Table 35-3)

Solitary fracture in the middle to distal third diaphysis of the radius with associated dorsal dislocation of the distal radioulnar joint (Galeazzi type) may be caused by direct blows to the

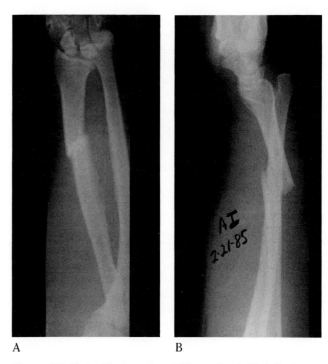

A   B

Figure 35-15 A. AP view of a middle to distal third diaphyseal fracture of the radius with dorsal dislocation of the radioulnar joint. **B.** Lateral view.

dorsolateral side of the wrist, as well as by a fall on an outstretched forearm (Fig. 35-15). Most injuries are closed, with a transverse fracture of the radius noted.[138] Galeazzi noted that the subluxation of the distal radioulnar joint may be immediately apparent, or may appear over a period of time.

TABLE 35-3   Fractures and Dislocations of the Radius and/or Ulna

Type	Eponym	Position of reduction/ immobilization	
		Wrist	Forearm
Radial styloid	Chauffeur's Hutchinson's Scaphoid impression	Ulnar deviation	Neutral
Mid to distal 1/3 diaphysis radius with dislocated R/U joint	Galeazzi Piedmont Reverse Monteggia	Neutral	Supination
Dorsal R/U* joint dislocation		Neutral	Supination
Volar R/U* joint dislocation		Neutral	Pronation

R/U = Radioulnar

Radioulnar joint symptoms may be noted. Careful roentgenographic analysis of both the wrist and the elbow joints using standard anteroposterior and lateral views will help make the diagnosis. If the radius is significantly shortened, one will usually find dorsal subluxation of the ulnar head.

Hughston's[88] classic article reported a 92 percent failure rate with closed treatment. Mikic[130] showed very good results in the open treatment of 125 patients. All adults with a true Galeazzi fracture should be treated by the open methods.[130,137] Moore[137] reported excellent results with radial compression plating of 36 Galeazzi fractures.

Treatment

Treatment of the distal radioulnar joint following fixation of the radius remains controversial. If the distal radioulnar joint can be reduced using closed methods and if it appears stable in supination, a long-arm cast with the forearm held in supination for a period of 6 weeks is mandatory.[138] If the radioulnar joint is unstable[4] then one or two transfixing K wires should be placed transversely across the joint. The extremity is then held for a 6-week period in a long-arm cast.

ULNAR STYLOID FRACTURES

Ulnar styloid fractures are relatively common injuries.[57,85] They are often seen in association with distal radius fractures and may also occur as an isolated entity.[173] Most are caused by forced radial deviation or dorsiflexion injuries.

The patients present acutely with tenderness at the ulnar styloid. Forearm supination and pronation may cause discomfort. Routine anteroposterior x-ray views allow one to determine whether a fracture is present. Occasionally, one can see an anomalous carpal bone called the *lunula, os styloides,* or *os triangulare.*

Treatment

Treatment of these injuries should be based on the amount of displacement. The triangular fibrocartilage complex (TFCC) attaches to the ulnar styloid.[154] Theoretically, significant displacement may lead to instability of the distal radioulnar joint. It is unclear how much displacement is significant. If the ulnar styloid is minimally displaced, a short-arm cast with the wrist in slight ulnar deviation relaxes the TFCC complex and will allow the fracture to heal. Healing should take place in 4 to 6 weeks. If the ulnar styloid is significantly displaced, and the distal radioulnar joint is subluxed, then open reduction and fixation of the ulnar styloid fracture with a Kirschner wire is recommended. The fracture should then be held for 4 to 6 weeks in a long-arm cast.

Occasionally one will see a patient with a painful nonunion of the ulnar styloid. Simple excision in selected patients provides excellent results.

RADIOULNAR JOINT DISLOCATIONS (TABLE 35-3)

The radioulnar joint is a trochoid, or pivot, joint. The radius rotates around the ulna, with stability achieved by the bony architecture, joint capsule, the pronator quadratus, and the triangular fibrocartilage complex.[154] This homogeneous complex is made up of the articular disc, the dorsal and volar radioulnar ligaments, the meniscus homologue, the ulnar collateral ligament, and the sheath of the extensor carpi ulnaris.[184] Radioulnar dislocations are not rare injuries.[155] They may be noted as radial fractures, and in ulnar styloid fractures. Isolated radioulnar joint dislocations are commonly referred to as ulnar dorsal or ulnar volar, although the ulna is truly the fixed forearm unit.[35,85,207] Dorsal dislocations are more frequently seen than volar dislocations. The mechanism of injury of dorsal dislocations is felt to be hyperpronation. Volar dislocations of the radioulnar joint are hypersupination injuries.

Most patients with these injuries present acutely with radioulnar joint pain. The pain is reproducible with downward pressure on the joint or by supination and pronation movements of the forearm. A painful "click" or "clunk" may be present. Difficulties in diagnosis may be encountered upon examining x-ray films. Anteroposterior (AP) and lateral films of both wrists are helpful for comparison. AP views in pronation and supination may help with the determination of injury. Recently, computed tomography has been noted to help make specific diagnoses.[131,132,177]

Treatment

Acute injuries, including sprains, are best held in the position that allows ligamentous healing. In dorsal sprains or dislocations, the patient is treated with a long-arm cast in supination for 6 weeks. In volar sprains, patient is treated in hyperpronation in a long-arm cast for 6 weeks. Postreduction films are mandatory. If there are any questions as to the position of the reduction, CT scan of the radioulnar joint is recommended. Although rare, a dorsal or volar dislocation may be unstable. An open reduction, followed by K-wire stabilization transversely into the radius, is carried out.[18] The arm is then held in the position of reduction for 6 weeks in a long-arm cast.

FRACTURES OF BOTH BONES OF THE FOREARM

The correct treatment of a fracture of both forearm bones demands some attention to the appropriate anatomy.[89] The demanding functional requirements of the human forearm make good results difficult to achieve. Sage[167] felt that the lateral bow of the radius was extremely important in achieving full pronation and supination and must be restored at reduction. He also showed how individual muscles caused deformity after forearm fractures.[168] Axial and rotational alignment must also be achieved.[120,197] For these reasons, open reduction and internal fixation of these fractures is now the most accepted form of management.[5,38,134,135,163]

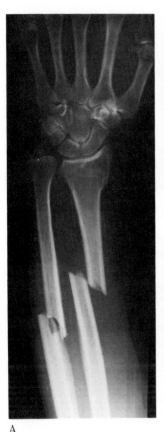
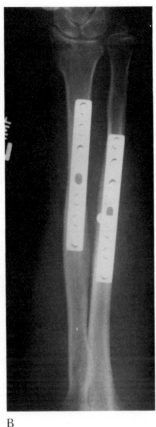

A   B

Figure 35-16 A. A 62-year-old female nurse sustained this fracture of both radius and ulna. Note the marked shortening. Additional views were taken to include the elbow joint. **B.** AP view of the forearm reveals anatomical reduction of a fracture that involved both bones of the forearm. Lateral view revealed a similar restoration of length and alignment.

Most of these fractures are caused by direct blows either in motor vehicle accidents or by blunt objects. They may be open or closed fractures. Careful emergency room assessment detailing the patient's upper extremity neurovascular exam is essential.

Routine anteroposterior and lateral roentgenograms, including views of the wrist joint and elbow, are mandatory. Evans[47] determined the amount of fracture fragment rotation by using a "tuberosity view" and observing the prominence of the bicipital tuberosity in various degrees of pronation and supination. This is important if one attempts to treat these injuries closed.

Treatment

Management of fractures of both bones is controversial. Numerous studies[105,173,174,186] have outlined the use of closed treatment[24] and have detailed many different types of open treatments. The uncommon undisplaced fractures of both bones of the forearm may be treated with a long-arm cast with the hand in neutral rotation and the elbow flexed at 90

degrees for 4 to 6 weeks. Routine roentgenographic evaluations are important weekly for 4 weeks. Functional braces may be used at 8 to 12 weeks, depending on the amount of healing.

Most series of displaced fractures of both bones of the forearm treated closed give unsatisfactory results. Sarmiento,[173,174] however, has described good functional results using closed treatment and functional braces.

Most displaced fractures of both bones of the forearm require open reduction. Several methods have been described to maintain this alignment including the use of Rush pins, K wires, Steinmann pins, Lottes nails, and Küntscher nails. The end results of these attempts were not encouraging. In 1959 Sage[167] introduced a new intramedullary nail for the treatment of forearm fractures. However, he did not recommend that fractures of the distal third of the radius be treated in this manner. He noted that for this injury, routine, autogenous iliac bone grafting should be performed but nonetheless obtained a delayed union in 4.9 percent and nonunion in 6.2 percent.[180] Open reduction and compression plating is now recommended for such distal third fractures (Fig. 35-16).[38,141,163,198]

Open Fractures

Open injuries of both bones of the forearm remain significant management problems.[34] Irrigation and thorough debridement of the wound in the operating room are essential. Antibiotics should be given intravenously in the emergency room after appropriate cultures are taken and tetanus prophylaxis is given. Most class I open injuries can be managed by wound management and delayed open reduction. Class II and class III open injuries, in which there is significant loss of soft tissue and bone, may require skin and bone grafting, immediate debridement, culture, and external fixation. Secondary debridement, bone grafting, and complex soft tissue coverage may also be required.

═══ **SECTION B** ═══

Ligament Injuries of the Wrist, Hand, and Elbow

Robert Y. Garroway and Frank C. McCue III

Ligament injuries to the wrist, hand, and elbow are common injuries. Conservative treatment is appropriate for most of them; however, some require primary operative repair, and a small percentage require a secondary reconstructive procedure.

LIGAMENT INJURIES OF THE WRIST

The ligament of the wrist and hand provide functional stability to the bony architecture. Table 35-4[24] reviews the intrinsic and extrinsic ligamentous supports of the wrist.

Ligaments are static structures. They may be taut, limiting the excursion of the joint system involved, or lax, not affecting joint motion. The wrist relies on both ligamentous and the contact surfaces of the bones as constraints during normal motion.[27]

The key ligaments of the wrist are volar and intracapsular. The palmar, or volar, radiocarpal ligaments consist of three strong intracapsular ligaments:[11] the radiocapitate, volar radiotriquetral, and radioscaphoid ligaments. These ligaments have an essential role in carpal instabilities.

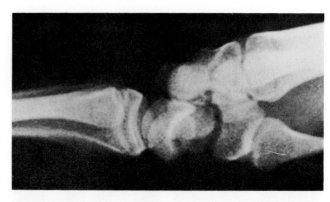

Figure 35-17 Lateral roentgenogram of a perilunate dislocation.

Perilunate Dislocation and Transscaphoid Perilunate Dislocation

These dislocations are usually the result of a direct force, and the distal carpus is dislocated dorsally to the lunate. In a simple perilunate dislocation (Fig. 35-17), the entire scaphoid is dislocated with the rest of the carpus. Frequently, the scaphoid is fractured through its midportion, and the proximal portion remains attached to the lunate. This transscaphoid perilunate dislocation is associated with extensive ligamentous disruption.[5,10]

After application of straight longitudinal traction, reduction may be obtained by pressing the lunate dorsally while

TABLE 35-4 Wrist Ligamentous Structures

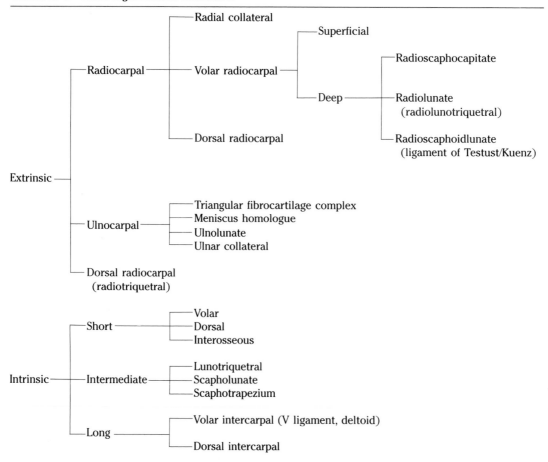

Source: American Society for Surgery of the Hand, *Regional Review Course in Hand Surgery—Manual,* 1984. Reproduced with permission.

the rest of the carpus is pressed volarly. Because of the magnitude of the ligamentous tears, the reduction is frequently unstable. If the scaphoid fragments are displaced, open reduction should be performed with pin or screw fixation to restore the wrist anatomy to as near a normal condition as possible.[3,16]

Rotary Subluxation of the Scaphoid

The scaphoid is the link between the proximal and distal carpal rows, and in rotary subluxation of the scaphoid its strong ligamentous attachments are disrupted. After reduction of a perilunate dislocation, residual scaphoid rotary subluxation is frequently overlooked and the patient will develop pain, clicking and weakness in the wrist.

In addition to the standard radiographic views of the wrist, a clenched-fist view in supination should be taken (Fig. 35-18). Frequently, the anteroposterior view will show a gap between the scaphoid and lunate. The normal gap is 1 to 2 mm, and a 3-mm gap is considered abnormal.[5,16] Because of the rotation, the scaphoid also appears shortened on the anteroposterior view. Lateral roentgenograms will show an increased volar rotation of the distal pole.[10]

Acute subluxations usually require open repair for the best results, and both a volar and dorsal approach should be used to repair the ligaments. In chronic cases with disability, reconstruction can be performed, but the results are not as good as primary repair. Chronic cases may require a limited wrist arthrodesis.

Lunate Dislocation

A lunate dislocation is seen more commonly than the perilunate dislocation; however, the lunate dislocation is itself probably secondary to a perilunate dislocation which spontaneously reduces. With the reduction, the lunate is rotated and pushed volarly where it may give symptoms of

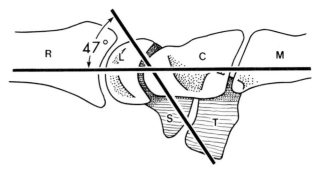

Figure 35-19 Normal carpal alignment in the lateral view is shown. Note that the longitudinal axes of the radius, lunate, capitate, and third metacarpal are in a straight line. The longitudinal axis of scaphoid makes a 47-degree angle (average) with this straight line. Up to 60 degrees is considered within normal limits, and 70 degrees or more is clearly pathological. *(From Beckenbaugh, R.D., Orthop Clin North Am 15(2):295, 1984. Reproduced with permission.)*

median nerve compression. The palmar radiolunate ligament remains intact, and this preserves the blood supply to the lunate. Diagnosis is easily made with lateral roentgenograms of the wrist, where the lunate is seen volar to the carpus in the carpal tunnel.

The lunate is reduced with longitudinal traction, extension of the wrist, and pressure on the lunate from the palmar surface toward the dorsum. It is not unusual to have to recreate a perilunate dislocation to reduce the lunate and then reduce the perilunate dislocation itself.

Normally, wrist dislocations are immobilized for 4 weeks in a cast with the wrist in slight flexion. At that time, we allow asymptomatic athletes to resume competition if they are protected for 4 more weeks in a silicone cast.

If a lunate dislocation is not diagnosed acutely, open reduction is usually necessary. Common complications of this injury are late rotary instability of the scaphoid, median nerve palsies, and late flexor tendon ruptures.

Carpal Instability

For accurate analysis of carpal instability, it is important to evaluate history, physical examination, and roentgenographic findings systematically.[1] Linscheid and Dobyns[10] emphasize the importance of the scapholunate axis which is formed by the angle of the longitudinal axis of the scaphoid and a line connecting the longitudinal axis of the radius, lunate, capitate, and metacarpals. This angle should be between 30 and 60 degrees, and is a key to carpal instability (Fig. 35-19).

Dorsal Intercalated Segment Instability

The dorsal intercalated segment instability (DISI) is the most common form of wrist instability. It is caused by the disruption of the scapholunate interosseous ligament and the volar

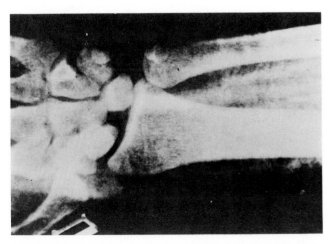

Figure 35-18 Rotary subluxation of the scaphoid is indicated by the gap between scaphoid and lunate.

radial scapholunate ligament. This results in the lunate axis pointing dorsally and the scaphoid rotating palmarly and the scapholunate axis measuring 60 degrees or more.[1]

Partial acute injuries can be treated with 6 to 12 weeks of casting.[1] Complete rupture of the above two ligaments requires operative repair and temporary stabilization with Kirschner's wires. When the instability is old and degenerative changes of the radioscaphoid and lunocapitate articulations are seen, treatment consists of wrist arthrodesis, proximal row carpectomy, or wrist arthroplasty. Intermediate instances where ligamentous atrophy has occurred but degenerative changes are not seen on roentgenograms may be treated with either ligamentous reconstruction using tendon grafts or limited carpal fusion.[1]

Volar Intercalated Segment Instability

Volar intercalated segment instability (VISI) is a result of disruption of the dorsal and /or ulnar stabilizing structures of the wrist. These include the lunotriquetral ligament or the dorsal ulnocarpal and dorsal ulnoradial ligaments. VISI may be recognized on a lateral roentgenogram by a downward tilt of the lunate and a scapholunate axis of 30 degrees or less.[1] Early treatment can usually be accomplished with closed reduction and casting with or without percutaneous wire fixation. Chronic lesions result in dorsal subluxation, and volar angulation of the lunate may be treated by various ligamentous reconstructions or intercarpal fusions as favored by the individual surgeon.

The results of any type of treatment of these instabilities of the wrist vary greatly, and there has been no proven method of treatment—including surgery—which gives any significant better results. Recurrences of the deformities are commonly found after any type of treatment.

Ulnocarpal Instabilities

Injuries of the triquetrolunate articulation were first discussed by Regan and associates who described a lunotriquetral ballottement test.[21] These injuries consist of triquetrolunate tears (sprains) or dislocation. The lunate is stabilized with the thumb and index finger of one hand while the other hand is used to attempt to displace the triquetrum and pisiform dorsally and then palmarly. A positive test detects excessive laxity associated with pain and crepitus. Treatment of this type of instability is a trial of immobilization, and if symptoms persist, reconstruction of the triquetrolunate ligaments using a free tendon graft or triquetrolunate arthrodesis.[1]

Distal Radioulnar Joint Instability

Palmer and Werner[20] introduced the term *triangular fibrocartilage complex (TFCC)*. The TFCC (Fig. 35-20) incorporates the dorsal and volar radioulnar ligaments, the ulnar collateral ligaments, and meniscus homologue, the anatomically definable articular disc, and the extensor carpi ulnaris sheath. The

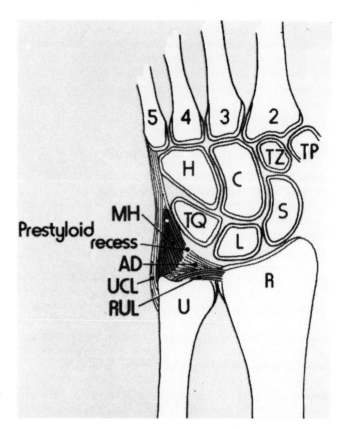

Figure 35-20 TFCC (triangular fibrocartilage complex). Components: RUL = radioulnar ligaments, ULC = ulnar collateral ligament, AD = articular disc, MH = meniscus homologue. Also shown are the radius (R), ulna (U), scaphoid (S), lunate (L), triquetrum (TQ), trapezium (TP), trapezoid (TZ), capitate (C) and hamate (H). *(From Palmer, A.K., Orthop Clin North Am 15(2):321–326, 1984. Reproduced with permission.)*

complex arises from the ulnar aspect of the lunate fossa of the radius and courses ulnarward to insert into the caput ulna. It flows distally and is joined by fibers arising from the ulnar styloid. It then becomes thickened (the meniscus homologue) and inserts distally into the triquetrum, the hamate, and the base of the fifth metacarpal.

A careful physical examination as described by Palmer[15] is essential in diagnosing instability associated with injury to the TFCC. This includes examination of forearm rotation, point tenderness, and clicking on motion or direct pressure. Computed tomography is becoming an important aid in the diagnosis of distal radioulnar instability.

Acute subluxation of the distal radioulnar joint is treated in a long-arm cast in supination for dorsal subluxations and pronation for volar subluxations. Partial acute tears of the TFCC complex can be treated with debridement. When these tears are explored late and there is ulnar or lunate chondromalacia, ulnar shortening must be performed.[16]

Carpometacarpal Sprains

Fractures and fracture dislocations of the carpometacarpal joint have been covered elsewhere. Ligamentous sprains occur in a group of patients without injury sufficient to dislocate or fracture the carpometacarpal joint who have minor luxations, pain during stressful occupations, or pain for no obvious reason at all. Few of these injuries are seen. Physical findings include point tenderness over the involved joint and reproduction of pain when the joint is stressed by the examiner. Temporary immobilization is the treatment of choice in the acute cases, but chronic cases usually require an arthrodesis of the involved joints.

LIGAMENT INJURIES OF THE FINGERS AND THUMB

Ligament structures of the hand include the collateral ligaments of the metacarpophalangeal (MP) and proximal interphalangeal (PIP) joints. Both consist of a cordlike collateral ligament proper and a membranous accessory ligament. The collateral ligaments at the MP joint are taut in flexion and lax in extension, and at the PIP joint the membranous portion is also tight in extension.

The MP joints of the thumb and finger are condyloid joints. The thumb MP joint is anatomically unique. On the ulnar aspect of the joint, the adductor pollicis muscle is inserted partly into the ulna sesamoid bone, partly into the volar plate, and partly through a powerful tendon directly into the proximal phalanx. Additional fibers contribute to the dorsal aponeurosis. This aponeurosis overlies the ulnar collateral ligament of the MP joint of the thumb and must be divided to provide operative exposure of the ligaments.

The PIP joint is particularly important, in that any fixed deformity, either flexion or extension, is extremely disabling. Because it is a small non-weight-bearing joint, there is a tendency to minimize the severity of its injuries. Patients, especially poorly supervised athletes, tend to return to unprotected uses long before adequate healing has taken place.

The PIP joint is particularly vulnerable because of the relatively long proximal and distal lever arms that transmit lateral and torque stress to this hinge-type joint, which has minimal lateral mobility. The anatomy of this joint is extremely complex. It is a hinged joint that has a range of motion between 0 and 120 degrees in the plane perpendicular to the palm. The lateral ligaments and volar plate are thick and strong. The dorsal central slip of the extensor tendon and the volar flexor tendons supplement these capsular ligaments. In addition, the lateral band and its various extensions, the oblique and transverse retinacular ligaments, and both Cleland's and Grayson's ligaments must move and glide freely to allow proper motion. The volar plate has a proximal cul-de-sac which must be free of scar, otherwise, during PIP joint flexion, the base of the middle phalanx cannot glide into the sac.

Ulnar Collateral Ligament Injuries of the Thumb

This injury is often overlooked, but it can lead to instability when the thumb is stressed in abduction, thus compromis-

ing pinch. It occurs frequently in football players, the mechanism of injury being forced abduction of the thumb; but it is also seen in hockey players, skiers, wrestlers, and baseball players.

In acute injuries, the following can occur: local tenderness to pressure over the ulnar collateral ligament, pain in the joint with abduction stress testing, swelling along the ulnar side of the metacarpal head, weakness of thumb-index pinch, and instability. Tests of stability should be compared to the uninvolved side and are performed with the MCP joint in extension and flexion. Stress x-ray views comparing both thumbs should be obtained if there is any doubt about the diagnosis.[2,5,15]

The ulnar collateral ligament usually tears at its distal attachment to the proximal phalanx. Most of these are partial tears in which there is soreness, but not complete disruption of the ligament on testing. To prevent further injury, these tears must be protected until they heal. In the incomplete lesions, immobilization may be accomplished by taping. In an individual who does not need to use this thumb for grasp, such as an offensive tackle, the thumb may be taped to the hand itself. However, in less severe injuries in athletes who use the thumb for grasp and extension, such as receivers and ball handlers, the thumb may be taped in a figure-of-eight fashion to the index finger. The tape acts as a checkrein to prevent hyperabduction.

Complete tears are more serious because of the clinical instability of the thumb MP joint. Laxity is at least 20 degrees greater than the opposite thumb. Roentgenograms may show a displaced, rotated avulsion fracture from the proximal phalanx. In complete ligament tears, the adductor pollicis aponeurosis can become interposed between the ends of the ulnar collateral ligament,[20] and the latter cannot heal. For this reason, we advocate operative repair when the tear is complete (Fig. 35-21). Surgical indications in acute cases include: significant involvement of the articular surface, displacement and/or rotation of the fracture fragment, gross clinical insta-

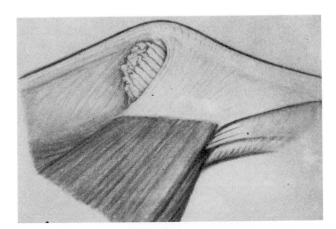

Figure 35-21 Ulnar aspect of the metacarpophalangeal joint of the right thumb. After distal rupture, the ulnar collateral ligament has been folded over. The torn end protrudes proximal to the adductor aponeurosis. *(From Flynn, J.D., ed: Hand Surgery. Baltimore, Williams & Wilkins, 1966.)*

bility, and inability to reduce the fractures secondary to soft tissue interposition.[25] The major indications for chronic repair are pain, functional instability, and weakness in pinch.

The initial step in the surgical repair is to divide the adductor aponeurosis, exposing the ulnar collateral ligament. The collateral ligament is reattached, using the pullout suture technique in the case of an avulsion injury. If the ligament is torn at its midportion, nonabsorbable braided sutures are placed with the metacarpophalangeal joint flexed 15 to 20 degrees during the repair. A splint or thumb spica is worn for 5 weeks.

In chronic reconstructions, a slip of the adductor pollicis still attached to the proximal phalanx can be advanced as a dynamic component of the repair.[16] In certain cases in which the ulnar collateral ligament is thin, atrophic, or missing, replace it with a slip of the abductor pollicis longus.

Collateral Ligament Injuries to Metacarpophalangeal Joints

Collateral ligament injuries of the MCP joints are less common and usually less disabling than those involving the PIP joint. Since radial and ulnar control are maintained by the intrinsics, usually lateral instability is not a problem. However, after an avulsion fracture, the distal attachment of the collateral ligament may become interposed in the joint, and this can be disabling. If the collateral ligament becomes interposed, open repair becomes necessary. Most other tears can be treated with a short course of splinting and then an 8 to 12-week course of buddy taping to protect the healing process.

Injuries to Proximal Interphalangeal Joints

Collateral Ligament

Injuries to PIP joints are most common on the radial side of the digit where the proximal attachment of the collateral ligament is avulsed. They are usually associated with partial or

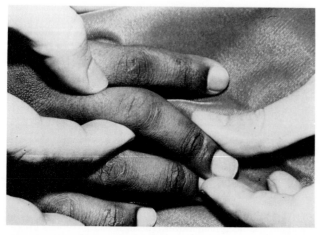

Figure 35-22 Stress roentgenograms confirmed a complete collateral ligament rupture suspected on physical examination.

complete rupture of the volar plate, depending upon the magnitude of the force applied. The injury, caused by a ball or other object striking the extended finger, causes severe pain and localized soft tissue swelling on the side of the injured ligament. Examination shows generalized tenderness over the collateral ligament. At this stage, it is necessary to determine whether the injury is a strain—probably the most common injury—or a complete disruption of the ligament. Complete rupture creates lateral instability. This can be demonstrated clinically and radiographically by stress films (Fig. 35-22). The examination can be performed under nerve block if indicated. Even without obtaining stress films, one may be able to make the diagnosis by routine radiograph if a small bony fragment is associated with ligament avulsion. It must be emphasized that too-rigorous stress may convert a partial collateral ligament rupture into a complete one.

The treatment for a mild strain of the collateral ligaments or for any other soft tissue injury is splinting the finger in a functional position until the pain has subsided and the range of motion can be restored.[15] For an athlete who needs protection during play, taping a mildly injured finger to the adjacent finger acts as a splint. This provides protection as well as mobility.

For injuries in which there is joint laxity and incomplete tearing of the ligament (a portion of the ligament intact, thereby preventing retraction), the finger should be splinted in 30 degrees of flexion.[12] Active motion exercises are begun in 10 to 14 days with protective splinting for at least 3 weeks. Active sports participation with the finger either in a splint or firmly taped to the adjacent finger is permitted in 4 to 6 weeks. An individually cut felt spacer between the two fingers affords additional protection. It is important to remember that inadequate protection of partial tears can lead to further injury involving complete tearing of the ligament.

There is a great deal of controversy concerning treatment of complete tears of the collateral ligament of the PIP joint. Many believe that conservative treatment is satisfactory. Others feel the optimal treatment in these cases is open inspection and repair of the torn ligament.[13] Conservative methods are prone to leave the patient with a swollen, tender joint that is unstable and susceptible to additional injury as well as to degenerative change. Unless the surgeon is experienced in techniques of hand surgery, increased damage may result. Often, reconstructive surgery is required in chronic cases, but the results are less satisfactory and less predictable than primary repair. In chronic repairs, frequently a free tendon graft or slip of the flexor sublimis may be used to reinforce the repair.

Volar Plate Injuries

The volar plate of the PIP joint is composed of a thin, membranous proximal portion attached to the head of the proximal base of the middle phalanx. It may be injured when an extended finger is hyperextended, such as after being struck by a baseball or basketball. The patient experiences acute onset of pain and swelling following the injury. Examination shows point tenderness over the volar aspect of the joint, usually at the distal attachment of the volar plate to the base of the middle phalanx in the proximal interphalangeal joint. A routine x-ray film may reveal a small bone chip associated with an avulsion injury.

As a result of the above anatomy, volar plate injuries may result in either hyperextension or flexion deformities of the PIP joint. In most cases, the hyperextension deformity is caused by rupture of the volar plate at its distal end. In the acute injury, protection by splinting in 25 to 30 degrees of flexion is indicated for 3 weeks followed by protected motion for 2 to 3 more weeks. Splinting prevents the digit from extending. Disruption of the volar plate distally can result in the swan neck deformity (Fig. 35-23). Secondary surgical reconstruction is indicated only when the PIP joint locks in hyperextension and subsequently interferes with normal hand function.

Disruption of the volar plate at its proximal membranous portion can result in a pseudoboutonniere deformity.[12,15] This resembles the true boutonniere, but disruption of the central slip is not present. The diagnostic features of pseudoboutonniere deformity are as follows: a flexion contracture of the PIP joint, which is more resistant to correction by passive extension than the typical boutonniere; slight hyperextension of the DIP joint; radiological evidence of calcification at the distal end of the proximal phalanx (proximal attachment of the volar plate), and a history of hyperextension or twisting injury to the middle joint rather than one of hyperflexion injury.

If the lesions are diagnosed early, extension is more easily obtained by conservative means, but the patient must be followed, since the deformity may recur. A mild deformity (less than 40 degrees of flexion) will respond to prolonged splinting. A "safety pin" splint (deriving the name from its appearance, which is similar to that of a horse blanket pin), together with active and passive finger exercises, is used to control the flexion contracture.

For severe injury with a flexion deformity of 45 degrees or more, surgical intervention is usually required for optimal function. Repair consists of release and distal advancement of the scarred proximal volar plate, gouging out the bone spur, and releasing the accessory collateral ligament. The proximal interphalangeal joint is maintained in extension for 3 weeks by the use of a transarticular Kirschner wire, along with an external splint.

LIGAMENT INJURIES OF THE ELBOW
Elbow Anatomy

The elbow is a relatively stable joint because of the articulation between the ulna and the distal end of the humerus. The articulation between the capitellum and the radial head adds further stability. The lateral side of the elbow is much weaker than the medial side; a weak lateral collateral ligament inserts into the annular ligament and does not contribute much to stability.[22] Stability laterally is achieved more by the anconeus and by the extensors of the forearm, which insert into the lateral epicondyle.

The medial side of the elbow has greater ligamentous stability.[23] The medial collateral ligament of the elbow is

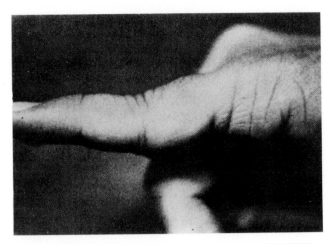

Figure 35-23 Disruption of the volar plate distally at the PIP point results in swan neck deformity.

composed of three parts.[22] The anterior oblique portion, with an origin from the medial epicondyle, and an insertion into the coronoid process, is tense throughout motion[23] and produces the greatest amount of stability. The middle portion of the ligament is weak and provides little stability. The posterior oblique portion is taut in flexion[9] but is relaxed when the elbow is extended. The flexor muscle mass also adds stability to the medial side of the elbow.

Little League Elbow

Little league elbow is the popular name given to overuse conditions of the elbow in the adolescent thrower.[22] These injuries result from the severe valgus stress and extensor thrust on the elbow inherent in the throwing mechanism.[4] The athlete complains of pain in the elbow, especially during throwing. Physical findings include medial tenderness, swelling, and slight restriction of motion.[22] Roentgenographic findings may show fragmentation, separation, and accelerated growth of the medial epicondyle as the result of constant traction on the open median epicondylar epiphysis.[4] Osteochondritis dissecans involving the radial head or the capitellum may also be seen.[4,22,26]

Treatment tends to be conservative. Before roentgenographic changes are seen, rest is usually all that is necessary. Frequently, correction of throwing mechanics is needed. When avascular changes are seen, restriction from throwing activity must be maintained until roentgenographic signs of revascularization are seen.[22,26] When loose bodies are seen in the elbow, they should be removed to prevent further deterioration of the joint.[4,22,26] Tivnon et al[26] have shown that excising the fragments and curetting the base has given the most satisfactory results for osteochondritis with loose bodies. However, the throwing career of a young athlete frequently is ended after such surgery. Possibly, arthroscopic removal may lead to less morbidity.

Lateral Epicondylitis

Irritation of the lateral epicondyle is common among tennis players but also present in many other athletic pursuits and occupations.[4,9,17] It is also commonly found in middle-aged women.[17] Frequently, the patient complains of pain at the lateral aspect of the elbow which comes on after activity. The pain often progresses to a point where it is difficult to lift a cup or turn a doorknob. Physical examination reveals tenderness over the lateral epicondyle. There is usually pain with resistance to extension of the wrist and/or extension of the index, ring, and long fingers.[4,22] Roentgenograms are usually negative but may reveal calcification at the origin of the extensor mass at the lateral epicondyle. Nirsch[17] believes that the major pathological process is located in the extensor carpi radialis brevis, with chronic repetitive trauma causing fibroangiomatous hyperplasia.[17,22]

Treatment involves measures to relieve acute and chronic inflammation, increase in forearm extensor power, and increase in flexibility and endurance.[17] Stroke or activity alteration may be necessary to decrease the force moments acting at the elbow.

Acute episodes should be treated by rest from the activity for at least 7 days, along with the use of nonsteroidal anti-inflammatories. With severe symptoms, injection into the inflamed area of 20 mg of triamcinolone acetate and 3 ml of 0.5% Xylocaine is necessary.[17,22] A forearm-elbow brace of a nonelastic material also may be beneficial in the relief of symptoms. After symptoms have subsided, an exercise program should be initiated to rebuild the strength of the extensor group as well as the forearm flexors.[17] Exercises should include full extension of the elbow with the forearm pronated and maximum dorsiflexion of the wrist and fingers for a count of 10 s repeated 30 times daily.[17,22]

In chronic resisted cases, surgical release should be performed. This is an extraarticular procedure that involves release of the extensor digitorum communis and extensor carpi radialis brevis aponeurosis from the lateral epicondyle.[17] Occasionally, in the triangular subaponeurotic space, small amounts of grey granulation tissue will be found that should be excised.[17,22] Postoperatively, splinting for 10 days, a strengthening program, and avoidance of the causative activity for 2 months are essential.

Medial Epicondylitis

Medial epicondylitis is an overuse syndrome of the common flexor-pronator muscle group.[4,22] This occurs from multiple microtears of the muscle. This occurs frequently in golfers as a result of hitting the ground prior to hitting the ball, and it may occur in baseball pitchers who use a great deal of forceful flexion when releasing their pitch. Conservative measures such as rest, ice, and anti-inflammatory agents are usually successful in treatment. Steroid injections are sometimes necessary at the site of maximum tenderness. A forearm-elbow band may be helpful. Attention should be given to correcting improper mechanics in sport or work. Chronic cases may develop a permanent flexion contracture of the elbow.[4]

Medial Ligamentous and Capsular Elbow Problems

Chronic repetitive trauma may cause overload syndromes to the ligamentous and capsular structures of the elbow. Acute ruptures of the medial ligamentous structures of the elbow are rare. Norwood et al[18] have reported on acute surgical repair of these injuries and the abduction stress test in 15 degrees of flexion is an essential part of the examination of an acutely injured elbow.[18] Ligamentous and capsular manifestations of medial overload syndromes are sequelae of chronic repetitive trauma. Long-term signs of chronic straining of the ulnar collateral ligament include painful calcium deposits, ulnar traction spurs, and loose bodies. Surgery in chronic cases include traction spur removal, loose body removal, and occasionally ulnar nerve transposition. In pitchers, chronic stretch of the ulnar collateral ligament may require ligamentous reconstruction that may require a tendon graft.

═══ **SECTION C** ═══

Fractures and Dislocations of the Elbow, Arm, and Shoulder Girdle of Adults

Craig Ordway, Roger Dee, and Enrico Mango

FRACTURES AND DISLOCATIONS AROUND THE ELBOW

Monteggia Fracture Dislocation

The Monteggia lesion,[131] as classically described, is a fracture of the proximal one-third of the ulna with anterior dislocation of the radial head (Fig. 35-24). This complex accounts for approximately 60 percent of this fracture type, and other patterns with posterior and lateral dislocations of the radius occur less commonly.[8,134] These are described in Bado's classification (Table 35-5).

The mechanism of the commonest type I injury is usually a fall on the outstretched hand with the forearm locked in full pronation.[54] Direct injury to the ulna is occasionally responsible for Monteggia fractures.

Disruption of the elbow joint in this manner will injure the radial nerve and its branches in as many as 20 percent of

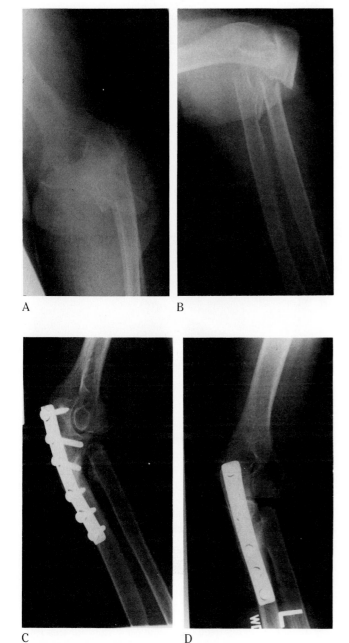

A   B

C   D

Figure 35-24 Monteggia fracture dislocation (type IV*b*). **A** and **B.** Anteroposterior and lateral views. There is anterior fracture dislocation of the radial head. **C** and **D.** Postoperative views. The radial head has been trimmed and fragments removed. The ulna fracture is reduced and fixed.

the cases.[25] Most authors agree, however, that the nerve injury is usually transient and should be treated expectantly.[23,93]

Although the diagnosis of the ulna fracture is seldom missed, the associated dislocation of the radial head may elude the examiner in as many as one-quarter of the cases.[23,66]

Treatment

Successful treatment of the Monteggia lesion depends on three factors: (1) rigid internal fixation of the ulnar fracture utilizing bone graft in the presence of severe comminution,[134] (2) anatomical reduction of the radial head with open reduction if necessary, and (3) sufficient immobilization in a long-arm cast to permit soft tissue healing—at least 6 to 8 weeks. Significant disability frequently follows even the most meticulous care of this lesion.[23,25]

Fractures of the Olecranon

Fracture of the olecranon commonly results from direct trauma to the point of the elbow. An indirect mechanism is thought to occur secondary to sudden violent contraction of the triceps as in an attempt to break a fall.[72,104] The first mechanism may be characterized by a high degree of comminution.[147] The second is usually associated with wide displacement of the fragments.[40]

Treatment

Several methods of treatment are generally recognized for olecranon fractures.[85] The undisplaced fracture complex may be treated with a posterior slab in 45 degrees of elbow flexion. Gentle motion is begun after 2 to 4 weeks.[53, 88]

Nonarticular displaced fractures are best-treated by internal fixation with one or more 4-mm AO cancellous screws.[3,85,86] Displaced fractures involving the articular surface of the olecranon should be treated either by tension band wiring[3,85] (Fig. 35-25) or by excision of the olecranon fragment with triceps reattachment to the ulna.[61]

Properly performed, the tension band wiring technique converts the tensile stresses on the posterior surface of the bone to compressive stresses on the articular side of the olecranon.[3] Open reduction is followed by immediate range-

TABLE 35-5   Bado's Classification of Monteggia Fracture Dislocations

Type   I
   a. Anterior radial head dislocation
   b. Fracture of the ulnar shaft at any level with anterior angulation

Type   II
   a. Posterior or posterolateral radial head dislocation
   b. Fracture of the ulnar shaft with posterior angulation

Type   III
   a. Lateral or anterolateral radial head dislocation
   b. Fracture of the ulnar metaphysis

Type   IV
   a. Anterior radial head dislocation
   b. Fracture of the proximal radius and ulna at the same level

Source: Bado, J.L., *Clin Orthop* 50:71-86, 1967. Reprinted with permission.

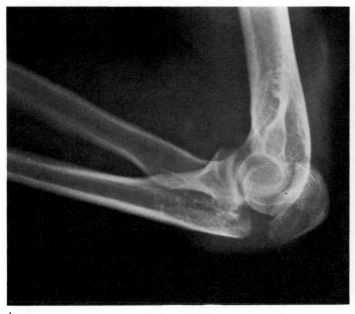

A

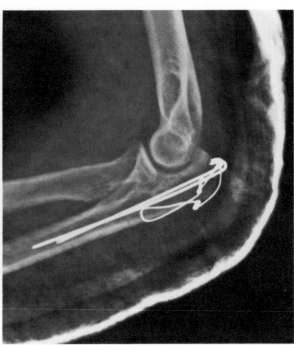

B

Figure 35-25 A. Displaced intraarticular fracture of the olecranon with disruption of the extensor mechanism. **B.** After open reduction and internal fixation with tension-band wiring.

of-motion exercises and a rapid return to full function. Some loss of elbow extension occurs more commonly than does loss of flexion.

Severe comminution of the fracture may necessitate excision of the olecranon[1,117] with triceps reconstruction.[133] This repair may require supplemental fixation in cases of comminution extending distally along the ulna.[43] Gartsman has reported good results with primary excision of the fracture fragment even if it is not comminuted.[61] These results were comparable to those found with open reduction and internal fixation. Many surgeons seem to prefer to save the noncomminuted proximal fracture fragment, but it is not necessary for elbow joint stability (except that portion to which is attached the medial collateral ligament).

Oblique fractures of the olecranon that propagate from the distal third of the joint surface distally can be rigidly fixed with interfragmentary compression additionally protected with a neutralization plate.[85,86,134]

Complications

Complications associated with tension-band wiring of olecranon fractures are usually minor and are usually related to loosening and migration of the K wires.[119] Careful attention to proper technique will minimize this complication.

Nonunion of the olecranon fracture occurs in approximately 5 percent of cases.[36,123] It is commonly the result of inadequate internal fixation of the initial fracture. Treatment of established nonunion of the olecranon consists of excision of the proximal fragment if it is less than 50 percent of the articular surface. If the proximal fragment includes greater than 50 percent of the articular surface, then debridement of the pseudoarthrosis site, internal fixation with either tension-band wiring or plate fixation, and cancellous grafting should be performed.[36]

Fracture of the Radial Head

Fracture of the radial head occurs as a solitary injury or in connection with dislocation or other fractures of the elbow joint.

Classification

The most frequently used classification system for this fracture complex was introduced by Mason.[122]

Type I Undisplaced fracture
Type II Marginal fracture with minimal displacement of a portion of the head
Type III Comminuted fracture involving the entire head
Type IV Fractures associated with dislocation of the elbow joint

The last category was added by subsequent authors[62,96] who recognized the importance of this complex fracture dislocation.

Treatment

Even the simple type II injury has historically been treated on occasion by radical excision of the head and proximal fragments.[50,178] Comminution and cartilaginous injury was thought to lead irrevocably to degenerative arthritis and late loss of function. Enthusiasm for the ablative procedure has been dampened somewhat by the subsequent late development of pain at the distal radioulnar joint with limited function and complaints of weakness of the extremity.[129] Recent thinking leans toward preserving the radial head by reconstruction of the displaced fracture fragments if possible.[133,142] A compression screw has been used successfully.[184] The decision whether to perform open reduction of a type II or type III fracture can be facilitated by range-of-motion testing after local aspiration and instillation of Xylocaine into the joint.[152] Open operation is recommended when full pronation and/or supination cannot be obtained following this procedure.[187] Preservation of the radial head or replacement with a Silastic spacer[118] to stabilize the elbow joint is of particular importance when the fracture is associated with total medial collateral ligament disruption or instability secondary to fracture dislocation of the elbow[50] (type IV).

Complications

Development of wrist pain may be associated with proximal migration of the radius following radial head excision. This has been used as an argument for always replacing the radial head with a spacer after excision. However correlation between the degree of migration and the incidence of wrist pain is poor. The wrist pain in many cases is probably related to associated primary damage to the inferior radioulnar joint at the original injury.

Extraarticular Fractures of the Distal Humerus (Table 35-6)

Supracondylar Fractures

Supracondylar fractures of the distal humerus are described as occurring from either hyperextension[26] or (rarely) forced flexion at the elbow. The fracture in children is discussed in detail in Chap. 36

TABLE 35-6 Classification of Fractures of the Distal Humerus

Extraarticular fractures
  Supracondylar
  Transcondylar
  Epicondylar
    Medial
    Lateral
  Supracondylar process

Intraarticular fractures
  Intercondylar (T and Y condylar)
  Lateral condylar
  Medial condylar
  Articular
    Capitellum
    Trochlea

Source: From Bryan, R.S., and Morrey, B.F, in *The Elbow and Its Disorders.* Philadelphia, Saunders, 1985. Reprinted with permission.

Treatment Manipulative reduction of the supracondylar fracture complex is most frequently employed. Manipulation requires longitudinal traction to overcome the pull of the triceps and biceps.[101,117] The fracture fragments must be completely distracted before flexion is used in the reduction maneuver. Failure to follow this rule places the neurovascular structures at significant risk.[172]

Postreduction care includes the use of a posterior slab with collar and cuff; this is employed for 4 to 6 weeks with protected motion as soon as clinical union is identified.[34] Forced, passive stretching exercises should be avoided because of the risk of heterotopic bone formation.[113]

Operative reduction may be indicated in the presence of vascular compromise, irreducible fracture complexes or in those fractures which are unacceptably unstable. Fixation can be accomplished in children through the percutaneous use of pins,[97] but in adults, plates and screws utilizing interfragmentary compression may be required.[26,133] Postoperative mobilization should be immediate. There is considerable debate concerning the type of exercise prescribed as there is evidence that passive stretching may encourage heterotopic bone formation.[59,115,171,51,131] On the other hand, this modality is felt to be helpful in brain-injured patients by some practitioners.[59] Devices which encourage constant passive motion should be used with care even in the neurologically normal population. Factors which appear to minimize heterotopic bone formation (see p. 272) are early operation, meticulous operative technique, the use of diphosphonates,[83,175] anti-inflammatory drugs, or low-dose radiation.[100]

Transcondylar ("Dicondylar") Fractures

This fracture is much less common than the supracondylar fracture. It differs from the supracondylar type in the more distal, intraarticular location of the fracture line which traverses the distal humeral condyles within the joint capsule.[26]

Transcondylar fractures can occur after a fall on the outstretched hand (extension type) or after a fall on the flexed elbow (flexion type). Often, the patients are elderly with osteoporotic bone. Nondisplaced, or minimally displaced, fractures appear to occur more frequently than displaced fractures.[44]

Treatment The treatment is similar to that for supracondylar fractures. Nondisplaced, or minimally displaced, fractures require simple cast immobilization. Displaced fractures are treated by closed reduction followed by casting unless the fracture is unstable and then percutaneous (or limited open) K-wire fixation should be employed.[26] Overhead olecranon pin traction will also achieve reduction in unstable or irreducible fractures, but the attendant complications of prolonged bed rest, especially in the elderly, are serious disadvantages of this form of treatment. The need for open reduction in transcondylar fractures is rare, and is usually necessary only for irreducible fractures in patients where the use of skeletal traction is undesirable.

Since this fracture is intraarticular, the most common complication is elbow stiffness, which may be the result of a bony block due to callus formation within the coronoid and/or olecranon fossa.[27]

Posada's fracture describes a rare type of transcondylar fracture that consists of complete anterior displacement of the distal condylar fragment with dislocation of this fragment from the proximal radius and ulna.[42] Closed reduction is extremely difficult to achieve; therefore, open reduction and internal fixation is the procedure of choice.[70]

Supracondylar Process Fractures

The supracondylar process, a congenital bony spur projecting from the anteromedial surface of the lower third of the humeral shaft, is present in less than 3 percent of elbow injuries.[108] The ligament of Struthers attaches to this process and to the medial epicondyle, forming an arch through which pass the median nerve and the brachial artery or one of its branches.[121]

Direct injury may produce a rare fracture of the supracondylar process, occasionally causing compression of the median nerve. Nondisplaced fractures usually heal well with cast immobilization. Excision of the fractured process with the surrounding periosteum should be considered for displaced fractures that either remain painful, or in cases where median nerve compression persists or develops after healing has occurred.[13] Myositis ossificans is a reported complication that may occur after excision.[63,108]

Fractures of the Epicondyles

Medial Epicondyle Isolated fracture of the medial epicondyle of the elbow is an uncommon injury in adults, and it is usually the result of a local direct blow. It more frequently occurs indirectly after a fall on the outstretched hand in association with other fractures or dislocations of the elbow.[102,189] In children or adolescents, an avulsion fracture occurs, especially in association with posterior dislocation, because the ossification center of the medial epicondyle does not fuse with the medial condyle until the late teens. The injury is discussed in more detail in the discussion of fractures of the elbow in children (Chap. 36).

Local swelling, tenderness, and painful limitation of elbow, and wrist motion are the usual findings on physical examination. The sensorimotor status of the ulnar nerve should be checked since the course of the ulnar nerve is just posterior to the medial epicondyle. Plain x-ray films will confirm the diagnosis, but displacement of the medial epicondylar fragment as far distal as the joint line should arouse concern for possible intraarticular entrapment, especially after reduction of a posterior elbow dislocation with an associated medial epicondylar fracture.[146]

Treatment Minimally displaced fractures should be treated by immobilization in a plaster splint or cast with the elbow flexed to 90 degrees.[26,42,186] Pronation of the forearm and flexion of the wrist will further reduce the distraction force of the attached flexor muscles. After 1 to 2 weeks of immobilization, early range-of-motion exercises should be instituted in order to minimize elbow stiffness, which is a frequent complication. Follow up radiographs often reveal a fibrous union that is usually compatible with painless, normal function of the elbow.[102] The treatment of displaced fractures remains controversial.[42,186] It is often difficult to obtain exact anatomical reduction by closed manipulation and casting, but less than optimal reduction appears to be compatible with a good func-

tional result.[18,172] Larger fragments, especially if displaced greater than 1 cm, should be reduced open and internally fixed with either a cancellous screw or K wire. Fragments that are too small for fixation can be excised, and the flexor tendon origin can be reattached to the medial condyle.

Intraarticular entrapment of the medial epicondyle usually requires arthrotomy to remove the fragment, but a single attempt at closed reduction is reasonable although it is only rarely successful. Applying a valgus force to the elbow with the wrist extended and the forearm supinated may result in release of the fragment.[26,146]

Complications Since the most common complication of this fracture is loss of elbow motion, range-of-motion exercises should be instituted as early as possible after closed or open treatment. Symptomatic nonunion after a displaced medial epicondylar fracture is rare.[18] In such cases, the ununited fragment should be excised and the flexor tendon origin reattached. Elbow instability and, later, ulnar neuropathy are also uncommonly seen after this fracture.[26,42]

Lateral Epicondyle A fracture of the lateral humeral epicondyle may follow a direct blow to the outer elbow. This is an extremely rare fracture. Treatment consists of immobilization in a posterior splint or cast until the pain and swelling subside, followed by early motion of the elbow joint.[26]

Intraarticular Fractures of the Distal Humerus

Intercondylar Fractures

Intercondylar fractures of the distal humerus are uncommon; they account for approximately 5 percent of all distal humeral fractures.[106] They occur more frequently in middle-aged or elderly persons. A fall on the outstretched hand, or a direct blow to the posterior elbow, wedges the coronoid process of the ulna into the intercondylar region of the distal humerus, usually at the trochlear sulcus.[29,44,172] A T or a Y condylar fracture pattern, often with comminution, is typically seen.

The most frequently quoted classification is Riseborough and Radin[156] which divides this fracture into four types:

Type I: Undisplaced intercondylar fracture
Type II: Displaced intercondylar fracture without significant rotational deformity
Type III: Displaced intercondylar fracture with significant rotatory deformity
Type IV: Severely comminuted and displaced intercondylar fracture (Fig. 35-26)

Except for the undisplaced type I fracture where the physical and x-ray findings may be less than obvious, the various types of intercondylar fractures are readily diagnosed on plain x-ray films. Additional radiographic views (such as oblique views), tomography, or computed tomography may assist in planning treatment, especially when open reduction with internal fixation is being considered for the comminuted type IV fracture pattern.

Treatment Undisplaced type I intercondylar fractures are treated by splint or cast immobilization for 3 weeks followed by early range-of-motion exercises.[26,42,156] The treatment of displaced fractures depends on the type of fracture, the age

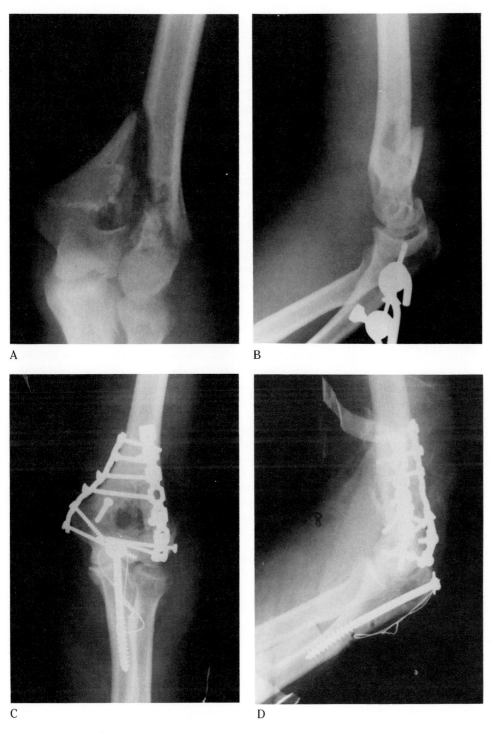

A B

C D

Figure 35-26 A and **B.** A comminuted intercondylar fracture of the distal humerus (type IV). **C** and **D.** Open reduction and internal fixation was performed by means of a transolecranon approach. Mobilization commenced immediately after surgery.

and activity level of the patient, the quality of bone, and the condition of the soft tissues surrounding the fracture.[79]

Closed reduction of type II intercondylar fractures by manipulation with bicondylar pressure and cast immobilization is an acceptable method of treatment in the younger patient if anatomical reduction is achieved and maintained.[26] Exact anatomical repositioning is less of a concern in the elderly patient, especially in one who is a poor candidate for surgery.

In type III fractures and when closed reduction is unsuccessful in type II fractures, open reduction with rigid internal fixation using AO technique is becoming an increasingly popular method of treatment. This is the case not only in younger patients but also in older active patients, provided there is good-quality bone stock.[29,99,185] A posterior approach with transolecranon osteotomy is preferred. This gives the best exposure in the more difficult cases where comminution of the articular surfaces extends on to the anterior surface of the condyles.[99] The keys to success with this method of treatment is that fixation be rigid and accurate, that the fossae be free of metal fixation or bone, and that early postoperative range-of-motion exercises be instituted. Open reduction and internal

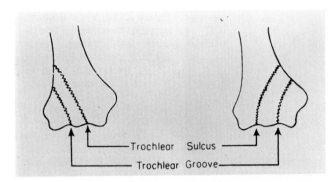

Figure 35-27 Milch classification of condylar fractures. At the left is a lateral condyle fracture. At the right is a medial condyle fracture. *(From Milch, H., J Trauma 4:592–607, 1964. Reproduced with permission.)*

fixation of severely comminuted, displaced type IV fractures is technically quite challenging. It has been well described by several authors.[3,95,99] It should be performed by those surgeons with sufficient experience in techniques of surgical fixation.[99]

Skeletal traction with an olecranon pin may still be an acceptable, although less popular, method of treatment for the comminuted fracture (particularly type IV) that does not appear to be reconstructible by open reduction and internal fixation.[26] Other appropriate indications for this technique include open fractures with severe soft tissue injury that precludes the immediate use of internal fixation. One of the main disadvantages of skeletal traction is the prolonged period of immobilization of the patient, which is undesirable for elderly persons. Early elbow motion must be instituted while the patient is still in traction.

An alternative method of treatment for the severely comminuted type IV fracture in the very elderly patient with osteopenia is the "bag of bones" technique of nonoperative treatment.[24] This technique involves placing the affected upper extremity in a collar and cuff with the elbow free. Early range-of-motion exercises are begun as soon as the initial swelling and pain have diminished and the patient is able to tolerate movement. Despite the nonanatomical radiographic appearance of the healed fracture, the clinical result is often quite satisfactory for the elderly patient with decreased functional demands.[124]

Complications Undoubtedly, the most common complication of intercondylar fractures of the elbow is elbow stiffness.[106] The institution of early range-of-motion exercise, whether it be following operative or nonoperative treatment is of paramount importance in attempting to minimize the loss of elbow motion. Nerve injury, especially of the ulnar nerve, has been reported in up to 15 percent of cases following surgery.[29]

Nonunion is rare, but when it occurs, it usually involves the supracondylar segment of the intercondylar fracture.[26,42,106]

Humeral Condylar Fractures

Fractures of the medial or lateral condyles and of the distal humerus account for less than 5 percent of distal humeral fractures in adults.[106] These intraarticular fractures have been classified into two types by Milch[130] (Fig. 35-27). The type I fracture of the lateral or medial condyle involves the smaller, outer margin of the humeral condyles. The elbow joint is inherently stable in this type of fracture unless the contralateral collateral ligament of the elbow has been disrupted. The type II fracture of either condyle is unstable since it includes the trochlear lip (or ridge), a bony prominence just lateral to the trochlear sulcus, which provides osseous stability to the elbow joint.[35,42]

Fractures of the humeral condyles result either from avulsion forces applied at the origin of the collateral ligaments of the elbow or by axial compressive loads that produce radial or ulnar impaction against the distal humeral condyles after a fall on the outstretched hand.[44,130,174]

Treatment The nondisplaced type I or II fractures of the medial or lateral condyles should be treated by splint or cast immobilization. Early range-of-motion exercise commences after initial healing has occurred, in approximately 3 weeks. Displaced type I fractures of either condyle may be reduced by closed methods, but anatomical restoration of the distal humeral articular surface can be difficult to achieve so that open reduction with internal fixation by pins or screws is often necessary.[26,27,65,106] Associated contralateral ligament disruption should also be repaired if the elbow joint is unstable.

Displaced type II fractures of the medial or lateral condyles are unstable injuries and are not amenable to closed treatment. Open reduction with internal fixation is recommended as soon as possible after injury.[42,130]

Complications In addition to elbow stiffness, the occurrence of degenerative arthritis and tardy ulnar neuropathy has been reported after fractures of each humeral condyle.[106,130,164] Malunion of a lateral condyle fracture, especially the type II fracture, may result in cubitus valgus deformity. A malunited medial condyle fracture may produce cubitus varus.[26,27,42]

Articular Fractures

Fractures occurring through the articular portion of the capitellum or trochlea are rare injuries. The lack of soft tissue attachment to these fracture fragments allows for significant displacement (usually anteriorly) within the elbow joint, making successful closed reduction often difficult to achieve.

Fractures of the Capitellum Fractures of the capitellum result from a shearing force inflicted by the radial head that may occur during a fall on the outstretched hand with the elbow semiflexed.[111] This fracture occurs far more commonly in women than in men possibly due to an increased valgus carrying angle or to a higher incidence of osteoporosis.[69] Three types of capitellar fractures are described:

Type I: Hahn-Steinthal fracture. This is the commonest type of capitellar fracture and includes not only the articular surface of the capitellum but also the underlying subchondral and cancellous bone. Occasionally, it may also consist of a portion of the lateral margin of the trochlea (Fig. 35-28).

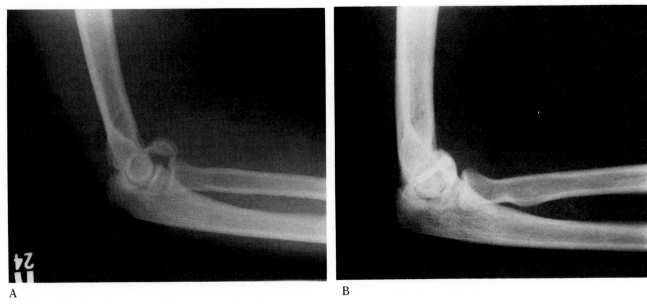

A   B

Figure 35-28 A. Displaced type I articular fracture of the capitellum in a 45-year-old female. **B.** Open reduction and internal fixation.

Type II: Kocher-Lorenz fracture. This is an articular slice fracture of the capitellum usually with minimal associated subchondral bone.

Type III: Impaction or comminution of the capitellar articular surface.

Moderate swelling, pain, crepitation, and limited motion of the elbow are the usual findings on physical examination. Anteriorly displaced fractures may be palpable in the antecubital fossa. An associated tear of the medial collateral ligament should be suspected if swelling and tenderness exist over the medial side of the elbow, or if valgus instability is present. Plain radiographs of the elbow joint, especially the lateral view, will establish the diagnosis, but the actual size of the articular fragment is never adequately estimated in this manner.

Treatment Opinions differ as to the appropriate treatment for type I fractures of the capitellum. Anatomical reduction of a displaced capitellar fracture is generally agreed upon as being of importance, and closed or open reduction is the chosen method of treatment.[42,44,69] The issue centers on whether to excise the larger type I fracture fragment or to internally fix it. Those who support closed reduction or open reduction with internal fixation believe that valgus instability of the elbow may result if the type I fracture fragment is excised.[102,172] Proponents of excision stress that valgus instability is a rare complication. They believe excision produces minimal morbidity and permits early mobilization.[48,69,111] Dushuttle recently performed cadaveric studies to determine the effect of excision of the capitellum on elbow instability. He found that valgus instability after capitellar fragment excision occured only if an associated rupture of the medial collateral ligament of the elbow was present.[48] Whenever this ligament was intact, valgus stability was not produced.

The choice of treatment of capitellar fractures should be made on an individual basis, depending on patient age, qual-

ity of the bone, and type of fracture.[69] Nondisplaced fractures of the capitellum should be treated by splint or cast immobilization for several weeks followed by early range-of-motion exercises. Displaced type II slice fractures can be satisfactorily treated by arthrotomy and excision of the fragment.[69]

An attempt at closed reduction of a displaced type I capitellar fracture is reasonable, but reduction must be anatomical or a bony block to elbow motion will occur.[42] After closed reduction, the elbow should be immobilized in a long-arm cast with the elbow flexed to at least 90 degrees and the forearm pronated to enable the radial head to assist in maintaining the reduction of the capitellar fracture.[44]

If closed reduction of the displaced type I fracture fails, then open reduction with rigid internal fixation (cancellous screws) or excision of the fragment can be performed with the expectation of a satisfactory result as long as early motion of the elbow is possible after surgery.[48,55,69,111,] The type I capitellar fragment should not be excised if the elbow is unstable due to a rupture of the medial collateral ligament of the elbow or if an associated radial head fracture is present which itself requires excision.[26,42]

Type III capitellar fractures involving comminution of the articular surface should be excised.[42,69]

Avascular necrosis of the capitellar fragment after either closed reduction or open reduction with internal fixation is an extremely rare complication, and for all practical purposes it should not be a concern when one decides upon the appropriate treatment of this fracture.

Fractures of the Trochlea An isolated fracture of the articular surface of the trochlea is much less common than an articular fracture of the capitellum except when it is found as part of a type II capitellar fracture.[26] The mechanism of injury is believed to be caused by an impingement of the ulna against the trochlea as may occur during a posterior dislocation of the elbow or by a direct blow to the posterior proximal ulna.[42]

TABLE 35-7 Classification of Elbow Dislocations in Adults

Dislocation of radius and ulna
Posterior dislocation
    Posterolateral
    Posteromedial
Medial dislocation
Lateral dislocation
Anterior dislocation
Divergent dislocation (with superior radioulnar joint disruption)
    Anteroposterior
    Mediolateral (transverse)

Isolated dislocation of the radius
Anterior
Posterolateral

Isolated dislocation of the ulna
Anterior
Posterior

Source: Adapted from Stimson, L.A.: *A Treatise on Fractures.* Philadelphia, Leas's, 1890. Reprinted with permission.

The clinical findings are similar to those seen for fractures of the capitellum. Nondisplaced fractures should be immobilized for several weeks, and then early motion of the elbow is begun. Small, or comminuted, displaced fractures can be safely excised. Large fragments require open, anatomical reduction with rigid internal fixation.[150] Early range-of-motion exercises are important in order to minimize elbow stiffness.

Dislocation of the Elbow (Table 35-7)

Dislocation of the elbow occurs in a predominantly male population under 30 years of age. The nondominant extremity is usually involved.[114,139,181] This injury is further discussed in the section on children's upper extremity injuries (Chap. 36).

Considerable debate concerns the position of the elbow at the time of the most common posterior or posterolateral type of dislocation of the elbow. The most commonly held opinion is that the joint is hyperextended and that initially there is rupture of the medial collateral ligaments.[165,180] Regardless of mechanism, the deformity involves posterior displacement of the radius and the ulna in relation to the distal humerus. The joint is held in the semiflexed position locked over the coronoid process. The magnitude of the soft tissue injury is indicated by frequent massive swelling.[38] Injury to the surrounding structures is reported to involve the brachial artery and its branches.[52,116,182] The ulna and median nerves are also at risk of injury from the original trauma, and entrapment of the median nerve can occur during the reduction procedure.[37,56,64,73,120,153,162,169]

Treatment

Reduction is accomplished by gentle longitudinal traction disengaging the coronoid process.[180] Muscular relaxation

with general anesthesia is frequently required. Although a considerable volume of literature recommends 3 weeks of posterior slab immobilization[114,115] excellent results are also reported using earlier active exercise while protecting the elbow from full extension.[161,172]

Indications for open treatment of the acute elbow dislocations include irreducibility, elbow joint instability after reduction, or the finding of loose bodies within the joint.[47]

Complications

The irreducible dislocation complex is extremely rare.[114] Entrapment of the radial head in the posterolateral tissues of the forearm has been found to be a cause of irreducibility.

Instability due to ligamentous laxity is manifested by subluxation or early recurrent dislocation. It occurs infrequently but must be considered during the follow-up of these injuries. Instability of the lateral side of the elbow joint has been found to be more common than medial instability by Durig and his associates.[47] Posterior subluxation or recurrent isolated dislocation of the radial head may occur associated with posterolateral instability. Alternatively these may be a true chronic, recurrent dislocation of the elbow joint.[5,67,98,144] Instability may also be due to bony insufficiency when there are associated intraarticular fractures, such as those involving the coronoid process of the ulna. Treatment may be directed toward reconstruction of the lateral ligamentous complex as recommended by Osborne.[75,144] This is particularly necessary if true medial dislocation occurs. Medial collateral ligament reconstruction will often stabilize posterior and posterolateral instability.[165,166]

Chronic, unreduced posterior dislocations of the elbow that are older than 3 weeks require open reduction. Naidoo reported satisfactory results in a series of 23 patients who underwent open reduction irrespective of the age of the patient or of the duration of the dislocation.[135]

Vascular injury is uncommon following elbow dislocation and is more common in open dislocations. The median nerve may then be injured. Usually it is the ulnar nerve that is damaged in closed elbow dislocation.

Fracture of the Diaphysis of the Humerus

Diaphyseal fractures of the humerus result from either torsional or bending forces of the bone.[94] Displacement secondary to these forces places the surrounding neurovascular structures at extreme risk both at the time of injury and during later stages of healing[158] (Fig. 35-29). Injuries to the brachial artery are reported in 0.6 percent to 3 percent of cases.[35,155] Radial nerve palsy, observed as motor dysfunction,[149] occurs in up to 16 percent of these fractures.[57,103,145,168]

Treatment

Nonoperative treatment alternatives of humeral shaft fractures include hanging cast,[30] coaptation and abduction splints,[33,45] shoulder spica, sling and swath, Velpeau sling[32] or functional bracing.[10,163,164] Accepted deformity of the shaft fractures may range up to 20 degrees anterior angulation and 30 degrees of valgus or varus.[89,105] Compared with lower limb fractures, shortening is also more permissible. Up to 1 in. will generally only require modification of the patient's shirt sleeves. Both neurological complications and nonunions appear to increase in frequency at the lower third of the shaft of the humerus when the fracture is treated in a closed manner.[84]

Satisfactory operative treatment of humeral shaft fractures utilizes plates,[133] intramedullary nails,[49,109] and external fixation devices.[71] Indications include persisting dysfunction in a previously normal radial nerve following manipulation. An unstable, severely displaced fracture with soft tissue interposition may also be an appropriate indication for open treatment. Pathologic fractures particularly from breast carcinoma also commonly require fixation. Fixation of humeral shaft fractures is increasingly employed in patients with multiple injuries as a part of a program involving their rapid mobilization. More conservative surgeons, however, usually will reserve fixation for those fractures which clearly show clinical and radiographic signs of delayed healing after 6 weeks immobilization.[151]

Use of Rush rod fixation as a form of intermedullary device has fallen from favor and is associated with a high complication rate. Stern and co-workers gave the startling figure of 67 percent of patients developing complications using this method![179] They also observed that the incidence of delayed union and nonunion was 39 percent following open reduction but was as high as 9 percent even when the nailing was done by closed or semiopen techniques. In many cases the pin was inserted adjacent to the shoulder joint and additional complications included symptomatic capsulitis necessitating early removal of the metal. The authors point out the importance of good three-point fixation and proper methods of nail insertion.

Closed retrograde nailing using multiple Ender's pins followed by immediate active mobilization of the upper limb give satisfactory results without the complication of painful capsulitis of the shoulder. Union occurred in 90 percent of patients treated in this way who had exhibited clinical or radiographic signs of delayed union after 6 weeks conservative treatment.[151] Stiffness of the elbow joint, which might be expected following retrograde insertion, does not seem to occur. An important technical point is that the smaller (3.2 mm in diameter) nails must be available since 4.5-mm nails are not suitable to this technique.[151] Use of a single intramedullary rod such as a K nail is less satisfactory in resisting rotation.

Excellent results can be achieved by plating fractures of the shaft of the humerus. This technique has been used successfully in patients with multiple injuries by Bell and co-workers.[15] All fractures save one of their 34 patients united primarily, and there was only one case of significant limitation of shoulder motion. All patients preserved elbow motion. There were no neurological complications as a result of surgery and only one case in which the fixation failed. Infection similarly was seen in only one patient. In pathologic fractures with considerable loss of bone substance, where methylmethacrylate may be necessary in addition to internal fixation, plating is probably the method of choice.

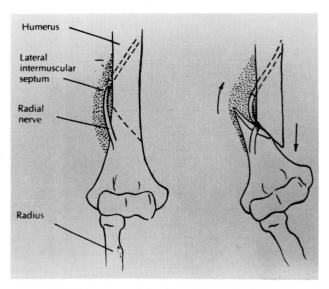

Figure 35-29 Fractures of the distal third of the humerus may contuse, lacerate, or entrap the radial nerve (before or after reduction) as it winds around the humeral shaft at this level. *(From Holstein, A., and Lewis, G.B., J Bone Joint Surg 45A:1382, 1963. Reproduced with permission.)*

Treatment of Radial Neuropathy

Individuals with fractures in the distal third of the humerus are most often at risk for radial nerve injury.[94] Complete return of function is usually to be expected. Pollack and co-workers[149] found 4 percent of their patients had an actual laceration of the nerve, and they observe that such was the case in 12 percent of those patients described in the literature. Late repair or decompression of the nerve which is entrapped in callus does not jeopardize the results, which are still excellent. Expectant treatment, therefore, should be adopted with careful clinical review together with appropriate electrodiagnostic tests. The absence of either sensory or motor sparing at the first examination does not necessarily mean a complete division.[149] If there is no improvement with careful clinical and electromyographic monitoring at 3½ to 4 months, the nerve should be explored.[149]

Fractures of the Proximal Humerus

Classification

Eighty-five percent of these fractures are designated minimal displacement fractures in that no segment is displaced more than 1 cm or angulated more than 45 degrees. Because they are undisplaced, further classification is unnecessary.

On the other hand, displaced fractures are severe and disabling injuries and commonly occur in the fifth and sixth decade when the residual disability is of great significance. The accurate classification by Neer[136,154] provides a basis for discussion of treatment and has been useful as a basis for comparison of clinical results. He initiated a four-segment terminology to be applied only to displaced fractures. One or all of the four major segments may be displaced. They are (1) the articular segment, (2) the lesser tuberosity segment,

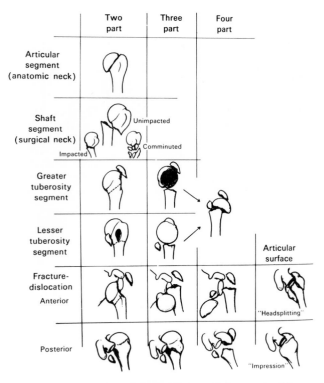

Figure 35-30 Classifications of fractures of the proximal humerus and also fracture dislocation of the shoulder joint. *(From Neer, C.S., II, Instr Course Lect 24:163, 1975. Reproduced with permission.)*

(3) the greater tuberosity segment, or (4) the shaft segment. Either two-part, three-part, or four-part fracture patterns are recognized and classified according to the key segment that is displaced. In addition, anterior or posterior fracture dislocations, which may be two-, three-, or four-part, are described in the classification (Fig. 35-30). The classification also identifies a fracture pattern in which the head is indented or crushed. This is the so-called *impression fracture*. Another variety exists in which the articular surface is split into a number of pieces, the so-called *head-splitting fracture*.

Radiological Procedures

Standard anteroposterior and tangential scapula x-ray films are taken. These are supplemented by an axillary view and also use of CT scan. A thorough appreciation of the precise anatomy of each fracture is critical for successful treatment.

Treatment

Undisplaced Fractures These fractures are inevitably treated nonoperatively by functional exercises. A good outcome is to be expected provided that a careful rehabilitation program is followed as outlined in the Chap. 49, on rehabilitation in the upper limb.

Displaced Fractures Neer recommends surgical reconstruction for the two-part greater tuberosity segment displacement in which the fragment is reattached with wire sutures and the cuff repaired. Surgery is also necessary for the displaced two-part articular segment, but the late results are

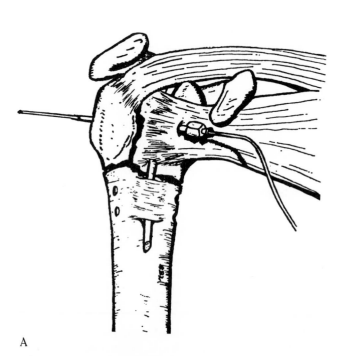

A

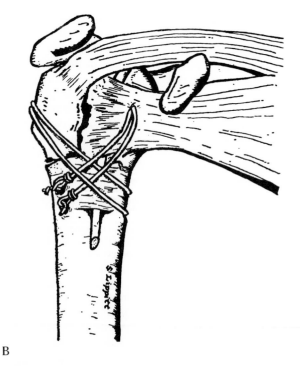

B

Figure 35-31 Surgical technique for fixation of a three-part displaced fracture of the proximal humerus. **A.** With the colpotomy needle in position pinning the fragments of the lesser and greater tuberosities, a free wire is passed and drill holes are prepared in the anterior aspect of the humeral shaft. **B.** The first wire is passed through the holes in the humeral shaft and tightened; with the fracture stabilized, a second wire is passed in a similar fashion. *(From Hawkins R.J., et al., J Bone Joint Surg 68A:1412, 1986. Reproduced with permission.)*

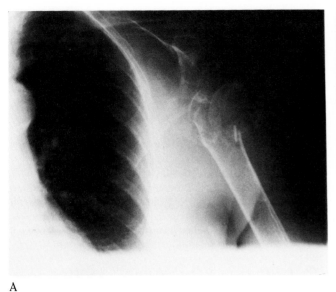

A

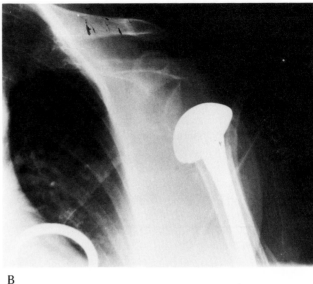

B

Figure 35-32 A. Four-part fracture dislocation of the shoulder joint. **B.** Endoprosthetic replacement of the humeral head and reattachment of the greater and lesser tuberosities performed.

not good since avascular necrosis commonly occurs. The two-part lesser tuberosity segment displacement may be treated by functional exercises.[136] In the three-part greater tuberosity segment displacement, the prognosis for survival of the head is good after its rotation is corrected at open reduction, the greater tuberosity segment being then reattached and the cuff repaired.[112,136] In the three-part lesser tuberosity segment displacement, Neer advises open surgery principally to correct the rotated articular segment which is rotated by the muscles still attached to the intact greater tuberosity.

Hawkins and his co-workers[77] have described the technique of maintaining the fragments of a three-part fracture in a reduced position using a colpotomy needle through which is passed the 20-gauge wire, which is then used to tension-band the fragments in position (Fig. 35-31). These authors also recommend the three-phase rehabilitation program, which is so important in the management of these cases. All authors agree that unless the patient is well motivated and the rehabilitation program is of high caliber, the results of surgery will be inferior.[77,136,177] Hawkins's patients had an average of 126 degrees of active elevation of the upper limb with good internal and external rotation following surgery for the displaced three-part fracture.[77]

Neer points out that, with four-part displacement, the detachment of the tuberosities deprives the humeral head of adequate circulation. He recommends that prosthetic replacement be performed at the same time that the tuberosities are reattached[136] (Fig. 35-32). Endoprosthetic replacement is also required when there is a head defect occupying more than 50 percent of the articular surface in the impression fracture and in the head-splitting variety. Manipulative treatment has little place in the management of these displaced multiple-part fractures, for even if it is possible to reduce them, redisplacement is certain.[190]

In patients who are very elderly, a conservative attitude has been recommended by some authors, but then only limited goals should be anticipated.[190,177] Stableforth pointed out that in his series of 32 patients treated nonoperatively for displaced four-part fracture, 25 were unable to get the hand of the injured limb either to the mouth or the buttocks. Many of them were totally dependent or needed active assistance for activities of daily living, and, in addition, two-thirds of them found their sleep disturbed by pain.[177] By contrast, in his hands, surgically treated patients had a consistently better range of motion and a fuller functional recovery with less long-term disability and pain. Stableforth also observed a 6.1 percent incidence of associated brachial plexus damage in displaced four-part fractures, the majority of which only made an incomplete recovery. Associated injuries included other ipsilateral fractures and chest complications such as pneumothorax associated with ipsilateral fractures of the upper ribs.

Dislocation of the Shoulder

Acute and chronic instability of the glenohumeral joint is discussed in Sect. D of this chapter.

FRACTURES AND DISLOCATIONS OF THE SHOULDER GIRDLE

Sternoclavicular Joint

Sternoclavicular fractures and dislocations occur uncommonly, representing approximately 3 percent of shoulder girdle injuries.[32,160] Force transmitted along the clavicle from the lateral tip of the shoulder causes the medial end of the clavicle to dislocate anteriorly or posteriorly. Anterior dislocations are by far the most common.

Posterior dislocation of the sternoclavicular joint may occur from a direct blow to the chest.[78,128] The medial end of the clavicle is driven retrosternally into the deeper structures of the chest, which may cause both immediate and delayed injury.[28] The patient should be supported by interscapular bolster.[32] The patient may complain of hoarseness, dyspnea, dysphagia, or numbness and weakness of the upper extremity.[167]

Radiological Procedures

The sternoclavicular joint may not be well seen on standard radiographs and CT scan is recommended.[167] The importance of the physical examination in the diagnosis of this dislocation cannot be overemphasized.

Treatment

Anterior dislocations can usually be treated with closed reduction. Traction is applied with the arm held between 70 degrees and 90 degrees of abduction. The surgeon presses directly downward to reduce the joint. Obtaining reduction is easy but maintaining it can be difficult. Figure-of-eight immobilization is applied, holding the shoulders back in a braced position for 6 weeks. Immobilization for up to 6 weeks may be followed by a gentle range-of-motion exercise program, the limb returning to function at 12 weeks. Failure of reduction or persisting instability may indicate the need for surgical stabilization. Unfortunately, most of the complications seen with this injury are iatrogenic.[125] Late surgical excision of the joint and meniscus can be accomplished without added loss of function.

Closed reduction is also performed for posterior dislocations utilizing traction through the adducted humerus. A towel clip is used to pull the proximal clavicle forward, yielding a stable reduction. Closed reduction should only be undertaken in the controlled setting of the operating room and with the patient under general anesthetic because of the risk of vascular or tracheal injury.[78] Failure of reduction may necessitate open exploration of the joint, a hazardous undertaking because of the proximity of the great vessels. An unstable reduction requires posterior capsular repair with heavy suture material which may also be used to anchor the clavicle to the first rib. The use of interosseous K wires is fraught with serious potential complications.[41,87] Wires have migrated from the joint as far as the liver[184] and spinal cord.[171]

Fractures of the Clavicle

Fractures of the clavicle are among the most common fractures.

Classification

Fractures of the clavicle have been subdivided into three groups by Allman.[6] Group 1 are the common middle third fractures; group 2 are fractures lateral to the coracoclavicular ligaments; and group 3 are medial third fractures, which are often undisplaced. Neer[137,138] has further classified fractures of the outer clavicle: *type I* fractures are undisplaced fractures in the region of the coracoclavicular ligaments and are held in place by these structures. *Type II* fractures of the distal clavicle are displaced fractures because the medial fragment is no longer attached to the retaining ligaments and consequently displaces superiorly (Fig. 35-33). In *type III* fractures of the

outer end of the clavicle, the fracture involves the articular surface of the acromioclavicular joint, which may subsequently lead to degenerative arthritis.

The mechanism of injury may be a direct blow to the bone or indirect trauma associated with a fall on the point of the shoulder.

Radiological Procedures

Standard anteroposterior and scapular views will usually show the displacement of the fragments. However, an anteroposterior view with weights attached to the wrists is useful for evaluating the integrity of the coracoclavicular ligament and will indicate whether there is ligamentous continuity between the medial fragment of the clavicle and the coracoid process. If the ligament is detached from the fragment or ruptured, then descent of the scapula will occur.

Treatment

Middle third fractures comprise 82 percent of these injuries.[92,159] Reduction is usually satisfactorily achieved by appropriate strapping with a figure-of-eight bandage for 4 to 6 weeks with a graded return to full activity after x-ray evidence of union is seen.[19,161] With an undisplaced fracture, sometimes, a simple sling is sufficient immobilization. Similar methods of treatment are satisfactory for fractures involving the medial third of the clavicle and for type I fractures of the outer third.

Controversy surrounds the treatment of Neer type II displaced fractures of the outer third of the clavicle with loss of integrity of the coracoclavicular ligaments. Attempting to strap the medial fragment downward in a reduced position using felt pads on the point of the acromion and over the medial fragment are rarely successful and invite skin problems. Nonunion may approach 40 percent if these fractures are treated nonoperatively.[148] Consequently Philips recommended open reduction and internal fixation using a transacromial wire which transfixes the two fragments of the clavicle.[148] It is important that the end of the wire be bent over at its outer margin so that the complications of wire migration

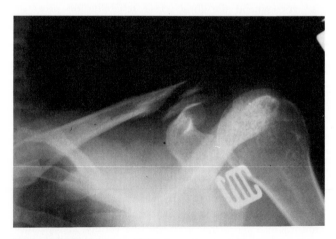

Figure 35-33 Neer type II fracture of outer clavicle adjacent to the coracoid process. The important coracoclavicular (conoid and trapezoid) ligaments may be disrupted.

are not seen. If union does not occur, wire breakage is a distinct possibility.[68] Some authors prefer a more substantial fixation using a Steinman pin or a Bosworth screw. Other favor using a sling of material such as Dacron connecting the medial clavicular fragment and the coracoid; this sling will take over the lost function of the coracoclavicular ligaments until the fracture heals.[39] In type II injuries, excision of the outer fragment should not be performed since it will make matters worse and will do nothing to stabilize the shoulder girdle. However, in type III injuries of the outer clavicle, where the fracture involves the acromioclavicular joint but the coracoclavicular ligaments are intact, excision of a small outer portion of the clavicle may be useful treatment for secondary degenerative arthritis.[101]

Complications

Immediate neurovascular compromise can occur with a clavicular injury.[11,14] Occasionally, open reduction is required for unacceptable deformity and in the rare case of irreducible fracture.[92] The rate of nonunion is 1 to 2 percent of all patients.[188] Refracture of a previously healed injury is of significance in promoting nonunion as is also trauma of such severity to completely displace the clavicular fragments and produce significant comminution.[188] Many patients with nonunion have associated multiple injuries.[188] Bone grafting with internal fixation is the best method of treatment for nonunion, since excision of the pseudarthrosis results in continuing symptoms. Exuberant callus associated with the pseudarthrosis will occasionally lead to compression of the neurovascular structures and a thoracic outlet syndrome. The overall failure rate for surgical procedure may be as high as 52 percent.[188]

Acromioclavicular Joint Injury

Injuries of the acromioclavicular joint occur predominantly in young athletic males and usually involve incomplete disruption of the joint. Dislocations of this region have been staged from type I to type VI by Rockwood[157] according to the degree of involvement of the acromioclavicular and coracoclavicular ligaments (Table 35-8).

Treatment

Complete disruption of the joint (type III and higher) has been treated with closed reduction.[17,20,141,176,183] Techniques attempt to support the weight of the arm and elevate the scapula to the clavicle, maintaining the acromioclavicular joint reduced until the coracoclavicular ligaments heal. Despite felt pads over the bony prominences of the outer clavicle and the point of the acromion to prevent skin complications, strapping techniques are poorly tolerated and inevitably fail to maintain position. Open reduction and reconstruction using fixation by acromioclavicular wiring[17] or coracoclavicular screws[21,30] fail because of the degree of the range of motion and stresses at this joint. The use of synthetic fiber to act as a scaffold for ligamentous healing (e.g., Dacron) has given more satisfactory results.[9,12,13,39,110] Other techniques use fas-

TABLE 35-8   Classification of Acromioclavicular Joint Dislocations

Type I: Sprain of acromioclavicular ligament but intact acromioclavicular joint

Type II:
  a. Complete tear of the acromioclavicular ligaments with upward subluxation of the acromioclavicular joint
  b. Sprain of the coracoclavicular ligaments
  c. Minor tear of the deltoid and trapezius muscles

Type III:
  a. Superior dislocation of the acromioclavicular joint
  b. Complete tear of the coracoclavicular ligaments with increased coracoclavicular interspace
  c. Detachment of the deltoid and trapezius muscles from the distal clavicle

Type IV: Superior and posterior dislocation of the acromioclavicular joint into or through the trapezius muscle

Type V: Severe superior dislocation of the acromioclavicular joint with extensive detachment of the deltoid and trapezius muscles from the distal half of the clavicle

Type VI: Severe inferior dislocation of the acromioclavicular joint with the clavicle displaced under the acromion or coracoid process

Source: Adapted from Rockwood, C.A., in Rockwood, C.A., and Green, D.P., eds: *Fractures in Adults.* Philadelphia, Lippincott, 1984. Reprinted with permission.

cia[4] or transferred biceps tendon.[110] Recently good results have been reported by immediate excision of the lateral end of the clavicle and transfer of the coracoacromial ligament into the cut end.[185a] Often in the nonathletic patient, there is remarkably little functional loss with an untreated complete separation,[46a] and some surgeons do not perform primary anatomical reconstruction.[182a] If the deformity is unacceptable, late ligament reconstruction can be combined with excision of the prominant lateral end of the clavicle.[76,140]

Fractures of the Scapula

Fractures of the scapula are rare, constituting 1 percent of all fractures and 5 percent of fractures involving the shoulder.[90,105] Since they are often associated with automobile accidents or other severe trauma, associated injury to the ipsilateral limb and to the thorax is common.

Classification

The various categories of injury are shown in Fig. 35-34. The injury may involve the body of the scapula, the rim of the glenoid or the fossa of the glenoid itself; the anatomical or the surgical neck of the scapula; the scapular spine, or the acromion or coracoid process. Combined fractures involving several of these regions may also be seen. There has also been an

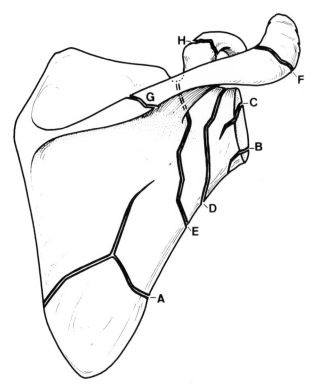

Figure 35-34 The various types of fractures seen in the scapula. Shown are fractures of the body (A), glenoid rim (B), glenoid fossa (C), anatomical neck (D), surgical neck (E), acromion (F), spine (G), and corocoid process (H). *(From Hardegger, F.H., et al, J Bone Joint Surg 66B:725–731, 1984. Reproduced with permission.)*

isolated report of an avulsion fracture of the superior border of the scapula.[91] It is important to distinguish this latter injury from a normal variant seen on x-ray film when there is a hole in the supraspinatous fossa giving the appearance of a separate bony rim to the superior border.[91]

Treatment

Fractures of the Body of the Scapula Hardegger and his co-workers have summarized the treatment of the various types of scapular injury. They point out that in fractures of the scapular body, surgical treatment is usually unnecessary because of the attached muscles, which reduce the degree of displacement of the fragments. Occasionally, they point out, the lateral margin of the body may be displaced and a sharp spike may enter the joint capsule, which will require operative reduction and fixation.

Fractures of the Glenoid Rim These fractures are usually associated with dislocation of the glenohumeral joint and may reduce with the dislocation following manipulation. Occasionally, open fixation is required to prevent recurrent dislocation of the shoulder.

Fractures of the Glenoid Fossa Open reduction may be required if there is a significant displacement of fragments.

Fractures of the Anatomical Neck of the Scapula The long head of the triceps may inferiorly displace the fragment which contains the glenoid. Traction through the olecranon may be successful; otherwise, open reduction is recommended.[74]

Fractures of the Surgical Neck of the Scapula Hardegger and co-workers point out that the degree of displacement with this fracture depends on the nature of any associated injury to either the clavicle or the coracoclavicular ligaments. If these are intact, the fracture will remain stable. If the suspension mechanism is interrupted, however, the neck fragment will become unstable due to the weight of the arm and operative treatment will be required (Fig. 35-35*B*).

Fractures of the Acromion Operative reduction may be indicated, fixation being achieved either with a screw or tension band if there is significant displacement and tilting of a fracture of the acromion. The acromion is particularly vul-

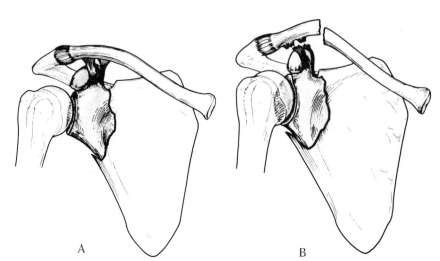

Figure 35-35 The two types of fracture of the surgical neck of the scapula. **A.** With an intact clavicle and coracoclavicular ligaments, the fracture remains stable. **B.** With an associated clavicular fracture and ligamentous disruption, the fracture is unstable. *(From Hardegger, F.H., et al, J Bone Joint Surg 66B:725–731, 1984. Reproduced with permission.)*

nerable to a direct blow to the shoulder region.[154] Acromionectomy should not be performed. Associated axillary nerve lesions have been documented.[124]

Fractures of the Spine of the Scapula The treatment for this injury is usually conservative.

Fractures of the Coracoid Process The coracoid process provides origin for the short head of the biceps, the coracobrachialis, and the pectoralis minor muscles. Most of the patients sustaining this injury are young.[155] The injury may be an isolated entity, or it may be associated with separation of the acromioclavicular joint or subglenoid dislocation of the shoulder.[16] If the coracoacromial and coracoclavicular ligaments are intact, the fracture is stable and will heal uneventfully.[46,55,74] Fractures of the tip of the coracoid represent avulsion fractures involving the attached muscles, and their surgical reattachment may be indicated in the young athletic individual.[46]

Conclusions

Hardegger and colleagues have summarized the treatment of these fractures and have also given details of the operative technique.[74] They point out that most fractures of the scapular body and also those of the scapular neck and the apophyses (coracoid process acromion, scapular spine) will have minimum displacement, and conservative treatment is usually sufficient. However, a second group of fractures, particularly glenoid fracture dislocations, unstable fractures of the scapular neck, and significantly displaced apophyseal fractures will usually require surgery, and surgery will be expected to give better results than conservative treatment in this second group.

Complications

Pneumothorax, which may be delayed in onset, is a serious and common condition associated with fractures of the scapula. An incidence of up to 62 percent has been reported in one series.[107,126,127] McLennan and Ungersma found associated pneumothorax in 16 of their 30 patients.[127] They point out that the association of decreased breath sounds, hyperresonance, rales, and rhonchi together with low values for arterial oxygen saturation in patients with a scapular fracture, particularly when the body of the left scapula is involved, should alert the examiner to the possibility of a delayed pneumothorax. They also recommend daily chest radiographs for the first 3 days following injury.

Neurovascular injury may accompany fractures of the scapula, given the proximity of the brachial plexus and the large vessels.

Traumatic Lateral Displacement of the Scapula

Complete closed separation of the scapula and the upper extremity from the thoracic attachment can occur in severe trauma.

Clinically, there may be massive swelling in the region of the shoulder girdle with acromioclavicular separation and associated avulsion injuries to the brachial plexus and the great vessels. The radiograph will confirm the diagnosis by showing a characteristic lateral displacement of the entire forequarter.[143] Attention must be given as a matter of urgency to the associated vascular injury, which may be life-threatening. Since there is avulsion of the brachial plexus, the prognosis for neurological recovery in the extremities is very poor, and glenohumeral arthrodesis and above-the-elbow amputation are usually required. To save this amount of the arm, however, it is often necessary to repair the injured artery.[143]

SECTION D

Glenohumeral Instability

Louis U. Bigliani and David S. Morrison

Instability of the glenohumeral joint is one of the earliest orthopaedic disorders to be identified. Descriptions of shoulder dislocations and various types of therapeutic intervention are prevalent in the ancient and medieval literature. The first reference to glenohumeral instability is found in the Edwin Smith papyrus[5] circa 3000 B.C., and the earliest analysis of the subject is credited to Hippocrates circa 450 B.C.[1] However, little was written about methods of reduction until the late eighteenth century and about surgical repair until the late nineteenth century. In the twentieth century, much has been written concerning pathological processes, causes, and methods of reduction and repair. The historical reviews of Rockwood[19] and Moseley[18] are recommended for a more in-depth presentation of the history of this disorder.

Glenohumeral instability can occur in different degrees from minor joint laxity and subluxation to true dislocation. Subluxation occurs when the humerus is partially and transiently displaced from the glenoid fossa. In dislocation, there is a complete loss of articular contact in the glenohumeral joint. A dislocation may become recurrent or chronic and may result in degeneration of the glenohumeral joint. In this discussion, glenohumeral instability will include both subluxations and true dislocations.

INCIDENCE

The shoulder is the most commonly dislocated major joint in the body because it is the most mobile. Instability of this joint is a very common orthopaedic condition affecting all age groups and both sexes. In a study by Hovelius in Sweden, 2092 random individuals were surveyed regarding shoulder dislocations.[11,12] He found that in the 18- to 70-year-old age group, the overall incidence was 1.7 percent, with a male-female ratio of 3:1. This sex ratio varies tremendously depending upon age. In the 21- to 30-year-old group, there is a 9:1 male predominance, whereas in the sixth and seventh decade, there is a female predominance of 3:1. If we consider conditions of partial dislocation or subluxation, the incidence of instability is probably 30 percent higher. Rowe found that the highest number of primary dislocations occurred between 10 and 20 years of age. The next-highest number occurred between 50 and 60 years of age.[27] Anterior dislocation is by far the most common with posterior dislocations accounting for only about 3.8 percent.[17] Multidirectional and inferior instability, previously believed to be rare, are now recognized as important considerations in the differential diagnosis of glenohumeral instability.[20] Recent data suggests that unrecognized multidirectional instability is responsible for a large percentage of failed surgeries for anterior instability.[21]

CAUSES OF SHOULDER INSTABILITY

Anatomical Considerations

Before considering the causes of shoulder instability, it is necessary to make some observations on the anatomy of the glenohumeral joint and its stabilizing structures.

Osseous Stability

The architecture of the glenohumeral joint is such that there is very little inherent osseous stability. The glenoid fossa is usually only slightly concave and has an articular surface only one-fourth the area of the humeral head. This allows for a tremendous range of motion but unfortunately compromises anterior and inferior stability. Posterior stability is somewhat enhanced by the 40-degree angulation of the scapula to the frontal plane. This places the posterior half of the glenoid and the spine of the scapula behind the humeral head and supports the head against posterior dislocation when a direct anteroposterior force is applied to the shoulder. Superior stability is enhanced by the acromion, which sits directly above the humeral head and blocks superior dislocation.

Because of this lack of significant bony stability, the glenohumeral joint must instead depend upon its capsular ligaments and glenoid labrum for static stability and on the rotator cuff muscles for dynamic stability.

Static Stabilizers

The joint capsule must be large and somewhat redundant in order to allow an unrestricted range of motion. The volume of the joint is second only to that of the knee. Along the anterior border of the glenohumeral joint, the capsule has developed four areas of reinforcement: the three glenohumeral ligaments and the coracohumeral ligament. The superior, middle, and inferior glenohumeral ligaments arise from the capsule and may only represent thickenings in it. However, they are

consistently present, though their size varies greatly. The largest and strongest of these ligaments is the inferior ligament which has been shown to effectively block anteroinferior dislocation when it is intact.[31] The site of its glenoid attachment often coincides with the area of a Bankart lesion in an unstable shoulder. The coracohumeral ligament lies above the superior glenohumeral ligament and acts to strengthen it and block excessive external rotation. Finally, the coracoacromial ligament, along with the coracoid and the acromion, forms the coracoacromial arch. This structure acts as a roof for the glenohumeral joint, and thus may provide some anterosuperior stability.

In addition to these ligaments, the joint also gains stability from the glenoid labrum. This fibrocartilaginous ring varies widely in size and in definition, and its overall function is a source of continuing controversy. The labrum increases the size and depth of the glenoid cavity, thus improving stability and favorably affecting the load distribution of the joint as indicated by Saha.[28] It lies at the junction of the capsule, the periosteum, and the glenoid neck, and is continuous with the inferior glenohumeral ligament.

Dynamic Stabilizers

The muscles which originate on the scapula and insert on the humerus act as dynamic stabilizers of the glenohumeral joint. The subscapularis acts anteriorly, the supraspinatus superiorly, and the infraspinatus and teres minor posteriorly. The coordinated action of these muscles allows for rotation with stability. An imbalance in these muscle forces can result in instability. The deltoid muscle can also be a factor in stability. With its contraction, the humerus is drawn superiorly. Simultaneously, the muscles of the rotator cuff act as depressors and stabilize the head in the glenoid fossa. If the cuff is deficient, there will be superior migration of the humeral head. The long head of the biceps may also act as a depressor. In addition, the coracoid muscles, the short head of the biceps, and the coracobrachialis may act to stabilize the joint in abduction and external rotation.

CLASSIFICATION

Glenohumeral instability can be classified according to four criteria: mechanism, direction, circumstance, and degree. (Table 35-9).

Acute trauma is the most common mechanism of instability. It occurs after a violent injury—either direct or indirect—to the upper extremity such as a fall in sports or a direct blow upon the shoulder. There is immediate, severe pain and deformity. Spontaneous reduction at the time of injury frequently occurs, making clinical and radiographic documentation difficult. Further, when acute, subluxations of the glenohumeral joint may have no objective clinical or x-ray findings. The patient may suffer a brief excruciating pain which becomes a dull ache in a very brief time but recurs with motion. Furthermore, there is prolonged loss of voluntary function of the entire limb—the so-called "dead arm syndrome."

TABLE 35-9 Classification of Glenohumeral Instability

1. Mechanism
   a. Traumatic
   b. Microtraumatic
   c. Atraumatic

2. Direction
   a. Anterior
   b. Posterior
   c. Inferior
   d. Superior
   e. Multidirectional
3. Circumstance
   a. Acute
   b. Recurrent
   c. Chronic
   d. Involuntary
   e. Voluntary
4. Degree
   a. Subluxation
   b. Dislocation

In both *subluxation* and *dislocation,* there must be some injury to the capsular ligaments, the labrum, or the muscles in order to allow the previously stable joint to sublux or dislocate. The extent of the injury varies. It may involve only a stretching of the capsule, or there may be an avulsion of the anterior capsule and labrum due to a dislocation or a Bankart lesion. It is therefore reasonable to assume that these acute instabilities, due to violent injury, may best be treated by a period of immobilization of at least 6 weeks in order to allow the injured structures to heal and, it is hoped, to stabilize the joint.

The *microtraumatic mechanism* of instability frequently is seen in athletes in whom shoulder instability occurs after apparently little or no trauma. However, if we look carefully at the sport in which the athlete is involved, frequently we see that the glenohumeral joint has been put through a tremendous amount of "microtrauma" for a prolonged period of time. Prime examples of this phenomenon are seen in swimming, gymnastics, wrestling, weight lifting, baseball pitching, javelin throwing, etc. All these sports (in particular the back and butterfly strokes in swimming) place repetitive stresses on the shoulder in the "apprehension" position. Thus, without any acute gross traumatic injury, the athlete develops an unstable glenohumeral joint. This instability may be recurrent subluxation or dislocation.

Because of the cause of this type of instability, it is doubtful that acute immobilization for any prolonged length of time in excess of that necessary for comfort would be helpful in gaining permanent stability. The lack of recognition of this minor subgroup of instability probably accounts for the discrepancy in the literature as to the usefulness of postdislocation immobilization in glenohumeral dislocations.

The *atraumatic mechanism* of instability is related more to anatomical considerations than to injury. As described earlier, there are multiple anatomical stabilizers of the glenohu-

meral joint, and if any of these are absent or attenuated, the joint may become unstable. The osseous structures may be abnormal or deficient. The most commonly cited examples are "malrotation" of the humerus and flattening or deficiency of the glenoid. These bony abnormalities are very rare but should be considered. Also, neuromuscular disorders which result in muscular imbalance or in loss of muscular integrity about the shoulder can result in atraumatic instability.

More commonly we see individuals, usually young females, who are hypermobile in many joints, in particular in the hands, the knees, and the elbows. These patients exhibit a range of motion in excess of the normal, and glenohumeral instability may be the result of such ligamentous and capsular laxity. It should also be noted that pregnancy is known to induce ligamentous laxity, and therefore the pregnant patient may experience new or worsened shoulder instability. This usually improves post partum.

An *acute dislocation* is seen within several days of its occurrence; otherwise it is chronic, or unreduced. A *locked dislocation* is one in which the humerus is impaled on the glenoid and suffers an impression fracture resulting in an irreducible or chronic dislocation. It is not infrequent to miss an acute posterior dislocation and see it go on to become a chronic situation, and over half are missed by the initial examiner.[19,25]

Recurrent instability usually means multiple episodes of documented subluxations or dislocations. However, it may be difficult to determine accurately how many times, or in what direction, a dislocation or subluxation occurs since the only evidence may be the patient's history. Furthermore, it may be impossible to differentiate between a subluxation and a dislocation. Although provocative maneuvers performed during the physical examination may reproduce the patient's symptoms, differentiating instability from impingement syndrome remains a problem that may require an examination under anesthesia, or an impingement "injection test," to solve.

Recurrent anterior instability of the glenohumeral joint occurs by way of two mechanisms: anterior and posterior. These terms do not refer to the direction of the instability, but rather to the location of the anatomical cause of the instability. In the anterior mechanism, we have an interruption of the anterior capsule ligament. This results in greatly increased laxity of the joint and the possibility of dislocation in any direction, although the anterior direction is by far the most common. The posterior mechanism of anterior instability is seen when there is a disruption in the musculotendinous rotator cuff. This disruption can be due to a tear in the rotator cuff or to a fracture of the greater tuberosity, the former being common in primary dislocations in persons over 40 years of age. Such a disruption of the rotator cuff and thus of the muscular balance about the shoulder may result in glenohumeral instability by the posterior mechanism.

As noted above, recurrent dislocation of the shoulder may be either involuntary or voluntary. When it is *involuntary,* it presents in individuals who have no desire, either consciously or subconsciously, to have the dislocation recur. These individuals may indeed be able to dislocate their shoulders at will, but they do not *wish* to do so.[20] The *voluntary* dislocator, on the other hand, has both the ability and the *desire* to dislocate the shoulder. This desire may be either a subconscious or a conscious motivation for secondary gain or for other psychiatric reasons. These patients are usually adolescents; many have generalized ligamentous laxity and may also have psychological problems. Surgical intervention in these patients should be undertaken with great caution.[27] Physical therapy can be useful to strengthen the rotator cuff muscles and the deltoid and to relieve the symptoms of instability; if appropriate, a full psychiatric evaluation may also be indicated.

CLINICAL DIAGNOSIS

Instability of the shoulder can be one of the most difficult diagnoses to make. At the time of examination the patient may be asymptomatic and have little clinical or radiological evidence of instability. This is particularly true with subluxation. Furthermore, instability may be difficult to differentiate from subacromial impingement. This is especially true of the microtraumatic mechanism of instability.

In considering the clinical diagnosis of instability, it is easiest to understand if we approach it from the aspect of direction (Table 35-9).

Anterior Instability

Patient history is most often that of trauma, from either a fall on, or a blow to, the abducted externally rotated arm. An anterior dislocation is by far the most frequent type. Moseley[18]

found that 47 percent of primary dislocations were spontaneously reduced or self-reduced; 24 percent were reduced by a physician without anesthetic; and the remaining 29 percent required anesthesia for reduction.

In the acute anterior dislocation (Fig. 35-36), the physical examination reveals a patient in severe pain with an alteration in the normal contours of the shoulder. The head is dislocated anteriorly beneath the coracoid (subcoracoid), with a posterior glenohumeral defect and a prominent acromion. If the head is dislocated more inferiorly, the subacromial area may appear to be empty, giving the shoulder a squared-off appearance. The humeral head creates a fullness anteriorly which, along with the swelling, makes it very difficult to palpate the coracoid process. The patient often assumes a position of slight abduction, with neutral or external rotation, and maintains this position with the help of the other arm. Any movement causes significant pain. A common complication of anterior dislocation is injury to the axillary nerve, and this should always be evaluated before and after reduction. In the case of recurrent dislocations, the clinical picture may be markedly different. Pain and swelling are often less, and the patient may tolerate some movement. Often they are able to reduce the dislocation themselves and do not require a maneuver by a physician or sedation.

In the radiographic examination of the unstable shoulder, there are three important findings: the location of the humeral head in relation to the glenoid; the configuration of the humeral head (i.e., fractures, defects), and the configuration of the glenoid. Numerous views have been described to

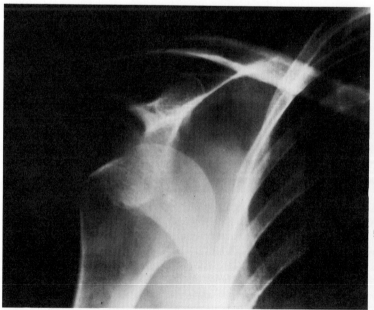

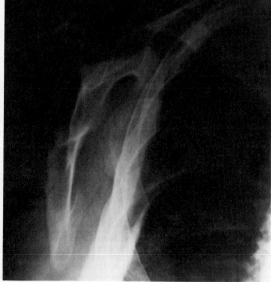

A

B

Figure 35-36 A. AP x-ray film of the shoulder in a patient with anterior subcoracoid dislocation. **B.** A lateral view in the scapular plane of same patient. The humeral head is completely dislocated anteriorly beneath the coracoid instead of sitting in the center of the Y formed by the body of the scapula, scapular spine, and coracoid.

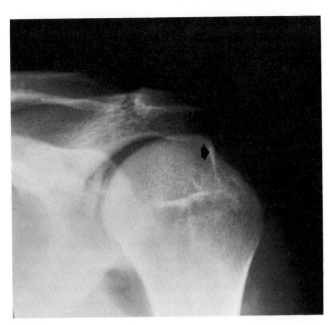

Figure 35-37 Internal rotation anteroposterior view of a patient with recurrent anterior dislocations. A large Hill-Sachs defect (arrow) is on the lateral aspect of the humeral head.

obtain this information, but for routine purposes few are ever used. The standard views should include

1. Anteroposterior in neutral, IR, and ER views in the scapular plane to define the glenohumeral relationship and the condition of the humeral head and glenoid.
2. A lateral view in the scapular plane to define the glenohumeral alignment.
3. True axillary view—to define the condition of the gle-

noid and the anterior-posterior location of the head, and the presence of a Hill-Sachs lesion[9] (which can also be seen in the IR view).

In addition to these views, several other useful views are helpful in establishing the diagnosis of recurrent anterior dislocation. The Stryker notch view[8] and an AP view with internal rotation can be very helpful in looking for a posterior humeral head defect (Fig. 35-37). The West Point axillary view can be used to more closely evaluate the anterior glenoid rim (Fig. 35-38).

If the diagnosis cannot be made by any of the above means, certain special tests may be of assistance. An arthrotomogram or an arthro-CT scan (Fig. 35-39) may be helpful in diagnosing a Bankart lesion as well as in evaluating the anterior and posterior glenoid and labrum for wear.

If the diagnosis remains unclear after physical and radiographic examinations, an examination under anesthesia may be necessary. Norris has used the C arm to fluoroscopically evaluate anterior and posterior instability.[21] Arthroscopy has also been a helpful diagnostic tool to demonstrate labrial fraying and detachment.

Posterior Instabililty

Posterior dislocations are far less common than anterior dislocations. They constitute only 1 to 3.8 percent of the dislocations seen in several large series.[25] However, over 60 percent of primary posterior dislocations are missed at the initial evaluation, with some series showing a rate of incorrect diagnosis as high as 79 percent.[25]

An acute posterior dislocation can result from an electric shock (either accidental or therapeutic) or from seizure. This is secondary to the spasmic contraction and pull of the larger

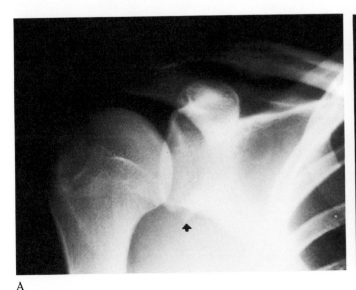

A

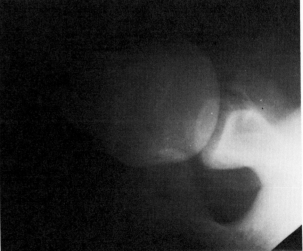

B

Figure 35-38 A. Anteroposterior view of shoulder of patient with a history of violent traumatic dislocation (anterior). Note small bone fragment at inferior aspect of glenoid. **B.** Axillary view of same patient shows a fracture of the anterior glenoid rim.

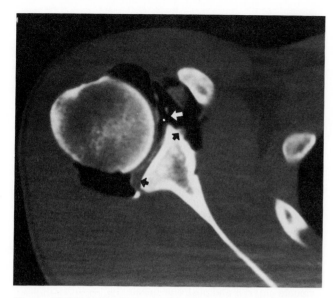

Figure 35-39 Arthro-CT scan of shoulder of patient with recurrent anterior dislocation, showing normal labrum posteriorly (lower arrow), disruption of anterior labrum, Bankart lesion (white arrow), and bone reaction on anterior glenoid rim (upper arrow).

and more numerous internal rotators (subscapularis, pectoralis major, teres major, latissimus dorsi) overpowering the weaker external rotators (infraspinatus, teres minor) and pushing the humerus out posteriorly. There is also a relationship between the Charcot shoulder and posterior dislocation.

Other causes of posterior dislocation include developmental disorders such as scapular aplasia, neuromuscular diseases including stroke and head injury, and connective tissue disorders such as Ehlers-Danlos Syndrome. Capsular laxity also contributes to posterior instability and is often seen in conjunction with multidirectional instability. Another important cause of posterior dislocation is the voluntary dislocator; such a person is able to use the superior strength of the internal rotators to sublux or dislocate the shoulders posteriorly at will. For this reason, extreme care must be taken in the evaluation of the posterior dislocator, and for that matter, any dislocator, so as to rule out any voluntary component, since this would be a contraindication to surgery.

The clinical diagnosis of posterior instability may be difficult to establish. Over 60 percent of all posterior dislocations are missed on initial evaluation, many of these being unrecognized on routine x-rays films. A good history can be a great assistance. A complete radiographic evaluation is essential, and should include an AP and a lateral view of the shoulder in the scapular plane (Fig. 35-40) and an axillary

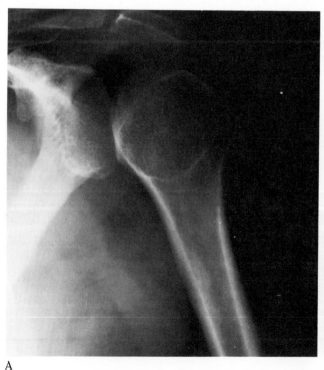

A

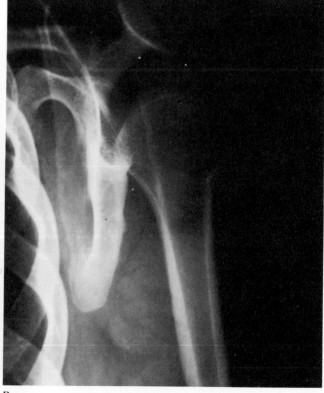

B

Figure 35-40 A. Anteroposterior view of posterior dislocation. May be read as normal, but vacant glenoid and "cystic" appearance of humeral head, due to fixed internal rotation, are sugges-

tive of posterior dislocation. **B.** Lateral scapular view of same patient shows complete posterior dislocation of humeral head (compare to Fig. 35-38*B*).

view if necessary. In the lateral scapular view, the humeral head is posterior to the glenoid in the acute dislocation; otherwise it may be only partially subluxed. The axillary view will help define the condition of the glenoid, reveal a fracture of the posterior glenoid, and show a reverse Hill-Sachs lesion if present. On physical examination, there may be a loss of the anterior contour of the shoulder with prominence of the coracoid and a loss of external rotation, the arm being fixed in internal rotation. Observation from the side may show the humerus to be angled posteriorly to the acromion when ordinarily it tends to have a slight anterior inclination.

There will also be a fullness posteriorly with the humeral head out the back. If the shoulder is not subluxed or dislocated at the time of presentation, a posterior apprehension test may be performed. This is done by placing the arm about 90 degrees anteriorly and pushing the humerus posteriorly by pressure on the flexed elbow while slowly internally and externally rotating the arm, a positive test result being pain and apprehension with or without a click or pop. Another useful test is the Fukuda sign. This sign is illustrated by placing the palms of each of the examiner's hands on the ipsilateral acromion from behind. Then with the patient relaxed, and with the thumbs extended along the scapular spines for counterpressure, an attempt is made to sublux both humeral heads posteriorly by the action of the four fingers of both hands. In this way, the laxity of the two shoulders can be compared. A positive test is one which demonstrates a posterior laxity or causes pain similar to an apprehension test. If the diagnosis cannot be made on clinical or radiological grounds, then an examination under anesthesia is indicated.

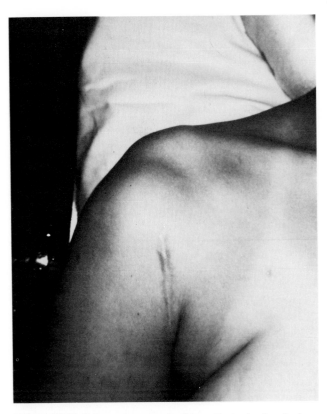

Figure 35-41 Sulcus sign seen in this patient who has had two previous failed anterior repairs for unrecognized multidirectional instability; both the Magnuson-Stack and Bristow repairs failed to reduce the volume of the redundant inferior capsule.

Inferior and Superior Instability

Isolated inferior instability exists very rarely, if at all. The exception to this is luxatio erecta, a traumatic dislocation with the humerus in nearly full forward elevation and the humeral head fully dislocated below the glenoid. The rarity of this true isolated inferior dislocation is surpassed only by superior dislocation.

Multidirectional Instability

Multidirectional instability is a relatively new concept, popularized by Neer in 1980.[20] It may be mainly anteroinferior, posteroinferior, or a combination of the two. This is an extremely important concept to understand when considering a surgical procedure for shoulder instability. Norris reported that a significant factor in failed repairs was the lack of appreciation of the scope of instability by the previous surgeon.[21] Rockwood found that in a series of failed repairs for dislocations, over 60 percent of the failures were secondary to multidirectional instability[23] (Fig. 35-41). The idea that one procedure is appropriate for all dislocations must be abandoned. Any surgical procedure for instability should be directed at correcting the pathological anatomy encountered at the time of surgery.

Multidirectional instability can be one of the most difficult clinical diagnoses to make since there may be signs of both anterior and posterior instability. The patient may have anterior and posterior apprehension as well as inferior apprehension. Downward traction on the involved arm usually demonstrates a *sulcus sign* (a dimple between the anterior acromion and the humeral head) (Fig. 35-41), and downward pressure on the proximal humerus with the arm abducted 90 degrees may produce pain and apprehension. It is often necessary to perform an examination under anesthesia to appreciate the full scope of the instability. A C-arm fluoroscopic examination is also helpful. The key is to recognize that the patient is not a pure anterior dislocator, and to be able to modify your treatment plan accordingly since the redundant inferior and/or posterior capsule must be addressed at the time of surgery. Failure to recognize this may result in an operation which corrects only one component of the instability and may seriously compromise the surgical result. A weighted AP x-ray picture of both shoulders is useful to demonstrate inferior subluxation of the humeral head (Fig. 35-42). The weight should not be held but rather strapped to the wrist, and 15 to 25 lb should be used. Arthro-CT scan has also been helpful to demonstrate glenoid wear.

Subluxation

Subluxation occurs when the humerus is briefly and partially displaced from its normal position in the glenoid fossa. The

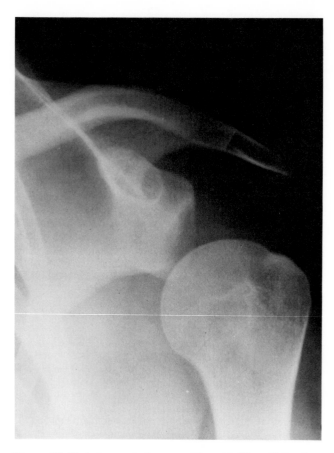

Figure 35-42 Anteroposterior x-ray film with 15 to 25 lb of weight strapped to the patient's wrist shows inferior instability.

true significance of subluxation as a pathological entity is unclear since it is such a difficult diagnosis to make, but it does exist, and is responsible for shoulder pain and disability. Except for the inferior subluxation seen with deltoid atony, subluxations rarely persist for more than an instant. Thus, radiographs are usually normal unless stress films are obtained. The physical examination is carried out as described above for dislocations. Findings of pain, apprehension, and laxity may or may not be found, and the examination may be confusing and seem to support the diagnosis of subacromial impingement. Since subluxation and dislocation exist in a continuum, their differential diagnosis overlaps, and we use the term *instability*. That is, depending upon the amount of laxity, a shoulder will either subluxate or dislocate, and it is difficult to determine the amount of laxity on clinical grounds alone. As with all forms of instability, an examination under anesthesia may be necessary.

One of the most difficult differential diagnoses to make in the shoulder is that between subluxation and subacromial impingement syndrome. The apprehension tests we perform are very likely to elicit pain and muscle guarding in a patient with impingement syndrome. X-ray films are usually of little help, and the history may at times be misleading. Frequently, rest and gentle physical therapy to strengthen the internal

and external rotators will relieve the patient's symptoms. The subacromial impingement injection test may be helpful and if the problem is long-standing and severe enough, an examination under anesthesia may be indicated. This examination is done with the understanding that the findings of the examination will determine the type of surgical procedure, if any, to be performed. As mentioned previously, C-arm fluoroscopy, as well as diagnostic arthroscopy, can be helpful.

TREATMENT

Nonoperative Treatment

Patients who have had several nonvoluntary dislocations and who present with pain or a shoulder disability which severely limits their lifestyle should be considered for early operative intervention. Others such as voluntary dislocators, subluxators, patients with mild instability symptoms, and true nonvoluntary dislocators who have not had a sufficient conservative trial should be placed on a strengthening exercise regimen. The program will vary with each patient, but there are basic principles to be followed. Such principles include avoiding provocative activities which cause the symptoms and at the same time, performing a closely supervised physical therapy program to strengthen the muscles about the shoulder. The therapy should be directed first at overcoming pain. In instability, pain can be due to three things: muscle weakness, subluxation of the glenohumeral joint, and joint surface incongruity. The first two are the target of the physical therapy program.

The patient with an unstable shoulder tends not to use the affected arm in daily activities or sports because of apprehension and the pain of subluxation. This leads to muscle weakness and easier subluxation. Sometimes patients are so apprehensive that they refuse to set their muscles at all, and this may lead to inferior humeral head subluxation. The aim of physical therapy is to regain muscle balance about the shoulder and thus stability. The recommended physical therapy program and the specific exercises used are presented in depth in the chapter on rehabilitation (see Chap. 49).

Operative Treatment

When conservative management has failed or when patients present with a severe disability which is not amenable to conservative therapy, operative intervention should be considered.

Surgical procedures for instability of the glenohumeral joint can be divided into five categories:

1. Capsulorrhaphy and repair of the Bankart lesion (Bankart repair, DuToit stapling, arthroscopic stapling)
2. Muscular advancements (Putti-Platt, Magnuson-Stack, and Boyd-Sisk procedures)
3. Bone blocks (Bristow, Eden-Hybbinette, and posterior bone blocks)
4. Osteotomies (anterior or posterior glenoplasty, derotational humeral osteotomy)
5. Capsular advancement and plication, inferior capsular shift, and anterior cruciate repair (Neer)

Capsulorrhaphy and Repair of the Bankart Lesion

This group of procedures seeks to repair the detachment of the anterior capsule from the glenoid and then to tighten up the capsular laxity, thus stabilizing the joint. These procedures tend to be aimed at restoring near-normal anatomy. In the Bankart repair,[26] drill holes are used to reattach the anterior capsule to the glenoid and then the capsule is overlapped on itself for reinforcement. In the staple capsulorrhaphy, as described by DuToit,[6] a metal staple is used to both reattach and tighten the capsule anteriorly. With the advent of the use of the arthroscope in shoulder surgery, methods of performing a closed repair using miniature staples are being developed.

Muscular advancements

These procedures rely on removing muscles from their normal attachments and placing them about the joint in such a way as to limit glenohumeral motion. In the Putti-Platt procedure,[22] the subscapularis tendon is divided 2.5 cm from its insertion and is used to reinforce the anterior capsule. The muscle itself is then advanced and attached laterally to the lesser tuberosity to limit external rotation. Some orthopaedists combine this with the repair of a Bankart lesion, if one is found. The Magnuson-Stack method[15,16] moves the insertion of the subscapularis from the lesser tuberosity to the greater tuberosity, thus greatly diminishing external rotation and, it is hoped, stabilizing the joint anteriorly. In the Boyd-Sisk operation,[4] the long head of the biceps is transferred laterally around the neck of the humerus and reattached to the posterior aspect of the glenoid so as to prevent posterior dislocation.

Bone blocks

The principle behind these procedures is to provide a bony block to dislocation. The Bristow procedure[10] moves the conjoined tendon as well as a piece of the coracoid to the raw anterior neck of the glenoid and secures the transfer with either sutures or a screw. It is believed that this will have a checkrein effect in keeping the humeral head properly located when the arm is abducted and externally rotated, since in this position the transferred muscles lie across the anterior aspect of the joint. At the same time, the extra bone acts to deepen or reinforce the anterior glenoid rim. The Eden-Hybbinette operation[3,7] consists simply of an anterior bone block without muscular transfers. In addition, bone blocks may be placed posteriorly either alone or in conjunction with other repairs. These bone blocks are intended to stabilize the joint mechanically, and should not come in contact with the articular surface of the humerus.

Osteotomy

The theory behind osteotomy is that there exists a component of abnormal osseous tissue in the unstable shoulder which contributes to the instability. Either the slope of the glenoid is abnormal or the humerus is malrotated. A posterior opening wedge osteotomy of the glenoid is intended to place more bone behind the humeral head and prevent posterior dislocation, whereas the opposite is true with an anterior wedge osteotomy.[30] A derotational osteotomy of the humerus[32] is meant to correct abnormal humeral version or compensate for humeral head defects. The efficacy of these procedures is controversial and difficult to evaluate since they are usually combined with capsular or muscle reconstruction.

Capsular advancement and plication

The inferior capsular shift was devised by Neer to treat multidirectional instability when the pathological process is a large redundant inferior capsule. It can be performed from either the anterior or the posterior side, depending on the major direction of instability. In essence, the volume of the joint is decreased because the inferior flap of capsule, which has been dissected around the neck of the humerus, is shifted superiorly and the superior flap of capsule is advanced inferiorly above this. If the direction is only anterior, then an anterior cruciate repair is performed in which the partially dissected inferior flap is advanced superiorly, and the superior flap brought down. If a Bankart lesion is present, it should be repaired. If the major direction is only posterior, then a capsular plication should be performed from a posterior approach.

Our preferred method of treatment is the anatomical approach described by Neer. With this approach, no single procedure is the "standard" technique. The goal is to restore the anatomy of the involved shoulder to as near-normal as possible and to correct any anatomical abnormalities which contribute to the instability.

The procedure begins with an examination under anesthesia. This is necessary if the surgeon is to understand the true scope of the instability. The range of motion is evaluated and a careful examination of anterior, posterior, and inferior instability is made. If it is clear that the patient is a purely posterior dislocator, then a posterior approach and repair is performed. If this is not the case, then an anterior approach is made with the understanding that a second incision may be necessary if severe posterior instability is found to be present later. Because it is often impossible to tell whether the humeral head is moving from a posterior dislocated position to a located position, or from a located position to an anterior dislocation, a second examination to determine the direction of instability is necessary at the time of exposure of the subscapularis. At this time, it is possible to better palpate the coracoid, anterior glenoid, and humeral head without the deltoid, the skin, and cutaneous fat intervening. A careful examination is necessary in order to rule out multidirectional instability because as mentioned previously, the major cause of failed repair for anterior instability is failure to recognize the scope of the instability. After this second exam, the subscapularis tendon is split and the superficial portion reflected medially with the anterior capsule reinforced by the deep portion of the tendon. The capsule is then incised in a T fashion to expose the joint.[20] With the joint now open and the anterior restraints removed, another examination for posterior and inferior instability is performed. At this time it is important to check for a large inferior and/or posterior pouch of the capsule. If posterior and/or inferior instability is found, an inferior capsular shift is performed from the anterior side. If it had been predetermined that the major direction was posterior, and a posterior approach was performed, then an inferior capsular shift is performed from the posterior side. If there is bone destruction of the anterior or posterior glenoid, then a bone block is performed using as a graft the tip of the coracoid anteriorly or a portion of the scapular spine posteriorly. If the instability is purely anterior, an anterior capsular cruciate repair is performed. If a Bankart lesion is found, it is repaired to raw bone through drill holes. If a huge Hill-Sachs or reverse Hill-Sachs lesion makes the shoulder unstable, then a bone graft is considered either primarily in the first case or in conjunction with a modified McLaughlin procedure[19] in the latter.

Postoperative immobilization is determined on the basis of the extent of the procedure and the scope of the instability. An inferior capsular shift or other repair for multidirectional instability requires that the part be placed in a brace in 10 degrees of external rotation at the side for 6 weeks. A simple anterior repair is immobilized for a period of 7 to 10 days, and the patient is allowed to use the arm at the side, perform isometrics, externally rotate to 10 degrees, and forward flex in a supine position to 90 degrees for 4 weeks. The patient is then allowed to "loosen up" by the performance of normal light activities. At 6 weeks, a progressive strengthening and stretching program is begun with isometrics and is advanced gradually as tolerated. No heavy lifting or contact sports are allowed for 9 months to 1 year. The long-term goal is a stable shoulder and near-normal range of motion.

The arthroscope has been used in the diagnosis of difficult shoulder problems. In addition, operative techniques for cartilage shaving, debridement of labrum, and percutaneous staple capsulorrhaphy are under development. The usefulness and long-term results of these procedures are not yet known.

The operative procedures outlined above are those most commonly used at the present time. Although there are many more which were not described, most of these fit into one or more of the categories above. In a review of the literature, Row[27] found that in 53 studies of 3332 operative repairs, there was an average recurrence of only 3.0 percent. Rates varied between 0 and 18 percent, with a mean of 2.0 percent.

COMPLICATIONS OF GLENOHUMERAL INSTABILITY

Nonoperative Complications

The major nonoperative complications of glenohumeral instability are neurovascular injury, fracture, rotator cuff tear, missed posterior dislocation, and arthritis of the dislocation.

With an anterior dislocation, the humeral head is situated beneath the coracoid and presses against the brachial plexus. The severity of the symptoms depends upon the violence of the injury, the length of time the shoulder is dislocated, and the local anatomy in relation to the humeral head. The axillary artery may be compromised and, in fracture dislocations, the sharp humeral calcar can lacerate nerves and

arteries. The incidence of neurovascular injuries varies between 2 and 25 percent, depending upon the study, with the incidence of isolated axillary nerve injuries being between 10 and 20 percent. For this reason, an assessment of the neurovascular status of the extremity is a must prior to reduction.

As mentioned in the section on posterior instability, 60 percent of posterior dislocations are missed at the initial evaluation. This can lead to severe posttraumatic arthritis with destruction of the posterior glenoid and the humeral head, often necessitating a glenohumeral replacement. If a posterior dislocation is not considered at the time of examination, it will not be found.

The arthritis of dislocations can be caused by recurrent dislocations or can appear as a result of surgery. Each time a shoulder dislocates, there is an injury, however small, to the glenohumeral articulation. If such a disturbance is allowed to continue unrestricted, it can result in classic degenerative changes.[29]

Operative Complications

The complications seen with operative intervention are all those generally seen with orthopaedic surgery as well as those specific problems seen with each repair. If a surgical procedure is too tight anteriorly and posteriorly, it may push the humeral head out the other side, resulting in chronic subluxation and degenerative changes. Operation on the "wrong side" of the joint, i.e., an anterior procedure for unrecognized posterior instability, will result in worsening the problem and in more rapid degeneration of the joint.

If the surgeon fails to recognize multidirectional instability, the chances for operative success are significantly diminished since the redundant inferior capsule is not corrected.

Also, repairs which do not open the capsule may miss a Bankart lesion. Any time that metal is used around the shoulder, there is a risk of articular destruction due to poor placement as well as loosening and migration.[33] Both of these problems are seen in Bristow and staple capsular repairs.

REFERENCES

Section A: Fractures and Dislocations of the Hand, Wrist, and Forearm

1. Abdon, P., et al. Subcapital fractures of the fifth metacarpal bone. Arch Orthop Trauma Surg 103:231–234, 1984.
2. Adler, J.B., and Shafton, G.W. Fractures of the capitate. J Bone Joint Surg 44A:1537–1543, 1962.
3. Agee, J.M. Unstable fracture dislocations of the proximal interphalangeal joint of the fingers: a preliminary report of a new treatment technique. J Hand Surg 3:386, 1978.
4. Alexander, A.H., and Lichtman, D.M. Irreducible distal radioulnar joint occurring in a Galeazzi fracture—Case report. J Hand Surg 6:258–261, 1981.
5. Anderson, L.D., Sisk, T.D., Tooms, R.E., and Parks, W.I., III. Compression-plate fixation in acute diaphyseal fractures of the distal radius and ulna. J Bone Joint Surg 57A:287–297, 1975.

6. Arzimanoglou, A., and Skiadaressis, S.M. Study of internal fixation by screws of oblique fractures in long bones. J Bone Joint Surg 34:219–223, 1952.

7. Bado, J.L. The Monteggia lesion. Clin Orthop 50:71–86, 1967.

8. Baird, D.B., and Friedenberg, Z.B. Delayed ulnar nerve palsy following a fracture of the hamate. J Bone Joint Surg 50A:570–572, 1968.

9. Beasley, R.W. Principles of managing acute hand injuries, in Littler, J.W. (ed): Reconstructive Plastic Surgery, vol 6. Philadelphia, Saunders, 1977, pp 3000–3102.

10. Beasley, R.W. Hand Injuries. Philadelphia, Saunders, 1981.

11. Belsky, M.R., Eaton, R.G., and Lane, L.B. Closed reduction and internal fixation or proximal phalangeal fractures. J Hand Surg 9A:725–729, 1984.

12. Bilos, Z.J., Pankovich, A.M., and Yelda, S. Fracture-dislocation of the radiocarpal joint: A clinical study of five cases. J Bone Joint Surg 59A:198–203, 1977.

13. Bora, F.W., and Didizian, N.H. The treatment of injuries to the carpometacarpal joint of the little finger. J Bone Joint Surg 56A:1459–1463, 1974.

14. Bora, F.W., Osterman, A.L., and Brighton, C.T. The electrical treatment of scaphoid nonunion. Clin Orthop 161:33–38, 1981.

15. Bowers, W.H. Mallet deformity of a finger after phalangeal fracture. J Bone Joint Surg 59A:525–526, 1977.

16. Bowers, W.H., and Fajgenbaum, D.M. Closed rupture of the volar plate of the distal interphalangeal joint. J Bone Joint Surg 61A:146, 1979.

17. Bowers, W.H., Wolf, J.W., Jr., Nehil, J., and Bittinger, S. The proximal interphalangeal joint volar plate. Part I: An anatomical and biomechanical study. J Hand Surg 5:79–88, 1980.

18. Bowers, W.H. The distal radio-ulnar joint, in Green, D.P. (ed): Operative Hand Surgery, 2d ed. New York, Churchill Livingstone, 1982.

19. Bryan, R.S., and Dobyns, J.H. Fractures of the carpal bones other than lunate and navicular. Clin Orthop 149:107–111, 1980.

20. Burton, R.I. Fractures of the proximal phalanx of the finger. Contemp Surg 11:32–37, 1977.

21. Carter, P.R., Eaton, R.G., and Littler, J.W. Un-united fractures of the hook of the hamate. J Bone Joint Surg 59A:583–588, 1977.

22. Carter, P.R. Common Hand Injuries and Infections. Philadelphia, Saunders, 1983.

23. Chapman, D.R., Bennett, J.B., Bryan, W.J., and Tullos, H.S. Complications of distal radial fractures: Pins and plaster treatment. J Hand Surg 7:509, 1982.

24. Charnley, J. The Closed Treatment of Common Fractures. Edinburgh, Livingstone, 1961.

25. Cole, J.M., and Obletz, B.E. Comminuted fractures of the distal end of the radius treated by skeletal transfixion in plaster cast: An end-result study of 33 cases. J Bone Joint Surg 48A:931, 1966.

26. Cooney, W.P., Linscheid, R.L., and Dobyns, J.H. External pin fixation for unstable Colles' fractures. J Bone Joint Surg 61A:840, 1979.

27. Cooney, W.P., Dobyns, J.H., and Linscheid, R.L. Fractures of the scaphoid: A rational approach to management. Clin Orthop 149:90–97, 1980.

28. Cooney, W.P., Dobyns, J.H., and Linscheid, R.L. Non-union of the scaphoid: Analysis of the results from bone grafting. J Hand Surg 5:343, 1980.

29. Cooney, W.P., Dobyns, J.H., and Linscheid, R.L. Complication of Colles' fractures. J Bone Joint Surg 62A:613, 1980.

30. Coonrad, R.W., and Pohlman, M.H. Impacted fractures in the proximal portion of the proximal phalanx of the finger. J Bone Joint Surg 51A:1291–1296, 1969.

31. Crawford, G.P. Screw fixation for certain fractures of the phalanges and metacarpals. J Bone Joint Surg 58A:487–492, 1976.

32. Dabezies, E.J., and Schutte, J.P. Fixation of metacarpal and phalangeal fractures with miniature plates and screws. J Hand Surg 11A:284–288, 1986.

33. Dameron, T.B. Traumatic dislocation of the distal radioulnar joint. Clin Orthop 83:55–63, 1972.

34. DeLee, J.C. External fixation of the forearm and wrist. Orthop Rev 6:43–48, 1981.

35. DeOliviera, J.C. Barton's fractures. J Bone Joint Surg 55A:586–594, 1973.

36. DePalma, A.F. Comminuted fractures of the distal end of the radius treated by ulnar pinning. J Bone Joint Surg 34:651, 1951.

37. Dingman, P.V.C. Resection of the distal end of the ulna (Darrach operation): An end-result study of 24 cases. J Bone Joint Surg 34A:893, 1952.

38. Dodge, H.S., and Cady, G.W. Treatment of fractures of the radius and ulna with compression plates. A retrospective study of one hundred and nineteen fractures in seventy-eight patients. J Bone Joint Surg 54A:1167–1176, 1972.

39. Dunn, A.W. Fractures and dislocations of the carpus. Surg Clin North Am 52:1513, 1972.

40. Eaton, R.G. Joint Injuries of the Hand. Springfield, IL, Thomas, 1971.

41. Eaton, R.G., and Littler, J.W. Ligament reconstruction for the painful thumb carpometacarpal joint. J Bone Joint Surg 55A:1655–1666, 1973.

42. Eaton, R.G., and Littler, J.W. Joint injuries and their sequelae. Clin Plast Surg 3:85–98, 1976.

43. Eaton, R.G., and Malerich, M.M. Volar plate arthroplasty of the proximal interphalangeal joint. A review of ten years experience. J Hand Surg 5:260–268, 1980.

44. Eddeland, A., Eiken, O., Hellgren, E., and Ohlsson, N.M. Fractures of the scaphoid. Scand J Plast Reconstr Surg 9:234–239, 1975.

45. Edwards, E.S., O'Brien, E.T., and Heckman, M.M. Retrograde cross-pinning of transverse metacarpal and phalangeal fractures. Hand 14:141–148, 1982.

46. Ellis, J. Smith's and Barton's fractures: A method of treatment. J Bone Joint Surg 47B:724–728, 1965.

47. Evans, E.M. Rotational deformity in the treatment of fractures of both bones of the forearm. J Bone Joint Surg 27:373–379, 1945.

48. Falkenberg, P. An experimental study of instability during supination and pronation of the fractured scaphoid. J Hand Surg 10B:211, 1985.

49. Farnborough, R.A., and Green, D.P. Tendon rupture as a complication of screw fixation in fractures of the hand. J Bone Joint Surg 61A:781–782, 1979.

50. Ferraro, M.C., Coppola, A., Lippman, K., and Hurst, L.C. Closed functional bracing of metacarpal fractures. Orthop Rev 12:49–56, 1983.

51. Fernandez, D.L. Correction of post-traumatic wrist deformity in adults by osteotomy, bone grafting and internal fixation. J Bone Joint Surg 64A:1164, 1982.

52. Fernandez, D.L. A technique for anterior wedge-shaped grafts for scaphoid non-unions with carpal instability. J Hand Surg 9A:733–737, 1984.

53. Fraker, W.H., Wray, R., and Weeks, P.M. Factors influencing final range of motion in the fingers after fractures of the hand. Plast Reconstr Surg 63:82–87, 1979.

54. Freeland, A.E., and Finley, J.S. Displaced vertical fracture of the trapezium treated with a small cancellous lag screw. J Hand Surg 9A:843–845, 1984.

55. Freeman, B.H., and Hay, E.L. Non-union of the capitate: A case report. J Hand Surg 10A:187–190, 1985.

56. Friedenberg, Z.B. Anatomical considerations in the treatment of carpal navicular fractures. Am J Surg 78:379, 1949.

57. Frykman, G. Fractures of the distal end of the radius, including sequelae—Shoulder, hand, finger syndrome, disturbance in the distal radioulnar joint and impairment of nerve function. Acta

Orthop Scand 108(Suppl):27, 1967.

58. Frykman, G.K., and Nelson, E.F. Fractures and traumatic conditions of the wrist, in Hunter, J.M., et al (eds): *Rehabilitation of the Hand,* 2d ed. St. Louis, Mosby, 1984, pp 165–179.

59. Fulkerson, J.P., and Watson, H.K. Congenital anterior subluxation of the distal ulna. Clin Orthop 131:179–182, 1978.

60. Gavel, A., et al. Bone scanning in the assessment of fractures of the scaphoid. J Hand Surg 4:540–543, 1979.

61. Garroway, R.Y., Hurst, L.C., Leppard, J., and Dick, H.M. Complex dislocations of the proximal interphalangeal joint—A pathoanatomic classification of the injury. Orthop Rev 13:490–497, 1984.

62. Gartland, J.J., and Werley, C.W. Evaluation of healed Colles' fractures. J Bone Joint Surg 33:895, 1951.

63. Gedda, K.O. Open reduction and osteosynthesis of the so-called Bennett's fracture in the carpo-metacarpal joint of the thumb. Acta Orthop Scand 22:249–257, 1953.

64. Gelberman, R.H., and Mann, J. The vascularity of the scaphoid. J Hand Surg 5:508, 1980.

65. Gelberman, R.H., Panagris, J.S., Taleisnik, J., and Baumgaertner, M. The arterial anatomy of the human carpus. Part I: The extra-osseous vascularity. J Hand Surg 8:367, 1983.

66. Gonclaves, D. Correction of disorders of the distal radio-ulnar joint by artificial pseudarthrosis of the ulna. J Bone Joint Surg 56B:462–463, 1974.

67. Goodman, M.L., and Pfenninghaus, N. Closed metacarpal fractures—A retrospective study excluding the thumb. Orthop Rev 9:69–78, 1980.

68. Grana, W.A., and Kopta, J.A. The Roger Anderson device in the treatment of fractures of the distal end of the radius. J Bone Joint Surg 61A:1234–1238, 1979.

69. Grazier, K.L., et al. *The Frequency of Occurrence, Impact and Cost of Musculoskeletal Conditions in the U.S.* Chicago, American Academy of Orthopedic Surgeons, 1984.

70. Green, D.P., and O'Brien, E.T. Fractures of the thumb metacarpal. South Med J 65:807, 1972.

71. Green, D.P., and Terry, G.C. Complex dislocation of the metacarpal-phalangeal joint. Correlative pathological anatomy. J Bone Joint Surg 55A:1480–1486, 1973.

72. Green, D.P., and Anderson, J.R. Closed reduction and percutaneous pin fixation of fractured phalanges. J Bone Joint Surg 55A:1651, 1973.

73. Green, D.P. Pins and plaster treatment of comminuted fracture of the distal end of the radius. J Bone Joint Surg 57A:304, 1975.

74. Green, D.P. Pisotriquetral arthritis. J Hand Surg 4:465–467, 1979.

75. Green, D.P., and Rowland, S.A. Fractures and dislocation in the hand, in Rockwood, C.A., and Green, D.P. (eds): *Fractures.* Philadelphia, Lippincott, 1984.

76. Green, D.P. *Operative Hand Surgery.* New York, Churchill Livingstone, 1982.

77. Green, D.P. Metacarpal fractures. Instr Course Lect 1984.

78. Green, D.P. The effect of avascular necrosis on Russe bone grafting for scaphoid non-union. J Hand Surg 10A:597–605, 1985.

79. Gunther, S.F. The carpometacarpal joints. Orthop Clin North Am 15:259–277, 1984.

80. Haddad, R.J., and Edmunds, J.O. The treatment of Bennett's fracture dislocation: An anatomic and clinical study. Presented at AAOS annual meeting, Anaheim, 1983.

81. Hall, T.D. Loose body in the pisotriquetral joint. J Bone Joint Surg 63A:498, 1981.

82. Hartwig, R.H., and Louis, D.S. Multiple carpometacarpal dislocations. J Bone Joint Surg 61A:906–908, 1979.

83. Hartz, C.R., and Beckenbaugh, R.D. Long term results of resection of the distal ulna for post-traumatic conditions. J Trauma 19:219–226, 1979.

84. Heim, U., and Pfeiffer, K.M. *Small Fragment Set Manual.* Berlin, Springer-Verlag, 1982.

85. Heiple, K.G., Freehafer, A.A., and Van't Hof, A. Isolated traumatic dislocation of the distal end of the ulna or distal radio-ulnar joint. J Bone Joint Surg 44A:1387–1394, 1962.

86. Herbert, T.J., and Fisher, W.E. Management of the fractured scaphoid using a new bone screw. J Bone Joint Surg 66B:114, 1984.

87. Hsu, J.D., and Curits, R.M. Carpometacarpal dislocations on the ulnar side of the hand. J Bone Joint Surg 52A:927, 1970.

88. Hughston, J.C. Fracture of the distal radial shaft. J Bone Joint Surg 39A:249–264, 1957.

89. Hughston, J.C. Fractures of the forearm, anatomical considerations. J Bone Joint Surg 44A:1664–67, 1962.

90. Hunter, J.M., and Cowens, N.J. Fifth metacarpal fractures in a compensation clinic population. A report of one hundred and thirty-three cases. J Bone Joint Surg 52A:1159–1165, 1970.

91. Imbriglia, J.E., and Sciulli, R. Open complex metacarpophalangeal joint dislocation. Two cases: Index finger and long finger. J Hand Surg 4:72–75, 1979.

92. Imbriglia, J.E. Chronic dorsal carpometacarpal dislocation of the index, middle, ring and little fingers: a case report. J Hand Surg 4:343–345, 1979.

93. Jabaley, M.E., and Freeland, A.E. Rigid internal fixation in the hand: 104 cases. Plast Reconstr Surg 77:288–289, 1986.

94. Jahss, S.A. Fractures of the proximal phalanges: Alignment and immobilization. J Bone Joint Surg 18:726–731, 1936.

95. James, J.P., and Wright, T.A. Fractures of the metacarpals and proximal and middle phalanges of the finger. J Bone Joint Surg 48B:181–182, 1966.

96. Jones, W.A., and Ghorbal, M.S. Fractures of the trapezium—A report on three cases. J Hand Surg 10B:227–230, 1985.

97. Jupiter, J.B., Koniuch, M.P., and Smith, R.J. The management of delayed union and non-union of the metacarpals and phalanges. J Hand Surg 10A:457–466, 1985.

98. Kaplan, E.B. Dorsal dislocation of the metacarpophalangeal joint of the index finger. J Bone Joint Surg 39A:1081–1086, 1957.

99. Kaye, J.J., and Lister, G.D. Another use for the Brewerton view. J Hand Surg 3:603, 1978.

100. Kim, W.C., Shaffer, J.W., and Idzikowski, C. Failure of treatment of ununited fractures of the carpal scaphoid—the role of noncompliance. J Bone Joint Surg 65A:985–991, 1983.

101. King, R.E. Barton's fracture dislocation of the wrist. Curr Pract Orthop Surg 6:133, 1975.

102. Kleinert, J.M., and Zenni, E.J. Non-union of the scaphoid—Review of literature and current treatment. Orthop Rev 13:125–141, 1984.

103. Kleinert, J.M. et al. Complications of scaphoid silicone arthroplasty. J Bone Joint Surg 67A:422–427, 1985.

104. Kleinman, W.B., and Grantham, S.A. Multiple volar carpometacarpal joint dislocation. J Hand Surg 3:377–382, 1978.

105. Knight, R.A., and Purvis, G.D. Fractures of both bones of the forearm in adults. J Bone Joint Surg 31A:755–764, 1949.

106. Knirk, J.L., and Jupiter, J.B. Intra-articular fractures of the distal end of the radius in young adults. J Bone Joint Surg 68A:647–659, 1986.

107. Lane, C.S. Detecting occult fractures of the metacarpal head: The Brewerton view. J Hand Surg 2:131–133, 1977.

108. Lankford, L.L., and Thompson, J.E. Reflex sympathetic dystrophy, upper and lower extremity: Diagnosis and management. Instr Course Lect 26:163, 1977.

109. Lazar, G., and Schulter-Ellis, F.P. Intra-medullary structure of human metacarpals. J Hand Surg 5:477–481, 1980.

110. Leslie, I.J., and Dickson, R.A. The fractured carpal scaphoid. Natural history and factors influencing outcome. J Bone Joint Surg 63B:225–230, 1981.

111. Levy, M., Fischel, R.E., Stern, G.M., and Goldberg, I. Chip fractures of the os triquetrum. J Bone Joint Surg 61B:355–357, 1979.

112. Lichtman, D.M., and Alexander, C.E. Decision making in scaphoid

non-union. Orthop Rev 16:55–67, 1982.

113. Lilling, M., and Weinberg, H. The mechanism of dorsal fracture dislocation of the fifth carpometacarpal joint. J Hand Surg 4:340–342, 1979.

114. Linscheid, R.L., Dobyns, J.H., Beabout, and Bryan, R.S. Traumatic instability of the wrist: Diagnosis, classification and pathomechanics. J Bone Joint Surg 54A:1612–1632, 1972.

115. Lohman, C.L. The use of fascia-lata in the repair of disability at the wrist. J Bone Joint Surg 12:400–402, 1930.

116. London, P.S. The broken scaphoid bone: The case against pessimism. J Bone Joint Surg 53B:237–244, 1961.

117. Lynch, A.C., and Lipscomb, P.R. The carpal tunnel syndrome and Colles' fracture. JAMA 185:363, 1963.

118. Mansoor, I.A. Fractures of the proximal phalanx of fingers. J Bone Joint Surg 51A:196–198, 1969.

119. Mack, G.R., Bosse, M.J., and Gelberman, R.H. The natural history of scaphoid non-union. J Bone Joint Surg 66A:504–509, 1984.

120. Matthews, L.S., et al. Effect on supination-pronation of angular malalignment of fractures of both bones of the forearm. J Bone Joint Surg 64A:14–17, 1982.

121. McCue, F.C., Honner, R., Johnson, M.C., Jr., and Geick, J.H. Athletic injuries of the proximal interphalangeal joint requiring surgical treatment. J Bone Joint Surg 52A:937–56, 1970.

122. McElfresh, E.C. Dobyns, J.H., and O'Brien, E.T. Management of fracture—Dislocation of the proximal interphalangeal joints by extension-block splinting. J Bone Joint Surg 54A:1705, 1972.

123. McElfresh, E.C., and Dobyns, J.H. Intra-articular metacarpal head fractures. J Hand Surg 8:383–393, 1983.

124. McLaughlin, H.L., and Parker, J.C. Fracture of the carpal navicular (scaphoid) bone. Gradations in therapy based upon pathology. J Trauma 9:311–319, 1969.

125. Melone, C.P. Scaphoid fractures. Clin Plast Surg 8:83–94, 1981.

126. Melone, C.P. Articular fractures of the distal radius. Orthop Clin North Am 15:217–236, 1984.

127. Meyer, V.E., Chiu, D.T., and Beasley, R.W. The place of internal skeletal fixation in surgery of the hand. Clin Plast Surg 8:51–64, 1981.

128. Milch, H. Treatment of disabilities following fracture of the lower end of the radius. Clin Orthop 29:157–163, 1963.

129. Milford, L. The hand, in Crenshaw, A.H. (ed): *Campbell's Operative Orthopaedics*, 6th ed. St. Louis, Mosby, 1980.

130. Mikic, Z. Galeazzi fracture-dislocations. J Bone Joint Surg 57A:1071–1080, 1975.

131. Mino, D.E., Palmer, A.K., and Levinsohn, E.M. The role of radiography and computerized tomography in the diagnosis of subluxation and dislocation of the distal radio-ulnar joint. J Hand Surg 8:23–31, 1983.

132. Mino, D.E., et al. Radiography and computerized tomography in the diagnosis of incongruity of the distal radio-ulnar joint. J Bone Joint Surg 67A:247–252, 1985.

133. Moberg, E. The shoulder-hand-finger syndrome. Surg Clin North Am 40:367–373, 1960.

134. Mueller, M.E., et al. *Technique of Internal Fixation of Fractures*. New York, Springer-Verlag, 1965.

135. Mueller, M.E., et al. *Manual of Internal Fixation*. New York, Springer-Verlag, 1979.

136. Monheim, M.S., et al. Radiocarpal dislocation classification and rationale for management. Clin Orthop 192:199–209, 1985.

137. Moore, T.M., et al. Results of compression plating of closed Galeazzi fractures. J Bone Joint Surg 67A:1015–1027, 1985.

138. Moore, T.M., Lester, D.K., and Sarmiento, A. The stabilizing effect of soft tissue constraints in artificial Galeazzi fractures. Clin Orthop 194:189–194, 1985.

139. Murakami, Y. Irreducible dislocation of the distal interphalangeal joint. J Hand Surg 10B:231–32, 1985.

140. Nance, E.P., Kaye, J.J., and Milek, M.A. Volar plate fractures. Diag Radiol 133:61–64, 1979.

141. Naiman, P.T., et al. Use of ASIF compression plates in selected shaft fractures of the upper extremity. Clin Orthop 71:208–216, 1970.

142. Nakata, R.Y., et al. External fixators for wrist fractures: A biomechanical and clinical study. J Hand Surg 10A:845–851, 1985.

143. Nielsen, P.T., et al. Bone scintigraphy in the evaluation of fracture of the carpal scaphoid bone. Acta Orthop Scand 54:303–306, 1983.

144. Norman, A., et al. Fractures of the hook of the hamate: Radiographic signs. Radiology 154:49–53, 1985.

145. Obletz, B.E., and Halbstein, B.M. Non-union of fractures of the carpal navicular. J Bone Joint Surg 20:424, 1938.

146. O'Brien, E.T. Fractures of the metacarpals and phalanges, in Green, D.P. (ed): *Operative Hand Surgery*. New York, Churchill Livingstone, 1982, pp 596–635.

147. O'Brien, E.T. Acute fractures and dislocations of the carpus. Orthop Clin North Am 15:237–258, 1984.

148. Ogunro, O. Fracture of the body of the hamate bone. J Hand Surg 8:353–355, 1983.

149. Osterman, A.L., and Bora, F.W. Injuries of the wrist, in Heppenstall, R.B. (ed): *Fracture Treatment and Healing*. Philadelphia, Saunders, 1980, p 504.

150. Palmer, A.K., and Linscheid, R.L. Irreducible dorsal dislocation of the distal inter-phalangeal joint of the finger. J Hand Surg 2:406–408, 1977.

151. Palmer, A.K., and Linscheid, R.L. Chronic recurrent dislocation of the proximal interphalangeal joint of the finger. J Hand Surg 3:95–97, 1978.

152. Palmer, A.K. Trapezial ridge fractures. J Hand Surg 561–564, 1981.

153. Palmer, A.K., Dobyns, J.H., and Linscheid, R.L. Management of post-traumatic instability of the wrist secondary to ligament rupture. J Hand Surg 3:507–532, 1978.

154. Palmer, A.K., and Werner, F.W. The triangular fibrocartilage complex of the wrist—Anatomy and function. J Hand Surg 6:153–162, 1981.

155. Palmer, A.K. The distal radio-ulnar joint. Orthop Clin North Am 15:321–325, 1984.

156. Peimer, C.A., Sullivan, D.J., and Wild, D.R. Palmar dislocation of the proximal interphalangeal joint. J Hand Surg 9A:39–47, 1984.

157. Pool, C. Colles' fracture: A prospective study of treatment. J Bone Joint Surg 55B:540–544, 1973.

158. Posner, M.A., and Wilenski, M. Irreducible volar dislocation of the proximal interphalangeal joint of a finger caused by interposition of an intact central slip: A case report. J Bone Joint Surg 60A:133–134, 1978.

159. Rand, J.A., Linscheid, R.L., and Dobyns, J.H. Capitate fractures. Clin Orthop 165:209–216, 1982.

160. Reckling, F.W. Unstable fracture—Dislocations of the forearm (Monteggia and Galeazzi lesions). J Bone Joint Surg 64A:857–863, 1982.

161. Riggs, S.A., and Cooney, W.P. External fixation of complex hand and wrist fractures. J Trauma 23:332–336, 1983.

162. Rolfe, E.B., et al. Isotope bone imaging in suspected scaphoid trauma. Br J Radiol 54:762–767, 1981.

163. Rosacker, J.A., and Kopta, J.A. Both bone fractures of the forearm: A review of surgical variables associated with union. Orthopedics 5:1353–1356, 1981.

164. Ruby, L.K., Stinson, J., and Belsky, M.R. The natural history of scaphoid non-union—A review of fifty-five cases. J Bone Joint Surg 67A:428–432, 1985.

165. Ruggeri, S., Osterman, A.L., and Bora, F.W. Stabilization of metacarpal and phalangeal fractures in the hand. Orthop Rev 9:107–110, 1980.

166. Russe, O. Fracture of the carpal navicular. J Bone Joint Surg 42A:759, 1960.

167. Sage, F.P. Medullary fixation of fractures of the forearm. A study

of the medullary canal of the radius and a report of fifth fractures of the radius treated with a prebent triangular nail. J Bone Joint Surg 41A:1489–1516, 1959.

168. Sage, F.P. Fractures of the shaft of the radius and ulna in the adult, in Adams, J.P. (ed): *Current Practice in Orthopaedic Surgery,* vol 1. St. Louis, Mosby, 1963, pp 152–173.

169. Salamon, P.B., and Gelberman, R.H. Irreducible dislocation of the interphalangeal joint of the thumb. J Bone Joint Surg 60A:400–401, 1978.

170. Sandzen, S.C. Complications of the skeleton system of the hand, in Sandzen, S.C. (ed): *The Hand and Wrist.* Baltimore, Williams & Wilkins, 1985.

171. Sarmiento, A. The brachioradialis as a deforming force in Colles' fractures. Clin Orthop 38:86–92, 1965.

172. Sarmiento, A., Pratt, G.W., Berry, N.C., and Sinclair, W.F. Colles' fractures. Functional bracing in supination. J Bone Joint Surg 57A:311, 1975.

173. Sarmiento, A., et al. Forearm fractures, early functional bracing, a preliminary report. J Bone Joint Surg 57A:297–304, 1975.

174. Sarmiento, A., Zagorski, J.B., and Sinclair, W.F. Functional bracing of Colles' fractures: A prospective study of immobilization in supination versus pronation. Clin Orthop 146:175, 1980.

175. Schenk, M. Long-term follow-up of treatment of comminuted fractures of the distal end of the radius by transfixing with Kirschner wires and cast. J Bone Joint Surg 44A:337, 1962.

176. Schulter-Ellis, F.P., and Lazar, G.T. Internal morphology of human phalanges. J Hand Surg 9A:490–495, 1984.

177. Sclafani, S.J.A. Dislocation of the distal radio-ulnar joint. J Comput Assist Tomogr 5:450, 1981.

178. Segmuller, G. *Surgical Stabilization of the Skeleton of the Hand.* Baltimore, Williams & Wilkins, 1977.

179. Smail, G.B. Long-term follow-up of Colles' fracture. J Bone Joint Surg 47B:80–85, 1965.

180. Smith, H., and Sage, F.B. Medullary fixation of forearm fractures. J Bone Joint Surg 39A:91–98, 1957.

181. Smith, R.J., et al. Silicone synovitis of the wrist. J Hand Surg 47: , 1985.

182. Smith, R.J. Management principles for fractures and dislocations of the hand. Presented at AAOS Summer Institute, New York City, 1985.

183. Spinner, M., and Choi, B.Y. Anterior dislocation of the proximal interphalangeal joint: A cause of rupture of the central slip of the extensor mechanism. J Bone Joint Surg 52A:1329–1336, 1970.

184. Spinner, M., and Kaplan, E.B. Extensor carpi ulnaris—Its relationship to stability of the distal radio-ulnar joint. Clin Orthop 68:124–129, 1970.

185. Stark, H.H. Troublesome fractures and dislocations of the hand. Instr Course Lect 19: , 1970.

186. Stark, H.H., and Jobe, F.W. Fracture of the hook of the hamate in athletes. J Bone Joint Surg 59A:575–582, 1977.

187. Stern, P.J., and Druvy, W.J. Complications of plate fixation of forearm fractures. Clin Orthop 175:25–29, 1983.

188. Stordahl, A., et al. Bone scanning of fractures of the scaphoid. J Hand Surg 9B:189–190, 1984.

189. Strickland, J.W., Steicher, J.B., Kleinman, W.B., et al. Phalangeal fractures: factors influencing digital performance. Orthop Rev 11:39–50, 1982.

190. Strickland, J.W., and Steichen, J.B. *Difficult Problems in Hand Surgery.* St. Louis, Mosby, 1982.

191. Stripling, W.D. Displaced intra-articular osteochondral fracture—Cause for unreducible dislocation of the distal interphalangeal joint. J Hand Surg 7:77–78, 1982.

192. Swanson, A.B. *Flexible Implant Resection Arthroplasty in the Hand and Extremities.* St. Louis, Mosby, 1973, pp 240–253.

193. Taleisnik, J., and Kelly, P.J. The extra-osseous and intra-osseous blood supply of the scaphoid bone. J Bone Joint Surg 48A:1125, 1966.

194. Taleisnik, J., and Watson, H.K. Midcarpal instability caused by fractures of the distal radius. J Hand Surg 9A:350, 1984.

195. Taleisnik, J. Complications of fractures, dislocations, and ligamentous injuries of the wrist, in Boswick, J.A. (ed): *Complications in Hand Surgery.* Philadelphia, Saunders, 1986.

196. Taleisnik, J. *The Wrist.* New York, Churchill Livingstone, 1985.

197. Tarr, R.R., Garfinkel, A.I., and Sarmiento, A. The effects of angular and rotational deformities of both bones of the forearm. J Bone Joint Surg 66A:65–70, 1984.

198. Teipner, W.A., and Mast, J.W. Internal fixation of forearm diaphyseal fractures: Double plating versus single compression (tension band) plating—A comparative study. Orthop Clin North Am 11:381–391, 1980.

199. Terry, D.W., and Ramin, J.E. The navicular fat stripe. A useful roentgen feature for evaluating wrist trauma. AJR 124:25-28, 1975.

200. Thomas, F.B. Reduction of Smith's fracture. J Bone Joint Surg 39B:463–470, 1957.

201. Thompson, J.S., and Eaton, R.G. Volar dislocation of the proximal interphalangeal joint. J Hand Surg 2:232, 1977.

202. Thompson, G.H., and Grant, T.T. Barton's fractures—Reverse Barton's fracture—Confusing eponyms. Clin Orthop 122:210–221, 1977.

203. Tubiana, R. *The Hand,* vol 11, secs 2 and 3. Philadelphia, Saunders, 1985, pp 763–1030.

204. Vance, R.M., Gelberman, R.H., and Evans, E.F. Scaphocapitate fractures: Patterns of dislocation, mechanism of injury, and preliminary results of treatment. J Bone Joint Surg 62A:271–276, 1980.

205. Van der Linden, W., and Ericson, R. Colles' fracture. How should its displacement be measured and how should it be immobilized? J Bone Joint Surg 63A:1285, 1981.

206. Vasilas, A., et al. Roentgen aspects of injuries to the pisiform bone and pisotriquetral joint. J Bone Joint Surg 42A:1317–1328, 1960.

207. Vesely, D.G. The distal radio-ulnar joint. Clin Orthop 51:75–91, 1967.

208. Wagner, C.J. Methods of treatment of Bennett's fracture-dislocation. Am J Surg 80:230–232, 1950.

209. Weber, E.R., and Chao, E.Y. An experimental approach to the mechanism of scaphoid waist fractures. J Hand Surg 3:142, 1978.

210. Weber, E.R. Biomechanical implications of scaphoid waist fractures. Clin Orthop 149:83–89, 1980.

211. Weber, S.C., and Szabo, R.M. Severely comminuted distal radial fractures as an unsolved problem: Complications associated with external fixation and pins and plaster technique. J Hand Surg 11A:157–165, 1986.

212. Weeks, P.M. *Acute Bone and Joint Injuries of the Hand and Wrist.* St. Louis, Mosby, 1981.

213. Weiss, C., Laskin, R.S., and Spinner, M. Irreducible radiocarpal dislocation: A case report. J Bone Joint Surg 52A:562–564, 1970.

214. Weissman, B.N., and Sledge, C.B. *Orthopaedic Radiology.* Philadelphia, Saunders, 1986.

215. Wilson, J.N., and Rowland, S.A. Fracture dislocations of the proximal interphalangeal joint of the finger. J Bone Joint Surg 48A:293, 1966.

216. Wood, M.B., and Dobyns, J.H. Chronic complex volar dislocation of the metacarpophalangeal joint. Report of three cases. J Hand Surg 6:73–76, 1981.

217. Woods, G.L., and Burton, R.I. Avoiding pitfalls in the diagnosis of the acutely injured proximal interphalangeal joint. Clin Plast Surg 8:95–105, 1981.

218. Zemel, N.P., et al. Treatment of selected patients with an ununited fracture of the proximal part of the scaphoid by excision of the fragment and insertion of a carved silicon-rubber spacers.

J Bone Joint Surg 66A:510–517, 1984.

219. Zook, E.G., Van Beek, A.L., and Wavak, P. Transverse volar skin laceration of the finger: A sign of volar plate injury. Hand 11:213–216, 1979.
220. Zook, E.G., Guy, R.J., and Russell, R.C. A study of nail bed injuries: Cause, treatment and prognosis. J Hand Surg 9A:247–252, 1984.

Section B: Ligament Injuries of the Wrist, Hand, and Elbow

1. Beckenbaugh, R.D. Accurate evaluation and management the painful wrist following injury: An approach to carpal instability. Orthop Clin North Am 15(2):289–306, 1984.
2. Bowers, W.H., and Hurst, L.C. Gamekeeper's thumb. J Bone Joint Surg 59A:519–524, 1977.
3. Campbell, R.D., et al: Indications for open reduction of lunate and perilunate dislocations of the carpal bones. J Bone Joint Surg 47A:915–937, 1965.
4. Deharen, K.E., and Evarts, C.M. Throwing injuries of the elbow in athletes. Orthop Clin North Am 1:801–808, 1973.
5. Dobyns, J.H., et al: Traumatic instability of the wrist. Instr Course Lect 24:182–199, 1975.
6. Frank, W.E., and Dobyns, J. Surgical pathology of collateral ligamentous injuries of the thumb. Clin Orthop 83:102–114, 1972.
7. Flynn, J.E. Acute trauma to the hand. Clin Orthop 13:124–134, 1959.
8. Flynn, J.E. (ed). *Hand Surgery.* Baltimore, Williams & Wilkins, 1966.
9. Garden, R.S. Tennis elbow. J Bone Joint Surg 43B:100–106, 1961.
10. Linscheid, R.L., Dobyns, J.H., Beabout, J.W., and Bryan, R.S. Traumatic instability of the wrist: Diagnosis, classification, and pathomechanics. J Bone Joint Surg 54A:1612–1632, 1972.
11. Mayfield, J.K. Wrist ligamentous anatomy and pathogenesis of carpal instability. Orthop Clin North Am 15(2)209–216, 1984.
12. McCue, F.C., and Abbot, J.L. The treatment of mallet finger and boutonniere deformities. Virginia Med Monthly 94:623–628, 1967.
13. McCue, F.C., Honner, R., Johnson, M.C., and Gieck, J.H. Athletic injuries of the proximal interphalangeal joint requiring surgical treatment. J Bone Joint Surg 52A:937–956, 1970.
14. McCue, F.C., Andrews, J.R., and Hakala, M.W. The coach's finger. Am J Sports Med 2:270–275, 1974.
15. McCue, F.C., Hakala, M.W., Andrews, J.R., and Gieck, J.H. Ulnar collateral ligament injuries of the thumb in athletes. Am J Sports Med 2:70–80, 1974.
16. McCue, F.C., Baugher, W.H., Dulund, D.N., and Gieck, J.H. Hand and wrist injuries in the athlete. Am J Sports Med 7:275–286, 1979.
17. Nirsch, R.P. Tennis elbow. Orthop Clin North Am 43:787–800, 1973. Hugston, J.C., Bowden.
18. Norwood, L.A., Shook, J.A., and Andrews, J.R. Acute medical elbow ruptures. Am J Sports Med 9(1):16–9, 1981.
19. Palmer, A.K. The distal radioulnar joint. Orthop Clin North Am 15(2):321–336, 1984.
20. Palmer, A.K., and Werner, F.W. The triangular fibrocartilage complex of the wrist—Anatomy and function. J Hand Surg 6:153–162, 1981.
21. Regan, D.S., Linscheid, R.L., and Dobyns, J.H. Lunotriquetral sprains. Presented at the 36th Annual Meeting of the American Society of Surgery of the Hand, Las Vegas, Nevada, 1981.
22. Schneider, R.C., Kennedy, J.C., and Plant, M.L. (eds) *Sports Injuries, Mechanisms, Prevention and Treatment.* Baltimore, Williams & Wilkins, 1985.
23. Schwab, G.H., Bennett, J.B., Woods, G.W., and Tullos, H.S. Biomechanics of elbow instability: The role of the medical collateral ligament. Clin Orthop 146:42–52, 1980.
24. Regional Review Course in Hand Surgery: Manual, 1984. Sponsored by the American Society for Surgery of the Hand.
25. Stener, B. Displacement of the ruptured ulna collateral ligament of the metacarpophalangeal joint of the thumb: A clinical and anatomical study. J Bone Joint Surg 44B:869–879, 1962.
26. Tivnon, M.C., Anzel, S.H., and Waugh, T.R. Surgical management of osteochondritis dessicans of the capitellum. Am J Sports Med 4:121–128, 1976.
27. Weber, E.R. Concepts governing the rotational shift of the intercalated segment of the carpus. Orthop Clin North Am 15(2):193–208, 1984.

Section C: Fractures and Dislocations of the Elbow, Arm, and Shoulder Girdle of Adults

1. Adler, S., et al. Treatment of olecranon fractures: Indications for excision of the olecranon fragment and repair of the triceps tendon. J Trauma 2:597-602, 1962.
2. Aitken, G.K., and Rorabeck, C.M. Distal humeral fractures in the adult. Clin Orthop 207:191–197, 1986.
3. Allgower, M., et al. *Manual of Internal Fixation,* 2nd ed. New York, Springer-Verlag, 1979.
4. Alldredge, R.H. The surgical treatment of acromioclavicular dislocations. J Bone Joint Surg 64B:597–599, 1982.
5. Allende, G., and Freytes, M. Old dislocation of the elbow. J Bone Joint Surg 26:691–706, 1944.
6. Allman, F.L. Fractures and ligamentous injuries to the clavicle and its articular relation. J Bone Joint Surg 49A:774–784, 1967.
7. Anderson, L.D. Fracture of the shafts of the radius and ulna, in Rockwood, C.A., and Green (eds): *Fractures in Adults,* 2nd ed. Philadelphia, Lippincott, 1975.
8. Bado, J.L. The Monteggia lesion. Clin Orthop 50:71–86, 1967.
9. Bailey, R.W., et al. A dynamic method repair for acute and chronic injuries of the acromioclavicular disruption. Am J Sports Med 4:58–71, 1976.
10. Balfour, G.W., Mooney, V., and Ashby, M. Diaphyseal fractures of the humerus treated with a ready-made fracture brace. J Bone Joint Surg 64A:11–13, 1982.
11. Bargar, W.L., et al. Late thoracic outlet syndrome secondary to pseudoarthrosis of the clavicle. J Trauma 24:857–859, 1984.
12. Bargren, J.H., et al. Biomechanics and comparison of two operative methods of treatment of complete acromioclavicular separation. Clin Orthop 130:267–272, 1978.
13. Barnard, L.B., and McCoy, S.M. The supracondyloid process of the humerus. J Bone Joint Surg 28A:845–850, 1946.
14. Bateman, J.E. Neurovascular syndromes related to the clavicle. Clin Orthop 58:75–84, 1968.
15. Bell, M.J. Beauchamp, C.G., et al. The results of plating humeral shaft fractures in patients with multiple injuries. J Bone Joint Surg 67B:283–295, 1985.
16. Benchetrit, E., et al. Fracture of the coracoid process associated with subglenoid dislocation of the shoulder. A case report. J Bone Joint Surg 61A:295–296, 1979.
17. Beorden, J.M., Hugston, J.C., and Whatley, G.S. Acromioclavicular dislocation: Methods and treatment. J Sports Med 1:5–17, 1973.
18. Bernstein, S.M., King, J.D., and Sanderson, R.A. Fractures of the medial epicondyle of the humerus. Contemp Orthop 3:637–642, 1981.
19. Billington, R.W. A new (plaster yolk) dressing for fracture of the clavicle. South Med J 24:667, 1931.
20. Bjerneld, H., et al. Acromioclavicular separations treated conservatively. A 5-year follow-up study. Acta Orthop Scand 54:743–745, 1983.
21. Bosworth, B.M. Acromioclavicular separation: New method of repair. Surg Gynecol Obstet 73:866–871, 1941.
22. Bosworth, B.M. Acromioclavicular dislocation end results of screw suspension treatment. Ann Surg 127:98–111, 1948.

23. Boyd, H.B., and Boals, J.C. The Monteggia lesion, a review of 159 cases. Clin Orthop 66:94–100, 1969.

24. Brown, R.F., and Morgan, R.G. Intercondylar T-shaped fractures of the humerus: Results in ten cases treated by early mobilization. J Bone Joint Surg 53B:425–428, 1971.

25. Bruce, H.C., Harvey, J.P., and Wilson, J.C. Monteggia fractures. J Bone Joint Surg 56A:1563–1576, 1974.

26. Bryan, R.S. Fractures about the elbow in adults. Instr Course Lect 30:200–223, 1981.

27. Bryan, R.S., and Bickel, W.H.T. Condylar fractures of the distal humerus. J Trauma 11:830, 1971.

28. Buckerfield, C.T., and Castle, M.E. Acute traumatic retrosternal dislocation of the clavicle. J Bone Joint Surg 66A:379–385, 1984.

29. Burri, C., Henkelmeyer, H., and Spier, W. Results of operative treatment of intra-articular fractures of the distal humerus. Acta Orthop Belg 41:227, 1975.

30. Caldwell, J.A. Treatment of fractures of the shaft of the humerus by hanging cast. Surg Gynecol Obstet 70:421, 1940.

31. Carothers, R.G., and Boyd, F.J. Thumb traction technique. Arch Surg 58:848–852, 1949.

32. Cave, E.F. *Fractures and Other Injuries.* Chicago, Year Book Medical, 1958.

33. Charnley, J. *The Closed Treatment of Common Fractures,* 3d ed. Baltimore, Williams & Wilkins, 1961.

34. Conn, J., and Wade, P.A. Injuries of the elbow (a ten year review). J Trauma 1:248–268, 1961.

35. Connolly, J. Management of fractures associated with arterial injuries. Am J Surg 120:3131, 1970.

36. Coonrad, R.W. Nonunion of the olecranon and proximal ulna, in Morrey, B.F. (ed): *The Elbow and Its Disorders.* Philadelphia, Saunders, 1985.

37. Cotton, F.J. Elbow dislocation and ulna nerve injury. J Bone Joint Surg 11:348–352, 1929.

38. Cromack, P.I. The mechanics and nature of the injury in dislocation of the elbow and a method of treatment. Aust J Surg 30:212–216, 1960.

39. Dahl, E. Vascular prosthesis in fractures and dislocations in the clavicular region. Chirurgia 53:120–122, 1982.

40. Daland, E.M. Fractures of the olecranon. J Bone Joint Surg 15:601–607, 1933.

41. Dameron, T.B., Jr. Complications of treatment of injuries of the shoulder, in Epps, C.H. (eds): *Complications in Orthopaedic Surgery.* Philadelphia, Lippincott, 1978.

42. DeLee, J.C., Green, D.P., and Wilkins, K.E. Fractures and dislocations of the elbow, in Rockwood, C., and Green, D. (eds): *Fractures in Adults,* 2nd ed. Philadelphia, Lippincott, 1975.

43. Deliyannis, S.N. Comminuted fracture of the olecranon treated by Weber-Vasey technique. Injury 5:19–24, 1973.

44. DePalma, A.F. *The Management of Fractures and Dislocations,* vol 1. Philadelphia, Saunders, 1959.

45. DePalma, A.F. *Surgery of the Shoulder.* 2d ed. Philadelphia, Lippincott, 1973.

46. DeRosa, G.P., et al. Fracture of the coracoid process of the scapula. Case report. J Bone Joint Surg 59A:696–697, 1977.

46a. Dias, J.J., Steingold, R.F., Richardson, R.A., et al. The conservative treatment of acromioclavicular dislocation. J Bone Joint Surg 69B:719–722, 1987.

47. Durig, M., Muller, W., Ruedi, T.P., and Gauer, E.F. The operative treatment of the elbow dislocation in the adult. J Bone Joint Surg 61A:239–244, 1979.

48. Dushuttle, R.P., Coyle, M.P., Zawadsky, J.P., and Bloom, H. Fractures of the capitellum. J Trauma 25:317–321, 1985.

49. D'Uthurbicle, B., et al. Closed intramedullary nailing of fracture of the shaft of the humerus. Int Orthop 7:195–203, 1983.

50. Edmonson, A.S., and Crenshaw, A.H. (eds): *Campbell's Operative Orthopaedics.* St. Louis, Mosby, 1980.

51. Edwards, H.C. Mechanism and treatment of backfire fracture. J Bone Joint Surg 8:701–717, 1926.

52. Eliason, E.L., and Broiwn, R.B. Posterior dislocation at the elbow with rupture of the radial ulna arteries. Ann Surg 106:1111–1115, 1937.

53. Eliot, E., Jr. Fracture of the olecranon. Surg Clin North Am 14:487–491, 1934.

54. Evans, E.M. Rotational deformity in the treatment of fractures of broken bones of the forearm. J Bone Joint Surg 27A:373–379, 1949.

55. Fromison, A.I. Fracture of the coracoid process of the scapula. J Bone Joint Surg 60A:710, 1978.

56. Galbraith, K.A., et al. Acute nerve injury as a complication of closed fracture or dislocation of the elbow. Injury 11:1959–1964, 1979.

57. Garcia, A., Jr., and Malch, B.M. Radial nerve injuries in fracture of the shaft of the humerus. Am J Surg 99:625, 1960.

58. Garland, D.E. Forceful joint manipulation in head injured adults with heterotopic ossification. Clin Orthop 169:133–138, 1982.

59. Garland, D.E. Fractures and dislocations about the hip in head injured adults. Clin Orthop 186:154–158, 1984.

60. Garland, D.E., and O'Hollaren, R.M. Fractures and dislocations about the elbow in the head-injured adult. Clin Orthop 168:38–41, 1982.

61. Gartsman, G.M., Sculco, T.P., and Otis, J.C. Operative treatment of olecranon fractures. J Bone Joint Surg 63A:718–721, 1981.

62. Gaston, S.R., Smith, F.M., and Bach, O.D. Adult injuries of the radial head and neck—Importance of time element in treatment. Am J Surg 78:631–635, 1949.

63. Genner, B.A. Fracture of the supracondyloid process. J Bone Joint Surg 41A:1333–1335, 1959.

64. Gessini, L., Jandolo, B., and Pietrangeli, A. Entrapment neuropathies of the median nerve at and above the elbow. Surg Neurol 19:112–116, 1983.

65. Ghawabi, M.H. Fracture of the medial condyle of the humerus. J Bone Joint Surg 57A:677–679, 1975.

66. Giustra, P.E., et al. The missed Monteggia fracture. Radiology 110:45–47, 1974.

67. Gosman, J.A. Recurrent dislocation of the ulna at the elbow. J Bone Joint Surg 25:448–449, 1943.

68. Grabski, R.S., et al. Intraosseous fixation of clavicular fractures with the Kirschner wire. Chir Narzadow Ruchu Otop Pol 49:1–3, 1984.

69. Grantham, S.A., Norris, T.R., and Bush, D.C. Isolated fracture of the humeral capitellum. Clin Orthop 161:262–269, 1981.

70. Grantham, S.A., and Tretzen, R. Tanscondylar fracture-dislocation of the elbow. J Bone Joint Surg 58A:1030–1031, 1976.

71. Green, S.A. *Complication of External Skeletal Fixation; Causes, Prevention and Treatment.* Springfield, IL, Thomas, 1981.

72. Guerna, A., et al. Transolecranon dislocations. Ital J Orthop Traumatol 8:175–181, 1982.

73. Hallet, J. Entrapment of the median nerve after dislocation of the elbow. A case report. J Bone Joint Surg 63B:408–412, 1981.

74. Hardegger, F.H., Simpson, L.A., and Weber, B.G. The operative treatment of scapular fractures. J Bone Joint Surg 66B:725–731, 1984.

75. Hassman, G.C., Brunn, F., and Neer, C.S. Recurrent dislocation of the elbow. J Bone Joint Surg 57A:1080–1084, 1975.

76. Hawkins, R.J. *The Acromioclavicular Joint.* A paper presented at the summer institute, A.A.O.S., Chicago, 1980.

77. Hawkins, R.J., Bell, R.H., and Gurr, K. The three-part fracture of the proximal part of the humerus. J Bone Joint Surg 68A:1410–1414, 1986.

78. Heining, C.F. Retrosternal dislocation of the clavicle: Early recognition, x-ray diagnosis and management. J Bone Joint Surg 50A:830, 1968.

79. Helfet, D.L. Bicondylar intraarticular fractures of the distal humerus in adults: Their assessment, classification, and operative management. Adv Orthop Surg 8:223–235, 1985.

80. Hejse-Moore, G.H., et al. Avulsion fractures of the scapula. Skeletal Radiol 9:27–32, 1982.

81. Henderson, N.J., et al. The management of complex forearm fractures. Injury 14:395–404, 1983.

82. Heppenstall, R.B. Fractures of the proximal humerus, in Heppenstall, R.B. (ed): *Fracture Treatment and Healing.* Philadelphia, Saunders, 1980.

83. Holmsen, H., et al. Myositis ossificans progressive clinical and metabolic observation in a case treated with diphosphonate and surgical removal of bone. Acta Orthop Scand 50:33–38, 1979.

84. Holstein, A., and Lewis, G.B. Fractures of the humerus with radial nerve paralysis. J Bone Joint Surg 45A:1382–1388, 1963.

85. Horne, J.G., et al. Olecranon fractures: A review of 100 cases. J Trauma 6:469–472, 1981.

86. Horne, J.G. Olecranon fractures: Classification and techniques of internal fixation. Techn Orthopaed 1:54–58, 1986.

87. Howard, F.M., and Shafer, S.J. Injuries to the clavicle with neurovascular complications. J Bone Joint Surg 61B:74, 1979.

88. Howard, J.L., and Urist, M.R. Fracture dislocations of the radius and ulna at the elbow joint. Clin Orthop 12:276–284, 1958.

89. Hunter, S.G. The closed treatment of fractures of the humeral shaft. Clin Orthop 164:192–198, 1982.

90. Imatani, R.J. Fractures of the scapula: A review of 53 fractures. J Trauma 15:473–478, 1975.

91. Isahizuki, M., Yamaura, I., et al. Avulsion fracture of the superior border of the scapula. J Bone Joint Surg 63A:820–822, 1981.

92. Jablon, M., Sutker, A., and Post, M. Irreducible fracture of the middle third of the clavicle. J Bone Joint Surg 61A: 296–298, 1979.

93. Jessing, P. Monteggia lesions and their complicating nerve damage. Acta Orthop Scand 46:601–609, 1975.

94. Johansson, D. Capsular and ligamentous injuries of the elbow joint. Acta Clin Scand 287, 1962.

95. Johansson, H., and Olerud, S. Operative treatment of intercondylar fractures of the humerus. J Trauma 11:836–843, 1971.

96. Johnston, G.W. A follow up of one hundred cases of fracture of the head of the radius with a review of the literature. Ulster Med J 31:51–56, 1962.

97. Jones, K.G. Percutaneous pin fixation of fractures of the lower end of the humerus. Clin Orthop 50:53–69, 1967.

98. Josefsson, P.O., Johnell, O., and Gentz, C.F. Long-term sequelae of simple dislocation of the elbow. J Bone Joint Surg 66A:927–930, 1984.

99. Jupiter, J.B., Neff, U., Holzach, P., and Allgower, M. Intercondylar fractures of the humerus: An operative approach. J Bone Joint Surg 67A:226–239, 1985.

100. Kenmore, P.I., and Kranik, A.D. chap 9, in Epps (eds): *Complications of Musculoskeletal Infections.* Philadelphia, Lippincott, 1978, pp 129–158.

101. Keon-Cohen, B.T. Fractures of the elbow. J Bone Joint Surg 48A:1623–1639, 1966.

102. Keon-Cohen, B.T. Fractures at the elbow. J Bone Joint Surg 48:1623–1630, 1966.

103. Kettelkamp, D.B., and Alexander, H. Clinical review of radial nerve injury. J Trauma 7:424–432, 1967.

104. Kiviluoto, D., et al. Fracture of the olecranon, analysis of 37 consecutive cases. Acta Orthop Scand 49:28–31, 1978.

105. Klenerman, L. Experimental fractures of the adult humerus. Med Biol Eng 7:357, 1969.

106. Knight, R.A. Fractures of the humeral condyles in adults. South Med J 48:1165, 1955.

107. Kobayashi, S. *Pneumothorax Occurring with Scapular Fractures.* Paper read at the Rocky Mountain Trauma Society Meeting, Aspen, CO, January 27, 1978.

108. Kolb, L.W., and Moore, R.D. Factures of the supracondylar process of the humerus. J Bone Joint Surg 49A:532–534, 1967.

109. Kuntscher, G.B. The Kuntscher method of intramedullary fixation. J Bone Joint Surg 40A:17–26, 1958.

110. Laing, P.G. Transplantation of the long head of the biceps in complete acromioclavicular separations. J Bone Joint Surg 51A:1677–1678, 1969.

111. Lansinger, O., and Mare, K. Fracture of the capitellum humeri. Acta Orthop Scand 52:39–44, 1981.

112. Lee, C.K., et al. Post traumatic avascular necrosis in displaced proximal humeral fractures. J Trauma 21(9):788–791, 1981.

113. Levy, R.N., and Sherry, H.S. Complications of treatment of fractures and dislocations of the elbow, in Epps, C.H. (eds): *Complications of Orthopaedic Surgery.* Philadelphia, Lippincott, 1978, 237–256.

114. Linscheid, R.L., and Wheeler, D.K. Elbow dislocations. JAMA 19:411–418, 1965.

115. Loomis, L.K. Reduction and after treatment of posterior dislocations of the elbow. Am J Surg 63:56–60, 1944.

116. Louis, D.S., Riccardi, J.E., and Spengler, D.M. Arterial injury: A complication of posterior elbow dislocation—A clinical and anatomical study. J Bone Joint Surg 56A:1631–1666, 1974.

117. MacAusland, W.R., Jr., and Wyman, E.T., Jr. Fractures of the adult elbow. Instr Course Lect 24:169–181, 1975.

118. MacKay, I., et al. Silastic replacement of the head of the radius in trauma. J Bone Joint Surg 61B:494–497, 1979.

119. Macko, D., and Szabo, R.M. Complications of tension-band wiring of olecranon fractures. J Bone Joint Surg 67A:1396–1401, 1985.

120. Malkawi, H. Recurrent dislocation of the elbow accompanied by ulnar neuropathy: A case report and review of the literature. Clin Orthop 161:270–274, 1981.

121. Mandruzzato, F. Patalogia E Chirurgia del processo supraepitrocleare dell'omero. Chir Organi Mov 24:123–132, 1938.

122. Mason, M.L. Some observations on fractures of the head of the radius with a review of one hundred cases. Br J Surg 42:123–132, 1954.

123. Mayer, P.J., and Evarto, C.M. Nonunion, delayed union, malunion and avascular necrosis, in Epps, C.H. (ed): *Complications in Orthopaedic Surgery.* Philadelphia, Lippincott, 1975.

124. McGahan, J.P., et al. Fracture of the acromion associated with an axillary nerve deficit. A case report and review of the literature. Clin Orthop 147:216–218, 1980.

125. McLaughlin, M.L. *Trauma.* Philadelphia, Saunders, 1959.

126-127. McLennan, J.G., and Ungersma, J. Pneumothorax complicating fracture of the scapula. J Bone Joint Surg 64A:598–599, 1982.

128. Mehta, J.C., Sachdev, A., and Collins, J.J. Retrosternal dislocation of the clavicle. Injury 5:79–83, 1973.

129. Mikic, Z.D., et al. Late results in fractures of the radial head treated by excision. Clin Orthop 181:220–228, 1983.

130. Milch, H. Fractures and fracture dislocation of the humeral condyles. J Trauma 4:592–607, 1964.

131. Monteggia, G.B. *Institujioni Chirrugiche.* Maspero, Milan, 1814.

132. Montgomery, S.P., et al. Avulsion fracture of the coracoid epiphysis with acromioclavicular separation. Report of two cases in adolescents and review of literature. J Bone Joint Surg 59A:963–965, 1977.

133. Muller, M.E., et al. *Manual of Internal Fixation,* 2d ed. New York, Springer-Verlag, 1979.

134. Mullich, S. The lateral Monteggia fracture. J Bone Joint Surg 59A:543–544, 1977.

135. Naidoo, K.S. Unreduced posterior dislocations of the elbow. J Bone Joint Surg 64B:603–606, 1982.

136. Neer, C.S., II. Four segment classification of displaced proximal humeral fractures. Instr Course Lect 24:160–168, 1975.

137. Neer, C.S., II. Fracture of the distal clavicle with detachment of

the coracoclavicular ligaments in adults. J Trauma 3:99–110, 1963.

138. Neer, C.S., II. Fractures of the distal third of the clavicle. Clin Orthop 58:43–50, 1968.

139. Neviaser, J.S., and Wickston, J.K. Dislocation of the elbow: A retrospective study of 115 patients. South Med J 70:172–173, 1977.

140. Nicol, E.E. Miners and mannequins: Editorial. J Bone Joint Surg 36B:171–172, 1954.

141. Norrell, H., Jr., and Llewellyn, R.C. Migration of a threaded Steinmann pin from an acromioclavicular joint into the spinal canal. A case report. J Bone Joint Surg 47A:1024–1026, 1965.

142. Odenheimer, K., et al. Internal fixation of fracture of the head of the radius. Two case reports. J Bone Joint Surg 61A:785–787, 1979.

143. Oreck, S.L., Burgess, A., and Levine, A.M. Traumatic lateral displacement of the scapula: A radiographic sign of neurovascular disruption. J Bone Joint Surg 66A:758–763, 1984.

144. Osborne, G.B., and Cotterill, P. Recurrent dislocation of the elbow. J Bone Joint Surg 48B:340–346, 1966.

145. Packer, J.W., et al. The humeral fracture with radial nerve palsy: Is exploration warranted? Clin Orthop 88:34–38, 1972.

146. Patrick, J. Fracture of the medial epicondyle with displacement into the elbow joint. J Bone Joint Surg 28A:143–147, 1946.

147. Perkins, G. Fractures of the olecranon. Br Med J 2:668–669, 1936.

148. Philips, H. Complications of displaced fractures (type II Neer) of the outer end of the clavicle. J Bone Joint Surg 67B:492–493, 1985.

149. Pollack, F.H., et al. Treatment of radial neuropathy associated with fractures of the humerus. J Bone Joint Surg 63A:239–243, 1981.

150. Potter, C.M. Fracture-dislocation of the trochlea. J Bone Joint Surg 36B:250–253, 1954.

151. Pritchett, J.W. Delayed union of humeral shaft fractures treated by closed flexible intramedullary nailing. J Bone Joint Surg 57B:715–718, 1985.

152. Quigley, T.B. Aspiration of the elbow joint in the treatment of fractures of the head of the radius. N Engl J Med 240:915–916, 1949.

153. Rappaport, N.H., Clark, G.L., and Bora, W.J., Jr. Median nerve entrapment about the elbow. Adv Orthop Surg 8:270–275, 1985.

154. Rask, M.R., et al. Fracture of the acromion caused by muscle forces. J Bone Joint Surg 60A:1146–1147, 1978.

155. Rich, N.M., et al. Acute arterial injuries in Vietnam: 1000 cases. J Trauma 10:359–369, 1970.

156. Riseborough, E.J., and Radin, E.L. Intercondylar "T" fractures of the humerus in the adult: A comparison of operative and non-operative treatment in twenty-nine cases. J Bone Joint Surg 51A:130–140, 1969.

157. Rockwood, C.A., Jr. in Rockwood, C., and Green, D. (eds): Fractures in Adults, 2d ed. Philadelphia, Lippincott, 1984.

158. Rose, S.H., et al. Epidemiologic features of humeral fractures. Clin Orthop 168:24–30, 1982.

159. Rowe, C.R. An atlas of anatomy and treatment of mid clavicular fractures. Clin Orthop 58:29–42, 1968.

160. Rowe, C.R. Symposium on surgical lesions of the shoulder. J Bone Joint Surg 44A:977–978, 1962.

161. Rowe, C.R., and Cave, E.F. Fractures of the clavicle. Fractures and Other Injuries. Chicago Year Book, 1958.

162. St. Claire Strange, F.G. Entrapment of the median nerve after dislocation of the elbow. A case report. J Bone Joint Surg 64B:224–225, 1982.

163. Sarmiento, A., et al. Functional bracing of fractures of the shaft of the humerus. J Bone Joint Surg 59A:596–601, 1977.

164. Sarmiento, A., and Latta, L. Closed Functional Treatment of Fractures. Berlin, Springer-Verlag, 1981.

165. Schwab, G.M., Bennett, J.B., Woods, G.W., and Tollos, H.S. Biome-

chanics of elbow instability—The medial collateral ligament. Clin Orthop 50:7–15, 1967.

166. Schwab, G.M., et al. Biomechanics of elbow instability. The role of the medial collateral ligament. Clin Orthop 146:42–56, 1983.

167. Selesnick, F.H., Jablon, M., Frank, C., and Post, M. Retrosternal dislocation of the clavicle. J Bone Joint Surg 66A:287–291, 1984.

168. Shah, J.J., et al. Radial nerve paralysis associated with fractures of the humerus: A review of 62 cases. Clin Orthop 172:171–176, 1983.

169. Sharma, R.K., et al. An unusual ulnar nerve injury associated with dislocation of the elbow. Injury 8:145–147, 1976.

170. Shmueli, G., et al. Compression screwing of displaced fractures of the head of the radius. J Bone Joint Surg 63B:535–538, 1981.

171. Silver, J.R. Heterotopic ossification: A clinical study of its possible relationship to trauma. Paraplegia 7:220, 1969.

172. Smith, F.M. Surgery of the Elbow, 2d ed. Philadelphia, Saunders, 1972.

173. Smith, H., and Sage, F.P. Medullary fixation of forearm fractures. J Bone Joint Surg 39A:91–98, 1957.

174. Speed, J.S. Surgical treatment of condylar fractures of the humerus. Instr Course Lect 7:187–194, 1950.

175. Spielman, G. Disodium etidronate: Its role in preventing heterotopic ossification in severe head injury. Arch Phys Med Rehabil 64:539–542, 1983.

176. Spigelman, L. A harness for acromioclavicular separation. J Bone Joint Surg 51A:585–586, 1969.

177. Stableforth, P.G. Four part fractures of the neck of the humerus. J Bone Joint Surg 66C: 104–109, 1984.

178. Stephen, I.B. Excision of the radial head for closed fracture. Acta Orthop Scand 52:409–412, 1981.

179. Stern, P.J., Mattingly, D.A., et al. Intramedullary fixation of humeral shaft fractures. J Bone Joint Surg 66A:639–646, 1984.

180. Stimson, L.A. A Practical Treatise on Fractures and Dislocations. Philadelphia, Lea Brothers, 1900.

181. Strauss, R.H., et al. Injuries among wrestlers in school and college tournaments. JAMA 248:2016–2019, 1982.

182. Storm, J.T., et al. Brachial artery disruption following closed elbow dislocation. J Trauma 18(5):364–366, 1978.

182a. Taft, T.N., Wilson, F.C., and Oglesby, J.W. Dislocation of the acromioclavicular joint. J Bone Joint Surg 69A:1045–1051, 1987.

183. Varney, J.M., Coker, J.K., and Cawley, J.J. Treatment of acromioclavicular dislocation by means of a harness. J Bone Joint Surg 34A:232–233, 1952.

184. Vashchenko, A.E., et al. Migration of a metal bone pin from left clavicle into the liver. Klin Khir 9:63, 1983.

185. Waddell, J.P. Supracondylar fractures of the humerus. Techn Orthop 1:44–50, 1986.

185a. Warren-Smith, C.D., and Ward, M.W. Operation for acromioclavicular dislocation. J Bone Joint Surg 69B: 715–718, 1987.

186. Watson-Jones, R. Fractures and Joint Injuries, 4th ed. Edinburgh, Livingstone, 1955.

187. Weseley, M.S., et al. Closed treatment of isolated radial head fractures. J Trauma 23:36–39, 1983.

188. Wilkins, R.M., and Johnston, R.M. Ununited fractures of the clavicle. J Bone Joint Surg 65A:773–778, 1983.

189. Wilson, J.N. The treatment of fractures of the medial epicondyle of the humerus. J Bone Joint Surg 42B:778–781, 1960.

190. Young, T.V., and Wallace, W.A. Conservative treatment of fractures and fracture dislocations of the upper end of the humerus. J Bone Joint Surg 67B:373–377, 1985.

Section D: Glenohumeral Instability

1. Adams, F. The Genuine Works of Hippocrates. Baltimore, Williams & Wilkins, 1939.

2. Bateman, J.E. The diagnosis and treatment of ruptures of the rota-

tor cuff. Surg Clin North Am 46(6):1523–1530, 1963.

3. Bateman, J.E. *The Shoulder and Neck,* 2d ed. Philadelphia, Saunders, 1978.

4. Boyd, H.B., and Sisk, T.D. Recurrent posterior dislocation of the shoulder. J Bone Joint Surg 54A:779–786, 1972.

5. Breasted, J.H. *The Edwin Smith Surgical Papyrus.* Chicago, University of Chicago Press, 1930.

6. DuToit, G.T., and Roux, D. Recurrent dislocation of the shoulder. A twenty-four year study of the Johannesburg stapling operation. J Bone Joint Surg 38A:1–12, 1956.

7. Eden, R. Zur Operation der habituellen Schyulterluxation unter Mitteilung eines neuern Verfahrens bei Abriss am inneren Pfannenrande. Dtsch Z Chir 144:269–280, 1918.

8. Hall, R.H., Isaac, F., and Booth, C.B. Dislocations of the shoulder with special reference to accompanying small fractures. J Bone Joint Surg 41:489–494, 1959.

9. Hill, H.A., and Sachs, M.D. The grooved defect of the humeral head. A frequently unrecognized complication of dislocation of the shoulder joint. Radiology 35:690–700, 1940.

10. Hovelius, L, Akermark, C., Albrektsson, B., Berg, E., Korner, L., Lundberg, B., and Wredmark, T. Bristow-Latarjet procedure for recurrent anterior dislocation of the shoulder. A 2-5 year follow-up study on the results of 112 cases. Acta Orthop Scand 54:284–290, 1983.

11. Hovelius, L. Incidence of shoulder dislocation in Sweden. Clin Orthop 166:127–131, 1982.

12. Hovelius, L., Eriksson, K., Fredin, H., Hagberg, G., Weckstrom, J., and Thorling, J. Incidence and prognosis of shoulder dislocation. A preliminary communication. In Bayley, I., and Kessel, L. (eds): *Shoulder Surgery.* New York: Springer-Verlag, 1982, pp 73–75.

13. Hybbinette, S. De la transplantation d'un fragment osseux pour remedier aux luxations recidivantes de l'epaule. Constatations et resultats operatoires. Acta Chir Scand 71:411–445, 1932.

14. Inman, V.T., Saunders, J.B.DeC., and Abbot, L.C. Observations on the function of the shoulder joint. J Bone Joint Surg 26:1–30, 1944.

15. Magnuson, P.B. Treatment of recurrent dislocations of the shoulder. Surg Clin North Am 251:14–20, 1945.

16. Magnuson, P.B., and Stack, J.K. Recurrent dislocations of the shoulder. JAMA 123:889–892, 1943.

17. McLaughlin, H.L. Posterior dislocation of the shoulder. J Bone Joint Surg 34A:584–590, 1952.

18. Moseley, H.F. *Recurrent Dislocation of the Shoulder.* Montreal, McGill University Press, 1961.

19. Neer, C.S., and Rockwood, C.A., Fractures and dislocations of the shoulder, in Rockwood, C.A., and Green, D.P. (eds): *Fractures,* 2d ed. Philadelphia, Lippincott, 1984, 675–985.

20. Neer, C.S., and Foster, C.R. Inferior capsular shift for involuntary inferior and multidirectional instability of the shoulder. A preliminary report. J Bone Joint Surg 62A:897–908, 1980.

21. Norris, T.R., and Bigliani, L.U. Analysis of failed repair for shoulder instability. A preliminary report, in Bateman, J.E., and Welsh, R.P. *Surgery of the Shoulder.* Philadelphia, Decker, 1984, 111–116.

22. Osmond-Clarke, H. Habitual dislocation of the shoulder. The Putti-Platt operation. J Bone Joint Surg 30B:19–25, 1948.

23. Rockwood, C.A. Personal communication.

24. Rikous, J.R., Feagin, J.A., and Abbott, H.G. Modified axillary roentgenogram. A useful adjunct in the diagnosis of recurrent instability of the shoulder. Clin Orthop 82:84–86, 1972.

25. Rowe, C.R., and Zarins, B. Chronic unreduced dislocations of the shoulder. J Bone Joint Surg 64A:494–505, 1982.

26. Rowe, C.R., Patel, D., and Southmayd, W.W.: The Bankart procedure. A long-term end-result study. J Bone Joint Surg 60A:1–16, 1978.

27. Rowe, C.R. Prognosis in dislocations of the shoulder. J Bone Joint Surg 83A:957–977, 1956.

28. Saha, A.K. *Theory of Shoulder Mechanisms; Descriptive and Applied.* Springfield, IL, Thomas, 1961.

29. Samilson, R.L., and Prieto, V. Dislocation arthrography of the shoulder. J Bone Joint Surg 65A:456–460, 1983.

30. Stamm, T.T. Para-gleonid osteotomy. J Bone Joint Surg 44B:228, 1962.

31. Turkel, S.J. Panio, M.W., Marshall, J.L., and Girgis, F.G. Stabilizing mechanisms preventing anterior dislocation of the glenohumeral joint. J Bone Joint Surg 63A:1208–1217, 1981.

32. Weber, B.G., Simpson, L.A., and Hardegger, F. Rotational humeral osteotomy for recurrent anterior dislocation of the shoulder associated with a large Hill-Sachs lesion. J Bone Joint Surg 66A:1443–1450, 1984.

33. Zuckerman, J.D. Matsen, F.A. Complications about the glenohumeral joint related to the use of screws and staples. J Bone Joint Surg 66A:175–180, 1984.

CHAPTER 36

Fractures and Dislocations of the Upper Extremity in Children

Stuart B. Polisner

FRACTURES OF THE DISTAL RADIUS AND ULNA

The radius is the most commonly fractured bone in the child.[9] Three-quarters or more of these fractures involve the distal third because of the relative weakness of the distal radial metaphyseal bone.[12,64]

These fractures differ from their adult counterpart in that they are rarely intraarticular. Additionally, they usually do not show the radial collapse or radioulnar joint dysfunction that often results from similar adult fractures.[64]

Osteological Characteristics

The distal radial epiphysis ossifies at 1 to 2 years and fuses at 16 to 18 years of age. The distal ulnar epiphysis ossifies at 5 to 7 years and fuses at 16 to 18 years of age.[55] Seventy-five percent of the radial and 80 percent of the ulnar longitudinal growth occurs at the distal end.[73]

Mechanism

The mechanism of injury is generally a fall on the outstretched hand with the wrist dorsiflexed.[8] Occasionally, the wrist is palmarflexed upon impact.[12,80]

Clinical Features

Nondisplaced torus or greenstick fractures exhibit tenderness over three-fourths the circumference of the distal radial metaphysis. Swelling is usually present, but it may be minimal. Displaced epiphyseal fractures are obvious and usually appear as a "silver fork" deformity, which may simulate a wrist dislocation. The skin should be carefully inspected for puncture wounds which may communicate with the fracture. The neurovascular status should be assessed, and documented prior to treatment.[64]

Radiological Characteristics

Subtle fractures may be difficult to diagnose. Soft tissue (pronator quadratus) fat pad swelling may be the only obvious radiological finding.[19] Torus fractures appear as a cortical bulge, often visible on only one x-ray view. Greenstick fractures may also reveal a mild cortical angulation on one view only. The x-ray views in undisplaced physeal fractures may demonstrate only a mild, asymmetrical widening of the physis (Fig. 36-1). If in doubt, oblique views and/or comparison x-ray views of the opposite wrist should be taken.

Treatment

Nondisplaced or nonangulated fractures are treated in a well-molded short arm cast for 6 weeks in teenagers (less in younger children). With infants, obese forearms, or potentially unstable fractures, a cast extending above the elbow is preferable.[41,65]

Fractures with an unacceptable degree of angulation (see Complications, below) are treated by closed reduction. Hematoma infiltration anesthesia is usually adequate. If one elects to break the intact cortex, controlled force is used to avoid displacement of the fragments.[64] If the displacement of the epiphysis is in a pronated position, it should be splinted in supination after reduction. Usually the converse is the case.

Displaced (overriding) fractures are treated by closed reduction, usually under general anesthesia with muscle relaxation. Gentle traction is applied while the deformity is exaggerated to hook the ends together.[64,65,72] When end-to-end contact is established, angulation can then be readily corrected. Displacement of less than 50 percent is acceptable. More should be reduced or the fracture will be prone to redisplacement. Somewhat more latitude is permissible in the child under 5 years of age, in whom general anesthesia is unwise and remodeling will occur.

Epiphyseal displacement should be reduced by applying gentle traction and then realigning the fragment utilizing thumb pressure to correct the dorsal displacement. Pronation of the fragment is helpful. A long arm cast in some pronation and mild wrist flexion with good three-point molding is indicated for 2 to 3 weeks followed by a short arm cast until the fracture is healed. Undisplaced physeal fractures are protected in a short arm cast until united.

Open reduction is rarely indicated. Occasional case reports of irreducible fractures have involved interposition of tendons (e.g., extensor pollicis longus)[85] and buttonholing of the distal radial metaphysis through the volar wrist supports.[54] These special fractures required open reduction and internal fixation.

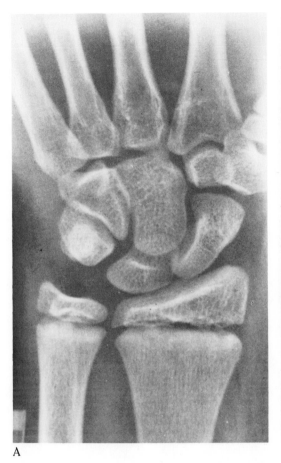
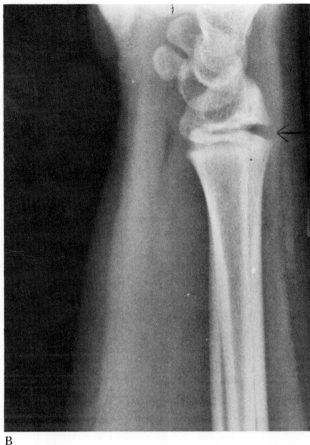

A   B

Figure 36-1 A. Anteroposterior x-ray view of a Salter I injury to the distal radial physis, which appears normal on this projection. The patient had pain, moderate swelling of the wrist, and ring tenderness over the distal radial physis. **B.** Widening of the dorsal aspect of the distal radial physis (*arrow*) on this lateral projection confirms the clinical diagnosis of a Salter I injury.

Complications

Strength and motion are usually restored with simple rehabilitation. Growth disturbances are rare.[87] Deformity in the plane of motion of the wrist joint usually remodels completely if less than 45 degrees in very young children, less than 30 degrees in prepubertal children,[87] and less than 15 degrees in growing teenagers.[65] Fractures of the distal radius correct at approximately 1 degree per month, or about 10 degrees per year as a result of epiphyseal realignment during growth. Radial or ulnar angulation has less remodeling capacity. Rotational deformities have little or no remodeling potential.[30,31,32] In summary, the younger the child and the closer the fracture to the physis, the greater the remodeling capacity.

FRACTURES OF THE RADIAL AND ULNAR SHAFTS

Mechanism

The mechanism of injury is usually a fall on the outstretched hand[48] often with a rotatory component. Direct contusion is a less common cause.[90] Propagation of diaphyseal fractures requires greater force than propagation of metaphyseal or physeal fractures.

Clinical Features

There is usually considerable pain and swelling. Clinical deformity is usually obvious. Undisplaced fractures, and those fractures caused by plastic deformation (bowing), may go undiagnosed.[48]

Radiological Characteristics

Care should be taken to assess the fracture site, as well as the adjacent joints. Ipsilateral fractures of the distal end of radius and ulna, or of the navicular, may be overlooked.[48,65]

The bicipital tuberosity reveals the rotational alignment of the proximal radius, while the distal radius can be assessed clinically or radiographically.[65,72] Dissimilar shapes and diameters of opposing bone ends suggest rotational malalignment.[48]

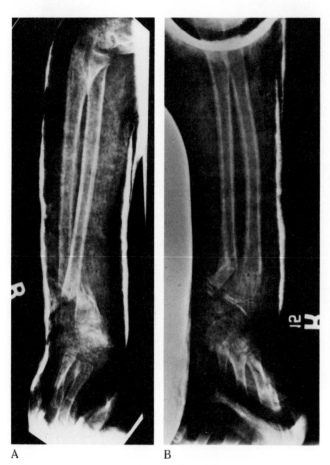
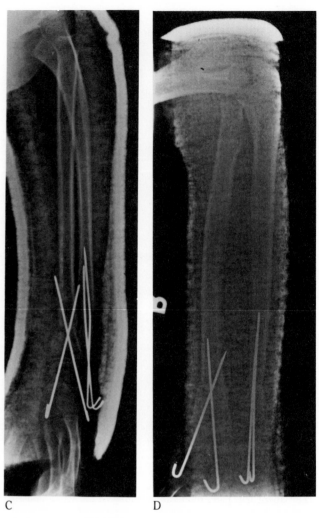

A   B   C   D

Figure 36-2 A and **B.** This 10-year-old patient was referred 3 weeks after reduction with fracture of both bones of the forearm. There is considerable volar displacement, and ulnar angulation exceeds 20 degrees. **C** and **D.** Additional closed manipulation at this stage was not indicated. Open reduction and percutaneous pinning maintained alignment, the pins being removed at 3 weeks. A cast was applied for a total of 6 weeks. Excellent forearm rotation was restored.

Treatment

Cosmesis and function are both important. Functional recovery includes full restoration of wrist and elbow motion, forearm rotation, and upper extremity strength.

Nondisplaced greenstick fractures require a well-molded long arm cast until healed. When firm, but cautious manipulation is used, the angulated greenstick fractures can be corrected without separating the remaining intact cortex and rendering the fracture unstable.[18,48,70,84] The cast must be applied with good three-point molding to prevent reangulation. The elbow is maintained at 90 degrees and the forearm supinated if the angulation is dorsal, or pronated if volar.

Complete fractures (overriding) require gentle traction and exaggeration of the deformity to hook the ends; then correction of the angulation and rotation is attempted. The distal fragments are rotated to match the rotation of the proximal fragments.[29,48] Adequate anesthesia with relaxation of the patient is essential. The normal radial curve must be maintained (the ulna is relatively straight) to provide forearm shape and rotation. Casts with a flat ulnar border avoid gravitational sag of the ulna.

In prepubertal children, bayoneted positioning is compatible with a satisfactory result, as long as alignment and rotation are normal[72] and the interosseous space is maintained on at least one view.[29] Adolescents, with little or no remaining growth, will lose some forearm rotation unless reduction is excellent. Weekly follow-ups with radiographs and excellent cast maintenance are necessary for this extremely unstable fracture.

If acceptable reduction is not achieved or maintained, open reduction and internal fixation are recommended in patients over the age of 10 years. Closed methods resulting in more than 10 degrees of malalignment will probably result in

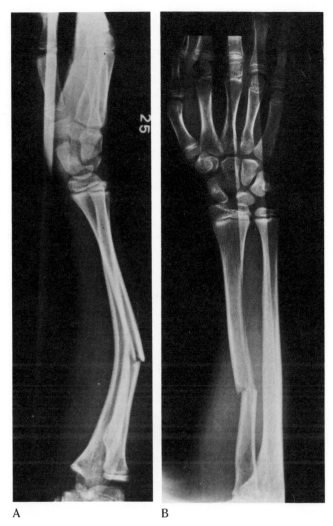

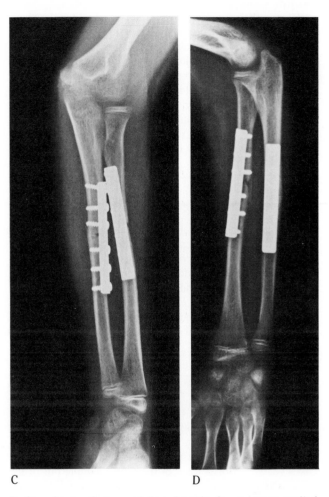

A B C D

Figure 36-3 A and **B.** Plastic deformation of the ulna associated with midshaft fracture of the radius in a 10-year-old. Note that ulna looks straight on the oblique AP view (B), but the radial fragments are rotated and the interosseous space is lost. **C** and

D. Closed osteoclasis consisting of gentle slow pressure applied for several minutes did not correct bowing. Open osteotomy and internal fixation were required.

significant loss of forearm rotation in patients beyond prepuberty (Fig. 36-2). There is a high incidence of failure of closed treatment beyond that age.[45]

In a heavily contaminated open fracture or in the presence of severe soft tissue loss, the external fixator is an alternative. When early stabilizing callus is present, the fixator may be removed and replaced with a well-molded long arm cast until healed. Recently, Amit et al presented a preliminary report on the successful use of closed intramedullary nailing of this fracture in adolescents[4]

SPECIAL TYPES OF FOREARM FRACTURES

Plastic Deformation

These "bent bones" without cortical buckling or obvious fracture only occur in prepubertal children and are often overlooked. Occasionally only one bone bows, the other bone

of the forearm remaining perfectly straight, or alternatively the accompanying bone is fractured (or the radial head dislocates).

The mechanism of injury is a fall creating a slowly applied, low-energy force causing the bone to bend beyond its elastic limits.[48] The force terminates prior to the propagation of a fracture line, resulting in an abnormally curved bone which deforms the forearm (Fig. 36-3).

Pain, tenderness, and subtle deformity of the forearm are typically present. Pronation and supination may be limited by pain or degree of deformity. Swelling may be minimal.

If one is in doubt, comparison views of the opposite forearm in the same rotation are helpful. X-ray views should include the elbow and wrist to rule out associated injuries. A positive bone scan differentiates an acute bowing from residual deformation following previous injury.[56] During healing, periosteal reaction may be minimal or absent. At 4 to 6 weeks, cortical thickening may be evident on the concavity of the bowed bone.

If the deformity is obvious or if there is restriction of forearm rotation, reduction is indicated. With the patient under anesthesia, a corrective force is applied progressively over several minutes, preferably over a firm fulcrum. Children under 4 years of age usually spontaneously remodel mild to moderate degrees of bowing.[74] Parents should be forewarned that fracturing the bone may be necessary in order to achieve a reduction. In older children osteotomy may rarely be required (Fig. 36-3). Usually correction can be achieved by osteotomizing at one level only, at the point of maximal bowing. A small wedge of bone is removed to correct the angulation, and internal fixation may be necessary.

Monteggia's Fracture-Dislocation

The lesion, described in 1814 by Monteggia, is a proximal ulnar fracture with an associated radial head dislocation.[72] The classification is described in the section on adult fractures. In children the Bado type I injury is most common.[28] Also a "Monteggia equivalent" injury has been reported in children; it consists of a proximal ulnar fracture associated with a lateral humeral condylar fracture.[74] Another equivalent consists of anterior radial head dislocation and plastic bowing of the ulna.

Treatment

If the ulnar fracture is transverse, closed reduction and above-elbow casting in the position of radial head stability is sufficient. Open reduction is necessary for oblique fractures which are unstable with plate or K-wire fixation.[28] In late cases corrective osteotomy of the ulna, cleaning out of the radial notch, annular ligament reconstruction, and K-wire stabilization of the radiocapitellar joint may be necessary.[28]

Galeazzi Lesion

The Galeazzi lesion is a fracture of the distal shaft of the radius with a dislocation of the distal radioulnar joint.

In young children, these fractures can generally be treated by closed reduction and casting, while open reduction is required in older teenagers and adults (see Chap. 34, Sect. A).[28]

Complications of Children's Forearm Fractures

Malunion of fractures is unfortunately a common complication. With adequate immobilization, and avoidance of rotational or angular malalignment, union may be expected without functional loss.[45] Refracture of both bones at the same site is common (7 percent) during the first 6 months after fracture.[90] Nerve injuries have been reported and are usually transitory. Compartment syndromes may occur and must be diagnosed and treated immediately.

FRACTURES OF THE PROXIMAL RADIUS

Fractures of the proximal radius usually involve the radial neck at the physis but may be greenstick fractures through the metaphysis in very young children. Several patterns are possible (Salter types I to IV), but a type II Salter fracture is most common.[95] Related fractures occur simultaneously about the elbow in 50 percent of cases.[72]

Osteological Characteristics

The proximal radial epiphysis ossifies at 4 to 5 years and fuses at 14 to 15 (female) and 15 to 17 (male) years of age. The proximal ulnar apophysis appears in the eighth to tenth and fuses at about 12 to 14 (female) and 14 to 15 (male) years of age.[88]

Mechanism

The mechanism of injury is generally a valgus force to the elbow, creating a radiocapitellar impaction. The resulting deformity of the head may be angulation or displacement. With this mechanism it tilts laterally and displaces outward. In another mechanism a posterior subluxation of the elbow occurs and then reduces, leaving the radial epiphysis behind the capitellum, often with a 90-degree backward tilt. Some fractures occur in association with other injuries such as damage to the medial collateral ligament of the elbow or medial humeral condyle. The whole injury and its mechanism must be carefully evaluated.

Clinical Features

Nondisplaced fractures are often diagnosed and treated late. The parents may be unimpressed with the appearance of the arm, or the magnitude of the complaints, and the pain is often referred to the wrist. Proximal radial pain is elicited while gently pronating and supinating the forearm or during active wrist dorsiflexion.

Radiological Characteristics

X-ray views should include the entire elbow, forearm, and wrist to rule out associated fractures and dislocations. Oblique and/or comparison views are often helpful in diagnosing undisplaced fractures.[34] When the radial head is nonossified, the only radiographic sign may be irregularity of the adjacent metaphyseal border.[63] If a displaced, unossified radial head fracture is suspected, an arthrogram using a few drops of dye may be indicated. Magnetic resonance imaging may prove useful in difficult cases.

Treatment

When the appropriate treatment is selected, the degree and type of displacement, presence of associated injuries, age of the patient, and time elapsed from injury should be taken into consideration.[63,82,92,95]

A long arm cast is adequate for most nondisplaced or nonangulated fractures. Slings, collar cuffs, and posterior splints are usually inadequate for immobilization in children.

Manipulative closed reduction is indicated for angulated (or translocated) fractures.[82] Although untreated fractures angulated up to 45 to 60 degrees will generally remodel to a remarkable degree in the prepubertal child,[12,93] angulations over 30 degrees should be manipulatively corrected.[65,95] Manipulative technique is based on application of a varus stress to open the lateral side of the joint. The forearm is pronated and supinated to palpate the radial head at its maximum prominence, and then digital pressure is applied to the radial head. A well-molded long arm cast is applied with the elbow at 90 degrees. The amount of pronation or supination is determined by the position of stability and the radiographic appearance of the radiocapitellar joint. When in doubt, one uses moderate pronation as this is the motion that is generally lost after healing.·

Open reduction is required for completely displaced fractures or when closed reduction is considered inadequate. Internal fixation can be avoided if a stable reduction is obtained. When required, oblique K wires which do not cross the radiocapitellar joint should be used.

Complications

Radial head excision should be avoided in growing children since complications include stiffness, proximal radioulnar synostosis, cubitus valgus, and distal radioulnar joint derangement.[65,82,93,95]

Other complications following this injury include growth abnormalities such as overgrowth or premature physeal closure. Posterior interosseous nerve palsy may follow use of K wire. Pin breakage or migration may follow use of radiohumeral transfixion wires to maintain reduction. Heterotopic calcification, myositis ossificans, and proximal radioulnar synostosis, have also been reported.

FRACTURES OF THE PROXIMAL ULNA

Fractures of the proximal ulna are extremely rare in isolation. They are usually associated with other fractures or dislocations at the elbow.

Osteological Characteristics

The proximal ulnar apophysis appears in the eighth to tenth year and fuses at 14 to 15 (female) and 15 to 17 (male) years of age.

Mechanism

The mechanisms of injury are direct trauma to the point of the elbow, and indirect forces that occur during a fall on the hand with the elbow extended.

Classification

Apophyseal fractures (Fig. 36-4) are rare since the triceps expansion protects this area, attaching distally beyond the apophysis. A Salter type II physeal separation may occur and not be visible radiographically before 10 years of age. Careful palpation may reveal the metaphyseal irregularity. The fracture line may extend through the cartilage of the proximal ulna so that the coronoid is also part of the proximal fragment.

The varieties of *metaphyseal* fracture depend on elbow position at injury.

In flexion, the triceps posteriorly and the brachialis anteriorly apply tension, while the distal humerus is the fulcrum over which the ulna breaks.

In extension, if an abduction or adduction force occurs with the olecranon locked in its humeral fossa, the proximal ulna may fail. With associated valgus stress, this olecranon fracture is associated with a radial neck or medial humeral epicondylar fracture. With varus stress in extension, an olecranon fracture occurs with radial head displacement.[95] The olecranon fracture is commonly an angulated greenstick fracture.

Coronoid fractures are rare in children. They are usually associated with elbow dislocations and are thus seen in older children. As an isolated fracture, they occur as a result of an avulsion of the brachialis tendon. Radiographically, the radial head may overlay the coronoid process, necessitating oblique views for diagnosis.

Clinical Features

Physical examination reveals a palpable olecranon gap if displacement has occurred. Extension may be weak or absent if the triceps tendon is injured or interrupted.

Radiological Characteristics

Associated elbow fractures and dislocations must be ruled out. Oblique x-ray and comparison views of the opposite elbow are helpful. When the olecranon apophysis is nonossified (before age 10 years), the diagnosis must be made clinically. A small metaphyseal spike may be palpable.

Treatment

Apophyseal fractures, if undisplaced or mildly displaced, are immobilized in a long arm cast in moderate extension (30 to

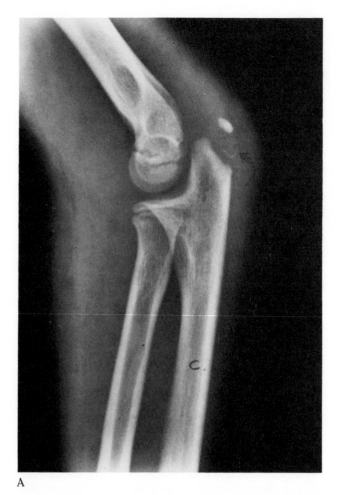

A

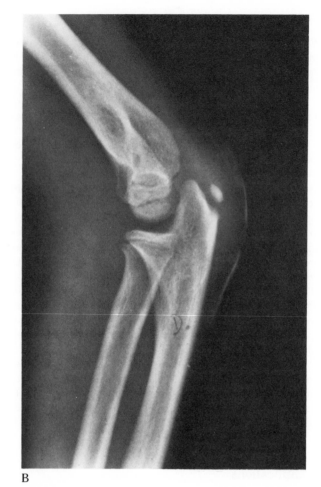

B

Figure 36-4 A. A young boy fell with his elbow extended and sustained an avulsion fracture of the olecranon apophysis. Despite some proximal displacement, triceps function remained intact. Note metaphyseal flake (*arrow*). **B.** The fracture was reduced by extension of the elbow with direct thumb pressure. A long arm cast was then applied with the elbow in mild flexion. A pressure pad was used over the tip of the olecranon within the cast.

45 degrees) to avoid triceps or capsular tension. If the fracture is displaced significantly, open reduction and internal fixation with axial pins and compression wires are indicated.

Metaphyseal fractures are treated with consideration given to the mechanism of injury. Flexion at the fracture reduces any greenstick angulation caused by hyperextension. Varus or valgus angulation is corrected by manipulation with the elbow in full extension locking the olecranon. Varus deformity and radial head dislocation have a tendency to recur, and close observation and follow-up are necessary. With moderate or no displacement, a well-molded long arm cast is applied with elbow flexion of no more than 60 degrees. Displacement of more than 2 mm at the joint surface requires open reduction and internal fixation. Repair of the aponeurosis and tension banding are sufficient to maintain reduction. Crossing the physis with fixation pins should be avoided.

Coronoid fractures are immobilized in a long arm cast with the arm at 90 degrees. This fracture may indicate the presence of a spontaneously reduced elbow dislocation. Careful watch for heterotopic new bone is indicated, and rehabilitation should be gentle and unhurried.

DISLOCATION OF THE ELBOW

Elbow dislocation is a common injury in children. Children rarely develop a pure dislocation of the elbow or radial head without an associated fracture. Most common is a fracture of the medial epicondyle, which may become entrapped in the joint, blocking reduction.

Classification

The most common mechanism of injury is a valgus force in extension. This disrupts the medial collateral ligament or avulses the medial epicondyle, permitting valgus angulation. Posterior dislocation then occurs, the forearm bones usually being displaced posterolaterally. There is associated stripping of the capsule from the posterior distal humerus.[61] Occasionally the elbow is disrupted by a varus or medial displacement force and the forearm bones lie posteromedially. In both types the lateral ligament complex and medial collateral ligament are disrupted.

Anterior dislocation is unusual but can occur and is associated with the highest incidence of complications. Dislocation of the elbow joint can occur associated with disruption of the superior radioulnar joint ("divergent" type).

Clinical Features

The elbow is held semiflexed. With posterior dislocation there is an undue prominence of the olecranon.[65] The dislocation is then obvious. Prior to radiological evaluation this may be confused with a displaced supracondylar fracture, especially when there is considerable swelling.

Radiological Characteristics

Pre- and postreduction x-ray views should be closely examined for associated avulsion fractures and fragments which have become trapped in the joint.[27,70] Increased joint space indicates probable interposed fragments.

These dislocations should be considered unstable, and weekly x-ray films should be taken for the first month to confirm reduction. The radial head must oppose the capitellum on all views, or subluxation is present (Fig. 36-16B and E).[53,68]

Treatment

Most elbow dislocations can be reduced closed with adequate anesthesia and relaxation. Reduction should be performed expeditiously to avoid vascular compromise. Open reduction may be required because of fragment entrapment or continuing instability.

Posterior dislocations are reduced by applying gentle traction with the forearm supinated, avoiding full extension, which may cause further soft tissue injury anteriorly. Digital pressure over the posterior olecranon may be added to help direct the ulna anteriorly onto the humerus, while distal humeral pressure is directed posteriorly. Finally, pronation and supination may assist in and confirm location of the radial head. Following reduction the elbow should be casted in flexion at 100 degrees.[70]

Anterior dislocations have the highest incidence of complications. Reduction is by flexing the elbow, applying gentle traction, and using the forearm as a lever to posteriorly reduce the proximal radius and ulna. Posterior support under the distal humerus is helpful. Postreduction immobilization is at minimal flexion (approximately 45 degrees) since this is a flexion injury.

True medial or lateral dislocations are extremely rare in children. Longitudinal traction is utilized to dislodge the proximal radius and ulna while regaining proper length. Medial or lateral force is then applied to restore proper positions. Correction is maintained by careful molding in the cast with the elbow at 90 degrees.

Divergent dislocations are also extremely rare in children. Reduction is effected by longitudinal traction on the semiextended elbow, correcting the divergence by gentle compression. The position is held with cast molding and the elbow at 90 degrees. Open reduction and internal fixation may be required.[16]

Meticulous casting techniques with close follow-up is important in order to maintain the reduction. The elbow is usually immobilized for 3 to 4 weeks, but a recent study has recommended a shorter period of immobilization.[16]

Complications[17,26,44,70,71,72,95]

Vascular injuries are uncommon in children. Recurrent dislocation is quite rare. Neurological injuries are common (particularly of the ulnar nerve). Myositis ossificans is fortunately uncommon but is a disastrous complication. Over enthusiastic physiotherapy and particularly manipulation and passive motion are traditionally thought to contribute in some cases. Such prescriptions are best avoided. Residual stiffness or posterior blocking of full extension by heterotopic new bone often improves dramatically with time and *gentle*, but active, use.

ISOLATED DISLOCATION OF THE RADIAL HEAD

Isolated dislocation of the radial head in children is uncommon, especially in those over the age of 10 years. The traumatic dislocation in children is usually anterior (Fig. 36-5).

Mechanism

The usual mode of injury is a fall on the outstretched hand with the forearm locked in pronation. Occasionally isolated radial head dislocation is produced by a direct blow to the proximal forearm. The common mechanism is believed to be similar to that which occurs during Monteggia's fracture-dislocation.[36] The anatomical studies of Wiley led him to believe that the annular ligament is the most important structure torn in isolated dislocations of the radial head.[94] There may be occult plastic deformation of the ulna, and some cases of "congenital" radial head dislocation are possibly sequelae of injuries overlooked in early childhood.

Clinical Features

Localized swelling and tenderness over the anterior or posterolateral aspect of the elbow are present depending on the direction of dislocation. Elbow motion may be limited, especially rotation of the forearm. The radial head may be palpable in the antecubital space in cases of anterior dislocation.

Radiological Characteristics

In the absence of an obvious fracture line, a radial head dislocation may easily be missed. A line through the radial shaft should normally pass through the capitellum on every x-ray

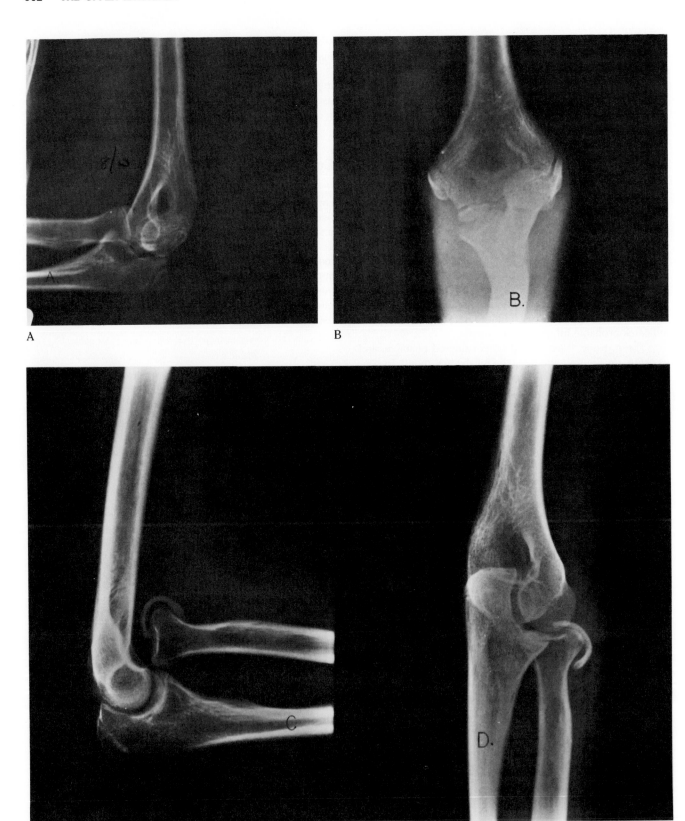

A

B

C

D

Figure 36-5 Anterior radial head dislocation in an 11-year-old girl who sustained a direct blow to the posterior aspect of the upper forearm and elbow. **A** and **B.** Anterior dislocation of the radial head was overlooked on these initial radiographs. If the radiocapitellar line were to be drawn through the radial shaft, it would cross superior to the capitellum. The patient was not seen by an orthopaedist until several months later and was minimally symptomatic. **C** and **D.** At 2 years after injury, the patient remained only mildly symptomatic. Note the ringlike calcification of the soft tissues overlying the dislocated radial head.

view.[53,68] If this radiocapitellar line is disrupted, a subluxation or dislocation of the radial head is present (Figs. 36-5C and D, and 36-16E). An associated occult fracture of the proximal ulna may not be apparent until healing callus is detected 2 to 3 weeks later.

Treatment

Acute anterior dislocation of the radial head is generally reducible by supination of the forearm with traction on the extended elbow. Downward (anterior to posterior) pressure against the radial head will assist a difficult reduction. The elbow should then be immobilized with the elbow flexed slightly less than 90 degrees, and the forearm supinated. In cases where treatment is delayed a week or more, open reduction is indicated if closed reduction fails. Open reduction is worth the attempt even late, at 6 to 8 weeks, but then annular ligament reconstruction may be required.

Complications

If the dislocation is untreated, restriction of joint motion may result, but often there is little functional loss. In preadolescents, shortening of the radial side of the forearm may occur, with distal radioulnar joint distortion. The anteriorly displaced radial head may articulate with the distal humerus creating a localized pseudarthrosis (Fig. 36-5C and D).

PULLED ELBOW

Pulled elbow, nursemaid's elbow, radiocapitellar subluxation, subluxation of radial head, and *temper tantrum elbow* are among 18 names for this entity as listed by Salter and Zaltz in 1971.[81] It is probably the commonest musculoskeletal injury in children under 5 years of age. It is found more commonly in boys and more often affects the left elbow.

Mechanism

The mechanism of injury is forcible traction on the pronated hand or wrist with the relaxed elbow extended. Frequently, the traction force occurs when the child suddenly decides to pull away from the parents or drop to the ground. Often a click or snap may be felt or heard.

Pathological Characteristics

Salter and Zaltz found experimentally that if traction is applied to a pronated forearm with the elbow extended, a transverse tear of the distal attachment of the annular ligament results, allowing partial escape of the radial head.[81] Subluxation of the radial head occurs only in pronation, which is the position where the diameter of the radial head is the narrowest in the anteroposterior plane. Supination of the forearm with some flexion of the elbow allows instantaneous reduction of the radial head.

Clinical Features

The child may be tearful, and the arm hangs limply with the elbow extended and the forearm pronated. Pain, if vocalized, is referred toward the wrist. There is tenderness over the radial head but no obvious swelling or deformity. Mild flexion and extension are painless, but supination is resisted.

Radiological Characteristics

X-ray studies are invariably negative but should still be obtained to rule out fracture or other abnormality.

Treatment

Frequently, pulled elbow reduces spontaneously when the elbow is placed in a sling, or when the x-ray technician attempts to position the forearm in extension. Reduction is accomplished by firmly supinating the forearm, applying downward (anterior to posterior) radial head pressure, then flexing the elbow to slightly beyond 90 degrees. If reduction is successful, within a few minutes when the child's confidence returns, full elbow motion and forearm rotation are present. In older children (e.g., 3 to 5 years), or when the elbow has been subluxed for many hours, a sling or cast should be applied in the position noted above for several days since all the discomfort will not immediately resolve. In a rare resistant case, the child does not respond in the predicted manner. Usually spontaneous reduction occurs within a few days, however, without further intervention.

In cases of recurrent subluxations, a splint or cast may be used for several weeks to encourage stability. The parents should be counseled to avoid longitudinal traction strains on the child's arms by not pulling on the hand or wrist.

Regardless of the number of recurrences, the ability to subluxate usually disappears by 5 or 6 years of age, leaving a normal elbow.[70] One may suspect an occult cartilaginous or bony fracture if the history, physical examination, or response to treatment is not typical.

SUPRACONDYLAR FRACTURES OF THE HUMERUS

A supracondylar fracture propagates transversely across the thin region of metaphysis proximal to the distal humeral transverse physis. Commonly occurring between 3 and 10 years of age, these troublesome fractures constitute 50 to 60 percent of children's elbow injuries.[65]

Mechanism

The mechanism of injury is a fall on the outstretched hand with transmission of indirect force to the distal humerus. Most commonly, since the elbow is in extension, the distal humeral fragment angulates or displaces posteriorly, with varying degrees of posterior tilt or displacement. Depending on the precise nature of the injury, there may be a pure exten-

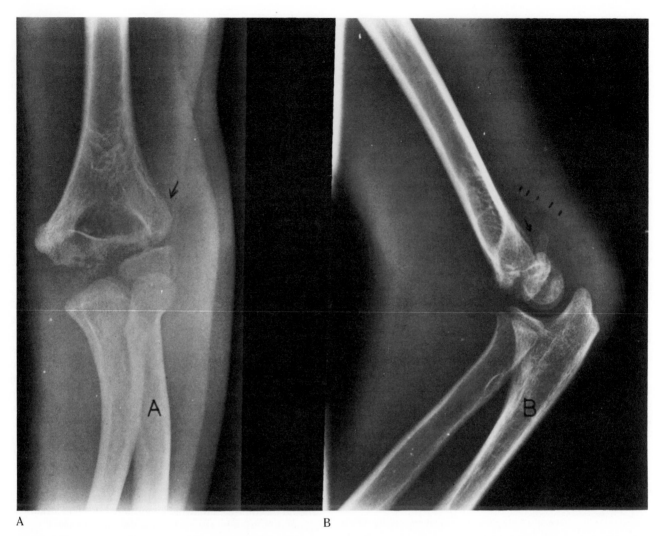

A   B

Figure 36-6 A and **B.** Mildly displaced extension type of supra-condylar fracture of the humerus. The humerotrochlear angle is reversed on the lateral view (*B*) (compare Fig. 36-7*A*). A large intraarticular effusion is present with a markedly enlarged poste-rior fat pad sign (*arrow*). A closed reduction with the elbow im-mobilized in 110 degrees of flexion restored the normal anterior inclination of the condyles.

sion deformity or alternatively associated abduction or ad-duction of the fragment. There is also the possibility of rota-tional deformity. The adducted fragments (posteromedial fracture pattern) are sometimes internally rotated, and ab-ducted fragments (posterolateral fracture pattern) are often externally rotated. If the elbow is in flexion, the distal humeral fragment angulates or displaces anteriorly. This uncommon type of supracondylar fracture may also have associated rota-tional or tilt deformity of the fragment, but usually neurovas-cular injury does not occur.

Classification

One may describe these injuries as being of the flexion or extension category. The extension fractures may be further subdivided into those showing a posterolateral fracture pat-tern and those with a posteromedial fracture pattern. Alterna-tively one may speak of type 1 (undisplaced), type 2 (angu-lated but with one intact cortex), or type 3 (completely displaced) fractures.

Clinical Features

If posteriorly displaced, there is an S-shaped or zigzag de-formity when viewed from the side, or in the lateral projec-tion. The anterior prominence represents the distal end of the humeral shaft. If this anterior spike approaches the skin, ec-chymosis appears in the antecubital space. An antecubital wound infers puncture by the distal humerus, and an open fracture. A dimple or puckering in the antecubital space in-dicates that the humeral shaft has penetrated the anterior compartment musculature and lies beneath the skin. These fractures are difficult to reduce closed.[65]

Swelling depends upon the severity of the displacement and the time elapsed between injury and presentation. The

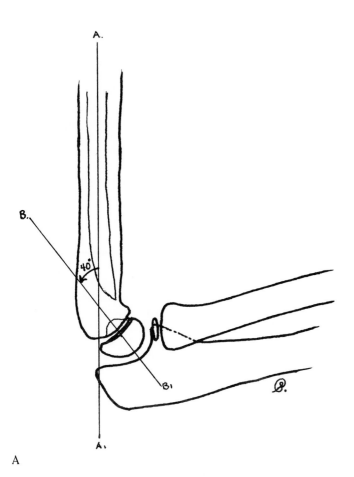

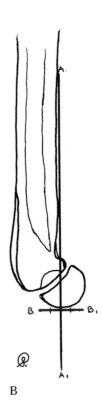

A

B

Figure 36-7 A. The humerotrochlear angle (more appropriately termed the condylar-humeral angle) is the angle formed between the longitudinal axis of the humerus (A–A1) and the axis of the condyles on the lateral x-ray via (B–B1). **B.** Anterior humeral line (AHL) is drawn along the anterior surface of the distal humerus (A–A1) extending through the capitellum. Another line (B–B1) is drawn perpendicular to AHL from the posterior to the anterior margin of the capitellum. This line is divided into thirds. AHL should normally pass through the middle third of the capitellum.

neurovascular status must be well documented prior to treatment. Also, associated fractures in the ipsilateral extremity must be ruled out before electing a plan of treatment.

A supracondylar fracture may be clinically differentiated from an elbow dislocation. An equilateral triangle, posteriorly, is formed between the tip of the olecranon and the humeral epicondyles. Following a supracondylar fracture, this triangle of relations is preserved.

Radiological Characteristics

In addition to standard views, oblique and comparison views may be required for full understanding of a fracture. A positive posterior "fat pad sign" on a true lateral x-ray view suggests the presence of a fracture in a child (Fig. 36-6B). Careful assessment of the mechanism and the nature of any tilt, rotation, or displacement is essential prior to reduction. Adequacy of reduction should be evaluated by measurement. The humerotrochlear angle and Baumann's angle (Figs. 36-6, 36-7, and 36-8) are recorded. The latter, which is around 15 degrees, varies with sex. It is related to, but not equal to, the carrying angle.[97] The angle is a good predictor of final carrying angle.[97] It is also useful to compare the member with the opposite elbow. However, care must be taken to align the x-ray tube not more than 10 degrees off the axis of the forearm, at right angles to the axis of the humerus and not tipped caudally.[98]

Treatment

Undisplaced fractures require a well-molded long arm cast with balancing collar and cuff, or a sling. Although some authors still recommend posterior splints,[42] the author has found them unreliable in children. Any complete cast above the elbow in a fresh injury must, however, be used with utmost care to avoid circulatory embarrassment, and it is prudent to widely monovalve (or bivalve) it down to skin. Antecubital pressure must be avoided.

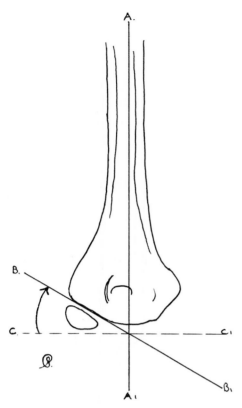

Figure 36-8 Baumann's angle. This measurement, which is obtained from an anteroposterior radiograph of the distal humerus, allows the determination of the alignment of a supracondylar fragment to the humeral shaft. Measurement of Baumann's angle of the injured elbow must be compared with that of the normal elbow in order to determine the exact degree of cubitus varus (or valgus). Baumann's angle is formed by a line (C–C1) perpendicular to the humeral shaft and a line parallel to the physis of the lateral condyle (B–B1).

Manipulative Reduction

Mild amounts of sagittal plane angulation (Fig. 36-6) have been reported to correct themselves during growth and remodeling but are nevertheless best corrected initially.[42] Severe posterior displacement (Fig. 36-9) requires a logical approach to treatment with attention to basic principles: (1) reduction must be adequate, (2) position must be maintained, and (3) neurovascular status must be closely observed for possible compromise. Reduction involves gradual gentle longitudinal traction with the elbow extended, while mildly exaggerating the deformity to hook the bone ends together. Posterior thumb pressure is applied to push the distal fragment anteriorly until hitched, and then the reduction is stabilized by gradually flexing the elbow. An assistant holding a posteriorly directed force against the distal shaft is helpful. Medial or lateral displacement and rotation are then corrected. The elbow is flexed to 90 or 100 degrees (providing circulation remains adequate) and the cast applied. The forearm is maintained in the pronated position if the distal fragment is displaced medially, or it is supinated if the distal fragment is displaced laterally.[95] Forearm position maintains tension on

the elbow ligaments and any intact periosteal hinge to maintain reduction and is therefore very important.

Anterior displacement, due to a flexion-type injury, is generally easier to reduce. Traction is applied in a 90 degree flexed position while using the forearm as a lever to push the distal fragment posteriorly. Thumb pressure may be assist in reduction. Any mediolateral displacement, or angulation, is then corrected. The long arm cast is applied in relative extension (around 30 degrees)[65,70] and should be well molded, taking care to avoid antecubital compression.

The period of immobilization for supracondylar fractures ranges from 3 weeks for toddlers, up to 6 weeks for teenagers.

Reduction Using Skeletal Traction

In severely displaced supracondylar fracture, reduction may be achieved by skeletal traction applied to a horizontal Kirschner wire or olecranon traction screw inserted at least 1 in. distal to the point of the olecranon to avoid the physis (in the case of the wire, great care is necessary to avoid the ulnar nerve). The humerus may be aligned horizontally (Dunlop's method) or vertically (overhead method) (Fig. 36-10). The elbow is maintained at the desired degree of flexion by skin traction applied to the forearm. Baumann's angle should be monitored. This is done by aligning the x-ray tube at 90 degrees to the humerus, staying no more than 10 degrees medial or lateral to the axis of the forearm.[97,98] This method gives very good results with minimal risk of cubitus varus providing the x-ray monitoring is performed.[98] It is particularly useful when there is soft tissue swelling or when after the fracture is reduced by closed methods, it is impossible to flex the elbow to a stable position without compromising the blood flow to the forearm. When the swelling is reduced, traction can often be discontinued, and cast immobilization then maintains the reduction. Alternatively traction may be maintained for 2 weeks until early callus has stabilized the fracture.[98]

Fixation with Percutaneous Pins

Another method of stabilizing an unstable reduction is the introduction of smooth pins percutaneously, transfixing the fragment crossing the fracture line and penetrating the proximal humerus.[13,38] The use of a fluoroscope is necessary. Careful avoidance of neurovascular penetration is essential and facilitated by the use of laterally placed pins (Fig. 36-11). This method has replaced open reduction and pinning under direct vision, which sometimes resulted in a stiff elbow.[35,46,67] Open reduction is still required with arterial compromise and for the occasional case in which the fracture is completely irreducible.

Complications

Vascular

Vascular compromise leading to Volkmann's ischemia is the most devastating complication of this injury. The vascular status of the arm assumes priority over all treatment. The presence of pulses does not rule out the presence of a com-

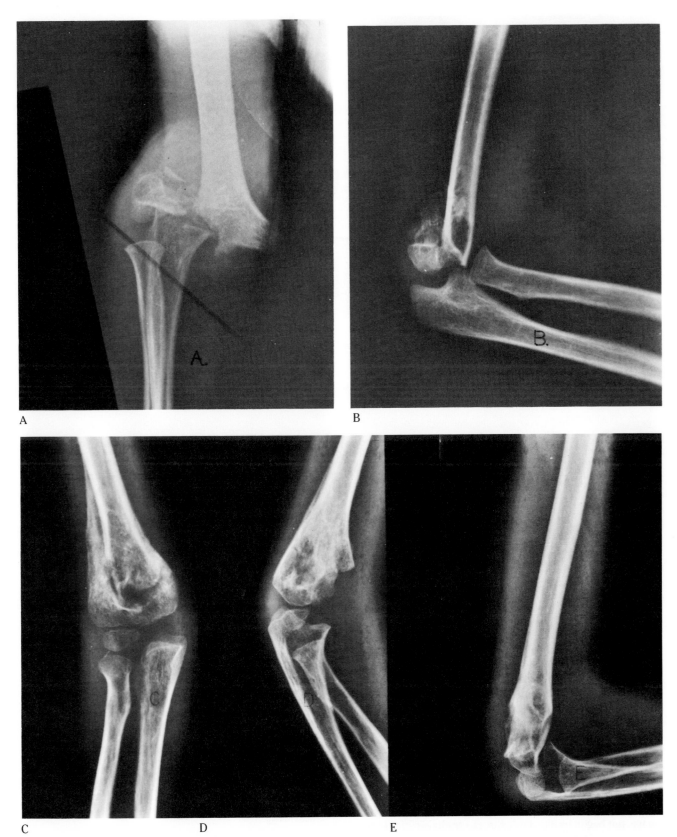

Figure 36-9 A and **B.** Severely displaced extension type of supracondylar fracture. The distal fragment is displaced posterolaterally. **C, D,** and **E.** The fracture was reduced closed under general anesthesia and immobilized in a long arm cast until healed. Traction or closed (or open) reduction with pin fixation is usually required to treat this fracture. Mild residual cubitus valgus deformity was present after the fracture healed, but elbow function was normal.

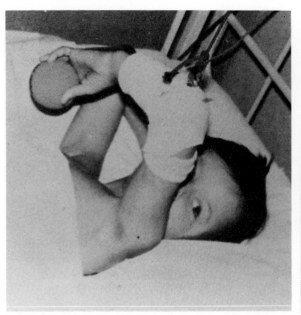

A

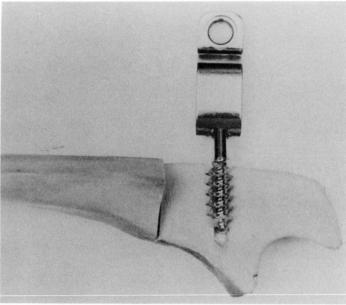

B

Figure 36-10 A. A child with a supracondylar fracture treated by overhead traction. Note the neutral position of the forearm. **B.** Ideal position of an olecranon traction screw. Several types of olecranon traction screws are commercially available. *(From Worlock, P.N., and Colton, C.L., Injury 15:316, 1984. Reproduced with permission.)*

partment syndrome. The presence of severe pain and swelling associated with active finger flexion or passive finger extension and poor nail bed capillary filling are important clinical indications for immediate action. The cast and all circumferential padding or stockinette must be split to skin and opened. If there is no immediate improvement, all cast should be removed, compartment pressures tested, the operating room prepared, and the vascular surgeon consulted. At surgery the brachial artery is inspected and lacerations or spasm treated locally. At the same time the fracture may be conveniently stabilized, and fasciotomy of the entire forearm with or without the carpal tunnel is performed.

Neurological

The incidence of nerve injuries after supracondylar fracture is approximately 5 to 10 percent.[42] The radial nerve is most often injured, especially with posteromedial displacement of the condyles. The median nerve is next in frequency of injury, such injury usually occurring with posterolateral displacement of the distal fragment. Ulnar nerve injuries, which are least common, are associated with flexion injuries. These injuries are most often related to improper use of olecranon pin traction.[22]

Nerve recovery is generally spontaneous and complete.[91] Signs of recovery are usually present by 6 to 8 weeks. If recovery has not begun by 3 to 4 months, electrodiagnostic studies are indicated. With no subsequent sign of early recovery, exploration should be considered; however, nerve transection in association with this fracture is rare.

Loss of Mobility

Given time for proper rehabilitation and growth, most children regain most or all of their motion. Fewer than 5 percent lose flexion or extension over 5 degrees. Few have flexion contractures or hyperextension up to 30 degrees.[39] Loss of flexion is due to posterior angulation or translocation of the distal fragment, or the result of rotational deformity leaving an anterior spike. Prepubertal children, through growth, remodel the fracture site, resulting in spontaneous improvement in motion for years after injury.[42]

Myositis ossificans is rare but has been reported to occur after either closed or open reduction. Repeated attempts at manipulative reduction may encourage its formation. Any attempts to force further motion by vigorous physiotherapy should cease if the condition is noticed and an expectant attitude be adopted since spontaneous improvement may occur.

Angular Deformities

Current authors agree that coronal plane or mediolateral (varus-valgus) angular deformities do not remodel to a significant degree. Mild amounts of sagittal plane or anteroposterior angulation do remodel, although the amount is perennially debated.[42,51,72] These deformities, although basically cosmetic rather than functional,[39] create much patient unhappiness and generate frequent litigation.

Cubitus Varus Cubitus varus, or gunstock deformity (Fig. 36-12), is the commonest deformity after supracondylar fractures in children, with a reported incidence ranging from zero

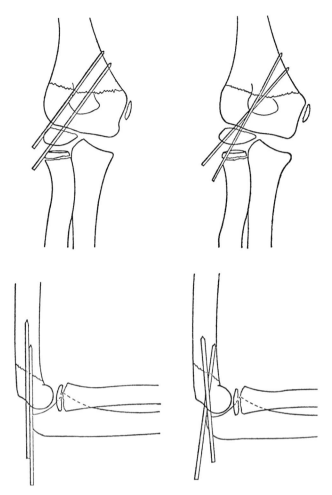

Figure 36-11 Internal fixation of a supracondylar fracture with parallel or crossed Kirschner's wires. A medial and lateral crossed-wire technique can also be used, but care should be taken to avoid injury to the ulnar nerve when inserting the medial pin. *(From Arino, V.L., et al, J Bone Joint Surg 59A:915, 1977. Reproduced with permission.)*

to 60 percent.[42] It is associated with a medially displaced fragment and does not occur with the posterolateral fracture pattern. The maximum amount of varus is often not appreciated until the elbow extends fully. Careful radiological monitoring is therefore crucial from the earliest moment whatever the treatment method.[98] However, in 40 percent of patients with this fracture, the carrying angle decreases with subsequent growth even after perfect reduction. Growth disorders are certainly responsible in some cases.[42] The role of uncorrected rotation is disputed but not as important as that of varus tilting. If the cubitus varus deformity is cosmetically unacceptable, surgical correction is performed by wedge[10] or dome supracondylar osteotomy with internal fixation. The procedure should be performed at skeletal maturity in order to eliminate the risk of physeal disturbance.

In some cases of cubitus varus there is a significant element of internal rotation. In such cases accurate assessment of the degree or rotation is necessary prior to surgical correc-

tion. A simple and useful clinical method has recently been described comparing the degree of internal humeral rotation bilaterally with the arm in the "arm lock" position behind the back.[99]

Cubitus Valgus Cubitus valgus is rare and associated with a posterolateral fracture pattern. Cosmetically less objectionable than cubitus varus, it accentuates the normal carrying angle. Functionally, it is frequently associated with loss of full extension. A late concern is the development of tardy ulnar nerve palsy. In contrast to cubitus varus, cubitus valgus has a much greater incidence of associated functional loss in the extremity. The treatment recommended by Langenskiold is a medial closing wedge osteotomy with anterior transposition of the ulnar nerve.[51]

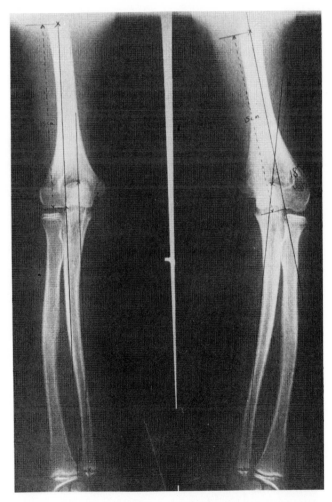

Figure 36-12 Anteroposterior x-ray view of a 12-year-old girl with cubitus varus deformity of her left elbow; both elbows in full extension and supination. The carrying angle is measured by the intersection of lines drawn through the humerus and ulna. The left elbow measures 18 degrees of varus malunion. *(From Kirz, P.H., and Marsh, H.O., Orthop Rev 10:85, 1981. Reproduced with permission.)*

Associated Ipsilateral Fractures

The average incidence of associated ipsilateral fracture is 10 percent (in 150 cases). Most involve the forearm or distal radius and occur with severe trauma with ipsilateral fractures. There is then a higher incidence of late cubitus varus, but the incidence of neurovascular complications does not appear to be increased.[75]

CONDYLAR AND EPICONDYLAR FRACTURES OF THE HUMERUS

Lateral Epicondylar Fracture

This fracture is relatively uncommon in children as an isolated injury.[60] It may occasionally be associated with an elbow dislocation.[72]

Osteological Characteristics

The lateral epicondyle ossifies at approximately 11 (female) to 12 (male) years of age and fuses with the lateral condyle during puberty.

Clinical Features

Since this structure is subcutaneous, local tenderness and swelling over the lateral epicondyle can be readily appreciated.

Radiological Characteristics

Prior to approximately 12 years of age, the lateral epicondyle is nonossified, rendering x-ray films unhelpful except to rule out adjacent injuries. Ossification is often irregular and may be confused with an avulsion fracture between the age of 12 and 14 years. Comparison views of the opposite elbow in the same projection may be helpful, but often the clinical evaluation makes the diagnosis.

Treatment

Generally 3 to 4 weeks of casting is adequate.[60] If displacement exceeds 3 mm, open reduction and internal fixation are indicated.[65]

The risk of growth arrest is minimal as these fractures occur near skeletal maturity. Fibrous union may occur. The fragment may be excised if the patient is symptomatic.

Lateral Condyle Fractures

These injuries usually occur between the ages of 3 and 14 years, with the peak between 6 and 10 years (Fig. 36-13). These fractures constitute about 18.5 percent of distal humeral fractures in children.[78]

Osteological Characteristics

The ossific nucleus of the lateral condyle and lateral ridge of the trochlea appear at approximately 4 to 5 months. The centers of ossification for the lateral epicondyle and medial trochlea fuse with that of the lateral condyle during puberty, and the common growth center fuses with the shaft in adolescence—14 (female) to 17 (male) years.[88]

Mechanism

The mechanism of injury is a varus stress combined with avulsion of the lateral condyle by the lateral ligament. The bone usually separates, but the articular cartilage remains intact or hinged to the trochlea. The fracture line extends to the articular cartilage of the trochlea, and the fragment does not therefore consist merely of the capitellum.[65] The fracture may be undisplaced (type 1) or there may be displacement on a cartilaginous hinge (type 2). Further force tears the hinge, allowing the fragment to displace through 90 degrees in two planes (type 3).[72]

Clinical Features

Generally, there is severe pain with marked swelling and tenderness over the lateral half of the elbow. Pronation and supination are usually normal, while flexion and extension movements are painful and limited.

Radiological Characteristics

This injury is usually a Salter type IV physeal injury (Fig. 36-13), although it may occasionally be a Salter type III injury. The diagnosis of a displaced fracture when the condyle is ossified is obvious. Nondisplaced fractures, or displaced fractures with a nonossified condyle, are difficult to diagnose. Oblique views, comparison x-ray views of the opposite elbow, and stress radiography may be helpful. In difficult cases, single-contrast arthrograms with only 0.5 ml of dye (to avoid pooling) visualize the joint surfaces and outline cartilaginous fragments.[2] The role of magnetic resonance imaging is being assessed in each diagnostic area.

Treatment

Undisplaced fractures may be immobilized in a long arm cast, with the elbow flexed to 90 degrees. A recent study recommends 6 to 8 weeks of immobilization to ensure union.[25] Displacement during healing is a distinct possibility, so frequent serial x-ray studies, and cast checks are indicated in the early stages of healing. Union should be confirmed by anteroposterior, lateral, and oblique x-ray views before mobilizing the limb.

If the lateral condyle fracture is displaced less than 2 mm, closed treatment appears to yield satisfactory results.[25] If there is more displacement, open reduction and internal fixation are indicated since the fracture involves a physis, epiphysis, and articular surface.[1] A Monteggia equivalent has been reported involving fractures of the lateral condyle and proximal ulna.[74]

Delayed union after 8 weeks is an indication for open reduction, internal fixation, and grafting. Established nonunions in good position are also treated by open reduction and bone grafting. For malunions, treatment should be deferred until after skeletal maturity.[25]

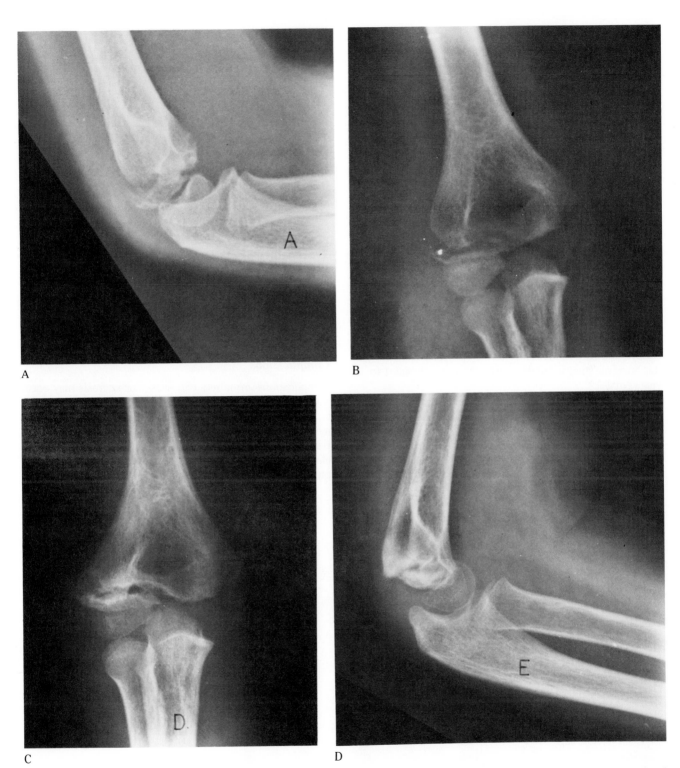

Figure 36-13 A and **B.** Lateral condyle fracture with minimal displacement (<2 mm) treated conservatively. Pin fixation merits consideration. **C** and **D.** At 3 months, fracture healing is delayed with union progressing slowly from the lateral margin of the fracture toward the center of the joint.

Complications

Fishtail deformity of the distal humerus occurs when malreduction is present.[78] Functional results are good, regardless of the radiographic or clinical findings.[25] Probable causes for delayed and nonunion include lack of immobilization, fracture gap with synovial bathing, soft tissue interposition, and, most important, inadequate reduction. Nonunions and growth arrests are more common in minimally displaced fractures than in markedly displaced ones.[70] Cubitus valgus may evolve slowly from proximal migration of the ununited fragment.[47,70] Tardy ulnar palsy may result.[47,60,70]

Premature physeal closure is common but usually occurs close to skeletal maturity. Thus deformity is not obvious.[72] Rutherford reviewed 39 cases with only 1 physeal closure, despite malreduction in 10.[78] Overgrowth, or enlargement, of the lateral side of the elbow is common. Rang reported 15 of 27 cases and observed that this cosmetic deformity is especially obvious in thin patients.

Medial Condyle Fractures

Medial condyle fractures are rare in children, constituting less than 3 percent of children's elbow fractures. Displaced fractures usually occur in older children.[11]

Osteological Characteristics

The medial condyle (and medial trochlea) ossifies at 8 years (female) to 9 years (male) of age and fuses with the lateral condyle during puberty. The entire epiphysis then fuses with the humeral shaft in adolescence—14 years (female) to 17 years (male).[88]

Mechanism

The mechanism of injury is generally considered to be an avulsion injury during a valgus force to the elbow. A second mechanism is a fall onto the point of the flexed elbow.

Clinical Features

Tenderness, swelling, and ecchymosis are present over the medial side of the elbow.

Radiological Characteristics

This fracture is generally a Salter type IV injury,[11] although Ogden observes that type III injuries may also occur.[65] During adolescence, the fracture may occur as part of a T-condylar type of fracture. In young children, whose medial condyle has yet to ossify, an arthrogram may be necessary to establish the diagnosis.

Treatment

Undisplaced fractures may be treated by immobilization in a long arm cast until the fracture is healed. Displaced fractures (more than 2 mm) require anatomic reduction, usually by open reduction and internal fixation.[11,65]

Complications

Complications are infrequent. Avascular necrosis may occur with extensive surgical dissection, so such dissection should be avoided during open reduction.[61] The blood supply to the medial condyle is of the terminal type.[11] Nonunion is a mild risk, especially in neglected fractures. Limited motion (especially flexion/extension) often resolves slowly and incompletely. Growth injury may occur, leading to cubitus varus.[11]

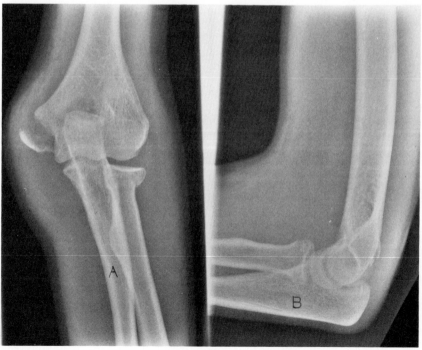

Figure 36-14 A and **B.** Adolescent female gymnast with displaced avulsion fracture of the medial epicondyle. Note the radial neck fracture. A closed reduction was performed by thumb pressure over the epicondylar fragment, flexion of the elbow and wrist, and long arm cast immobilization (with a medial pressure pad). The fracture went on to fibrous union, but the patient was asymptomatic, and the elbow joint is clinically stable.

A   B

Medial Epicondyle Fractures

Medial epicondyle fractures (Fig. 36-14) usually occur in patients from 7 to 15 years of age. They constitute about 10 percent of children's elbow fractures.[65]

Osteological Characteristics

The medial epicondyle ossifies at about 5 years (female) to 7 years (male) of age. It remains separate from the common growth center and fuses to the shaft in adolescence—15 years (female) to 18 years (male).[88]

Mechanism

The mechanism of injury is a valgus strain combined with forceful contraction of the flexor muscles. Fifty percent of these fractures occur with an elbow dislocation (Fig. 36-14).[60,70,72]

Clinical Features

The physical findings of tenderness, swelling, ecchymosis, and crepitation over the medial prominence of the lower humerus strongly suggest the diagnosis of a medial epicondyle fracture. If this injury occurs in association with an elbow dislocation, the area may be markedly swollen, thereby obscuring the diagnosis.

Radiological Characteristics

Radiographic diagnosis can be difficult before ossification of the apophysis. Comparison x-ray views may be helpful. Associated fractures and dislocations are common and should be anticipated. Clinical correlation is critical in children under the age of 5 years. The epicondyle should be sought on all appropriate x-ray views, particularly following severe trauma such as dislocation. Its apparent absence may be explained by its entrapment within the joint. In young children, the only radiographic sign may be joint widening, compared with the opposite elbow. In older children, oblique views may provide needed information. An arthrogram is useful in difficult cases.[2]

Treatment

Undisplaced and minimally displaced fractures require a long arm cast for protection until healed.[70,72] A trapped intraarticular medial epicondylar fragment can occasionally be disimpacted by a valgus stress to the elbow while supinating the forearm. Closed reduction is often unsuccessful, indicating the need for arthrotomy to remove the epicondyle, and then open reduction with internal fixation. With fragment entrapments, displacement over 5 mm, or associated medial instability of the elbow joint, open reduction is indicated.[65] Stabilizing the fragment also restores function of the medial collateral ligament of the elbow joint. Sutures or pins are used for fixation.

Complications

Motion often recovers slowly, and some degree of permanent stiffness may result. Nonunion occurs, and fragments may be excised if symptomatic. Median nerve entrapment may occur, requiring surgical extrication.[72] Ulnar entrapment may develop months or years later.[65]

T-Condylar Fractures of the Distal Humerus

T-Condylar fractures of the distal humerus are rarely seen in the pediatric age group. However, it has been pointed out that the nature of the injury may be overlooked in very young children.[69] In younger children the fracture line is vertical and extends through the epiphysis but may not extend completely through the thick articular cartilage. Near skeletal maturity the fracture fragments completely separate as in adults. Open reduction via a posterior triceps-splitting approach and fixation with K wires is recommended and achieves good results if reduction is accurate.[69] Rehabilitation may be difficult and prolonged.

Transphyseal Separation

Transphyseal separation is relatively uncommon in children, although many feel that this fracture may be occasionally mislabeled as elbow dislocation. It can also be confused with fracture of the lateral condyle. The injury is usually a Salter type I or type II injury (Figs. 36-15 and 36-16C). Diagnosis is particularly difficult in the first year of life if the ossification center for the lateral condyle has not yet appeared.

Mechanism

The mechanism of injury may be a direct blow or an indirect transmitted force from a fall on the hand. It may be associated with child abuse.[61] Two newborn cases associated with difficult delivery were also recently reported.[6]

Clinical Features

Physical findings vary according to the severity of the trauma and the degree of swelling or displacement. There is usually deformity, crepitus, and instability.[57] As with other intraarticular fractures, elbow flexion and extension are limited and painful.

Radiological Characteristics

This injury can be difficult to differentiate from other pediatric elbow injuries, especially since it more commonly occurs at an age prior to appearance of the condylar ossification centers. Multiple x-ray views, and comparison x-rays of the opposite elbow, may help establish the diagnosis (see also Fig. 36-16), but an arthrogram is commonly needed for definitive diagnosis (Figs. 36-15C and 36-16D).[2] The distal epiphysis may be displaced posteriorly, laterally, or anteriorly. With an elbow dislocation, the relation between the radial head and the lateral condylar ossification center are altered since the

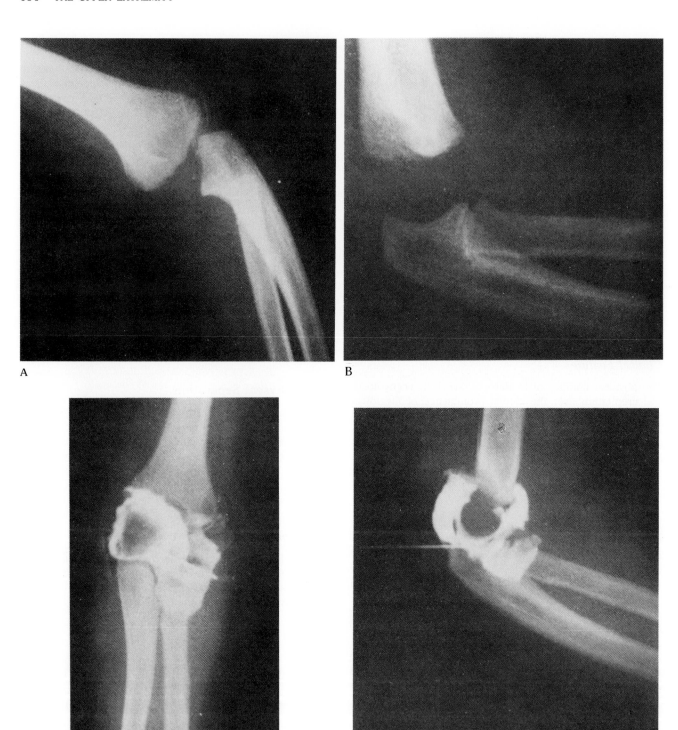

A

B

C

D

Figure 36-15 Fracture separation of the distal humeral physis of an infant. **A** and **B.** An 11-month-old boy after a 4-day history of a painful right elbow. These x-ray views demonstrate a lateral metaphyseal flake (Thurston-Holland sign). At this age, the capitellum has yet to ossify, thereby making it difficult to arrive at a precise diagnosis. **C** and **D.** An elbow arthrogram was performed. The anteroposterior x-ray view demonstrates dye in the cleft between the lateral metaphyseal flake and the remainder of the metaphysis, with extension medially across the humerus. The lateral view completely outlines the trochlea, which is displaced posteriorly. This arthrogram confirmed the diagnosis of a distal humeral fracture separation (type II physeal injury) and ruled out the existence of the more serious type IV physeal injury. *(From Hansen, P.E., Barnes, D.A., and Tullos, H.S., J Pediatr Orthop 2, 569, 1982. Reproduced with permission.)*

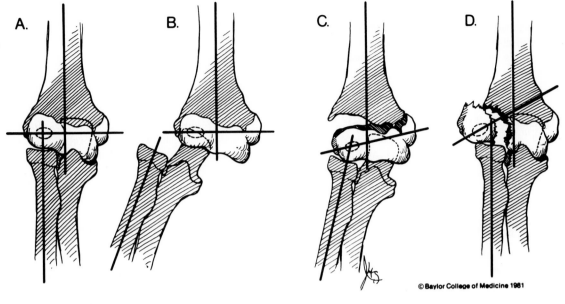

© Baylor College of Medicine 1981

Axis of radius

E

Figure 36-16 Radiographic method of differentiating a fracture separation of the distal humeral epiphysis from other pediatric elbow injuries that may occur in a very young child before the distal humeral epiphysis ossifies. Lines are drawn through the longitudinal axis of the humerus and the radial shaft, and a transverse line is drawn through the distal humeral epiphysis. The capitellum can be used as a reference point if it is ossified. **A.** Unaffected elbow. Normal radiocapitellar and humerocapitellar alignment. **B.** Elbow dislocation. Normal humerocapitellar alignment, altered radiocapitellar alignment. **C.** Salter type II epiphyseal injury. Normal radiocapitellar alignment, altered humerocapitellar alignment. **D.** Salter type IV epiphyseal injury. Altered radiocapitellar and humerocapitellar alignment. **E.** The radiocapitellar line. (A–D *are from Hansen, P.E., et al, J Pediatr Orthop 2:569, 1982.* E *was modified from Lee, J., et al, J Bone Joint Surg 62A:46, 1980. Reproduced with permission.)*

radius and ulna are usually displaced laterally. In an epiphyseal separation, the radius and ulna are usually displaced medially (Fig. 36-16C) but the radiocapitellar line on the lateral x-ray view remains intact.[21,57] With displaced fractures of the lateral condyle, the relation of the condylar center to the radial head is altered, but the axial relations of the long bones are normal (Fig. 36-16D).[57]

Treatment

Closed reduction is performed with initial traction, followed by correction of the medial tilt and varus angulation of the distal fragment. Any residual rotational deformity should then be bimanually corrected. Utilizing the intact medial periosteal hinge for stability, the elbow is flexed to 90 degrees and the forearm is pronated.[65] A long arm cast is applied with three-

point molding, creating a mild valgus force at the elbow. If the swelling is extensive, the circulation precarious, or the family unreliable, hospitalization is indicated for circulatory observation for the first few days. In extreme cases, with marked swelling, overhead traction may be utilized initially. Because of the degree of swelling, some authors recommend posterior splinting, but the author has found this extremely unreliable in children.

Most authors consider that open reduction is rarely necessary. However, it has been advocated as the treatment of choice by Mizuna et al.[57] Medial and lateral K wires are appropriate for fixation, augmented by postoperative casting.

If there is a treatment delay of 2 or more weeks, significant healing will already have occurred. Reduction should not then be attempted since iatrogenic physeal damage may occur. Subsequent supracondylar osteotomy may be necessary to correct deformity.

Complications

Cubitus varus occurs less frequently than after supracondylar fractures. Growth disturbances have not been reported as a consequence of this injury. Neurovascular complications are infrequent.[65]

FRACTURES OF THE HUMERAL SHAFT

These fractures are uncommon in children and are usually associated with severe trauma, or occasionally fracture through cystic lesions.

Osteological Characteristics

Ossification begins at about 42 days in utero, and the entire diaphysis is ossified at birth.[20]

Mechanism

The most common mechanism of injury is direct, severe trauma, creating a transverse or short oblique fracture. A heavy fall on the outstretched hand occasionally produces torsional forces which create a spiral fracture.[72]

Clinical Features

Infants usually present with irritability and pseudoparalysis of the upper arm. Older children with undisplaced fractures may be remarkably free of symptoms. With displaced or angulated fractures, the diagnosis is obvious. The neurovascular status, especially radial nerve function, should be carefully evaluated prior to manipulative treatment.

Radiological Characteristics

Birth fractures show callus at 1 to 2 weeks. Metaphyseal fractures should be evaluated for underlying cysts.

Standard radiographic views usually confirm the diagnosis. In cases with equivocal x-ray findings, or if a metaphyseal fracture is suspected near the proximal or distal humeral growth plates, comparison x-ray views of the opposite extremity are indicated.

Treatment

Closed treatment is generally indicated. Posterior splints, U or sugar-tong splints, and long arm casts with collar and cuff are all reportedly adequate methods of treatment. In recumbent patients, skin or skeletal traction may be used.[67] The use of a shoulder spica is generally excessive and unnecessary. Hanging casts, if used, should be fabricated of lightweight synthetic casting material to avoid distracting the fracture. As the pain subsides, isometric exercises assist humeral realignment and healing.

Open reduction and internal fixation are indicated rarely to maintain position but occasionally are required for soft tissue interposition with complete displacement in an adolescent.

Complications

Healing and remodeling are excellent in these fractures. Associated radial nerve injuries usually recover spontaneously. Vascular complications are uncommon. Overgrowth of 1 cm can be expected.

FRACTURES OF THE PROXIMAL HUMERAL METAPHYSIS

The proximal humeral metaphysis is particularly susceptible in the 5- to 11-year-old age group.[65] Compression type (torus) and greenstick fractures occur. Closed treatment is the rule, and displacement requiring reduction is rare. Pathologic fractures through benign cystic lesions (e.g., simple bone cyst) are treated identically to ordinary fractures, definitive treatment of the lesion being delayed until union has occurred.

FRACTURES OF THE HEAD OF THE HUMERUS

Fractures and traumatic epiphyseal separations of the proximal humerus represent only 3 percent of all epiphyseal injuries.[62]

Osteological Characteristics

Ossification of the humeral head appears between birth and 6 months of age; the greater tuberosity ossifies between 7 months and 3 years of age; and the lesser tuberosity ossifies approximately 2 years after the greater tuberosity. The physes close by the age of 17 (females) or 18 (males) years. The proximal physis accounts for 80 percent of the growth of the humerus. The medial portion of the physis and a few millimeters of the medial metaphysis are intraarticular.[20]

Classification

Fractures in this region are usually Salter type I or type II, the latter producing a medial metaphyseal spike of variable size attached to the head fragment. Neer and Horowitz' classification is based upon the degree of displacement of the epiphysis.[62]

Grade 1—less than 5 mm of displacement
Grade 2—displacement up to 1/3 the width of the shaft
Grade 3—displacement up to 2/3 the width of the shaft
Grade 4—displacement over 2/3 the width of the shaft (and complete displacement)

Mechanism

The mechanism of injury is generally a fall backward onto the outstretched arm with the elbow extended and the wrist dorsiflexed. Neonates usually sustain a Salter type I fracture while older children develop Salter type II fractures. The fracture line involves only the metaphysis in 90 percent. In 10 percent it is metaphyseodiaphyseal.[49] The metaphyseal spike may entrap the long head of the biceps and render the fracture irreducible. Salter types III and IV fractures are very rare[7] and are usually due to direct trauma. Salter type V injuries have not been reported.[7,20]

Clincial Features

In young children, pseudoparalysis of the upper extremity is a common presentation. Painful limitation of shoulder motion, swelling, and deformity (in displaced fractures) are seen in older children.

Radiological Characteristics

The diagnosis is difficult in neonates since 80 percent of these children have an unossified epiphysis. They are often diagnosed as having a birth palsy, or shoulder dislocation.

Treatment

About 70 percent of children sustain grade 1 or 2 fractures and require only simple support such as a sling and swathe, or Velpeau's bandage, for 3 to 4 weeks followed by early motion and rehabilitation.[72] Even with severe displacement the capacity for remodeling enables excellent functional results. The same is true for moderate degrees of varus. Severe varus can be corrected by gentle manipulation under general anesthesia. However, Baxter and Wiley found that manipulation of displaced fresh fracture did not improve the final outcome in their hands.[7] The manipulative maneuver involves longitudinal traction combined with abduction of the arm. For varus angulation, Kohler and Trilland recommend abduction greater than 90 degrees with flexion and external rotation, followed by traction. For valgus angulation they recommend reduction in adduction.[49]

"Statue of Liberty" spica casting to control the fracture has been used[19] but is awkward and may create complications including prolonged stiffness and nerve injury.[72] Others recommend the salute position with abduction to 130 degrees for 4 to 5 weeks.[49] If the arm cannot be immobilized at the side of the body after reduction since the reduction is unstable, inpatient traction in the abducted position is preferred by some authors. This may achieve reduction and maintain it long enough for the arm to be brought down without losing position. Hanging plasters are not recommended.[49]

Surgery consisting of open reduction with internal fixation (with K wires or screws) is rarely indicated.[20] It should be reserved for those nonimpacted irreducible fractures which are completely unstable and with suspected bicipital tendon interposition.[20,49] Surgery should only be done in an adolescent at the end of the growth period.[49]

Complications

This fracture usually heals and remodels well with full return of motion, strength, and appearance. The physis may occasionally close prematurely.[20] Neer found up to 3 cm of shortening in 10 percent of cases with undisplaced fractures, and in 40 percent with severely displaced fractures.[62] Smith reported shortening in 20 percent of cases, regardless of the method of treatment, but the discrepancy usually remains unnoticed by the patient.[20] Others have observed the final shortening at about 2 cm.[7]

FRACTURES OF THE CLAVICLE

Clavicular fractures are among the commonest fractures in children. They almost always heal well, without complications or disability.

Osteological Characteristics

The clavicle is the first bone to ossify. Primary ossification centers appear at about day 42 in utero (19 mm). One occurs at the junction of the middle and lateral third of the bone; the second is at the junction of the middle and medial third. The shaft is established by membranous bone formation.[20]

The ends of the clavicle develop by endochondral ossification centers at each end. The acromial end often remains nonossified, or appears briefly before fusing at about 19 years of age. The sternal end appears variably at 12 to 19 years of age. Fusion occurs at 22 to 35 years of age. This epiphysis is difficult to see on plain x-ray films.

Mechanism

The mechanism of injury may be direct or indirect. Indirect injury is the more frequent, occurring by a fall on the hand or against the outer shoulder.

Birth fractures occur in about 0.5 percent of vertex and 16 percent of breech deliveries, when the shoulders are compressed during passage through the narrow pelvic inlet. They are generally greenstick fractures and are more common in babies with high birth weights, and with forceps usage.[20]

Clinical Features

In infants and young children symptoms may be minimal. The diagnosis is often made days later when the parent notices swelling over the clavicle. Neonates may present with pseudoparalysis due to pain or associated birth palsies. This injury must be differentiated from proximal humerus injury, septic shoulder, and osteomyelitis.

Physical examination reveals localized tenderness, swelling, and often ecchymosis or crepitus. The subcutaneous location of the clavicle greatly facilitates diagnosis.

Fractures of the Medial End of the Clavicle

Until the age of 25 years, the medial physis may separate at the time of injury with the sternoclavicular ligaments remaining intact. Displacement may be anterior, posterior, or superior. A Rockwood view (45° upshot), AP x-ray views, tomograms, CT, or an MRI scan assist in diagnosis, which is often obvious on clinical examination. Reduction and its maintenance are difficult. Only rarely is displacement significant and are open reduction and suturing, or internal fixation, required. Posteriorly displaced fragments are adjacent to the great vessels. A vascular surgeon should be in attendance.

Fractures of the Outer End of the Clavicle

This lesion is often mistaken for acromioclavicular dislocation, which, however, is uncommon except in adolescents. In young children the outer end of the clavicular can sustain Salter type I or II epiphyseal separation since the acromioclavicular and coracoclavicular ligaments are stronger than the physis. Fracture healing occasionally produces reduplication of the clavicle in the inferiorly displaced periosteal sleeve. Infrequently, it may be necessary to trim away the excess of the "old" clavicle.[66] These displaced distal clavicular physeal injuries can be reduced and percutaneously pinned if detected early.[66] The author has found that excellent healing and remodeling generally makes pinning unnecessary.

Differential Diagnosis of Clavicular Injury

Congenital pseudarthrosis occurs in the lateral end of the middle third of the clavicle. A history of trauma is absent. The pseudoarthrosis is often asymptomatic. It is usually discovered between 2 and 4 years of age because of the bony prominence at the pseudarthrosis site. Usually occurring on the right side, it is presumed to be due to prenatal compression of the clavicle by the subclavian artery, which is more cephalad on the side opposite the heart. If the lesion is left-sided, one may suspect the presence of dextrocardia. Bilateral cases are associated with cervical ribs. Cleidocranial dysostosis should also be considered in the differential diagnosis.[20,33,83]

Treatment

A figure-of-eight harness is adequate for immobilization of the majority of these fractures. It may be fabricated or purchased. This basically provides protective padding over the fracture site and diminishes shoulder-clavicle motion during healing. Axillary care with powder and absorbent pads avoids chafing. Bilateral hand (gripping) exercises minimize swelling and maintain forearm strength. A sling may also be used for added comfort during the early painful period and for protection around other children.

Complications

The clavicle heals well in spite of respiratory and upper extremity movement. Healing may occur with displacement and angulation, which remodels in children within 1 to 2 years. The family should be forewarned of the possibility of a visible "bump" over the healed fracture site.

Superior angulation is common, and any effort to depress the bone should be avoided since the major neurovascular structures are directly subjacent. Rarely, subclavian vein compression (with upper extremity edema) occurs because of an inferiorly angulated fracture of the clavicle. It may be treated by closed reduction with or without a spica cast, or by bed rest with the arm comfortably elevated. Open reduction is rarely required in children. Infection and nonunion only occur after open reduction.

Occasionally, a comminuted fracture spikes into the subcutaneous tissue, tenting the skin. If an attempt at cautious closed reduction is unsuccessful, the safest treatment is to allow the fracture to heal and to remove the spike electively, under local anesthesia, if the patient remains symptomatic.[20]

DISLOCATION OF THE ACROMIOCLAVICULAR JOINT

Acromioclavicular joint dislocations, for practical purposes, do not occur in preadolescents. The clavicle usually fails first. If the fracture line is not visible, it has propagated through the cartilaginous lateral epiphysis, which is radiolucent. Adolescents sustaining acromioclavicular separations should be treated as adults.

DISLOCATIONS OF THE STERNOCLAVICULAR JOINT

Sternoclavicular joint dislocations are rare in children and adolescents as the medial epiphysis may fuse as late as the age of 25 years. Before fusion, the physis fails before the sternoclavicular ligaments, creating a fracture with or without displacement. Fractures generally heal and remodel satisfactorily, while true medial dislocations require attempted closed reduction, with possible open reduction if not successful.

A recent study of retrosternal clavicular dislocations concluded that all cases under age 25 should be considered displaced Salter type I fractures. If closed reduction was unsuccessful, open reduction and suturing was indicated. Pin fixation is dangerous because of potential migration into the chest.[83]

DISLOCATIONS OF THE GLENOHUMERAL JOINT

Dislocations of the glenohumeral joint are extremely rare in prepubertal children, but the condition becomes more prevalent in adolescence. The force that dislocates an adult shoulder fractures the child's proximal humerus. One should be alert for congenital anomalies of the articular surfaces or for the presence of predisposing factors such as joint laxity, Ehlers-Danlos syndrome, or neuromuscular disease. The treatment is similar to that described for adults elsewhere in this book.

Voluntary shoulder dislocation is occasionally encountered, especially in pubertal females and nervous children. Treatment should remain within the realm of counselling, as surgery is often unsucessful.[77]

REFERENCES

1. Agins, H.J., and Marcus, N.W. Articular cartilage sleeve fracture of the lateral humeral condyle capitellum: A previously undescribed entity. J Pediatr Orthop 4:620–622, 1984.

2. Akbarnia, B., Siberstein, M.J., Rende, R.J., Graviss, E.R., and Luisiri, A. Arthrography in the diagnosis of fractures of the distal end of the humerus in infants. J Bone Joint Surg [Am] 68:599–601, 1986.

3. Almquist, E.E., Gordon, L.H., and Blue, A.I. Congenital dislocation of the head of the radius. J Bone Joint Surg [Am] 51:1118–1127, 1969.

4. Amit, Y., Salai, M., Chechik, A., Blankstein, A., and Horoszowski, H. Closed intramedullary nailing for the treatment of diaphyseal forearm fractures in adolescence: A preliminary report. J Pediatr Orthop 5:143–146, 1985.

5. Barnett, L.S. Little league shoulder syndrome: Proximal humeral epiphysealysis in adolescent baseball pitchers: J Bone Joint Surg [Am] 67:495–496, 1985.

6. Barrett, W., Almquist, E.A., and Staheli, L.T. Fracture separation of the distal humeral physis in the newborn: A case report. J Pediatr Orthop 4:617–619, 1984.

7. Baxter, M.P., and Wiley, J.J. Fractures of the proximal humeral epiphysis. J Bone Joint Surg 68B:570–573, 1986.

8. Bayne, O., and Rang, M. Medial dislocation of the radial head following breech delivery: A case report and review of the literature. J Pediatr Orthop 4:485–487, 1984.

9. Beekman, F., and Sullivan, J.E. Some observations on fractures of the long bones in children. Am J Surg 51:722–728, 1941.

10. Bellemore, G.C., Barrett, I.R., Middleton, R.W.D., Scougall, J.S., and Whiteway, D.W. Supracondylar osteotomy of the humerus for correction of cubitus varus. J Bone Joint Surg [Br] 66:566–572, 1984.

11. Bensahel, H., Csukonyi, Z., Badelon, O., and Badaoui, S. Fractures of the medial condyle of the humerus in children. Pediatr Orthop 6:430–433, 1986.

12. Blount, W.P. Fractures in Children, vol 75. Baltimore, Williams & Wilkins, 1964, pp 58–59.

13. Bohler, J. Wire osteosynthesis of supracondylar humerus fractures in children, in Chapchal, G. (ed): Fractures in Children. New York, Thieme-Stratton 1983, p 147.

14. Buckerfield, C.T., and Castle, M.E. Acute traumatic retrosternal dislocation of the clavicle. J Bone Joint Surg [Am] 66:379–384, 1984.

15. Buhl, O., and Hellberg S. Displaced supracondylar fractures of the humerus in children. Acta Orthop Scand 53:67–71, 1982.

16. Carey, R.P.H. Simultaneous dislocation of the elbow and the proximal radio-ulnar joint. J Bone Joint Surg [Br] 66:254–256, 1984.

17. Carlioz, H., and Abobs, Y. Posterior dislocation of the elbow in children. J Pediatr Orthop 4:8–12, 1984.

18. Catterall, A. Fractures in children, in Wilson, J.N. (ed): Watson-Jones Fractures and Joint Injuries, 5th ed. Edinburgh, Churchill Livingstone, 1976.

19. Curtis, D.J., et al.: Importance of soft tissue evaluation in hand and wrist trauma. Am J Radiol 142:781–788, 1984.

20. Dameron, T.B., Jr., and Rockwood, C.A., Jr. Fractures and dislocations of the shoulder, vol 3, in Rockwood, C.A., Wilkins, K., and King, R.E. (eds): Fractures in Children. Philadelphia Lippincott, 1984, pp 577–607.

21. De Lee, J.C., et al. Fracture separation of the distal humeral epiphysis. J Bone Joint Surg 62A:46–51, 1980.

22. Edman, P., and Lohr, G. Supracondylar fractures of the humerus treated with olecranon traction. Acta Chir Scand 126:505–516, 1963.

23. Erne, P., Fricker, U., Muller, H.P., et al. Late results of supracondylar fractures of the humerus in children, in Chapchal, G. (ed): Fractures in Children. New York, Thieme-Stratton, 1981.

24. Evans, E. Pronation injuries of the forearm with special attention to the anterior Monteggia fractures. J Bone Joint Surg [Br] 31:578–588, 1949.

25. Foster, D.E., Sullivan, A., and Gross, R.H. Lateral humeral condylar fractures in children. J Pediatr Orthop 5:16–22, 1985.

26. Fowles, J.V., Kassab, M.T., and Douik, M. Untreated posterior dislocation of the elbow in children. J Bone Joint Surg [Am] 66:921–926, 1984.

27. Fowles, J.V., Kassab, M.T., and Moula, T. Untreated intra-articular entrapment of the medial humeral epicondyle. J Bone Joint Surg [Br] 66:562–565, 1984.

28. Fowles, J.V., Sliman, N., and Kassab, M. The Monteggia lesion in children: J Bone Joint Surg [Am] 65:1276–1283, 1983.

29. Freuler, F., Weber, B.G., and Brunner, C.H. Shaft fractures in the forearm, in Weber, B.G. (ed): Treatment of Fractures in Children and Adolescents. New York, Springer-Verlag, New York, 1980, pp 179–202.

30. Friberg, K.S.I. Remodeling after distal forearm fractures in children: I. The effect of residual angulation on the spatial orientation of the epiphyseal plates. Acta Orthop Scand 50:537–546, 1979.

31. Friberg, K.S.I. Remodeling after distal forearm fractures in children: II. The final orientation of the distal and proximal epiphyseal plates of the radius. Acta Orthop Scand 50:731–739, 1979.

32. Friberg, K.S.I. Remodeling after distal forearm fractures in children: III. Correction of residual angulation in fractures of the radius. Acta Orthop Scand 50:741–749, 1979.

33. Gibson, D.A., and Carroll, N. Congenital pseudarthrosis of the clavicle. J Bone Joint Surg [Br] 52:629–652, 1970.

34. Greenspan, A., and Norman, A. The radial head, capitellum view: Useful technique in elbow trauma. Am J Radiol 138:1186–1188, 1982.

35. Gruber, M., and Hudson, O. Supracondylar fractures of the humerus in childhood. End result study of open reduction. J Bone Joint Surg [Am] 46:1245–1252, 1964.

36. Hamilton, W., and Parkes, J.C. Isolated dislocation of the radial head without fracture of the ulna. Clin Orthop 97:94–96, 1973.

37. Harvey, S., and Tchelebi, H. Proximal radio-ulnar translocation. J Bone Joint Surg [Am] 61:447–449, 1979.

38. Hellinger, J. Supracondylar fractures of the humerus, in Chapchal, G. (ed): Fractures in Children. New York, Thieme-Stratton, 1981, pp 141–147.

39. Henrikson, B. Supracondylar fractures of the humerus in children. Acta Chir Scand (suppl): 369, 1966.

40. Howorth, M.B., and Baab, O. Orthopaedic disorders: Fractures involving the elbow, in Howorth, M.D. (ed): Orthopaedic Conditions due to Trauma, Sec III, chap 15, p 571.

41. Hughston, J.C. Fractures of the forearm in children. J Bone Joint Surg [Am] 44:1678–1693, 1962.

42. Ippolito, E., Caterini, R., and Scola, E. Supracondylar fractures of

the humerus in children. J Bone Joint Surg [Am] 68:333–344, 1986.

43. Jarvis, J.G., and D'Astous, J.L. The pediatric t-supracondylar fracture. J Pediatr Orthop 4:697–699, 1984.

44. Jaefsson, P.O., Johnell, O., and Gentry, C.F. Long-term sequelae of single dislocation of the elbow. J Bone Joint Surg [Am] 66:927–930, 1984.

45. Kay, S., Smith, C., and Oppenheim, W.L. Both bone midshaft forearm fractures in children. J Pediatr Orthop 6:306–310, 1986.

46. Kekomaki, M., Luoma, R., Rikalainen, H., and Vilkki, P. Operative reduction and fixation of difficult supracondylar extension fractures of the humerus. J Pediatr Orthop 4:13–15, 1984.

47. Keyl, W., Wirth, C.J., and Munchen,. Residual deformities after supracondylar humeral fractures, in Chapchal, G. (ed): *Fractures in Children.* New York, Thieme-Stratton, 1981, pp 179–183.

48. King, R.E. in Rockwood, C.A., Wilkins, K., and King, R.E. (eds): *Fractures in Children,* vol 3, chap 5, Philadelphia, Lippincott, 1984.

49. Kohler, R., and Trilland, J.M. Fracture and fracture separation of the proximal humerus in children: Report of 136 cases. J Paediatr Orthop 3:326–332, 1983.

50. Kuhn, D., and Rosman, G. Traumatic, nonparalytic dislocation of the shoulder in a newborn infant: Case report. J Pediatr Orthop 4:121–122, 1984.

51. Langenskiold, A., and Kirilaakaso, R. Varus and valgus deformity of the elbow following supracondylar fracture of the humerus. Acta Orthop Scand 38:313–321, 1967.

52. Last, R.J. *Anatomy: Regional and Applied.* J. and A. Churchill, Radius and Ulna-Artic. 1963, pp 164–165.

53. Lusted, L.B., and Keats, T.E. Elbow measurements, in *Atlas of Roentgenographic Measurement,* 2d ed. Chicago, Year Book, 1967, pp 119–121.

54. Manoli, A., II. Irreducible fracture-separation of the distal radial epiphysis. J Bone Joint Surg [Am] 64:1095–1096, 1982.

55. McRae, R., and Freeman, P.A. The lesion in pulled elbow. J Bone Joint Surg [Br] 47:808.

56. Miller, J.H., and Osterkamp, J.A. Scintigraphy in acute plastic bowing of the forearm. *Radiology* 142:742, 1982.

57. Mizuno, K., et al. Fracture separation of the distal humeral epiphysis in young children. J Bone Joint Surg 61A:570–573, 1979.

58. Morrissy, R., and Wilkins, K.E. Deformity following distal humeral fracture in childhood. J Bone Joint Surg [Am] 66:557–562, 1984.

59. Moseley, H.F. The clavicle: Its anatomy and function. Clin Orthop 58:17–27, 1968.

60. Muller, H.P., and Erne, P. Condylar fractures of the elbow region, in Chapchal, G. (ed): *Fractures in Children.* New York, Thieme-Stratton, 1981, pp 166–68.

61. Neviaser, R.J., and LeFeure, W. Irreducible isolated dislocation of the radial head. Clin Orthop 80:72–74, 1971.

62. Neer, C.S., and Horowitz, B.S. Fractures of the proximal humeral epiphyseal plate. Clin Orthop 41:24–31, 1965.

63. Nussbaum, A. The off-profile proximal radial epiphysis: Another potential pitfall in the x-ray diagnosis of the elbow trauma. J Trauma 23:40–46, 1983.

64. O'Brien, E.T. in Rockwood, C.A., Wilkins, K., and King, R.E. (eds): *Fractures in Children,* vol 3. Philadelphia, Lippincott, 1984.

65. Ogden, J.A. *Skeletal Injury in the Child.* Philadelphia, Lea Febiger, 1982.

66. Ogden, J.A.: Distal clavicular physeal injury. Clin Orthop 188:68–73, 1984.

67. Osterwalder, C., Thur, C.H., Wagener, G., et al. Open reduction and fixation with two crossed pins in supracondylar fractures of the humerus in children. Indications, technique, results, in Chapchal, G. (ed): *Fractures in Children.* New York, Thieme-Stratton, 1981, pp 178–179.

68. Ozonoff, M.D. *Pediatric Orthopaedic Radiology.* Philadelphia, Saunders, 1979.

69. Papavasiliou, V.A., and Beslikas, T.A. T-condylar fractures of the distal humerus during childhood. J Pediatr Orthop 6:302–305, 1986.

70. Pollen, A.G. *Fractures and Dislocations in Children.* Baltimore, Williams & Wilkins, 1973.

71. Pritchett, J.W. Entrapment of the medial nerve after dislocation of the elbow. J Pediatr Orthop 4:752–753, 1984.

72. Rang, M. *Children's Fractures,* 2d ed. Philadelphia, Lippincott, 1982.

73. Rang, M. *The Growth Plate and Its Disorders.* London, Livingstone, 1969.

74. Ravessoud, F.A. Lateral condylar fracture and ipsilateral ulnar shaft fracture: Monteggia equivalent lesions? J Pediatr Orthop 5:364–366, 1985.

75. Reed, F.E., and Apple, D.F. Ipsilateral fractures of the elbow and forearm. South Med J 69:149–151, 1976.

76. Riordan, D.C., and Bayne, L.G. The upper limb, in Lovell, W.W., and Winter, R.B. (eds): *Pediatric Orthopedics,* 2d ed. Philadelphia, Lippincott, 1986, pp 649–702.

77. Rowe, C.R., Pierce, D.S., and Clark, J.G. Voluntary dislocation of the shoulder. J Bone Joint Surg [Am] 55:445–459, 1973.

78. Rutherford, A. Fractures of the lateral humeral condyle in children. J Bone Joint Surg [Am] 67:851–856, 1985.

79. Rydholm, V., and Nilsson, J.E. Traumatic bowing of the forearm. Clin Orthop 139:121–124, 1979.

80. Salter, R.B. *Textbook of Disorders and Injuries of the Musculoskeletal Structure,* 2d ed. Baltimore, Williams & Wilkins, 1983.

81. Salter, R.B., and Zaltz, C. Anatomic investigations of the mechanism of injury and pathologic anatomy of "pulled elbow" in young children. Clin Orthop 77:134–143, 1971.

82. Schubert, J. Dislocation of the radial head in the newborn infant. J Bone Joint Surg [Am] 47:1019–1023, 1965.

83. Selesnick, F.H., Jablon, M., Frank, C., and Post, M. Retrosternal dislocation of the clavicle. J Bone Joint Surg [Am] 66:287–291, 1984.

84. Sharrard, W.J.W. *Paediatric Orthopaedics and Fractures,* vol 2. London, Blackwell Scientific, 1979.

85. Shinley, J.L., and Lesnick, D.S. Distal radius fracture with tendon entrapment. Orthopaedics 5:1330–1332, 1982.

86. Stimson, L. A. *A Practical Treatise on Fractures and Dislocations.* Philadelphia, Lea Brothers, 1900.

87. Stuhmer, K.G. in Weber, B.G. (ed): *Treatment of Fractures in Children and Adolescents.* New York, Springer-Verlag, 1980, pp 201–217.

88. Tachdjian, M.O. *Pediatric Orthopedics,* vol 2. Philadelphia, Saunders, 1972.

89. Tarr, R.R., Gardinkel, A.S., and Sarmiento, A. The effects of angular and rotational deformities of both bones of the forearm. J Bone Joint Surg [Am] 66:65–70, 1984.

90. Tredwell, K., Van Peteghem, K., and Clough, M. Pattern of forearm fractures in children. J Pediatr Orthop 4:604–608, 1984.

91. Von Laer, L. Fractures and luxations around the elbow in children and adolescents, in Chapchal, G. (ed): *Fractures in Children.* New York, Thieme-Stratton, 1981, pp 149–54.

92. Von Laer, L. The fracture of the proximal end of the radius in adolescence. Arch Orthop Trauma Surg 99:167–174, 1982.

93. Wedge, J.H., and Robertson, D.E. Displaced fractures of the neck of the radius. J Bone Joint Surg [Br] 64:256, 1982.

94. Wiley, J.J., Pegington, J., and Horwich, J.P. Traumatic dislocation of the radius in the elbow. J Bone Joint Surg [Br] 56:501–507, 1974.

95. Wilkins, K. in Rockwood, C.A., et al (eds): *Fractures in children,* vol. 3. Philadelphia, Lippincott, 1984, pp 363–575.

96. Worlock, P.H. and Colton, C. Displaced supracondylar fractures of the humerus in children treated by overhead olecranon traction. Injury 15:316–321, 1984.
97. Worlock, P. Supracondylar fractures of the humerus. Assessment of cubitus varus by the Baumann angle. J Bone Joint Surg 68B: 755–757, 1986.
98. Worlock, P.H., and Colton, C. Severely displaced supracondylar fractures of the humerus in children: A simple method of treatment. J Paediatr Orthop 7:49–53, 1987.

99. Yamamoto, I., Ishii, S., Usui, M., Ogino, T., and Kameda, K. Cubitus varus deformity following supracondylar fracture of the humerus. Clin Orthop 201:179–185, 1985.
100. Yates, C., and Sullivan, J.A. Arthrographic diagnosis of elbow injuries in children. J Paediatr Orthop 7:54–60, 1987.
101. Zimmerman, H. Fractures of the elbow, in Weber, B.G. (ed): *Treatment of Fractures in Children and Adolescents.* New York, Springer-Verlag, 1980, pp 158–178.

CHAPTER 37

Miscellaneous Degenerative Disorders of the Shoulder

Louis U. Bigliani and David S. Morrison

SECTION A

Rheumatologic and Degenerative Disorders

Louis U. Bigliani

This chapter discusses some common degenerative disorders of the shoulder joint and their surgical management. The incidence of degenerative disease in the shoulder is less than that in other major joints such as the hip and knee, but it is still a significant problem. Through the years, orthopaedic surgeons have tended to ignore the shoulder because it is not a weight-bearing joint and in many instances, restricted shoulder motion can be compensated for by the elbow and scapula. This is especially true in rheumatoid arthritis, where the hip, knee, hand, and wrist have had more emphasis than the shoulder. Recently, with the development of new surgical techniques, especially total shoulder replacement,[21] most degenerative disorders can be successfully treated. Therefore, the shoulder should not be ignored or treated by skillful neglect since pain and disability can be improved.

However, total shoulder arthroplasty is more than just resurfacing the articular surface of the glenohumeral joint with metal and plastic components. The soft tissues, adjacent joints, subacromial space, and postoperative rehabilitation must all be considered. The deltoid must not be scarred or weakened, and the rotator cuff must be preserved. Adhesions and contractures of the cuff must be recognized and released or lengthened to stabilize the implant. Furthermore, a painful acromioclavicular joint can hinder postoperative rehabilitation and compromise a glenohumeral replacement. Less frequently the sternoclavicular joint may be involved. Also, subacromial impingement can cause pain in forward elevation and restrict motion. A well-organized rehabilitation program is a key factor for success of a shoulder arthroplasty. Passive motion must be achieved in the early postoperative period or the arthroplasty will fail. Without adequate passive motion, strengthening is difficult and pain persists.

The degenerative disorders which affect the shoulder discussed in this chapter include primary and secondary osteoarthritis, rheumatoid arthritis, cuff tear arthropathy, avascular necrosis, and calcific tendonitis.

PRIMARY OSTEOARTHRITIS

Primary osteoarthritis is one of the more common degenerative disorders to affect the shoulder. However, it is significantly less common than osteoarthritis of the hip, spine, or knee, but more common than osteoarthritis of the elbow and ankle.[26] The etiology of osteoarthritis in the shoulder is probably the same as in other joints. It is not a systemic disease such as rheumatoid arthritis, nor have any specific chemical abnormalities or genetic factors been identified. Rather it is a mechanical problem in which abnormal forces across the shoulder slowly deform the articular surfaces. The characteristic picture is cartilage degradation with secondary hypertrophic cartilage and bony remodeling leading to joint failure.[26] The disease is called primary when no known predisposing factor is present.

Shoulder osteoarthritis usually presents in the sixth and seventh decades and is the result of a slow ongoing process. There is a gradual increase in pain and limitation of motion. Males are affected more often than females. It has been reported that laborers and persons involved in heavy lifting are more susceptible to osteoarthritis.[12,26]

The differential diagnosis for primary osteoarthritis includes rheumatoid arthritis, avascular necrosis, rotator cuff tear, cuff tear arthropathy, posttraumatic or septic arthritis, and metabolic and neuropathic disorders.

Rheumatoid arthritis is a systemic disease and usually involves multiple joints.[6,12,22] Avascular necrosis involves the humeral head and only secondarily causes glenoid degeneration.[11] There is a characteristic radiographic picture of the humeral head. An arthrogram differentiates a cuff tear, and in cuff tear arthropathy, there is a massive cuff tear with weakness and riding up of the humerus.[20] A detailed history or previous surgery differentiates posttraumatic and septic arthritis. Metabolic diseases such as gout and pseudogout rarely involve the shoulder and are easily diagnosed by joint fluid analysis.[12] In a neuropathic joint, there is excessive destruction with debris and, in many instances, an absence of pain. This condition must always be ruled out prior to joint replacement since replacements in this disorder are doomed to failure.

In osteoarthritis, there is progressive joint space narrowing with bony deformity. The humeral head becomes flattened with sclerosis and subchondral cyst formation as well as an inferior osteophyte (Fig. 37-1A). The bone on the articular surface is hard and marblelike without cartilage. Loose bodies may also be present. Occasionally, the acromioclavicular joint is also involved. The glenoid is usually worn posteriorly, and there may also be inferior osteophyte formation. The rotator cuff is usually intact in osteoarthritis.[8,21] There may be a contracture of the subscapularis with loss of external rotation as well as adhesions and thickening of the subacromial bursae.

Gradually progressive pain and stiffness are the outstanding clinical characteristics. There is difficulty sleeping on the affected side. The restriction of motion is severe with a decreased range in all directions, especially external rotation. A comprehensive examination of the cervical and lumbar spine is essential since arthritic involvement of these areas can add to pain and stiffness, thus hindering rehabilitation. A true AP view in the scapular plane and an axillary view are the important radiographic views. The true AP view reveals the joint space narrowing, sclerosis, subchondral cyst formation in the upper part of the head, and the inferior osteophyte (Fig. 37-1A). The axillary view best demonstrates glenoid wear and deformity (Fig. 37-1B). An arthrogram is not needed since the cuff is intact. Blood tests are usually normal, although the sedimentation rate may be slightly elevated.

Conservative treatment consists of rest, hot packs, and antiinflammatory agents. Physiotherapy should be avoided since it tends to increase discomfort. However, gentle

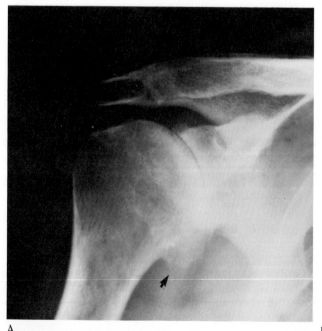

A

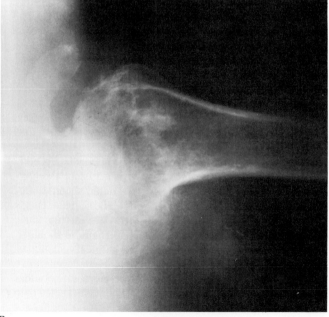

B

Figure 37-1 A series of radiographs of a 68-year-old woman with primary osteoarthritis of the shoulder. **A.** An AP radiograph reveals a narrowed joint space with sclerosis and flattening of the humeral head and a large inferior osteophyte. **B.** An axillary radiograph reveals head deformity and joint space narrowing and also allows evaluation of the glenoid for wear and deformity.

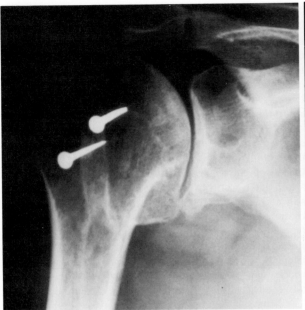

A

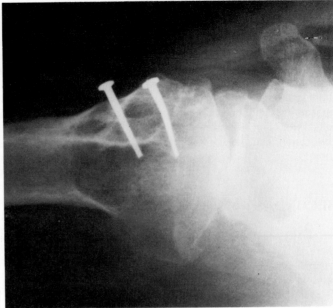

B

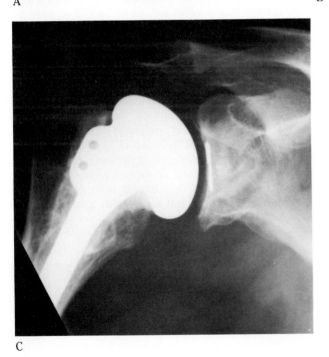

C

Figure 37-2 A series of radiographs of a 52-year-old man with secondary arthritis 29 years following Nicola and Magnuson-Stack procedures. The repairs made the shoulder too tight and limited external rotation, pushing the head posteriorly. **A.** An AP radiograph reveals joint space narrowing and inferior osteophytes on the humeral head and glenoid. **B.** An axillary radiograph reveals posterior subluxation and posterior glenoid wear. **C.** A Neer total shoulder replacement 2 years postoperatively. The patient is pain-free and works as a furniture mover.

stretching may be necessary to help maintain motion. Through the years, several different types of operative procedures have been performed to treat osteoarthritis. A resection arthroplasty[15] may relieve some of the pain but should be avoided since it weakens and deforms the shoulder, greatly compromising function.[9] Furthermore, there may be residual pain. Debridement and exostectomy usually result in a painful stiff shoulder. Benjamin has reported adequate pain relief in a small series of patients with double osteotomy of the humerus and glenoid, but motion was only slightly improved.[3] Several authors[2,9] have reported that shoulder arthrodesis is a reliable procedure to relieve pain and improve function.[2,9]

However, there is loss of all glenohumeral motion and restriction of overhead and behind-the-back activities. In 1974, Neer reported good results with hemiarthroplasty,[23] but considering that the glenoid is usually involved, total shoulder replacement is the procedure of choice.[21]

Osteoarthritis of the glenohumeral joint is an ideal indication for a conforming surface, unconstrained type of replacement since the articular surfaces are deformed, but the muscles about the shoulder are intact. There is no need for a fixed-fulcrum or constrained prosthesis that would replace the cuff. Neer has reported over 80 percent good or excellent long-term results in 40 patients having total shoulder replacement for osteoarthritis.[23] Pain relief was excellent, and the average increase in forward elevation was 77 degrees, and in external rotation, 55 degrees. Cofield has also reported good long-term results using the Neer total shoulder prothesis.[8,10] Since the soft tissues are constricted and the joint is stiff preoperatively, a meticulous postoperative rehabilitation program is essential to get early motion. Radiolucent lines have appeared around the glenoid cavity, but have not been correlated with clinical loosening.[8] Infection, humeral loosening, dislocation, and mechanical breakage have not been common.

SECONDARY OSTEOARTHRITIS

Secondary osteoarthritis is differentiated from primary in that there is a clearly defined underlying condition such as trauma, metabolic disease, or inflammatory arthritis contributing to its cause.[26] However, sometimes the differentiation can be quite arbitrary and confusing. In reference to the shoulder, the most common cause is posttraumatic, from fracture or dislocation. Metabolic causes are uncommon but do occur.[12] The age range is younger in the posttraumatic group, especially in arthritis of dislocation.[21] Trauma as a cause occurs secondary to an unstable shoulder which continues to subluxate or dislocate. Also there can be degenerative arthritis from a failed repair. In addition, hardware complications may cause joint degeneration.

Total shoulder replacement is also the treatment of choice for the type of arthritis but is more technically difficult because of bone deformity and soft tissue contractures (Fig. 37-2). There may be glenoid deficiencies which require bone grafting, and malunion of the tuberosities which requires osteotomy. Also, there may be a nonunion of the tuberosities or neck of the humerus. Soft tissue contractures, especially in the subscapularis, may be severe and require releases or lengthening procedures to gain equilibrium of soft tissues about the shoulder. Great care must be taken not to injure the axillary nerve during replacement. Whenever there has been previous surgery, infection must be ruled out. Postoperative physiotherapy is essential to maintain motion, as these patients may be quite stiff.

RHEUMATOID ARTHRITIS

Rheumatoid arthritis affecting the shoulder joint is not infrequent and can be a painful, disabling problem.[6,14,16,22] In the past, attention has been focused on the hip, knee, hand, wrist, and cervical spine, which are probably all more frequently involved. The reasons for this lack of attention are that the shoulder is usually covered with clothes and less obvious than the hand and wrist; the shoulder is not a weight-bearing joint like the hip and the knee; restriction in shoulder motion can be compensated for by the elbow and scapula; and surgical reconstruction of the shoulder is more difficult because it involves not only a reliable implant but also complex soft tissue reconstruction and prolonged postoperative rehabilitation.

The clinical course can vary from a mild low-grade involvement with only minor restrictions in activity to a severe, destructive involvement which is totally incapacitating secondary to pain, stiffness, and instability. The progression of the disease is subtle since the episodes of involvement are often subacute and transitory, and the resultant disability minimal. However, with each attack, there is a tendency to splint the shoulder close to the chest to avoid pain, and stiffness follows. Eventually, there is a stiff, painful shoulder with severe restriction of motion. Neer has stressed the importance of identifying the specific pattern of involvement since this affects the surgical reconstruction.[22] There may be a dry, a wet, and a resorptive pattern. The dry type, although quite stiff and sclerotic, has preservation of bone stock and soft tissue. Surgical reconstruction is more reasonable. The wet type is more severe with greater bone destruction and erosion. The rotator cuff is thinned out or torn. Degenerative changes are even more advanced in the resorptive type, which may be associated with vasculitis. In the resorptive forms, surgical reconstruction is more difficult since there is less bone stock and poor quality soft tissue.

It must be remembered that rheumatoid arthritis is a systemic disease that involves soft tissue as well as bone and cartilage. There is generalized osteoporosis, and in severe cases the bone can become extremely fragile and fracture easily. The joint surfaces become narrowed, and there is degeneration of joint cartilage with marginal erosions (Fig. 37-3). In addition to the cartilage degeneration, there may be significant erosion of the subchondral bone of the glenoid cavity. This erosion may extend into the adjacent base of the coracoid. The rotator cuff is not always deficient in rheumatoid arthritis, and in many instances may be quite good. Neer[21] reported an incidence of 42 percent rotator cuff tears in his series of 69 patients.[21] Furthermore, only 17 percent of the tears were massive. Therefore, in most rheumatoid patients, there is a rotator cuff for reconstruction. It must be remembered that the acromioclavicular joint may also be

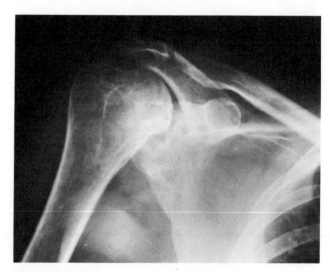

Figure 37-3 An AP radiograph of rheumatoid arthritis showing severe joint destruction with sclerosis, riding up of the humerus, and glenoid wear.

involved in rheumatoid arthritis, and this is frequently a source of pain. Occasionally, the sternoclavicular joint may also be involved.

Today, the surgical treatment of choice for the majority of shoulders severely affected by rheumatoid arthritis is an unconstrainted total shoulder replacement.[14,22] However, through the years, other procedures have been used, and some still do have a place in certain instances. If the involvement of the shoulder is primarily in the bursa and not the glenohumeral joint, bursectomy and release of adhesions should be considered.[22] If there is an element of subacromial impingement, an anterior acromioplasty should also be performed. Frequently, the acromioclavicular joint is involved and causes significant pain. Humeral head replacement has been used in the past,[16] but the glenoid is usually involved and should also be resurfaced. Also, Ferlic has reported glenoid erosion with humeral head replacement.[14] Clayton and Ferlic have also recommended the use of a subacromial spacer in cases with large rotator cuff tears.[6] However, these have not been used since the availability of total shoulder prosthesis. Glenohumeral arthrodesis,[2,9] humeral head resection,[15] double osteotomy,[3] and constrained total shoulder replacement[27,28] have all been used but are no longer recommended.

There is a greater incidence of complications following surgery in patients with rheumatoid arthritis. Often they have been treated with steroids or other systemic medication which weakens resistance. Therefore, these patients must be considered compromised hosts, with increased incidence of infection. Also, the skin is attenuated and very fragile, which often delays wound healing. Soft tissue contractures may limit motion and result in residual stiffness. A painful acromioclavicular joint may be overlooked and be a source of pain which may spoil the result of a perfectly good implant. The bone is quite soft, and postoperative fractures may occur. Also the rotator cuff is often quite attenuated and must be protected.

CUFF TEAR ARTHROPATHY

Cuff tear arthropathy is the end stage of a subacromial impingement process where there is glenohumeral joint degeneration secondary to a long-standing neglected rotator cuff tear.[20] Cuff tear arthropathy has only recently been described, and the incidence of this lesion is quite low; it is estimated that roughly 4 percent of all complete thickness rotator cuff tears go on to cuff tear arthropathy. In this process, there is malnutrition of the cartilage surface because there is loss of compression of joint fluid, secondary to a large or massive cuff tear. This leads to collapse of the humeral head and degeneration of the glenohumeral joint (Fig. 37-4A and B). This process occurs in stages, with a precollapse stage in which there is thin, atrophic cartilage and rounding of the greater tuberosity followed by ascent of the head. In the later stages, there is loss of cartilage with collapse of subchondral bone and further ascent of the head with erosion into the acromion, acromiclavicular joint, glenoid, and even coracoid. There is gross instability of the joint. This condition is similar to the condition described as Milwaukee shoulder,[17] which has many of the same pathological characteristics.[4]

The pain is significant and usually worse at night and with activity. There is weakness of the external rotator with atrophy of the spinati muscles and inability to elevate or abduct the arm. In addition to a massive rotator cuff tear, the biceps tendon is ruptured or dislocated, further contributing to the ascent of the humeral head. There is crepitus and a fluid sign, which is a fullness over the shoulder, secondary to joint fluid in the bursa. There are no specific laboratory tests for this condition, and no chemical abnormalities. The radiographic picture is severe, with riding up of the humeral head, rounding of the greater tuberosity, degeneration of the humeral head and glenoid, and, in more advanced cases, wear into the acromion, glenoid, and coracoid.

Conservative treatment consists of limiting activity and supportive measures to decrease pain such as anti-inflamma-

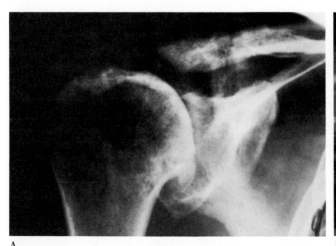

A

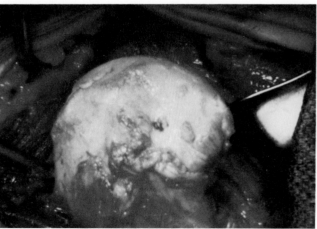

B

Figure 37-4 A. An AP radiograph of cuff tear arthropathy in which there has been a long-standing massive rotator cuff tear. The humeral head, riding up, has caused wear in the acromion and acromioclavicular joint. Sclerosis and joint degeneration are present. **B.** An operative photograph of cuff tear arthropathy revealing cartilage degeneration, collapse of the head, and a massive rotator cuff tear.

tory agents, warm soaks, and pain medication. The surgical treatment is total shoulder replacement but with limited goals.[20] Adequate pain relief can usually be achieved, but functional improvement is less certain. This depends on the status of the remaining rotator cuff, which is usually attenuated, shortened, and of poor quality. However, some patients do have enough cuff left to achieve a good functional result. In most instances, fusion is not as appropriate as total shoulder replacement.

OSTEONECROSIS (AVASCULAR NECROSIS)

Osteonecrosis of the humeral head is a painful degenerative lesion caused by an interruption of the blood supply to the bone. The humeral head is a frequent site of involvement, with the femoral head probably being the only site more commonly involved. There are many causes of osteonecrosis, including systemic corticosteroids, metabolic diseases, sickle cell disease, trauma, alcoholism, caisson disease, radiation, and Gaucher disease.[5,11,13,24] Sometimes a specific cause cannot be identified, and the lesion is idiopathic. It is not the scope of this chapter to discuss the pathological process in depth; however, the subchondral bone is involved, becoming necrotic and soft, allowing the articular surface to be deformed (Fig. 37-5A and B). A fracture into the articular surface can occur followed by collapse of the head. The degenerative process is primarily in the humeral head, but in long-standing cases, there can be secondary arthritis of the glenoid articular surface.

A thorough radiographic evaluation is essential to establish the degree of involvement and to determine if the humeral head is still a concentric conforming surface. An AP view of the shoulders in different rotations is helpful, and an axillary view often better depicts the amount of humeral head flattening and may reveal glenoid wear. Tomograms or a CT

scan may also be required to further delineate deformity. In the early stages when the x-ray films are negative, a bone scan may be needed to make the diagnosis.

The surgical treatment depends on the degree of involvement. If the condition is at an early stage and the head is still concentric, core decompression and/or bone grafting may be appropriate. When the head is deformed and the glenoid is spared, a humeral head replacement is indicated.[23] The deltoid approach should be used, and the only muscle that needs to be cut is the subscapularis. The rotator cuff is usually intact and should be preserved. The subscapularis may need to be lengthened if it is contracted and scarred down. A press fit of the humeral prosthesis should be attempted so that cement may be avoided. If there is wear on the glenoid cavity or cartilage degeneration, a glenoid replacement should be used.[21] The rehabilitation is outlined in Chap. 49.

CALCIFIC TENDONITIS

Calcific deposits can frequently occur in the rotator cuff tendons and bursa.[1,4,7,18,19,25,29] Calcific tendonitis usually occurs during the fifth and sixth decades, and there is an equal sex ratio. The specific etiology is unclear, but it is generally believed to be secondary to local avascular changes in the rotator cuff tendon without systemic involvement. Excessive trauma may even play a role. There is degeneration of the collagen in the tendons, with calcium salt deposition in necrotic tissue and focal inflammation. The calcium can be in two forms: a semiliquid, gel-like substance usually seen in the acute phase and a granular, chalklike deposit seen in the more chronic phase. A calcium deposit can be dormant for years and not cause symptoms. The most common location for calcium is in the supraspinatus and then the infraspinatus tendon. Less frequently, there can be deposits in the subscapularis and teres minor. The calcium is situated superficially on the tendons next to the bursa and can also involve the

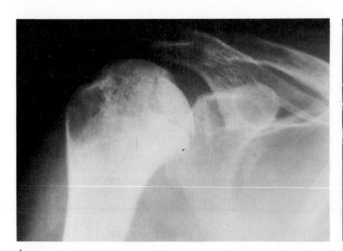

A

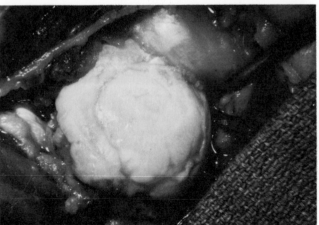

B

Figure 37-5 A. An AP radiograph of avascular necrosis with a subchondral fracture and significant head deformity. **B.** An operative photograph of the same patient at the time of total shoulder replacement, revealing the head deformity and irregularity.

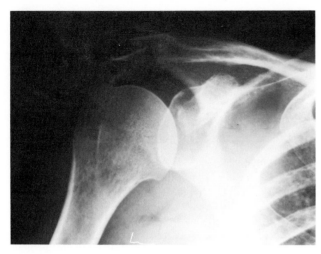

Figure 37-6 An AP radiograph showing a large calcium deposit in the area of the supraspinatus tendon.

bursa (Fig. 37-6). Perforation into the bursa can be beneficial as it decompresses the blisterlike swelling in the rotator cuff tissue. The calcium deposit does not rupture into the joint. There is no relationship between full-thickness rotation cuff tears and calcium except that occasionally the two may coexist.

Clinically, there are two stages: acute and chronic. The acute stage is characterized by excruciating pain which may radiate down the arm. The patient holds the arm close to his or her side and is fearful of making even the slightest movement. Therefore, it is very difficult to perform an examination. There is a great deal of local tenderness to palpation, and inflammation may also be present. In the chronic phase, the pain is usually less intense. There is a longer history of pain and of discomfort which is more gradual in onset. The patient can have a stiff shoulder which severely limits mobility. In fact, sometimes the frozen shoulder may be the problem which brings the patient to the physician. If the calcium deposit is large enough, it can click with motion and impinge against the undersurface of the acromion or coracoacromial ligament (Fig. 37-6). Radiographic evaluation of the shoulder for calcium requires a complete series of shoulder views in different rotations and planes to properly locate the calcium.

Treatment in the acute stage consists of steroid injection, pain medication, and an anti-inflammatory agent. In this stage, the calcium may be liquid and an attempt should be made to aspirate the calcium prior to injection of cortisone. A narcotic pain medication is usually indicated for brief period of time, as well as an anti-inflammatory agent. The arm should be protected in a sling, and range-of-motion exercises should be started when the patient becomes more comfortable. A second cortisone injection may be indicated, but multiple injections are not recommended. If after several months these measures fail, which is rarely the case, then surgical excision is indicated. This is performed through a small 2-in. deltoid-splitting incision so that minimal deltoid is cut. If there is an element of impingement from a prominent acromion, or anterior acromial spur, an anterior acromioplasty

should be performed. The bursa is usually thickened and fibrotic and should routinely be excised. Active physiotherapy should be started early to alleviate any stiffness. In the chronic stage, one or two steroid injections are also indicated as well as an anti-inflammatory agent.

SECTION B

Subacromial Impingement Syndrome

Louis U. Bigliani and David S. Morrison

In recent years, it has become apparent that anterior subacromial impingement is a leading cause of shoulder pain and disability. The acromion offers protection, stability, and mechanical advantage to the glenohumeral joint because it lies directly above the humeral head and provides the origin of the large deltoid muscle, a prime mover in forward elevation and overhead activity. Because of this relation between the acromion and the humeral head, the intervening rotator cuff tendons, the biceps tendon, and the subacromial bursa may be impinged during elevation. Pain and disability from persistent impingement causing wear on the rotator cuff will occur.

The functional arc of elevation of the extremity is in the forward plane, and therefore subacromial impingement is usually between the anterior undersurface of the acromion and the superior aspect of the greater tuberosity.[40] This has been described by several authors as the critical zone[6,32] or area of impingement.[40] Besides the anterior acromion, the area of impingement may extend to involve the acromioclavicular joint and coracoacromial ligament.

In the early stages of impingement there is edema, inflammation, and hemorrhage which can progress to fibrosis and tendonitis. These changes are usually reversible. In the later stages, there is progressive wear with bony changes (Fig. 37-7), tendon thinning, and eventual tearing of the rotator cuff, all of which is not reversible. A classification of subacromial impingement lesions was developed by Neer[35] to help better understand, diagnose, and treat this problem; it is presented in Table 37-1.

INCIDENCE AND ETIOLOGY

Subacromial impingement is a common problem affecting all age groups and both sexes, with a slight predominance in

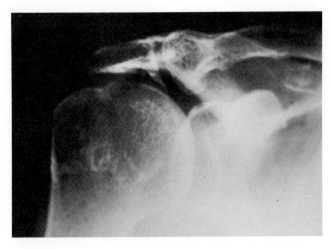

Figure 37-7 An AP radiograph of a right shoulder showing advanced changes, secondary to impingement. Present are an excrescence of the greater tuberosity, an anterior acromial spur, riding up of the humeral head, and acromioclavicular arthritis with an inferior distal clavicular osteophyte.

males. There is an increased incidence in those over 40 years of age[15] and in individuals involved in overhead activity. Wilson[55] noted a 20 percent incidence of supraspinatus tears in a necropsy study of patients over 32 years of age.

Several causes have been proposed for subacromial impingement lesions and rotator cuff tears. These include avascular changes in the supraspinatus tendon, mechanical wear, and trauma.

Through the years, several authors[23,26,32,46,48,49,72] have studied the vascularity of the shoulder joint and have noticed an avascular zone in the distal part of the supraspinatus tendon, just proximal to its insertion in the greater tuberosity. This avascular area seems to correspond with the area of tendon degeneration and rupture. Lindholm[25,26] and Mosely[32] felt that this decreased vascularity in the critical zone represents an area of anastomosis between the vessels derived from bone and those derived from the muscle belly. Rathburn and MacNab[46] proposed that with the arm in a neutral and adducted position, there is constant pressure by the humeral head against the supraspinatus tendon. This compression more or less wrings the blood out of the tendon at the critical area. They maintain that the avascular zone precedes, and is not the result of, degenerative changes.

Neer[39,40] has felt that subacromial impingement is a mechanical process secondary to progressive wear over a period of time and in his experience is the cause of 95 percent of rotator cuff tears. The tendons undergo degeneration, thinning, and finally full-thickness tears. The impingement is centered on the supraspinatus as it inserts on the greater tuberosity but may extend to include the long head of the biceps,[38] and infraspinatus tendons. An anterior acromial traction spur (Fig. 37-8A) is usually present in the coracoacromial ligament, and the acromioclavicular joint may be involved with an inferior osteophyte on the distal clavicle. Another predisposing factor may be either a prominent anterior acromion or an excessive downward slope to the anterior part of the acro-

TABLE 37-1 Classification of Subacromial Impingement (Neer)

Stage I

Pathological findings	Edema, hemorrhage
Age	<25 years
X-ray findings	Negative
Differential diagnosis	Subluxation, acromioclavicular arthritis
Clinical course	Reversible, 1 or 2 short episodes
Treatment	Conservative physiotherapy, heat, anti-inflammatory agents, rest from sports if sports-related, biomechanical analysis of arm motion

Stage II

Pathological findings	Fibrosis and tendonitis
Age	25 to 40 years
X-ray findings	Negative
Differential diagnosis	Acromioclavicular arthritis, frozen shoulder, calcific tendonitis
Clinical course	Recurrent pain and disability with activity
Treatment	Conservative as in stage I; also one or two steroid injections, NOT MORE. Consider bursectomy, coracoacromial ligament resection, and anterior acromioplasty, if needed.

Stage III

Pathological findings	Bone spurs and tendon ruptures
Age	40 years
X-ray findings	Anterior acromial spur, greater tuberosity excrescence plus positive arthrogram with complete tear
Differential diagnosis	Calcific tendonitis, cervical radiculitis, osteoarthritis, rheumatoid arthritis, neoplasm
Clinical course	Progressive disability
Treatment	Anterior acromioplasty and cuff repair; acromioclavicular arthroplasty if needed

mion. Mechanical impingement by the acromion has been recognized for years, but it was felt that the entire or lateral aspect of the acromion is the offending part.[1,7,17,28,29] Subsequently, different parts of the acromion, including the lateral edge, lateral half, and entire acromion, were removed to relieve impingement. These procedures either removed too much acromion, weakening the deltoid, or missed the offend-

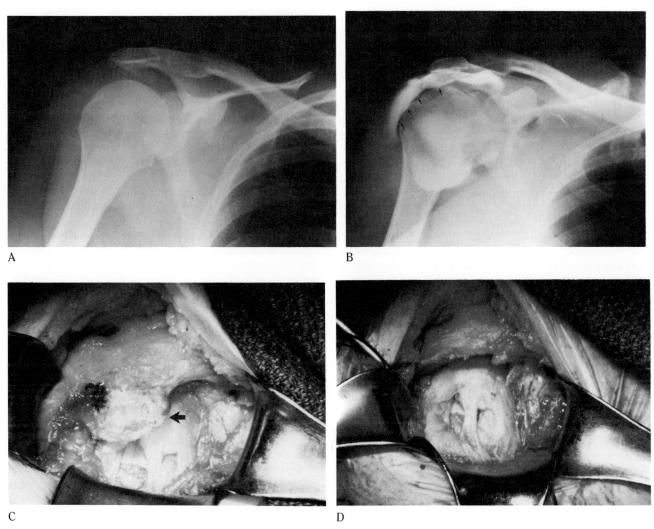

A

B

C

D

Figure 37-8 A 57-year-old woman with light shoulder pain which is more severe with activity and at night. Her impingement sign was markedly positive. **A.** An AP radiograph of the right shoulder showing an anterior acromial spur projecting into the subacromial space. **B.** An arthrogram revealing a full-thickness rotator cuff tear with dye extravasating into the bursa from the joint. **C.** At surgery, a full-thickness tear of the supraspinatus was revealed. The spur (arrow) is directly above the tear and with forward elevation, impinges on the cuff and tuberosity. **D.** After anterior acromioplasty, there is decompression of the subacromial space and relief of impingement.

ing part, the anterior one-third. Neer[40] observed that the position the shoulder is most used in is forward, not lateral. The critical area of impingement on the greater tuberosity then passes under the anterior edge of the acromion and acromioclavicular joint, not the lateral or posterior edge. Because of this fact, anterior acromioplasty was developed to decompress the subacromial space and relieve impingement.

Trauma may also be cause of impingement lesion and cuff tears and can be divided into sudden violent incidents (macrotrauma) or more subtle, repetitive motions (microtrauma) resulting in an overuse syndrome. A single violent event resulting in a cuff tear is unusual, but a tear can occur, especially in older persons who fall on an outstretched hand or who dislocate their shoulder. However, 50 percent of patients with documented rotator cuff tears usually do not re-

call a traumatic episode.[35] Furthermore, many of the patients with a positive history of trauma have a prior history of shoulder pain and disability. Therefore, the trauma may have extended a preexisting partial tear to a complete tear or a small tear to a larger tear.

Microtrauma is a very common cause in sports-related impingement problems.[18,22] Impingement occurs in sports that require repetitive throwing or overhead motions, such as baseball, tennis, and swimming. During an overhead activity, the greater tuberosity and rotator cuff move beneath the acromion as the arm is rotated to reach horizontal abduction and external rotation in a stroking or throwing motion. Faulty biomechanics or a sudden, improper, forceful action during the motion can create strain and wear between the cuff and acromion leading to an impingement lesion. Impingement can occur at any age in an athlete from a competitive teenaged pitcher or swimmer to a middle-aged weekend tennis player.

DIFFERENTIAL DIAGNOSIS

The differential diagnosis of impingement lesions differs with the various stages as well as with the age of the patient. During the early stages, one of the most difficult differential diagnoses to make is that of impingement as opposed to subluxation (Table 37-1). The patient is usually a young athlete involved in repetitive overhead activity. It may be difficult to localize pain or tenderness at the greater tuberosity or the inferior glenoid region. Testing in abduction and external rotation can cause pain from impingement as well as from anterior subluxation. The impingement injection test is extremely useful in this instance since it relieves pain secondary only to impingement and not to subluxation. Patients with subluxation may also have excessive external rotation, laxity of other joints, and an audible or a palpable click which may help in making a diagnosis of instability. However, it should be kept in mind that the precise localization of clicks and pops about the shoulder may be difficult.

Posttraumatic acromioclavicular arthritis is another problem which must be identified. Usually there is direct tenderness over the acromioclavicular joint and degenerative radiographic changes. Selectively injecting lidocaine only into the acromioclavicular joint and not into the subacromial space helps make this diagnosis. An impingement lesion may be present in addition to acromioclavicular arthritis. Acute traumatic bursitis is usually the result of a violent blow, either direct or indirect, which causes edema and hemorrhage. This usually resolves in a short period of time, 3 to 6 weeks, with rest and conservative treatment. However, such an incident may initiate an impingement lesion or in older individuals cause a cuff tear.

Calcific tendonitis occurs usually in the fifth and sixth decades and can be confused with impingement.[20] A calcific density is seen on x-ray views, but multiple views in different rotations may be required. The pain and tenderness are usually more intense than with impingement, and there may be a frozen shoulder. Also, a cervical radiculitis can radiate pain to the shoulder, and this may mimic an impingement lesion. If there is any doubt, cervical spine films, electromyographic studies, and a complete neurological examination are helpful in distinguishing calcific tendonitis. Entrapment of the suprascapular nerve can be confused with a cuff tear because it involves weakness of the supraspinatus and the infraspinatus tendons.[13] Entrapment is a rare condition which must be confirmed by an electromyogram. It may occur following scapula fractures involving the suprascapular notch and base of coracoid.

In older patients, metastatic lesions to the proximal humerus must always be considered, especially if there is a lucent area on the x-ray film. Osteoarthritis is usually differentiated by x-ray evaluation and a markedly restricted range of motion. Rheumatoid arthritis is a systemic disease which usually involves several joints. When the shoulders are involved, there are full-thickness rotator cuff tears in approximately one-third of the cases.

PATHOLOGICAL CHARACTERISTICS

The pathological changes present in impingement lesions vary with the different stages (Table 37-1). Younger patients tend to have stage I lesions while older patients tend to have stage III lesions. However, the age of the patient may not always directly correlate with the exact stage of impingement. For example, a 45-year-old patient with only one episode of pain secondary to impingement may have only a stage I lesion. Also, a stage II lesion can exist in an individual less than 25 years of age if there are repeated episodes of impingement. In the past, there has been confusion because it was felt that the age and stage of impingement must directly correspond. The age ranges for impingement lesions are arbitrary, and exceptions do exist.

The pathological changes in the first stage consist of edema, inflammation, and hemorrhage. There is less room in the subacromial space for the cuff to pass under the acromion. There is irritation of the bursa, making it less compliant and increasing the friction across the subacromial space. These changes are completely reversible and respond well to rest and avoidance of harmful or provocative activities. It is important to remember that the proximal aspect of the long head of the biceps may also be involved in the impingement process.[38] There are no radiological changes present in the bone or soft tissues about the shoulder in this stage.

In stage II lesions, there is fibrosis and tendonitis. These are more chronic and are secondary to repeated episodes of impingement. The bursa is not only irritated but becomes thickened and fibrotic, further decreasing its compliance. There is irritation and scarring and possible fiber dissociation in the superficial rotator cuff. These lesions are less apt to be completely reversible, and there is usually some residual damage. There are still no radiological changes present in most instances; however, there may be some sclerosis and subtle excrescence visible on the greater tuberosity.

Stage III lesions are characterized by the formation of bone spurs and excrescences as well as tears in the substance of the rotator cuff tendons. The tears may be either full-thickness, which extend into the glenohumeral joint, or partial-thickness tears, which are usually on the superficial surface. However, there can be a deep surface blister which is a separation of an inferior portion of the tendon communicating with the joint. Full-thickness tears usually start in the supraspinatus tendon at the critical zone. This is the area which is subject to the most wear. There is direct communication between the subacromial bursa and the joint cavity. A small tear can enlarge by "acute extension" into the infraspinatus teres minor and subscapularis. This may occur after a violent trauma or just a trivial motion if the tendon edges are sufficiently attenuated and weakened. If enough of the infraspinatus is involved, there may be sudden weakness of external rotation.

One of the most popular ways to categorize a cuff tear is by measuring its longest diameter in centimeters.[8] A small tear is less than 1 cm, a medium tear is less than 3 cm, a large tear is less than 5 cm, and a massive tear is over 5 cm. In massive tears there is scarring and retraction. The entire supraspinatus and infraspinatus are usually involved.

The bony changes which can occur are squaring and excrescence formation of the greater tuberosity as well as an anterior traction spur in the substance of the coracoacromial ligament. These are usually early changes. Further changes include osteophyte formation on the inferior surface of the acromioclavicular joint on both the acromial and clavicular sides as well as an excrescence on the undersurface of the anterior acromion. Cuff tear arthropathy,[37] which is discussed in depth in Sect. A, is the end stage of the impingement process.

The long head of the biceps can also be involved in impingement, with inflammation, wear, and finally rupture of the long head. The rupture may occur before or after a tear in the supraspinatus tendon. The depressor function of the biceps tendon is lost, and the impingement process can be accelerated.

There is also an association with failure of fusion of the distal acromial epiphysis, os acromiale, and rotator cuff tears.[4,34] The unfused distal part of the acromion is loose and protrudes inferiorly into the subacromial space, causing impingement.

CLINICAL DIAGNOSIS

The most significant symptom in the subacromial area is pain. It is usually centered on the greater tuberosity but can extend down in the area of the deltoid muscle. There may be radiation of pain down the arm to the elbow, medially to the chest wall, or superiorly in the area of the trapezius muscle. If the acromioclavicular joint is arthritic or involved in impingement, this may also be a source of pain. Night pain is very common and either interrupts sleep or does not allow the patient to lie on the affected shoulder. The intensity and duration of pain vary. The pain can be a dull, toothache-like type which lingers for a long time, or a sharp, burning type which is not well tolerated and requires treatment. Patients may complain of weakness and loss of function. They are usually unable to participate in sporting activities such as tennis and swimming or perform overhead motion. They may be unable to do activities of daily living such as reaching to an overhead cabinet, combing hair, and lifting objects to the side.

On physical examination, there may be palpable tenderness about the shoulder, but its location varies. It is usually centered about the greater tuberosity but may involve the acromioclavicular joint, bicipital groove, coracoid area, or posterior aspect of the shoulder. The most reliable physical sign is the impingement sign.[35] In this sign, there is pain beneath the anterior acromion with passive elevation of the arm in the forward plane. The examiner should stand behind the patient and stabilize the scapula with one hand. With the other hand, the arm is elevated in the forward plane. Impingement may occur anywhere between 70 and 180 degrees. An extremely helpful diagnostic tool is the impingement injection test. If the impingement sign is positive, 10 ml of lidocaine can be injected beneath the acromion and the impingement sign repeated. If the pain is significantly diminished, this is a positive sign and indicates a subacromial cause. The impingement test is very helpful in ruling out pain referred from other areas such as the neck, chest, or glenohumeral joint. It

is also a very good indication of the type of pain relief that can be achieved from subacromial decompression.

The arc of pain is another useful test, but not quite as consistent as the impingement sign. There is pain between 120 and 70 degrees as the arm is slowly, actively lowered from overhead to the side; also the arm may be internally rotated, moving the greater tuberosity under the acromion, and then raised. There may be weakness of active external rotation which is secondary either to pain or to a complete-thickness tear of the infraspinatus tendon. The fluid sign, which is fullness in the bursa secondary to joint fluid, and spinati atrophy are signs consistent with a full-thickness rotator cuff tear. As a rule, there is very little restriction of passive motion, especially in full-thickness tears, where joint fluid readily leaks into the bursa and lubricates it. A frozen shoulder may be seen in patients with partial-thickness tears and rarely in those with full-thickness tears. Patients with large or massive tears may have weakness of forward elevation as well as external rotation and may not be able to raise their arm above the horizontal.

The radiographic changes in impingement lesions usually do not begin until stage III. The most subtle change is a squaring off of the greater tuberosity which can develop into an excrescence. Also early in the impingement process, an anterior acromial spur can develop in the substance of the coracoacromial ligament, and as impingement progresses, there may be osteophyte formation at the distal clavicle and excrescences beneath the acromion (Fig. 37-7). Furthermore in a full-thickness tear, there may be riding up of the humerus with a decrease in the acromiohumeral interval.[54] An axillary view is helpful to evaluate for a persistent unfused acromial epiphysis.

The most reliable radiographic procedure to demonstrate a full-thickness rotator cuff tear is arthrography (Fig. 37-8B).[47] This has been the standard since Codman[6] and Lindblom first described its usefulness in diagnosing tears of the supraspinatus. Some authors[12,14] feel that double-contrast arthrography is superior since it can better outline the cuff, and in some instances, define the size of a cuff tear. Tomography has been used in conjunction with this technique to further detail the size of the tear and the quality of the tissue. However, the reproducibility and accuracy of these tests vary, and they require an interested radiologist. The indications for an arthrogram include: unresponsiveness to conservative treatment for 12 weeks in patients over 40 years of age; sudden marked weakness of external rotation and forward elevation after an injury; rupture of the long head of the biceps when there are shoulder symptoms; and glenohumeral dislocations followed by shoulder symptoms in a patient older than 40 years of age.[35] Recently, sonography, a noninvasive technique, has been used to outline the rotator cuff and define both partial- and full-thickness tears. Bursography[24,52,53] has also been used with some success to outline partial-thickness tears on the superficial surface of the cuff that are not diagnosed by arthrography. Arthroscopy is another procedure which can be performed to diagnose a cuff tear, but with the accuracy and availability of the arthrogram, this procedure seems less appropriate. There are no specific diagnostic laboratory tests for the impingement syndrome. However, a complete blood cell count, erythrocyte sedimentatation rate, SMAC, and latex fixation should be routine in the workup to rule out systemic infection or metabolic disease. In patients with radicular neck pain or sudden marked weakness, cervical spine films and electromyography are indicated.

TREATMENT

The treatment of the impingement syndrome differs with the stages. Stage I and II lesions can generally be treated conservatively, while stage III lesions usually require operative repair. Stage I lesions are reversible and respond well to rest and physiotherapy. Some stage II lesions are reversible, but others can become sufficiently disabling that they require decompression. The coracoacromial ligament is transected, and if the anterior aspect of the acromion is prominent or sloped downward, this should be beveled. Some stage III lesions respond to conservative therapy, and some authors[11,50] have recommended conservative treatment of rotator cuff tears in the past, but the patient usually stops using the involved extremity for most activities. This rest and disuse decrease the pain, but the patient has limited function with the involved extremity and may even switch hand dominance. This accommodation of lifestyle may be acceptable for older, inactive patients, but active patients require operative treatment.

Conservative treatment consists of rest and avoidance of harmful or provocative motions, but not inactivity. This is especially true with athletes, who must stop the offending motion but must maintain flexibility, strength, and conditioning.[39] The mechanics of the overhead motion must be analyzed to correct any obvious imperfections which create friction and wear. For example, a pitcher with impingement must stop pitching but should maintain a full range of motion, maintain the strength of the muscles involved in throwing, and continue cardiovascular fitness. The specific approach to physiotherapy will be discussed in Chap. 49 for both athletic and nonathletic rehabilitation. Anti-inflammatory agents are useful to help decrease edema and inflammation. No one drug seems to be particularly effective in the treatment of impingement lesions. Multiple injections of steroids into the bursa or cuff area should be avoided since this can lead to degeneration of tendinous tissue. One, possibly two, steroid injections followed by a rest period should be the limit.

Surgery is indicated in patients with a painful impingement lesion when there is a full-thickness rotator cuff tear or when a partial-thickness tear is resistant to conservative measures for a considerable amount of time (more than 9 months). Recently, good results have been reported with arthroscopic subacromial decompression for stage II impingement lesions. Long-term results are not available, but this technique is a promising alternative to open acromioplasty in selected patients without full-thickness cuff tears. Open operative repair should consist of two steps: decompression of the subacromial space and repair of full-thickness rotator cuff tears (Fig. 37-8C–D). For years, authors[5,7,9,25,31] diagnosed tears in the supraspinatus tendon as a cause of shoulder pain and recognized the acromion as the offending structure in impingement lesions.[1,17,30] However, too much acromion or the wrong part was removed until Neer proposed that the anterior one-third is the part involved in subacromial impingement.[40] Several authors described complete acromionectomy for relief,[1,17] but this procedure seriously weakens the deltoid and deforms the shoulder. A large portion of deltoid insertion is removed, and the leverage needed for strength in overhead activity is lost.[36] This procedure should never be performed. Radical lateral acromionectomy also removes too much acromion and significantly weakens the deltoid. McLaughlin[28,29,30,46] described the modified lateral acromionectomy, but this procedure does not remove the offending anterior acromion and there is residual impingement. The transacromial approach does not remove any acromion but divides it, which can weaken the acromion and result in a nonunion.[43] Furthermore it does not allow exposure of the anterior acromion, which must be removed. The same is true for posterior approaches. Stamm has proposed paraglenoid osteotomy,[51] but this procedure does not consider the offending part, the acromion. The procedure of choice for decompression of impingement lesions is the anterior acromioplasty approach described by Neer in 1972.[40] This procedure has provided consistently excellent results with respect to pain relief.[19,35,45] It not only achieves decompression but provides adequate exposure for cuff repair with only minimal removal of the deltoid insertion (Fig. 37-8). The technique of this surgery has been described previously and will not be discussed here. It should be remembered that acromioclavicular arthroplasty is part of the decompression if the acromioclavicular joint is involved. A complete acromioclavicular arthroplasty is performed only if there is preoperative joint tenderness. If the joint is asymptomatic preoperatively but found to be arthritic with osteophytes at surgery, a modified acromioclavicular arthroplasty is performed. Only the undersurface of the distal clavicle is removed. This maneuver avoids weakening the deltoid. The distal clavicle has also been removed to gain more exposure in repair of massive tears, but the indication for this is rare. The second step in the procedure is to repair the rotator cuff defect. Most authors recommend cuff repair.[2,3,11,21,28,33,35,45,56,57] Small and medium-sized cuff tears are usually amenable to direct suture or reattachment to the greater tuberosity. A trough is made in the sulcus between the head and tuberosity, nonabsorbable nylon sutures are placed through drill holes, and the cuff is reattached. It is in the larger and massive tears where there is scarring, retraction, and possible loss of substance that cuff repair becomes more difficult. Various techniques have been proposed. McLaughlin described a procedure in which the cuff is mobilized as far as possible and the freshened edge is sutured into a trough made in the head.[30] Fascia lata and coracoacromial ligament have been used to bridge large defects. Different methods have been proposed to use the long head of the biceps tendon as either a free graft or an intact interpositional stint between tendons.[41] Neviaser has reported on the use of freeze-dried allograft to bridge large defects, as well as transfer of the teres minor and subscapularis.[42] Cofield has reported good results with transfer of the upper portion of the subscapularis tendon into a large defect.[8] Debeyre[10] and Ha'eri[16] have described advancement of the supraspinatus from a posterior approach. Various synthetic materials have been used, such as mersilene, nylon mesh, and carbon fiber, but such techniques are still developmental.[44] Most large and massive tears can be closed with careful mobilization of the torn cuff edges supplemented with transfer of the upper subscapularis and biceps interposition when needed. An abduction brace may be required to relieve tension across the cuff repair. This should be maintained for 5 to 6 weeks. Whether the patient is in a sling or a brace, passive exercises are started on the fifth day, and active exercises at 6 weeks.

COMPLICATIONS

There are several complications which can occur after anterior acromioplasty and rotator cuff repairs. One of the most common is a stiff shoulder from insufficient postoperative rehabilitation.

Another common problem may be residual impingement from an incorrectly performed acromioplasty or a failure to recognize that acromioclavicular arthritis is also present and adding to the impingement. Postoperative radiography is mandatory whenever bone is removed. It must always be remembered that a cuff repair can retear as a result of either overzealous physiotherapy or a traumatic incident. If a retear is suspected, arthrography should be performed without delay. Also, if there is a traumatic incident, the deltoid repair may also be involved. Infection is a very rare complication following anterior acromioplasty and cuff repair.

REFERENCES

Section A: Rheumatologic and Degenerative Disorders

1. Arner, O., Lindvall, N., and Rieger, A. Calcific tendinitis (tendinitis calcarea) of the shoulder joint. Acta Chir Scand 114:319–331, 1958.
2. Barton, N.J. Arthrodesis of the shoulder for degenerative conditions. J Bone Joint Surg 54A:1759–1764, 1972.
3. Benjamin, A., Hirschowitz, D., and Arden, G.P. The treatment of arthritis of the shoulder by double osteotomy. Int Orthop 3:211–216, 1979.
4. Bosworth, B.M. Calcium deposits in the shoulder and subacromial bursitis. A survey of 12,122 shoulders. JAMA 116:2477–2482, 1941.
5. Chung, S.M.K., and Ralston, E.L. Necrosis of the humeral head associated with sickle cell anemia and its genetic variants. Clin Orthop 80:105–117, 1971.
6. Clayton, M.L., and Ferlic, D.C. Surgery of the shoulder in rheumatoid arthritis. A report of nineteen patients. Clin Orthop 106:166–174, 1975.
7. Codman, E.A. *The Shoulder: Rupture of the Supraspinatus Tendon and Other Lesions in or About the Subacromial Bursa.* Boston, Thomas Todd, 1934.
8. Cofield, R.H. Total shoulder arthroplasty with the Neer prosthesis. J Bone Joint Surg 66A:899–906, 1984.
9. Cofield, R.H. Arthrodesis and resectional arthroplasty of the shoulder, in Evarts, C.M. (ed): *Surgery of the Musculoskeletal System.* New York, Churchill Livingstone, 1983.
10. Cofield, R.H. Unconstrained total shoulder prosthesis. Clin Orthop 173:97–108, 1983.
11. Cruess, R.L. Steroid-induced avascular necrosis of the head of the humerus. Natural history and management. J Bone Joint Surg 58B:313–317, 1976.
12. Curran, J.F., Ellman, M.H., and Brown, N.L. Rheumatologic aspects of painful conditions affecting the shoulder. Clin Orthop 173:27–37, 1983.
13. Diggs, L.W. Bone and joint lesions in sickle-cell disease. Clin Orthop 52:119–143, 1967.
14. Ferlic, D.C., and Clayton, M.L. Rheumatoid arthritis of the shoulder, in Evarts, C.M. (ed): *Surgery of the Musculoskeletal System.* New York, Churchill Livingstone, 1983.
15. Jones, L. The shoulder joint. Observations on the anatomy and physiology. With an analysis of reconstructive operation following extensive injury. Surg Gynecol Obstet 75:433–444, 1942.
16. Marmor, L. Hemiarthroplasty for the rheumatoid shoulder joint. Clin Orthop 122:201–203, 1977.
17. McCarty, D.J., Halverson, P.B., Carrera, G.F., Brewer, B.J., and Kozin, F. "Milwaukee shoulder." Association of microspheroids containing hydroxyapatite crystals, active collagenase, and neutral protease with rotator cuff defects. Arthritis Rheum 24:464–473, 1981.
18. McLaughlin, H.L. The selection of calcium deposits for operation. The technique and results of operation. Surg Clin North Am 43(6):1501–1504, 1963.
19. McLaughlin, H.L. Lesions of the musculotendinous cuff of the shoulder. III. Observations on the pathology, course and treatment of calcific deposits. Ann Surg, 124:354–362, 1946.
20. Neer, C.S., Craig, E.V., and Fukuda, H. Cuff-tear arthropathy. J Bone Joint Surg 65A:1232–1244, 1983.
21. Neer, C.S., Watson, K.C., and Stanton, F.J. Recent experience in total shoulder replacement. J Bone Joint Surg 64A:319–337, 1982.
22. Neer, C.S. Reconstructive surgery and rehabilitation of the shoulder, in Kelley, W.U., Harris, E.D., Ruddy, S., and Sledge, C.B. (eds): *Textbook of Rheumatology.* Philadelphia, Saunders, 1981, pp 1944–1959.
23. Neer, C.S. Replacement arthroplasty for glenohumeral osteoarthritis. J Bone Joint Surg 56A:1–13, 1974.
24. Neviaser, R.J. Painful conditions affecting the shoulder. Clin Orthop 173:63–69, 1983.
25. Pedersen, H.E., and Key, J.A. Pathology of calcareous tendinitis and subdeltoid bursitis. Arch Surg 62:50–63, 1951.
26. Peyron, J.G. Epidemiologic and etiologic approach of osteoarthritis. Semin Arthritis Rheum 8:288–306, 1979.
27. Post, M., and Jablon, M. Constrained total shoulder arthroplasty. Long-term follow-up observations. Clin Orthop 173:109–116, 1983.
28. Post, M., Haskell, S.S., and Jablon, M. Total shoulder replacement with a constrained prosthesis. J Bone Joint Surg 62A:327–335, 1980.
29. Rogers, M.H. A study of one hundred cases of subdeltoid bursitis. J Bone Joint Surg 16:145–150, 1934.

Section B: Subacromial Impingement Syndrome

1. Armstrong, J.R. Excision of the acromion in treatment of the supraspinatus syndrome. Report of ninety-five excisions. J Bone Joint Surg 31B:436–442, 1949.
2. Bateman, J.E. The diagnosis and treatment of ruptures of the rotator cuff. Surg Clin North Am 46(6):1523–1530, 1963.
3. Bayne, O., and Bateman, J.E. Long term results of surgical repair of full thickness rotator cuff tears, in Bateman, J.E., and Welsh, R.P. (eds): *Surgery of the Shoulder.* Philadelphia, Decker, 1984, pp 167–171.
4. Bigliani, L.U., Norris, T.R., Fischer, J., and Neer, C.S. The relationship between the unfused acromial epiphysis and subacromial impingement lesions. Orthop Trans 7:138, 1983.
5. Codman, E.A. *The Shoulder; Rupture of the Supraspinatus Tendon and Other Lesions in or About the Subacromial Bursa.* Boston, Thomas Todd, 1934.

6. Codman, E.A. Rupture of the supraspinatus, 1834–1934. J Bone Joint Surg 19:643–652, 1937.

7. Codman, E.A. Complete rupture of the supraspinatus tendon. Operative treatment with report of two successful cases. Boston Med Surg J 164:708–711, 1911.

8. Cofield, R.H. Subscapular muscle transposition for repair of chronic rotator cuff tears. Surg Gynecol Obstet 154:667–672, 1982.

9. Cotton, R.E., and Rideout, D.F. Tears of the humeral rotator cuff. A radiological and pathological necropsy survey. J Bone Joint Surg 46B:314–328, 1964.

10. Debeyre, J., Patte, D., and Elmelik, E. Repair of ruptures of the rotator cuff of the shoulder. With a note on advancement of the supraspinatus muscle. J Bone Joint Surg 47B:36–42, 1965.

11. DePalma, A.F. *Surgery of the Shoulder,* 2d ed. Philadelphia, Lippincott, 1973.

12. DesMarchais, J.E., and Vezina, J. Diagnosis of rotator cuff tears by double contrast arthrotomography. Reliability study, in Bateman, J.E., and Welsh, R.P. (eds): *Surgery of the Shoulder.* Philadelphia, Decker, 1984, pp 126–128.

13. Donovan, W.H., and Kraft, G.H. Rotator cuff tear versus suprascapular nerve injury. A problem in differential diagnosis. Arch Phys Med Rehabil 55:424–428, 1974.

14. Ghelman, B., and Goldman, A.B. The double contrast shoulder arthrogram. Evaluation of rotary cuff tears. Radiology 124:251–254, 1977.

15. Grant, J.C.B., and Smith, G.C. Age incidence of rupture of the supraspinatus tendon. Anat Rec 100:666, 1948.

16. Ha'eri, G.B., and Wiley, A.M. Advancement of the supraspinatus muscle in the repair of ruptures of the rotator cuff. J Bone Joint Surg 63A:232–238, 1981.

17. Hammond, G. Complete acromionectomy in the treatment of chronic tendinitis of the shoulder. A follow-up of ninety operations on eighty-seven patients. J Bone Joint Surg 53A:173–180, 1971.

18. Hawkins, R.J., and Hobeika, P.E. Impingement syndromes in the athletic shoulder. *Clin Sports Med* 2(2):391–405, 1983.

19. Hawkins, R.J., and Brock, R.M.: Anterior acromioplasty. Early results for impingement with intact rotator cuffs. Orthop Trans 3:274, 1979.

20. Hollinshead, W.H. *Anatomy for Surgeons,* vol 3: *The Back and Limbs,* 3d ed. New York, Harper & Row, 1982.

21. Jobe, F.W. Serious rotator cuff injuries. Clin Sports Med 2(2):407–412, 1983.

22. Jobe, F.W., and Jobe, C.M. Painful athletic injuries of the shoulder. Clin Orthop 173:117–124, 1983.

23. Laing, P.G. The arterial supply of the adult humerus. J Bone Joint Surg 38A:1105–1116, 1956.

24. Lie, S., and Mast, W.A. Subacromial bursography. Technique and clinical application. Radiology 144:626–630, 1982.

25. Lindblom, K., and Palmer, I. Ruptures of the tendon aponeurosis of the shoulder joint. The so-called supraspinatus ruptures. Acta Chir Scand 82:133–142, 1939.

26. Lindblom, K. On pathogenesis of ruptures of the tendon aponeurosis of the shoulder joint. Acta Radiol 20:563–577, 1939.

27. Lindblom, K. Arthrography and roentgenography in ruptures of the tendons of the shoulder joint. Acta Radiol 20:548–562, 1939.

28. McLaughlin, H.L. Repair of major cuff ruptures. Surg Clin North Am 43(6):1535–1540, 1963.

29. McLaughlin, H.L. Rupture of the rotator cuff. J Bone Joint Surg 44A:979–983, 1962.

30. McLaughlin, H.L. Lesions of the musculotendinous cuff of the shoulder. I. The exposure and treatment of tears with retraction. J Bone Joint Surg 26:31–51, 1944.

31. Meyer, A.W. Spontaneous dislocation and destruction of tendon of long head of biceps brachii. Fifty-nine instances. Arch Surg 17:493–506, 1928.

32. Moseley, H.F., and Goldie, I. The arterial pattern of the rotator cuff of the shoulder. J Bone Joint Surg 45B:780–789, 1963.

33. Moseley, H.F. Ruptures of the rotator cuff. Br J Surg 38:340–369, 1951.

34. Mudge, M.K., Wood, V.E., and Frykman, G.K. Rotator cuff tears associated with os acromiale. J Bone Joint Surg 66A:427–429, 1984.

35. Neer, C.S. Impingement lesions. Clin Orthop 173:70–77, 1983.

36. Neer, C.S., and Marberry, T.A. On the disadvantages of radical acromionectomy. J Bone Joint Surg 63A:416–419, 1981.

37. Neer, C.S., Craig, E.V., and Fukuda, H. Cuff-tear arthropathy. J Bone Joint Surg 65A:1232–1244, 1983.

38. Neer, C.S., Bigliani, L.U., and Hawkins, R.J. Rupture of the long head of the biceps related to subacromial impingement. Orthop Trans 1:111, 1977.

39. Neer, C.S., and Welsh, R.P. The shoulder in sports. Orthop Clin North Am 8(3):583–591, 1977.

40. Neer, C.S. Anterior acromioplasty for the chronic impingement syndrome in the shoulder. A preliminary report. J Bone Joint Surg 54A:41–50, 1972.

41. Neviaser, R.J., and Neviaser, T.J. Reconstruction of chronic tears of the rotator cuff, in Bateman, J.E., and Welsh, R.P. (eds): *Surgery of the Shoulder.* Philadelphia, Decker, 1984, pp 172–179.

42. Neviaser, J.S., Neviaser, R.J., and Neviaser, T.J. The repair of chronic massive ruptures of the rotator cuff of the shoulder by use of a freeze-dried rotator cuff. J Bone Joint Surg 60A:681–684, 1978.

43. Niebauer, J.J. The acromial splitting incision for repair of the shoulder capsule. J Bone Joint Surg, 45A:661, 1963.

44. Ozaki, J., Fujimoto, S., and Masuhara, K. Repair of chronic massive rotator cuff tears with synthetic fabrics, in Bateman, J.E., and Welsh, R.P. (eds): *Surgery of the Shoulder.* Philadelphia, Decker, 1984, pp 185–191.

45. Post, M., Silver, R., and Singh, M. Rotator cuff tear. Diagnosis and treatment. Clin Orthop 173:78–91, 1983.

46. Rathbun, J.B., and Macnab, I. The microvascular pattern of the rotator cuff. J Bone Joint Surg 52B:540–53, 1970.

47. Reeves, B. Arthrography of the shoulder. J Bone Joint Surg, 48B:424–435, 1966.

48. Rothman, R.A. Vascular anatomy of the rotator cuff. Clin Orthop 44:280, 1966.

49. Rothman, R.A., and Parke, W.W. The vascular anatomy of the rotator cuff. Clin Orthop 41:176–186, 1965.

50. Rowe, C.R. Ruptures of the rotator cuff. Selection of cases for conservative treatment. Surg Clin North Am 43(6):1531–1534, 1963.

51. Stamm, T.T. Para-glenoid osteotomy. J Bone Joint Surg 44B:228, 1962.

52. Strizak, A.M., Danzig, L., Jackson, D.W., Greenway, G., Resnick, D., and Staple, T. Subacromial bursography. An anatomical and clinical study. J Bone Joint Surg 64A:196–201, 1982.

53. Uthoff, H.K., Sarkar, K., and Hammond, D.I. The subacromial bursa. A clinicopathological study, in Bateman, J.E., and Welsh, R.P. (eds): *Surgery of the Shoulder.* Philadelphia, Decker, 1984, pp 121–125.

54. Weiner, D.S., and Macnab, I. Superior migration of the humeral head. A radiological aid in the diagnosis of tears of the rotator cuff. J Bone Joint Surg 52B:524–527, 1970.

55. Wilson, C.L., and Duff, G.L. Pathologic study of degeneration and rupture of the supraspinatus tendon. Arch Surg 47:121–135, 1943.

56. Wolfang, G.L. Rupture of the musculotendinous cuff of the shoulder. Clin Orthop 134:230–243, 1978.

57. Wolfang, G.L. Surgical repair of tears of the rotator cuff of the shoulder. Factors influencing the result. J Bone Joint Surg 56A:14–26, 1974.

CHAPTER 38

Rheumatologic and Degenerative Disorders of the Elbow

Roger Dee

PHYSICAL EXAMINATION

Inspection of the elbow will reveal gross malalignment of the arm plus any obvious swelling, erythema, scarring, etc. The attitude in which the patients hold the arm, particularly if they support the limb with the other arm, may give important clues as to the degree of discomfort or loss of function.

Palpation of the medial and lateral epicondyles and the tip of the olecranon should confirm the normal equilateral triangle, which is their configuration at 90 degrees of elbow flexion. Joint subluxation or dislocation may disrupt this triangle. With the elbow in extension, these three points approximate a straight horizontal line.

The ulnar nerve can be directly palpated or gently percussed for tenderness. It may be felt to move out of its bed if it is subluxing. Careful palpation also identifies the humeroulnar joint line posterolaterally and gives important evidence about joint line tenderness, synovial thickening, and the presence or absence of small amounts of joint fluid. The posterior aspect of the joint should not be neglected since the joint is close to the surface on either side of the triceps and can easily be palpated.

Medial and lateral gapping of the joint can be detected clinically where there is gross instability. Volz and Morrey recommend testing for valgus instability with the humerus externally rotated at the shoulder and for varus instability from the posterior aspect of the joint whilst fully internally rotating the shoulder. In both cases the elbow is flexed 15 degrees during the test to unlock the olecranon.[74] If the arm is x-rayed in extension and full supination with a fulcrum under the upper arm, gapping which may not be clinically obvious is often seen on the radiograph from the weight of the forearm opening up the lateral joint. A Lachman type of test performed at 90 degrees and also at 15 degrees of flexion detects anteroposterior instability.

When the range of motion is assessed, it is important to realize that full extension is 0 degrees and an elbow flexed at right angles is 90 degrees. Pronation/supination is best assessed with the elbow at 90 degrees with the upper arm in contact with the thorax to prevent shoulder motion. Pronation and supination measure a little less than 90 degrees in normal subjects. The midposition of pronation/supination is recorded as 0 degrees. A normal range of flexion-extension may be taken as 0 to 145 degrees. Use of a goniometer is recommended.

RHEUMATOID ARTHRITIS OF THE ELBOW

One may conveniently classify rheumatoid arthritis of the elbow joint into *grade 1,* in which osteoporosis and soft tissue changes only are present; *grade 2,* in which there are mild or moderate degrees of erosion and a moderate reduction of joint space, not less than 1 mm; *grade 3,* a more advanced situation in which the joint space is markedly narrowed to 1 mm or less with extensive erosions; and *grade 4,* in which there is subluxation and ankylosis. This classification[62] is a useful starting point from which to discuss the indication and results of surgery of the elbow in rheumatoid arthritis.

Synovectomy

Synovectomy has long been recognized as a useful procedure for the relief of rheumatologic pain.[6] In the 1971 Hospital for Special Surgery report of 28 elbows that had undergone synovectomy for rheumatoid arthritis, it was observed that all patients fell into grade 3 or grade 4.[30] The operation was performed through a transolecranon approach, but the complication of separation and nonunion of olecranon fragments was noted in two patients. Although 18 of the 28 elbows were classified as good and 6 as satisfactory and they observed only 4 failures, the follow-up period was only 3½ years. Synovectomy did not render the joint unstable.

Porter, Richardson, and Vainio noted that 70 percent of 154 synovectomies (primarily grade 3 and grade 4 cases) could be rated as "good" using the patients' judgment alone.[49] The indication for surgery was pain, and most patients had failed drug and other conservative treatment. Radiological deterioration was seen to be progressive, especially after the third postoperative year, but there was no particular relation between radiological deterioration and recurrence of symptoms. This was confirmed by a recent series of 35 patients with grade 3 and grade 4 disease treated by synovectomy at Rancho Los Amigos.[5]

Copeland and Taylor[11] also noticed that radiological deterioration occurs in early cases (grade 2 and grade 3).[4] They concluded that radiographic assessment is essential for selecting elbows for synovectomy because it enables one to grade patients but pointed out it is not much help in evaluating results of surgery. Most authors report use of an extended lateral incision or a combination of medial and lateral incisions to perform the synovectomy rather than the trans-olecranon approach.

The results of synovectomy in children with juvenile rheumatoid arthritis are less favorable than those in adults.[31] In joints without radiographic change at the time of an early synovectomy there is little if any retardation of the progress of the disease. In cases of more advanced joint disease and preexisting radiographic changes, deterioration seems to continue and the authors noted that there are few if any benefits from the operation with reference to pain or improvement of range of motion. The only improvement seems to be to provide permanent relief of joint swelling.[22]

If preoperative assessment indicates painful crepitus in the radiohumeral joint during pronation and supination, synovectomy may conveniently be combined with excision of the radial head. Indeed some authors consider it should be performed in all cases.[1,52] Swanson has recommended inserting a Silastic implant at the time of synovectomy to replace the excised radial head and has reported a clinical and radiological study of 105 cases with a follow-up period of up to 10 years.[65] He concluded that the implant can provide stability in rheumatoid elbows following radial head removal and so avoid the main complications of the procedure, which include bone formation at the resection site and proximal migration of the radial shaft. The latter may cause pain at the elbow and wrist in rheumatoid patients following the loss of the important loading mechanism across the radiocapitellar joint. Occasionally, excision of the radial head is combined with a Darrach subperiosteal excision of the distal inch of the ulna. This is indicated when it is considered that the distal radioulnar joint contributes to loss of pronation/supination which can thereby be restored.

The degree of proximal migration of the radius following radial head excision for fracture is only 1 or 2 mm.[4] This degree of migration of the radial head cannot be correlated with the quality of the functional result or used to justify routine replacement. It seems unlikely that migration alone can account for the wrist symptoms sometimes seen to cause disability following radial head excision.[42] Replacement of the radial head seems to be indicated to enhance stability when the fracture of the radial head has been associated with damage to the medial collateral ligament in unstable fracture dislocations, and its replacement helps stabilize an otherwise unstable elbow. Replacement is also appropriate in those patients in whom a fracture of the radial head is associated with radioulnar disassociation at the wrist joint. Replacement then contributes some stability at its proximal end to a very unstable radius.

Arthroplasty of the Elbow Joint

Although synovectomy would seem to be a useful procedure for early disease, an alternative in grade 4 disease and advanced grade 3 disease is some form of arthroplasty.

Excision Arthroplasty

Removing a large piece of the distal humerus together with its periosteum and ligament attachments obviously produces

instability, and it is not surprising that it was condemned a century ago by Ollier.[48] Ollier was primarily concerned with immobilizing tuberculous joints rather than those of rheumatoid arthritis. He proposed instead a subperiosteal subcapsular excision of the joint. Following this procedure he applied a hinged splint and was able to make use of the remodeling characteristics of regenerating subperiosteal bone and refashion a reasonably stable joint in these young patients. Kirkaldy-Willis achieved acceptable results in an African population using this type of subperiosteal procedure.[37]

However, excision arthroplasty for rheumatoid arthritis can lead to serious instability.[13] Occasionally some functional stability is achieved when the patient is able to use the support of the upper arm muscles,[28] but usually this is not enough, since at 90 degrees the fulcrum collapses and the muscles are unable to support the limb. Following this operation, the patient can rarely bear weight on crutches.[7] The unmodified operation should not be attempted in rheumatoid arthritis since there are now preferred options.

Anatomical Arthroplasty

As first described by DeFontaine[18] in 1887, it is possible to refashion the articular contours of a diseased joint while maintaining the ligaments of the joint and thus its stability. Fashioning a crest on the olecranon and a notch in the trochlea also helps maintain mediolateral stability. However, the loss of joint surfaces and the considerable erosion commonly seen in this disease ensure that the ligaments are relatively lax and the joint consequently unstable. Also since further destruction is likely, some form of interposition material is now recommended.

All authors agree that the best results are achieved when the operation is performed for ankylosis and that the penalty for too little resection of bone is reankylosis, though this is much more likely if there is no interposition membrane. Post-

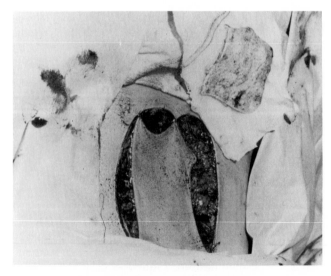

Figure 38-1 Method of obtaining a dermal graft for cutis arthroplasty. The epidermis has been returned to the graft bed and resuturing has commenced. The dermal graft is seen on the gauze (*top right*).

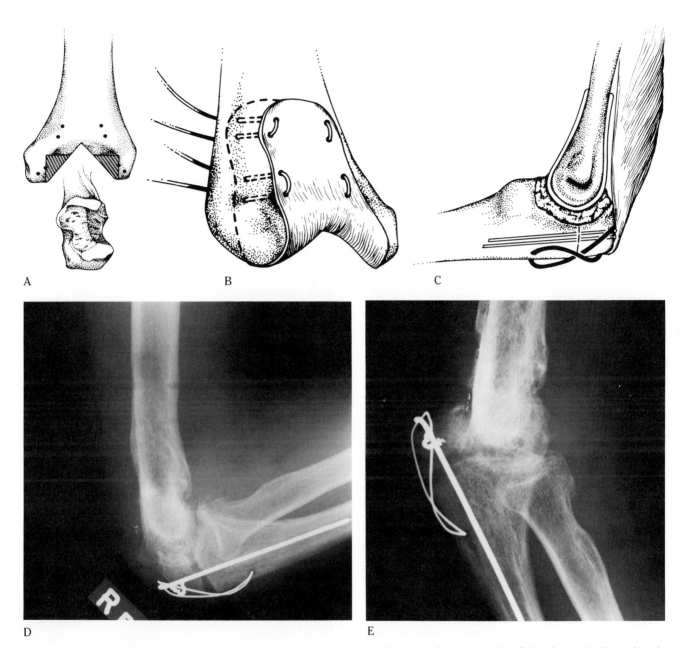

A   B   C

D   E

Figure 38-2 A. Preparation of the bone for cutis arthroplasty. Note that a portion of the coronoid and also the tip of the olecranon have been removed and a central crest fashioned in the ulna. An inverted V shape is created within the contour of the eroded humerus, and drill holes are made to receive the graft. **B.** The dermal graft is sutured in position, deep surface to the bone. **C.** The completed cutis arthroplasty. Bone chips have been interposed between the cutis graft and the ulnar articular surface (a useful technique where severe erosion occurs in rheumatoid arthritis). **D** and **E.** Two x-ray views of posttraumatic arthritis in a 24-year-old man treated by cutis arthroplasty. Note the excellent range of motion. There is fibrous union of the olecranon (a complication of the surgical approach).

operative subluxation is a notable complication recorded by Knight and VanZandt.[35,36] These authors recommend excision of the head of the radius to reduce the risk of lateral epicondylar erosion.

One can also use the classic fascial arthroplasty developed by Campbell[8] and MacAusland[41] or the deep dermal layer of the skin for interposition according to the technique described by Froimson and his coauthors.[24] The fascia lata graft is applied to the humerus with its deep surface applied

to the bone. A fold is made in the flap of fascia to mimic the posterior recess of capsule. The flap is of sufficient length to be then applied continuously over the floor of the olecranon and is sutured to the margins of the articular surface of that bone and anteriorly to the coronoid process. In this method there are two gliding surfaces of fascia in contact at the conclusion of the arthroplasty.

In the technique of cutis arthroplasty, a thin epidermal layer of skin is raised with a dermatome and left attached at the margin of the donor site. The deep dermal layer is then excised from the underlying fat with a sharp scalpel and used as a graft, being sutured snugly over the distal humerus with the fat side toward the bone. The epidermal flap is resutured back into position or excised (Fig. 38-1). When there is considerable erosion of the olecranon, Vainio has used bone chips beneath a cutis graft to replace the eroded olecranon (Fig. 38-2).

Following synovectomy and arthroplasties of the elbow, rehabilitation must be gentle since overenthusiastic "passive" manipulative physical therapy can be counterproductive. Since lack of extension rather than loss of flexion seems to be the biggest postoperative problem, it is my practice to put these elbows up at 35 degrees of flexion postoperatively rather than 90 degrees. A padded dressing with a posterior mold is used for a few days, and then active exercises are instituted.

Interposition arthroplasty can be performed either through a transolecranon approach or through an extended lateral (Kocher) incision, but in both instances it is important to preserve the collateral ligaments. Early postoperative mobilization is critical, and the surgical approach should be planned so that a long period of postoperative immobilization is not necessary.

Prosthetic Replacement

However good the techniques of interposition arthroplasty, one may expect a failure rate of between 20 and 30 percent in rheumatoid arthritis and considerably more if one performs excision arthroplasty.[7,8,13,19,24,27,28,35,41] Consequently, since the mid 1960's, efforts have been made to devise a successful replacement prosthesis which will give a higher proportion of acceptable results without the described complications of instability, reankylosis, bone erosion, and subluxation seen in the nonprosthetic operations.

Prosthetic Hemiarthroplasty

There are numerous case reports of replacement of the lower end of the humerus[3,41,43,56,73] or the proximal end of the ulna[32] by custom-made anatomic prostheses. Abrasive wear has caused rapid deterioration of these prostheses when they are made of inappropriate materials such as Teflon, but even when they are made of metal, problems of erosion of bone on the host side of the joint, subluxation, and prosthetic loosening have been seen. They do not give such complete pain relief as one achieves by resurfacing both sides of the joint.

Fully Constrained Prosthesis

Early results with the author's fully constrained hinge were encouraging,[14] but by 5 years 25 percent of the joints were loose and the loosening was accompanied by serious salvage problems. The intrusion of large stems into the medullary cavities of the ulna and humerus and the fragmenting cement mantle caused considerable damage to the bone when loosening occurred. The bone often ballooned and eroded and at revision was often seen to be paper thin (Fig. 38-3). Other

early constrained joint designs suffered a similar fate and were eventually abandoned.[6,10,44,45,46,69]

Following the failure of totally constrained hinged joints, the field of elbow prosthetics moved toward the development of two separate kinds of elbow joint systems. One kind is a totally unconstrained surface replacement, which is biomechanically preferable since it is least likely to loosen. Another kind of joint is semiconstrained and usually allows some rotation plus varus-valgus laxity. It is for use in low-demand situations where the bone stock may be deficient and unsuitable for surface replacement and where some kind of linkage mechanism is required (Fig. 38-4). Semiconstrained joints are less likely to loosen than constrained joints, but large mechanical forces are transmitted across the linkage so that component breakage and some instance of loosening are common.

Semiconstrained Prosthesis

Semiconstrained prostheses are only used in severe rheumatoid arthritis. They are probably technically a little easier to insert than unconstrained prostheses since tissue balancing

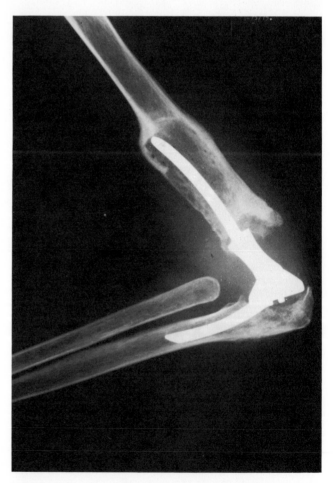

Figure 38-3 An early Dee hinge which was rigidly constrained. Note the ballooning of the humeral cortex, a consequence of long-term loosening. The cement is not visible since it did not contain barium.

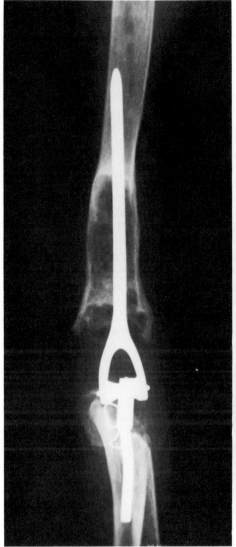

A

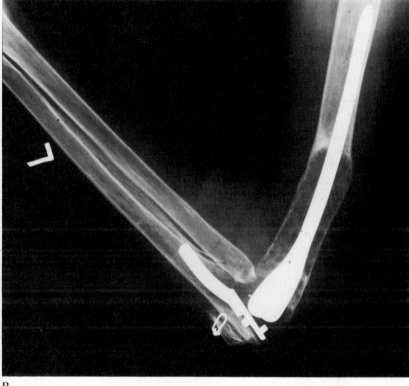

B

Figure 38-4 The same patient as in Fig. 38-3 after reconstruction using a semi-constrained linking type of endoprosthesis. **A.** Anteroposterior view. **B.** Lateral view.

to avoid subluxation is not so critical. The short-term results seem to indicate that designing to permit some varus-valgus motion and rotation results in an acceptable trade-off in terms of loosening. This has been the experience with the modified Coonrad and Dee prostheses,[10,17] the triaxial prosthesis of Inglis,[30] the designs from the Mayo Clinic,[45,46] and the Volz AHSC prosthesis.[6]

There have been some component failures in most series[5,30,46] and consequently some need for redesign.

Fracture of the humeral shaft or condyles during insertion can occur.[5,30] Conservative treatments seems to be sufficient to stabilize the interoperative fracture. Careful surgery together with good preoperative radiographic evaluation and implant selection should prevent this complication.

Unconstrained Prosthesis

Unconstrained prostheses are the prostheses of choice in rheumatoid arthritis, and in experienced hands they probably give results marginally superior to those of interposition arthroplasty, but this is disputable. Good minimally eroded bone stock and intact collateral ligaments are necessary for successful result.

Early reports in the literature indicate that the incidence of loosening in these prostheses is acceptably low. Thus, Kudo reported that in 24 patients with rheumatoid arthritis there was only one case of loosening and one case of instability.[38] Loosening certainly seems to be more common in the humeral component than on the ulnar side.[39] Where there is severe erosive disease the lower end of the humerus is represented by a wishbone-shaped piece of bone. Then a stem seems to be necessary for secure fixation even in an unconstrained design. Soni and Cavendish noted that changing the design so that the humeral component was stemmed reduced their loosening problem in the humeral component of the Liverpool prostheses to acceptable levels.[60]

It is critically important to preserve the anterior oblique portion of the medial collateral ligament at surgery, and for this reason use of the extended lateral Kocher approach is stressed.[12,27] Authors report postoperative instability as occurring in 5.7 percent,[21] 13.3 percent,[12] and 14.3 percent[50] using Ewald's capitellocondylar design, with which they achieved good or satisfactory results in 80 percent of cases with rheumatoid arthritis (Fig. 38-5). They found an average residual flexion contraction of a little over 30 degrees.[12,21,50]

At the present time it is difficult to obtain a stable unconstrained elbow prosthetic replacement and achieve full extension. Sophisticated jigging systems are not currently available for the elbow joint. Perfect balancing of soft tissues and appropriate geometry of bone cuts remain our immediate goal for the future. The problem is complex because of the requirement to resurface the radiocapitellar joint at the same time, which adds great complexity to the jigging system. If the lateral side is not reconstructed appropriately, even with an intact medial collateral ligament, supination of the forearm subluxes the ulnar component off the humeral component, to which it is not linked. This instability is difficult to prevent without accurate repair of the lateral ligament complex. The matter is made worse if the ulnar component is not correctly

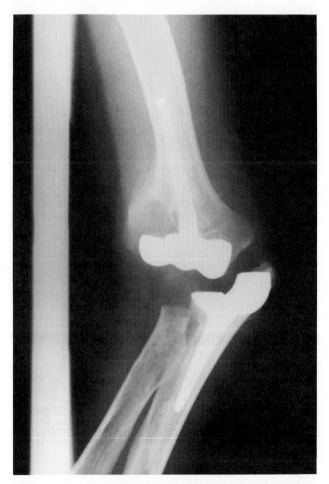

Figure 38-5 The medial collateral ligament is especially important when inserting unconstrained elbow prostheses. Here a capitellocondylar prosthesis has dislocated postoperatively, probably because the medial collateral ligament was not preserved during its insertion.

aligned in the appropriate position of axial rotation relative to the shaft of the ulna and if there is restriction of motion in the radioulnar joints. All these factors produce a tendency to rotatory subluxation across the new joint. Complications of these operations include high risk of infection. For semiconstructed joints the incidence of infection ranges from 3.2[29] to 8.8.[45] In the three reported series of capitellocondylar (Ewald) joints, an average infection rate of 8 percent has been reported in 127 cases.[12,21,50] For the Liverpool elbow prosthesis, which is an unconstrained design, an infection rate of 5 percent was reported.[60]

Complications involving the ulnar nerve range from neuropraxia with some temporary loss of function to irritating ulnar nerve paresthesias and local tenderness following elbow arthroplasty. The incidence of ulnar nerve complications averaged 12 percent using the capitellocondylar prosthesis.[12,21,50] In Ewald's own series approximately 50 percent of the ulnar nerve lesions recovered. A 21 percent incidence of ulnar nerve complications was reported using the Liverpool prosthesis,[60] but the surgical approach was not described by the authors. It seems that using the lateral incision and preserving the medial collateral ligament at the same time offers the best method of preventing traction lesions to the ulnar nerve.

RECONSTRUCTION OF THE ELBOW FOLLOWING SEVERE TRAUMA

These patients are often young, and the commonest trauma is severe open fracture. Primary internal fixation may have been unsatisfactory because of infection, or there may have been severe loss of bone stock. Similar problems in elbow reconstruction follow removal of a failed hinge endoprosthesis or tumor.

Where the articular surface of a joint has been severely damaged but there is no major bone deficiency, a surface replacement (unconstrained prosthesis) may be considered. However, these patients are often young and unlike patients with rheumatoid arthritis may impose high demand upon their elbow joint. In many cases the medial collateral ligament is not intact. Under these conditions, to restore function it is probably safer to perform an interposition anatomic-type arthroplasty as described using either cutis or fascia as an interposition membrane. Certainly in the author's experience simple lysis of interarticular adhesions is not sufficient to obtain motion in fibrous ankylosis. It is possible to successfully mobilize an elbow with solid intraarticular bony ankylosis using interposition arthroplasty and approaching the joint through the transolecranon osteotomy.

In the presence of loss of bone stock on one side of the joint, it is necessary to restore length to that segment so that stability is restored and the muscles may work efficiently at their normal resting length. Under these conditions one may be tempted to insert a semiconstrained prosthetic hinge, but the long-term durability of these devices is still questionable, especially in a young patient with high functional demands. To inject large quantities of methylmethacrylate into the humeral or ulnar shaft in young patients is to risk a difficult

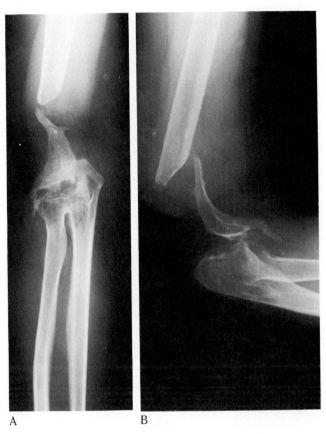

A   B

Figure 38-6 Two x-ray views of a flail elbow following a severe open fracture in a young woman. The loss of bone stock was due to a combination of destruction caused by the initial injury and subsequent surgical debridement for infection.

long-term salvage problem, but semiconstrained hinge devices may soon be sufficiently sophisticated to use in a press-fit manner so that cement can be omitted.

An alternative option which restores bone stock is the use of freeze-dried allografts.[17] These can be plated directly to the shaft of the host bone in an operation which is not technically demanding (Fig. 38-6 and 38-7A). Even though erosion of the articular surface and the metaphysis occurs (with time with some loss of stability), more than 50 percent of the implant is usually incorporated permanently into the host bone so that there is permanent gain of bone stock (Fig. 38-7B). By contrast, in the case of implant failure, the situation is worse off than when one started reconstruction. A worthwhile consideration may be prosthetically resurfacing the allograft (with a small uncemented stem protecting the metaphysis during the period of graft incorporation).

REVISION OF THE FAILED TOTAL ELBOW JOINT

The principles underlying revision surgery and the various procedures available have been described.[17] It is not good practice to remove a loose prosthesis of the hinged variety and reimplant one with a similar design. A prosthesis that is

biomechanically flawed in that situation will repeatedly fail. Removal of the cement mantle can be extremely difficult, and the technique includes the use of a headlight and some form of specialized tool (for example, a Midas Rex tool). Visualizing the external cortex of that portion of bone being cleared of cement or the use of fluoroscopy reduces the risk of perforation.

A failed unconstrained joint can be revised to a stemmed unconstrained prosthesis or a semiunconstrained joint. The failure may be due to malalignment of components, which causes a persistent instability that cannot be corrected by attention to the ligamentous structures, and revision may be more appropriate.

Where there is considerable thinning of the bone stock of the host bone, it is unlikely that a cemented prosthesis of any design will succeed, and under the circumstances the correct option may be to bone graft with allograft to the shaft and allow the host bone to reconstitute before performing a definitive reconstruction procedure.[17]

OSTEOARTHRITIS

Osteoarthritis involving the humeroulnar compartment is relatively uncommon in the elbow joint. By contrast degenerative changes in the radiocapitellar joint are common, especially following radial head injury. For severe disease of the whole joint, interposition arthroplasty or unconstrained endoprosthetic arthroplasty is to be considered after failed conservative therapy. One must take care to exclude the following alternative diagnoses:

1. *Spondyloarthropathies.* This is a group of joint diseases characterized by spondylitis. They often present with sacroiliac, ocular, or genital involvement. Included are psoriatic arthropathy, Reiter's disease, and ankylosing spondylitis. The HLA-B27 antigen is detectable in a high proportion of these patients, which together with the clinical features of the disease may suggest the appropriate diagnosis.

2. *Gout and pseudogout.* The area of the olecranon is a common site for rheumatoid nodule formation and also for sodium urate deposition in tophaceous gout. The synovial fluid may show sodium urate crystals present and causing a synovitis. These crystals are often within phagocytes and are identified using a polarizing microscope (with a first-order red compensator), which reveals them as needle-shaped negatively birefringent crystals.

   Calcium pyrophosphate deposition disease (CPDD) can present as an acute monarticular arthritis involving the elbow. Radiological examination may reveal the typical linear pattern of calcification in the capsule and the normally unseen articular cartilage. The examination of fresh synovial fluid under the polarizing microscope reveals positively birefringent rhomboid-shaped calcium pyrophosphate crystals in this condition.

3. *Septic arthritis.* Septic arthritis of the elbow is uncommon but does occur in patients who are drug abusers because of the proximity of the elbow joint to the common site of injection in the antecubital fossa. Occasionally sepsis in

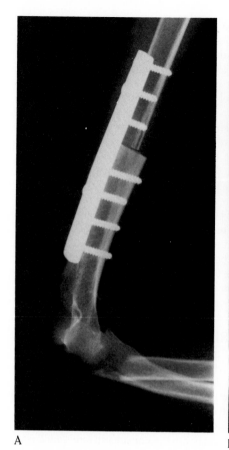

A

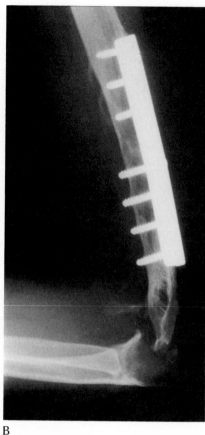

B

Figure 38-7 Same patient as shown in Fig. 36-6. **A.** Skeletal length and muscle balance have been restored by replacement of the distal humerus with a fresh frozen allograft. Union to the host bone was achieved in 6 months. **B.** Three years later there is considerable erosion in the region of the elbow joint not only of the allograft but also of the host bone. Sufficient stability persists, however, for useful function without a brace.

an olecranon bursa spreads to involve the elbow joint, especially if not promptly treated. Rheumatoid patients on steroids are also at risk for septic arthritis, which may involve this joint. One should always be aware that septic change may have occurred in any joint in this disease. In the young patient, differentiation from acute hematogenous osteomyelitis is important since the metaphysis of the distal humerus is not intracapsular and involvement of the joint is not therefore inevitable. Careful physical examination and accurate determination of the maximum site of tenderness together with diagnostic technetium and gallium scans should help to differentiate a true arthritis from humeral osteomyelitis with a sympathetic effusion. Blood cultures and diagnostic aspiration should support the diagnosis.

Septic arthritis is usually accompanied by severe pain and distress upon the slightest attempt to move the joint. Presentation may be subacute in a patient with rheumatoid arthritis, and the diagnosis can therefore be overlooked. Appropriate antibiotic treatment is based on the identification of the organism involved, which is commonly *Staphylococcus aureus.* A wide variety of other organisms may be identified in patients who are drug abusers.

The use of the arthroscope permits lavage of the joint to reduce the intraarticular bacterial count by dilution. This is a technique which avoids the need for open surgical drainage in most cases. Arthroscopy, early lavage and

drainage, and well-managed blood levels of appropriate antibiotics enable controlled assisted active motion to be recommenced as soon as the infection is under control. Early diagnosis and therapeutic motion are necessary for a good result.

THE ELBOW JOINT AND BLEEDING DIATHESES

In hemophilia the elbow joint ranks only second to the knee joint in the frequency of involvement.[25] Treatment of this disease is discussed in Chap. 21. Although in acute hemarthrosis the treatment is primarily appropriate factor replacement, recurrent hemarthrosis may be alleviated by synovectomy.[34]

In chronic arthropathy, spontaneous intraarticular hemorrhages have produced deterioration in the joint surfaces, and at this stage there is a virtually ankylosed joint which unfortunately remains painful and liable to bleed. A major side effect of the loss of function (which affects most commonly the dominant side) is an increased stress on the ipsilateral shoulder and the contralateral elbow, which leads to progressive arthropathy in these joints, which may have been only slightly affected.[57] A modified interposition arthroplasty using silicon rubber sheet as the interposition membrane has been successfully used to relieve pain, improve motion, and reduce the subsequent incidence of spontaneous hemorrhage into the elbow joint. Patients with hemophilia A received operative cover with factor VIII concentrates, while patients with von Willebrand's disease received factor VIII concentrate combined with cyroprecipitate.[57]

Attention has been drawn to the difficulty in interpreting an acute synovitis in a patient with sickle cell disease. The patients at risk are homozygous for this disease, which is due to the presence of a hemoglobin molecule which sickles in the deoxygenated state. Gilchrist points out that acute gouty arthritis has been described in this disease, and serum uric acid levels are often elevated.[26] Aspiration of joint fluid may show very high polymorphonuclear leukocyte counts and may lead to suspicion of infection. Infection is common in sickle cell patients, so the possibility of septic arthritis certainly exists. However, the fluid from the uninfected joint may be purulent in uncomplicated cases of sickle cell arthropathy, so confirmation by culture is essential.[25,26]

OSTEOTOMY AROUND THE ELBOW JOINT

Osteotomy has not been used in the region of the elbow joint in the treatment of either osteoarthrosis or rheumatoid arthritis. For gunstock deformity following malunion of a supracondylar fracture, valgus osteotomy is occasionally indicated. Premature fusion of the capitellum or damage to the epiphysis may cause overgrowth on the medial side leading to a cubitus valgus with tardy ulnar palsy, but usually the treatment of choice is transplantation of the ulnar nerve anteriorly.

When corrective osteotomy is performed, fixation can be achieved by use of a small plate or external pins, but when using the latter one must take care that the position not be lost. French has described a method of inserting two screws, from the lateral side above and below the osteotomy, in such a way that they lie parallel after the wedge has been removed and then fixing the heads of the screws together with wire.[23] A lateral cortical spike can be fashioned on the proximal fragment to impale the metaphyseal fragment. The screw is then passed through the lateral cortex of the metaphyseal fragment which transfixes the cortical spike from the proximal fragment and then penetrates the rest of the distal fragment. This gives secure fixation, and the screw may easily be removed.

ARTHRODESIS OF THE ELBOW

Arthrodesis of the elbow is rarely performed and has a high failure rate where there is loss of bone stock. It is seldom indicated in rheumatoid arthritis since for these patients loss of any mobile joint throws additional stresses on proximal and distal joints which are already diseased. Following trauma there are now adequate methods of reconstruction without arthrodesis. Tuberculous arthritis was thought to be an indication for arthrodesis. This disease is infrequently

seen and if treated early can be appropriately handled by appropriate drug therapy following confirmatory diagnosis by synovial biopsy. With early treatment one may expect to obtain a mobile joint. In more advanced tuberculous arthritis, where the articular cartilage is destroyed, joint clearance that removes debris and disease is combined with appropriate drug therapy. In an elbow rendered ankylosed by burned out tuberculosis, interposition arthroplasty or some such mobilizing procedure is certainly feasible, and there is no longer the need to perform arthrodesis on the joint to render it "safe." Of course, no major reconstructive procedure on the joint should be performed with any possibility of continuing active infection. When there is no major bone loss, arthrodesis can be achieved by fashioning the olecranon via a square cut into a flat surface to approximate to the humerus between the epicondyles. Additional fixation may be by means of a posterior plate at right angles fixing both humerus and ulna, alternatively by the use of transfixing screws passing from one bone to another (Fig. 38-8*A* and *B*). Appropriately placed external fixators using either transfixion pins or half pins or combinations thereof together with bilateral triangular or trapezoidal external fixator frames are a great help in immobilizing the joint and increase the chances of a successful fusion. Bone graft is placed between the joint surfaces and supplemented by extraarticular bone graft. Extraarticular fixation is preferable in the presence of recent infection. The appropriate angle of fusion may be decided after careful consideration of the patient's employment.[59] It may be decided that a position other than 90 degrees is preferable in individual patients.

OLECRANON BURSITIS

Swelling and erythema over the point of the elbow may indicate bursitis in the olecranon bursa. This can be occupational due to mechanical irritation directly in the region of the olecranon tip or it can arise spontaneously. If unaccompanied by overlying cellulitis or pyrexia, the inflammation may be sterile. A period of rest is then usually enough to cause the fluid-filled cavity to shrink. However, such attacks frequently become chronic, and one is left with a permanent fluctuant swelling with some thickening in the bursal tissue. Under these conditions surgical removal is justified. One should clearly indicate to the patient the risk of recurrence, though recurrence can be minimized by careful operative technique. The proximity of the ulnar nerve makes removal of the bursa without identification and mobilization of the nerve difficult and hazardous. Both an adequate excision and a clear visualization of the nerve can easily be obtained through a midline incision. The floor of the bursa may be removed with a lining of periosteum or a very fine sliver of the bone, particularly if there is an associated exostosis.

Aspiration of synovial bursae in unsanitary conditions or with careless technique can lead to an infected bursa, and a bursa can similarly become infected without any obvious predisposing cause such as a skin abrasion. The patient may be toxic and ill with a high fever and leukocytosis. In the presence of frank pus, surgical drainage and appropriate immobi-

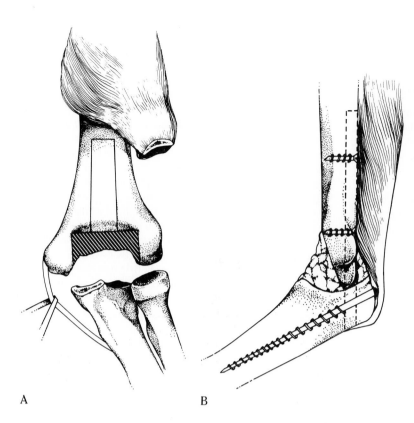

A   B

Figure 38-8 **A.** One of many available techniques for arthrodesing the elbow. The figure shows the area of bone (cross-hatched) removed to stabilize the construct. Note the rectangular area of posterior cortical bone outlined by the saw cut and ready to be used as a sliding bone graft. **B.** The posterior cortical graft is slid distally and transfixed by a long screw, which also reattaches the olecranon. The graft is fixed to the humerus in its new position. Autogenous bone is packed around.

lization of the elbow in a windowed cast is recommended. Irrigation of the bursa at the time of surgery is helpful. Appropriate antibiotic therapy should then resolve the situation. Several months later when the acute attack is settled and the wound is dry, definitive removal of the bursa can be entertained.

REFERENCES

1. Allison, N., and Coonse, G.K. Synovectomy in chronic arthritis. Arch Surg 18:824–840, 1929.
2. Amis, A.A., Dowson, D., and Wright, V. Elbow joint force predictions for some strenuous isometric actions. J Biomech 13:765–775, 1980.
3. Barr, J.S., and Eaton, R.G. Elbow reconstructions with a new prosthesis to replace the distal end of the humerus. J Bone Joint Surg 47A:1408–1413, 1965.
4. Basmajian, J.V., and Griffin, W.R. Function of anconeus muscle. J Bone Joint Surg 54A:1712–1714, 1972.
5. Brumfield, R.G., and Resnick, C.T. Synovectomy of the elbow in rheumatoid arthritis. J Bone Joint Surg 67A:16–20, 1985.
6. Brumfield, R.H., Jr., Volz, R.G., and Green, J.F. Total elbow arthroplasty, a review of 30 cases employing the Mayo and the A.H.S.C. prosthesis. Clin Orthop 158:137–141, 1981.
7. Buzby, B.F. End results of excision of the elbow. Ann Surg 103:625, 1936.
8. Campbell, W.C. Mobilization of joints with bony ankylosis. JAMA 83:976, 1924.
9. Cofield, R.H., Morrey, B.F., and Bryan, R.S. Total shoulder and total elbow arthroplasties; the current state of development, Part II J Contin Educ Orthop 17–25, 1979.
10. Coonrad, R.W. *Coonrad Total Elbow Replacement.* Presented at the Annual Meeting of the American Orthopaedic Association, June 27, 1978.
11. Copeland, S.A., and Taylor, J.G. Synovectomy of the elbow in rheumatoid arthritis. J Bone Joint Surg 61B:69–73, 1979.
12. Davis, R.F., Weiland, A., Hungerford, D.S., et al. Nonconstrained total elbow arthroplasty. Clin Orthop 171:156–160, 1982.
13. Dee, R. Arthroplasty of the elbow. Proc Soc Med 62:1031, 1969.
14. Dee, R. Total replacement arthroplasty of the elbow for rheumatoid arthritis. J Bone Joint Surg 54B:88–95, 1972a.
15. Dee, R. Total replacement of the elbow joint. Mod Trends Orthop 6:250, 1972b.
16. Dee, R. Total replacement of the elbow joint. Orthop Clin North Am 4:415, 1973.
17. Dee, R. Reconstructive surgery following failed total elbow endoprosthesis. Clin Orthop 170:196–203, 1982.
18. DeFontaine, L. Osteotomie Trochleiforme (1887). Rev Chir (Paris) 6:716, 1887.
19. Dickson, R.A., Stein, H., and Bentley, G. Excision arthroplasty of the elbow in rheumatoid disease. J Bone Joint Surg 58B:227–229, 1976.
20. Ewald, F.C. Reconstructive surgery and rehabilitation of the elbow, in Kelley, W.N. et al. (eds): *Textbook of Rheumatology,* vol II. Philadelphia, Saunders, 1981, pp 1921–1943.
21. Ewald, F.C., Scheinberg, F.D., Poss, R., et al. Capitellocondylar total elbow arthroplasty. J Bone Surg, 62A–63:1259, 1980.
22. Fink, C.W., Baum, J., Paradies, L.H., Carrell, B.C. Synovectomy in juvenile arthritis. Ann Rheum Dis 28:612–618, 1969.
23. French, P.R. Varus deformity of the elbow following supra condylar fractures of the humerus in children. Lancet 2:439, 1959.
24. Froimson, A.I., Silva, J.E., and Richley, W.G. Curtis arthroplasty of the elbow joint. J Bone Joint Surg 58A:963–965, 1976.
25. Gilchrist, G.S. Hematologic arthritis, in Morrey, B.F. (ed): *The Elbow and its Disorders.* Philadelphia, Saunders, 1985, pp 674–681.

26. Gilcrest, G.G., Espinoza, L.R., Spillburg, I., and Osterland, C.K. Joint manifestations of sickle cell disease. Medicine 53:295, 1974.

27. Hass, J. Functional arthroplasty. J Bone Joint Surg 26:297–306, 1944.

28. Hurri, L., Pulkki, T., and Vainio, K. Arthroplasty of the elbow in rheumatoid arthritis. Acta Chir Scand 127:459–465, 1964.

29. Inglis, A.E., and Pellicci, P.M. Total elbow replacement. J Bone Joint Surg 62A:1252–1258, 1980.

30. Inglis, A.E., Ranawat, C.S., and Straub, L.R. Synovectomy and debridement of the elbow in rheumatoid arthritis. J Bone Joint Surg 53A:652–622, 1971.

31. Jacobsen, S.T., Levinson, J.E., and Crawford, A.H. Late results of synovectomy in juvenile rheumatoid arthritis. J Bone Joint Surg 67A:8–15, 1955.

32. Johnson, E.W., Jr., and Schlein, A.P. Vitallium prosthesis for the olecranon, and proximal part of the ulna. J Bone Joint Surg 52A:721–724, 1970.

33. Kampner, S.L., and Ferguson, A.B., Jr. Efficacy of synovectomy in juvenile rheumatoid arthritis. Clin Orthop 88:94–109, 1972.

34. Kaye, L., Stainsby, D., Buzzard, B., Fearns, M., Hamilton, P.J., Owen, P., and Jones, P. The role of synovectomy in the management of recurrent hemarthrosis in hemophilia. Br J Haematol 49:53, 1981.

35. Knight, R.A., and Van Zandt, I.L. Arthroplasty of the elbow. N Eng J Med 236:97, 1947.

36. Knight, R.A., and Van Zandt, I.L. Arthroplasty of the elbow. An end result study. J Bone Joint Surg 34A:610–615, 1952.

37. Kirkaldy-Willis, W.H. Excision of the elbow joint. Lancet 1:53, 1948.

38. Kudo, H., Iwano, K., and Watanabe, S. Total replacement of the rheumatoid elbow with a hingeless prosthesis. J Bone Joint Surg 62A:277–285, 1980.

39. Lowe, L.W., Miller, A.J., Allum, R.L., and Higginson, D.W. The development of an unconstrained elbow arthroplasty; a clinical review. J Bone Joint Surg 66B:243–247, 1984.

40. MacAusland, W.R. Arthroplasty of the elbow. N Engl J Med 236:97, 1947.

41. MacAusland, W.R. Replacement of the lower end of the humerus with a prosthesis. A report of four cases. West J Surg Gynecol Obstet 62:557, 1954.

42. McDougall, A., and White, J. Subluxation of the inferior radioulnar joint. Complication fracture of the radial head. J Bone Joint Surg 39B:278–287, 1957.

43. Mellen, R.H., and Phalen, G.S. Arthroplasty of the elbow by replacement of the distal portion of the humerus with acrylic prosthesis. J Bone Joint Surg 29:348–353, 1947.

44. Morrey, B.F., and Bryan, R.S. Total joint arthroplasty. Mayo Clin Proc 54:507–512, 1979.

45. Morrey, B.F., Bryan, R.S., Dobyns, J.H., and Linscheid, K.L. Total elbow arthroplasty. J Bone Joint Surg 63A:1050–1063, 1981.

46. Morrey, B.F., and Bryan, R.S. Complications of total elbow arthroplasty. Clin Orthop 170:204–212, 1982.

47. Morrey, B.F., Chao, E.Y., and Hui, F.C. Biomechanical study of the elbow following examination of the radial head. J Bone Joint Surg 61A:63–68, 1979.

48. Ollier, L. *Traité des Resections et des Operations Conservatrices qu'on peut Practiquer sur le Systéme Osseaus.* Paris, Masson, 1885.

49. Porter, B.B., Richardson, C., and Vainio, K. Rheumatoid arthritis of the elbow. The results of synovectomy. J Bone Joint Surg 56B:427–437, 1974.

50. Rosenberg, G.M., and Turner, R.H. Nonconstrained total elbow replacement. Clin Orthop 187:154–162, 1984.

51. Rosenfeld, S.R., and Anzel, S.H. Evaluation of the Pritchard total elbow arthroplasty. Orthopaedics 5(6):713, 1982.

52. Rymasewski, L.A., Mackay, I., Amis, A.A., and Miller, J.H. Long term effects of excision of the radial head in rheumatoid arthritis. J Bone Joint Surg 66B:109–113, 1984.

53. Schlein, A.R. Semiconstrained total elbow arthroplasty. Clin Orthop 121:222–229, 1976.

54. Schwabe, G.H., Bennett, J.B., Woods, G.W., and Tullios, H.S., The role of the medial collateral ligament. Clin Orthop 146:42–52, 1980.

55. Scudder, C. Arthroplasty for complete ankylosis of the elbow. Ann Surg 48:711, 1908.

56. Silva, J.F. Arthroplasty of the elbow. Singapore Med J 8:222, 1967.

57. Smith, M.A., Savidge, G.F., Fountaine, K.J. Interposition arthroplasty in the management of advanced hemophilic arthropathy of the elbow. J Bone Joint Surg 65B:436–440, 1983.

58. Smith-Peterson, M.N., Aujrane, O.E., and Larson, C.B. Useful surgical procedures for rheumatoid arthritis. Arch Surg 46:764–770, 1943.

59. Snider, W.J., and DeWitt, H.J. Functional studies for optimum position for elbow arthrodesis ankylosis. J Bone Joint Surg 55A:1305, 1973.

60. Soni, R.K., and Cavendish, M.E. A review of the Liverpool elbow prosthesis from 1974–1982. J Bone Joint Surg 66B:248–253, 1984.

61. Souter, W.A. Arthroplasty of the elbow. Orthop Clin North Am 4:395, 1973.

62. Steinbrocker, O., Taeger, C.H., and Batterman, R.C. Therapeutic criteria in rheumatoid arthritis. J Am Med Assoc 140:659–662, 1949.

63. Street, D.M., and Stevens, P.S. A humeral replacement prosthesis for the elbow. J Bone Joint Surg 56A:1147–1158, 1974.

64. Swanson, A.B. *Flexible Implant Resection Arthroplasty in the Hand and Extremities.* St. Louis, Mosby, 1973.

65. Swanson, A.B., Percinel, A., and Herndon, J.H. Long term follow-up of implant arthroplasty following radial head excision in rheumatoid arthritis. Presented at the 45th meeting of the AAOS in Dallas, 1978.

66. Swett, P.P. Synovectomy in chronic infective arthritis. J Bone Joint Surg 5:110–121, 1923.

67. Taylor, A.R., Muberijea, S.K., and Rana, N.A. Excision of the head of the radius in rheumatoid arthritis. J Bone Joint Surg 58B:485–487, 1976.

68. Taylor, K.F., and O'Connor, B.T. The effect upon the inferior radioulnar joint of excision of the head of the radius in adults. J Bone Joint Surg 46B:83–88, 1964.

69. Tenner, R.H., Englert, H.M., Bush, W.H., and Krauss, F.J. Roentgenology of total elbow joint replacement arthroplasty. Orthop Rev 5, 12:17, 21, 1976.

70. Tullos, H.S., Schwab, G., Bennett, J.B., and Woods, G.W. Factors influencing elbow instability. Instr Course Lect 32:185, 1983.

71. Unander-Scharin, L., and Karlholm, S. Experience of arthroplasty of the elbow. Acta Orthop Scand 36:54, 1966.

72. Vainio, K. Arthroplasty of the elbow and hand in rheumatoid arthritis. A study of 131 operations, in Chapchal, G. (ed): *Synovectomy and Arthroplasty in Rheumatoid Arthritis.* Stuttgart, Thieme-Verlag, 66–70. 1967.

73. Venable, C.S. An elbow and an elbow prosthesis: Case of complete loss of the lower third of the humerus. Am J Surg 83:271, 1952.

74. Volz, R., and Morrey, B.F. Physical examination of the elbow, in Morrey, B.F. (ed): *The Elbow and Its Disorders.* Philadelphia, Saunders, 1985, pp 62–72.

75. Walker, P.S. Deflection of the radio-humeral joint, in *Human Joints and Their Artificial Replacements.* Springfield, IL, Thomas, 1977, pp 190–194.

CHAPTER 39

Rheumatoid Disorders of the Hand and Wrist

Jerry L. Ellstein and James W. Strickland

The primary target of rheumatoid arthritis in the hand and wrist is the synovium of tendon and joints. Chronic involvement of peritendinous and periarticular tissues results in the loss of capsular and ligamentous support; joint instability; contractures; and functional impairment. All tissues may be affected including skin and local blood vessels, the latter leading to secondary vasculitis and Raynaud's phenomenon. Muscle involvement may produce wasting, contracture, and weakness.

Synovial proliferation in the form of tenosynovitis about tendons and pannus formation in the joints of the hand and wrist results in hyperemia, increased fluid production, and thickening of the synovial joint lining. Tendons may be eroded, attenuated, or ruptured by direct synovial invasion; by ischemic changes created by pressure within compartments such as the flexor tendon sheath in the palm and digit, under the extensor retinaculum, and within the carpal canal; or by erosion from bony spurs created by the invasive disease process. Joint changes ultimately occur in the many diarthrodial joints of the hand and wrist. The earliest changes occur at the joint margins, where synovial reflections are located. Synovial proliferation results in increased fluid production and joint pressure, which reduce cartilage nutrition. Direct invasion of the cartilage by pannus formation also contributes to the loss of the normal smooth joint surface. Capsular and ligament support are slowly lost because of chronic distension and direct invasion. Ultimately deformities occur which are characterized by erosions; periarticular osteoporosis; and cyst and spur formation leading to joint destruction, collapse, subluxation, dislocation, fibrous adhesions, or ankylosis.

Rheumatoid nodules (granulomas), which consist of fibrinoid necrosis, cellular debris, and monocytes, are probably secondary to small vessel vasculitis. They occur in 20 percent of the patients and are frequently located over the extensor surface of the elbow and the dorsum of digits. Vasculitis with injury to vessel intima may also be the cause of Raynaud's phenomenon and peripheral neuropathy. Chronic myositis leads to muscular atrophy, weakness, and contracture, with lymphocyte accumulation in the tissues.

No one area of the hand or wrist is immune to the effects of rheumatoid arthritis. A wide variety of dysfunction and deformity may develop, and, although certain recurring patterns are said to be characteristic of the disease, the clinical presentation is highly variable. The particular deformity that develops is dependent on the site, intensity, and duration of the synovitis and may often result in neighboring digits exhibiting different deformities.

TABLE 39-1 Common Deformities and Tendon Involvement in Rheumatoid Arthritis of the Hand and Wrist

Hand Deformities

Swan-neck ⎫
Boutonniere ⎭ digits and thumb
Joint subluxations
Joint dislocations
Ulnar deviation of digits (ulnar drift)
Radial deviation of the hand
Volar subluxation and supination of the hand and wrist with apparent distal ulna dorsal subluxation
Digital flexion contractures
Ankylosed joints
Unstable or floppy joints
Stiff joints

Tendon Involvement

Vaughan-Jackson syndrome (rupture of extensors to ring and/ or small fingers)
Caput ulnae syndrome
Rupture of extensor pollicis longus
Ruptured wrist extensors associated with volar wrist subluxation and dislocation
Subluxation or dislocation of the extensor carpi ulnaris
Extensor tenosynovitis
Triggering digit, palm, wrist
Flexor tenosynovitis
Digital or flexor tendon ruptures (Mannerfelt syndrome)
Nerve involvement
Carpal tunnel syndrome
Posterior interosseous syndrome
Cubital tunnel syndrome

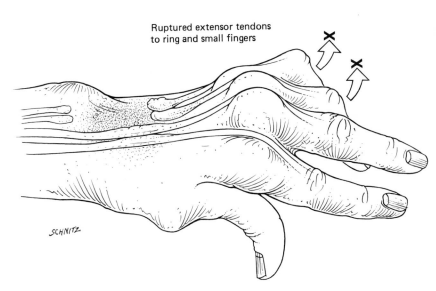

Ruptured extensor tendons to ring and small fingers

Figure 39-1 Tendon ruptures are not infrequent occurrences in rheumatoid arthritis. Extensor tendon ruptures (Vaughan-Jackson syndrome[151]) most often involve the common extensors to the fourth and fifth digits and the extensor digiti quinti. This most often occurs in association with the caput ulnae syndrome, in which the tendons are eroded over the dorsally prominent distal ulna. *(Reprinted with permission from Manus.)*

CLINICAL DIAGNOSIS AND EXAMINATION

The diagnosis of rheumatoid arthritis is discussed in Chap. 19. Examination of the hands and wrists reveals increased warmth over affected joints, tenderness, swelling, and palmar erythema. Synovitis presenting as boggy swelling over joints and fullness of the flexor tendon sheaths or dorsum of the wrist is both visible and palpable. Rheumatoid nodules occur in 20 percent of patients. Decreased muscle strength with atrophy frequently accompanies joint involvement and may lead to progressive loss of motion and deformity.

Table 39-1 lists the more common deformities which develop in the hand and wrist in rheumatoid arthritis. Instability or collapse of a single joint may have an untoward effect on the entire balance of the hand. As Landsmeer has shown, the collapse of an intercalated segment of the osseous chain of the hand produces at contiguous segments deformity which is often opposite in direction and of equal severity.[73] For example, in the rheumatoid hand, palmar subluxation and ulnar translocation of the carpus result in radial deviation and dorsal displacement of the metacarpals and ulnar deviation and flexion of the digits.[121] Similarly, lateral dislocation of the base of the first metacarpal secondary to basilar joint disease leads to adduction of the first ray, hyperextension of the metacarpophalangeal joint, and a reciprocal hyperflexion of the interphalangeal joint. Correction or stabilization of impending deformity of a joint whose collapse may initiate a multilevel deformity is one of the important considerations for the management of rheumatoid arthritis affecting the wrist and hand.

Sensory and motor neuropathy presenting as carpal tunnel syndrome frequently occur due to vasculitis of the vasa nervorum or from entrapment resulting from the increased volume produced by flexor tenosynovitis in the carpal canal. Rheumatoid patients should be specifically questioned about symptoms of carpal tunnel syndrome as this may be an easily overlooked cause of hand discomfort.

Tendon ruptures are not infrequent and may be secondary to attrition over bony spurs or from direct invasion by the diseased synovium. Extensor tendon ruptures (Vaughan-Jackson syndrome[151,153]) most often involve the common extensors to the fourth and fifth digits and the extensor digiti quinti in association with the *caput ulnae syndrome,* in which the tendons are eroded over the dorsally prominent distal ulna (Fig. 39-1). The extensor pollicis longus may rupture at Lister's tubercle when it becomes eroded by the rheumatoid process (Fig. 39-2). Involvement of flexor tendons may produce triggering or digital motion loss, and chronic tenosynovial invasion may result in attenuation or rupture of the profundus or superficialis tendons, or both. Rupture may also result from attrition over palmar carpal bony irregularities (Mannerfelt syndrome)[81] and most commonly involves the flexor pollicis longus, which ruptures over a prominent trapezial ridge.

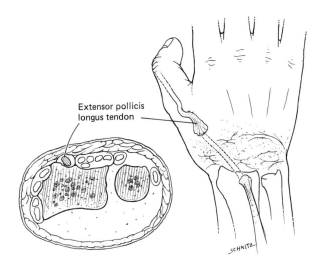

Extensor pollicis longus tendon

Figure 39-2 The extensor pollicis longus may rupture at Lister's tubercle when it becomes eroded by the rheumatoid process. *(Reprinted with permission from Manus.)*

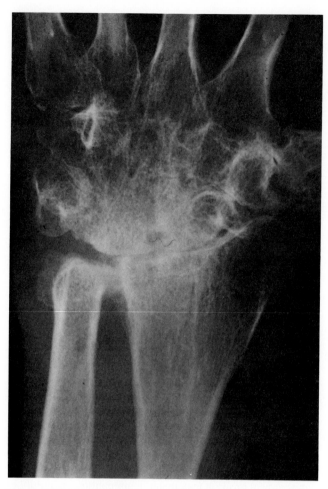

Figure 39-3 Carpal coalition may be seen in both advanced cases of rheumatoid arthritis and in juvenile rheumatoid arthritis. *(Reprinted with permission from Manus.)*

Radiographs of the hands and wrists early on may show soft tissue swelling, periarticular osteoporosis, joint space narrowing, and bony erosions of the metacarpal necks as best seen on the Brewerton view.[17,21] Late findings include progression of the bony erosions from the joint margins to complete joint surface destruction and articular incongruity. Ulnar and radial styloid erosions are characteristic.[116] As the disease progresses, loss of joint space, subluxations, and dislocations can be expected to follow. Partial or complete carpal coalition is seen in advanced cases and in juvenile rheumatoid arthritis (Fig. 39-3). Loss of bone stock with digital shortening and telescoping may be seen in the advanced stages of rheumatoid arthritis mutilans and in psoriatic arthritis.[103] Bone erosion, often associated with tendon rupture, includes the distal ulna, trapezial ridge, and Lister's tubercle.

The various clinical findings and radiographic features of rheumatoid arthritis in the upper limb can be divided into a staging system which may be helpful in planning treatment (Table 39-2).[35,92]

TREATMENT
Nonsurgical Treatment

Nonsurgical treatment of rheumatoid arthritis consists of medical management of the disease, including the use of salicylates, steroids, gold injections, antimalarial and immunosuppressant drugs, occasional and judicious use of steroid injections, and an individualized therapy program. The hand therapist can be helpful to patients with rheumatoid arthritis in all stages of disease. Splinting programs may be designed to rest joints, to strengthen the hand, to provide assistance or modification of the use of the hand in activities of daily living, to assist in the evaluation and treatment of individual patient needs, and to provide the means to maintain or improve joint motion and strength.[35] It is unlikely, however, that splinting will prevent the development of deformity in patients with chronic and progressive rheumatoid involvement.

Surgical Considerations in the Rheumatoid Patient

The goals of hand surgery in the rheumatoid patient are to help control the medically resistant inflammatory process and to either preserve function prior to the onset of deformity or restore function and correct established deformity. This is accomplished by procedures designed to excise chronic synovial accumulations and to reestablish joint alignment, congruity, and stability. Static stability, dynamic stability, and motor balance should be carefully evaluated, and the surgeon must recognize that surgery cannot eliminate the underlying systemic disease and that many procedures may be more palliative than curative. Surgery can be helpful in rheumatoid patients who have severe pain, chronic synovitis unresponsive to medical treatment, tendon ruptures, nerve entrapment, and deformities associated with compromised hand function. Surgical candidates should be well-motivated and healthy enough to undergo surgery and the strenuous postoperative rehabilitation program. Patients must thoroughly understand the specific goals of surgery and the expected result. Although multiple surgical procedures may be combined at one operation, it is often impossible to complete all indicated procedures at one sitting due to the time constraints or to noncomplementary postoperative therapy requirements. The patient must be aware of the possible need for additional surgery.

Finally, the timing of hand surgical procedures for the rheumatoid patient must be carefully planned with consideration for the patient's needs for reconstructive surgery in other anatomic sites. Preference is usually given to lower extremity reconstruction in view of the excessive demands which may be placed on the hands by the need to use crutches and other walking aids. The status of the shoulders and elbows must also be considered. A functionally reconstructed hand will do the patient little good if the patient cannot adequately position it in space (Table 39-3).[30]

Operative procedures for the hand and wrist in the rheumatoid patient should be individually designed for each patient dependent upon the stage of disease and functional limi-

TABLE 39-2 Staging of Rheumatoid Arthritis of the Upper Limb

Stage	Tendon rupture	Syno-vitis	Teno-syno-vitis	Loss of ROM	Muscle weak-ness or atrophy	Deform-ity	Insta-bility	Destruc-tive osse-ous chan-ges	Medical management including steroid use
I	−	+	+	None or mild	−	−	−	−	+
II	+/−	++	++	+	+	Mild	−	−	+/−
III	+/−	+/−	+/−	+	++	Fixed	+	+	−
IV	+/−	+/−	+/−	++	++	Fixed	++	++	−

Source: Davis, J., et al, Orthop Clin North Am 9:559, 1978. Reproduced with permission.

tations present. Surgery should not be reserved for the severely deformed hand (Table 39-2). Often, better functional preservation or restoration may be provided for a longer period of time if surgical intervention is performed earlier in the course of the disease. Procedures which can help preserve function and relieve pain prior to the onset of deformity include synovectomy, nerve decompression, trigger finger release, and intrinsic releases. Additional procedures which can be used to help restore function after the onset of deformity include soft tissue reconstruction of joints and tendons, arthroplasty, arthrodesis, and combinations of these techniques.

THE RHEUMATOID WRIST

Initial involvement of the wrist in rheumatoid arthritis is unusual (2.7 percent), with the hand affected five times more frequently. However, with time and continuance of the disease,

TABLE 39-3 Preferred Surgical Sequence in Treatment of Rheumatoid Patient

Priority	Site
1	Cervical spinal column
2	One upper extremity (only if needed for activities of daily living)
3	Lower extremities if walking is a reasonable goal Forefoot Hip Hindfoot
4	Upper extremities Positioning—elbow before shoulder End organ Wrist fusion Thumb stabilization Metacarpophalangeal arthroplasties Digital surgery

Source: Cooney, W.P., and Bryan, R.S., AAOS ICL 28:247, 1979. Used with permission.

synovitis affects the hand and wrist in 95 percent of cases.[124] While the characteristic digital deformities that occur in rheumatoid arthritis (Table 39-1) including ulnar drift and swan neck deformities are not directly the result of rheumatoid wrist collapse, wrist deformity may contribute to their development, worsen preexistent deformity, and compromise their surgical correction.[85,122] Most authors, therefore, recommend treating the wrist imbalance prior to or simultaneous with the treatment of finger deformities.[63,76,112,123,129,144]

The carpus is suspended in position by ligamentous attachments to both volar radial and dorsal ulnar aspects of the distal radius, including the ulnocarpal complex (Fig. 39-4).[142] Additional wrist stability is provided by the two radial wrist extensors and a single ulnar wrist extensor tendon. The radial ligamentous sling stabilizes the lateral carpal column (scaphoid), and the ulnar sling supports the medial carpal column (triquetrum).[117,142,143] Synovitis of the carpus, in the closed extensor compartments of the wrist, and in the carpal tunnel may locally invade and weaken the ligamentous and tendinous support of the wrist joint (Fig. 39-5).

Development of Deformities

On the radial side of the wrist, attenuation of the radioscapholunate and radiocapitate ligaments causes instability of the scaphoid proximal pole, leading to rotary subluxation of the scaphoid and scapholunate dissociation (Fig. 39-6). This produces radiocarpal shortening and contributes to a radial shift of the metacarpals when accompanied by the changes occurring in the ulnar aspect of the wrist.[144] In the ulna, synovitis attacks the ligamentous support, including the triangular fibrocartilage which extends from the dorsum of the ulna to the volar wrist capsule. The disease also results in attenuation of the ulnolunate and ulnotriquetral ligaments. Palmar collapse of the ulnar carpus follows, producing a relative supination of the carpus and an increased metacarpal descent (Fig. 39-7).[160] This palmar displacement and supination of the carpus creates a prominent appearance of the distal ulna, which may actually be in its normal anatomic position.[144] Synovitis affecting the distal radioulnar joint may further contribute to the deformity by producing radioulnar dissociation and a true dorsal displacement of the ulna. The distal radioulnar joint

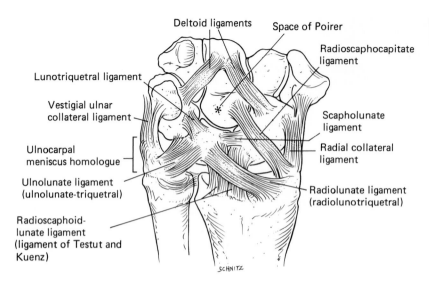

Deltoid ligaments — Space of Poirer — Radioscaphocapitate ligament — Lunotriquetral ligament — Vestigial ulnar collateral ligament — Scapholunate ligament — Ulnocarpal meniscus homologue — Radial collateral ligament — Ulnolunate ligament (ulnolunate-triquetral) — Radiolunate ligament (radiolunotriquetral) — Radioscaphoid-lunate ligament (ligament of Testut and Kuenz)

SCHNITZ

Figure 39-4 The volar wrist ligaments. *(Reprinted with permission from Manus.)*

becomes painful because of persisting synovitis and crepitus, and the condition has been referred to as the *caput ulnae syndrome*.[10]

With the loss of radiocarpal height and collapse of the carpus,[85] there is a relative excess length of the distal ulna, causing impingement and pain. The clinical manifestations are pain along the ulnar border of the wrist, mostly with forearm rotation.

As the wrist moves in a volar and relatively supinated position, the extensor carpi ulnaris moves with it, becoming volar to the axis of wrist motion, and contributing to further carpal displacement (Fig. 39-8) encouraged by the unopposed radial wrist tendons.[4]

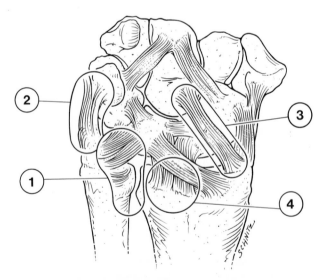

Figure 39-5 Most frequent sites for synovial involvement in the rheumatoid wrist: (1) ulnolunate, ulnotriquetral ligaments, distal radioulnar joint including the triangular fibrocartilage complex; (2) ulnocarpal meniscal homologue and vestigial ulnar collateral ligament; (3) radioscaphocapitate ligament; and (4) radioscapholunate and radiolunate ligaments. *(Reprinted with permission from Manus.)*

Tendon Rupture at the Wrist

Impending rupture may often be recognized by pain along the course of the involved tendon. Apparent tendon rupture, with loss of extension of the metacarpophalangeal joints of the index through small finger, may mimic true tendon rupture. This phenomenon may be caused by two different problems. The first is subluxation of the extensor tendons from their dorsal biomechanically efficient location atop the metacarpal heads into the valleys or sulcus between the metacarpal heads, where they become volar to the axis of rotation of the metacarpophalangeal joint and become flexors rather than extensors.[20] Careful examination demonstrates subluxation of the extensor tendons to the ulnar side of the metacarpal shafts, ulnar drift of the digits, or even metacarpophalangeal joint dislocation. A complete loss of extension at the metacarpophalangeal joints does not always accompany extensor tendon rupture because of the presence of tendinous interconnections between the finger extensors known as *juncturae tendinum* (connexus intertendineus). Often, when the juncturae alone extend the metacarpophalangeal joint, extension is weak, painful, or incomplete. The second cause of apparent tendon rupture may be a partial or complete posterior interosseous nerve syndrome secondary to rheumatoid synovitis of the elbow and compression of the motor branch of the radial nerve as it passes through the two layers of the supinator muscle at the arcade of Frohse.[97] Electrodiagnostic tests may be helpful in making the proper diagnosis, although the tenodesis effect which produces digital extension when the wrist is flexed may help demonstrate that the tendons are intact. Fixed joint deformities which limit tendon excursion may also compromise the ability to clinically evaluate tendon integrity.

Rupture of the extensor pollicis longus may be easily overlooked since the thumb intrinsics may continue to extend the interphalangeal joint. True extensor pollicis longus function may be tested by placing the affected hand flat on a table with the patient extending or lifting the thumb off the table surface while the examiner palpates the extensor pollicis longus distal to Lister's tubercle.

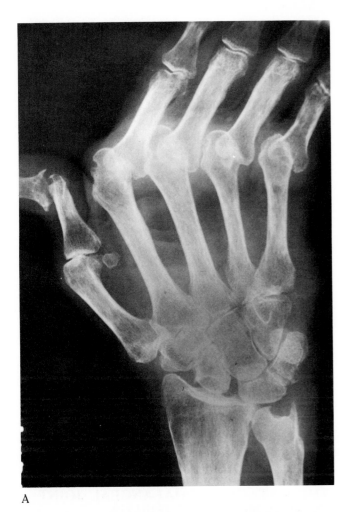

A

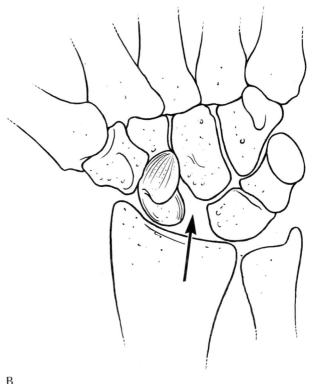

B

Figure 39-6 Rotatory subluxation of the scaphoid due to rheumatoid synovitis weakening the extrinsic (radioscapholunate and radioscaphocapitate) ligaments and intrinsic (scapholunate) wrist ligaments, contributing to radiocarpal shortening. In **B**, the arrow points to the scapholunate gap (diastasis) and sometimes is referred to as the Terry Thomas sign. *(Reprinted with permission from Manus.)*

Surgery for the Rheumatoid Wrist

Indications for surgery of the rheumatoid wrist include chronic synovitis of the extensor tendons, flexor tendons, and carpus when the synovitis is unresponsive to medical management after 3 to 6 months, or with impending tendon rupture or demonstrably ruptured tendons. Because the results of tendon transfer are inversely proportional to the number of tendon ruptures, prompt diagnosis and early treatment should be carried out.[104] While synovial inflammation may recur following synovectomy, it rarely returns to the extent present preoperatively, and tendon rupture seldom occurs.[86] Without surgical intervention, a single tendon rupture is often followed rather rapidly by additional ruptures. When ruptures have occurred an early surgery is indicated to correct loss of function, prevent additional ruptures, and preserve joint function.

Carpal tunnel syndrome is frequently seen in association with flexor tenosynovitis. Patients should be specifically questioned about symptoms from median nerve embarrass-

ment in an effort to separate that entity from the pain associated with arthritic joints. Surgical decompression of the carpal tunnel is a simple procedure which may often provide considerable benefit to the rheumatoid patient.

Surgery for caput ulnae syndrome with ulnar wrist pain may be of value with or without angulation, subluxation, or frank dislocation of the wrist. Finally, pain with loss of function due to severe arthritis of the radiocarpal or intercarpal joints may be an indication for surgical intervention in the rheumatoid wrist (Fig. 39-9).

The surgical procedures utilized in the management of the rheumatoid wrist may be divided according to whether they are employed early or late in the course of the disease. Prior to the onset of deformity, the following procedures may be appropriate:

1. Synovectomy of the extensor and flexor tendons[68,92,94,100,107]
2. Synovectomy of the dorsal and volar carpus[144]
3. Carpal tunnel release[26]

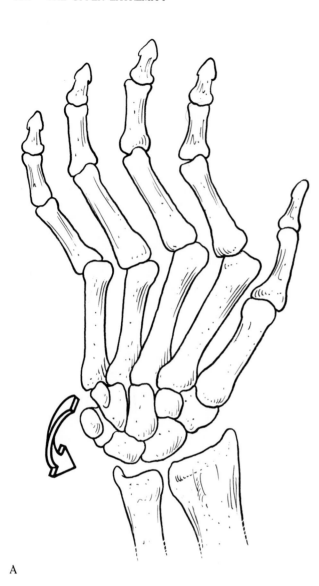

A

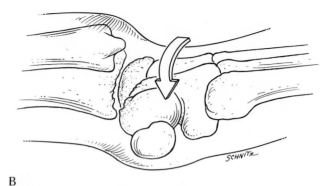

B

Figure 39-7 Ulnar wrist translocation with palmar collapse of the ulnar carpus produces a relative supination of the carpus and an increasing metacarpal descent. **A.** AP view. **B.** Lateral view. *(Reprinted with permission from Manus.)*

6. Total wrist arthroplasty.
   a. Articulated prosthesis[11,12,77,88,90,154]
   b. Flexible implant arthroplasty[36,51,138]
7. Wrist arthrodesis[38,71,132]
   a. Steinmann pin without bone graft (Nalebuff)[26,80]
   b. Steinmann pin with bone graft[22]
   c. Closed arthrodesis with Steinmann pin[95]

THE METACARPOPHALANGEAL JOINT IN RHEUMATOID ARTHRITIS

The metacarpophalangeal joints are the keystones of both the longitudinal and the transverse skeletal arches of the hand.[45] They are frequently the site of intense rheumatoid synovitis which ultimately results in ulnar deviation of the digits and volar subluxation of the proximal phalanx.[57] Dislocation of the metacarpophalangeal joint is the final stage of this de-

4. Restoration of ruptured tendons
   a. Tendon transfer
   b. End-to-side repair and free tendon graft[20,45,62,93,101,134,153]
5. Wrist rebalancing
   a. Tendon transfer[15,28,29,112]
   b. Dorsal stabilization techniques[71]

After the onset of deformity or late in the course of the disease, procedures which may improve function include

1. Darrach excision of the distal ulna (or its modifications)[27,31]
2. Hemiresection arthroplasty of the distal radioulnar joint[14]
3. Silicone capping of the distal ulna[136,139,140]
4. The Sauve-Lauenstein ulnar pseudarthrosis operation[50]
5. Arthroplasty of the radiocarpal joint
   a. Soft tissue interposition
   b. Shelf procedures[1]

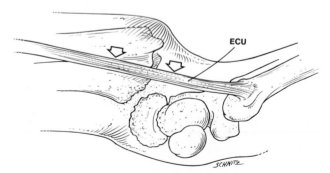

Figure 39-8 Volar displacement of the extensor carpi ulnaris contributes to volar carpal displacement in the rheumatoid wrist. *(Reprinted with permission from Manus.)*

forming progression, and the consequent disruption of the continuity of the longitudinal arch creates an imbalance of forces which in turn leads to a reciprocal distal joint collapse (Fig. 39-10).[45]

Many authors have implicated various factors which contribute to the deformities that occur at the metacarpophalangeal joint in rheumatoid arthritis. These factors have been categorized by Smith and are listed in Table 39-4.[126]

Surgical Treatment of the Rheumatoid Metacarpophalangeal Joint

Procedures for the surgical management of rheumatoid arthritis of the metacarpophalangeal joint may be placed into two categories: those procedures that can be performed early in the course of disease, and reconstructive procedures that are reserved for later or advanced stages.

In the early stages of disease, before deformity has occurred, synovectomy and soft tissue procedures including intrinsic transfer have been recommended.[3] Chemical syno-

vectomy has been tried, but no ideal substance has yet been identified.[45] Various agents have been tried, including beta-emitter isotopes and alkylating agents such as nitrogen mustard and thiotepa. Because of the risk of skin necrosis, only beta emitters of low energy and shallow penetration such as erbium 169 can be used in the fingers, and they have been reported to offer an alternative to early surgical synovectomy.[87] The response of a given joint to the use of intraarticular thiotepa with or without the addition of steroids is unpredictable, and this treatment has been reserved for poor surgical candidates or some patients who have single-joint involvement.[32,42,45,56,119,148,157,161]

The indications for surgical synovectomy of the metacarpophalangeal joint include marked synovial proliferation which has not responded well to systemic treatment, has persisted for at least 6 months, is painful, and appears to be progressing to inevitable deformity. Contraindications include joint destruction with articular erosion, instability, irreducible dislocation, or fixed deformity.[20] Synovectomy has not been uniformly successful and is often disappointing

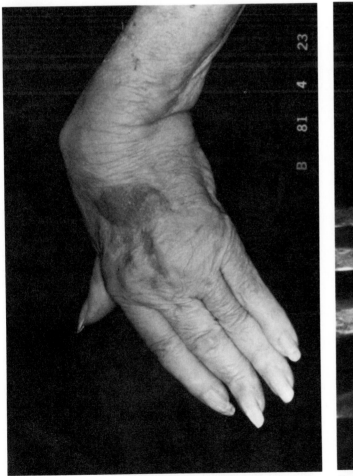

A

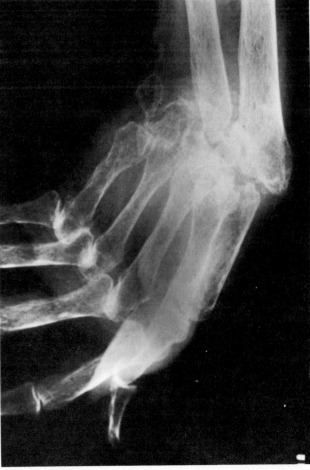

B

Figure 39-9 The final stage of deformity in the rheumatoid wrist—volar dislocation. **A.** Clinical appearance. **B.** X-ray appearance.

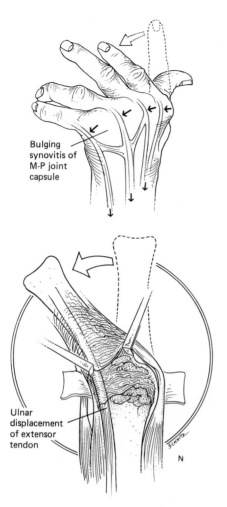

Bulging synovitis of M-P joint capsule

Ulnar displacement of extensor tendon

A

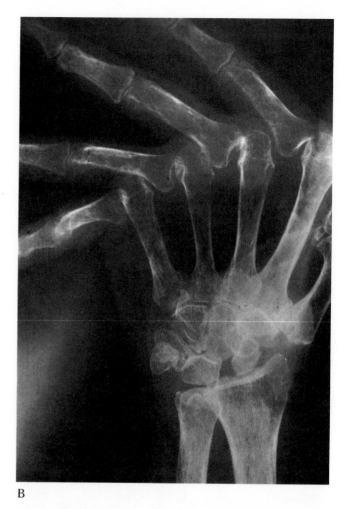

B

Figure 39-10 A. Synovitis of the metacarpophalangeal joints and ulnar subluxation of the extensor tendons. **B.** X-ray appearance confirms the metacarpophalangeal joint dislocations. *(Part A reprinted with permission from Manus.)*

because of the rapid return of diseased synovium. It may, however, offer a satisfactory alternative in carefully selected patients who are early in the course of their disease and have no radiographic changes.[6,16,41,49,75,110,114,131,145] Synovectomy may also be combined with extensor tendon relocation and intrinsic release when indicated. The reader is referred to surgical texts on hand surgery for a description of the surgical techniques.[96]

In the late stages of rheumatoid involvement of the metacarpophalangeal joint, resection-interposition arthroplasty utilizing soft tissue or silicone rubber, rebalancing procedures including extensor relocation, intrinsic release, and transfer or arthrodesis have been described.[3] Arthrodesis of the metacarpophalangeal joint in the fingers is not commonly performed because of the importance of maintaining motion at this joint in order to retain satisfactory hand function. However, in some situations, when there is good mobility at both the proximal and the distal interphalangeal joints, stabilization of the metacarpophalangeal joint of a finger may be of value.[45]

Prior to the advent of silicone interpositional techniques, excision arthroplasty of the metacarpophalangeal joint was employed to improve finger alignment, mobility, and function. A popular technique involved the excision of the metacarpal head, reduction of the proximal phalangeal base, and stabilization by the use of the extensor tendon interposed as a support mechanism.[59,147,149] Another method utilized the volar plate interposed between the resected joint ends with or without the reconstruction of the radial collateral ligament.[146] The results of excisional soft tissue interpositional arthroplasty procedures were often quite good, with a range of motion up to 60 degrees and overall improvement in alignment and balance of the digits.[66,156] Unfortunately, the techniques were quite demanding and, depending on the variable nature of individual tissue healing, produced very unpredictable motion and stability. In recent years the procedures have been largely abandoned.

Replacement arthroplasty of the metacarpophalangeal joint using the Swanson silicone rubber or Niebauer silicone-Dacron implants (spacers) has become more popular because of more predictable pain relief, motion, and stability. Although true hinged implants have been employed using cemented or noncemented devices, none has provided the technical ease, predictable results, and low complication

TABLE 39-4 Factors Leading to Deformities at the Metacarpophalangeal Joints in Rheumatoid Arthritis

I. Forces normally acting on the hand that may promote ulnar deviation of the digits in rheumatoid arthritis
   A. Gravity[150]
   B. Lateral pinch pressure[150]
   C. Power grasp[74]

II. Normal anatomy that may contribute to ulnar deviation of the finger
   A. Asymmetrical shape of metacarpal heads (smaller sloping ulnar condyle)[57]
   B. Unequal collateral ligament length, and their differing orientations[57,72]
   C. Asymmetry of the intrinsic muscles to the small finger (hypothenars are stronger than third volar interosseous)

III. Rheumatoid involvement which can lead to ulnar deviation and volar subluxations of the metacarpophalangeal joint
   A. Decreased joint stability due to bony erosions of the metacarpal head and base of proximal phalanx[37,150]
   B. Attrition and stretching of the collateral ligaments by rheumatoid synovitis allowing the volarly directed flexor tendon force on the proximal phalanx to go unheeded[125]
   C. Stretching of the accessory collateral ligaments by rheumatoid synovitis allowing ulnar and palmar displacement of the palmar plate and flexor tendons at the base of the finger
   D. Flexor tenosynovitis with resultant stretching of the flexor tendon sheath pulley system resulting in ulnar and volar displacement of the flexor tendons
   E. Ulnar dislocation of the extensor digitorum communis due to attenuation and stretching of the radial sagittal band
   F. Rupture of the extensor digitorum communis creating an unopposed imbalance at the metacarpophalangeal joint[152]
   G. Contracture of the intrinsic muscles with volar subluxation and ulnar deviation of the digits[82]
   H. Flexion of the fourth and fifth metacarpal bases with grip
   I. Rheumatoid deformities at the wrist which contribute to radial deviation at the wrist which contribute to ulnar deviation of the fingers and increase the ulnar-directed extensor and flexor tendon forces at the metacarpophalangeal joint including
      1. Attenuation of the dorsal-radial support system against the strong palmar-ulnar forces[159]
      2. Increased metacarpal descent associated with volar subluxation of the ulnar carpus[160]
      3. Ulnar translocation of the carpus
      4. Radial deviation of the metacarpals[122,123]

Source: Smith, R.J., Kaplan, E.B., J Bone Joint Surg 49A:31, 1967. Reproduced with permission.

rates that have been demonstrated with the silicone spacers.[79,108,137,140] Complications of these procedures include infection, implant fracture, and a progressively decreased range of motion. Synovial infiltration by silicone particles has recently been reported, and cyst formation and local bone resorption have also been described, with carpal implants being most frequently incriminated.[5,9,23,52,113,158]

RHEUMATOID ARTHRITIS OF THE PROXIMAL INTERPHALANGEAL JOINT

The proximal interphalangeal joint of the rheumatoid hand may develop either flexion or hyperextension patterns which are commonly referred to as boutonniere and swan-neck deformities, respectively. Swan-neck deformities, which Bunnell

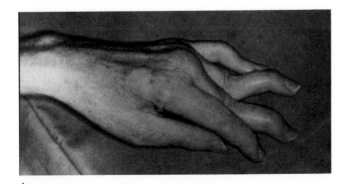

A

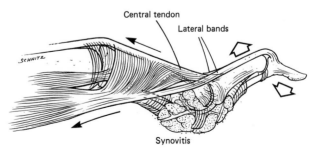

B

Figure 39-11 Swan-neck deformity in the hand of a patient with rheumatoid arthritis. **A.** Clinical appearance. **B.** Volar synovitis about the proximal interphalangeal joint is one possible cause (see text). *(Reprinted with permission from Manus.)*

TABLE 39-5 Swan-Neck Deformities

Type	PIP* joint flexibility	Treatment
I	Flexible in all positions	Flexor tenosynovectomy
II	Limited with metacarpophalangeal joint extension (intrinsic tightness)	Flexor tenosynovectomy, intrinsic release, tenodesis, dermodesis
III	Limited in all positions of the metacarpophalangeal joint (articular/pararticular problems)	Manipulation, lateral band mobilization, capsulectomy, extensor lengthening, palmar arthroplasty
IV	PIP joint stiff with advanced radiographic changes	Arthroplasty (resection) flexible implant, arthrodesis

*PIP = proximal interphalangeal.
Source: Nalebuff, E.A., and Millender, L.H., Orthop Clin North Am 6:733, 1975. Reproduced with permission.

has also called the intrinsic plus deformity[19] and Steindler has called pill roller's hand,[130] are common, occurring in 28 percent of all patients with rheumatoid arthritis, whereas boutonniere deformities occur in 15 percent.[3] Each deformity may also be associated with lateral displacement or subluxation due to either bone erosion or the loss of soft tissue support. Hand function may be greatly compromised as these deformities increase and become fixed.

Swan-Neck Deformity

Swan-neck deformity is a hyperextension deformity of the proximal interphalangeal joint with a concomitant extensor lag of the distal interphalangeal joint, often associated with some degree of metacarpophalangeal joint flexion (Fig. 39-11). Landsmeer defined this deformity as a terminal imbalance of an intercalated segment in a bimuscular biarticular system.[73] Nalebuff and Millender[105] have developed a system which classifies this deformity into four types based on the flexibility of the proximal interphalangeal joint, the amount of intrinsic tightness, and the radiographic changes. (Table 39-5).

Multiple factors may contribute to the development of swan-neck deformity of the proximal interphalangeal joint in rheumatoid arthritis. These factors include intrinsic muscle contracture or adhesion, intrinsic muscle shortening secondary to metacarpophalangeal joint synovitis or contracture, intrinsic muscle shortening secondary to mallet deformity of the distal interphalangeal joint, proximal interphalangeal joint synovitis or effusion, flexor tenosynovitis (wrist, palm, or digital sheath), distal profundus entrapment, extensor tendon contracture or adhesion, collateral ligament contracture or adhesion, palmar plate adhesion to bone, capsular contracture, retinacular ligament contracture or adhesion, bony block, joint fibrosis, ankylosis or articular incongruity, dorsal skin contracture,[33,34,60,65,69,70,98,105,118] and proximal migration of the carpal-hand unit with the "extrinsic minus" phenomenon resulting in muscle imbalance.[122]

The surgical treatment selected for the management of swan-neck deformity is dependent upon the stage of involvement. Early deformities may be amenable to flexor tenosynovectomy and intrinsic release, while later stages are treated by procedures which include manipulation, mobilization of lateral bands, capsulectomy, extensor tendon lengthening, arthroplasty, or arthrodesis (Table 39-5).

Boutonniere Deformity

Boutonniere deformities exhibit flexion at the proximal interphalangeal joint and hyperextension at the distal interphalangeal joint. To some extent, the deformity may also involve some degree of metacarpophalangeal joint hyperextension, and synovitis is again the initiating factor (Fig. 39-12). Chronic dorsal synovitis with capsular swelling results in a gradual attenuation of the central extensor tendon and the more distal triangular ligament. As the extensor tendon lengthens, there is progressive loss of the ability to actively extend the proximal interphalangeal joint. The lateral bands eventually sublux palmarward and lose their mobility. They come to lie volar to the axis of the proximal interphalangeal joint, where they act as flexors instead of extensors of the joint. The lateral bands gradually tighten in their subluxed position and produce a secondary hyperextension deformity of the distal interphalangeal joint. This terminal hyperextension is further aggravated by shortening of the oblique retinacular ligaments, which further limit active flexion of the distal interphalangeal joint. The retinacular component of the deformity may be demonstrated by extending the proximal interphalangeal joint to its maximum and demonstrating the passive loss of distal joint flexion (intrinsic-intrinsic tightness test). This test may not be entirely reliable in advanced boutonniere deformities, when the shortened and displaced lateral bands produce the same phenomena. As the synovial invasion persists, joint changes ensue, contributing to further stiffness. The metacarpophalangeal joint may become secondarily involved with some degree of compensatory hyperextension, as

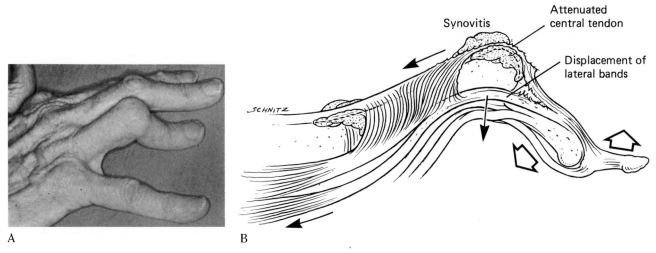

Figure 39-12 Boutonniere deformity in rheumatoid arthritis. **A.** Clinical appearance. **B.** Pathomechanics, showing dorsal synovitis with central slip attenuation and displacement of lateral bands. *(Reprinted with permission from Manus.)*

the extensor tendon, unable to extend the proximal interphalangeal joint, increases its proximal pull at the metacarpophalangeal level. Intrinsic tightness of metacarpophalangeal joint disease, however, may negate this metacarpophalangeal extension influence. Millender and Nalebuff have developed for boutonniere deformities a classification system which aids in selecting the proper treatment for each stage of the process (Table 39-6).[96] It should be made clear, however, that the presence of the deformity does not necessarily mean that significantly compromised hand function has occurred.

DISTAL INTERPHALANGEAL JOINT INVOLVEMENT

Rheumatoid arthritis directly involves the distal interphalangeal joint much less frequently than the proximal two digital joints and must not be confused with coexisting degenerative arthritis involvement. As rheumatoid synovitis erodes the distal finger joint surfaces and attenuates the capsule and liga-

ments about the joint, pain and limited motion result, often associated with joint instability. Mallet deformity occurs with rupture of the terminal extensor tendon (Fig. 39-13), or hyperextension deformity may result from rupture or stretching of the volar plate and long flexor tendon.

In many instances, no treatment is necessary for distal interphalangeal joint involvement in rheumatoid arthritis. Severe deformity, instability, or pain are best managed by simple arthrodesis. This procedure restores distal joint stability and may improve function at the more proximal finger joints as strength of the extensor and flexor mechanism is concentrated at those levels.

THE THUMB IN RHEUMATOID ARTHRITIS

The thumb is often considered to represent 40 percent of the value of the hand.[2] In rheumatoid arthritis, as a consequence

TABLE 39-6 Staging and Treatment for the Rheumatoid Boutonniere Deformity

Stage	Deformity	PIP* joint	DIP* joint	Treatment
I	Mild	10–15° lag	± hyperextension with positive intrinsic-intrinsic tightness test	Extensor tenotomy over middle phalanx
II	Moderate	30–40° lag	Hyperextended (+) intrinsic-intrinsic tightness test	Central slip shortening, mobilization of lateral bands and tenotomy
III	Severe	Fixed flexion posture	Hyperextended	Release of contracture, splint or surgery and then central slip shortening, mobilization of lateral bands, tenotomy, arthroplasty, PIP joint fusion

*PIP = proximal interphalangeal; DIP = distal interphalangeal.
Source: Millender, L.H., Nalebuff, E.A., and Feldon, P.G., in Green, D.P., ed: *Operative Hand Surgery,* New York, Churchill Livingstone, 1982. Adapted with permission.

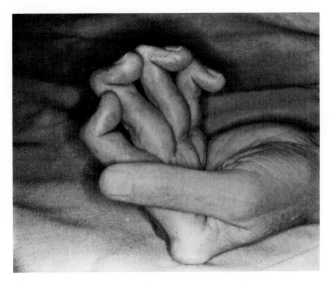

Figure 39-13 Mallet deformities due to rupture of the terminal extensor tendons in rheumatoid arthritis.

of joint destruction, instability, or muscle imbalance, the thumb loses its ability to act as a strong opposition post. As grasp-and-pinch function decreases, hand function becomes seriously compromised. The rheumatoid thumb deformities have been classified by Nalebuff,[96,99] and Table 39-7 provides a summary of the rheumatoid thumb deformities and their treatment based on this classification system (Fig. 39-14). An

additional type of rheumatoid thumb deformity, described by Ratcliff,[115] has been added to Nalebuff's classification (type V in Table 39-7). There can be no question that stabilization procedures such as metacarpophalangeal joint or interphalangeal joint arthrodesis rank at the top of the list rheumatoid procedures with regard to their ability to restore strong, pain-free thumb function, particularly when good basilar joint motion remains or can be preserved by arthroplasty.

FLEXOR TENOSYNOVITIS AND TENDON RUPTURE

Flexor tenosynovitis has been briefly discussed as a causative factor in many of the deformities of the individual joints of the hand and wrist in rheumatoid arthritis. The significance of this problem cannot be overemphasized and must be carefully searched for at the level of the wrist, palm, and digits in rheumatoid patients. Because of the depth of the deep transverse carpal ligament, flexor tenosynovitis of the wrist may be less obvious than its extensor counterpart (Fig. 39-15). Symptoms of carpal tunnel syndrome should be carefully sought out in addition to an observation of any fullness of the volar wrist or palm, catching (triggering) of the flexor tendons at the wrist level, or digital dysfunction resulting from ruptured or attenuated flexor tendons. Although steroid treatment may occasionally be beneficial, wrist flexor tenosynovectomy and carpal tunnel release are often indicated.

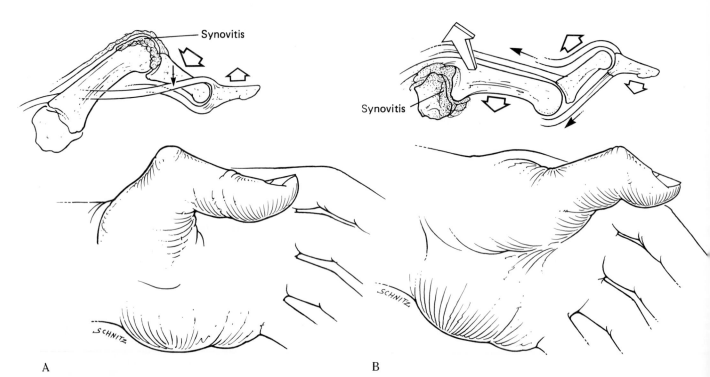

A

B

Figure 39-14 Boutonniere and swan-neck deformities may also occur in the rheumatoid thumb. Frequently, one joint is predominately affected by reciprocal changes at the contiguous joints (see text). **A.** Boutonniere deformity of the thumb with synovitis affecting predominantly the metacarpophalangeal joint. **B.** Swanneck deformity of the thumb. Synovitis affects predominantly the carpometacarpal joint. *(Reprinted with permission from Manus.)*

TABLE 39-7   Rheumatoid Thumb Deformities and Their Treatment

Type thumb deformity	Deformity	Joint involved by synovitis	CMC* joint	MP* joint	IP* joint	Treatment
I	Boutonniere (A + B + C = 57% of rheumatoid thumb deformities)	MP	—	Flexed	Extended	—
I_A (mild)			—	Flexed, passively corrects	Hyperextended, passively corrects	MP joint synovectomy extensor mechanism reconstruction
I_B (moderate)		MP		Fixed in flexion with or without joint destruction	Hyperextended, passively corrects	MP joint arthrodesis or arthroplasty
I_C (severe)		MP	—	Fixed in flexion	Fixed in hyperextension	Depending on joint status, IP joint: capsulotomy vs. fusion; MP joint: synovectomy, extensor reconstruction, arthroplasty vs. fusion

(continued on next page)

Fullness in the distal palm and digits with evidence of triggering or crepitus is seen in rheumatoid arthritis patients with digital flexor tenosynovitis. When they are sufficiently symptomatic, treatment consists of flexor tenosynovectomy. Although incising the proximal A-1 pulley is still the most frequent technique for decompression of the flexor tendon sheath, some authors have advocated decreasing the bulk of the flexor tendon system by excising one slip of the flexor digitorum superficialis.[43] This method may be biomechanically helpful by not increasing the ulnar approach of the flexor tendons and the resultant ulnar drift of the digits. Nalebuff has described four types of rheumatoid trigger finger problems based on the location of the tendon nodule and whether or not diffuse tenosynovitis is present.[100] For all four types, flexor tenosynovectomy and excision of flexor tendon nodules is the recommended treatment.

Unattended flexor tenosynovitis may contribute to flexor tendon rupture. The most commonly affected tendon is the flexor pollicis longus with attrition occurring at the level of the trapezial crest or scaphoid.[81] The tendon rupture may be in the wrist, palm, or digit, often requiring surgical exploration to determine the exact site. Care must be made to distinguish between a flexor tendon rupture and a stenosing teno-

synovitis with the digit locked in extension. Flexor tendon ruptures may be treated by tendon graft or tendon transfer.[101,102] On occasion, arthrodesis of the terminal joint for profundus or flexor pollicis longus rupture may be a simpler alternative.

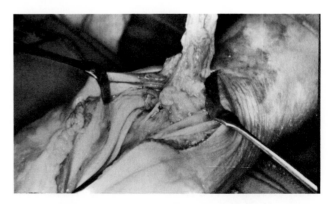

Figure 39-15 Surgical exposure demonstrating volar wrist synovectomy and depth of tenosynovium. Flexor tenosynovitis of the wrist is usually less clinically apparent than its dorsal counterpart.

TABLE 39-7 (*Continued*)

Type thumb deformity	Deformity	Joint involved by synovitis	CMC* joint	MP* joint	IP* joint	Treatment
III	Swan-neck (a + b + c = 9% of rheumatoid thumb deformities)	CMC	Dorsal and radial subluxation to frank dislocation	Hyperextended 2° metacarpal adduction contracture		
III_a (mild)		CMC	Minimal subluxation and deformity	—	Reciprocal flexion	Conservative management vs CMC hemiarthroplasty
III_b (moderate)		CMC	Subluxation and deformity	Passively correctable joint hyperextension	Reciprocal flexion	CMC hemiarthroplasty or resection arthroplasty, volar tenodesis of MP joint or MP joint fusion
III_c (severe)		CMC	Dislocation with fixed adduction contracture (of MC)	Fixed hyperextension deformity	Reciprocal flexion	CMC hemiarthroplasty MP joint fusion
IV	Gamekeeper's	MP	—	Abduction deformity with 2° adduction deformity of MC	—	MP joint synovectomy collateral ligament reconstruction vs. MP joint fusion and adductor fascia release
II	Combination types I and III (rare)	MP, CMC	Subluxation or dislocation	Flexed	Hyperextended	As types I and II
V^{115}	Instability of IP or MP joints due to joint destruction as seen with arthritis mutilans	IP, MP		Multidirectional instability	Multidirectional instability	Joint fusion using bone graft

*CMC = carpal metacarpal; MP = metacarpophalangeal; IP = interphalangeal; MC = metacarpal.
Source: Millender, L.H., Nalebuff, E.A., and Feldon, P.G., in Green, D.P., ed: *Operative Hand Surgery.* New York, Churchill Livingstone, 1982, pp 1241–1256. Adapted with permission.

MULTIPLE-LEVEL INVOLVEMENT OF THE RHEUMATOID HAND AND WRIST

Some surgeons experienced in the surgical management of the rheumatoid hand favor an aggressive multilevel surgical approach to the complex rheumatoid hand. Complementary reconstructive procedures must be carefully selected and must not present conflicting rehabilitation requirements.[135]

General guidelines for the reconstruction of the rheumatoid hand with multiple-level involvement suggest surgical correction of more proximal joints such as the wrist and metacarpophalangeal joints before proceeding further distally. When severe deformities exist, it may be most practical to try to achieve improved motion at one joint level and to stabilize adjacent joints. The benefit of each surgical procedure may be maximized by combining those procedures which are complementary in terms of the postoperative therapy requirements. Above all, the patient's needs, expectations, and motivation must be considered. The mere existence of deformity is not an indication for surgery. The specific reconstructive program must be tailored to the individual rheumatoid patient.[128]

SYSTEMIC LUPUS ERYTHEMATOSUS (SLE)

Muscular pain and atrophy as well as joint pain are frequent symptoms in this systemic multisystem disease.[18]

Although the hallmark of the disease as it affects the hands and wrists are deformities which appear rheumatoid-like, the joint changes are nonerosive.[55] Radiographic findings have been reported to include joint erosion, destruction, effusion, narrowing, juxtaarticular demineralization, subluxation or dislocation, bone infarction, aseptic necrosis, and abnormal calcification. Joint destruction, even in long-standing cases with severe joint disease, is usually scant.[111] Other authors have reported that articular destruction and ankylosis do not occur unless there is coexistent rheumatoid arthritis.[13]

The common hand lesions seen in SLE include migratory polyarthralgias, flexor tenosynovitis, metacarpophalangeal and proximal interphalangeal arthritis, skin rash, Raynaud's phenomenon, and avascular necrosis of carpal bones.[7] The pathophysiological mechanisms producing deformities differ slightly from those of rheumatoid patients in that distension of soft tissue rather than direct destruction and fibrosis of supporting elements appears to be the primary offender. Although both diseases exhibit synovitis, the pannus is not as aggressive in producing deformity in SLE. The synovitis results in stretching of supporting structures, allowing normal muscle-tendon forces to deform the joint.[7]

Surgical treatment of hand involvement with SLE is primarily designed to rebalance the affected soft tissue structures.[13,61] Some authors have reported the inadequacy of soft tissue rebalancing alone and recommend selected joint fusion and implant arthroplasty in combination with soft tissue rebalancing.[18,120]

JUVENILE RHEUMATOID ARTHRITIS (JRA)

Several distinctions set JRA apart from rheumatoid arthritis seen in the adult and merit consideration. Children affected with JRA in general have a much milder course, resulting in less disability than in adults, with 50 to 70 percent of cases achieving remission.[58] The disease may, however, result in greater joint stiffness and ankylosis than its adult counterpart. Although surgery may play a minor role in the early management of the JRA patient, conservative treatment consisting of splinting and exercises is most often recommended.[53] In growing children, reconstructive procedures often used in adults are not appropriate, as epiphyseal arrest

may ensue. Even as afflicted children with active disease pass through puberty, their bones are often too narrow and medullary canals too small to make them acceptable candidates for many procedures such as arthroplasty.[8,40,67,112]

In the child with JRA, ulnar deviation of the hand (metacarpals) with radial deviation of the fingers associated with a short ulna may occur.[74] This is opposite to the deformity which occurs most frequently in adults. Boutonniere finger deformities are common as well as fixed flexion deformities of the interphalangeal joints. Swan-neck deformities are seen infrequently.[24] At the metacarpophalangeal joint level, in addition to radial deviation, loss of flexion without loss of extension is seen as contrasted to adult-onset rheumatoid arthritis in which ulnar drift and extension deficits are present with the maintenance of reasonable metacarpophalangeal flexion. Intrinsic tightness, so often seen in the adult, was not seen at all in a large reported series of JRA patients.[54] Finally, in the adult with rheumatoid arthritis, dorsal tenosynovitis of the wrist is frequently seen early, while in JRA early clinical signs are a mild loss of complete wrist extension prior to the presence of palpable synovitis or other clinical findings.[54]

The primary function of the surgeon is to follow patients afflicted with JRA closely and detect joint imbalance prior to the development of fixed deformities. The key to the early management is physical therapy with exercise, splinting, and occasional steroid injections.[54] In neglected or unresponsive cases, wedging casts can help bring the subluxed or volar-flexed wrist into a functional position, with the hope that this position can then be maintained in an orthosis.[44] Immobilization in this manner may permit spontaneous intercarpal or radiocarpal fusion to take place with the wrist in a functional position.[78] Reconstructive surgery for the wrist can then be reserved for the adult patient.

ARTHRITIS MUTILANS

Arthritis mutilans, main en lorgnette, and opera-glass hand are terms used to denote a severe form or variant of rheumatoid arthritis often associated with psoriasis.[25,47,109] It is manifested by extreme resorption of the ends of bones but with sparing of the vessels, nerves, and tendons. In the hand there is severe shortening, telescoping, and instability of the digits. It has been distinguished from Charcot's neuropathy by the presence of normal nerve conduction.[141] The deformities may be quite severe and are frequently seen about the wrist, elbow, and shoulder joints as well as the ribs, ankles, and toes.[127] In the hand and wrist, significant disability may result and include unequal shortening of adjacent digits, decreased grasp due to loss of digital length, instability, and angular deformity.[103] The goal of treatment is to preserve or restore length. Early treatment may be more successful than late salvage procedures accomplished with intercalary iliac bone grafts and joint fusions.[103]

PSORIATIC ARTHRITIS

Approximately 5 to 10 percent of patients with rheumatoid disease have psoriasis. According to Flatt, the diagnosis of psoriatic arthritis rather than rheumatoid disease is considered when the seronegative, nodule-free patient has psoriasis and when the disease appears patchy and less symmetrical in distribution.[45] It also may be less progressive in its course. In addition to the usual rheumatoid hand involvement, the distal interphalangeal joint in particular is affected in psoriatic arthritis. Although there may be less synovial proliferation, bone and joint destruction occur. The surgical treatment is much the same as in the rheumatoid patient, although arthrodesis may be more difficult to achieve.

GOUT

Gout may affect the hand and wrist but usually presents earlier and in other locations. Large tophi composed of urate crystals and draining sinuses are occasions for surgical intervention; however, the mainstay of treatment is medical management.[133]

OSTEOARTHRITIS

Osteoarthritis is common in the hands of both men and post-menopausal women. All men and women over the age of 60 years show some physical or radiological evidence of osteoarthritis, but only 25 percent of the women and 15 percent of the men are symptomatic.[45] The joints most frequently involved are the basilar joints of the thumbs and proximal and distal interphalangeal joints, which exhibit Bouchard's and Heberden's nodes respectively.

Patients with osteoarthritis can be subdivided into those presenting with Heberden's nodes only, those with generalized osteoarthritis with hand involvement of the thumb basilar joint and distal interphalangeal joints, and those with osteoarthritis affecting both proximal and distal interphalangeal joint levels.[91] Radiographs may show joint space narrowing, subchondral sclerosis, and osteophyte formation. Most patients are best managed medically with aspirin or the nonsteroid antiinflammatory drugs.

Painful instability of the thumb carpometacarpal joint is frequently seen in women and may be evaluated with the grind and circumduction tests.[39] Care must be taken to distinguish this condition from more proximal arthritic involvement of the scaphoid, trapezium, and trapezoid articulations. The arthritic process may also be pantrapezial, affecting not only the carpometacarpal joint but also the surrounding trapezial articulations to the trapezoid and scaphoid. Another area of the wrist frequently affected in osteoarthritis is in scaphoradial joint. The SLAC wrist, or scapholunate advanced collapse pattern, presents with significant degenerative changes at the scaphoradial articulation with sparing of the radiolunate joint.[155] This may also be seen in calcium pyrophosphate deposition disease.

Surgical treatment for osteoarthritis in the hand and wrist is reserved for cases unresponsive to medical management. Fusions and joint arthroplasties have both been recommended for cases that do not respond satisfactorily to medical management.

REFERENCES

1. Albright, J.A., and Chase, R.A. Palmar-shelf arthroplasty of the wrist in rheumatoid arthritis: A report of nine cases. Bone Joint Surg 52A:896–906, 1970.
2. American Medical Association. *Guide to the Evaluation of Permanent Impairment,* 2d ed. American Medical Association 1984, p 4.
3. American Society for Surgery of the Hand. Hand Review Course, 1982, p 178.
4. American Society for Surgery of the Hand. Regional Review Course in Hand Surgery, chapter on Rheumatoid Arthritis of the Hand and Wrist, 1982, p 172.
5. Aptekar, R.G., Davie J.M., and Cattell, H.S. Foreign body reaction to silicone rubber; complications of the finger-joint implant. Clin Orthop 98:231, 1974.
6. Aptekar, R.G., and Duff, I.F. Metacarpophalangeal joint surgery in rheumatoid arthritis. Clin Orthop 83:123–127, 1972.
7. Aptekar, R.G., Lawless, O.J., and Decker, J.L. Deforming non-erosive arthritis of the hand in systemic lupus erythematosus. Clin Orthop 100:120–124, 1974.
8. Athreya, B.H. The hand in Juvenile rheumatoid arthritis. In Proceedings of the First ARA Conference on the Rheumatoid Diseases of Childhood. Arthritis Rheum 20 (suppl 2):573–574, 1976.
9. Atkinson, R.E., Smith, R.J., and Jupiter, J.B. Silicone Synovitis of the Wrist. Read at the Annual Meeting of the American Society for Surgery of the Hand, Las Vegas, January 23, 1985.
10. Backdahl, M. The caput ulnae syndrome in rheumatoid arthritis. A study of the morphology, abnormal anatomy and clinical picture. Acta Rheumatol Scand 5 (suppl):1, 1963.
11. Beckenbaugh, R.D., and Linscheid, R.L. Total wrist arthroplasty: A preliminary report. J Hand Surg 2:337–344, 1977.
12. Beckenbaugh, R.D. Total joint arthoplasty—the wrist. Mayo Clin Proc 54:513–515, 1979.
13. Bleifeld, C.J., and Inglis, A.E. The hand in systemic lupus erythematosus. J Bone Joint Surg 56A:1202–1215, 1974.
14. Bowers, W. Distal radio-ulnar joint, in Green, D.P. (ed): *Operative Hand Surgery,* chap 19. New York, Churchill Livingstone, 1982, p 765.
15. Boyce, T., Youm, Y., Sprague, B.L., and Flatt, A.E. Clinical and experimental studies on the effect of extensor carpi radialis longus transfer in the rheumatoid hand. J Hand Surg 3:390, 1978.
16. Branemark, P.I., Ekholm, R., and Goldie, I. Physiologic aspects on the timing of synovectomy in rheumatoid arthritis, in Hijmans, W., Paul, W.D., and Herschel, H. (ed.): *Early Synovectomy in Rheumatoid Arthritis.* Amsterdam, Excerpta Medica, 1969, pp 11–19.
17. Brewerton, D.A. The tangential radiographic-projection for demonstrating involvement of metacarpal heads in rheumatoid arthritis. Br J Radiol 40:233–234, 1967.
18. Brumfield, R.H., Patzakis, M.J., Conaty, P., Monagan, E.H., and Kitridov, R.C. Surgery of the hand in systemic lupus erythematosus: A preliminary study. Contemp Orthop 1:5:42–45, 1979.
19. Bunnell, S., Soherty, E.W., and Curtis, R.M. Ischemic contracture located in the hand. Plast Reconstr Surg 3:424, 1948.
20. Burton, R.I. The rheumatoid hand, in Kilgore and Graham (eds): *The Hand, Surgical and Nonsurgical Management.* Philadelphia, Lea & Febiger, 1977, p 408.
21. Bywaters, E.G.L. The early radiological signs of rheumatoid arthritis. Bull Rheum Dis 2:231, 1960.
22. Carroll, R.E., and Dick, H.M. Arthrodesis of the wrist for rheumatoid arthritis. J Bone Joint Surg 53A:1365, 1971.
23. Carter, P.S., and Benton, L.J. Late Osseous Complications of Carpal Silastic Implants. Read at the Annual Meeting of the American Society for Surgery of the Hand, Las Vegas, January 23, 1985.
24. Chaplin, D., Pulkki, T., Sacrimoa, A., and Vaninio, K. Wrist and

finger deformities in juvenile rheumatoid arthritis. Acta Rheum Scand 15:206–233, 1969.

25. Clarke, O. Arthritis mutilans associated with psoriasis. Lancet 1:249, 1950.

26. Clayton, M.L. Surgical treatment of the wrist in rheumatoid arthritis. A review of 37 cases. J Bone Joint Surg 47(A):741, 1965.

27. Clayton, M.L. The caput ulnae syndrome: Update, in Strickland, J.W., and Steichen, J.B. (eds): *Difficult Problems in Hand Surgery,* chap 23. St. Louis, Mosby, 1982, p 199.

28. Clayton, M.D., and Ferlic, D.C. Tendon transfer for radial deviation of the wrist in rheumatoid arthritis. Clin Orthrop 100:176, 1974.

29. Clayton, M.L., and Ferlic, D.C. The wrist in rheumatoid arthritis. Clin Orthop 106:192, 1975.

30. Cooney, W.P., III, and Bryan, R.S. Rheumatoid arthritis in the upper extremity: Treatment of the elbow and shoulder joints. Instr Course Lect 27:247, 1979.

31. Cracchilo, A., III, and Marmor, L. Resection of the distal ulna in rheumatoid arthritis. Arthritis Rheum 12:415, 1969.

32. Currey, H.L.F. Intra-articular Thiotepa in rheumatoid arthritis. Ann Rheum Dis 24:382, 1965.

33. Curtis, R.M. Capsulectomy of the interphalangeal joints of the fingers. J Bone Joint Surg 26:1219–1232, 1954.

34. Curtis, R.M. Management of the stiff proximal interphalangeal joint. Hand 1:32–37, 1979.

35. Davis, J. et al: Rehabilitation of the rheumatoid upper limb. Orthop Clin of North Am 9(2):559–568, April 1978.

36. Davis, R.F. Weiland, A.J., and Dowling, S.V. Swanson implant arthroplasty of the wrist in rheumatoid patients. Clin Orthop 166:132, 1982.

37. Duncan, H., Frost, H.M., Villanueva, A.R., and Sigler, J.W. Osteoporosis of rheumatoid arthritis. Arthritis and Rheum 8:943, 1965.

38. Dupont, M., and Vanio, K. Arthrodesis of the wrist in rheumatoid arthritis. A study of 140 cases. Ann Chir Gynecol 57:513–519, 1968.

39. Eaton, R.G., and Littler, W. Ligament reconstruction for the painful thumb carpometacarpal joint. J Bone Joint Surg 55A:1655–1666, 1973.

40. Edstrom. G., and Gedda, P.O. Clinic and prognosis of rheumatoid arthritis in children. Acta Rheum Scand 3:129–153, 1957.

41. Ellison, M.R., Kelly, K.J., and Flatt, A.E. The results of surgical synovectomy of the digital joints in rheumatoid disease. J Bone Joint Surg 53A:1041–1060, 1971.

42. Fearnley, M.E. Intra-articular Thiotepa therapy in rheumatoid arthritis. Ann Phys Med 7:294–298, 1964.

43. Ferlie, D.C., and Clayton, M.L. Flexor tenosynovectomy in the rheumatoid finger. J Hand Surg 3(3):292, 1978.

44. Findley, T.W., Halpern, D., and Easton. J.K.M. Wrist subluxation in juvenile rheumatoid arthritis: Pathophysiology and management. Arch Phys Med Rehabil 64:69–74, 1983.

45. Flatt, A. *Care of the Arthritic Hand,* 4th ed. St. Louis, Mosby, 1983.

46. Flatt, A.E. Some pathomechanics of ulnar drift. Plas Reconstru 37:295–303, 1966.

47. Froimson, A.I. Hand reconstruction in arthritis mutilans. J Bone Joint Surg 53A:1377, 1971.

48. Gilliland, B.C., and Mannik, M. Rheumatoid arthritis, in Thorn, G.W. et al (eds): *Harrison's Principles of Internal Medicine,* 8th ed. New York, McGraw-Hill, 1977, pp 2050–2058.

49. Goldie, I., and Wellisch, M. The presence of nerves in original and regenerated synovial tissue in patients synovectomised for rheumatoid arthritis. Acta Orthop Scand 40:143–152, 1969.

50. Goncalves, D. Correction of disorders of the distal radio-ulnar joint by artificial pseudarthrosis of the ulna. J Bone Joint Surg 56(B):462–463, 1974.

51. Goodman, M.J., Millender, L.H., Nalebuff, E.A., and Phillips, C.A. Arthroplasty of the rheumatoid wrist with silicone rubber: An early evaluation. J Hand Surg 5:114–121, 1980.

52. Gordon, M., and Bullough R.G. Synovial and osseous inflammation of failed silicone-rubber prostheses: A report of 6 cases. J Bone Joint Surg 64:574–588, 1982.

53. Granberry, W.M., and Brewer, E.J. Early synovectomy in juvenile rheumatoid arthritis. Instr Course Lect 27–32, 1974.

54. Granberry, W.M. and Mangum, G.L. The hand in the child with juvenile rheumatoid arthritis. J Hand Surg 5:105–113, 1980.

55. Green, N., and Osmer, J.C. Small bone changes secondary to systemic lupus erythematosus. Radiology 90:118–120, 1968.

56. Gristina, A.G., Pace, N.A., Kantor, T.G., and Thompson, W.A. Intra-articular Thiotepa compared with Depo-Medrol and procaine in the treatment of arthritis. J Bone Joint Surg 52A:1603–1610, 1970.

57. Hakstan, R.W., and Tubiana, R. Ulnar deviation of the fingers, the role of joint structure and function. J Bone Joint Surg 49A:299, 1967.

58. Hansen V., Konreich, H., Bernstein, B., King, K.K., and Singsen, B. Prognosis of juvenile rheumatoid arthritis. In Proceedings of the 1st ARA Conference on the Rheumatic Disease of Childhood. Arthritis Rheum 20 (suppl 2):279–284, 1976.

59. Harrison, H. Excision arthroplasty of the metacarpophalangeal joints, in Tubian, R. (ed): *La Main Rheumatoid, Groupe d'Etude de la Main,* monograph no. 3. Paris, L'Expansion Scientifique Française, 1969, pp 159–164.

60. Harrison, S.H. The proximal interphalangeal joint in rheumatoid arthritis. Hand 3:125–130, 1971.

61. Hastings, D.E. and Evans, J.A. The lupus hand: A new surgical approach. J Hand Surg 3:179–183, 1978.

62. Hastings, D.E., and Evans, J.A. The rheumatoid wrist deformity and its surgical correction. Orthop Rev 9:61, 1980.

63. Hastings, D.E., and Evans, J.A. Rheumatoid wrist deformities and their relations to ulnar drift. J Bone Joint Surg [Am] 57:930, 1975.

64. Helal, B.H. Distal profundus entrapment in rheumatoid disease. Hand 2:48–51, 1970.

65. Helal, B.H. Extra-articular causes of proximal interphalangeal joint stiffness in rheumatoid arthritis. Hand 7:37–40, 1975.

66. Jackson, I.T. Surgical treatment of the hand in rheumatoid arthritis. Gaz Sanitaria, 19:84–91, 1970.

67. Jakobowski, S., and Roszczynska, P. The possibility of surgical treatment in cases of juvenile rheumatoid arthritis. Acta Rheumatol Scand 13:113–118, 1967.

68. Kessler, L., and Vainio, K. Posterior (dorsal) synovectomy for rheumatoid involvement of the hand and wrist. A follow-up study of sixty-six procedures. J Bone Joint Surg 48:1048, 1966.

69. Klein, M.J. Classification and Pathogenesis of Arthritis Related to the Upper extremities. Read at the Surgery for Upper Extremity Arthritis Course, New York University, New York, 1980.

70. Kuczynski, F. The proximal interphalangeal joint. J Bone Joint Surg 50:656–663, 1968.

71. Kulick, R.G., DeFiore, J.C., Straub, L.R., and Ranawat, C.S. Long term results of dorsal stabilization of the rheumatoid wrist. J Hand Surg 6:272, 1981.

72. Landsmeer, J.M.F. Anatomical and functional investigations of the articulation of the human fingers. Acta Anat 25 (suppl):24, 1955.

73. Landsmeer, J.M.F. Studies in the anatomy of articulation: I. The equilibrium of the "intercalated" bone. Acta Morphol Neerl Scand 3:287, 1961.

74. Landsmeer, J.M. Power grip and precision handling. Ann Rheum Dis 21:164–170, 1962.

75. Lipscomb, P.R. Is early synovectomy of the small joints of the hand worthwhile? in Cramer, L.M., and Chase, R.A. (eds): *Symposium on the Hand,* vol 3. St. Louis, Mosby, 1971, pp 29–32.

76. Lipscomb, P.R. Surgery of the arthritic hand: Sterling Bunnell Memorial Lecture. Proc Mayo Clin 40:132, 1965.

77. Linscheid, R.L., and Beckenbaugh, R.D. Total arthroplasty of the

wrist to relieve pain and increase motion. Geriatrics 31:48–52, 1976.

78. Maldonado-Cocco, J.A., Garcia-Morteo, O., Spindler, A.J., Hubscher, O., and Gagliardi, S. Carpal ankylosis in juvenile rheumatoid arthritis. Arthritis Rheum 23:1251–1255, 1980.

79. Mannerfelt, L., and Andersson, K. Silastic arthroplasty of the metacarpophalangeal joints in rheumatoid arthritis. Long term results. J Bone Joint Surg 57A:484, 1975.

80. Mannerfelt, L., and Malmsten, M. Arthrodesis of the wrist in rheumatoid arthritis. A technique without external fixation. Scand J Plast Reconstr Surg 5:124, 1971.

81. Mannerfelt, L., and Normal O. Attrition ruptures of flexor tendons in rheumatoid arthritis caused by bony spurs in the carpal tunnel. J Bone Joint Surg 51B:270–277, 1969.

82. Marmor, L. The role of hand surgery in rheumatoid arthritis. Surg Gynecol Obstet 116–335, 1963.

83. Martel, W. The pattern of rheumatoid arthritis in the hand and wrist. Radiol Clin North Am 2:221, 1964.

84. Martel, W., Hayes, J.T., and Duff, I.F. The pattern of bone erosion in the hand and wrist in rheumatoid arthritis. Radiology 84:204, 1965.

85. McMurtry, R.Y., Youm, Y., Flatt, A.E., and Gillespie, T.E. Kinematics of the wrist: II. Clinical applications. J Bone Joint Surg [AM] 60:955, 1978.

86. Melone, C. Wrist synovitis and tendon ruptures in *Surgery for Upper Extremity Arthritis Course,* New York University, 1980, p 79.

87. Menkes, C.J., Tubian, R., Galmiche, B., and Del Barre, F. Intra-articular injection of radioisotopic beta emitters. Orthop Clin North Am 4:1113–1125, 1973.

88. Meuli, H.C. Alloarthroplastick des Handgelenks. Z Orthop 113:476–478, 1975.

89. Meuli, H.C. Arthroplastic due Poignet. Ann Chir 27:527–530, 1973.

90. Meuli, H.C. Reconstructive surgery of the wrist joint. Hand 4:88–90, 1972.

91. Millender, L.H. Surgery of the hand in osteoarthritis. Orthop Rev 9:73–81, 1980.

92. Millender, L.H., and Nalebuff, E.A. Evaluation and treatment of early rheumatoid hand involvement. Orthop Clin North Am 6:697–708, 1975.

93. Millender, L.H., Nalebuff, E.A., Albin, R., Ream, J., and Gordon, M. Dorsal tenosynovectomy and tendon transfer in the rheumatoid hand. J Bone Joint Surg 56A:601, 1979.

94. Millender, L.H., and Nalebuff, E.A. Preventative surgery—Tenosynovectomy and synovectomy. Orthop Clin North Am 6:765, 1975.

95. Millender, L.H., and Nalebuff, E.A. Arthrodesis of the rheumatoid wrist. An evaluation of sixty patients and a description of a different surgical technique. J Bone Joint Surg 55A:1026, 1973.

96. Millender, L.H., Nalebuff, E.A., and Felton, P.G. Rheumatoid Arthritis, in Green, D.P. (ed): *Operative Hand Surgery.* New York, Churchill Livingstone, 1982, pp 1161–1262.

97. Millender, L.H., Nalebuff, E.A., and Holdsworth, D.E. Posterior interosseous nerve syndrome secondary to rheumatoid synovitis. J Bone Joint Surg 55A:753, 1973.

98. Millis, M.B., Millender, L.H., and Nalebuff, E.A. Stiffness of the proximal interphalangeal joints in rheumatoid arthritis. J Bone Joint Surg 58:801–805, 1976.

99. Nalebuff, E.A. Diagnosis, classification and management of rheumatoid thumb deformities. Bull Joint Dis 29:119–137, 1968.

100. Nalebuff, E.A. Surgical treatment of rheumatoid tenosynovitis in the hand. Surg Clin North Am 49:799–809, 1969.

101. Nalebuff, E.A. Surgical treatment of tendon rupture in the rheumatoid hand. Surg Clin North Am 49:811–822, 1969.

102. Nalebuff, E.A. The recognition and treatment of tendon ruptures in the rheumatoid hand. *AAOS Symposium on Tendon Surgery in the Hand.* St. Louis, Mosby, 1975, pp 255–269.

103. Nalebuff, E.A., and Garrett, J. Opera-glass hand in rheumatoid arthritis. J Hand Surg 1:210–220, 1976.

104. Nalebuff, E.A., and Millender, L.H. Reconstructive surgery and rehabilitation of the hand, in Resnick and Newayand (ed): *Diagnosis of Bone and Joint Disorders,* vol 2. Philadelphia, Saunders, 1981.

105. Nalebuff, E.A., and Millender, L.H. Surgical treatment of the swan-neck deformity in rheumatoid arthritis. Orthop Clin North Am 6:733–752, 1975.

106. Nalebuff, E.A., and Patel, M.R. Flexor digitorum sublimis transfer for multiple extensor tendon ruptures in rheumatoid arthritis. Plast Reconstr Surg 52:530, 1973.

107. Nalebuff, E.A., and Potter, T.A. Rheumatoid involvement of tendons and tendon sheaths in the hand. Clin Orthop 59:147, 1968.

108. Neibauer, J.J. Dacron-silicone prosthesis for the metacarpophalangeal and interphalangeal joints, in Cramer, L.H., and Chase, R.A. (eds): *Symposium of the Hand,* vol 3. St. Louis, Mosby, 1971, pp 96–105.

109. Nelson, L.S. The opera-glass hand in chronic arthritis. "La main enlorgnette" of Marie and Leri. J Bone Joint Surg 20:1045, 1938.

110. Nicolle, F.V., Holt, P.J.L., and Calnan, J.S. Prophylactic synovectomy of the joints of the rheumatoid hand. Ann Rheum Dis 30:476–480, 1971.

111. Noon, C.D., Odone, D.T., Engleman, E.P., and Splitter, S.D. Roentgenographic manifestations of joint disease in systemic lupus erythematosus. Radiology 80:837–843, 1963.

112. Pahle, J.A., and Raunio, P. The influence of wrist position on finger deviation in the rheumatic hand. A clinical and radiological study. J Bone Joint Surg [Br] 51:669–696, 1969.

113. Peimer, C.J., Medige, J., Eckert, B.S., and Wright, J.R. Invasive Silicone Synovitis of the Wrist. Read at the Annual Meeting of the American Society for Surgery of the Hand, Las Vegas, January 23, 1985.

114. Preston, R.L. Early synovectomy in rheumatoid arthritis: Introductory paper on the orthopaedic aspects, in Hijmans, W., Paul, W.D., and Herschel, H. (eds). Amsterdam, Excerpta Medica, 1969,

115. Ratcliff, A.H.C. Deformities of the thumb in rheumatoid arthritis. Hand 3:138–143, 1971.

116. Resnick, D. Rheumatoid arthritis of the wrist: Why the ulnar styloid? Radiology 112:29–35, 1974,

117. Scaramuzza, R.F.J. El movimiento de rotacion en el carpo ye su relacion con las fisiopathlgical de sus lesiones traumaticas. Bol Trab Soc Argent Ortop Traumatol 39:337, 1969.

118. Scott, F.A., and Boswick, J.A. Palmar arthroplasty for the treatment of the stiff swan-neck deformity. J Hand Surg 8:267–272, 1983.

119. Scherbel, A.L., Schucker, S.L., and Weyman, J.S. Intra-articular administration of nitrogen mustard alone and combined with corticosteroid for rheumatoid arthritis. Cleve Clin Q 24:78–89, 1957.

120. Shomacker, H.R., Zweiman, B., and Bora, F.W. Corrective surgery for the deforming hand arthropathy of systemic lupus erythematosus. Clin Orthop 117:292–295, 1976.

121. Shapiro, J.S. Ulnar drift. A report of related findings. Acta Orthop Scand 39:346, 1968.

122. Shapiro, J.S. Wrist involvement in rheumatoid swan-neck deformity. J Hand Surg 7:484–491, 1982.

123. Shapiro, J.S., Heijna, W., Nasatir, S., and Ray, R.S. The relationship of the wrist motion to ulnar phalangeal drift in the rheumatoid patient. Hand 3:68, 1971.

124. Short, C.L., Bauer, E., and Reynolds, W.E. *Rheumatoid Arthritis—A Definition of the Disease and a Clinical Description Based on a Numerical Study of 293 Patients and Controls.* Cambridge, Harvard University Press, 1957.

125. Smith, E.M., Juvinall, R.C., Bender, L.F., and Pearson, J.R. Role of

the finger flexors in rheumatoid deformities of the metacarpophalangeal joints. Arthritis and Rheum 7:467–480, 1964.

126. Smith, R.J., and Kaplan, E.B. Rheumatoid deformities of the metacarpophalangeal joints of the finger, a correlative study of anatomy and pathology. J Bone Joint Surg 49(A):31, 1976.

127. Soloman, W.M., and Stecher, R.M. Chronic absorptive arthritis or opera-glass hand. Report of eight cases. Ann Rheum Dis 9:209, 1950.

128. Souter, W.A. Planning treatment of the rheumatoid hand.

129. Stack, H.G., and Vaughan-Jackson, O.J. The zig-zag deformity in the rheumatoid hand. Hand 3:62, 1971.

130. Steindler, A. Arthritic deformities of the wrist and fingers. J Bone Joint Surg 33(A):849, 1951.

131. Strang, R.F.A., and Heuston, J.T. Healing of bony rheumatoid lesions after synovectomy of metacarpophalangeal joints Med J Aust 1:809, 1968.

132. Straub, L.R., and Ranawat, C.S. The wrist in rheumatoid arthritis. J Bone Joint Surg [Am] 51:1–20, 1969.

133. Straub, L.R., Smith, J.W., Carpenter, G.K., and Deitz, G.H. Surgery of gout in the upper extremity. J Bone Joint Surg 43(A):731–752, 1961.

134. Straub, L.R., and Wilson, E.H., Jr. Spontaneous rupture of extensor tendons in the hand associated with rheumatoid arthritis. J Bone Joint Surg 38A:1208, 1956.

135. Strickland, J.W., and LaSalle, W.B. The surgical management of multiple-level deformities of the rheumatoid hand, a practical approach, in Strickland, J.W., and Steicher, J.B. (eds): *Difficult Problems in Hand Surgery.* St. Louis, Mosby, 1982, pp 224–240.

136. Swanson, A.B. Flexible implant arthroplasty for arthritic finger joints. J Bone Joint Surg 54A:435, 1972.

137. Swanson, A.B. *Flexible Implant Resection Arthroplasty in the Hand and Extremities.* St. Louis, Mosby, 1973.

138. Swanson, A.B. Flexible implant arthroplasty for arthritic disabilities of the radiocarpal joint. A silicone-rubber intramedullary stemmed flexible hinge implant for the wrist joint. Orthop Clin North Am 4:383–394, 1973.

139. Swanson, A.B. Implant arthroplasty for disabilities of the distal radioulnar joint. Use of a silicone-rubber capping implant following resection of the ulnar head. Orthop Clin North Am 4:373, 1973.

140. Swanson, A.B. Silicone-rubber implants for replacement of arthritic or destroyed joints in the hand. Surg Clin North Am 48:113, 1968.

141. Swezey, R.L., Bjarnason, N., and Austin, E.S. Nerve conduction studies in resorptive arthropathies. Opera-glass hand. J Bone Joint Surg 55(A):1680, 1973.

142. Taleisnik, J. The ligaments of the wrist. J Hand Surg 1:110, 1976.

143. Taleisnik, J. Post-traumatic carpal instability. Clin Orthop Related Res 149:73, 1980.

144. Taleisnik, J. Rheumatoid synovitis of the volar compartment of the wrist joint—Its radiological signs and its contribution to wrist and hand deformity. J Hand Surg 4:526–534, 1979.

145. Thompson, M., Douglas, G., and Davidson, E.P. Evaulation of synovectomy in rheumatoid arthritis. Proc R Soc Med 66:197–199, 1973.

146. Tupper, J.W. The volar plate arthoplasty for rheumatoid arthritis. *Proceedings of the Fifteenth Annual Meeting of the Japanese Society for Surgery of the Hand.* Niigota, 1972, p 24.

147. Vainio, K.: Arthrodesis and arthroplasties in the treatment of the rheumatoid hand, in *La Main Rheumatoide.* Paris, Expansion Scientifique Francaise, 1966, pp 30–35.

148. Vainio, K., and Julkunen, H. Intra-articular nitrogen mustard treatment of rheumatoid arthritis. Acta Rheumatol Scand 6(1):25–30, 1960.

149. Vainio, K., Reiman, I., and Pulkki, T. Results of arthroplasty of the metacarpophalangeal joints in rheumatoid arthritis. Reconst Surg Traumatol 9:1–7, 1967.

150. Vainio, K., and Oka, M. Ulnar deviation of the fingers. Ann Rheum Dis 12:122–124, 1953.

151. Vaughan-Jackson, O.J. Attrition ruptures of tendons in the rheumatoid hand. J Bone Joint Surg 40A:1431, 1958.

152. Vaughan-Jackson, O.J. Rheumatoid hand deformities considered in the light of tendon imbalance. J Bone Joint Surg 44(B):764–775, 1962.

153. Vaughan-Jackson, O.J. Rupture of extensor tendons by attrition of the inferior radio-ulnar joint: Report of two cases. J Bone Joint Surg 30(B):528–530, 1948.

154. Volz, R.G. Total wrist arthroplasty. A new approach to wrist instability. Clin Orthop 128:180–189, 1977.

155. Watson, H.K., and Ballet, F.L. The SL AC wrist: Scapholunate advanced collapse pattern of degenerative arthritis. J Hand Surg 9(A):358–365, 1984.

156. Weilby, A. Resection arthroplasty of the metacarpophalangeal joint; A.M. Tupper using interposition of the volar plate. Scand J Plast Reconstr Surg 11:239–242, 1977.

157. Wenley, W.G., and Glick, E.N. Medical synovectomy with Thiotepa, Ann Phys Med 7:287–293, 1964.

158. Worsing, R.A. Engber, W.D., and Lang, T.A. Reactive synovitis of particulate silastic. J Bone Joint Surg 64:581–585, 1982.

159. Zancolli, E.—Correction of the arthritic ulnar drift before cartilage destruction—An operation to rebalance the metacarpophalangeal forces, in Cramer, L.M., and Chase, R.A. (eds): *Symposium on the Hand.* St. Louis, Mosby, pp 73–95, 1971.

160. Zancolli, E. *Structural and Dynamic Basis of Hand Surgery.* Philadelphia, Lippincott, pp 51–84, 1968.

161. Zuckner, J., et al. Evaluating intra-articular Thiotepa in rheumatoid arthritis. Ann Rheum Dis 25:178–183, 1966.

CHAPTER 40

Peripheral Nerve Injuries and Entrapments

Lawrence C. Hurst, Marie A. Badalamente,
Seth Paul, and Michael P. Coyle, Jr.

SECTION A

Nerve Injuries in the Upper Extremity

Lawrence C. Hurst, Marie A. Badalamente, and Seth Paul

Peripheral nerve injuries constitute a major source of chronic disability. The introduction of the operative microscope as well as refinement of microsurgical techniques have advanced the treatment of these injuries. However, these advances have not readily translated into improved clinical results.[56,63] This chapter deals with the biological process of nerve regeneration following injury and repair, the technical aspects of nerve repair, and the results of nerve repair. A discussion of brachial plexus injuries and obstetrical palsy is also included.

CLASSIFICATION OF NERVE INJURY

Seddon[52] and Sunderland[59] have both proposed classification schemes for nerve injuries. In 1943 Seddon classified nerve injuries into three groups: neuropraxia, axonotmesis, and neurotmesis. *Neuropraxia* represents a physiological block of nerve function in which anatomical continuity of the nerve is preserved, but there is selective demyelination of large fibers without distal axon degeneration. *Axonotmesis* represents a disruption of nerve function based on the disruption of the axon and its myelin sheath without disruption of the epineurium, perineurium, or endoneurium. In axonotmesis wallerian degeneration does occur distally and recovery of the nerve is dependent on a regeneration process. *Neurotmesis* is the most severe injury, being a complete discontinuity between the distal portion of the nerve and its cell body either because of a complete transection of the nerve or because of extensive peripheral nerve damage that represents a complete functional degeneration.

Sunderland[59] classified the severity of nerve injuries according to degrees ranging from first-degree to fifth-degree injury. The first degree in Sunderland's classification corresponds to neuropraxia. This is a physiological interruption of nerve function due to local demyelination of nerve fibers without division of the axon. Motor paralysis occurs and may or may not be accompanied by anesthesia. There is no wallerian degeneration, and spontaneous recovery within a few days to several weeks is expected. Neuropraxis may be caused by compression leading to intussusception of axons through the nodes of Ranvier resulting in prolonged nerve conduction block.[7] Most closed injuries are either neuropraxia or neurotmesis.

Second-degree injury or axonotmesis is transection of the axon which leaves the endoneurium intact. Wallerian degeneration occurs distal to the level of the axon transection. Motor, sensory, and autonomic nerve dysfunction is complete. Recovery is slow, occurring within 2 or 3 months. The third degree in Sunderland's classification overlaps the axonotmesis and the clinical neurotmesis of the Seddon classification: endoneurial damage occurs, but the fascicular pattern remains intact. This reversible lesion corresponds to a more severe form of axonotmesis. Some lesions are irreversible because such a large number of axons are damaged that there is an extensive fibrotic process within the fasciculi following the injury.[59]

Sunderland's fourth-degree injury is fascicular disorganization with no gross retraction of nerve ends. The epineurium remains intact. It is similar to a neuroma-in-continuity. Spontaneous recovery is not expected. This fourth degree injury corresponds to clinical neurotmesis.[59]

Fifth-degree injury is complete severance of the nerve fiber with retraction of the ends and loss of anatomical continuity.[59]

NERVE REGENERATION

The response of a peripheral nerve to injury depends upon the severity of the initial trauma. In mild neuropraxic lesions, axons generally respond by focal demyelination and remyelination.[63] Axon degeneration and regeneration occurs in the more severe classes of nerve injuries.[63] Further, ischemia is a complicating factor in either mild or severe nerve injuries, especially in entrapment injuries.

In focal demyelination, a length of the axon is denuded. Histologically, this demyelination appears as rounded myelin ovoids. These ovoids are subsequently phagocytized by Schwann cells and macrophages. The denuded axons are then repaired by the process of Schwann cell remyelination. This type of axonal damage produces localized slowing or blocking of conduction over the demyelinated region. Conduction is restored by the process of remyelination.[63]

In the more severe nerve injuries, which include crush or transection, Waller's classic work[68] has shown that distal axon degeneration occurs and death of the cell body can also occur. Sunderland has quite correctly stated that the essential feature of regeneration in the nerve fiber is the outgrowth of the axon to replace the portion that perishes distally as a result of the injury. The great complexity of the regenerative process has been summarized by Sunderland[59] in simplified terms as progressing as follows: (1) the recovery of the axon from retrograde effects and the onset of regeneration at the axon tip; (2) the growth of the axon tip to the site of injury; (3) the passage of the axon across the zone of injury; (4) the growth of the axon down the endoneural tube below the injury; (5) the restoration of appropriate end organ relationships; (6) the functional maturation of newly reinnervated endoneural tubes; (7) the recovery of sufficient number of axons in appropriate patterns to give a response to voluntary effort or to a sensory stimulus; (8) finally, restoration of function.[59]

It is becoming increasingly apparent that the degenerative events in the distal stump after a nerve injury are linked to the regenerative events listed above. The classic wallerian changes, occurring distal to a nerve injury, are well-established and include fragmentation of the axon, retraction of the myelin sheath, and subsequent myelin and axonal breakdown and degradation.[68] Evidence is accumulating that the influx of calcium ions into injured nerve may be one of the first events in the triggering of wallerian degeneration.[51] The more recent finding that the enzyme *calcium-activated neutral protease* (CANP) is present in axons from a variety of species[24,49] lends credence to the hypothesis that calcium ions may trigger the protease to contribute to nerve degeneration, especially of neurofilaments. An analogous situation appears to exist in vertebrate skeletal muscle. Calcium ion has been implicated in triggering the atrophic process after muscle injury such as denervation.[55] The enzyme CANP is reported to be present in myofibers, especially in association with Z lines. The regenerative process occurs concomitantly with this enzymatic breakdown.[10] After nerve repair, Schwann cells proliferate and migrate toward the severed ends of the nerve to form the classic bands of Büngner. These columns of Schwann cells serve as guides for the axons as they grow toward the severed stump.

Ramon ý Cajal[45] definitively showed that nerve outgrowth occurs from the proximal stump. Following injury, there is a variable latent period of 6 to 36 h before outgrowth of sprouts of the cut axon tips. This latent period is generally shorter in younger animals. Subsequently, axon tips swell into cones of growth.

The growth cones of regenerating axons contain abundant agranular endoplasmic reticulum, large mitochondria, microtubules, microfilaments, lysosomes, and amorphous vacuolar structures.[53] Clinically, the growth-cone region may be localized in a general manner by eliciting Tinel's sign. This region is hyperexcitable, such that mechanical tapping stimulates sensory axons to produce Tinel's sign.[58]

Forward growth occurs by advancement of the cone by a sprouting of collaterals from the growth-cone tip and from the nodes of Ranvier several segments proximal to the tip.[53] Growth through scarred connective tissue at a nerve repair site may be slow, that is, about 0.25 mm/day. The rate of distal regeneration for most axons is 1 to 3 mm/day.

The success or failure of the regenerative process is influenced by various factors. The neurotropic factors, produced by both distal segments of the injured peripheral nerves and the denervated muscle, are an important aspect of the neural microenvironment of regenerating axons. These factors play a major role in the success or failure of regeneration. The microenvironmental stages of differentiation in neurons of the peripheral nervous system has been reviewed by Varon and Bunge.[66] These authors characterize stage I of neural development as axonal growth proceeding toward a prescribed periphery but cell survival as being independent of the potential availability of target tissue (as in embryogenesis); stage II is characterized by a state of vulnerability of the nerve fiber, leading to death unless connection is made (again as in embryogenesis); stage III is reached after nerve fiber target connections have been made, during which cell stability may persist indefinitely; finally, stage IV may be imposed following disconnection of the nerve fiber from its peripheral target, as in axotomy. The most widely supported hypothesis to explain the stability of stage III and the tropic influence in stage IV is the existence of tropic agents supplied by the peripheral targets.

It is now becoming apparent that the distal segments of crushed or cut peripheral nerve are an important part of the peripheral target which can exert tropic influence.[37] It has been recently reported that these segments show increased synthesis of a 37-kilodalton (kd) protein identified as apolipoprotein E.[37] It has been postulated that this protein is involved in debris removal and lipid transport necessary for formation of regenerating neural membranes. Interestingly, this protein accumulates only in the peripheral nervous system after injury, not in the central nervous system after injury. This may represent one of the critical molecular differences between the abilities of the peripheral nervous system and of the central nervous system to regenerate. It is well known that denervated muscle also exerts a tropic influence on regenerating axons,[54] but this molecular signal has not yet been fully determined.

Despite the regenerative ability of the axon tips and the tropic influence of distal nerve segments and denervated muscle, there is at present no exogenous mechanism that can be employed to guide regenerating axons to their peripheral targets. Reinnervation occurs randomly and thus the extent to which appropriate connections are made, or not made, determines ultimate neuromuscular recovery. It is apparent that the neurobiology of the nerve repair process will require continued scrutiny before we achieve the understanding necessary to influence neuromuscular recovery favorably.

BLOOD SUPPLY TO NERVES

The vascular supply of peripheral nerves consists of intrinsic and extrinsic systems.[23,30,57] Recent work on vascularized nerve grafts has delineated the different vascular patterns that exist between the extrinsic vascular system and the nerve trunk proper.[4] These range from nerve trunks supplied by multiple extrinsic vessels to nerves with no documented extrinsic vessel. The intrinsic system is composed of a longitudinal vascular plexus coursing through the epineurium, perineurium, and endoneurium. Short vessels, called the vasa nervorum, connect the extrinsic and intrinsic systems. Nutrient vessels, the arteriae nervorum, pass through the mesoneurium in an arcade distribution. Theoretically, the mesoneurium, with its multiple anastomoses, allows movement of the extremities without interruption of neural blood supply. This complex intraneural microcirculation ensures an adequate supply of oxygen, which is essential for nerve function. Intraneural blood flow is affected by compression or by excessive tension on the nerve.[36] The endoneural blood vessels have certain barrier properties, constituting a "blood-nerve" barrier similar to the blood-brain barrier of the central nervous system. Thus, the local environment of nerve fibers in their endoneurium is controlled by the dual action of the perineural plexus and the blood-nerve barriers.[47]

NERVE REPAIR

The goal of nerve repair is to provide an environment which will maximize axonal regeneration with optimal fascicular orientation. The advent of microsurgical technique ushered in a new era of nerve repair. The operative microscope allows better identification of nerve structures and facilitates more detailed suture technique.[22] The various methods of microsurgical repair include epineural repair, group fascicular or bundle repair, and epineural plus group fascicular repair (Fig. 40-1). Numerous reports have appeared in the literature advocating specific suture techniques for treating peripheral nerve injuries.[24,64,65]

Epineural repair involves placement of sutures through the epineural sheath. It is the most universally used repair technique. Repair of the epineurium alone; however, may allow for improper alignment of endoneural tubes and fascicles.

Group fascicular repair is the alignment of matching groups of fasciculi. Fascicular identification is achieved by one of several methods. First, referring to the neural topography maps of Sunderland[59] and Jabaley[22] can be helpful in identifying the fascicular patterns. The second method involves acetylcholinesterase staining.[14] However, this staining requires a 48-h delay for identification of fascicular patterns. A third technique for identifying fascicular groups is the intraoperative electrical stimulation of the proximal nerve trunk in awake patients for the identification of sensory fascicular groups.[15] Stimulation of distal nerve trunks, prior to the onset of wallerian degeneration, allows for identification of the motor fasciculi. Alignment of the vascular pattern of the proximal and distal nerve trunks also allows for gross orientation.

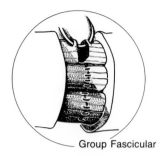 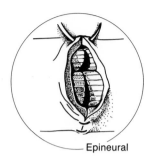

Group Fascicular   Epineural

Figure 40-1 Group fascicular nerve repair and epineural nerve repair are shown.

A review of the clinical and experimental work concerning the efficacy of epineural as opposed to perineural suture techniques reveals an end result in which there is little functional difference between these techniques.[42] It is clear that the suturing technique is not as important as strict adherence to atraumatic technique and to optimizing fascicular realignment by use of magnification, epineural vessel markings, cross-sectional pattern, and possibly fascicular electrical studies. In addition, tension at the suture site should be avoided. Several studies have demonstrated that tension at the nerve repair site has an adverse effect on nerve regeneration.[3,31,48]

The poor results seen after end-to-end repairs with excessive tension has led to the use of nerve grafting.[33,34,35] However, nerve grafting should be reserved for those cases where immobilization of the nerve ends, transposition of the nerve, or joint flexion will not allow for primary neurorrhaphy without undue tension at the suture site. Gaps of 2.5 to 7 cm or greater will often require nerve grafting to avoid tension at the suture site. Tension at the suture site results in a high degree of fibrosis and may cause axon sprouts to undergo axonolysis. Nerve grafting may also allow for immediate joint motion. However, regenerating axons must cross two suture lines. Although this technique deals with the tension problem, the new dilemma of multiple suture sites means that conventional nerve grafting does not completely solve the problem of traumatic nerve gaps.

Vascularized Nerve Grafts

Recognition of the importance of nerve graft blood supply has lead to the development of free vascularized nerve grafts. These have been used in scarred recipient beds with large nerve gaps and in proximal nerve lesions. Vascularized grafts may be able to act as carriers for the unvascularized nerve graft.[17] Comparison of vascularized nerve grafts with unvascularized grafts is under study, and the clinical usefulness of the technique has not been well defined.[7,44,46]

Timing of Nerve Repair: Primary versus Secondary Repair

As in tendon surgery, debate continues concerning the efficacy of primary as opposed to secondary repair in nerve injuries. Primary repair or delayed primary repair is advocated in clean wounds where fascicular group orientation and alignment is easier to delineate and there is less retraction of nerve stumps. Dissection is also facilitated by the absence of mature scar. Following crush or avulsion injuries or other untidy wounds, delayed primary repair or secondary repair has certain advantages. There is less chance of infection, and there is also a better demarcation of normal fasciculi as opposed to severely damaged neural tissue that must be resected. Yet, Millesi and Dieter Buck-Gramcko[7,33] believe they have demonstrated that early repairs have better functional results than late repairs.

In addition to timing, there are many other factors that influence the results of nerve repair: The type of injury, age of the patient, length of the defect, and the status of the surrounding tissue are all important factors. Sensory or pure motor nerve repairs consistently give better results than repairs in mixed nerves. Distal lesions fare better than more proximal lesions. Associated injuries to joints and soft tissues as well as loss of recipient integrity in the muscle or skin will also compromise the result of neurorrhaphy. Adults never achieve perfectly normal function. Cortical reorientation may explain the better clinical results seen in children. However, in adults the result can be improved following nerve repair if sensory reeducation techniques are employed.[12,71] In children this is a more natural process.[11]

Anatomical motor and sensory reinnervation does not necessarily ensure a functional recovery. Recovery following nerve injury and repair proceeds in three phases. The first phase is a period of axon regeneration with the establishment of neural connections between the proximal stump of the nerve and the periphery. The second phase is the return of function in its simplest form as demonstrated by the reappearance of contractions in individual muscle fibers or by the return of protective sensation. The third and last phase is the return of complex movements requiring the coordinated activity of groups of muscles and the return of the more discriminate aspects of sensation. This last phase is termed *useful functional recovery.*[58]

Results of nerve repair may be evaluated using the British Medical Research Council Nerve Injury Committee classification scheme for sensory recovery and motor recovery (Table 40-1). In this scheme SO is the absence of sensation and S4 signifies complete recovery. MO is complete motor paralysis without any evidence of muscle contraction. M5 is the contraction against powerful resistance or normal power.

Digital neurorrhaphy is associated with the best results of any type of nerve repair. Despite this, widely differing reports have appeared in the literature regarding recovery after digital nerve neurorrhaphy. Dieter Buck-Gramcko[7] reported a series of 154 digital nerve repairs in which 51.4 percent of the patients achieved an S3, or greater, sensory level. Using the dorsal sensory branch of the ulnar nerve for digital nerve grafting, Green and Stockin reported that 11 of 12 patients recovered two-point discrimination in the area supplied by the involved digital nerve.[19]

Sullivan did not achieve similarly impressive results.[56] In 42 cases, one-half of his patients were left with moderate to marked hypesthesia but most did achieve protective sensation. He concluded that "severed digital nerves must still carry a guarded prognosis in the adult."

Results of repair for both median and ulnar nerves in different series revealed that the level of injury and the age of the patient were the most important determinants of the outcome. Buck-Gramcko reported on 25 patients with median nerve injuries. Thirty-six percent of these patients recovered their sensation to an S3, or greater, level. In 21 median nerve repairs, 42.8 percent of the patients achieved an M4, or greater, level of motor function. In 17 repairs of the ulnar nerve, however, only 29.4 percent of the patients recovered at the level of the S3, or greater. Also, motor recovery was achieved in only 34.3 percent of the patients at a level of M4, or greater.[7]

Millesi reported on the results of median nerve repair by nerve grafting.[33] In 39 patients, 19 achieved S3 sensory level and an M4 to M5 motor level. Gaul reported on 41 patients with ulnar nerve lacerations.[16] In 14 adult patients, only 1 of the 14 showed useful intrinsic motor recovery after 1 year. Six of the adult patients recalled 26 to 51 months after the nerve repair showed surprisingly good intrinsic motor recovery in the involved hand. Twelve young patients showed favorable intrinsic motor recovery after lower-level ulnar nerve injuries. In high-level injuries, two of the five patients recovered good key pinch power by 1 year. Two of the remaining three recovered near-normal key pinch power on lateral examinations. None of the 10 adult patients, however, with high-level

TABLE 40-1 End-Result Grading System

Motor Recovery:

M10	No contraction
M1	Return of perceptible contraction in the proximal muscles
M2	Return of perceptible contraction in both proximal and distal muscles
M3	Return of function in both proximal and distal muscles of such degree that all important muscles are sufficiently powerful to act against resistance
M4	Return of function as in stage M3 with the addition that all synergic and independent movements are possible
M5	Complete recovery

Sensory Recovery:

S0	Absence of sensibility in the autonomous area
S1	Recovery of deep cutaneous pain sensibility within the autonomous area of the nerve
S2	Return of some degree of superficial cutaneous pain and tactile sensibility within the autonomous area of the nerve
S3	Return of superficial cutaneous pain and tactile sensibility throughout the autonomous area with disappearance of any previous overreaction
S3+	Return of sensibility as in stage S3 with the addition that there is some recovery of two-point discrimination within the autonomous area
S4	Complete recovery

Source: Introduced by the Nerve Injuries Committee of the (British) Medical Research Council (MRC) 1954.

ulnar lesions showed any significant recovery in intrinsic motor function.

Recent reports on the results of nerve repair using microsurgical techniques demonstrate a slight improvement over the earlier series of nerve repairs that were done without magnification.[48,50,72] However, long-term follow-up of these patients will be needed before the degree of improvement provided by microneural techniques can be quantitated.

NEUROMAS

Following transection, peripheral nerves form neuromas at their cut ends. Fortunately, relatively few neuromas become symptomatic. The subsequent distortion in the injured nerve is the result of regenerating axons escaping a Schwann cell–endoneural barrier and of severe collagen proliferation. This proliferation produces a neuroma scar that contains myofibroblasts and fibroblasts.[2] Common clinical situations which lead to symptomatic neuromas are amputations, inadvertent transection of the radial sensory nerve during treatment of de Quervain disease, or excision of dorsal carpal ganglia. Reports also showed that the severity of the neuroma symptoms varies with personality types.[70]

Many surgical procedures have been proposed for treatment of painful neuroma.[13,18,21,60] The number of treatment methods suggests the lack of a universally successful method for this difficult clinical problem. Among the treatment methods proposed has been nerve capping,[60] fasciculectomy, epineural sleeves, or a combination of all these methods.[18] Interosseous transposition has been recommended. Transposition or translocation of the neuroma to a tension- and friction-free or vascularized bed has been proved most effective.[13,21]

The neuroma-in-continuity is a separate complicated problem which usually results from the incomplete transection of a nerve. Intraoperative electrophysiological assessment may be useful in the treatment.[25,67]

BRACHIAL PLEXUS INJURIES

The brachial plexus consists of the anterior rami of C5, C6, C7, C8, and T1 nerve roots (Fig. 40-2).[59] These nerve roots lie between the scalenus anterior and scalenus medius muscles beneath the floor of the posterior triangle of the neck. At the lateral border of the scalene muscles three trunks are formed. These trunks lie in the lower part of the posterior triangle of the neck. Each trunk divides into an anterior and a posterior

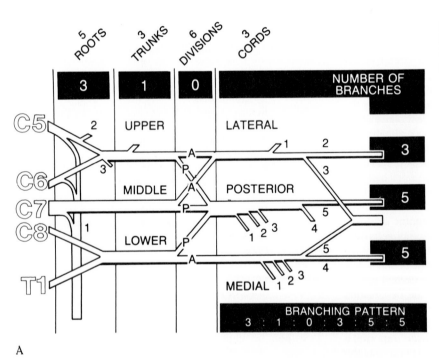

Figure 40-2 A. Brachial plexus starting from roots C5, C6, C7, C8, and T1. **B.** The branching pattern of brachial plexus nerves.

BRANCHING PATTERN

3	1	0	3	5	5
1 Long thoracic n. 2 Dorsal scapular n. 3 Subclavian n.	1 Suprascapular n.		1 Lateral pectoral n. 2 Musculocutaneous n. 3 Lateral head of Median n.	1 Upper subscapular n. 2 Thoracodorsal n. 3 Lower subscapular n. 4 Axillary n. 5 Radial n.	1 Medial pectoral n. 2 Medial cutaneous nerve of arm 3 Medial cutaneous nerve of forearm 4 Ulnar n. 5 Medial head of Median n.

B

division, supplying the flexor and extensor muscle groups respectively. As divisions enter the axilla, the cords are found. The anterior divisions of the upper and middle trunks form the lateral cord which lies lateral to the axillary artery. The anterior division of the lower trunk forms a medial cord which lies medial to the axillary artery. Posterior to the axillary artery is the posterior cord, which is formed from the union of all three posterior divisions.[59] Nerve branches from the brachial plexus are arranged according to the 3:1:0:3:5:5 rule (an extension of Last's 3:5:5 rule).[28] There are three branches from the roots, one from the upper trunk, none from the divisions, three from lateral cord, five from posterior cord, and five from medial cord. Three branches of the roots are the long thoracic nerve (C5, C6, and C7), the nerve to the subclavius muscle (C5, C6) and the dorsal scapular nerve (C5). The single branch from the trunk is the suprascapular nerve. Three branches from the lateral cord are the lateral pectoral nerve, the musculocutaneous nerve, and the lateral contribution of the median nerve. The medial cord gives off five branches including the medial cutaneous nerve of the arm, medial cutaneous nerve of the forearm, medial pectoral nerve, median nerve, and ulnar nerve. The posterior cord has five branches: the radial nerve, axillary nerve, thoracodorsal nerve, subscapular nerve, and lower subscapular nerve (Fig. 40-2B).[28]

A prefixed brachial plexus consists of contributions from the anterior rami of C4, C5, C6, C7, and C8. A postfixed brachial plexus contains contributions from C6, C7, C8, T1, and T2. Prefixation is more common than postfixation. Sympathetic fibers are distributed to each of the roots in the brachial plexus. The greatest number of postganglionic sympathetic fibers are contributed to the eighth cervical and first thoracic nerve roots. Forty to seventy percent of the postganglionic fibers in the brachial plexus are contained in the lower trunk.[59]

The fourth, fifth, sixth, and seventh cervical nerves are securely attached to a posterior bar of the transverse process as they leave the neural foramen. They maintain this position with the aid of the epineural sheath, by reflection of the prevertebral fascia, and through musculotendinous attachments to the transverse processes and vertebral artery. The eighth cervical and first thoracic nerves do not have these attachments as they leave their intervertebral foramina.[59] The absence of these features predisposes the eighth cervical and first thoracic nerves in lower trunk to injury. The eighth cervical and first thoracic spinal nerves unite behind the Sibson's fascia to form the lower trunk. The nerves thus have a direct relation with the neck of the first rib.[28,59]

Brachial plexus injuries are most commonly seen today following motorcycle accidents.[29] Direct traction on the plexus is caused by increasing the angle between the neck and the shoulder. Traction injuries are often characterized by widespread mixed lesions of the nerves and trunks. The fifth, sixth, and seventh nerve roots in the upper and middle trunks are more susceptible to lesions-in-continuity. The eighth cervical and first thoracic nerve roots are most vulnerable to avulsion injuries.[29]

Closed traction injuries may be divided into supraclavicular and infraclavicular lesions. Supraclavicular lesions have a less favorable prognosis then infraclavicular lesions. Preganglionic, or root avulsion, and postganglionic injuries are further subdivisions of supraclavicular injuries.

Evaluation of the patient with brachial plexus injury requires the taking of a careful history and detailed clinical examination. Initially it is difficult to determine the level of the injury and the potential for recovery. On clinical examination the distribution of the motor and sensory deficit must be carefully documented and followed at regular intervals. Preganglionic lesions are characterized by Horner syndrome (enophthalmos, miosis, and ptosis) and paralysis of the levatores, scapula, and rhomboids. Electromyographic studies and sensory nerve conduction studies are useful in delineating supraganglionic injuries. Cervical myelography can document nerve root avulsion at the level of the neural foramen. Normal axon reflexes, as manifested by the histamine flare response or cold vasodilatation test, are present in preganglionic injuries. The sensory parent cell in the dorsal root ganglion is left intact, allowing for these changes in preganglionic injuries. Somatosensory evoked potentials[27] from the cervical spine and the sensory cortex response to stimulation of peripheral nerves are being used to evaluate traction injuries of the brachial plexus.[27]

The management of brachial plexus injuries has changed somewhat with the evolution of microsurgery. Poor results in the 1950s and 1960s caused many investigators to wonder whether exploration of the plexus was worthwhile. Some patients had spontaneous recovery, making surgery unnecessary; others had clinical findings indicating such severe damage that prognosis was poor. Today, there are several centers with microsurgical teams operating on brachial plexus injuries.[6,9,32,38,39,40]

In situations of closed injury, there is no indication for immediate surgery. First-degree and second-degree lesions can undergo spontaneous recovery many months after the original injury. Examination of the patient at frequent intervals enables evaluation of the status of the lesions. Where there is no improvement or where there is evidence of nerve root avulsion, the timing of exploration ranges from as early as possible to 4 months.[32,38,39] Several different techniques are available for repair of the plexus. Neurolysis is advocated by some for lesions-in-continuity. Neurorrhaphy is possible in rare cases of clean transection. Nerve grafting is necessary in most cases.

Neurotization of peripheral nerves in brachial plexus avulsion injuries has been performed using the intercostal nerves,[6] the anterior nerves of the cervical plexus,[49] and the spinal accessory nerve.[40] In neurotization the donor nerves must supply a comparable number of motor or sensory fibers to achieve acceptable reinnervation of the receptor nerve. Evaluation by fiber counts of the donor nerve in comparison with fiber counts of the roots of brachial plexus and peripheral nerves reveals a gross mismatch in fiber counts. One intercostal nerve contains approximately 12,000 fibers as compared to an estimated 14,000 to 41,000 fibers in the C8 root or 16,000 nerve fibers in the ulnar nerve. The results of brachial plexus reconstructive surgery reveal that the results of nerve transfers are disappointing when complex functions such as shoulder abduction or finger motion need to be restored. There is no series of brachial plexus reconstructions in which patients regained good hand control.

Obstetrical Palsies of the Brachial Plexus

Obstetrical brachial plexus paralysis is often associated with traumatic deliveries. Brachial plexus birth palsies occur at a rate of 0.4 to 2.5/per 1000 live births.[5] The upper roots of the brachial plexus are usually injured during delivery when shoulder dystocia necessitates excessive lateral flexion in order to free the shoulder from the public arch. During breech deliveries the upper roots are also more commonly affected. Obstetrical paralysis is more common in multiparous rather than primiparous mothers. Improved obstetrical technique has decreased, but not eliminated, the incidence of plexus palsies.[5]

The majority of patients show a predominance of upper root C5 and C6 damage, which is a classic Erb-Duchenne palsy. Clinically there is loss of shoulder abduction and external rotation, loss of elbow flexion, and loss of forearm supination. The upper extremity assumes a "porter's tip" position. There is sensory loss in the C5 dermatome along the shoulder. The next most frequent type of injury is a complete lesion in which there is some damage to the entire brachial plexus. Klumpke's paralysis involves the C8 and T1 roots and clinically results in poor hand function with a good shoulder. Klumpke's paralysis is often associated with Horner syndrome.[29]

Diagnosis of brachial plexus injuries is suspected in a newborn when there is absence of active upper extremity motion but retention of full passive motion. The differential diagnosis of brachial plexus palsy includes fractures of the proximal humeral epiphysis or clavicle, osteomyelitis, congenital dislocation, or arthrogryposis. Frequent examination is necessary to confirm the diagnosis. X-ray views should be taken of the cervical spine, upper extremities, and diaphragm. Electromyography is not well tolerated but can be an important prognostic tool. Electromyography can provide evidence of reinnervation at least a month in advance of the clinical examination.[29]

The extent and rate of recovery following obstetrical and brachial plexus palsy is difficult to determine. More recent studies relate good to excellent recovery in the majority of cases.[20,61] This contrasts sharply with earlier reports by Adler and Patterson,[1] who found full recovery in only 7 percent and Wickstrom,[65] who found full recovery in only 13.4 percent. Two poor prognostic signs are lower paralysis and total paralysis. The persistence of pupillary signs is also a very negative sign.

The length of time during which spontaneous recovery will occur affects the decision for surgical intervention. Spontaneous recovery may occur until 18 to 24 months of age. Several authors feel that if recovery is going to occur, it will happen prior to 6 months. Taylor in 1920 stated that if complete recovery were to occur, it would do so by 3 months of age.[62] Anatomic motor and sensory reinnervation does not necessarily ensure functional recovery. Infants with brachial plexus birth palsy may have good "clinical recovery" but refuse to use the arm. On the other hand, a study by Tada, Tsyuguchi, and Kawai[61] documents useful sensory recovery in 70.4 percent and useful motor recovery in 33.3 percent of patients with documented nerve root avulsions. This is related to the plasticity of the nervous system in the newborn infant and possible collateral sprouting from intact neurons.

The major complication of unresolved brachial plexus palsies is the development of contractures. Range-of-motion exercises are advocated to completely prevent or to diminish the severity of such contractures. No association has been demonstrated between physical therapy and recovery of motor function.

Splinting for shoulder abduction is not recommended.[1] Functional bracing has been effective in some children.[43]

Surgical treatment of unresolved brachial plexus palsy involves releases, tendon transfers, and osteotomies.

= SECTION B =

Nerve Entrapment Syndromes in the Upper Extremity

Michael P. Coyle, Jr.

Nerve entrapment lesions are a major cause of peripheral neuropathy. Although they may involve any nerve at any level, these lesions are usually found at predictable locations and share common elements of pathogenesis and neural pathophysiology.

PATHOGENESIS OF PERIPHERAL NERVE ENTRAPMENT

The pathogenesis of peripheral nerve entrapment is multifaceted:[33]

1. *Anatomic.* Normal anatomic structures (transverse carpal ligament, pronator teres, supinator arcade of Frohse) may thicken, hypertrophy, or fibrose.
2. *Postural.* Constant repetitive motions or positioning of an extremity at its extremes of motion are found in many occupations, recreations, and sporting hobbies.
3. *Developmental.* Anomalous or aberrant muscle bellies and fibrous bands.
4. *Inflammatory.* Synovitis and tenosynovitis may limit the available space in a tight compartment.
5. *Metabolic and endocrine.* Pregnancy and the premenstrual phase cause bodily fluid retention. Diabetes mellitus, hypothyroidism, acromegaly, gout, and pseudogout may also be associated with entrapment neuropathies.
6. *Tumors.* Any mass lesion (ganglion, lipoma) may compress a peripheral nerve.

7. *Trauma.* A nerve may be entrapped within a fracture, such as the radial nerve in an oblique fracture of the distal one-third of the humerus or within an acute compartment syndrome. Delayed entrapment may result from trauma having occurred years previously, such as ulnar nerve palsy following a supracondylar fracture of the elbow.

8. *Iatrogenic.* Injections into the nerve, retraction on a nerve during surgical procedures, and faulty positioning of an anesthetized patient may all produce a nerve compression lesion.

NEUROPATHOPHYSIOLOGICAL PROCESSES

Peripheral nerves are mixed motor and sensory nerves, each consisting of varying proportions of large heavily myelinated, small thinly myelinated, and very small unmyelinated axons. Large myelinated axons innervate the extrafusal muscle fibers and carry the sensory input of light touch, two-point discrimination, position, and vibratory sensation. Thinly myelinated and unmyelinated axons carry the small intrafusal muscle spindle fibers and the epicritic sensation of sharp pain and temperature.

Mechanical deformation and ischemia are the causes of nerve damage seen in entrapment syndromes.[55] Mechanical deformation of a nerve may be produced by compression, friction, traction, and angulation, and each nerve fiber type demonstrates differing susceptibility to the effects of these factors. Sensory fibers are more susceptible to stretch injury, whereas motor fibers are more susceptible to both pressure and ischemia. Both direct pressure and ischemia affect the larger nerve fibers before smaller ones, and the superficial fibers before the deeper ones. Nerves composed of large funiculi with scanty perineurium are more susceptible to compression and stretch injury than those with multiple small funiculi surrounded by abundant perineurium.

When a nerve is stretched, its microcirculation begins to diminish at 8 percent elongation.[55] Axons begin to disrupt at approximately 15 percent elongation. Friction produces a mechanical irritation leading to a fibrosis of the nerve and localized restrictive adhesions which interfere with its physiological excursion in the extremity.

Proximal entrapment of a nerve may render it more susceptible to the effects of a more distal entrapment (double-crush phenomenon).[57] This may be due to a diminished axoplasmic flow distally caused by the proximal lesion.

Ischemia will impair nerve function and produce a localized segmental conduction block by disrupting the intraneural circulation. Experimentally applied pressures to the surface of a nerve demonstrate that 30 mmHg pressure begins to impair intraneural venous flow, 50 mmHg diminishes intrafascicular arterial flow, and 60 to 80 mmHg stops endoneural capillary flow.[49] Entrapped nerves are more sensitive to the effects of ischemia. Sensory fibers tend to fail before motor fibers in pure ischemia.

Mechanical compression produces actual structural changes within the nerve fibers as a result of the applied pressure and shear forces.[41] An acute compression lesion causes an intussusception of one internodal segment of both the axon and its attached myelin into the adjacent internodal segment, producing a pinching-off effect on nerve function. Chronic pressure, however, produces a differential shearing effect on the multiple lamellae of myelin, squeezing the myelin away from the area of compression and forming a bulbous myelin lesion (tadpole configuration) with a segmental tapering of the internodal segments. Varying degrees of segmental demyelinization of the nerve occur in the area of entrapment.

The degree of nerve damage is more related to the severity of the compression than to its duration.[55] Permanent nerve damage can occur within a relatively short time span. Mild compression may cause only a minimal demyelinization, such as a widening of the nodal areas with a resultant slowing of the nerve conduction velocity across that segment. Chronic severe pressure will produce complete intranodal segmental demyelinization with a complete nerve conduction block.

Most nerve entrapment lesions may be either a neuropraxia or an axonotmesis, or more likely a combination of the two,[14] with different fibers damaged to varying degrees. Consequently some elements of the lesion will show relatively rapid recovery, and others will be delayed.

Current evidence favors the mechanical factors as the critical causative agents in chronic nerve entrapment neuropathy.[14] Histological specimens of chronic nerve entrapment lesions in both animals and humans have demonstrated myelin abnormalities in the entire region of nerve entrapment with bulbous myelin thickness irregularities in a tadpole configuration within the area of entrapment, as well as severe localized demyelination. Chronic low-pressure compression and friction appear to be the dominant mechanical factors in producing these lesions.

MEDIAN NERVE INVOLVEMENT

Although the median nerve may be entrapped at any point along its peripheral course, three distinct entrapment neuropathies have been emphasized: carpal tunnel syndrome, pronator teres syndrome, and anterior interosseous syndrome. In spite of the many differentiating points on clinical presentation and examination, the similarities they possess in common often confuse the physician.

Carpal Tunnel Syndrome (CTS)

Compression of the median nerve at the wrist in the carpal tunnel is the most common entrapment neuropathy in the upper extremity. The carpal canal is an open-ended, but rigid, compartment whose floor and walls are the bony carpus and whose roof is a thick rigid flexor retinaculum or transverse carpal ligament which attaches radially to the tubercle of the scaphoid and the ridge of the trapezium and ulnarly to the hook of the hamate and the pisiform. The volar carpal ligament, a less substantial, but still constricting structure, forms the most proximal portion of the roof of the carpal canal. The flexor pollicis longus, the flexor digitorum superficialis, and flexor digitorum profundus tendons accompany the median nerve in its passage through the carpal canal. The median nerve lies directly beneath the transverse carpal ligament with the flexor tendons deep to it. The flexor tendons are encased by the synovium of the radial and ulnar bursae.

Causes of CTS

Even though the carpal canal is open-ended, physical forces applied within the rigid confines of the canal will mechanically deform the nerve and interfere with its local blood supply (Fig. 40-3). Strong flexion and extension of the wrist and fingers forces the nerve against the transverse carpal ligament. With flexion and extension of the wrist and fingers, there is a normal excursion of the median nerve of approximately 20-mm, permitting friction against both the tendons and transverse carpal ligament.[55] A significant reduction in cross-sectional area of the carpal canal as evaluated by CT scan has been reported in patients with carpal tunnel syndrome.[15] Wick catheter studies have documented significantly increased pressures within the carpal canal (32 mmHg compared with normal values of 2.5 mmHg) in carpal tunnel syndrome, with further significant increases by wrist positional changes to the extremes of flexion and extension.[20]

Any factor which decreases the space available within the carpal canal will cause pressure against the median nerve.[14,33,55] Far and away the most common cause is a nonspecific tenosynovitis of the flexor tendons. Trauma, such as Colles' fracture and fracture dislocations of the carpal bones and carpometacarpal joints may alter the carpal canal itself or cause posttraumatic scarring and fibrosis. Inflammatory conditions, such as rheumatoid arthritis, gout, pseudogout, amyloidosis, and granulomatous infections can also induce a proliferative tenosynovitis. Tumors such as ganglions, lipomas, or hemangiomas and tumors of the median nerve itself (neurilemmomas, lipofibromas, hamartomas) can encroach

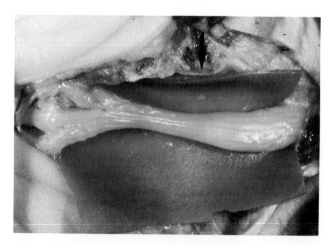

Figure 40-3 Median nerve in the carpal tunnel. Cut transverse carpal ligament is seen below the arrow. A piece of sterile rubber is behind median nerve. Note the motor branch distally, extreme narrowing of median nerve just proximal to the branching, and the large pseudoneuroma proximal to the constriction.

upon the carpal canal. Systemic conditions such as acromegaly, hypothyroidism, pregnancy, the postmenopausal state, diabetes mellitus, and lupus erythematosus and the use of the contraceptive pill affect the nerve presumably by increasing extracellular fluid retention and causing soft tissue swelling. Developmental conditions, such as a persistent median artery, distally lying superficialis muscle belly, hypertrophied lumbrical, and anomalous muscles (palmaris profundus) may also encroach upon the carpal tunnel.

Differential Diagnosis

A significant number of other medical conditions may mimic carpal tunnel syndrome and produce the common symptoms of numbness and tingling in one or both hands.[14,46,55] It is precisely because CTS is so common and has such a broad spectrum of clinical symptoms and findings that these other diagnoses must be kept in mind. Differential diagnosis must look at cervical radiculopathy, particularly the sixth cervical root, stenosis, central nervous system lesions (minor stroke, transient ischemic attack, atypical migraine), lesions of the spinal cord (tumor, syringomyelia, multiple sclerosis), Raynaud's phenomenon, reflex sympathetic dystrophy, peripheral neuropathy (toxic, alcoholic, uremic, diabetes, Déjerine-Sottas), and collagen vascular disorders (periarteritis nodosa, lupus erythematosus, rheumatoid arthritis). Other sites of peripheral entrapment must be considered (pronator syndrome, anterior interosseous syndrome).

Clinical Diagnosis

CTS is chiefly a condition of the middle-aged (40 to 65 years) although it has been reported in early childhood and may be seen in the elderly. Women are much more frequently affected than men (between 3 and 5 to 1).[46]

Pain and numbness are the most frequent complaints. The classic, burning nocturnal pain usually awakens the patient 2 to 4 h after retiring and is relieved by vigorously shaking the hand, exercising the wrist and fingers or hanging the arm in a dependent position. Vague complaints such as swelling of the fingers upon arising or the patient's description that the fingers feel like pieces of wood are not uncommon. Activities such as driving a car, reading a book or newspaper, knitting, or doing needlepoint as well as more vigorous physical activities may precipitate symptoms. Pain may radiate to the forearm or even to the shoulder.[8]

Classically, patients complain of numbness in the thumb, index and middle fingers and in the radial half of the ring finger. In early or mild cases, numbness may be noted only at the tip of the middle and/or index fingers. Patients may complain that their entire hand feels numb, although clinical examination shows the ulnar digits to have normal sensation. The complaint of clumsiness may be due to the loss of tactile sensation, thenar muscle weakness, or a combination of the two.[33]

Most of the nerve fibers of the median nerve within the carpal canal are sensory,[55] explaining the predominance of sensory symptoms and findings. Sensory findings range from a minimal hypesthesia to complete anesthesia of the median nerve–innervated field of the hand, which includes the thumb, index, middle, and radial half of ring fingers and the distal half of the radial palm. The most proximal portion of the palm, particularly at the base of the thenar eminence, is innervated by the palmar cutaneous branch of the median nerve, which has its origin proximal to the carpal canal. Light touch, two-point discrimination, and vibratory testing are more sensitive indicators of sensory disturbances than pin touch. The sensory comparison should be made with the tip of the ipsilateral little finger, as well as with the same digits in the opposite hand. Bilateral carpal tunnel syndrome is not infrequent.

Muscle atrophy is a late finding in CTS. Abductor pollicis brevis is usually the first muscle involved. Loss of thenar muscle tone and strength are easily assessed by examination.

Nerve entrapment and irritability may be demonstrated by a positive Tinel's sign just proximal to the carpal tunnel,[46] Phalen's wrist palmar flexion test, a reverse Phalen's test (wrist dorsiflexion), tourniquet compression test, and a direct median nerve compression test performed by placing the examiner's thumb directly over the median nerve at the proximal end of the carpal tunnel. The time interval required to reproduce paresthesias or hypesthesia is an indicator of the severity of nerve entrapment.

In the majority of cases, the diagnosis of CTS can be made with confidence on the basis of a careful clinical history and physical examination. In those cases where the clinical diagnosis is unclear or where there is a need to exclude coexisting conditions or a double-crush syndrome or to evaluate the clinical course of patients treated conservatively, electrophysiological studies should be considered. Prolongation of the distal median nerve sensory conduction is the most sensitive criteria for establishing an electrophysiological diagnosis of CTS. Although figures may vary slightly, in general, prolongation of sensory conduction beyond 3.5 ms and distal motor latency beyond 4.0 ms will confirm the diagnosis. Current electrodiagnostic accuracy in CTS is approximately 85 to 90 percent, with a 10 to 15 percent false-negative rate. However, this depends greatly upon the sophistication and technical ability of the electromyographer. Intact conduction in a small percentage of axons will give normal conduction velocities for the whole nerve. A normal study, therefore, does not rule out the clinical diagnosis. These studies are often of greatest value in localizing the site of nerve entrapment.

Treatment of CTS

Patients with mild intermittent, sensory symptoms without any evidence of neurological deficit may be treated with conservative measures. Such measures would include the use of neutral wrist splints at night, nonsteroidal anti-inflammatory agents, intermittent diuretics, and vitamin B6 (pyridoxine) in pharmacological doses. Neurotoxicity has been reported with massive doses of pyridoxine.

Local injection of corticosteroid into the carpal canal has given a high percentage (75 to 81 percent) of short-term relief of symptoms but has provided full relief of symptoms over a 1-year duration in a much smaller percentage of patients (11–22 percent).[21] Interestingly, those patients obtaining short-term relief following corticosteroid injection had a much bet-

ter response to surgical decompression than those who did not.

Those patients with progressing persistent symptoms and particularly those with objective neurological deficits (marked sensory loss and thenar weakness or atrophy) or significant functional impairment of the hand, are candidates for surgical decompression of the carpal tunnel. A complete release of the transverse carpal ligament should be carried out on its ulnar aspect as well as a release of the volar carpal ligament more proximally (Fig. 40-1). Variations in the takeoff of the motor branch to the thenar muscles, as well as anomalies of the median nerve, such as bifid nerve, must be kept in mind. A thickened, scarred epineurium may be a source of focal nerve compression, and consideration should be given to an epineurotomy of the nerve.[12,14,17] Excessive proliferation of the tenosynovium surrounding the flexor tendons may require a localized tenosynovectomy.[14,17]

Acute CTS, associated with trauma, is a special problem.[14] An acute compartmentlike syndrome involving the median nerve in the carpal tunnel may follow severe fractures of the wrist, dislocation of the carpus, burns, and hemorrhage. Immediate closed reduction of any fracture and/or dislocation should be performed with the wrist positioned as close to neutral as stability will allow. For severely comminuted or unstable fractures, pins and plaster or the use of an external fixator may be preferred. Increasing pain (particularly if dysesthetic in nature), worsening of carpal tunnel symptoms, or progression of the neurological deficits are all indications for immediate surgical release of the carpal tunnel. A delayed surgical release in the presence of a significant compression of the median nerve can result in a permanent loss of median nerve function.

Results of the surgical release of the carpal tunnel reflect the degree of preoperative neurological damage.[12,45] In most cases, the nocturnal pain that awakens the patient is immediately relieved. Those patients with intermittent or mild persistent symptoms obtain an immediate relief. Those with moderate sensory deficits will usually obtain normal return of sensation, but over a longer period. Lastly, those with long-standing, severe sensory loss associated with pain and with muscular atrophy, will obtain relief of pain with less than full sensory recovery. The return of thenar muscle function is similar to that of sensation.

Complications Associated with Surgery

Complications from surgical release of CTS may be more common than currently realized. A recent review has found an incidence of complications of 12 percent.[36] Complications reported include reflex sympathetic dystrophy, tender hypertrophic surgical scar, damage to the palmar cutaneous branches of both the median and ulnar nerves with resulting neuromas in the proximal palm, postsurgical tenosynovitis, and flexor tendon adhesions, and bowstringing of the flexor tendons out of the carpal canal. Inadequate release of the transverse carpal ligament has frequently been reported, but this represents not a complication but rather an inadequate surgical operation.[30] The use of a volar splint to hold the wrist in neutral or slight dorsiflexion has been advocated to prevent bowstringing and scarring of the flexor tendons as well as to provide constant pressure against the wound to inhibit reflex sympathetic dystrophy and encourage early finger motion.

Pronator Teres Syndrome

Entrapment of the median nerve in the proximal forearm has been loosely termed *pronator syndrome*.[50] There are three general areas of possible entrapment, the lacertus fibrosus, the pronator teres muscle, and the fibrous arcade of the flexor digitorum superficialis muscle. It is probably appropriate to also include entrapment underneath the ligament of Struthers, which originates from a supercondylar bony process on the anteromedial aspect of the distal humerus in approximately 1.5 percent of the population.

Causes of Pronator Teres Syndrome

Fracture and fracture dislocations about the elbow, anterior dislocation of the radial head, proximal forearm fractures, and acute intercompartmental hemorrhage within the forearm may all compress the median nerve. More commonly, repetitive minor trauma or repetitive use of the elbow and forearm lead to the development of symptoms. A tight or scarred lacertus fibrosus, tendinous bands within the pronator teres muscle, abnormalities in the presence or origin of the heads of the pronator teres muscle, a tight fibrous arch at the proximal level of the flexor digitorum superficialis, and hypertrophy of the pronator teres and other volar forearm muscles have all been reported as causative factors.[27]

Differential Diagnosis

The major differential point is distinguishing pronator syndrome from carpal tunnel syndrome. A double crush may exist with the median nerve compressed at both the proximal forearm and wrist levels. Other problems to be differentiated include cervical radiculopathy (especially C6 or C7 root compression), thoracic outlet syndrome, muscle strains of the flexor pronator mass, and musculoskeletal overuse syndromes of the forearm and elbow.

Clinical Diagnosis

An aching pain, fatigue, or tiredness in the proximal forearm is the most frequent subjective complaint.[14,24,55] Heavy or repetitive use of the arm causes an increase in symptoms. Repetitive elbow and forearm motions—such as occur in hammering or playing tennis or in using a screwdriver, wrench, or pliers—are likely to aggravate symptoms. Pain radiation down the forearm and up into the upper arm is common. The patient may complain of clumsiness and weakness in the use of the arm and often has great difficulty in describing and localizing those symptoms because the nerve entrapment is minimal and often intermittent. Paresthesias may occur with more severe degrees of entrapment, but persistent numbness

in the median nerve distribution is not a common finding. In contrast to carpal tunnel syndrome, nocturnal paresthesias are rare and wrist position does not exacerbate symptoms.[24]

Local tenderness to deep pressure is found over the site of nerve entrapment. Such pressure will reproduce the patient's pain and complaints and may also produce radiating paresthesias proximally and distally down to the wrist and digits. Tinel's sign may be present over the site of entrapment. Measurable weakness is usually not found on isolated muscle examination, and thenar atrophy is uncommon.

Muscle stressing tests have been described to help localize the area of compression and entrapment.[52] Pain and/or paresthesias evoked by the resisted pronation of the forearm with the elbow extended implicates the pronator teres, simultaneous resisted flexion of the elbow and supination of the forearm implicates the lacertus fibrosus, while symptoms evoked by the resisted flexion of the proximal interphalangeal joint of the middle finger implicates the arch of the flexor digitorum superficialis muscle belly.

Electrophysiological studies are frequently of little help.[24] Since the entrapment is often intermittent, the nerve conduction studies will usually not demonstrate a conduction delay in the forearm. Electromyographic studies may show some evidence of median nerve–innervated muscle denervation. These electrophysiological studies are usually more helpful in excluding other mimicking conditions in the differential diagnosis, particularly carpal tunnel syndrome.

Treatment of Pronator Teres Syndrome

Since the majority of pronator syndromes are intermittent and mild, conservative treatment should be utilized initially.[14,24,52,55] Avoidance of activities which necessitate repetitive flexing of the elbow and supination and pronation of the forearm is important. Changes in work habits and the way one functionally uses the extremity may provide lasting relief. The use of nonsteroidal anti-inflammatory drugs, as well as splintage of the upper extremity with the elbow and wrist gently flexed and the forearm pronated, may be of benefit. Conservative treatment and observation for 3 months is reasonable.

Persistent or progressive symptoms suggest the need for surgical exploration and neurolysis of the median nerve. Wide exposure of the proximal forearm is needed so that each of the possible offending structures can be identified and released, and the median nerve neurolysed throughout this area. If preoperative x-ray or local physical findings suggest a supracondylar process, the incision and exploration must be carried above the elbow to release the ligament of Struthers. The median nerve is identified just medial to the biceps tendon, and in sequence the lacertus fibrosus, any constricting portion of the pronator teres muscle, or fibrous bands within that muscle; finally the arch of the flexor digitorum superficialis muscle belly are released so that the median nerve has free passage through the proximal forearm (Fig. 40-4). Rarely is it necessary to completely transsect the pronator teres or to anteriorly transpose the median nerve volar to the pronator teres.

The majority of patients show improvement in symptoms following surgery.[14,24,52,55] Results of treatment obviously are dependent upon the degree of preexisting nerve damage and proper diagnosis.

Anterior Interosseous Syndrome

The anterior interosseous nerve arises from the dorsoradial aspect of the median nerve 5 to 8 cm distal to the lateral epicondyle, usually at the upper margin or just below the su-

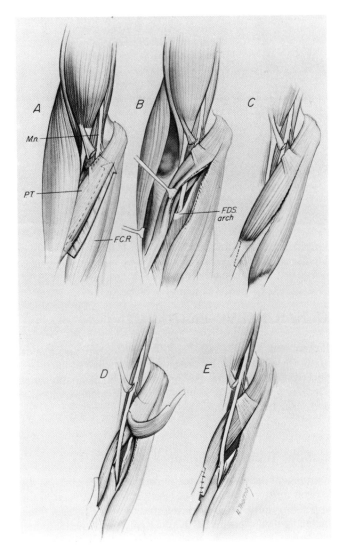

Figure 40-4 Pronator teres syndrome and repair. Mn (median nerve), PT (pronator teres), FCR (flexor carpi radialis), FDS arch (flexor digitorum superficialis arch). **A.** Note that the median nerve is found initially just medial to the biceps tendon; the lacertus fibrosus is cut and the interval between the pronator teres and flexor carpi radialis is opened. (Arrow shows direction of exposure.) **B.** The open interval between the pronator teres and flexor carpi radialis; the FDS arch is also exposed. **C.** Z-plasty of the anterior head of the pronator teres. **D.** Anterior head of the pronator teres taken off the median nerve. **E.** If needed, the anterior head of the pronator teres is placed behind the median nerve and the FDS arch is left open. (*From Spinner, M.: Injuries to the Major Branches of the Peripheral Nerves of the Forearm. Philadelphia, Saunders, 1978. Reproduced with permission.*)

perficial head of the pronator teres (Fig. 40-5). Although described as a purely motor nerve innervating the flexor pollicis longus, the flexor digitorum profundus to index and middle fingers, and the pronator quadratus, it does carry afferent sensory fibers from the deep capsular ligamentous structures of the wrist and distal radioulnar joints. Compression of this nerve produces a distinct entrapment syndrome.[28,55]

Causes of Anterior Interosseous Syndrome

Specific injuries such as fractures, deep lacerations, gunshot wounds, open reduction of forearm fractures, hemorrhage after venous cutdowns, attempted arterial punctures, and drug injections by addicts have all been implicated as causes of paralysis.[52,55] Anatomic variations such as tendinous bands within the deep head of the pronator teres or flexor digitorum superficialis or accessory muscles and tendons, vascular lesions (thrombosis of ulnar collateral vessels), and aberrant arteries have also been implicated.[52] Onset of paresis has been correlated with occupations requiring repetitive elbow flexion and forearm pronation. The effects of prolonged external pressure, such as might be sustained by an arm constantly draped over the side railing of a bed, or encased in a tight cast, or frequently leaning over a beam, have also been reported. Usually a preexisting anatomical variation must be present to provide a focus of entrapment.

Differential Diagnosis

An atypical presentation of the anterior interosseous syndrome may occur presenting isolated paralysis or paresis of either flexor pollicis longus or flexor digitorum profundus to index.[26] A brachial plexus neuritis can present an identical clinical picture, but there is usually coexisting involvement of muscles of the shoulder girdle.[43] Attritional rupture of flexor pollicis longus (Mannerfelt syndrome) at the scaphoid tubercle, chronic stenosing tenosynovitis with locking of the thumb in extension, and a partial laceration of the proximal median nerve must all be considered. The presence of a Martin-Gruber communication (said to occur in approximately 15 percent of forearms), bringing median nerve fibers over to the ulnar nerve distally, can further confuse the picture. Half of these Martin-Gruber communications have been reported to arise from the anterior interosseous nerve.[52] These fibers have been shown to innervate the ulnar intrinsic muscles of the hand, and so the anterior interosseous syndrome picture may be compounded with that of a partial ulnar palsy of the intrinsics of the hand.

Clinical Diagnosis

Spontaneous, vague proximal forearm pain is the most common presenting symptom. Often the symptom lasts for a short period and then resolves, leaving the patient with a loss of strength and dexterity in the radial digits and a weakness of pinch.[52]

Fine tip-to-tip pinch is impossible due to the inability to flex the distal joints of the thumb and index finger.[53] The patient is capable only of a weak pulp-to-pulp pinch between

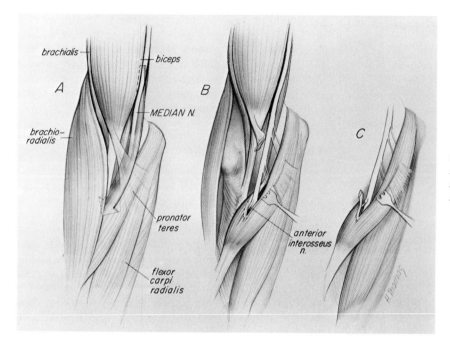

Figure 40-5 Anterior interosseous syndrome and repair. Exposure of the anterior interosseous nerve. **A.** Arrow shows direction of exposure starting over the median nerve medial to the biceps tendon. **B.** Lacertus fibrosus is released, exposing the median nerve and its branches. Pronator teres is cut, exposing the anterior interosseous nerve. **C.** A portion of the pronator teres is left cut. (*From Spinner, M.: Injuries to the Major Branches of the Peripheral Nerves of the Forearm. Philadelphia, Saunders, 1978. Reproduced with permission.*)

the thumb and index finger. No sensory deficit is present. Weak-to-absent flexion against resistance is found with the flexor pollicis longus and flexor digitorum profundus to index and less commonly to middle finger. Pronator quadratus weakness may be elicited by testing for forearm pronation with the elbow flexed.

Direct pressure over the nerve produces deep pain and tenderness, but Tinel's sign is usually negative.

Electrophysiological studies are not usually helpful unless electromyographic findings of denervation are present in the affected muscles. Increased distal motor latency from the elbow to pronator quadratus has been reported.

Treatment of Anterior Interosseous Syndrome

In the absence of a penetrating wound or an acute compartment syndrome, initial conservative treatment is advocated for recent syndrome onset.[52] The usual modalities of avoiding aggravating forearm motions, nonsteroidal anti-inflammatory medication, and the occasional use of forearm splintage has been advocated. A trial of conservative treatment for a period of at least 8 to 12 weeks is advocated by most authors. If there is no improvement or if symptoms persist, surgical exploration is a reasonable alternative. Although spontaneous recovery after 18 months' observation has been reported, most surgical series show a more rapid return of nerve function following exploration than after prolonged conservative therapy.[26,52,55]

The most common compressing structure has been the tendinous origin of the deep head of the pronator teres which crosses the anterior interosseous nerve at its hilum from the median nerve.[52]

Results of surgery, again, are related to the degree of nerve damage present. Most surgical series have reported good recovery of nerve function. Motor recovery may be prolonged (6 to 9 months). Persistence of symptoms or failure of functional motor recovery may be due to incorrect diagnosis.

ULNAR NERVE ENTRAPMENT

Entrapment of the ulnar nerve occurs at two major sites, about the elbow and the wrist, with entrapment at the elbow approximately 10 times more common than at the wrist. Ulnar nerve entrapment includes cubital tunnel syndrome and ulnar tunnel syndrome.

Cubital Tunnel Syndrome

Entrapment neuropathy of the ulnar nerve at the elbow is the second most common site of nerve entrapment seen in the upper extremity. It has been referred to under various titles, including ulnar neuritis, tardy ulnar palsy, and cubital tunnel syndrome.

Causes of Cubital Tunnel Syndrome

Anatomic features have a major causative role. The ulnar nerve passes from the anterior compartment of the brachium into the posterior compartment passing over the medial intermuscular septa and may course beneath the thick fibrous arcade of Struthers. This bridge of fibrous tissue between the medial intermuscular septum and medial head of the triceps may be present in up to 70 percent of upper extremities. Individual triceps muscle fibers may also course over the ulnar nerve at this point. This arcade is located approximately 8 cm above the medial epicondyle. The nerve then travels distally to lie behind the medial epicondyle in the postcondylar groove, where it enters the cubital tunnel, whose roof is formed by the triangular arcuate ligament which extends from the medial epicondyle to the medial border of the olecranon and serves as the common tendinous origin of both the humeral and ulnar heads of the flexor carpi ulnaris muscle.

The ulnar nerve has a normal excursion of approximately 12 mm at the elbow. The ulnar nerve also elongates approximately 4.7 mm during elbow flexion, and the medial head of the triceps can push the nerve 7 mm medially, adding traction.[1] As the elbow flexes, the arcuate ligament must stretch, and at 90 degrees of elbow flexion, the proximal edge of the ligament becomes taut. At the same time, the medial collateral ligament, which forms one of the borders of the cubital tunnel, tends to relax and bulge inward. These physical changes obviously compress the cubital tunnel and place stretch on the nerve. Cadaver studies on the cubital tunnel have demonstrated increased compartment pressures from 7 mmHg in elbow extension up to 24 mmHg at 90 degrees of flexion.[44]

Recurrent subluxation or dislocation of the ulnar nerve out of its postcondylar groove, potentially generating friction on the nerve and exposing it to repetitive minor trauma, has been demonstrated in 16.2 percent of an asymptomatic population.[9] A direct blow may obviously injure the nerve. Late sequelae from previous trauma may produce cubitus valgus deformity or irregularities of the postcondylar groove.

Arthritis of the elbow joint may produce a proliferative compressing synovitis and bony osteophytes. Multiple loose bodies and synovial chondromatosis may produce similar results. Tumor masses—such as ganglion, perineural cyst, lipoma—and anomalous muscles (anconeus epitrochlearis) may rarely encroach upon the nerve.[52]

Differential Diagnosis

Although the elbow is the most common site, entrapment may also occur more proximally (arcade of Struthers) as well as distally within the forearm (hypertrophied flexor carpi ulnaris and anomalous fibrous bands).[14,33,52,55] Entrapment at the wrist and hand level will be discussed later. Other conditions to be excluded are cervical radiculopathy (C8 to T1 involvement), thoracic outlet syndrome, spinal cord pathology (syringomyelia, tumor), cervical spondylosis, superior sulcus tumor (Pancoast tumor), amyotrophic lateral sclerosis, and localized peripheral neuropathy (Déjerine-Sottas interstitial neuritis, leprosy).

Clinical Diagnosis

Initial symptoms are usually a vague, dull, aching discomfort about the medial elbow and proximal forearm, accompanied by intermittent paresthesias down the medial forearm into the ulnar border of the hand. A popping or clicking sensation may be noted about the medial epicondyle, and prolonged flexion of the elbow exacerbates symptoms of pain, paresthesias, and numbness. Within the ulnar nerve at the elbow level, the sensory fibers to the ring and little finger lie superficial, and so they are more vulnerable than the deeper-lying motor branches. This helps explain the predominance of sensory symptoms in early entrapment. Awkwardness with fine hand movement, weakness of grasp and pinch, and loss of dexterity are later complaints of motor involvement. Patients may be awakened by severe nocturnal lancinating pain involving the elbow, medial forearm, and ulnar border of the hand, and they obtain relief not by shaking the hand but by extending the elbow. This complaint may obviously be confused with carpal tunnel syndrome, but careful questioning should distinguish the two.

Sensory examination will show hypesthesia over the ulnar aspect of both the palm and dorsum of the hand as well as the entire little finger and the ulnar half of the ring finger. Because of anomalous innervation, as many as 20 percent of patients have ulnar nerve sensation over the entire ring finger and ulnar half of middle finger. The medial forearm should have normal sensation as it is innervated by the medial cutaneous nerve of the forearm derived directly from the brachial plexus. Hypesthesia of the medial forearm implicates a much more proximal lesion.

Tinel's sign is usually present over the ulnar nerve behind the medial epicondyle or over the cubital tunnel. Dynamic flexing of the patient's elbow with the examiner's thumb behind the medial epicondyle may sublux or dislocate the ulnar nerve out of its postcondylar groove and reproduce the patient's symptoms. Likewise, extreme flexion of the elbow maintained for several minutes may reproduce the pain, paresthesias, and dysesthesia. Motor examination may reveal weakness of grasp and pinch and of flexor carpi ulnaris and flexor digitorum profundus to the ring and little fingers. The ulnar intrinsic muscles are more likely to be affected than the ulnar forearm muscles owing to the topographical location of their fibers within the ulnar nerve. Atrophy of the intrinsic muscles, clawing of the ring and little fingers, and Froment's sign may be present in severe cases.

Nerve conduction velocity of the ulnar nerve will be reduced across the elbow. Electromyographic studies may show the presence of denervation potentials in the affected muscles. These studies are of help in localizing the level of the lesion as well as in helping to determine the need for or urgency of surgical decompression. Unfortunately, these studies are not of great help in determining the presence of a thoracic outlet syndrome.

Treatment of Cubital Tunnel Syndrome

Conservative treatment is advised for patients with intermittent mild symptoms who show no significant neurological deficits.[14,33,52,55] However, repetitive flexion and extension of the elbow and prolonged flexion of the elbow in extreme positions should be avoided. A plaster splint or a pillow wrapped around the elbow may be used at night to maintain elbow extension. Nonsteroidal anti-inflammatory medication may be used, but steroid injections should be avoided as there is no tenosynovium within the cubital tunnel.

Surgical treatment is indicated for those with persistent significant symptoms or neurological deficit. Anterior transposition of the ulnar nerve has been the most common technique to alleviate the entrapment. Extensive mobilization of the nerve to accomplish this and placement of the nerve anterior to the elbow joint axis of motion can eliminate most of the causative factors. Following its transposition, the nerve is left either subcutaneously superficial or placed submuscularly (Learmonth procedure) beneath the flexor pronator mass.[31,32]

A medial epicondylectomy removes the pivot point of the ulnar nerve and decompresses the cubital tunnel by removing its floor.[11,19] The nerve migrates somewhat anteriorly and is left in a subcutaneous position next to the bony structures of the medial elbow where it is subject to repetitive trauma. However, good relief of sensory symptoms and some improvement in motor deficits have been reported with this procedure.

Simple surgical decompression of the ulnar tunnel with release of the arcuate ligament which forms the roof of the cubital tunnel and bridges the two heads of the flexor carpi ulnaris is quite effective if this is the only site of entrapment abnormality.[42] Unfortunately, it does not address any of the other factors seen with this complex syndrome.

In general, the postoperative relief of paresthesias and dysesthesias is good.[38] Overall, the return of sensation is better than that of motor function. The more severe the preexisting neurological deficits and the longer their duration, the less likely that treatment will provide full functional recovery. Functional recovery may continue slowly to proceed over a 3- to 5-year period. Higher success rates are found with transpositions and medial epicondylectomy than with simple decompression.[11,19,32] The submuscular transposition of Learmonth provides the best relief of symptoms.[32]

Complications Associated with Surgery

Complications from any of these procedures include painful hypertrophic surgical scar, painful neuromas of the medial antebrachial cutaneous nerve or medial brachial cutaneous nerve, and reflex sympathetic dystrophy. Persistent or recurrent symptoms may be due to a kinking of the nerve, an intact medial intermuscular septum or unreleased arcade of Struthers, a scarring of the nerve to the medial epicondyle, or a dislocation of the nerve back into the postcondylar groove following anterior transposition.[5] A subcutaneously transposed nerve in a patient with little protective subcutaneous fatty tissue may be the source of painful paresthesias and dysesthesias due to repetitive minor irritation and trauma.

Ulnar Tunnel Syndrome

Entrapment neuropathy of the ulnar nerve as it enters the wrist through Guyon's canal is called *ulnar tunnel syndrome.*[18] Compared to the carpal tunnel, Guyon's canal is a much smaller structure whose floor is the ulnarwood continuation of the transverse carpal ligament to the pisiform; its proximal ulnar wall, the pisiform; its radial distal wall, the hook of the hamate; and its roof the volar carpal ligament and pisohamate ligament (Fig. 40-6). In contrast to the carpal tunnel, only the ulnar artery and ulnar nerve course through Guyon's canal. There are no tendons or synovium present. Shortly after entering the canal, the ulnar nerve bifurcates

into a superficial sensory branch which innervates the ulnar palm, the little finger, and ulnar half of ring digit; continues into a deep motor branch which loops around the hook of the hamate; and innervates all the hypothenar- and ulnar-innervated intrinsic muscles of the hand except the palmaris brevis, which receives its innervation from the sensory branch. The flexor brevis and opponens digiti quinti hypothenar muscles take their origin from a common tendinous band stretching between the pisiform and hook of hamate which divides the nerve into its superficial and deep components. Lastly, the ulnar dorsum of the hand is innervated by the dorsal sensory branch of the ulnar nerve, which branches from the nerve approximately 5 cm proximal to the ulnar styloid; therefore, sensation over the dorsum of the hand along its ulnar border should be intact with an ulnar tunnel compression syndrome.

Causes of Ulnar Tunnel Syndrome

Guyon's canal is less rigid than the carpal tunnel, but since it is a closed space, any space-occupying lesion will compromise the ulnar nerve. The ganglion has been found as the most common tumor mass,[51] although a lipoma, a neurilem-

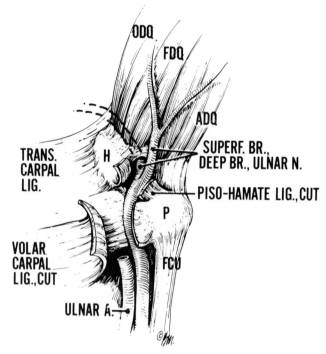

Figure 40-6 Guyon's canal. Note structures that compose the canal: transverse carpal ligament (trans. carpal lig.), pisohamate ligament (cut in this view), hook of the hamate (H), and the pisiform (P). Other structures noted are the ulnar artery, superficial and deep branches of the ulnar nerve passing through Guyon's canal, the flexor carpi ulnaris (FCU), and the hypothenar muscles, opponens digiti quinti (ODQ), flexor digiti quinti (FDQ), and adductor digiti quinti (ADQ). (*From Eversman, in Green, David P., ed: Operative Hand Surgery. New York, Churchill Livingstone, 1982. Reproduced with permission.*)

moma, anomolous muscles, and fascial or tendinous bands have also been reported. Pisiform instability, pisotriquetral joint arthritis,[7] and ulnar artery thrombosis have been noted. Although direct trauma to the nerve or fracture of the wrist or carpus (hook of hamate, pisiform) is occasionally found, indirect trauma on a repetitive basis (hypothenar hammer syndrome)[10] is probably the most common overall cause of ulnar tunnel syndrome today. A wide variety of people involved in numerous occupations and recreational activities use the hypothenar eminence, the heel of the hand, as a pressure counterpoint against tools, apparatus, and other physical objects. Examples include plumbers, carpenters, pipe cutters, metal polishers, gardeners, cyclists, weight lifters, and crutch and cane users. Thrombosis of the ulnar artery may result from this chronic repetitive trauma.

Differential Diagnosis

The differential diagnosis is essentially the same as that for cubital tunnel syndrome. Sensory disturbances over the ulnar dorsum of the hand should direct one's attention to the ulnar nerve above the wrist level.[51] Disturbance of sensation along the border of the medial forearm indicates a pathological process in the area of the brachial plexus, thoracic outlet, and neck or spinal cord level.

Clinical Diagnosis

Depending upon the level of entrapment within Guyon's canal, the patient may complain of a vague, ill-defined, aching discomfort in the ulnar region of the wrist and hand, with varying combinations of weakness, atrophy, paresthesias, and hypesthesia, with patients having a pure sensory deficit or a pure motor deficit, or a combination of both. Careful sensory evaluation is critical in that abnormal sensation over the ulnar dorsum of the hand implies that the nerve entrapment is proximal to Guyon's canal and the takeoff of the dorsoulnar sensory branch.

A pure motor deficit involving only the ulnar intrinsic muscles implicates entrapment of the deep motor branch at or distal to the hook of hamate, whereas involvement of both the hypothenar and intrinsic muscles would mean a more proximal canal entrapment.[51] The common fibrous origin of the hypothenar muscles between the hook of hamate and pisiform may be the offending agent.[25] A mixed motor and sensory deficit indicates entrapment within the proximal portion of the canal, whereas isolated sensory deficit may occur at any level.[56]

Cold intolerance and Raynaud's phenomenon may be noted.[14] Local tenderness to deep pressure, a positive Tinel's sign, positive Phalen's (wrist flexion) test, palpable swelling or a mass, and callused skin over the hypothenar eminence space may be found on careful examination. A positive Allen test (no arterial filling) may be present with an ulnar artery thrombosis. A discrete distal fingertip subcutaneous infarct and subungual splinter hemorrhages may result from distal thrombotic emboli.

Electrophysiological studies most often show a delayed distal motor latency from the ulnar nerve at the wrist to the first dorsal interosseous muscle. Denervation fibrillations will usually be found in the ulnar intrinsic hand muscles.

Treatment of Ulnar Tunnel Syndrome

As in all nerve entrapment syndromes, treatment of ulnar tunnel syndrome depends upon the cause, severity, and duration of the problem. Mild symptoms and neurological deficits resulting from either a single traumatic episode or from repetitive chronic trauma over a reasonably short period of time may be treated with rest, splinting of the wrist, and avoidance of the repetitive trauma. Those who fail to improve with conservative care or those with more severe neurological deficits should undergo surgical decompression with complete neurolysis of the nerve and of both its motor and sensory branches.[22,29] Coexisting contributory abnormalities should be simultaneously excised (nonunion hook of hamate fracture, pisiform excision for contributing pisotriquetral arthritis, ulnar artery segmental resection, or vascular reconstruction for thrombosis).

Complications of Ulnar Tunnel Syndrome

Injury to the palmar cutaneous branch of the ulnar nerve may produce a painful postoperative neuroma. Entrapment of the deep motor branch may occur distal to the hook of hamate by a deep ganglion or by the common tendinous origin of the hypothenar muscles and may go undetected in a limited surgical neurolysis. Resection of a nonunion of the hook of hamate or of the pisiform does not result in any functional disability.

RADIAL NERVE INJURY

Since the radial nerve, as it courses around the midshaft of the humerus, and its major motor branch the posterior interosseous nerve, as it winds around the proximal radius, are both in close proximity to bone, it is not surprising that trauma is the most common cause of radial nerve injury. Entrapment neuropathy of the radial nerve does occur, although far less frequently, and is noted at three distinct levels.

As the radial nerve winds posteriorly along the spiral groove of the humerus, it passes through a fibrous arch under the lateral head of the triceps about 2 cm distal and just posterior to the insertion of the deltoid on the humerus. Onset of symptoms may follow vigorous exercise or strenuous physical effort, and patients may present with a complete radial nerve palsy.[35] These palsies usually resolve spontaneously over the course of several weeks. The lateral head of the triceps without a fibrous arch or band has also been reported as a compression lesion in a high radial nerve entrapment.[37]

After coursing through the lateral head of the triceps, the radial nerve pierces the lateral intermuscular septum approximately 10 cm proximal to the lateral epicondyle. It then travels between the brachialis and biceps medially and the brachioradialis laterally and innervates the brachioradialis, extensor carpi radialis longus, and the lateral portion of the brachialis muscles. Passing anteriorly to the elbow joint, the nerve bifurcates into the superficial sensory radial nerve and the posterior interosseous motor nerve. It is here that chronic radial neuropathy entrapment most frequently occurs. Although two distinct syndromes have been described[47]—one causing pain only (radial tunnel syndrome), the other producing paresis (posterior interosseous nerve syndrome)—they are probably expressions of varying degrees of progressive nerve compression, one mild and intermittent, the other constant.

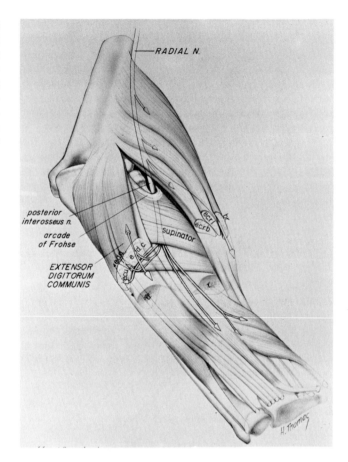

Figure 40-7 After the internervous plane between the extensor carpi radialis brevis (e.c.r.b.) and the extensor digitorum communis (e.d.c.) is developed, the posterior interosseous nerve is identified just proximal to the arcade of Frohse. It can be traced through the supinator, where distally its multiple terminal branches can be visualized (br., brachioradialis; e.c.r.l., extensor carpi radialis longus; e.c.u., extensor carpi ulnaris; r., radius; u., ulna). (*From Spinner, M.: Injuries to the Major Branches of the Peripheral Nerves of the Forearm. Philadelphia, Saunders, 1978. Reproduced with permission.*)

Posterior Interosseous Nerve Syndrome

Entrapment of the posterior interosseous nerve can be caused by a variety of etiologic factors. Anatomic anomalies are commonly implicated, the most common being a fibrous tendinous band (arcade of Frohse) at the proximal origin of the supinator muscle, which is seen in approximately 30 percent of the population (Fig. 40-7).[54] If present, the nerve must pass under this band as it courses through the supinator muscle. A similar fibrous band has also been reported at the distal edge of the supinator. Other less convincing anatomic anomalies, such as fibrous bands from the radiocapitellar joint, radial recurrent vessels, and a tendinous origin of the extensor carpi radialis brevis, have been mentioned as compressing factors.[34,47] Mass lesions (such as rheumatoid synovitis of the elbow and bicipital tendon bursitis at the radial tubercle) have also been noted. Trauma, such as dislocation of the elbow or Monteggia fracture with dislocation of the radial head, is a frequent cause, and the onset of the posterior interosseous nerve palsy may be delayed following trauma. Lastly, iatrogenic factors, such as injections in the area of the elbow, surgical resection of the radial head, and compression plating of fracture of the proximal radius have been implicated.

Clinical Diagnosis

Pain occurs in half the patients. It is often deep and aching and may resolve within several days or weeks. Weakness of the wrist and fingers is then noted and either a partial or complete palsy of the posterior interosseous nerve is found. In a partial paresis, the sequential order of muscle involvement may vary, although, commonly, the common extensors to the ring and little fingers are first affected. The patient is unable to extend the metacarpophalangeal joints of the ring and little fingers, producing a pseudo–ulnar claw hand.[52] This differs dramatically from a true ulnar claw hand in which the metacarpophalangeal joints are extended or hyperextended and in which the interphalangeal joints cannot be actively extended because of the ulnar nerve paresis. With complete paralysis, there is weak but persisting wrist extension in radial deviation since the extensor carpi radialis longus is innervated by the radial nerve before its bifurcation. The extensor carpi radialis brevis is supplied by the superficial sensory branch of the radial, the posterior interosseous nerve, or any

combination of these. The extensor carpi ulnaris is paralyzed and offers no counterbalance in extension. The metacarpophalangeal joint of all five digits cannot be extended beyond 45 degrees, although the interphalangeal joints of all the digits can be extended by the intact ulnar intrinsic muscles, giving the appearance of an intrinsic plus hand. Of great importance is the fact that sensation over the radial dorsum of the hand is normal. Localized tenderness to deep palpation is frequently found over the posterior interosseous nerve just before or just as it enters the arcade of Frohse of the supinator muscle.

Electrophysiological nerve studies may show an increased distal motor latency across the arcade of Frohse, as well as denervation fibrillations of the affected muscles.

Differential Diagnosis

Differentiation from a high radial nerve lesion is made by observance of the lack of any sensory disturbance and the presence of a normal brachioradialis, radial wrist extensors, and supinator muscles. Lead poisoning typically produces a full radial palsy without any sensory loss, although initially only the inability to extend the metacarpophalangeal joints of the middle and ring fingers may be seen. Lead neuropathy is usually bilateral, but may start unilaterally. Conversion reaction (hysterical wrist drop) may be differentiated by the inability of the patient to extend the interphalangeal joints, which are moved by the ulnar intrinsic muscles. Polyarthritis has been reported to produce an isolated paralysis of the posterior interosseous nerve which is usually transient.

Treatment

Posterior interosseous nerve palsy in the presence of a mass lesion should be surgically explored and the mass removed. In the absence of a mass lesion, a period of observation of 8 to 12 weeks to see if spontaneous recovery of the nerve paralysis occurs is reasonable.[21] Electromyographic studies of the affected muscles will show electrical evidence of recovery prior to clinical recovery.

Radial Tunnel Syndrome

As emphasized before, the *radial tunnel syndrome* is a mild compression entrapment syndrome of the posterior interosseous nerve causing pain without any muscular paresis. Its differentiation from the posterior interosseous nerve syndrome may be only a matter of degree of severity of nerve compression.[34,47]

Causes of Radial Tunnel Syndrome

Four anatomic features can cause compression of the posterior interosseous nerve in radial tunnel syndrome:[34,47] fibrous bands of adhesions which tether the nerve through the radiohumeral joint, a fibrous medial edge along the extensor carpi radialis brevis, a radial recurrent leash or fan of vessels overlying the nerve, and lastly, the fibrous arcade of Frohse. No space-occupying mass lesions have been reported with this syndrome.

The differential diagnosis does include lateral epicondylitis (tennis elbow), which, however, may occur simultaneously with radial tunnel syndrome.[59]

Clinical Diagnosis

Dull aching pain located deep in the extensor muscle mass is the main symptom. Pain is usually absent upon awakening, but often the patient develops a persistent aching soreness by day's end.[39] Weakness of grip strength is a frequent complaint, particularly with repetitive or prolonged gripping movements. The most important point of physical diagnosis is the localized tenderness directly over the posterior interosseous nerve approximately 5 cm distal to the lateral epicondyle. Increased pain may be elicited by resisted active supination of the forearm; similarly passive full pronation of the forearm may produce pain. In both cases the pain is caused by a tightening of the proximal edge of the supinator across the nerve. The "middle finger test" may aggravate pain symptoms.[34] The patient is asked to maintain the elbow, wrist, and all fingers in full active extension while counterpressure is exerted by the examiner over each finger dorsally, pushing it volarly. Symptom aggravation will usually be most severe while stressing the extended middle finger since the extensor carpi radialis brevis inserts into the base of the third metacarpal, and this stress test tenses the medial edge of that muscle against the nerve.

Electrophysiological studies of this condition have been confusing. Recently, increased motor latencies have been shown in patients during active forceful supination of the arm as the study is being performed.[48]

Treatment of Radial Tunnel Syndrome

In this pain syndrome without neurological deficit, conservative measures are the first form of treatment. Such measures include rest of the elbow and wrist from repetitive stressful activity and a course of anti-inflammatory medication. Surgical exploration with neurolysis of the posterior interosseous nerve is indicated if conservative treatment fails. Several authors have reported good to excellent results in a high percentage of patients.[23,34,39,47,59]

Whartenberg Syndrome

Whartenberg[58] in 1932 described an isolated neuritis of the superficial sensory branch of the radial nerve that produces persistent, severe dysesthetic pain on the radial dorsal surface of the wrist and distal third of the forearm radiating onto the dorsum of the hand. An exquisitely sensitive Tinel's sign is often present at the site of entrapment with numbness over the radial dorsum of the hand.

Because of its superficial location, the nerve is frequently injured. Lacerations, surgery for de Quervain's tenosynovitis, tight jewelery or wristwatch bands, snug-fitting casts, handcuffs, and the insertion of intravenous needles or dialysis shunts have all been reported as causative agents.

Complications from this entrapment syndrome or injury can be devastating. The patient may be left with a florid reflex sympathetic dystrophy.

Treatment consists in the relieving of any physical external compression over the nerve. Symptoms may take several months to resolve. Local steroid injections may be beneficial.

For persistent, severe symptoms, surgical exploration is warranted.[4,16] If found entrapped in scar tissue, the nerve should be very meticulously externally neurolysed and good healthy skin and subcutaneous tissue should be placed over the nerve. If a neuroma is found, the prognosis is much more guarded. A more proximal resection of the nerve underneath the brachioradialis, neurorrhaphy of the ends of the radial nerve, capping the nerve with silicone, and transposing the neuroma deeper in the forearm have all been advocated.

MISCELLANEOUS NERVE ENTRAPMENTS IN THE UPPER EXTREMITY

Musculocutaneous Nerve

Entrapment of the musculocutaneous nerve has been reported to occur at two distinct levels. After arising from the lateral cord of the brachial plexus, the musculocutaneous nerve courses beneath the coracobrachialis muscle and enters the upper arm, passing between the brachialis and biceps muscles distally. It supplies motor innervation to those three muscles and may occasionally travel deep to the brachialis and be in close contact with the anterior shaft of the humerus, where it is susceptible to injury in fracture.

Acute entrapment of the musculocutaneous nerve with a paresis of the three muscles has been reported after very strenuous physical exercise,[3] such as after building a rock wall or exercising with barbells. The entrapment is thought to occur under the edge of a hypertrophied coracobrachialis muscle. The muscle may be injured during retraction of this muscle in shoulder surgery.

The lateral antebrachial cutaneous nerve, which is the sensory branch continuation of the musculocutaneous nerve, may be entrapped by the lateral border of the biceps tendon where the nerve pierces the antebrachial fascia of the arm.[40] This may produce pain in the proximal forearm and elbow with hypesthesias and paresthesias down the radial aspect of the forearm. Elbow pain is markedly exacerbated by moving the forearm from supination into pronation with the elbow fully extended. Several such patients have faulty tennis strokes.

Patients with entrapment of the musculocutaneous nerve underneath the coracobrachialis recovered spontaneously.[3] In another series, approximately half the patients with a more distal sensory entrapment recovered spontaneously; the other half did not and required surgical neurolysis to free the nerve where it was compressed by the distal biceps tendon and lacertus fibrosus against the brachialis fascia.[40]

Axillary Nerve

Traumatic injury of the axillary nerve is commonly seen. This may occur following a direct blow to the posterior shoulder, such as in contact sports, or it may occur after a fall or following a dislocation of the glenohumeral joint.[2] Spontaneous entrapment of the axillary nerve by a fibrous band or muscle in the quadrilateral space may occur.[6] Pain and localized tenderness to deep pressure over the posterior shoulder, along with inability to actively adduct the arm, are noted.

Differentiation from a C5 cervical root lesion and a brachial plexus neuritis are important diagnostic concerns.

The majority of axillary nerve lesions resolve spontaneously.

SECTION C

Thoracic Outlet Syndrome

Lawrence C. Hurst and Seth Paul

Upper extremity dysfunction may result from compression of any of the neurovascular structures in the thoracic outlet. This symptom complex is called *thoracic outlet syndrome*. It has a wide variety of clinical presentations, depending on exactly which neurovascular structures are compressed.

The term "thoracic outlet syndrome" was first used in 1956 by Peet[26] at the Mayo Clinic. However, more than a century earlier, Sir Ashley Cooper[8] described the symptom complex itself. Surgery for this was performed by Coote[9] in 1861 when he excised the first cervical rib. The presence of cervical ribs in 1 percent of the population was established in 1913, but only 10 percent of these are symptomatic.[25] The scalenus anticus syndrome and Adson's maneuver were described in 1927.[1] Falconer and Weddell[11] described the costoclavicular syndrome in 1943. Wright[37] identified the hyperabduction syndrome in 1945.

The anatomy of the thoracic outlet has been well established.[23,24] The subclavian artery and brachial plexus leave the thorax by arching over the first rib posterior to the scalenus anticus muscle and anterior to the scalenus anticus muscle. The subclavian vein passes anterior to the scalenus anticus muscle. The vein, artery, and plexus then pass under the subclavian muscle and clavicle in the costoclavicular space and enter the axilla posterior to the pectoralis minor muscle. Abnormal structural variations may compress or cause friction on the nerves or vessels at the level of the intervertebral foramina, the interscalene triangle, costoclavicular space, or in the axilla (Fig. 40-8).[24] Dynamic factors such as neck motion, shoulder motion, and respiratory movements can also alter the capacity of the thoracic outlet. Fibrous bands have been separated into seven types which cause thoracic outlet obstruction.[29] Scalene musculature anomalies have been divided into five types and help account for upper thoracic outlet syndrome.[29] Types I and II are ligamentous bands associated with a cervical rib or a broad seventh cervical transverse process. Bonney[2] felt that Sibsen's fascia was responsible for trapping the lower elements of the brachial plexus. Congenital etiologies like a cervical rib (Fig. 40-9) and traumatic etiologies must also be considered.[8,24]

Thoracic outlet syndrome is most frequently found in young and middle-aged people, especially females[17] who have lead active lives without previous symptoms. Symptoms are usually of gradual onset and due to trauma, to job activities (especially those requiring overhead use of the arms), or to emotional stress, which can lead to chronic muscle spasm in the neck or shoulders.

Different patterns of clinical manifestations are seen depending on the neurovascular structures compressed. The majority of patients' symptoms are created by neurological

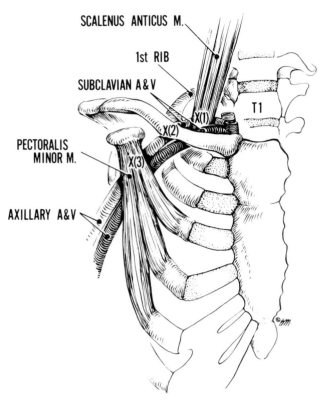

Figure 40-8 Three sites of potential compression are located at X(1), X(2), and X(3). X(1) is the interscalene triangle. X(2) is the costoclavicular space. X(3) is area posterior to the pectoralis minor. *(Reproduced with permission from Green, D.P., ed: Operative Hand Surgery. New York, Churchill Livingstone, 1982, p 1718.)*

compression. Typical symptoms are pain, numbness, or paresthesias. Sensory loss and muscle atrophy are rare but can occur. Arterial compression causes coldness, muscle fatigue, ischemic pain, and numbness. The symptoms may be aggravated with exercise or with exposure to cold. Arterial lesions may also produce a bruit in the supraclavicular region, but these bruits can be present in normal subjects.[14] Venous system involvement can also produce pain and swelling and can lead to distal edema and cyanosis.

A number of diagnostic maneuvers have been described to elicit signs of neurovascular compression. Adson's sign is the obliteration of the radial pulse when the patient turns the head to the affected side and extends the neck while holding her or his breath.[1] The hyperabduction maneuver and the "at-attention" test also have the end point of radial pulse obliteration.[11,37] Unfortunately, these pulse obliteration maneuvers can also bring about positive results in normal subjects[10,28,33,37] and probably should be considered positive only if they reproduce the patient's symptoms as well as obliterate the radial pulse. Symptoms can also be reproduced by Roos's 3-min elevated arm stress test.[29] Despite the shortcomings of these maneuvers, a careful history and physical exam remains the best method of establishing a diagnosis of thoracic outlet syndrome.[21,22] The workup must exclude the more common components of the differential diagnosis. In a differ-

ential diagnosis, cervical disc disease, cervical arthritis, a tumor originating from or compression of the plexus (such as a Pancoast tumor), ulnar or median nerve entrapment (carpal tunnel syndrome), aneurysms, and brachial plexitis must all be considered.[4,24] Infiltration of the cervical disc[20] or the scalene muscle[31,32] with local anesthetic has also been described as confirmatory tests in the workup for thoracic outlet syndrome.

Thoracic outlet syndrome can be broadly divided into vascular and neurogenic types. The classic true motor neurogenic thoracic outlet syndrome is very rare.[35,36] It is usually found in adult women who have a history of chronic arm pain followed by hand wasting, especially in the thenar eminence area.[12,13,17] Electrophysiological findings in these patients include a low-amplitude median motor response, low ulnar sensory potential, low ulnar motor potential, and normal median sensory potential.[5,13,34–36]

In the large series (300 or more cases) reported by vascular surgeons[15,18,31,34,39] there is no agreement on the specific indications for surgical treatment. Although an arteriogram may be a reliable way to diagnose an aneurysm, intimal arterial irregularities, and thrombosis, changes in the vessel's appearance during the Adson's maneuver, the hyperabduction maneuver, and the costoclavicular maneuver are not necessarily diagnostic of thoracic outlet syndrome.[4,30] Because arteriogram results are not pathognomonic for thoracic outlet syndrome, Urschel[34] popularized the ulnar motor conduction velocity across the thoracic outlet (UMCV-TO) test, but this test is not done in other centers. On the other hand, Roos's[27,28,29] elevated arm stress test is unique in his series. Thus, there are a large number of patients who have undergone surgery whose main complaint was upper extremity dysfunction without specific objective findings of thoracic outlet syndrome.[35,36] Many of these patients with presumed thoracic outlet syndrome may have, in fact, carpal tunnel syndrome. Although several people believe that this is evidence of a double-crush phenomenon, Carroll and Hurst[4] have shown that the coexistence of thoracic outlet syndrome and carpal tunnel syndrome approaches zero.

Much work has been done in the electrodiagnostic study of these patients. Previous assessment with nerve conduction studies and electromyography has proved to be unreliable and inconsistent.[16,35,36] Somatosensory evoked potentials combined with dynamic stress testing may increase the specificity of electrodiagnostic assessment of these patients.[6,38]

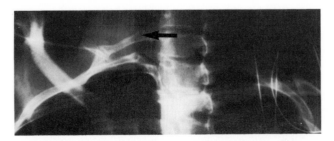

Figure 40-9 X-ray view demonstrating a cervical rib at arrow.

Despite this, thoracic outlet syndrome is still a controversial diagnosis.[35,36] In many patients a specific cause is usually lacking. Therefore, thoracic outlet syndrome should be a diagnosis of exclusion.

Initial management of patients with thoracic outlet syndrome begins with an exercise and weight reduction program[17] designed to diminish the soft tissue mass, increase the flexibility of the shoulder musculature, and improve posture. This regime may provide partial or complete relief for the majority of symptomatic patients with moderate neurological complaints.[3,26]

Patients with significant neurological or vascular involvement that does not respond to physical therapy may need surgery. Roos[27] achieved decompression of the thoracic outlet initially by first-rib resection through a transaxillary approach. However, first-rib resection alone was not sufficient in a number of patients. Thus, Sanders,[31,32] Roos,[29] and others now have combined transaxillary first-rib resection with scalenotomies to decompress the thoracic outlet more adequately. In recurrent cases Kline[19] advocates the subscapular approach originally described by Clagett.[7] Unlike the transaxillary approach, the subscapular approach permits direct inspection of the roots from the point where they exit the vertebral foramina and course distally to form the trunks, divisions, and cords of the brachial plexus. Intraoperative nerve testing can be performed when this approach is used.

In summary, the thoracic outlet syndrome encompasses a wide array of clinical manifestations of neurovascular compression or irritation. Despite a lack of specific diagnostic tests, a detailed examination may enable the physician to carefully select those patients who will benefit from surgical treatment.

REFERENCES

Section A: Nerve Injuries in the Upper Extremity

1. Adler, J.B., and Patterson, R.L. Erb's palsy, long term results of treatment in 88 cases. J Bone Joint Surg 49A:1052–1064, 1967.
2. Badalamente, M.A., Hurst, L.C., Ellstein, J.E., McDevitt, C.A. The pathobiology of human neuromas, an electron microscopic and biochemical study. J Hand Surg 10B(1):49–53, February 1985.
3. Bora, F.W., Richardson, S., and Black, J. The biomechanical responses to tension in peripheral nerve. J Hand Surg 5(1):21–25, January 1980.
4. Breidenbach, W., and Terzis, J.K. The anatomy of free vascularized nerve grafts. Clin Plast Surg 11:1:65–72, January 1984.
5. Brown, K.L.B. Review of obstetrical palsies: Nonoperative treatment. Clin Plast Surg 11(1):181–187, 1984.
6. Brunell, G. Neurotization of avulsed roots of brachial plexus by means of anterior nerves of cervical plexus. Clin Plast Surg 11(1):149–152, 1984.
7. Buck-Gramcko, D. Evaluation of perineural repair with nerve injuries, in Flynn, J.E. (ed): Hand Surgery, 3d ed. Baltimore, Williams & Wilkins, 1982, pp 433–442.
8. Castoldo, J.E., and Ochoa, J.L. Mechanical injury of peripheral nerves, fine structure and dysfunction. Clin Plast Surg 11(1):9–11, 1984.
9. Colenc, V.V. Intercostal neurotization of the peripheral nerves in avulsion plexus injuries. Clin Plast Surg 11(1):143–147, 1984.
10. Dayton, W.R., and Schollmeyer, J.V. Localization of Ca++ activated neutral protease in skeletal muscle. Biochem 87A:267, 1980.
11. Dellon, A.L. Evaluation of sensibility and reeducation of sensation of the hand. Baltimore, Williams & Wilkins, 1981, pp 193–202.
12. Dellon, A.L., Curtis, R.M., and Edgerton, M.T. Re-education of sensation in the hand following nerve injury. J Bone Joint Surg 53A:813, 1971.
13. Dellon, A.L., Mackinnon, S.E., and Pestronk, A. Implantation of sensory nerve into muscle: Preliminary clinical and experimental observations on neuroma formation. Ann Plast Surg 12:30–40, 1984.
14. Engel, J., Gonel, A., Melomed, R., et al: Choline acetyltransferase for differentiation between human motor and sensory nerve fibers. Ann Plast Surg 4:376–380, 1979.
15. Gaul, J.S. Electrical fascicle identification as adjunct to nerve repair. J Hand Surg 8(3):289–296, 1983.
16. Gaul, J.S. Intrinsic motor recovery—The long term study of ulnar nerve repair. J Hand Surg 7(5):502–508, 1982.
17. Gilbert, A. Vascularized sural nerve graft. Clin Plast Surg 11(1):73–77, 1984.
18. Goldstein, S., Sturan, H. Interosseous nerve transposition for treatment of painful neuromas. J Hand Surg 10A(2):270–274, March 1985.
19. Greene, T.L., and Steichen, J.B. Digital nerve grafting using the dorsal sensory branch of the ulnar nerve. J Hand Surg 10B:37–40, 1985.
20. Greenwald, A.G., Schute, P., and Shivgley, J. Brachial plexus birth palsy: A 10-year report on the incidence and prognosis. J Pediatr Orthop 4(6):689–692, 1984.
21. Herndon, J.H., Eaton, R.G., and Littler, J.W. Management of painful neuromas in the hand. J Bone Joint Surg 58A:369–373, 1976.
22. Jabaley, M.E. Technical aspects of nerve repair. J Hand Surg 9B(1):14–19, 1984.
23. Jabaley, M.E., Wallace, W.H., and Hechler, F.R. Internal topography of major nerves of the forearm and hand: A current review. J Hand Surg 5:1–18, 1980.
24. Kamakura, K., Ishiura, S., Sugita, H., and Toyokura, Y. Identification of Ca++ activated neutral protease and its effect on neurofilament degeneration. J Neurochem 40(4):908–913, 1983.
25. Kline, D.G., and Nulsen, F.E. The neuroma-in-continuity: Its preoperative and operative management. Surg Clin North Am 52:189–1209, 1972.
26. Kutz, J.E., Shealy, G., and Lubbers, L. Interfascicular nerve repair. Ortho Clin North Am 12(2):277–286, 1981.
27. Landi, A., Copeland, S.A., Wynn Parry, C.B., and Jones, S.J. The role of somatosensory evoked potentials and nerve conduction studies in the surgical management of brachial plexus injuries. J Bone Joint Surg 62B:492–496, 1980.
28. Last, R.J. Anatomy, Regional and Applied, 7th ed. New York, Churchill Livingstone, 1984, pp. 52–125.
29. Leffert, R.D. Brachial Plexus Injuries. New York, Churchill Livingstone, 1985.
30. Lundborg, G. Ischemic nerve injury. Experimental studies on intraneural microvascular pathophysiology and nerve function in a limb subjected to temporary circulatory arrest. Scand J Plast Reconstr Surg 6(suppl):1, 1970.
31. McCarroll H., and Rodkey, R.W. Epineural and perineural repair in cats with and without tension, in Nerve Repair: Its Clinical and Experimental Basis. Symposium, San Francisco, November 3–5, 1977.
32. Millesi, H. Brachial plexus injuries, management and results. Clin Plast Surg 11(1):115–120, 1984.
33. Millesi, H. Nerve grafting. Clin Plast Surg 11:105, 1985.
34. Millesi, H., Meissl, G., and Berger, A. Further experience with interfascicular grafting of the median, ulnar and radial nerves. J Bone Joint Surg 58A:209–218, 1976.

35. Millesi, H., Meissl, G., and Berger, A. The interfascicular nerve grafting of the median and ulnar nerves. J Bone Joint Surg 54A:727–750, 1972.

36. Miyamoto, Y., Watari, S., and Tsuge, K. Experimental studies and effects of tension on intraneural microcirculation and sutured peripheral nerves. Plast Reconstr Surg 63:398–403, 1979.

37. Muller, H.W., Gebicke-Harter, P.J., Hangen, D.H., and Shoter, E.M. A specific 37,000 dalton protein that accumulates in regenerating but not in nonregenerating mammalian nerves. Science 228:499–501, 1985.

38. Narakas, A. Brachial plexus surgery. Orthop Clin North Am 12:303–323, 1981.

39. Narakas, A. Surgical treatment of traction injuries of the brachial plexus. Clin Orthop 133:71–90, 1978.

40. Narakas, A. Thoughts on neurotization: Nerve transfers in irrepairable nerve lesions. Clin Plast Surg 11(1):153–159, 1984.

41. Nicholson, O.R., and Seddon, H.J. Nerve repair in civil practice: Results of treatment of median and ulnar nerve lesions. Br Med J 2:1065–1071, 1957.

42. Orgel, M.G. Epineural vs. Perineural repair of peripheral nerves. Clin Plast Surg 11:101, 1984.

43. Perry, J., Hsu, J., Barber, L., and Huffer, M.M. Orthoses in patients with brachial plexus injuries. Arch Phys Med Rehabil 55:134–137, 1974.

44. Pho, R.W.H., Lee. Y.S., Rujiwetpongstorn, V., and Pang, M. Histological studies of vascularized nerve graft and conventional nerve graft. J Hand Surg 10B:1:45–48, February 1985.

45. Ramon ý Cajal, S. Degeneration and regeneration of the nervous system, in May, R.M. (ed): New York, Oxford University Press, 1928.

46. Restrepo, Y., Merle, M., Mischon, J., Folliguet, B., and Barrat, E. Free vascularized nerve grafts: An experimental study in a rabbit. Microsurgery 6:78–84, 1985.

47. Ritovek, B., Brown, M., and Lundborg, G. Pathoanatomy and pathophysiology of nerve root compression. Spine 9(1):7–15, 1984.

48. Rodkey, W.G., Cabaud, E., and McCarroll, H.R. Neurorrhaphy after loss of a nerve segment: Comparison of epineural suture under tension vs. multiple nerve grafts. J Hand Surg 5(4):366–371, January 1980.

49. Roots, B.I. Neurofilament accumulation induced in synapses by leupeptin. Science 221:971–972, 1983.

50. Sahellarides, H. A follow-up study of 172 peripheral nerve injuries in the upper extremity in civilians. J Bone Joint Surg 44A:140–148, 1962.

51. Schlaepfer, W.W., and Hasler, M.B. Characterization of the calcium induced disruption of neurofilaments in rat peripheral nerve. Brain Res 168:299–309, 1979.

52. Seddon, H.J. Surgical Disorders of the Peripheral Nerves. Baltimore, Williams & Wilkins, 1972.

53. Selzer, M.E. Regeneration of peripheral nerve, in Sumner, A.J. (ed): The Physiology of Peripheral Nerve Disease. Philadelphia, Saunders, 1980, pp 358–431.

54. Slack, J.R., Hopkins, W.G., and Pockett, S. Evidence for a motor nerve growth factor. Muscle Nerve 6:243–252, 1983.

55. Stracher, A. Proteinase inhibitors and muscle degeneration. Muscle Nerve 5:494–496, 1982.

56. Sullivan, D.J. Results of digital neurorrhaphy in adults. J Hand Surg 10B(1):41–44, 1985.

57. Sunderland, S. Blood supply of the peripheral nerves. Arch Neurol Psychiatry 54:283–289, 1945.

58. Sunderland, S. Nerve Repair and Regeneration. St. Louis, Mosby, 1980, pp 337–355.

59. Sunderland, S. Nerves and Nerve Injuries, 2d ed. New York, Churchill Livingstone, 1978.

60. Swanson, A.B., Boeve, N.R., and Lumsten, R.M. Prevention and treatment of amputation neuroma by silicone capping. J Hand Surg 2:70–78, 1977.

61. Tada, K., Tsuyuguchi, Y., and Kawai, H. Birth palsy: Natural recovery course and combined root avulsion. J Pediatr Orthop 4(3):279–284, 1984.

62. Taylor, A.S. Brachial birth palsy and injuries of similar type in adults. Surg Gynecol Obstet 30:494–502, 1920.

63. Terzis, J.K. Neural microsurgery, in Daniel, R.K., Terzis, J.K. (eds): Reconstructive Microsurgery. Boston, Little, Brown, 1977, p 387.

64. Tupper, J. Fascicular nerve repair. AAOS Symposium on Microsurgery. St. Louis, Mosby, 1979, p 215.

65. Urbaniak, J.R. Fascicular nerve sutures. Clin Orthop 163:57–64, 1982.

66. Varon, S.S., and Bunge R.P. Trophic mechanisms in the peripheral nervous system. Ann Rev Neurosci 1:327–361, 1978.

67. VanBeek, A., Hubble, B., and Kinkead, L. Clinical use of nerve stimulation and recording techniques. Plast Reconstr Surg 71:225–238, 1983.

68. Waller, A. On the sensory, motory, and vaso-motory symptoms resulting from the refrigeration and compression of the ulnar and other nerves in man. Proc Soc Lond 12:89, 1905.

69. Wickstrom, J. Birth injuries of the brachial plexus. J Bone Joint Surg 42A:1448–1449, 1960.

70. Williams, H.B. The painful stump neuroma and its treatment. Clin Plast Surg 11(1):79–84, 1984.

71. Wynn-Parry, C.B., and Salter, M. Sensory reeducation after median nerve lesions. Hand 8:250–257, 1976.

72. Zachary, R.B. Results of nerve future, in Seddon, H.J. (ed): Peripheral Nerve Injuries. London, Her Majesty's Stationery Office, 1954, pp 354–388.

Section B: Nerve Entrapment Syndromes in the Upper Extremity

1. Apfelberg, D.B., and Larson, S.J. Dynamic anatomy of the ulnar nerve at the elbow. Plast Reconst Surg 51:76, 1973.

2. Blom, S., and Dahback, L.O.: Nerve injuries in dislocations of the shoulder joint and fracture of the neck of the humerus. Acta Chir Scand 136:461–466, 1970.

3. Braddom, R., and Wolfe, C. Musculocutaneous nerve injury after heavy exercise. Arch Phys Med Rehabil 59:290–293, 1978.

4. Braidwood, A.S. Superficial radial neuropathy. J Bone Joint Surg 57B:380–383, 1975.

5. Brody, A.S., Leffert, R.D., and Smith, R.J. Technical problems with ulnar nerve transposition at the elbow: Findings and results of reoperation. J Hand Surg 3:85–89, 1978.

6. Cahill, B.R., and Palmer, R.E. Quadrilateral space syndrome. J Hand Surg 8:65–69, 1983.

7. Carroll, R.E., and Coyle, M.P. Dysfunction of the pisotriquetral joint: Treatment by excision of the pisiform. J Hand Surg 10A:703–707, 1985.

8. Cherington, M. Proximal pain in carpal tunnel syndrome. Arch Surg 108:69, 1974.

9. Childress, H.M. Recurrent ulnar nerve dislocation at the elbow. J Bone Joint Surg 38A:978–984, 1956.

10. Conn, J., Bergan, J., and Bell, J. Hypothenar hammer syndrome: Post-traumatic digital ischemia. Surgery 68:1122–1128, 1970.

11. Craven, P.R., and Green, D.P. Cubital tunnel syndrome: Treatment by medial epicondylectomy. J Bone Joint Surg 62A:986–989, 1980.

12. Cseuz, K.A., Thomas, J.E., Lamberg, E.H. Long term results of operation for carpal tunnel syndrome. Mayo Clin Proc 41:232, 1966.

13. Curtis, R.M., and Eversmann, W.W. Internal neurolysis as an adjunct to the treatment of carpal tunnel syndrome. J Bone Joint Surg 55A:733–740, 1973.

14. Dawson, D.M., Hallett, M., and Millender, L.H. Entrapment Neuropathies. Little, Brown, Boston, 1983.

15. Dekel, S., and Coates, R. Primary carpal stenosis as a cause of

"idiopathic" carpal tunnel syndrome. Lancet 2:1024, 1979.

16. Dellon, A.L., and Mackinnon, S.E. Radial sensory nerve entrapment in the forearm. J Hand Surg 11A:199–205, 1986.

17. Doyle, J.R., and Carroll, R.E. The carpal tunnel syndrome: A review of 100 patients treated surgically. California Med 108:263, 1968.

18. Dupont, C., Cloutier, G.E., Prevost, Y., and Dion, M. Ulnar tunnel syndrome at the wrist. J Bone Joint Surg 47A:757–761, 1965.

19. Froimson, A., and Zahrawi, F. Treatment of compression neuropathy of the ulnar nerve at the elbow by epicondylectomy and neurolysis. J Hand Surg 5:391–395, 1980.

20. Gelberman, R.H., Hergenroeder, P.T., Hargens, A.R., Lundborg, G.N., and Akeson, W.H. The carpal tunnel syndrome—Study of carpal canal pressures. J Bone Joint Surg 63A:380–383, 1981.

21. Green, D.P. Diagnostic and therapeutic value of carpal tunnel injection. J Hand Surg 9A:850–854, 1984.

22. Grundberg, A.B. Ulnar tunnel syndrome. J Hand Surg 9B:72–74, 1984.

23. Hagert, C.G. Entrapment of the posterior interosseous nerve causing forearm pain. J Hand Surg 2:486, 1977.

24. Hartz, C.R., Linscheid, R.L., Gramse, R.R., and Daube, J.R. The pronator teres syndrome: Compressive neuropathy of the median nerve. J Bone Joint Surg 63A:885–890, 1981.

25. Hayes, J.R., Mulholland, R.C., and O'Connor, B.T. Compression of the deep palmar branch of the ulnar nerve. J Bone Joint Surg 51B:469–472, 1969.

26. Hill, N.A., Howard, F.M., and Huffer, B.R. The incomplete anterior interosseous nerve syndrome. J Hand Surg 10A:4–16, 1985.

27. Johnson, R.K., Spinner, M., and Shrewsbury, M.M. Medial nerve entrapment syndrome in the proximal forearm. J Hand Surg 4:48–61, 1970.

28. Kiloh, L.G., and Nevin, S. Isolated neuritis of the anterior interosseous nerve. Br Med J 1:850, 1952.

29. Kleinert, H.E., and Hayes, J.E. The ulnar tunnel syndrome. Plast Reconstr Surg 47:21, 1971.

30. Langloh, N.D., and Linscheid, R.L. Recurrent and unrelieved carpal tunnel syndrome. Clin Orthop 83:41–47, 1972.

31. Learsmonth, J.R. A technique for transplanting the ulnar nerve. Surg Gynecol Obstet 75:792, 1942.

32. Leffert, R.D. Anterior submuscular transposition of the ulnar nerve by the Learmonth technique. J Hand Surg 7:147–155, 1982.

33. Lister, G. The Hand: Diagnosis and Indications, 2d ed. Edinburgh, Churchill Livingstone, 1984.

34. Lister, G.D., Belsole, R.B., and Kleinert, H.E. The radial tunnel syndrome. J Hand Surg 4:52–59, 1979.

35. Lotem, M., Fried, A., Levy, M., Solzi, P., Najenson, T., and Nathan, H. Radial palsy following muscular effort. J Bone Joint Surg 53B:500–506, 1971.

36. MacDonald, R.I., Lichtman, D.M., Hanlon, J.J., and Wilson, J.N. Complications of surgical release for carpal tunnel syndrome. J Hand Surg 3:70–76, 1978.

37. Manske, P.R. Compression of the radial nerve by the triceps muscle. J Bone Joint Surg 59A:835–836, 1977.

38. McGowan, A.J. The results of transposition of the ulnar nerve for traumatic ulnar neuritis. J Bone Joint Surg 32B:293–301, 1950.

39. Moss, S.H., and Switzer, H.E. Radial tunnel syndrome: A spectrum of clinical presentations. J Hand Surg 8:414–420, 1983.

40. Nunley, J.A., and Bassett, F.H. Compression of the musculotendinous nerve at the elbow. J Bone Joint Surg 64A:1050–1052, 1982.

41. Ochoa, J. Nerve fiber pathology in acute and chronic compression, in Omer, G.E., and Spinner, M. (eds): Management of Peripheral Nerve Problems. Saunders, Philadelphia, 1980.

42. Osborne, G.V. Compression neuritis of the ulnar nerve at the elbow. Hand 2:10, 1970.

43. Parsonage, M.J., and Turner, J.W. Neuralgic amyotrophy: The shoulder girdle syndrome. Lancet 1:973, 1948.

44. Pechan, J., and Julis, I. The pressure measurement in the ulnar nerve: A contribution to the pathophysicology of the cubital tunnel syndrome. J Biomech 8:75–79, 1975.

45. Phalen, G.S. The carpal tunnel syndrome. Clin Orthop 83:29–40, 1972.

46. Phalen, G.S. The carpal tunnel syndrome: Seventeen years' experience in diagnosis and treatment of 654 hands. J Bone Joint Surg 48A:211–228, 1968.

47. Roles, N.C., and Mandsley, R. Radial tunnel syndrome: Resistant tennis elbow as a nerve entrapment. J Bone Joint Surg 54B:499–508, 1972.

48. Rosen, I., and Werner, C.O. Neurophysiological investigation of posterior interosseous entrapment causing lateral elbow pain. EEG Clin Neurophysiol 50:125–133, 1980.

49. Rydevik, B., Lundborg, G., and Bagge, U. Effects of graded compression on intraneural blood flow. J Hand Surg 6:3–12, 1981.

50. Seyffarth, H. Primary myoses in the M. pronator teres as cause of lesion of the N. medianus (the pronator syndrome). Acta Psychiatr Scand 74(suppl):251, 1951.

51. Shea, J.D., and McClain, E.J. Ulnar nerve compression syndrome at and below the wrist. J Bone Joint Surg 51A:1095–1103, 1969.

52. Spinner, M. Injuries to the Major Branches of Peripheral Nerves of the Forearm, 2d ed. Philadelphia, Saunders, 1978.

53. Spinner, M. The anterior interosseous nerve syndrome. J Bone Joint Surg 52A:84–94, 1970.

54. Spinner, M. The arcade of Frohse and its relationship to posterior interosseous nerve paralysis. J Bone Joint Surg 50B:809–812, 1968.

55. Sunderland, S. Nerves and Nerve Injuries, 2d ed. London, Churchill Livingstone, 1978.

56. Uniburu, I.J.F., Morchio, F.J., and Marin, J.C. Compression syndrome of the deep motor branch of the ulnar nerve (piso-hamate hiatus syndrome). J Bone Joint Surg 58A:145–147, 1976.

57. Upton, A.R.M., and McComas, A.J. Double crush in nerve entrapment syndromes. Lancet 2:359–361, 1973.

58. Wartenberg, R. Cheiralgia paresthetica (isolierte neuritis des ramus superficialis nervi radialis). A Ges Neurol Phychiatr 141:145, 1932.

59. Werner, C.O. Lateral elbow pain and posterior interosseous nerve entrapment. Acta Orthop Scand 174(suppl):1–62, 1979.

Section C: Thoracic Outlet Syndrome

1. Adson, A.W., and Coffey, J.R. Cervical rib, a method of anterior approach for relief of symptoms by division of the scalenus anticus. Ann Surg 85:839–857, 1927.

2. Bonney, G. Some lesions of the brachial plexus. Ann R Coll Surg Engl 59:298–306, 1977.

3. Britt, L.P. Nonoperative treatment of thoracic outlet syndrome symptoms. Clin Orthop 51:45–48, 1967.

4. Carroll, R.E., and Hurst, L.C. The relationship of the thoracic outlet syndrome and carpal tunnel syndrome. Clin Orthop 164:149–153, 1982.

5. Cherington, M. Ulnar conduction velocity in thoracic outlet syndrome. Letter to the editor. N Engl J Med 294:1185–1186, 1974.

6. Chodoroff, G., Lee, D.W., and Nonet, J.C. Dynamic approach in the diagnosis of thoracic outlet syndrome using somatosensory evoked responses. Arch Phys Med Rehabil 66:3–6, 1985.

7. Claggett, O. Research and prosearch (presidential address). J Thorac Cardiovasc Surg 44:153–166, 1962.

8. Cooper, A. On exostosis, in Cooper, B.B., Cooper, A., and Travers, B. (eds): Surgical Essays, 1st Am. ed. Philadelphia, James Webster, 1821, p 128.

9. Coote, H. Exostosis of the left transverse process of the seventh cervical vertebra surrounded by blood vessels and nerves: Successful removal. Lancet 1:360, 1861.

10. Dale, W.A., and Lewis, M.R. Management of thoracic outlet syn-

drome. Ann Surg 181:575–585, 1975.

11. Falconer, M.A., and Weddell, G. Costoclavicular compression of the subclavian artery and vein: Relation to scalenus anticus syndrome. Lancet 2:539–544, 1943.

12. Gilliatt, R.W., LeQuesne, P.M., Logue, V., et al: Wasting of the hand associated with a cervical rib or band. J Neurol Neurosurg Psychiatry 33:615–624, 1970.

13. Gilliatt, R.W. The classical neurological syndrome associated with a cervical rib or band, in Geep, J.M., Lemens, H.A., Roos, D.B., and Urschel, N.C. (ed): *Pain in Shoulder and Arm.* The Hague, Martinus Nijhoff, 1979, pp 173–183.

14. Halstead, W.S. An experimental study of circumscribed dilation of an artery immediately distal to partially occluding band and its bearing on the dilation of the subclavian artery observed in certain cases of cervical rib. J Exp Med 24:271–286, 1916.

15. Hempel, G.K., Rusher, A.H., Jr., and Wheeler, C.G. Supraclavicular resection of first rib for thoracic outlet syndrome. Am J Surg 141:213–215, 1981.

16. Jerrett, S.A., Cuzzone, L.J., and Pasternak, B.M. Thoracic outlet syndrome: Electrophysiologic reappraisal. Arch Neurol 41:960–963, 1984.

17. Kaye, B.L. Neurologic changes with excessively large breasts. South Med J 65(2):177–180, 1972.

18. Kelly, T.R. Thoracic outlet syndrome. Ann Surg 190:657–662, 1979.

19. Kline, D.G., Hackett, E.R., and Happel, L.H. Surgery for lesions of the brachial plexus. Arch Neurol 43:170–181, 1986.

20. Kofoed, H. Thoracic outlet syndrome: Diagnostic evaluation by analgesic cervical disk puncture. Clin Orthop 156:145–148, 1981.

21. Leffert, R. Thoracic outlet syndrome, in Omer, G.E., and Spinner, M. (eds): *Management of Peripheral Nerve Problems.* Philadelphia, Saunders, 1980.

22. Leffert, R.D. Thoracic outlet syndrome and the shoulder. Clin Sports Med 2:439–452, 1983.

23. Lord, J.W., and Rosati, L. Neurovascular compression syndrome of the upper extremity. Clin Symp 10:35–62, 1958.

24. Lord, J.W., and Rosati, L.M. Thoracic outlet syndromes. Clin Symp 23(2):1–32, 1971.

25. Nelson, R.M., and Davis, R.W.T. Thoracic outlet syndrome. Ann Thorac Surg 8:437–451, 1969.

26. Peet, R.M., Hendriksen, J.D., Anderson, T.P., and Martin, G.M. Thoracic outlet syndrome: Evaluation of therapeutic exercise program. Mayo Clin Proc 31:281–287, 1956.

27. Roos, D.B. Experience with first rib resection for thoracic outlet syndrome. Arch Surg 173:429, 1971.

28. Roos, D.B. Congenital anomalies associated with thoracic outlet syndrome. Am J Surg 132:771–778, 1976.

29. Roos, D.B. The place for scalenectomy and first rib resection in thoracic outlet syndrome. Surgery 92:1078, 1982.

30. Saldler, T.R., Rainer, W.G., and Twombley, G. Thoracic outlet compression application of positional arteriographic and nerve conduction studies. Am J Surg 130:704–706, 1975.

31. Sanders, R.J., Monsour, J.W., and Baer, S.B. Transaxillary first rib resection for the thoracic outlet syndrome. Arch Surg 97:1014–1023, 1968.

32. Sanders, R.J., Monsour, J.W., Gerber, W.F., Adams, W.R., and Thompson, N. Scalenectomy versus first rib resection for treatment of the thoracic outlet syndrome. Surgery 85(1):109–121, 1979.

33. Telford, E.D., and Mottershead, S. Pressure at the cervico-brachial junction: An operative and anatomical study. J Bone Joint Surg 30B:249–265, 1948.

34. Urschel, H.C., et al: Reoperation for recurrent thoracic outlet syndrome. Ann Thorac Surg 21:19–26, 1976.

35. Wilbourn, A.J. Slowing across the thoracic outlet with thoracic outlet syndrome: Fact or fiction. Neurology 34(suppl):1, 1984 p 143.

36. Wilbourn, A.J., and Lederman, R.J. Evidence for conduction delay in thoracic outlet syndrome is challenged. N Engl J Med 310:1052–1053, 1984.

37. Wright, I.S. The neurovascular syndrome produced by hyperabduction of the arms. Am Heart J 29:1–19, 1945.

38. Yiannikas, C., and Walsh, J.C. Somatosensory evoked responses in the diagnosis of thoracic outlet syndrome. J Neurol Neurosurg Psychiatry 46:234–240, 1983.

39. Youmans, C.R., and Smiley, R.H. Thoracic outlet syndrome with negative Adson's and hyperabduction maneuvers. Vasc Surg 14:318–329, 1980.

CHAPTER 41

Neuromuscular Disorders in the Upper Extremity

Donald K. Bynum

CEREBRAL PALSY

Surgery of the upper extremity has a definite, but limited, role in the management of cerebral palsy. The degree of involvement of the upper extremity runs the gamut from essentially none in diplegia to severe in the total-care spastic quadriplegic. Thus, the goals of surgery may range from improving function to merely enhancing cosmesis. Occasionally, a procedure is indicated for hygienic reasons. The key to successful surgical treatment is a good matchup of treatment goals, expectations of parents and patient, and surgical procedures. Achieving this matchup may be harder with these patients than in any other field of orthopaedics. This chapter is not intended to go into the details of operative procedures but is intended to serve as a general guide to understanding.

General Principles and Preoperative Evaluation

There are few hard and fast rules to guide the selection process, but some principles have gained general acceptance. Tendon lengthening gives a more predictable outcome than tendon transfer.[18] Lengthening both weakens the muscle and diminishes the stretch reflex and will not result in a reverse deformity. Muscles that are overactive during opposite functions, i.e., during both grasp and release, may cause a reverse deformity if transferred[18] and should be released or lengthened[18,26] rather than transferred. Tendon transfers should be performed using muscles which the patient can voluntarily control or using muscles which function synergistically.[26] Rigid joint or bony deformities cannot be corrected by tendon transfers alone.[47] Joints which cannot be controlled by voluntary muscle actions should be tenodesed or arthrodesed prior to tendon transfer.[19] The surgeon should bear in mind, however, that the tenodesis effect of a movable wrist joint is extremely important[18,19,58] and should usually be preserved. Arthrodesis is the last resort in management of the wrist.[18,34]

When the goal is improved hand function, the hemiplegic or quadriplegic is more likely to reap significant gains[19,61] than the already minimally involved diplegic. However, the better the hand is preoperatively, the better the end result.[58] Therefore, if a diplegic has a specific definable problem, it should certainly be addressed. The concept of improvement is relative. A poor hand can be improved to fair, and a good hand can be made better, but none will be made normal. The ultimate defect is not in the hand but in the central nervous system and is not currently amenable to our manipulations.

The outcome of surgery in patients with athetosis is unpredictable. In general, surgery should be avoided in athetosis. A possible exception is arthrodesis of a joint in which the arthrodesis has been preoperatively simulated by precise long-term casting, splinting, or pin fixation. However, there is insufficient support of this criterion in the literature to recommend it without reservation.

The factors which correlate best with a successful outcome are intelligence or cognition, sensibility, voluntary muscle control in the hand, motivation, placement of the hand in space, and age of the patient.[18,26,29,58]

Average intelligence is not necessary for a successful surgical result.[58] However, an IQ of 70 or above is desirable[18,61] if the patient is to cooperate with a postoperative rehabilitation regimen. The success of a hygienic procedure usually does not depend on the patient's IQ.

Most authors agree that good sensibility in the hand is a prerequisite for a good result in which improved function is the goal of surgery.[18,26,29] Gross sensibility is almost always present. Two-point discrimination, stereognosis, graphesthesia, and texture discrimination are useful tests[18,26] to assess sensory impairment. Of these, two-point discrimination is probably the most reliable[50] when the patient is old enough and intelligent enough to cooperate with the test. If two-point discrimination is not better than 10 to 12 mm, there is probably insufficient sensory input to control the hand except by visual cues.[50] There is no documentable improvement in sensory function following surgery.[20] Hand function may be improved by surgery, but this will not be because of, or lead to, any improvement in sensory feedback.

As might be expected, the quality of voluntary muscle control the patient exhibits is a good correlate in predicting the success of an operation.[29] Although the need for control in the hand is obvious, the need for control of placement is just as important. The hand cannot be used if it cannot be placed at the point of application. The ability to place the involved hand on the head and then to the opposite knee within 5 s is considered a favorable indicator of achieving improved function.[25] Where primitive mass reflexes (tonic neck reflex, etc.) interfere with motor control, there is poor functional potential.[26]

Age is important, but less so than the above considerations. Older patients may have disassociated themselves from the disabled limb and thus would not be good candidates for functional improvement; cosmetic improvement, however, could be achieved.[58] The pattern of functional deformity can be reliably determined by age 3,[18] and so surgery should be performed over the next few years.[61] The patient will not likely gain more selective muscle control when surgery is performed early, but may learn to use the new pattern more readily than if the change is delayed until the child is older.

Candidates for functional improvement should have favorable assessments in at least two, preferably three, of the above areas. Cosmetic and hygienic improvement are readily achieved and the decision for surgery rests with those special considerations, not with the other factors mentioned above.

One final parameter which can be used preoperatively to judge the likelihood of success is motivation. Some authors[58,64] consider motivation to be the most important factor and point out that intelligence is usually but not always a prerequisite to motivation. There is no reliable means of measuring motivation, but all orthopaedic surgeons recognize that its presence or absence can make or break the outcome of a surgical procedure. Good motivation cannot ensure a good outcome in cerebral palsy surgery; on the other hand, if improved function is the goal, absence of motivation will result in complete failure.

Muscle testing of patients with cerebral palsy is very complicated. Preoperatively, the surgeon must determine not only the strength of a muscle but also the degree of voluntary control of the muscle; the level of activity of the muscle during each separate functional task (phasic activity) such as grasp, release, and pinch; and finally whether the muscle is subject to pathologic reflexes such as the stretch reflex, clonus, or retained infantile reflexes.[18,26,61] This type of examination is difficult, but with experience it can be fairly reliable. An electromyogram can be used to supplement manual muscle testing.[18,28] Preoperative and postoperative evaluation with EMG is becoming more widespread and is providing exciting new insights into surgical and nonsurgical treatment of cerebral palsy.

Another adjunct to the preoperative evaluation is myoneural blockade of the spastic muscles with alcohol or local anesthetic.[6] Alcohol blockade will last for several weeks. This gives some time for the uninjected muscles to show their true strength.[18] Thus the patient and surgeon will have a better idea of what to expect from tendon lengthening or release.

Treatment of Specific Regions

Shoulder

Surgical correction is seldom required at the shoulder. Typical posturing includes adduction and internal rotation. If this position limits hand placement, lengthening of the pectoralis major and subscapularis is the recommended procedure[61] and should be augmented by aggressive physical therapy postoperatively. Rotational osteotomy of the humerus is rarely indicated.

Elbow

The usual deformity at the elbow is flexion, either as contracture or dynamic "overflow," or as a combination of both. When elbow flexion limits hand placement, appropriate correction should be attempted.[58] This will usually occur at 45 degrees or greater contracture.[61] Excessive spasticity may result in worsened elbow flexion during walking, and this is another indication for release at the elbow. Surgical correction is directed at the primary elbow flexors.[48] The lacertus fibrosus should be released, the biceps tendon Z-lengthened, and the brachialis lengthened by incision of its distal aponeurosis. Anterior capsulotomy of the elbow may be required in more severe cases or in older children. This procedure results in an average improvement of 40 degrees of extension, retains active elbow flexion sufficient to enable patients to place the hand to the mouth, and it provides lasting correction. Loss of supination has not been a problem with this procedure.

Forearm

Pronation contracture of the forearm is common in cerebral palsy.[61] This may be reduced by releasing the pronator teres from its insertion or by rerouting it to act as a supinator.[56] Occasionally the pronator quadratus will require release.[61] Some improvement in supination may follow a flexor-pronator slide or transfer of flexor muscles around the ulnar border of the forearm to the dorsum of the hand or wrist.[21] Neutral rotation is the optimum position and excessive supination should be avoided.[18]

Wrist and Hand

In the wrist and hand, the usual problems are flexed position of the wrist, flexed fingers, and thumb-in-palm deformity. These deformities result from the flexor muscles being stronger and more spastic than the extensors. Functionally, the impairments include a poor release of grasp because of the finger flexor spasticity, a weak opening of the hand due to weak finger extensors, a weak grasp because the wrist is held in flexion during grasp, and an inability to open the hand with the thumb retracted out of the palm. An occasional patient will have swan neck deformity of the fingers. Surgical procedures to improve function are generally aimed at diminishing flexor spasticity, augmenting extensor strength, or creating a more stable joint by arthrodesis, tenodesis, or capsulodesis. Cosmetic and hygienic procedures involve releasing tight contractures and stabilizing joint position by arthrodesis.

The majority of patients who are candidates for functional reconstruction have weak finger extension.[28,64] Surgery may be directed either at weakening the flexor tightness or strengthening finger extension, or both. The flexor-pronator slide has been used successfully in the past as a utilitarian procedure to provide improved function, control, and cosmesis.[32,55,62,64] Objections to this procedure are that some patients may lose too much grip strength or may develop a reverse deformity and that the procedure is not selective enough in patients who already have some selective control.[18,26] Another observation is that when the flexor pollicis longus origin is released as part of the flexor-pronator slide, the existing balance of the thumb-in-palm deformity is changed. Correction of the thumb deformity must then be delayed until the effects of this rebalancing can be determined.

A more selective approach would combine the clinical classification of Zancolli and Zancolli[67–69] with the use of preoperative EMG evaluation[28] to determine whether lengthening or specific transfers would be appropriate. Patients can be grouped into three categories. In group 1, mild, the patient can fully extend the fingers while the wrist remains flexed 20 degrees or less. Group 2 patients can extend the fingers only while the wrist is flexed more than 20 degrees. This group is also assessed on the basis of whether any degree of active wrist extension is possible while the fingers are held flexed. The group 2A patients have selective wrist extension, whereas the group 2B patients do not. Group 3 patients are severely involved and lack any active extension of either wrist or fingers. Present EMG and clinical data indicate that muscles which are active during a desired activity can be reliably transferred whereas those that are active during all phases of the grasp-release cycle or when the limb is at rest should be lengthened or released. Muscles with isolated activity in grasp should be transferred preferentially to improve grasp whereas those with isolated activity in release should be preferentially transferred to improve release.[28] Thus, if the flexor carpi ulnaris (FCU) is overactive during release, it can be tenotomized or lengthened in the mild (group 1) patient or transferred[21] (Green and Banks) to the extensor digitorum communis (EDC) to augment finger extension in the group 2A patient. If the patient's release is adequate but wrist extension is poor (group 2B), the FCU can be transferred to the extensor carpi radialis brevis (ECRB). This will also enhance grip strength by placing the wrist into a more extended position. The surgeon should confirm preoperatively, however, that the patient has active finger extension when the wrist is passively held in the desired degree of extension (usually neutral). Transfer of the FCU to the EDC is the more reliable procedure.[28,58]

When strengthening of a weak grasp is desired, several alternatives bear consideration. If the FCU is overactive in grasp but not in release, it is logical to transfer it to the ECRB. This transfer should not be performed when the FCU is overactive in release and the patient lacks finger extension. Alternatively, a flexor digitorum superficialis (FDS) can be transferred to the ECRB as a synergistic transfer.

Another alternative for improving hand function is to use a muscle such as the brachioradialis, extensor carpi ulnaris, extensor carpi radialis longus, or flexor carpi radialis to augment finger or thumb extension.[18,19,29,33,34,49,50,60] These transfers can be used to take advantage of the tenodesis effect of wrist motion and do not depend on the phasic activity of the transferred muscle if there is adequate wrist motion to produce the desired tenodesis.

In the severely involved hand, the EMGs will show overactivity in all attempted phases of grasp. In that instance, lengthening of all the flexors by proximal muscle slide or Z lengthening at the wrist will provide cosmetic and hygienic improvement. Some surgeons prefer Z lengthening because the degree of lengthening can be more precisely controlled, thus lessening the chance of overcorrection. The superficialis-to-profundus (STP)[1] procedure is also used for this purpose. In the STP procedure the tendons of the FDS are transected distally, the tendons of the FDP are transected proximally, and then the proximal tendons of the FDS are sutured to the distal tendons of the FDP. The net result is a substantial lengthening, but not complete release, of the finger flexors. Carpectomy or proximal-row carpectomy[54] is an alternate method of effectively weakening tight flexors and retaining wrist motion for its tenodesis effect. This procedure is useful when wrist contracture is so severe that neurovascular structures limit the amount of extension which might be obtained with muscle-tendon lengthenings. Transfers can be combined with proximal row carpectomy to provide additional balance.

Some patients with spastic cerebral palsy will have swan neck deformities of the fingers. This occurs when there is significant wrist and metacarpophalangeal joint flexion combined with sufficient tenodesis of the extensor digitorum communis to hyperextend supple PIP joints.[63] Tenodesis of the PIP joint into flexion using a slip of the flexor digitorum superficialis[63] provides reliable, durable correction of this problem.

Thumb

The usual deformity of the thumb is referred to as the thumb-in-palm deformity. The functional problems this imposes include small grip span and ineffective grip because the thumb blocks access to the palm. Pinch may be impossible. There are several components of this deformity, any of which can occur in combination with the others. These are an adduction contracture of the thumb–index finger web space, malposition of the metacarpophalangeal joint consisting of either flexion contracture or hyperextension, tightness of the flexor pollicis longus, and/or weakness of the extrinsic extensors of the thumb. The exact deformity depends on the severity of the imbalance between the intrinsic and extrinsic muscles. Treatment must be individualized using any of several accepted procedures. Correction of the thumb-in-palm deformity is usually reserved until other upper extremity deformities have been corrected[33] but may be combined with other procedures when the surgeon has enough experience and confidence to do so.[18]

In the mildly involved patient adduction contracture may be the only significant deformity of the thumb. Release of the insertion of the adductor pollicis and the metacarpal origin of the first dorsal interosseous muscle and its fascia has been considered the "classical" release. Myotenotomy of the entire adductor insertion can result in complete loss of adduction and thus loss of any ability to pinch. This complication may be avoided if only the metacarpal origins of the adductor are released[39,40,67] or, alternatively, if the tendon of insertion of the transverse head alone is released.[27] EMGs correlated with clinical follow-up confirm that grip span can be improved, pinch retained, and overcorrection avoided in mildly involved patients if only the transverse fibers of the adductor are released.[27] If the adduction involves other components of the thumb-in-palm deformity, a partial release of the adductor may be inadequate. Z-plasty of the thumb–index finger web space is usually required in all but mild cases. Bone block fusion of the thumb and index metacarpals into an abducted position has been successfully performed[35] but has not gained universal acceptance because the lack of some residual thumb adduction is felt to impair pinch too severely.[58,60]

The metacarpophalangeal (MP) joint may be held in flexion by overactive intrinsics, or it may be in hyperextension. The latter occurs when there is ligamentous laxity, the adduction contracture is severe, and the flexor pollicis longus is not as spastic as the other muscles.[29] The MP joint is then pulled into hyperextension by the extrinsic extensors.

Release of the flexion deformity requires releasing or recessing the intrinsic insertions or releasing the intrinsic origins. If the intrinsic insertions are released, the MP joint should be stabilized to prevent hyperextension. Reattaching the insertions along the metacarpal neck[12] will preserve some flexion strength to the thumb metacarpal, thus helping preserve active grasp and pinch. Release of the origins of the flexor brevis and part of the abductor brevis as well as the adductor can be performed through a volar-thenar crease incision.[39,40] This approach is intended to avoid overcorrection of the MP joint. When stabilization of the MP joint is necessary, either arthrodesis or capsulodesis[14,67] is effective. Arthrodesis of the MP joint should place the thumb in position for pulp-to-pulp pinch with the index and long fingers. This is usually about 20 degrees flexion and 20 degrees opposition.[61] Spasticity of the flexor pollicis longus (FPL) may be mild, or it may be the main deforming force. The FPL must be released in all but the mildest cases.[18,39] Frequently, the contribution of the FPL to the deformity is overlooked until correction of wrist flexion increases the tightness of the FPL. Either Z lengthening of the FPL tendon or fractional lengthening at the musculotendinous junction will relieve the excessive tightness. It is important to avoid overlengthening since instability of the interphalangeal (IP) joint may result.

Weakness of the thumb extensors is variable. Alcohol myoneural blockade of the FPL, FPB, and adductor pollicis may provide clues as to whether reinforcement of extension will be necessary to correct the thumb-in-palm deformity. Several options are available. A prerequisite to strengthening extrinsic extension is that the MP joint is stable. Combination extension and abduction is provided when the EPL is rerouted to the radial-volar aspect of the radius[18,19,33] and augmented by transferring the brachioradialis, flexor carpi radialis, palmaris longus, or a flexor digitorum superficialis to the FPL.

The desired abduction component of the correction can be enhanced by rerouting the extensor pollicis longus through the origin of the abductor pollicis brevis.[33] In some instances the surgeon may prefer to augment the extensor pollicis brevis or the abductor pollicis longus[34] as there may be less tendency for these procedures to destabilize the MP joint into hyperextension.[60] The procedure chosen will depend on the exact positions of the thumb and wrist and upon the stability of the MP and trapeziometacarpal joints.

Correction of the thumb-in-palm deformity has been classified and approached systematically[29,49] but remains the most difficult aspect of the upper extremity in cerebral palsy in which to correct deformity and yet maintain function. The least satisfactory results are from attempts to attain opposition by means of opponensplasty.[33] The goals of treatment in the thumb should be to correct the deformity, to maintain useful grip, to attain pulp-to-pulp pinch (not necessarily tip-to-tip pinch), and, as in all aspects of upper extremity surgery in cerebral palsy, to avoid overcorrection.

ARTHROGRYPOSIS

Treatment of the upper extremities of patients with arthrogryposis should begin immediately after birth. Splinting and active and passive range-of-motion programs are the initial modes of treatment. Early surgery may occasionally be indicated but is usually deferred until at least 2 years of age.[2,13,17,22] This allows time for the parents, therapists, and physicians to carefully assess not only the obvious deformities but also to assess the child's functional attributes as well as deficits. In addition, muscle testing becomes more reliable as the child gets older and more cooperative. Patients' adaptations may make surgery unnecessary, and potentially detrimental procedures can be avoided.[13,38]

Typical deformities in arthrogryposis include internal rotation and adduction contractures or posturing at the shoulders, elbows in either flexion or extension with a limited arc of motion, forearms in pronation, wrists in flexion and ulnar deviation, hands with thumb-in-palm, and stiff fingers with varying degrees of flexion contracture.[2,17] Fortunately, the thumb, although adducted, is frequently relatively spared and has some functioning intrinsic muscles. Skin creases are poorly developed, probably reflecting the lack of joint motion.

Associated anomalies in the upper extremities include dislocation of the radial head, radioulnar synostosis, cubital recurvatum, simian hands, syndactyly, constriction bands, and bilateral radial nerve palsy.[13,17]

Since each patient is unique, treatment should be individualized. Nonetheless, certain goals and principles should guide the therapeutic plan. The two primary functional goals in the upper extremity are self-feeding and independent toilet care.[12] Patient should not be deprived of one of these functions in an effort to provide the other.[2]

Recurrence of corrected deformities is common especially when muscle balancing alone or osteotomy alone is used.[38] Recurrent deformity "results principally from the rigid and thick capsule and periarticular tissues, which do not stretch as the limb grows. These structures seem to be the key to the successful treatment of arthrogryposis in the growing child."[13] Combinations of soft tissue and bony procedures also seem more durable than either alone. Some specific recommendations are discussed in the paragraphs below and in Table 41-1.

Shoulder

In spite of the frequency of internal rotation contracture of the shoulder, surgical correction is rarely required.[2,13] This is because most activities of personal care and hygiene are performed with the shoulder internally rotated to varying degrees. In fact, most tasks of daily living and jobs are per-

TABLE 41-1 Summary of Recommended Surgical Treatment in the Arthrogrypotic Upper Extremity

Joint	Problem	Procedure(s)
Shoulder	Internal rotation contracture	Derotational osteotomy; lengthen subscapularis and pectoralis; internal fixation; spica cast
Elbow	Extension contracture, no active flexion	Posterior elbow capsule release, triceps lengthening; pectoralis or triceps flexorplasty
Wrist	Excessive flexion, ulnar deviation	Volar capsule release, transfer FCU to ECRB; also carpectomy, fusion, or osteotomy if severe
Thumb	Thumb-in-palm deformity	Web deepening plus skin graft or flap; MP fusion; fractional lengthening of FPL; tendon transfers for abduction and extension when indicated and feasible
Digits	PIP flexion deformity	Volar release plus skin graft if active motion is present; PIP arthrodesis if severe; no surgery if deformity mild

formed in front of the body, and thus the shoulders are in internal rotation. Occasionally, however, shoulder internal rotation is so severe that the hand cannot be brought to the mouth when the elbow is flexed.[3] In such cases, correction of the rotary malalignment should be performed.

Carroll and Hill[8] report performing shoulder fusion prior to triceps transfer for elbow flexion. Most authors recommend derotational osteotomy combined with release or lengthening of the pectoralis major and subscapularis. Soft tissue release alone has failed to provide good lasting correction.[2,13,38] The radial nerve may be located more anteriorly than expected and extra caution is advisable.[13] Failure to maintain the desired derotation is likely unless a spica cast and/or internal fixation is used to prevent the arm from resting in an internally rotated position during healing.

The staging of shoulder and elbow procedures should be carefully considered in each case. Usually correction of shoulder malrotation is performed prior to tendon transfers to give elbow flexion. However, if extension contracture of the elbow makes it difficult to judge the axis of elbow flexion, the surgeon might prefer to perform the elbow release first. If the pectoralis major is to be transferred for elbow flexion, it should not be released at the shoulder because subsequent myostatic contracture would reduce its effectiveness as a transfer. In such a case a controlled lengthening of the pectoralis might be preferable or shoulder and elbow correction could be performed simultaneously.

Elbow

The elbow is the critical factor in upper extremity function in the arthrogrypotic. Most patients have bilateral fixed extension contractures. Only occasional patients have fixed flexion deformity.[2] The goals of treatment at the elbow are to enable patients to actively oppose both hands in a two-handed grip, to enable them to get at least one hand to the mouth and one to the perineum, and to enable them to push themselves out of a chair.[12,13] In order to achieve these goals, existing elbow

motion must be placed into a more functional arc or the motion must be increased, and usually it must be reinforced by a tendon transfer to provide flexion power. The pitfall to avoid is any accidental removal of extension power from both elbows by performing bilateral triceps to biceps transfers.[8]

Probably more benefit is derived from a successful elbow flexorplasty than from any other procedure in an arthrogrypotic's upper extremity. The shoulder should be addressed first if necessary, then the elbow extension contracture released, and then, or simultaneously, the flexorplasty performed. Posterior elbow release must be performed prior to the development of secondary changes in the bony architecture and is achieved most reliably by posterior capsulotomy combined with triceps tendon lengthening.[2,17] Extension deformity recurs following flexion osteotomy alone.

Pectoralis Transfer

Transfer of the pectoralis major seems to be the best elbow flexorplasty in arthrogrypotics.[13] Several variations have been described, but transferring the entire muscle seems superior to transferring only the sternal head.[2,12]

Pectoralis transfer can achieve a 90-degree arc of active motion.[2] This procedure allows preservation of extensor (triceps) function if present and may augment shoulder flexion.[9] The pectoralis transfer can be performed bilaterally since active elbow extension is not sacrificed; however tension on the transfers should be adjusted to allow sufficient elbow extension on at least one side for the hand to reach the perineum (Fig. 41-1).

The reader is referred to the works of Clark,[10] Carroll and Kleinman,[9] and Brooks and Seddon[5] for details of the pectoralis transfer.

Triceps Transfer

Anterior transfer of the insertion of the triceps is an alternative elbow flexorplasty. Whereas this procedure can provide a good arc of motion in posttraumatic and paralytic cases, the

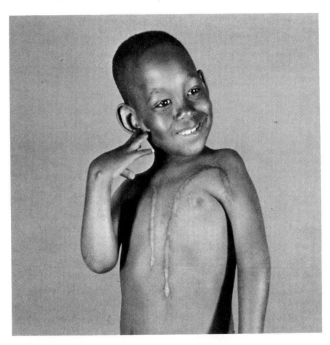

Figure 41-1 This patient has had bilateral pectoralis major transfers for elbow flexion. Active motion is 50 to 105 degrees on the right and 20 to 70 degrees on the left. These arcs allow both hands to function together in bimanual tasks, but they also allow the right hand to reach the mouth and the left hand to reach the perineum. Active elbow extension is preserved, although weak.

average arc of motion in arthrogrypotics is quite limited, averaging only 43 degrees in one series.[8] Still, some arc of elbow motion is better than none, and any improvement can help the arthrogrypotic patient tremendously. Most patients require release of the elbow extension contracture prior to triceps transfer. The average flexion contracture of the elbow after completion of the triceps transfer is approximately 60 degrees; thus, this procedure should not be performed bilaterally.

The details of the triceps transfer are described by Carroll.[7,8]

Steindler Flexorplasty

The Steindler technique of flexorplasty transplants the common flexor-pronator origin proximally and laterally on the humerus. This usually results in a flexion contracture and some active flexion. In the arthrogrypotic patient this is a weak transfer and in fact tends to aggravate flexion deformity of the wrist and fingers because wrist and finger extension are so weak or absent.[13] Although the Steindler flexorplasty is easier to perform than the pectoralis transfer, it is a less desirable procedure because it provides relatively weak flexion power and aggravates hand deformity.

Wrist

The typical deformity at the wrist is flexion and ulnar deviation. Wrist, finger, and thumb extension are weak or absent.

Correction of the deformities may be desirable to improve opposition of the hands and also to improve appearance. Before attempting complete correction, the surgeon should bear in mind that many functions of personal care (perineal hygiene, clothing fastening, etc.) are best performed with the wrist in slight flexion. In general, grip is stronger with the wrist in dorsiflexion, but severe arthrogrypotics lack sufficient wrist extensors or muscles for transfer to gain a good arc of wrist motion, and finger extensor power is too weak to extend the digits against tight finger flexors with the wrist dorsiflexed. In the mildly involved patient, wrist dorsiflexion and power grip can be attained, but this is probably the exception rather than the rule. Those patients with poor elbow motion, especially those with fixed extension, will actually require wrist flexion for optimum function.[2] Finally, neurovascular structures are frequently the limiting factor and may not allow dorsiflexion unless sufficient bone is removed.

There is a high recurrence rate when either soft tissue release or osteotomy is performed alone.[2,38] As mentioned previously, a key component of correcting these deformities is complete release of the restricting portions of the capsule, but this must be augmented by other measures. Functioning wrist flexors, if present, should be transferred to the dorsum.[2,59] Osteotomy can be combined with soft tissue release. Proximal-row carpectomy or wrist fusion can be used in older children,[59] but, again, supplemental soft tissue balancing will help prevent recurrence. Long-term night splinting is an integral part of the postoperative regimen and may need to be continued to skeletal maturity.

Although there are problems with recurrent deformity, the benefits to be gained make the effort worthwhile. It has been stated that "correction of the wrist deformity by carpectomy has done more to improve the position of the fingers than any single procedure performed in the hand itself."[13]

Hand

The principal problems in the hand are thumb-in-palm deformity and flexion contractures in the fingers. Despite these problems, arthrogrypotics show remarkable adaptability of hand function. A careful, cautious preoperative evaluation is vital so that only as little surgery as necessary is done in the hand.[13,65] When judiciously selected for surgery, patients can expect some improved function 75 percent of the time.[2]

Thumb function fortunately is frequently better spared than that of the other digits. If the thumb-in-palm deformity requires treatment, a variety of procedures are known to be successful. All approaches require a web space deepening. In the vast majority, the addition of skin (graft or flap) is essential to reduce recurrence. Adductor release, metacarpophalangeal fusion, metacarpal osteotomy, lengthening of flexor pollicus longus, and tendon transfer for extension-abduction should be performed as necessary to achieve correction.[2,13,46,59]

Attempts to improve the total arc of joint motion in the fingers have been unsuccessful but the functional position of the fingers can be improved. Skin grafting is recommended if contracture release is attempted. If useful grasp is blocked by severely flexed digits, the procedure of choice is probably proximal interphalangeal (PIP) joint arthrodesis in a more functional position.

TETRAPLEGIA

The recovery of upper extremity function is the restoration most desired by most tetraplegics.[36] Nonetheless, the surgeon must maintain a realistic perspective and not rush, force, or overstate the value of surgery. The goal of surgery is to maximize residual function; it cannot restore the hand to normality. When appropriately selected, 75 percent or more of tetraplegics can be significantly improved by reconstructive hand surgery.[23,24,36,52,66] Suitable criteria include: (1) sensibility with two-point discrimination less than 10 mm in at least part of the median nerve distribution, (2) plateau of neurological recovery—this usually means no sooner than one year after injury, (3) grade 4 (Medical Research Council[45]) or better muscles available for transfer, (4) no uncontrolled spasticity, (5) no excessive pain in the hand, and (6) psychological stability and motivation.[44,45] Success depends on proper detailed preoperative evaluation, selection of procedures and postoperative rehabilitation.[24,51,52] Advances in microcomputer technology coupled with electrical stimulation will probably significantly alter treatment and surgical indications in the next decade.

Historically, tetraplegia injuries have been referred to by the level of injury to the spinal column, i.e., C5–C6, C7, etc. Neurological level, however, frequently does not correspond to vertebral level because of asymmetry, incomplete lesions, ascending vascular lesions, and anatomical anomalies. In 1978, an international conference in Edinburgh, Scotland, brought about worldwide acceptance of a classification scheme based on (1) presence or absence of useful cutaneous sensibility, (2) lowest functioning muscle with MRC grade 4 strength, and (3) rating each extremity separately. Table 41-2 lists this classification as subsequently modified in 1984 in Giens, France.[42] Shoulder and elbow function are evaluated independently of the International Classification.

Surgical Goals

In general terms, realistic goals are to improve the performance of daily activities and to minimize or eliminate the need for splinting. The priority should be to first establish elbow control and then reconstruct the hand.[44,51,52] If the hand is reconstructed first, its rehabilitation or use will be interrupted by the immobilization necessary following triceps reconstruction. Function of the brachioradialis is enhanced by elbow extension; thus triceps reconstruction should be accomplished first so that the tension of the brachioradialis transfer can be set accordingly.

Patients in the lower groups of the International Classification (higher levels of cord injury) are candidates for procedures designed to enhance simple tenodesis grip. Those in the intermediate categories can achieve stronger grasp with some finger intrinsic balance, whereas thumb control can be refined in those in the higher categories. The better hand should be reconstructed first.[52] This would be the dominant hand in the event that both hands are neurologically equal. If neurologically unequal, the better hand should be addressed first regardless of previous hand dominance.

Elbow

When the deltoid and biceps are functioning but the triceps is weak, the patient may be a candidate for reconstruction of

TABLE 41-2   International Classification for Surgery of the Hand in Tetraplegia (Edinburgh 1978; Modified in Giens, France, 1984)

Sensibility:* O or CU	Group*	Motor Characteristics	Description of function
	0	No muscle below elbow suitable for transfer	Flexion of the elbow
	1	BR	May have weak wrist extension
	2	+ ECRL	Extension of the wrist (weak or strong)
	3	+ ECRB	Extension of the wrist (weak or strong)
	4	+ PT	Extension of the wrist (strong)
	5	+ FCR	Flexion of the wrist
	6	+ Finger extensors	Extrinsic extensors of the fingers
	7	+ Thumb extensors	Extrinsic extensor of the thumb
	8	+ Partial digital flexors	Extrinsic flexors of the digits (weak)
	9	Lacks only intrinsics	Extrinsic flexors of the digits
	X	Exceptions	

*Motor grouping assumes that all listed muscles are grade 4 (MRC) or better and a new muscle is added for each group; for example, a group 3 patient will have BR, ECRL, and ECRB rated at least grade 4 (MRC). If 10-mm or less "two-point" discrimination in the thumb and index finger, the correct classification would be CU 3 where the CU stands for the fact that the patient has adequate cutaneous sensibility. If "two-point" discrimination was greater than 10 mm (meaning inadequate cutaneous sensibility), the designation 0 would precede the motor group (for example, 0 3).

elbow control. Patients who have undergone both elbow and hand reconstruction feel that they have benefitted the most from reconstruction of triceps function.[59,62] The best procedure for this seems to be transfer of the posterior one-third of the deltoid to the triceps.[51,52] The posterior one-third of the deltoid is elevated from its insertion, mobilized from the middle third, and elongated using toe extensors,[51,52] tibialis anterior,[15] or fascia lata,[24] as graft material. Reinsertion is accomplished both through the distal triceps tendon[51,52] and the olecranon.[24] Postoperative rehabilitation should rigidly adhere to Moberg's guidelines of graduated increases in motion for 6 weeks, lest the transfer stretch out. This reliable procedure provides the active antagonist for elbow control needed to accurately position the hand in space. Even if the hand cannot be reconstructed, this improves the patient's ability to operate power controls such as those on a wheelchair. Lastly, if elbow extension is strong enough, the patient's ability to transfer himself or herself may be improved.

Hand

Prior to Nickel's[53] introduction of the flexor-hinge hand in the 1960s, tenodesis was usually the full extent of treatment offered to patients who fell into groups 1, 2, and 3. The concept of the flexor-hinge hand involved creating a tripod pinch and concentrating power at the finger MP joints by arthrodesing the IP joints. The thumb was shortened and fused into an opposition post. Thus, strong pinch became possible in those patients who had active wrist extension. Although a variation of this reconstruction is still used by Beasley[1] and gives good strength, technically this approach is exceedingly difficult and has largely been abandoned.

Current opinion is based primarily on Moberg's work and favors maintaining a more flexible hand because it is more emotionally acceptable to patients and is also more versatile.[51,52] Key pinch (see Chap. 45, Sect. B) is preferred because it is easier to achieve than tripod pinch, it provides a broader surface contact area which enhances stability of pinch, and it minimizes the problem of an opposed thumb acting as an obstruction to grasping objects. The tenodesis effect is an integral component of the reconstruction; therefore, wrist fusion is rarely indicated, especially for the purpose of obtaining a wrist motor for transfer.

Review of Groups

Group 0 patients have no active motors below the elbow which are suitable to function independently as transfers. Brachioradialis function may be sufficiently enhanced by restoration of elbow extension that it can be converted to a wrist extensor to activate a wrist-driven flexor splint.[43]

Groups 1, 2, and 3 patients are candidates for simple hand procedures. These reconstructions depend on strong active wrist extension and create tenodeses to achieve key pinch and simple grasp. The brachioradialis can be transferred to effect wrist extension or to provide limited finger or thumb power.[16] Moberg has developed a widely accepted and reliable procedure which involves pinning the thumb IP joint, releasing the A1 pulley, tenodesing the FPL to the radius,

tenodesing the thumb MP joint to prevent excessive flexion, and releasing the extensor retinaculum to improve the mechanical advantage and strength of wrist extension. Some surgeons[24] prefer to fuse the IP joint rather than to pin it because of a high incidence of pin breakage. Brand[3] describes a rerouting of the FPL which improves its mechanical advantage without sacrificing the A1 pulley.

When the ECRB is strong enough to act alone for wrist extension (confirmation requires testing under local anesthesia at the time of surgery), more complicated reconstructions can be entertained using the ECRL as a finger flexor (FDP) transfer. Finger flexor strength introduces an element of clawing to the tenodesis release action unless an intrinsic tenodesis or transfer is added. Zancolli's two-stage reconstruction exemplifies this concept. His "lasso"[52,66] procedure is a utilitarian intrinsic transfer which works somewhat in the group 3 patients, even though the FDS is not active.[43]

Reconstruction in groups 4 and 5 patients is similar to group 3 patients except that two more muscles are available for transfer. Digital flexor, extensor, and intrinsic functions must be balanced. This usually requires at least two stages because the flexor and extensor transfers must be immobilized in different positions. Curtis,[11] House,[30] and Henderson and Lipscomb,[23] among others, have described various combinations of transfers which give good results.

In group 6, the EPL can be attached to the EDC to provide active extension of all the digits. Group 7 patients have all extensors intact. The extensor indicis proprius may be suitable for transfer.

Patients in groups 8 and 9 have FDP and FDS function, respectively. They can be approached as if for low median and ulnar nerve palsies.

House[31] has stabilized the thumbs of patients in groups 4 to 7 by means of opponens-adductor-plasty in one hand and carpometacarpal arthrodesis in the other. The hands with the transfer had stronger lateral pinch, whereas those fused had stronger grasp. The patients showed no preference for one over the other but felt the differences were complementary. Either technique alone is acceptable, thus illustrating both the acceptability and desirability of using different procedures for different goals.

REFERENCES

1. Beasley, R.W. Surgical treatment of hands for C_5-C_6 tetraplegia. Orthop Clin North Am 14:893–904, 1983.
2. Bennett, J.B., Hansen, P.E., Granberry, W.M., and Cain, T.E. Surgical management of arthrogryposis in the upper extremity. J Pediatr Orthop 5:281–286, 1985.
3. Brand, P.F. Clinical Mechanics of the Hand. St. Louis, Mosby, 1985.
4. Braun, R.M., Vise, G.T., and Roper, B. Preliminary experience with superficialis to profundus tendon transfer in the hemiplegic upper extremity. J Bone Joint Surg 56A:466–472, 1974.
5. Brooks, D.M., and Seddon, H.J. Pectoral transplantation for paralysis of flexors of the elbow. A new technique. J Bone Joint Surg 41B:35–43, February 1958.
6. Carpenter, E.B., and Mikhail, M. The use of intramuscular alcohol as a diagnostic therapeutic aide in cerebral palsy (abstract). Dev Med Child Neurol 14:113–114, 1972.

7. Carroll, R.E. Restoration of the flexor power to the flail elbow by transplantation of the triceps tendon. Surg Gynecol Obstet 95:685–688, 1952.

8. Carroll, R.E., and Hill, N.A. Triceps transfer to restore elbow flexion. J Bone Joint Surg 52A:239–244, 1970.

9. Carroll, R.E., and Kleinman, W.B. Pectoralis major transplantation to restore elbow flexion to the paralytic limb. J Hand Surg 4:(6):501–507, 1979.

10. Clark, J.P.M. Reconstruction of biceps brachii by pectoral muscle transplantation. Br J Surg 34:180–181, 1946.

11. Curtis, R.M. Tendon transfers in the patient with spinal cord injury. Orthop Clin North Am 5:415–423, 1974.

12. DeBenedetti, M. Restoration of elbow extension power in the tetraplegic patient using the Moberg technique. J Hand Surg 4:86–89, 1979.

13. Doyle, J.R., James, P.M., Larsen, L.J., and Ashley, R.K. Restoration of elbow flexion in arthrogryposis multiplex congenita. J Hand Surg 5:149–151, 1980.

14. Drummond, D.S., Siller, T.N., and Cruess, R.L. Management of arthrogryposis multiplex congenita. Instr Course Lect 23:79–95, 1974.

15. Filler, B.C., Stark, H.H., and Boyes, J.H. Capsulodesis of the metacarpophalangeal joint of the thumb in children with cerebral palsy. J Bone Joint Surg 58A:667–670, 1976.

16. Freehafer, A.A, Kelly, C.M., and Peckham, P.H. Tendon transfer for the restoration of upper limb function after a cervical spinal cord injury. J Hand Surg 9:887–893, 1984.

17. Frehafer, A.A., and Mast, W.A. Transfer of brachioradialis to improve wrist extension in high spinal-cord injury. J Bone Joint Surg 49A:648–652, 1967.

18. Friedlander, H.L., Westin, G.W., and Wood, W.L. Arthrogryposis multiplex congenita. J Bone Joint Surg 50A:89–112, 1968.

19. Goldner, J.L. Upper extremity surgical procedures for patients with cerebral palsy. Instr Course Lect 28:36–66, 1979.

20. Goldner, J.L. Upper extremity tendon transfers in cerebral palsy. Orthop Clin North Am 5:389–414, 1974.

21. Goldner, J.L., and Ferlic, D.C. Sensory status of the hand as related to reconstructive surgery of the upper extremity in cerebral palsy. Clin Orthop 46:87–92, 1966.

22. Green, W.T., and Banks, H.H. Flexor carpi ulnaris transplant and its use in cerebral palsy. J Bone Joint Surg 44A:1343–1352, 1962.

23. Hansen, O.M. Surgical anatomy and treatment of patients with arthrogryposis. J Bone Joint Surg 43B:855, 1961.

24. Henderson, E.D., Lipscomb, P.R., Elkins, E.C., Auerbach, A.M., and Magness, J.L. Review of the results of surgical treatment of patients with tetraplegis. Proceedings of the American Society for Surgery of the Hand. J Bone Joint Surg 52A:1059, 1970.

25. Hente, V.R., Brown, M., and Keshian, L.A. Upper limb reconstruction in quadriplegia: Functional assessment and proposed treatment modifications. J Hand Surg 8:119–131, 1983.

26. Hoffer, M.M. Cerebral palsy, in Green, D.P. (ed): *Operative Hand Surgery.* New York, Churchill Livingstone, 1982.

27. Hoffer, M.M. The upper extremity and cerebral palsy, in Fredericks, S., and Brody, G. (eds): *Neurological Aspects of Plastic Surgery,* vol 17. St. Louis, Mosby, 1978.

28. Hoffer, M.M., Perry, J., Garcia, M., and Bullock, D. Adduction contracture of the thumb in cerebral palsy: A pre-operative electromyographic study. J Bone Joint Surg 65A:755–759, 1983.

29. Hoffer, M.M., Perry, J., and Melkonian, G.J. Dynamic electromyography and decision-making for surgery in the upper extremity of patients with cerebral palsy. J Hand Surg 4:424–431, 1979.

30. House, J.H., Gwathmey, F.W., and Fiddler, M.O. A dynamic approach to the thumb-in-palm deformity in cerebral palsy: Evaluation and results in 56 patients. J Bone Joint Surg 63A:216–225, 1981.

31. House, J.H., and Shannon, M.A. Restoration of strong grasp and lateral pinch in tetraplegia due to cervical spinal cord injury. J Hand Surg 1:152–159, September, 1976.

32. House, J.H., and Shannon, M.A. Restoration of strong grasp and lateral pinch in tetraplegia: A comparison of two methods of thumb control in each patient. J Hand Surg 10:22–29, 1985.

33. Inglis, A.E, and Cooper, W. Release of the flexor-pronator origin for flexion deformities of the hand and wrist in spastic paralysis: A study of 18 cases. J Bone Joint Surg 48A:847–857, 1966.

34. Inglis, A.E., Cooper, W., and Bruton, W. Surgical correction of thumb deformities in spastic paralysis. J Bone Joint Surg 52A:253–268, 1970.

35. Keats, S. Surgical treatment of the hand in cerebral palsy: Correction of thumb-in-palm and other deformities. Report of nineteen cases. J Bone Joint Surg 47A:274–284, 1965.

36. Lam, S.J.S. A modified technique for stabilizing the spastic thumb. J Bone Joint Surg 54B:522–525, 1972.

37. Lamb, D.W., and Chan, K.M. Surgical reconstruction of the upper limb in traumatic tetraplegia. J Bone Joint Surg 65B:291–298, 1983.

38. Lee, B.S., and Horstmann, H. The brachioradialis for restoration of abduction and extension of spastic thumb in children. Orthopaedics 7:1445–1448, 1984.

39. Lloyd-Roberts, G.C., and Lettin, A.W.F. Arthrogryposis multiplex congenita. J Bone Joint Surg 52B:494–508, 1970.

40. Matev, I.B. Surgical treatment of flexion-adduction contracture of the thumb in cerebral palsy. Acta Orthop Scand 41:439–445, 1970.

41. Matev, I.B. Surgical treatment of spastic "thumb-in-palm" deformity. J Bone Joint Surg 45B:703–708, 1963.

42. McCue, F.C., Honner, R., and Chapman, W.C. Transfer of the brachioradialis for hands deformed by cerebral palsy. J Bone Joint Surg 52A:1171–1180, 1970.

43. McDowell, C.L., Moberg, E.A., and House, J.W. The second in conference on surgical rehabilitation of the in tetraplegia (quadriplegia). J Hand Surg 11A:604–608, 1986.

44. McDowell, C.L. Tetraplegia, in Green, D.P. (ed): *Operative Hand Surgery.* New York, Churchill Livingstone, 1982, pp 1109–1127.

45. McDowell, C.L., Moberg, E.A., and Graham-Smith, A. International conference on surgical rehabilitation of the upper limb in tetraplegia. J Hand Surg 4:387–390, 1979.

46. Medical Research Council. *Aids to the Investigation of Peripheral Nerve Injuries, War Memorandum No. 7,* 2nd rev ed. London, His Majesty's Stationery Office, 1943.

47. Meyn, M., and Ruby, L. Arthrogryposis of the upper extremity. Orthop Clin North Am 7:501–509, 1976.

48. Milford, L. The hand, in Edmonson, A.S., and Crenshaw, A.H. (eds): *Campbell's Operative Orthopaedics,* 6th ed. St. Louis, Mosby, 1980.

49. Mital, M.A. Lengthening of the elbow flexors in cerebral palsy. J Bone Joint Surg 61A:515–522, 1979.

50. Mital, M.A., and Sakellarides, H.T. Surgery of the upper extremity in retarded individual with spastic cerebral palsy. Orthop Clin North Am 12:127–141, 1981.

51. Moberg, E. Reconstructive hand surgery in tetraplegia, stroke and cerebral palsy: Some basic concepts in physiology and neurology. J Hand Surg 1:29–34, 1976.

52. Moberg, E. Surgical treatment for absent single hand grip and elbow extension in quadriplegia. J Bone Joint Surg 57A:196–206, 1975.

53. Moberg, E. *The Upper Limb in Tetraplegia.* Stuttgart, Thieme, 1978.

54. Nickel, V.L., Perry, J., and Garrett, A.L. Development of useful function in the severely paralyzed hand. J Bone Joint Surg 45A:933–952, 1963.

55. Omer, G.E., and Capen, D.A. Proximal row carpectomy with muscle transfers for spastic paralysis. J Hand Surg 1:197–204, 1976.

56. Page, C.M. An operation for the relief of flexor contracture in the

forearm. J Bone Joint Surg 5:233, 1923.

57. Sakellarides, H.T., Mital, M.D., and Lenzi, W.D. Treatment of pronation contractures of the forearm in cerebral palsy by changing the insertion of the pronator radii teres. J Bone Joint Surg 63A:645–652, 1981.

58. Samilson, R.L., and Hoffer, M.M. Problems and complications in orthopaedic management of cerebral palsy, in Samilson, R.L. (ed): *Orthopaedic Aspects of Cerebral Palsy, Clinics in Developmental Medicine,* no. 52/53, Philadelphia, Lippincott, 1975, pp 258–274.

59. Samilson, R.L., and Morris, J.M. Surgical improvement of the cerebral-palsied upper limb. Electromyographic studies and results of 128 operations. J Bone Joint Surg 46A:1203–1216, 1964.

60. Sharrard, W.J.W. *Pediatric Orthopaedics and Fractures,* vol 2. London, Blackwell, 1979, pp 861–875.

61. Silver, C.M., Simon, S.D., Litchman, H.M., and Motamed, M. Surgical correction of spastic thumb-in-palm deformity. Dev Med Child Neurol 18:632–639, 1976.

62. Skoff, L., and Woodbury, D.F. Current concepts review: Management of the upper extremity in cerebral palsy. J Bone Joint Surg 67A:500–503, 1985.

63. Swanson, A.B. Surgery of the hand in cerebral palsy and muscle origin release procedures. Surg Clin North Am 48:1129–1138, 1968.

64. Swanson, A.B. Surgery of the hand in cerebral palsy and the swan-neck deformity. J Bone Joint Surg 42A:951–964, 1960.

65. White, W.F. Flexor muscle slide in the spastic hand: The Max Page operation. J Bone Joint Surg 54B:453–459, 1972.

66. Williams, P. The management of arthrogryposis. Orthop Clin North Am 9:67–88, 1978.

67. Zancolli, E.A. *Structural and Dynamic Bases of Hand Surgery,* 2d ed. Philadelphia, Lippincott, 1979.

68. Zancolli, E.A., Goldner, J.L., and Swanson, A.B. Surgery of the spastic hand in cerebral palsy: Report of the committee on spastic hand evaluation. J Hand Surg 8:766–772, 1983.

69. Zancolli, E.A., and Zancolli, E.A., Jr. The infantile spastic hand. Surgical indications and management. (In French and English.) Ann Chir Main 3:66–75, 1984.

70. Zancolli, E.A., and Zancolli, E.A., Jr. Surgical management of the hemiplegic spastic hand in cerebral palsy. Surg Clin North Am 61:395–406, 1981.

=== CHAPTER 42 ===

Tendon Injuries in the Upper Extremity

Peter C. Amadio

Tendon injuries in the distal portion of the arm may be caused by either acute trauma or cumulative stress. The orthopaedist must be continually aware of the anatomy, physiology, and biomechanics of tendon function in order to formulate rational plans of repair, reconstruction, and rehabilitation for the injured upper extremity.

TENDON ANATOMY, BIOMECHANICS, AND HEALING

Anatomy

Tendons consist primarily of longitudinally organized collagen fibers interspersed with spindle-shaped tenocytes. The fibers may be oriented in a linear, helical, or cruciate fashion.[46,66] These fibers are usually grouped in bundles that are separated by a less organized fibrocellular matrix, the *endotenon.* Superficially, the tendon is coated by a single layer of cells, the *epitenon,* which is confluent with the vascular

mesentery of the tendon, or *mesotenon.* Arteries are clearly present in the mesotenon. Some investigators, unable to identify veins within the digital fibrous sheath, have postulated that the vasculature of that area has a glomerularlike function.[127] Where tendons cross the concavity of a joint during part of its arc of motion, their displacement away from the center of motion may be restrained by one or more fibrous pulleys, which hold the tendon closer to the axis of motion and thus translate tendon excursion into greater angular movement.[32,55,74,103,155] If pulleys are present, the tendons may undergo various degrees of fibrocartilaginous metaplasia, produce sulfated mucopolysaccharides, and disperse multiple small collagen fibers in a manner similar to that seen in articular cartilage.[43,54]

The Flexor Surface

The distal one-third of the forearm contains the musculotendinous junctions and proximal tendons of all the extrinsic flexors of the wrist and hand. These are, in the superficial group: the flexor carpi radialis, palmaris longus, and flexor carpi ulnaris; in a slightly deeper location: the four tendons of the flexor digitorum superficialis; and, in the deepest layer: the four tendons of the flexor digitorum profundus and the flexor pollicis longus.

At the wrist, the flexor carpi radialis and the flexor carpi ulnaris insert into the second and fifth metacarpals, respectively. The palmaris longus inserts into the palmar fascia. All these muscles function as wrist flexors, the flexor carpi ulnaris being the most powerful. The other nine tendons pass beneath the transverse carpal ligament into the palm: the superficialis to the index and little fingers is the most superficial; next in depth is the superficialis to the middle and ring fingers; and deepest are the flexor pollicis longus and the four profundus tendons. In this region, a synovial sheath surrounds the tendons, usually with a separate sheath for the flexor pollicis longus and a combined sheath for the other tendons. Occasionally, the flexor pollicis longus and flexor digitorum profundus of the index finger may be connected by muscular, tendinous, or fibrous synovial bands in this region.[90] Such tethering may inhibit independent flexion of flexor pollicis longus when the flexor digitorum profundus is extended, as may occur in some manipulating and grasping activities. Attritional ruptures may also occur in this zone, either from arthritic changes in the carpal joints or from fractures of the hook of the hamate.[30,58,101,154,160]

Distal to the transverse carpal ligament, the lumbrical muscles arise from the flexor digitorum profundus. Classically, one arises from the radial aspect of each tendon, but actually they often arise from one or even two adjacent tendons as well, particularly on the ulnar side of the hand.[68] The sheaths of flexor pollicis longus and flexor digitorum profundus and superficialis to the little finger are usually continuous across this zone, but the lumbrical tendons cause a gap in the sheath system for the other digits. For this reason, pyogenic flexor tenosynovitis frequently coexists in the thumb and lit-

tle finger, whereas involvement of the other digits tends to be more independent.[122]

At the level of the metacarpophalangeal (MP) joint, the finger flexors enter the digital fibroosseous sheath system. The close tolerance of this system, which holds the tendons close to the finger joints to maximize the arc of motion per unit of excursion, does not allow for the voluminous, accordionlike, highly vascular sheath that is present proximally and that has multiple circumferential vascular connections to the tendon. Instead, vascular connections are limited to a few long dorsal branches termed the *vincula*. Each tendon has a single short vinculum at its insertion and a variable number of long vincula along its course (Fig. 42-1).[97,127] One long vinculum to the profundus at the level of the proximal interphalangeal (PIP) joint is usual. Occasionally, an additional long vinculum to the profundus is present in the proximal phalanx. The long vincula to the superficialis are highly variable. They are less frequently found in the middle and ring fingers and decrease in occurrence with age.[111] The thumb has its own distinct vincular system, usually one long and one short vinculum.[8]

The pulley system of the fingers maintains maximal proximity between the tendons and the axes of joint motion, so that 3 cm of profundus excursion can provide 270 degrees of combined total angular motion for the MP, PIP, and distal interphalangeal (DIP) joints. To provide a rigid restraint against bowstringing and yet permit flexibility, the portions of the pulley system over the phalangeal shafts and directly over the axes of joint motion are tough, fibrous, annular structures, whereas the sections that intervene are cruciform.[8,11,38,39] With flexion, the cruciate pulleys fold up. At maximum flexion, the annular pulleys are nearly in contact with one another. The fingers have five annular and three cruciate pulleys (Fig. 42-2). The thumb has two annular pulleys and one oblique pulley (which can be thought of as a combination cruciate and annular pulley).

As the flexor profundus passes through the finger, it be-

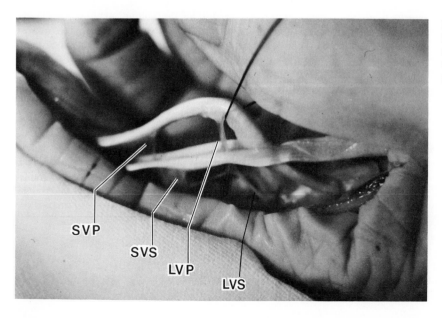

Figure 42-1 Anatomical dissection showing short vinculum to profundus (SVP) and superficialis (SVS) and long vinculum to profundus (LVP) and superficialis (LVS).

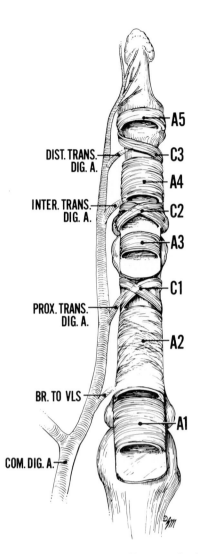

Figure 42-2 Pulley system of fingers. Between the A1 and A2 pulleys is a variable cruciate fiber area sometimes called "C-0" (C zero). (*From Schneider, L.H., and Hunter, J.M., in Green, D.P., ed: Operative Hand Surgery, vol 2. New York, Churchill Livingstone, 1982. Reproduced with permission.*)

gins deep to the superficialis, but it must gain volar access to reach the fingertip. It does so by passing between the two tendons of insertion of the flexor superficialis, which separate to form the chiasma tendinum, first described by Pieter Camper in 1760 and thus often called *Camper's chiasm.* The spiral course of the decussating fibers of superficialis as they pass around the profundus and insert on the middle phalanx in this region maximizes proximity of the profundus to the PIP joint; the superficialis itself acts as an auxiliary pulley to the profundus at this location.[68] This spiral pattern must be remembered during repair of superficialis lacerations at this level; malrotation at the suture line may limit tendon excursion.[91]

Bunnell[20] was the first to call widespread attention to the high rate of surgical complications with repair of tendon injuries within this fibroosseous sheath. He called this area "no-

man's-land." Verdan[168] divided the tendon sheath system into several zones on the basis of anatomical characteristics. The distal area, with a single tendon within a fibroosseous sheath, is generally called zone I; the proximal sheath, with two tendons—Bunnell's no-man's-land—is zone II; the zone of lumbrical origin is zone III; the carpal tunnel is zone IV; and the distal portion of the forearm is zone V (Fig. 42-3). The thumb has no lumbrical and only one tendon; there is no general agreement on the zone nomenclature for the thumb. The author believes it is consistent with the nomenclature to consider that in the thumb, zone I merges proximally with zone IV, as shown in Fig. 42-3. Additional classification based on tendon anatomy within the digital sheath may have further prognostic value. Within zone II, some surgeons additionally distinguish between the zone in the region of Camper's chiasm (zone IIa) and the zone proximal to it (zone IIb).[162] Subzones based on vascular anatomy and vincula insertion may also be useful.[5]

The Extensor Surface

The extensor tendons follow a similar, progressively more complex path from the forearm to the fingertip. Again, tendons form in the distal part of the forearm. A superficial layer consists of the abductor pollicis longus, extensor pollicis brevis, brachioradialis, extensor carpi radialis longus, extensor carpi radialis brevis, extensor digitorum communis, and extensor carpi ulnaris. A deeper layer is composed of extensor indicis proprius, extensor pollicis longus, and extensor digiti quinti. Only two tendons of insertion (brachioradialis and triceps) do not cross the wrist.

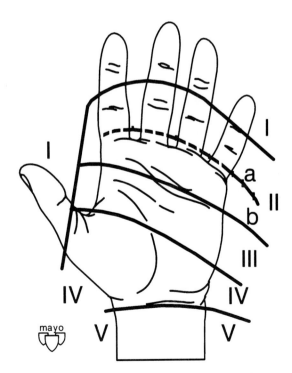

Figure 42-3 Zones of flexor tendon injury (see text).

At the wrist, six separate compartments are present, which usually are numbered from radial to ulnar.

The first compartment contains abductor pollicis longus and extensor pollicis brevis. Usually, extensor pollicis brevis has at least a partially separate sheath. This may trap the unwary, because the abductor pollicis longus often has multiple slips, one of which may be mistaken for an extensor pollicis brevis.

The second compartment contains the tendons of the extensor carpi radialis longus, which inserts on the second metacarpal, and of the extensor carpi radialis brevis, which inserts on the third metacarpal. These tendons not only pass under a fibroosseous tunnel at the wrist but also pass under the muscle bellies of abductor pollicis longus and extensor pollicis brevis in the distal part of the forearm. At this intersection, a bursa is present.[57]

The third compartment contains the extensor pollicis longus, which has a bony pulley at Lister's tubercle, where it angles toward the thumb. This is a frequent zone for attritional rupture from repetitive injury ("drummer boy palsy"), a complication of fracture of the distal radius, or rheumatoid synovitis.[61,136,142]

The fourth compartment contains extensor indicis proprius and extensor digitorum communis. This compartment is also frequently involved in rheumatoid tenosynovitis, and finger extensor ruptures in this zone are frequent.[26,166]

The fifth compartment contains extensor digiti quinti, which frequently has a double tendon. This compartment overlies the distal radioulnar joint. Attritional rupture of the extensor digiti quinti may follow injury to the distal radioulnar joint, particularly, again, in rheumatoid arthritis.[26]

The sixth compartment contains the extensor carpi ulnaris. It is located almost in the midaxial line along the ulnar border of the wrist and primarily acts as an ulnar deviator rather than as an extensor.[79] It moves dorsad to the wrist axis with supination and more volarad with pronation. A twisting injury into pronation may cause a recurrent painful volar subluxation of this tendon.[21] Spastic flexor-pronator contracture may also displace the tendon to a volar position, where it may add to the deforming forces.

On the dorsum of the hand, the thumb extensors usually have no special interconnections as they travel distally from the wrist retinaculum. The finger extensors are linked by intertendinous slips traditionally called *juncturae tendinum* or, in the more recent anatomical nomenclature, *conexus intertendineus.* The connection between the common extensors of the index and middle fingers is usually transverse; the other connections are oblique.[171] Often, there is no true common extensor of the little finger, but a large intertendinous slip connects the extensor digitorum communis of the ring finger and the extensor hood of the little finger at the level of the MP joint. Although the exact function of the intertendinous connections is not known, the oblique ones certainly help to transmit extensor force to adjacent tendons, and all help to hold the extensor tendons in place on the dorsum of the hand, thereby preventing lateral translation with finger movement and proximal retraction when a tendon is lacerated distal to the connection.

At the level of the metacarpal heads, the extensor apparatus becomes more complex (Fig. 42-4). The tendon is cen-

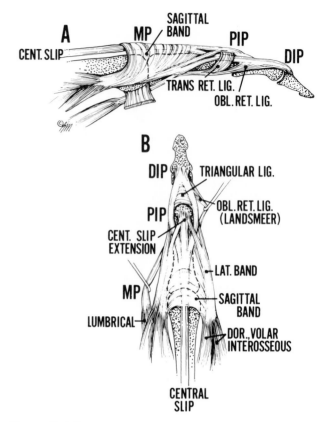

Figure 42-4 Extensor mechanism. **A.** Lateral view. **B.** Dorsal view. (*From Doyle, J.R., in Green, D.P., ed: Operative Hand Surgery, vol 2. New York, Churchill Livingstone, 1982. Reproduced with permission.*)

tered by sagittal bands, which insert into the deep transverse metacarpal ligament and volar plate complex. This circumferential sling helps the extensor digitorum communis to extend the MP joint. The extensor digitorum communis has no direct insertion into the proximal phalanx. It has an indirect insertion through its connection to the joint capsule and by the volar sling formed by the sagittal bands to the volar plate.

Distal to the sagittal bands and deep to the transverse metacarpal ligament, the interosseous tendons attach to the extensor mechanism. The dorsal interossei, which abduct the fingers, have two heads; one inserts directly into the base of the proximal phalanx and the other into the extensor expansion. For the special case of the little finger, the abductor digiti quinti has two heads, as do the other dorsal interossei; the flexor digiti quinti inserts directly onto the volar base of the little finger and does not contribute to the extensor expansion. The opponens digiti quinti also inserts directly into bone.

In the thumb, again, the flexor pollicis brevis inserts on the volar aspect of the proximal phalanx, as does one head of the adductor pollicis. The other head of adductor pollicis and abductor pollicis brevis attaches into the extensor expansion.

Over the proximal phalanx, the intrinsic tendons converge obliquely on the central extensor. Those fibers which are more transverse course over the dorsal aspect of the proximal phalanx and act as a dorsal sling to assist metacarpophalangeal flexion. The more oblique fibers meet the central tendinous slip of the extensor digitorum communis at the interphalangeal (IP) joint.

For the thumb, the interphalangeal joint is the terminal attachment of the oblique interosseous fibers and the central tendinous slip of the extensor pollicis longus; the extensor pollicis brevis attaches primarily to the MP joint capsule, and the abductor pollicis longus attaches to the base of the metacarpal. In the fingers, lateral fibers from the central tendinous slip and the intrinsic tendons converge to form the lateral bands which then insert at the base of the distal phalanx. The triangular ligament is located dorsally between the lateral bands and prevents them from subluxating volarly. The transverse retinacular ligament connects the lateral bands with the volar plate and flexor sheath and prevents dorsal displacement of the bands with finger extension. The oblique retinacular ligament also connects the proximal phalanx volar plate with the lateral bands but more distally; because this ligament is volar to the PIP joint, but attaches dorsal to the DIP joint, it is tightened as the PIP joint extends and acts to assist DIP joint extension.[84]

The extensor surface can also be divided into zones that roughly separate areas in which different principles or methods of treatment need to be considered. There is no general agreement on zone nomenclature for the extensor surface. The classification scheme shown in Fig. 42-5 is consistent with the nomenclature for the flexor surface. Zone V includes the distal third of the forearm up to the extensor retinaculum; zone IV is the region under the extensor retinaculum, including all six compartments; zone III is the level of the dorsum of the hand; zone IIc is the level of the MP joint; zone IIb is the level over the proximal phalanx; zone IIa is the region of the PIP joint; and zone I is the region distal to the PIP joint.

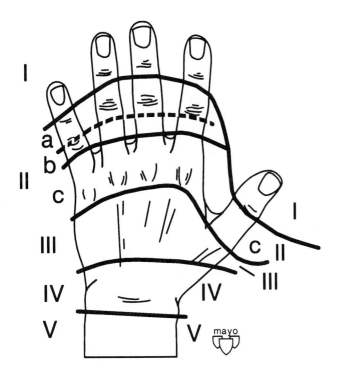

Figure 42-5 Zones of extensor injury (see text).

The blood supply of the extensor mechanism is not really as complex as that of the flexors. Except at the wrist, there is no synovial sheath system, and the tendons are generally well vascularized by adjacent circumferential paratenon.[105] None of the extensor tendons has a vincular system.

Tendon Biomechanics (See also Chap. 33, Sect. C)

In the forearm and hand, pulleys are present both volarly and dorsally at the wrist in the form of flexor and extensor retinacula and in the fingers on the flexor surface as the digital pulley system. Mechanically, these pulleys function as restraints against tendon bowing across a joint concavity. The pulleys are of three types: annular fibrous bands directed over the joint; annular bands, usually paired, at a distance from a joint; and cruciate pulleys. The first type, annular bands directly over a joint, include the dorsal wrist retinaculum and the A1, A3, and A5 digital pulleys. These are effective restraints against bowing, working in the most efficient spot, directly over the area of maximal potential bowing.[11] Probably because of the extensive degree of flexion possible at the PIP joint, there are additional annular pulleys in the fingers. These pulleys function as paired proximal and distal restraints to tendon bowing and augment the action of the joint-centered annular pulleys. The transverse carpal ligament and the forearm fascia probably function as a similar pair of pulleys for wrist flexion. There is evidence that the palmar fascia may also serve as a proximal pulley for the finger MP joints, with the proximal portion of the A2 pulley as the distal MP joint restraint.[106] Similarly, the distal A4 pulley may serve as a proximal restraint to the DIP joint, with the profundus insertion acting as the distal restraint.

It is important that the system remain balanced. If the proximal and distal restraints are asymmetrically placed, either in their distance from the joint axis or in the amount of bowing they permit, stress will concentrate on the "tighter" or closer, pulley, and the pulley may rupture.[74] It is particularly important, therefore, when one repairs or reconstructs the flexor mechanism, to keep in mind the concept of balanced pulleys. It is also important to remember that the long, phalanx-based A2 and A4 pulleys work mostly at their proximal and distal edges. During elective pulley resection or incision, one should take this fact into consideration and avoid interference to those areas, preferring instead the midportion of these pulleys. Reconstruction should by contrast concentrate on restoration of the proximal and distal portions of these pulleys, possibly even with two separate reconstructions for the A2 pulley, rather than on reconstructing the pulley at the center of the phalanx, where it has the least mechanical advantage to restrain bowing.[70,74]

Tendon Healing

In general, tendon healing is no different from the healing of ligament or any other soft connective tissue.[42,78,102,179] Hematoma forms at the site of injury and is organized. Vascular invasion occurs, bringing fibroblasts and capillaries, and a dense, disorganized matrix of types I and III collagen is then laid down. Over time, and in response to mechanical forces, type I collagen predominates and organizes into bundles parallel to the lines of tension, replacing but never exactly duplicating, the original structure[6,52,78,98] and material properties.[153] Tendons, of course, must glide and in most cases are enmeshed in a loose areolar tissue that permits such movement. This situation can usually be reproduced adequately after wound healing, provided that there has not been extensive associated fibrosis and that the normal length-tension relationship of the muscle-tendon unit is preserved. In the hand, this sort of generally favorable healing situation exists in flexor zones III and V and in all the extensor zones except at the wrist.

A significantly different situation exists for the extensors at the wrist, for flexor zone II, also for flexor zones I and IV, to some extent. Here the tendons are encased not in a loose, areolar paratenon but in a fibrous synovial sheath. The tendons are in close proximity to one another, and cross-adhesions may significantly impair differential gliding. They are also immediately superficial to periosteum in these areas. Lacerations that injure tendon also frequently injure periosteum or bone, with the potential then for deep binding adhesions to the bone itself.

In flexor zone II, the most treacherous environment for healing exists. The segmental vincular blood flow creates hypovascular watershed zones between the vincula (Fig. 42-6).[97,127] Tendon injury frequently implies associated vincular or other local vascular injuries; whole tendon segments may become ischemic or even infarct;[111–114,130] the adhesions that then form may be dense enough to preclude even the slightest movement.

The work of Mason and Allen[108] and later of Potenza[130,131]

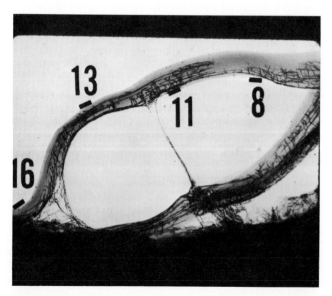

Figure 42-6 Injection specimen of human flexor tendon. Note hypovascular zone between markers 8 and 11. (*From Amadio, P.C., et al, in Hunter, J.M., et al, eds: Rehabilitation of the Hand, 2d ed. St. Louis, Mosby, 1984. Reproduced with permission.*)

in an experimental canine model of tendon injury and repair concluded that such adhesions were inevitable. At that time, however, the nutritional pathways to dog tendon were unknown. Evidence by Manske and Lesker[104,107] and others[63,116,144] has shown that canine tendons within the digital sheath probably rely almost exclusively on synovial fluid for nutrition. Uptake of nutrients from the fluid has been shown to be assisted by active finger motion.[96,169] Repair, sheath resection, and immobilization in the dog model of Mason, Allen, and Potenza all conspired to rob the tendon of its only nutritional support. It was the model, not the injury, that made the adhesions inevitable. In the human, it is likely that a combination of vascular and synovial nutrition pathways functions to maintain tendon homeostasis.[5,6] Manske et al[52,102,104] have clearly shown that the proportion of vascular contribution varies in different species: it is greater in primates and chickens and less in dogs and rabbits. In addition, the proliferative response induced in tendon by injury decreases as one moves up the evolutionary ladder. Extrapolation of animal data on tendon healing to the human situation must therefore be done with caution.

Given appropriate nutritional support, tendons within the digital sheath can heal with acceptable adhesion formation.[10,51,53,116] To some extent, the nature of the injury will determine if such healing is possible. Tendons with vincular injuries seem to do less well than those with intact vincula.[5] The principles governing the provision of adequate nutrition are based on the observations cited above. Care must be taken to avoid unnecessary injury to vincular and other vascular structures. The localization of digital artery feeders to the vincular system must be kept in mind. These vessels usually enter at the level of the cruciate pulleys.[68] Additional tissue trauma must be minimized at surgery by means of delicate technique and the use of suture material of small caliber and low reactivity. Potenza[131] has shown that all areas of exposed tendon collagen or disruption of the epitenon will lead to adhesions at that point. Surgical exposure and manipulation must be minimized. A tendon should not be grasped except during cutting; an intratendinous grasping suture should be used. Tenorrhaphy should be completed with a running inverting epitendinous suture to fold in the cut ends of collagen bundles exposed at the cut surface.[91,94] The synovial sheath system should be preserved and be repaired to restore continuity if at all possible.[93,94] Some authors have even recommended grafting of sheaths if segmental loss exists.[43] Synovial membranes recellularize rapidly, however, so that this may be unnecessary. To facilitate the diffusion of synovial nutrients into the injured tendon, early motion is appropriate.[51,83,159] Continuous passive motion devices may have special application in this area, although no clinical data at this time support the use of continuous passive motion in flexor tendon injuries.

For tendons injured in proximity to other tendons, especially other injured tendons, passive differential gliding exercises will limit development of restricting intertendinous adhesions and should be started early.[41] Finally, since tendons within the fibrous osseous sheath have less nutritional support than tendons elsewhere, an extended period of protected activity is necessary to prevent rupture or gap formation at the healing site.[44,80,83,94,126,135]

ACUTE TENDON INJURIES

Diagnosis

The diagnosis of acute tendon laceration may be difficult, even in the patient who is awake and cooperative. Tendon laceration must be suspected in any patient with an open wound in the forearm or hand who has pain on motion, weakness, or inability to move the wrist or one of the digits.

Clues may be sought even before the wound is actually inspected or the injured parts are manipulated. There is a normal resting posture of the digits, which depends on the viscoelastic properties of intact muscle-tendon units. This is the commonly observed *tenodesis effect,* in which wrist flexion causes passive finger extension and wrist extension causes passive finger flexion (the cascade). Normally, the resting posture of the hand is one of mild thumb and finger flexion, with the degree of flexion increasing from the radial to the ulnar side of the hand. Any alteration in this normal flexion cascade from radial to ulnar should make one suspect a tendon interruption (Fig. 42-7).

The main confusion in differential diagnosis of tendon injury comes from motor nerve injury, which also produces failure of active motion of a part. Nerve injury does not, however, affect the normal viscoelastic properties of the muscle-tendon unit. Examination of resting posture, the tenodesis effect, and the result of proximal milking of the muscle bellies of the forearm (which will produce finger motion if the muscle-tendon unit is intact) are all helpful in making the correct diagnosis. It is important to remember that the terminal motor branches of the radial, median, or ulnar nerve may be lacerated, and so absence of a sensory defect is not helpful in ruling out nerve injury.

Management of Tendon Injuries

In all suspicious cases, surgical exploration in a bloodless field should be carried out. Even if immediate definitive treatment is not anticipated, the wound should be debrided. Injured structures can then be identified and the wound closed or given a sterile dressing. These procedures will lessen the urgency of definitive treatment, permit stabilization of other serious injuries, and allow transfer of the patient to an appropriate facility for definitive care. It is generally accepted that delay in primary repair up to 3 weeks after injury will not impair the result of a flexor tendon injury.[140]

Surgical exploration almost always requires an extension of the laceration for identification of major tendons, nerves, and other vital structures at an undamaged level and then dissection back into the zone of injury. These incisions should follow the general principles of extensibility and avoid narrow or distally based skin flaps; they should not cross skin creases at a right angle. In the digit, the volar zigzag incision described by Bruner[18] and the midaxial approach[20] are commonly preferred.

The best results are obtained after early, direct repair of complete tendon injuries.[94,139,158] This is true at all levels and for all tendons. The definition of "early" has undergone some revision recently. Although initially restricted to injuries

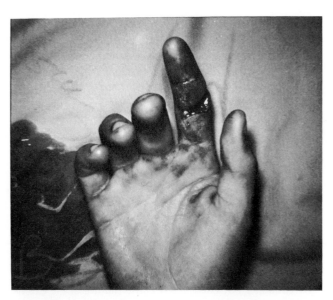

Figure 42-7 Clearly abnormal posture of index finger. Both profundus and superficialis tendons were lacerated in zone II. The normal resting posture of the hand with increasing interphalangeal flexor tone from index to little finger (the cascade) has been disrupted.

treated definitively within 8 to 24 h, the grace period is generally accepted to extend to at least 3 weeks after injury and in selected cases even longer.[87,110,140]

Partial Tendon Injuries

For partial tendon injuries, a controversy exists about treatment. Some favor suture of all partial injuries,[138] others favor debridement only,[180] and some advocate a mixture of the two approaches.[173] What evidence there is suggests that for partial injuries involving less than 60 percent of a tendon, debridement and early protective motion are the most appropriate actions;[35] lacerations of greater than 60 percent are more likely to rupture and may be best-treated like a complete laceration, with suture and postoperative rehabilitation.

Closed Tendon Injuries

Closed tendon injuries are frequent and are usually secondary to a forceful injury in the direction opposite to the line of pull of the tendon in question, often when the tendon itself is already under tension. The most common examples include "jersey finger," or avulsion of a profundus tendon, in a football player who has hooked an opponent's jersey with his fingertips and tries to hold on while the opponent pulls away;[24,88] the mallet, or baseball, finger, when a direct dorsal blow on the actively extended DIP joint causes rupture of the insertion of the terminal extensor tendon, an injury frequently seen in baseball catchers;[1,150] and rupture of the biceps tendon from the distal radius after forcible extension or extreme resistance to the actively flexed elbow.[9,64] Other injuries may occur after a direct blow, such as a crush injury to the PIP joint that causes rupture of the central slip or triangular ligament with the subsequent inability to actively extend the PIP joint[2] (the boutonniere, or buttonhole, deformity, so-called because the head of the proximal phalanx protrudes through the extensor mechanism like a button in its hole). Other, less common, closed injuries include rupture of a sagittal band[81] and rupture of a tendon from its muscle belly proximally.[50]

The third class of closed tendon rupture is not associated with acute trauma. This is attritional rupture, of which five locations are most frequent, with classic descriptions. The most common is probably the caput ulnae lesion, frequently seen in rheumatoid arthritis, in which synovitis and bony erosions around a prominent ulnar head may cause attritional rupture of the finger extensors.[166] An analogous lesion volarly has also been described, with the radial finger flexors jeopardized by osteophytes and synovitis of the scaphotrapezial joint.[101] Either Colles' fracture or repetitive use ("drummer boy palsy") may cause rupture of the extensor pollicis longus at Lister's tubercle.[142] Ancient fracture of the hook of the hamate can cause the ulnar finger flexors to rupture.[30] Finally, repeated steroid injection at a single location is associated with a recognized risk of tendon rupture at that location.[59,77]

Tendon Injury from Cumulative Trauma

Repetitive use may also cause tendon injury without rupture. Tenosynovitis is extremely common. In the hand and forearm, the most common tendons involved are the finger flexors (trigger finger and thumb) and the abductor pollicis longus and extensor pollicis brevis (usually called *de Quervain's tenosynovitis*). Proximal extension of de Quervain's tenosynovitis produces the extensor intersection syndrome. The areas of involvement are also vascular watershed zones; relative hypovascularity may render these zones less able to respond to repetitive stress by work hypertrophy.[6] These syndromes can usually be diagnosed by the presence of local tenderness and crepitus with active tendon motion, and there may be a palpable snap or click with tendon motion if triggering is truly present. The most common confusion in differential diagnosis is between de Quervain's tenosynovitis and extensor intersection syndrome, which occur in close proximity and may occur simultaneously; careful localization of points of maximal tenderness and crepitus is necessary.[57] The Finkelstein test (forced wrist ulnar deviation with the thumb clenched firmly within the fist) is considered diagnostic of de Quervain's tenosynovitis but may also be positive in cases of extensor intersection syndrome. The classic sign of extensor intersection syndrome is a leatherlike rub or squeak with wrist flexion and extension, palpable or even sometimes audible in the region of the intersection of the radial wrist extensors and the first dorsal compartment muscle belly.[34]

At the elbow, tenosynovitis of the common flexor and extensor origins is also extremely common. This, too, is usually secondary to cumulative trauma, from either sports or work activity. Finally, an additional area of tenosynovitis is receiving increasing attention. Linburg and Comstock[90] reported a high incidence of conjunction of the flexor profun-

dus of the index finger and the flexor pollicis longus. Overuse may cause an adhesive tenosynovitis further restricting separate use. Patients frequently complain of aching or burning pain in the distal forearm and hand. This condition may be confused diagnostically with carpal tunnel syndrome. The classic diagnostic test is to ask the patient to hold the fingers extended and then to flex the thumb across the palm and particularly to flex the interphalangeal joint.[90] If this maneuver reproduces the patient's pain, the diagnosis is made. If the patient has weakness of flexion of his thumb IP joint with the index finger extended and the thumb flexed across the palm but has no weakness of IP joint extension either with the index finger flexed or with the thumb extended, a presumptive diagnosis of a positive Linburg connection can be made.

One uncommon cumulative trauma problem about the elbow deserves mention because it can also be confused with a nerve compression lesion. The medial expansion of the triceps tendon may occasionally snap over the medial border of the humerus and the medial intermuscular septum. This anomaly can be painful in some patients who are required to perform repetitive elbow flexion and extension activities at work.[40] The painful palpable snap may be confused with subluxation of the ulnar nerve in this location. The fact that many patients have hypersensitivity of the ulnar nerve in the region of the elbow may add to the difficulty of establishing the diagnosis. In questionable cases, surgical exploration using local anesthesia may be necessary to confirm the diagnosis. Release or excision of the medial triceps expansion is usually successful in resolving the symptoms and permitting a return to full activity.

Treatment of cumulative trauma disorders can be difficult. Initial management should include rest, local heat, and anti-inflammatory or analgesic medication. Local steroid injection is often helpful in relieving the acute symptoms. Frequently, at least a temporary modification of the repetitive activity implicated in the cause is necessary. If symptoms are detected early, a brief period of rest can usually be followed by resumption of normal activities. If diagnosis is late or if the symptoms have been chronic, a prolonged period of rest followed by an extended period of rehabilitation and gradual strengthening should be instituted.[62,123] In some cases, it may be necessary to require a permanent change in either work or avocational activity. Finally, for chronic symptoms that do not respond to nonsurgical therapy, surgery may be indicated. In most cases of cumulative tendon trauma, some sort of debridement or release of the damaged area is in order. In stenosing tenosynovitis, local synovectomy and sheath release are usually curative.[47] Debridement of granulation tissue at the extensor and flexor origins, as recommended by Nirschl and Pettrone,[124] can also be of benefit.

Postoperatively, these patients may again require extensive rehabilitation before resuming their work or hobby activities. Recovery time is often measured in months, and it is usually advisable to begin with limited or modified activity and gradually progress up to unrestricted activity as strength and endurance improve.[123]

Tenosynovitis may be secondary to causes other than repetitive use. These are beyond the scope of this chapter, but rheumatoid arthritis, gout, and infection are all in the differential diagnosis. They can usually be identified by the patient's history, additional physical findings, and, in questionable cases, laboratory testing and radiographs.

TENOLYSIS

In some cases of primary tendon repair or graft, an unsatisfactory range of motion remains at the conclusion of postoperative rehabilitation. Tenolysis should be considered in such cases. First, however, it is important to be certain that no further gain can be expected from therapy alone and that enough time has been allowed for sound tendon healing. Most hand surgeons wait 3 to 6 months before considering tenolysis. One should be prepared, at the time of tenolysis, to proceed to staged tendon grafting if the condition of the tendon bed pulleys and of the tendon itself are poor.

Whenever possible, tenolysis is performed with local anesthesia so that the patient can actively flex and extend the digit at intervals during the procedure (Fig. 42-8).[73] An alternative measure is to begin with intravenous regional anesthesia; then, at the conclusion of the procedure, the tourniquet is deflated[156] to dissipate the anesthetic and allow testing of the active range of motion. Only by testing active range of motion can the surgeon be certain that all the restricting adhesions have been divided after tenolysis.

Postoperative pain control is critical during the first few days after tenolysis so that an uninhibited active exercise program can be carried out.[73] Continuous nerve block by either indwelling catheter or transcutaneous electrical nerve stimulation has the advantage of providing analgesia without sedation.[141] When early, vigorous active exercises can be pursued postoperatively, tenolysis is often successful in improving range of motion.[76,158,176,181]

Postoperative Tendon Rupture

Postoperative tendon rupture as a complication of primary repair, tendon grafting, or tenolysis is more likely to occur with early mobilization programs. Acute ruptures of primarily repaired tendons and tendon grafts should be explored and rerepaired as soon as possible after diagnosis. A recent study suggests that if a postoperative rupture after primary tendon repair is repaired again, the prognosis of the initial repair is not affected.[3] If a tendon that has undergone tenolysis ruptures, staged tendon reconstruction usually is necessary to salvage the situation.

Effect of Age on Results of Tendon Injury

Age is a strong determinant of the result of tendon injury. Injuries in children have, in general, a good prognosis;[165] tendon injuries, especially flexor injuries, in patients over the age of 40 do less well than those in patients who are younger.[134,162] This poorer result in older patients may be due to changes in tendon vascularity and healing potential with age. Most cumulative stress disorders related to tendon also occur in older patients,[47,124] a finding that again suggests decreased vascularity and healing potential for these injuries.

Assessment of Tendon Injury

The result of tendon injury is measured by active range of motion. In the hand, finding the total active motion of each injured finger is the method recommended by the American

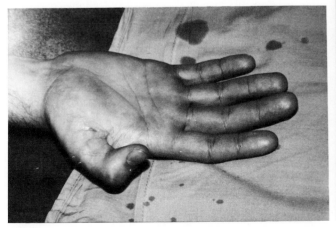

A

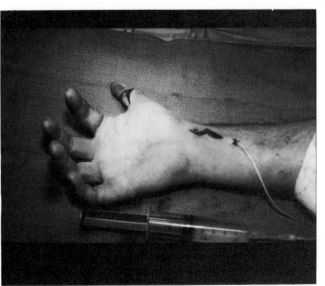

B

Figure 42-8 A. Fixed flexion contracture of thumb after primary repair of flexor pollicis longus. **B.** Intraoperative view of active extension. Note syringe on catheter. Syringe contains 0.5% bupivacaine, and catheter leads to median nerve. Postoperatively, patient had satisfactory pain relief from continuous median nerve block. Avoidance of sedation permitted better cooperation with therapy program.

Society for Surgery of the Hand.[83] Total active motion is determined by measurement of the angle of flexion of each finger joint as the patient tries to make a fist and then by subtraction of any flexion contracture as the patient extends the finger. This is a more accurate means of measurement than testing each joint individually with the proximal joints blocked. Many profundus repairs work very well with the metacarpophalangeal and proximal interphalangeal joints held in extension but do not produce distal interphalangeal joint flexion when these proximal joints are also flexed. Some authors prefer to measure only the total active motion at the proximal and distal interphalangeal joints when reporting the results of zone II flexor tendon lacerations,[159] since in those cases MP joint motion is almost always normal and can be assumed to contribute 85 to 90 degrees of total active motion. When the MP joint is included, the normal total active motion of a finger is generally considered to be 240 degrees or more. Total active motion of less than 180 degrees is generally considered unsatisfactory.[94,135,159,162]

For the special case of the thumb, total active motion of the MP and interphalangeal (IP) joints is also measured, but there is less general agreement on its definition, because MP and IP motion vary considerably from person to person. Flexion lag from the head of the fifth metacarpal is also a commonly performed measure; thumb extension can be measured as web span or as extension lag from the plane of the first metacarpal, or both.

IMMEDIATE TREATMENT OF FLEXOR TENDON INJURIES

Elbow and Forearm

In this zone, most injuries involve muscle bellies and not tendons. Muscle does not hold suture well, and surgical treatment is often limited to debridement and wound closure. If the tendon of the pronator teres is lacerated, it should be repaired, and the forearm should be immobilized with elbow flexion and forearm pronation for 3 to 4 weeks, followed by active range-of-motion exercises. Unless there is extensive muscle damage or denervation, prognosis for complete recovery in this area is good.

If the tendon of the biceps is lacerated, it should be repaired, the forearm should be immobilized with elbow flexion and forearm supination, and treatment should be as described above. Closed rupture of the biceps tendon is also possible after strong resistance or forcible extension of the actively flexed elbow. If the diagnosis is made early, the tendon should be reattached to the bicipital tuberosity of the radius by direct suture into bone. A two-incision approach is recommended.[9,64,119] In late rupture, the amount of functional impairment must be assessed. For many patients, the amount of elbow flexion provided by the brachialis and the amount of supination provided by the supinator are sufficient, and reconstruction is unnecessary. For patients who are disabled by distal biceps rupture, reconstruction with prolongation of the biceps tendon by tendon graft is recommended.[118]

Zone V

All finger and wrist flexor tendons begin in zone V. In this zone, they are still covered by a loose areolar tenosynovium in a bed that is fatty superficially, and muscular and well-vascularized deeply. This is an excellent bed for tendon healing. In clean lacerations, direct suture of all injured tendons, with the possible exception of palmaris longus, should usually be carried out. Rupture of a tendon from its muscle belly may also be treated by transfer of the ruptured tendon to an intact muscle-tendon unit.

With associated injury to bone, nerve, or vessels, primary repair of injured tendons is still advisable at this level because of the favorable soft tissue bed. With increasing severity of injury, the prognosis becomes less favorable, but even in replantation at this level, satisfactory tendon excursion can often be achieved.[137]

Postoperatively, zone V tendon lacerations can usually be treated with early mobilization, with the wrist held in 30 to 40 degrees of flexion. Many authors recommend active extension and passive flexion exercises that begin within a few days of surgery.[41,94,159,182] Rubber-band traction from the fingernail to the postoperative dressing or splint along the volar surface of the forearm helps relax the flexors during active extension and lessens the risk of rupture. It is important to remember that of the 6 to 7 cm of finger flexor excursion, fully half occurs as the wrist goes from maximal flexion to maximal extension and the other half when the fingers are put through a full range of motion.[74] For this reason, when active motion begins, the wrist and fingers should be exercised separately at first and later by combined gentle active motion of both fingers and wrist simultaneously. Strengthening and dynamic stretching of contractures complete the rehabilitation program, and results in this area are generally good.[158]

Zone IV

Although some authors recommend repair of the flexor pollicis longus and flexor digitorum profundus only,[139] the author believes that in zone IV, as in zone V, all injured flexors should be repaired. Unlike zone V, zone IV does not have a good soft tissue bed. The tendons are in close proximity within the synovial sheath, and a pulley, the transverse carpal ligament, is present. For tendon repair, incision of the transverse carpal ligament usually is necessary. Repair or preservation of at least a portion of the ligament is recommended to prevent tendon bowstringing postoperatively.[139] Whereas in the proximal forearm any of a variety of grasping and weaving tendon sutures provides sufficient holding power for the tendon repair, in zone IV one must begin to think about not only the holding power but also about the bulk and reactivity of the suture.[80,163,173] For this reason, an intratendinous grasping suture is most appropriate. Examples of this type of suture include the classic Bunnell,[20] the Kessler and its modifications,[94] and the Tsuge suture (Fig. 42-9).[162]

In patients with another associated injury, repair of injured tendons in zone IV is still usually advisable. As in zone V, however, the prognosis becomes less favorable with increasing severity of injury.

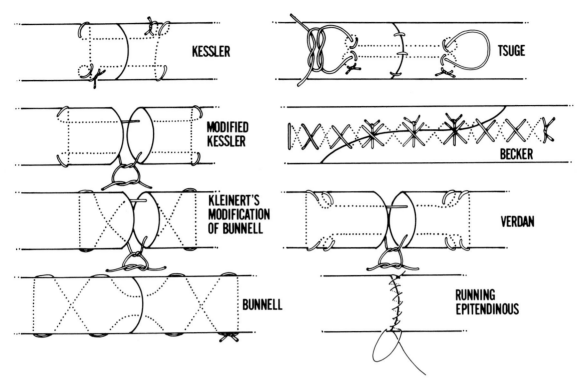

KESSLER

TSUGE

MODIFIED KESSLER

BECKER

KLEINERT'S MODIFICATION OF BUNNELL

VERDAN

BUNNELL

RUNNING EPITENDINOUS

Figure 42-9 Some intratendinous grafting sutures used in flexor tendon repair. (*From Leddy, J.P., in Green, D.P., ed: Operative* *Hand Surgery, vol 2. New York, Churchill Livingstone, 1982. Reprinted with permission.*)

Tendon rupture may occur in zone IV. Usually, it is attritional rupture due to arthritis[101] or, in some cases, fracture of the hook of the hamate.[30] If the diagnosis is made early, debridement and primary repair may be possible. If not, tendon grafting or transfer of the ruptured tendon to an adjacent intact tendon is advisable.[143,164]

Postoperatively, zone IV tendon lacerations can usually be treated with early mobilization. Wrist flexion needs to be minimized, however, because of the possibility of bowstringing or binding adhesions between the transverse carpal ligament and the repaired tendons. For relaxation of the tendons after repair, therefore, somewhat less wrist flexion and somewhat more metacarpophalangeal joint flexion are indicated in zone IV lacerations than in zone V. Although placing the IP joints in flexion to further relax the tendons is advisable, these joints should usually be kept close to full extension when at rest because of the risk of IP joint flexion contracture. Early protected passive mobilization followed by protected active motion exercises and finally by resisted exercises is recommended.[94,139,157]

Details of the postoperative rehabilitation program will obviously vary with specific cases. The reader is referred to the works of Lister et al,[94] Duran et al,[41] and others[23,45,159] for further information.

Zone III

Injuries in the region of lumbrical origin are analogous in some ways to zone V injuries because tendon blood supply is circumferential and a fairly good gliding bed exists. Again, primary repair of all injured structures is generally indicated in clean wounds. For untidy wounds, debridement and delayed primary repair often is possible. In selected cases, one may elect not to repair an isolated superficialis laceration, because the profundus will provide full finger motion alone. There will, however, be some loss of strength and independence of the digits. Consequently, such treatment is usually best-reserved for those patients medically or psychiatrically unsuited for surgery or, more commonly, for instances of laceration of an effete superficialis to the little finger.

In zone III, the area of adhesions is likely to be over the metacarpals. Protected mobilization of the joints distal to these injuries helps minimize adhesion formation. Tension on the repair can be relieved by a postoperative dressing with proximal flexion at the wrist, relatively less flexion at the metacarpophalangeal joint level, and, in order to reduce the risk of contracture, zero degrees of flexion of the interphalangeal joints. Early mobilization with passive flexion, dynamic flexion traction, and active protected extension are recommended.[157]

Zone II

In the past, zone II has been the controversial no-man's-land where primary tenorrhaphy was not recommended.[20] Today, primary repair is recommended even in the "worst-case" situation, that of digital replantation.[157,161] Again, in this zone, the bulk of the repair is critical. An intratendinous grasping suture is recommended. Many authors also advocate a running epitendinous suture to smooth the line of repair as well as closure of the digital sheath.[5,93] Such measures not only lessen the risk of a bulbous repair catching on the unrepaired edge of the sheath but also close the synovial fluid nutrition support system and may permit it to work more effectively.

In the past, excision of the superficialis was recommended to "make room" for the profundus repair. Excision, in fact, gives less satisfactory results than superficialis repair and is no longer recommended.[83,94,130,157] It is important to remember that the superficialis represents the smooth gliding bed for the profundus over the proximal interphalangeal joint and, further, that the blood supply to the profundus comes through the superficialis at this level. For both these reasons, superficialis excision is more likely to provide a profound adhesion reaction,[130] and it should be avoided.

In acute isolated laceration of the profundus within zone II, the profundus should be repaired. This injury often has a good prognosis, because the failure of the laceration to involve the more deeply situated superficialis suggests a wound of lesser violence. Frequently, the vincula are intact, providing better nutritional support for tendon healing.[5] Acute rupture in zone II is uncommon. Because of fraying of tendon ends, primary repair of a tendon rupture in zone II usually is not possible. Tenodesis of a distal superficialis stump to the proximal phalanx helps prevent swan neck deformity, which may occur after superficialis rupture.[146] Tendon grafting usually is necessary for combined profundus and superficialis rupture in zone II.

Postoperative therapy is somewhat more controversial in zone II than in other areas, some authors recommending early controlled mobilization[41,94] and others an initial 3-week period of immobilization.[29] A recent study by Strickland and Glogovac[159] compared the two methods directly, and early mobilization produced clearly superior results. Most hand surgeons are currently treating zone II lacerations postoperatively with early mobilization of some sort.[83,157]

Zone I

In zone I, by definition, only the flexor profundus or flexor pollicis longus is damaged. If the injury occurs within 1 cm of the tendon insertion, some authors recommend advancement into bone rather than primary repair.[133] Because the tendon insertion at this level is rather oblique and extends over roughly 1 cm of distal phalanx, the distal measuring point is somewhat subjective. There are good reasons not to consider advancement of the flexor profundus, the two most important of which are the risk of producing flexion contracture by an advancement under too great a tension and, along the same lines, a slackening of the conjoined adjacent profundus tendons, the *quadriga phenomenon.*[167] The quadriga phenomenon is named after the four-horse chariot of Roman times that was controlled by a single four-tailed leash. If one horse pulled ahead, the other three tails of the leash would become slack. Similarly, the profundus tendons usually share a single muscle belly. If one tendon is proportionately shorter than the others, it will pull into the palm ahead of its neighbors and cause flexion deficit in neighboring, uninjured digits. For avoidance of the tandem problems of contracture and quadriga, a good general rule is to repair the profundus end to end in zone I if technically possible. If the distal stump is too small to hold a suture, advancement usually is safe.

Rupture of the profundus or the flexor pollicis longus from the point of their insertion is not uncommon. A classification system for these injuries has been proposed by Leddy.[87] These injuries can usually be repaired primarily. In Leddy's type I injury, the tendon is retracted into the palm and should be repaired promptly. Such injuries frequently initiate a severe inflammatory response, probably because the avulsed tendon is ischemic distally, having lost not only its vincular but also its synovial nutritional support.[114] After 7 to 10 days, primary repair of the inflamed, retracted tendon usually is not possible. Type II ruptures remain in the digit and are usually supported by an intact vinculum and maintained in a synovial bed. This good nutritional system seems to inhibit inflammatory response, and these tendons can frequently be repaired directly, even beyond 3 weeks.[87] A small bony fleck, representing the tendon insertion, occasionally is seen at the PIP joint level on the lateral preoperative radiograph in type II rupture. Type III injuries, which are rare, include an associated major intraarticular fracture of the distal phalanx. Because of the size of the fracture fragment, the tendon in type III injuries also usually remains in the digit. Both tendon and bone injuries are treated by open reduction and internal fixation of the large fracture fragment.

Rehabilitation in zone I generally follows that of zone II, but the prognosis is better.

DELAYED RECONSTRUCTION OF FLEXOR TENDON INJURIES

Elbow and Forearm

Late reconstruction of biceps tendon injury is occasionally necessary. Prolongation of biceps with a tendon graft is usually necessary in late cases, with insertion to bone at the bicipital tuberosity. An alternative is to suture the distal biceps tendon to brachialis. This maneuver will augment flexion but not supination. Since many patients with chronic distal biceps rupture have little functional deficit, a careful clinical assessment should be undertaken before any reconstruction is recommended.[118]

Zone V

Late reconstruction of tendon injury in zone V involves either tendon transfer or tendon grafting. The critical tendons are the flexor digitorum profundus and the flexor pollicis longus, without which full finger motion is not possible. In addition, preservation of at least one wrist flexor is desirable to maintain independent wrist and finger flexion. Beyond this, reconstruction depends on the particular need of the patient and on the skill and interest of the surgeon.

Tendon transfer is a popular reconstructive option at this level. Depending on the specific injury, a number of transfer options are available. Most common, perhaps, is transfer of a damaged profundus to its adjacent intact neighbor. The tendon bed in zone V is generally good, and bulk of repair is usually not a problem. A weaving type of suture is preferred because it is stronger than an end-to-end grasping suture.[163]

In some cases of zone V injury, repair may be best effected by tendon grafting. If the injury is limited to zone V, an intercalary graft may be all that is necessary.[151]

Zone IV

In zone IV, the minimal essential requirements are, again, the flexor pollicis longus and the flexor digitorum profundus. Because of the poorer prognosis in this area, reconstruction of the flexor digitorum superficialis is not often indicated. As in zone V, transfer to an adjacent intact tendon unit and intercalary grafting are possible alternatives. The weave repairs are less often indicated because of space considerations. Although less strong, end-to-end grasping suture is usually necessary here. One available option is end-to-end transfer of an adjacent intact superficialis to a nonfunctional profundus.[139]

If the flexor superficialis is intact, as in cases of closed rupture, it may be advisable to debride, but not reconstruct, the profundus, for fear of compromising superficialis function.[24] This is a clinical decision that depends on the needs of the patient and the abilities of the surgeon.

Postoperative rehabilitation may include protected mobilization or an initial period of immobilization that is followed by active exercises.

Zone III

In zone III, reconstruction is generally limited to the flexor profundus if both tendons are injured. At this level, an isolated profundus injury is unlikely.

If tendon grafting is indicated at this level, some authors recommend a bridge, or intercalated graft.[149] Others favor a fingertip-to-palm,[16] or even fingertip-to-wrist,[139] graft. Occasionally, either end-to-side or end-to-end transfer of an adjacent intact tendon is indicated.[139] If this is considered, however, it is important to be sure that the graft does not impinge on the A1 pulley with finger extension.

During reconstruction of zone III injuries, excision of local palmar fascia may be indicated to allow a less restrictive bed.

Zone II

Reconstruction of zone II tendon injury remains the most challenging area of tendon surgery for the hand surgeon. Because of the difficulties involved, reconstruction of both the flexor superficialis and flexor profundus is not considered.

Reconstruction of the flexor profundus in the presence of an intact flexor superficialis must be considered very seriously.[24,72,132] In many, if not most, cases, stabilization of the distal interphalangeal joint proves sufficient treatment for an isolated profundus injury for which reconstruction is being considered.[24,88,133]

Tendon transfer is not advisable at this level, since the juncture would be in zone II. One-stage tendon grafting is indicated if the bed is good, the pulleys are intact, and the patient is cooperative.[16] At the time of surgery, profundus and superficialis remnants should be excised, care being taken to preserve all annular pulleys. The distal graft juncture is to bone at the distal phalanx and proximally to either the superficialis or the profundus in the palm or distal part of the forearm. For grafting to the palm, the palmaris longus makes a satisfactory donor; for longer grafts, the plantaris or toe extensor is necessary.

If the tendon bed is scarred, the pulleys are damaged, or other parts of the digit are damaged (skin, nerve, bone, joint, blood vessels), one-stage tendon grafting is unreliable in restoring active movement to the digit.[16,67,72,86] Two-stage tendon grafting improves the predictability of the procedure. A flexible silicone rubber tendon spacer is used to preserve a channel through the scarred bed while pulley are repaired and associated injuries and contractures are corrected. The details of this procedure are well described elsewhere.[67,70–72,170,175]

Briefly, pulleys that are not intact are reconstructed[70,82,92] with tendon or retinacular graft. A silicone rubber rod is used as a spacer to preserve a channel for later tendon grafting. The rod is fixed distally by a screw or suture so that passive finger motion causes the rod to move like a piston within the reconstructed sheath system. The friction of this motion induces a synovial sheathlike reaction and a bed better-suited for gliding of the subsequent tendon graft.[67,69–72] Usually, passive motion exercises continue for about 3 months after stage-one implantation of the passive tendon implant and pulley reconstruction.

After rehabilitation of the digit with a silicone tendon spacer, the spacer is removed and a conventional tendon graft is passed through the channel created by the spacer. An alternative technique, described by Paneva-Holevich[128] and Winspur et al,[178] involves end-to-end suture of the proximal profundus and superficialis stumps in zone III at the time of stage-one surgery. At stage two, the superficialis is cut proximally in the forearm and passed distally to the fingertip, where it is repaired to bone. As the profundus-superficialis juncture in the palm heals, in essence the profundus is recreated with a pedicled superficialis graft. The advantages of the Paneva-Holevich procedure are that only one juncture, at the fingertip, needs to be protected after stage two and the diameter of the superficialis more closely approximates profundus than the palmaris longus or the plantaris. The disadvantages are that the proximal juncture must be in the palm, which may be scarred, and the large superficialis may be less able than a thinner palmaris longus or plantaris graft to survive on synovial nutrition alone within the flexor sheath. Adhesions, bringing vascularity and nourishment, may thus be more likely to form with a superficialis than with a finer graft. Results of the Paneva-Holevich technique have been reported to be good,[128] but the procedure has gained only limited acceptance to date.

Another reconstructive option has remained tantalizingly attractive over the horizon for years, i.e., an active tendon prosthesis. An active model of the Hunter passive tendon implant is now available, but use at present must be considered investigational.[69]

Late salvage of the finger with zone II tendon injury operated on more than once is particularly challenging. Many patients are better off with amputation than with further attempts at reconstruction. A compromise that may be helpful in some cases is amputation or arthrodesis through the distal interphalangeal joint and staged tendon grafting to the proximal interphalangeal joint.[25] In a hand with multiple severely injured or absent digits, a superficialis finger reconstruction is worthy of consideration.

Rehabilitation after zone II tendon grafting may begin either with a period of immobilization or with controlled early mobilization.[99] Results of the two postoperative methods have not been directly compared but are generally thought to be similar. The recent trend is in favor of early protected mobilization.[157]

Zone I

Zone I injuries include all those of the flexor pollicis longus in the thumb and those of the flexor profundus distal to the superficialis. Late reconstruction options include tenodesis or arthrodesis of the terminal IP joint,[133] one-[115,132,151] or two-stage[177] tendon grafting, or tendon transfer. Transfer of an intact superficialis into the distal phalanx of the thumb is an excellent alternative to a tendon graft in treatment of late cases of flexor pollicis longus loss.[129,143,164] As in zone II, extreme caution must be exercised when reconstruction of a profundus tendon in the presence of an intact superficialis is considered.

IMMEDIATE TREATMENT OF EXTENSOR TENDON INJURIES

Elbow and Forearm

At the elbow, the triceps tendon is susceptible to laceration and, rarely, rupture. Direct suture is usually possible and is recommended.[48,89,118] Associated fracture of the radial head is not uncommon and may also require treatment. A period of immobilization, usually 3 to 4 weeks, followed by active exercises generally provides a satisfactory result. Triceps avulsion associated with fracture of the olecranon is more appropriately dealt with in the section on olecranon fractures.

Zone V

In extensor zone V, treatment is the same as that in flexor zone V: primary or delayed primary repair of all injured structures is generally recommended when the nature of the injury

makes this possible. Since the bed is of good quality unless there has been severe crushing or other associated injury, the prognosis is also usually good. The injured tendon should be protected postoperatively by 3 to 4 weeks of immobilization with the wrist held in extension; after that, active motion exercises are usually begun.

Rupture of extensors in zone V is rare. Treatment, again, is the same as that for flexor injuries in zone V.

Zone IV

Extensor zone IV, like flexor zone IV, is a zone of fibroosseous pulleys and synovial fluid[105] with many tendons in close proximity. As each tendon has a unique function not duplicated by its neighbor, repair of all injured tendons in this area is indicated. Multiple compartments make possible the tailoring of compartment release to just those that have been injured. Complete release of the compartments in which zone V extensor injuries have occurred is not advisable, since it may increase limitation of motion produced by postoperative bowstringing. For prevention of recurrent subluxation of the extensor carpi ulnaris, at least a portion of the sheath of that tendon must be left intact.

Ruptures are uncommon in the first two compartments, but the extensor pollicis longus in compartment three is a frequent victim. Rupture may be due to repetitive use (drummer boy palsy), underlying fractures, or rheumatoid tenosynovitis.[142] If fracture is the cause, the fracture is likely to have been undisplaced. In undisplaced radial fracture, therefore, complaints of pain with thumb motion should be taken seriously. For tenderness that persists along the course of the extensor pollicis longus, some surgeons have recommended early exploration, compartment release, and tenosynovectomy as prophylactic measures.[19] If extensor pollicis longus rupture in zone IV is diagnosed early, primary repair may be possible, even after debridement of frayed tendon ends, particularly if the tendon is transposed away from Lister's tubercle. If not, immediate reconstruction with tendon transfer is preferable. The extensor indicis proprius makes an excellent donor, and reliably satisfactory results have been reported in the literature.[142]

In the fourth compartment, extensor digitorum communis and extensor indicis proprius ruptures usually occur secondary to rheumatoid tenosynovitis or synovitis of the distal radial ulnar joint.[76,117,120,121,166]

The fifth compartment, which lies directly over the distal radial ulnar joint, is a frequent victim of closed rupture due to attrition over a protruding, deformed ulnar head in patients with rheumatoid arthritis—the caput ulnae, or Vaughan-Jackson, syndrome.[166] These lesions are described further in Chap. 39.

In the sixth compartment, rupture of the tendon is not as frequent a problem as rupture of the sheath and subsequent recurrent subluxation of extensor carpi ulnaris over the ulna with forearm rotation.[21] Usually, the injury is caused by a forcible pronation of the forearm, and symptoms are produced by twisting motion, such as swinging a golf club.

Zone II

Extensor zone II also parallels the flexor zone designation. Just as subzones are being recognized on the flexor surface, subdivisions are appropriate on the extensor side, where intrinsic and extrinsic tendons interweave in a complex biomechanical relationship.

Zone IIc is the zone of the metacarpophalangeal joint. Open injury may consist of laceration of the central extensor tendon or the sagittal band, including the special case of the barroom brawler's human bite injury.[37,100]

One other injury deserving mention in zone IIc is closed sagittal band rupture, which may occur with resisted finger extension. The unbalanced sagittal band mechanism that results usually leads to dislocation of the central extensor to the side of intact sagittal band, with either a recurrent painful subluxation as the finger moves from flexion to extension or the inability to actively extend the finger from the flexed position due to the displacement of the extensor completely into the valley between the metacarpal heads. Some of these injuries require suture of the sagittal band, but those diagnosed early often benefit from extension splinting for 3 to 4 weeks followed by active range-of-motion exercises.[22,81] My practice has been to treat these patients without surgery if they are able to actively extend the finger from the flexed position when first seen. If they cannot do so, surgical exploration and repair of the sagittal band are clearly indicated.

Postoperatively, zone IIc injuries can be treated either with immobilization or early controlled mobilization. If immobilization is chosen, one must be careful to relax the extensor mechanism by wrist extension and permit MP joint flexion of 30 to 45 degrees to avoid postoperative joint extension contracture.[95] If uncomplicated by MP joint infection, most zone IIc injuries have a good prognosis.[95]

Zone IIb is the region over the proximal phalanx. In this region, the intrinsic tendons insert into the extensor apparatus. Thus, there are actually three extensors in this zone: the radial and ulnar intrinsics and the central common extensor. Because of tethers at the MP and PIP joints, the tendons usually do not retract appreciably when lacerated. Direct repair followed by immobilization in MP joint flexion and PIP joint extension is the usual treatment for acute lacerations.[14,95]

Zone IIa injuries are perhaps the most complex and challenging on the extensor surface. These injuries involve the region about the insertion of the central tendon into the middle phalanx. Open injuries, as elsewhere, are best-treated with primary or delayed primary repair and immobilization of the PIP joint in extension for 4 weeks and then by protected active mobilization. Closed injuries present particular problems at this level because of failure of diagnosis.[2] Indirect trauma to the fingertip can result in rupture of the central tendon. Direct trauma to the dorsum of the PIP joint may also result in rupture of the central tendon. If only the central tendon is injured, active PIP joint extension will be possible for a time via the lateral bands. Eventually, these displace volarly, however, and a flexion deformity develops. The volar displacement limits distal excursion of the lateral bands, and a reciprocal DIP joint extension contracture results, yielding the classic boutonniere deformity.[145]

Since reconstruction of an established boutonniere deformity often permanently impairs motion, prevention is the best treatment. Closed injuries to the dorsum of the PIP joint that result in pain or swelling, particularly if the pain is to resisted active extension, should be assumed to involve the central slip mechanism. A period of 2 to 4 weeks of continuous extension splinting followed by carefully monitored active motion exercises should permit satisfactory healing in most cases.[37] If an acute closed injury causes a clear deficit of active extension (not merely due to pain or swelling) but full passive extension is possible, early exploration and anatomical repair[56] of the extensor mechanism should be considered. In such cases, the lateral bands may have been acutely displaced volarly with combined injury to the central slip and triangular ligament.

Zone I

Zone I extensor injuries involve DIP joint extension only. These injuries may be the result of either a laceration or a direct blow on the extended fingertip with closed injury. Such injuries may occur with or without avulsion fracture on the dorsum of the distal phalanx. Open laceration should be treated by suturing and splinting in extension for 4 to 6 weeks and then by active motion exercises. Closed injuries can usually be treated by continuous extension splinting for 6 to 8 weeks and then by protected active flexion exercises.[1,28,33,125] Although some permanent extension lag frequently persists, the deformity is usually not disabling.[172] Except in cases associated with large fracture fragments and actual DIP joint subluxation, open treatment of acute closed injuries is rarely indicated.[75,85,172]

LATE RECONSTRUCTION OF EXTENSOR TENDON INJURIES

Elbow and Forearm

If reconstruction of the triceps mechanism is necessary, recreation of the triceps tendon with a graft of fascia from the proximal portion of the forearm may be necessary.[12] In unusual cases with loss of triceps muscle substance or denervation of the triceps muscle, transfer of the latissimus dorsi provides an excellent triceps substitute as well.[65]

Zone V

In cases of zone V injury which are recognized late or which require reconstruction for other reasons, treatment options include transfer of the distal stump of the injured tendon to an uninjured muscle-tendon unit and intercalary grafting. As on the flexor surface, the results are generally good. Even if adhesions develop, a functional range of wrist extension is often possible, because the tendon excursion required for this is not great and finger extension can be achieved by the tenodesis effect.

Zone IV

In general, reconstruction by transfer of adjacent tendon units and intercalary grafting provides a satisfactory substitute for extensor tendon function after zone IV injury. In extensive scarring of the dorsum, such as that after a burn injury or severe crush injury, two-stage tendon reconstruction may be required.[13] Again, because the excursion required for satisfactory function of the extensor side is less than that required on the flexor side, results are generally better than those which could be expected for reconstruction of flexor zone IV.

Some special cases of reconstruction in zone IV deserve particular reference. Rupture of the extensor pollicis longus can be repaired by grafting,[60] but transfer of the extensor indicis proprius is a reliable reconstructive option.[142] Since the common digital extensor to the index finger is frequently independent, there is usually no loss of independent index extension, even after transfer of the extensor indicis proprius.[174] As mentioned in the section on acute injury, reconstruction for fourth and fifth compartment tendons is frequently necessary in patients with rupture secondary to rheumatoid arthritis. Transfer of the injured tendon to an intact neighbor or transfer of an intact superficialis tendon either through the interosseous membrane or around the forearm usually provides satisfactory reconstruction in these cases. Excision of the head of the ulna may be necessary for persistent distal radioulnar joint synovitis and subluxation.

Zone III

In extensor zone III, reconstruction is usually required because of severe associated injury secondary to burn or crush. Transfer or repair of a tendon beneath a skin graft or burn scar of poor quality is not advisable. In these cases, wound excision and flap coverage may be necessary. At the time of flap coverage, insertion of silicone rubber tendon spacers is helpful to provide channels through which later tendon grafts can be threaded without the necessity of reelevating the flap.[13] Rehabilitation after tendon transfer or grafting is the same as that used after acute injuries.[95]

Zone II

Reconstruction in zone IIc may be necessary in some cases. If a segmental gap exists in the common extensor, a tendon graft may be necessary.[27] Late treatment of sagittal band rupture may also require tendon graft, because the ruptured edges of the sagittal band usually retract and atrophy.[81]

Reconstruction in zone IIb usually takes the form of tenolysis, since these injuries may form adhesions to underlying bone or overlying skin that limit proximal interphalangeal and dorsal interphalangeal flexion.

Reconstruction after zone IIa injuries that have resulted in an established boutonniere deformity is not completely satisfactory, and often a permanent impairment of motion persists. Usually, anatomical reconstruction is possible by shortening the central slip mechanism and relocating the lateral bands more dorsally.[31,56] The central slip can be shortened by imbrication or by division and reattachment into the middle phalanx. Release of the transverse retinacular ligament is necessary to permit the lateral bands to reposition dorsally, and the triangular ligament can be re-created with suture. If significant shortening of the lateral bands has occurred, transection of the lateral bands between the proximal and distal interphalangeal joints will release their effect on the DIP joint and permit them to act as auxiliary PIP joint extensors, as advocated by Fowler and others.[36,147,148] In cases complicated by severe soft tissue loss, such as that seen in burns and severe crush or avulsion injury, additional skin cover may be necessary, and reconstruction may require either tendon graft woven through the extensor mechanism proximally and through drill holes in the middle phalanx distally or it may require the lateral band tendon transfer described by Matev.[109]

In late cases of boutonniere deformity, there may be a fixed volar capsular contracture, and flexor tendon adhesions may have developed. A separate volar release may also be necessary, either before or during reconstruction. After reconstruction, the PIP joint should be splinted or pinned in full extension for approximately 4 weeks and then active motion exercises begun. Finally, in late cases with severe associated injury or after multiple attempts at reconstruction, arthrodesis of the PIP joint should be considered.[152]

Zone I

Reconstruction for extensor tendon injuries in zone I is not often indicated. Tendon graft to the remnants of the terminal tendon is not reliable. If disabling flexion deformity at the fingertip develops without reciprocal hyperextension at the PIP, arthrodesis should be considered. Cases with associated hyperextension of the PIP joint can be treated either by reconstruction distally or by sectioning of the central slip as it inserts on the base of the middle phalanx.[15] This treatment permits a general proximal retraction of the extensor mechanism and increases the extensor tone at the DIP joint. Because dorsal fixation of the lateral bands at the PIP joint level already exists in these cases and is the cause of the hyperextension at the PIP joint, late development of a boutonniere deformity is rare.

For patients who do not have reciprocal hyperextension of the PIP joint and for whom arthrodesis is an unsatisfactory alternative, tenodermadesis, as described by Iselin et al,[75] is an additional treatment option.

REFERENCES

1. Abouna, J.M., and Brown, H. The treatment of mallet finger: The results in a series of 148 consecutive cases and a review of the literature. Br J Surg 55:653–667, 1968.
2. Aiche, A., Barsky, A.J., and Weiner, D.L. Prevention of boutonniere deformity. Plast Reconstr Surg 46:164–167, 1979.
3. Allen, B.N., and Leslie, M.S. Repeat Repair of Ruptured Flexor

Tendons in Zone 2 Which Had Been Previously Repaired. Presented at the Annual Resident's Meeting of the American Society for Surgery of the Hand, Atlanta, Georgia, February 6–8, 1984.

4. Allieu, Y., Asencio, G., Gomis, R., Teissier, J., and Rouzaud, J.C. Suture des tendons extenseurs de la main avec mobilisation assistée. A propos de 120 cas. Rev Chir Orthop 70 (suppl 2):69–73, 1984.

5. Amadio, P.C., Hunter, J.M., Jaeger, S.H., Wehbe, M.A., and Schneider, L.H. The effect of vincular injury on the results of flexor tendon surgery in Zone 2. J Hand Surg [Am], 10:626–632, 1985.

6. Amadio, P.C., Jaeger, S.H., and Hunter, J.M. Nutritional aspects of tendon healing, in Hunter, J.M., Schneider, L.H., Mackin, E.J., and Callahan, A.D. (eds): *Rehabilitation of the Hand,* 2d ed. St. Louis, Mosby, 1984, pp 255–260.

7. Method of Measuring and Recording Joint Motion. Chicago, American Academy of Orthopedic Surgeons, 1965.

8. Azar, C.A., Fleegler, E.J., and Culver, J.E. Dynamic anatomy of the flexor pulley system of the fingers and thumb [abstract]. Orthop Trans 8:122, 1984.

9. Baker, B.E., and Bierwagen, D. Rupture of the distal tendon of the biceps brachii: Operative versus non-operative treatment. J Bone Joint Surg [Am] 67:414–417, 1985.

10. Banes, A.J., Enterline, D., Bevin, A.G., and Salisbury, R.E. Effects of trauma and partial devascularization on protein synthesis in the avian flexor profundus tendon. J Trauma 21:505–512, 1981.

11. Barton, N.J. Experimental study of optimal location of flexor tendon pulleys. Plast Reconstr Surg 43:125–129, 1969.

12. Bennett, B.S. Triceps tendon rupture: Case report and a method of repair. J Bone Joint Surg [Am] 44:741–744, 1962.

13. Bevin, A.G., and Hothem, A.L. The use of silicone rods under split-thickness skin grafts for reconstruction of extensor tendon injuries. Hand 10:254–258, 1978.

14. Blue, A.I., Spira, M., and Hardy, S.B. Repair of extensor tendon injuries of the hand. Am J Surg 132:128–132, 1976.

15. Bowers, W.H., and Hurst, L.C. Chronic mallet finger: The use of Fowler's central slip release. J Hand Surg [Am] 3:373–376, 1978.

16. Boyes, J.H., and Stark, H.H. Flexor-tendon grafts in the fingers and thumb: A study of factors influencing results in 1000 cases. J Bone Joint Surg [Am] 53:1332–1342, 1971.

17. Browne, E.Z., Jr., Teague, M.A., and Snyder, C.C. Prevention of extensor lag after indicis proprius tendon transfer. J Hand Surg [Am] 4:168–172, 1979.

18. Bruner, J.M. The zig-zag volar-digital incision for flexor-tendon surgery. Plast Reconstr Surg 40:571–574, 1967.

19. Bunata, R.E. Impending rupture of the extensor pollicis longus tendon after a minimally displaced Colles fracture: A case report. J Bone Joint Surg [Am] 65:401–402, 1983.

20. Bunnell, S. Repair of tendons in the fingers. Surg Gynecol Obstet 35:88–97, 1922.

21. Burkhart, S.S., Wood, M.B., and Linscheid, R.L. Posttraumatic recurrent subluxation of the extensor carpi ulnaris tendon. J Hand Surg [Am] 7:1–3, 1982.

22. Burton, R.I. Extensor tendons—Late reconstruction, in Green, D.P. (ed): *Operative Hand Surgery,* vol 2. New York, Churchill Livingstone, 1982, pp 1465–1505.

23. Cannon, N.M., and Strickland, J.W. Therapy following flexor tendon surgery. Hand Clin 1:147–165, 1985.

24. Carroll, R.E., and Match, R.M. Avulsion of the flexor profundus tendon insertion. J Trauma 10:1109–1117, 1970.

25. Chuinard, R.G., Dabezies, E.J., and Mathews, R.E. Two-stage superficialis tendon reconstruction in severely damaged fingers. J Hand Surg [Am] 5:135–143, 1980.

26. Clayton, M. The caput ulnae syndrome, in Strickland, J.W., and Steichen, J.B. (eds): *Difficult Problems in Hand Surgery.* St. Louis, Mosby, 1982, pp 199–202.

27. Clayton, M.L., Thirupathi, R., Ferlic, D.C., and Goldberg, B. Extensor tendon rupture over the metacarpal heads. Hand 15:149–150, 1983.

28. Crawford, G.P. The molded polythene splint for mallet finger deformities. J Hand Surg [Am] 9:231–237, 1984.

29. Creekmore, H., Bellinghausen, H., Young, V.L., Wray, R.C., Weeks, P.M., and Grasse, P.S. Comparison of early passive motion and immobilization after flexor tendon repairs. Plast Reconstr Surg 75:75–79, 1985.

30. Crosby, E.B., and Linscheid, R.L. Rupture of the flexor profundus tendon of the ring finger secondary to ancient fracture of the hook of the hamate: Review of the literature and report of two cases. J Bone Joint Surg [Am] 56:1076–1078, 1974.

31. Curtis, R.M., Reid, R.L., and Provost, J.M. A staged technique for the repair of the traumatic boutonniere deformity. J Hand Surg [Am] 8:167–171, 1983.

32. Delattre, J.F., Ducasse, A., Flament, J.B., and Kénési, C. The mechanical role of the digital fibrous sheath: Application to reconstructive surgery of the flexor tendons. Anat Clin 3:187–197, 1983.

33. Din, K.M., and Meggitt, B.F. Mallet thumb. J Bone Joint Surg [Br] 65:606–607, 1983.

34. Dobyns, J.H. Personal communication, 1983.

35. Dobyns, R.C., Cooney, W.C., and Wood, M.B. Effect of partial lacerations on canine flexor tendons. Minn Med 65:27–32, 1982.

36. Dolphin, J.A. Extensor tenotomy for chronic boutonnière deformity of the finger: Report of two cases. J Bone Joint Surg [Am] 47:161–164, 1965.

37. Doyle, J.R. Extensor tendons—Acute injuries, in Green, D.P. (ed): *Operative Hand Surgery,* vol 2. New York, Churchill Livingstone, 1982, pp 1441–1464.

38. Doyle, J.R., and Blythe, W.F. The finger flexor tendon sheath and pulleys: Anatomy and reconstruction, in *Symposium on Tendon Surgery in the Hand.* St. Louis, Mosby, 1975, pp 81–109.

39. Doyle, J.R., and Blythe, W.F. Anatomy of the flexor tendon sheath and pulleys of the thumb. J Hand Surg [Am] 2:149–151, 1977.

40. Dreyfuss, U., and Kessler, I. Snapping elbow due to dislocation of the medial head of the triceps: A report of two cases. J Bone Joint Surg [Br] 60:56–57, 1978.

41. Duran, R.J., Houser, R.G., and Stover, M.G. Management of flexor tendon lacerations in zone 2 using controlled passive motion postoperatively, in Hunter, J.M., Schneider, L.H., Mackin, E.J., and Bell, J. (eds): *Rehabilitation of the Hand.* St. Louis, Mosby, 1978, pp 217–224.

42. Eiken, O., Hagberg, L., and Lundborg, G. Evolving biologic concepts as applied to tendon surgery. Clin Plast Surg 8:1–12, January 1981.

43. Eiken, O., Holmberg, J., Ekerot, L., and Sälgeback, S. Restoration of the digital tendon sheath: A new concept of tendon grafting. Scand J Plast Reconstr Surg 14:89–97, 1980.

44. Ejeskär, A. Finger flexion force and hand grip strength after tendon repair. J Hand Surg [Am] 7:61–65, 1982.

45. Ejeskär, A. Flexor tendon repair of no-man's-land: Results of primary repair with controlled mobilization. J Hand Surg [Am] 9:171–177, 1984.

46. Enna, C.D., and Ruby, J.R. Scanning electron microscopic study of long flexors in human fingers. J Hand Surg [Am] 6:329–335, 1981.

47. Fahey, J.J., and Bollinger, J.A. Trigger-finger in adults and children. J Bone Joint Surg [Am] 36:1200–1218, 1954.

48. Farrar, E.L., III, and Lippert, F.G., III. Avulsion of the triceps tendon. Clin Orthop 161:242–246, 1981.

49. Frère, G., Moutet, F., Sarorius, Ch., and Vila, A. Controlled postoperative mobilization of sutured extension tendons of the longer fingers. Ann Chir Main 3:139–144, 1984.

50. Gainor, B.J. Closed avulsion of the flexor digitorum superficialis origin causing compartment syndrome: A case report. J Bone

Joint Surg [Am] 66:467, 1984.

51. Gelberman, R.H., and Manske, P.R. Factors influencing flexor tendon adhesions. Hand Clin 1:35–42, February 1985.

52. Gelberman, R.H., Manske, P.R., Vande Berg, J.S., Lesker, P.A., and Akeson, W.H. Flexor tendon repair in vitro: A comparative histologic study of the rabbit, chicken, dog, and monkey. J Orthop Res 2:39–48, 1984.

53. Gelberman, R.H., Woo, S.L.-Y., Lothringer, K., Akeson, W.H., and Amiel, D. Effects of early intermittent passive mobilization on healing canine flexor tendons. J Hand Surg [Am] 7:170–175, 1982.

54. Gillard, G.C., Reilly, H.C., Bell-Booth, P.G., and Flint, M.H. The influence of mechanical forces on the glycosaminoglycan content of the rabbit flexor digitorum profundus tendon. Connect Tissue Res 7:37–46, 1979.

55. Goldstein, S.A., Greene, T.L., Ward, W.S., and Matthews, L.S. A biomechanical evaluation of the function of the digital pulleys [abstract]. Orthop Trans 8:354, 1984.

56. Grundberg, A.B. Anatomic repair of boutonnière deformity. Clin Orthop 153:226–229, 1980.

57. Grundberg, A.B., and Reagan, D.S. The pathologic anatomy of intersection syndrome [abstract]. Orthop Trans 8:124–125, 1984.

58. Hallett, J.P., and Motta, G.R. Tendon ruptures in the hand with particular reference to attrition ruptures in the carpal tunnel. Hand 14:283–290, 1982.

59. Halpern, A.A., Horowitz, B.G., and Nagel, D.A. Tendon ruptures associated with corticosteroid therapy. West J Med 127:378–382, 1977.

60. Hamlin, C., and Littler, J.W. Restoration of the extensor pollicis longus tendon by an intercalated graft. J Bone Joint Surg [Am] 59:412–414, 1977.

61. Helal, B., Chen, S.C., and Iwegbu, G. Rupture of the extensor pollicis longus tendon in undisplaced Colles' type of fracture. Hand 14:41–47, 1982.

62. Hochberg, F.H., Leffert, R.D., Heller, M.D., and Merriman, L. Hand difficulties among musicians. JAMA 249:1869–1872, 1983.

63. Hooper, G., Davies, R., and Tothill, P. Blood flow and clearance in tendons: Studies with dogs. J Bone Joint Surg [Br] 66:441–443, 1984.

64. Hovelius, L., and Josefsson, G. Rupture of the distal biceps tendon: report of five cases. Acta Orthop Scand 48:280–282, 1977.

65. Hovnanian, A.P. Latissimus dorsi transplantation for loss of flexion or extension at the elbow: A preliminary report on technic. Ann Surg 143:493–499, 1956.

66. Hueston, J.T., and Wilson, W.F. The aetiology of trigger finger: Explained on the basis of intratendinous architecture. Hand 4:257–260, 1972.

67. Hunter, J.M. Staged flexor tendon reconstruction. J Hand Surg [Am] 8:789–793, 1983.

68. Hunter, J.M. Anatomy of flexor tendons—pulley, vincular, synovial, and vascular structures, in Spinner, M. (ed): *Kaplan's Functional and Surgical Anatomy of the Hand,* 3d ed. Philadelphia, Lippincott, 1984, pp 65–92.

69. Hunter, J.M. Tendon salvage and the active tendon implant: A perspective. Hand Clin 1:181–186, February 1985.

70. Hunter, J.M., and Amadio, P.C. Two-stage tendon reconstruction using gliding implants, in Birch, R., and Brooks, D., (eds): *The Hand,* 4th ed. London, Butterworth's, 1984, pp 149–167.

71. Hunter, J.M., and Jaeger, S.H. Tendon implants: Primary and secondary usage. Orthop Clin North Am 8:473–489, April 1977.

72. Hunter, J.M., and Salisbury, R.E. Flexor-tendon reconstruction in severely damaged hands: A two-stage procedure using a silicone-Dacron reinforced gliding prosthesis prior to tendon grafting. J Bone Joint Surg [Am] 53:829–858, 1971.

73. Hunter, J.M., Seinsheimer, F., and Mackin, E. Tenolysis, in Strickland, J.B., and Steichen, J.B., (eds): *Difficult Problems in Hand Surgery.* St. Louis, Mosby, 1982, pp 312–318.

74. Idler, R.S. Anatomy and biomechanics of the digital flexor tendons. Hand Clin 1:3–11, February 1985.

75. Iselin, F., Levame, J., and Godoy, J. A simplified technique for treating mallet fingers: Tenodermodesis. J Hand Surg [Am] 2:118–121, 1977.

76. James, J.I.P. The value of tenolysis. Hand 1:118–119, 1969.

77. Karpman, R.R., McComb, J.E., and Volz, R.G. Tendon rupture following local steroid injection: Report of four cases. Postgrad Med 68:169–176, July 1980.

78. Ketchum, L.D. Primary tendon healing: A review. J Hand Surg [Am] 2:428–435, 1977.

79. Ketchum, L.D., Brand, P.W., Thompson, D., and Pocock, G.S. The determination of moments for extension of the wrist generated by muscles of the forearm. J Hand Surg [Am] 3:205–210, 1978.

80. Ketchum, L.D., Martin, N.L., and Kappel, D.A. Experimental evaluation of factors affecting the strength of tendon repairs. Plast Reconstr Surg 59:708–719, 1977.

81. Kettelkamp, D.B., Flatt, A.E., and Moulds, R. Traumatic dislocation of the long-finger extensor tendon: a clinical, anatomical, and biomechanical study. J Bone Joint Surg [Am] 53:229–240, 1971.

82. Kleinert, H.E., and Bennett, J.B. Digital pulley reconstruction employing the always present rim of the previous pulley. J Hand Surg [Am] 3:297–298, 1978.

83. Kleinert, H.E., and Verdan, C. Report of the Committee on Tendon Injuries. J Hand Surg [Am] 8:794–798, 1983.

84. Landsmeer, J.M.F. The anatomy of the dorsal aponeurosis of the human finger and its functional significance. Anat Rec 104:31–44, 1949.

85. Lange, R.H., and Engber, W.D. Hyperextension mallet finger. Orthopedics 6:1426–1431, 1983.

86. LaSalle, W.B., and Strickland, J.W. An evaluation of the two-stage flexor tendon reconstruction technique. J Hand Surg [Am] 8:263–267, 1983.

87. Leddy, J.P. Avulsions of the flexor digitorum profundus. Hand Clin 1:77–83, February 1985.

88. Leddy, J.P., and Packer, J.W. Avulsion of the profundus tendon insertion in athletes. J Hand Surg [Am] 2:66–69, 1977.

89. Levy, M., Fishel, R.E., and Stern, G.M. Triceps tendon avulsion with or without fracture of the radial head—a rare injury? J Trauma 18:677–679, 1978.

90. Linburg, R.M., and Comstock, B.E. Anomalous tendon slips from the flexor pollicis longus to the flexor digitorum profundus. J Hand Surg [Am] 4:79–83, 1979.

91. Lister, G. Pitfalls and complications of flexor tendon surgery. Hand Clin 1:133–146, February 1985.

92. Lister, G.D. Reconstruction of pulleys employing extensor retinaculum. J Hand Surg [Am] 4:461–464, 1979.

93. Lister, G.D. Incision and closure of the flexor sheath during primary tendon repair. Hand 15:123–135, 1983.

94. Lister, G.D., Kleinert, H.E., Kutz, J.E., and Atasoy, E. Primary flexor tendon repair followed by immediate controlled mobilization. J Hand Surg [Am] 2:441–451, 1977.

95. Lovett, W.L., and McCalla, M.A. Management and rehabilitation of extensor tendon injuries. Orthop Clin North Am 14:811–826, October, 1982.

96. Lundborg, G., Holm, S., and Myrhage, R. The role of the synovial fluid and tendon sheath for flexor tendon nutrition: an experimental tracer study on diffusional pathways in dogs. Scand J Plast Reconstr Surg 14:99–107, 1980.

97. Lundborg, G., Myrhage, R., and Rydevik, B. The vascularization of human flexor tendons within the digital synovial sheath region—structural and functional aspects. J Hand Surg [Am] 2:417–427, 1977.

98. Lundborg, G., and Rank, F. Experimental intrinsic healing of flexor tendons based upon synovial fluid nutrition. J Hand Surg

[Am] 3:21–31, 1978.

99. Mackin, E.J., and Maiorano, L. Postoperative therapy following staged flexor tendon reconstruction, in Hunter, J.M., Schneider, L.H., Mackin, E.J., and Bell, J. (eds): *Rehabilitation of the Hand.* St. Louis, Mosby, 1978, pp 247–261.

100. Mann, R.J., Hoffeld, T.A., and Farmer, C.B. Human bites of the hand: Twenty years of experience. J Hand Surg [Am] 2:97–104, 1977.

101. Mannerfelt, L., and Norman, O. Attrition ruptures of flexor tendons in rheumatoid arthritis caused by bony spurs in the carpal tunnel: A clinical and radiological study. J Bone Joint Surg [Br] 51:270–277, 1969.

102. Manske, P.R., Gelberman, R.H., and Lesker, P.A. Flexor tendon healing. Hand Clin 1:25–34, February 1985.

103. Manske, P.R., and Lesker, P.A. Strength of human pulleys. Hand 9:147–152, 1977.

104. Manske, P.R., and Lesker, P.A. Comparative nutrient pathways to the flexor profundus tendons in Zone II of various experimental animals. J Surg Res 34:83–93, 1983a.

105. Manske, P.R., and Lesker, P.A. Nutrient pathways to extensor tendons within the extensor retinacular compartments: An experimental study in dogs. Clin Orthop 181:234–237, 1983b.

106. Manske, P.R., and Lesker, P.A. Palmar aponeurosis pulley. J Hand Surg [Am] 8:259–263, 1983c.

107. Manske, P.R., Whiteside, L.A., and Lesker, P.A. Nutrient pathways to flexor tendons using hydrogen washout technique. J Hand Surg [Am] 3:32–36, 1978.

108. Mason, M.L., and Allen, H.S. The rate of healing of tendons: An experimental study of tensile strength. Ann Surg 113:424–456, 1941.

109. Matev, I. Transposition of the lateral slips of the aponeurosis in treatment of long-standing "boutonnière deformity" of the fingers. Br J Plast Surg 17:281–286, 1964.

110. Matev, I., Karagancheva, S., Trichkova, P., and Tsekov, P. Delayed primary suture of flexor tendons cut in the digital theca. Hand 12:158–162, 1980.

111. Matsui, T., Merklin, R.J., and Hunter, J.M. [A microvascular study of the human flexor tendons in the digital fibrous sheath—normal blood vessel arrangement of tendons and the effects of injuries to tendons and vincula on distribution of tendon blood vessels (author's trans.)]. Nippon Seikeigaka Gakkai Zasshi 53:307–320, 1979.

112. Matthews, J.P. Vascular changes in flexor tendons after injury and repair: An experimental study. Injury 8:227–233, 1977.

113. Matthews, P., and Richards, H. The repair potential of digital flexor tendons: An experimental study. J Bone Joint Surg [Br] 56:618–625, 1974.

114. Matthews, P., and Richards, H. Factors in the adherence of flexor tendon after repair: An experimental study in the rabbit. J Bone Joint Surg [Br] 58:230–236, 1976.

115. McClinton, M.A., Curtis, R.M., and Wilgis, E.F.S. One hundred tendon grafts for isolated flexor digitorum profundus injuries. J Hand Surg [Am] 7:224–229, 1982.

116. McDowell, C.L., and Snyder, D.M. Tendon healing: An experimental model in the dog. J Hand Surg [Am] 2:122–126, 1977.

117. Millender, L.H., and Nalebuff, E.A. Evaluation and treatment of early rheumatoid hand involvement. Orthop Clin North Am 6:697–708, July 1975.

118. Morrey, B.F. (ed): *The Elbow and Its Disorders.* Philadelphia, Saunders, 1985, pp 452–463.

119. Morrey, B.F., Askew, L.J., An, K.N., and Dobyns, J.H. Rupture of the distal tendon of the biceps brachii: A biomechanical study. J Bone Joint Surg [Am] 67:418–421, 1985.

120. Nalebuff, E.A. Surgical treatment of tendon rupture in the rheumatoid hand. Surg Clin North Am 49:811–822, August, 1969.

121. Nalebuff, E.A., and Patel, M.R. Flexor digitorum sublimis transfer for multiple extensor tendon ruptures in rheumatoid arthritis. Plast Reconstr Surg 52:530–533, 1973.

122. Neviaser, R.J. Closed tendon sheath irrigation for pyogenic flexor tenosynovitis. J Hand Surg [Am] 3:462–466, 1978.

123. Nirschl, R.P. Rehabilitation of the athlete's elbow, in Morrey, B.F. (ed): *The Elbow and Its Disorders.* Philadelphia, Saunders, 1985, pp 523–529.

124. Nirschl, R.P., and Pettrone, F.A. Tennis elbow: The surgical treatment of lateral epicondylitis. J Bone Joint Surg [Am] 61:832–839, 1979.

125. Nunley, J.A., and Urbaniak, J.R. Treatment of extensor tendon injuries of the hand. Orthop Surg (Update Series) 2:2–8, 1982.

126. Nyström, B., and Holmlund, D. Separation of sutured tendon ends when different suture techniques and different suture materials are used: An experimental study in rabbits. Scand J Plast Reconstr Surg 17:19–23, 1983.

127. Ochiai, N., Matsui, T., Miyaji, N., Merklin, R.J., and Hunter, J.M. Vascular anatomy of flexor tendons. I. Vincular system and blood supply of the profundus tendon in the digital sheath. J Hand Surg [Am] 4:321–330, 1979.

128. Paneva-Holevich, E. Two-stage tenoplasty in injury of the flexor tendons of the hand. J Bone Joint Surg [Am] 51:21–32, 1969.

129. Posner, M.A. Flexor superficialis tendon transfers to the thumb—An alternative to the free tendon graft for treatment of chronic injuries within the digital sheath. J Hand Surg [Am] 8:876–881, 1983.

130. Potenza, A.D. Tendon healing within the flexor digital sheath in the dog: An experimental study. J Bone Joint Surg [Am] 44:49–64, 1962.

131. Potenza, A.D. Prevention of adhesions to healing digital flexor tendons. JAMA 187:187–191, 1964.

132. Pulvertaft, R.G. The treatment of profundus division by free tendon graft. J Bone Joint Surg [Am] 42:1363–1371, 1960.

133. Reid, D.A.C. The isolated flexor digitorum profundus lesion. Hand 1:115–117, 1969.

134. Richards, H.J. Factors affecting the healing and return of function in the repaired digital flexor tendon. Aust NZ J Surg 50:258–263, 1980a.

135. Richards, H.J. Repair and healing of the divided digital flexor tendon. Injury 12:1–12, 1980b.

136. Riddell, D.M. Spontaneous rupture of the extensor pollicis longus: The results of tendon transfer. J Bone Joint Surg [Br] 45:506–510, 1963.

137. Russell, R.C., O'Brien, B.McC., Morrison, W.A., Pamamull, G., and MacLeod, A. The late functional results of upper limb revascularization and replantation. J Hand Surg [Am] 9:623–633, 1984.

138. Schlenker, J.D., Lister, G.D., and Kleinert, H.E. Three complications of untreated partial laceration of flexor tendon—entrapment, rupture, and triggering. J Hand Surg [Am] 6:392–396, 1981.

139. Schneider, L.H. *Flexor Tendon Injuries.* Boston, Little, Brown, 1984.

140. Schneider, L.H., Hunter, J.M., Norris, T.R., and Nadeau, P.O. Delayed flexor tendon repair in no man's land. J Hand Surg [Am] 2:452–455, 1977.

141. Schneider, L.H., and Mackin, E.J. Tenolysis, in Hunter, J.M., Schneider, L.H., Mackin, E.J., and Bell, J. (eds): *Rehabilitation of the Hand.* St. Louis, Mosby, 1978, pp 229–234.

142. Schneider, L.H., and Rosenstein, R.G. Restoration of extensor pollicis longus function by tendon transfer. Plast Reconstr Surg 71:533–537, 1983.

143. Schneider, L.H., and Wiltshire, D. Restoration of flexor pollicis longus function by flexor digitorum superficialis transfer. J Hand Surg [Am] 8:98–101, 1983.

144. Simonet, W.T., Weidman, K.A., Wood, M.B., Cooney, W.P., III, and Ilstrup, D.M. Quantification of blood flow to canine cruciate liga-

ments [abstract]. Orthop Trans 8:78, 1984.

145. Smith, R.J. Balance and kinetics of the fingers under normal and pathological conditions. Clin Orthop 104:92–111, 1974a.

146. Smith, R.J. Hyperextension injuries at the proximal interphalangeal joints of the fingers. Ann Chir 28:297–307, 1974b.

147. Souter, W.A. The boutonnière deformity: A review of 101 patients with division of the central slip of the extensor expansion of the fingers. J Bone Joint Surg [Br] 49:710–721, 1967.

148. Souter, W.A. The problem of boutonniere deformity. Clin Orthop 104:116–133, 1974.

149. Stark, H.H., Anderson, D.R., Boyes, J.H., Zemel, N.P., Rickard, T.A., and Ashworth, C.R. Bridge grafts of flexor tendons [abstract]. Orthop Trans 7:44, 1983.

150. Stark, H.H., Boyes, J.H., and Wilson, J.N. Mallet finger. J Bone Joint Surg [Am] 44:1061–1068, 1962.

151. Stark, H.H., Zemel, N.P., Boyes, J.H., and Ashworth, C.R. Flexor tendon graft through intact superficialis tendon. J Hand Surg [Am] 2:456–461, 1977.

152. Steichen, J.B., Strickland, J.W., Call, W.H., and Powell, S.G. Results of surgical treatment of chronic boutonniere deformity: An analysis of prognostic factors, in Strickland, J.W., and Steichen, J.B., (eds): *Difficult Problems in Hand Surgery.* St. Louis, Mosby, 1982, pp 62–69.

153. Steiner, M. Biomechanics of tendon healing. J Biomech 15:951–958, 1982.

154. Stern, P.J. Multiple flexor tendon ruptures following an old anterior dislocation of the lunate: A case report. J Bone Joint Surg [Am] 63:489–490, 1981.

155. Storace, A., and Wolf, B. Kinematic analysis of the role of the finger tendons. J Biomech 15:391–393, 1982.

156. Strickland, J.W. Flexor tenolysis. Hand Clin 1:121–132, February 1985a.

157. Strickland, J.W. Opinions and preferences in flexor tendon surgery. Hand Clin 1:187–191, February 1985b.

158. Strickland, J.W. Results of flexor tendon surgery in Zone II. Hand Clin 1:167–179, February 1985c.

159. Strickland, J.W., and Glogovac, S.V. Digital function following flexor tendon repair in Zone II: A comparison of immobilization and controlled passive motion techniques. J Hand Surg [Am] 5:537–543, 1980.

160. Takami, H., Takahashi, S., and Ando, M. Rupture of flexor tendon associated with previous fracture of the hook of the hamate. Hand 15:73–76, 1983.

161. Tamai, S., Michon, J., Tupper, J., and Fleming, J. Report of subcommittee on replantation. J Hand Surg [Am] 8:730–732, 1983.

162. Tsuge, K., Ikuta, Y., and Matsuishi, Y. Repair of flexor tendons by intratendinous tendon suture. J Hand Surg [Am] 2:436–440, 1977.

163. Urbaniak, J.R. Tendon suturing methods: Analysis of tensile strengths, in Hunter, J.M., and Schneider, L.H. (eds): *Symposium on Tendon Surgery in the Hand.* St. Louis, Mosby, 1975, pp 70–80.

164. Urbaniak, J.R., and Goldner, J.L. Laceration of the flexor pollicis longus tendon: Delayed repair by advancement, free graft or direct suture; a clinical and experimental study. J Bone Joint Surg [Am] 55:1123–1148, 1973.

165. Vahvanen, V., Gripenberg, L., and Nuutinen, P. Flexor tendon injury of the hand in children: A long-term follow-up study of 84 patients. Scand J Plast Reconstr Surg 15:43–48, 1981.

166. Vaughan-Jackson, O.J. Rupture of extensor tendons by attrition at the inferior radio-ulnar joint: Report of two cases. J Bone Joint Surg [Br] 30:528–530, 1948.

167. Verdan, C. Syndrome of the quadriga. Surg Clin North Am 40:425–426, April 1960.

168. Verdan, C.E. Primary repair of flexor tendons. J Bone Joint Surg [Am] 42:647–656, 1960.

169. Weber, E.R., Hardin, G., and Haynes, D. Synovial Fluid Nutrition of Flexor Tendons. Presented at the 36th Annual Meeting of the American Society for Surgery of the Hand, February 23, 1981.

170. Weeks, P.M., and Wray, R.C. Rate and extent of functional recovery after flexor tendon grafting with and without silicone rod preparation. J Hand Surg [Am] 1:174–180, 1976.

171. Wehbé, M. Personal communication, 1984.

172. Wehbé, M.A., and Schneider, L.H. Mallet fractures. J Bone Joint Surg [Am] 66:658–669, 1984.

173. Weidman, K.A., Malo, D.S., and Levine, R. The Influence of Tenorrhaphy on the Healing and Strength of Partial Lacerations of Canine Flexor Tendons. Presented at the Annual Resident's Meeting of the American Society for Surgery of the Hand, Atlanta, Georgia, February 6–8, 1984.

174. Weiland, A., and Naiman, J. Independent Index Extension Following Extensor Indicis Proprius Transfer. Presented at the 40th Annual Meeting of the American Society for Surgery of the Hand, Las Vegas, Nevada, January 21–23, 1985.

175. Weinstein, S.L., Sprague, B.L., and Flatt, A.E. Evaluation of the two-stage flexor-tendon reconstruction in severely damaged digits. J Bone Joint Surg [Am] 58:786–791, 1976.

176. Whitaker, J.H., Strickland, J.W., and Ellis, R.K. The role of flexor tenolysis in the palm and digits. J Hand Surg [Am] 2:462–470, 1977.

177. Wilson, R.L., Carter, M.S., Holdeman, V.A., and Lovett, W.L. Flexor profundus injuries treated with delayed two-staged tendon grafting. J Hand Surg [Am] 5:74–78, 1980.

178. Winspur, I., Phelps, D.B., and Boswick, J.A., Jr. Staged reconstruction of flexor tendons with a silicone rod and a "pedicled" *sublimis* transfer. Plast Reconstr Surg 61:756–761, 1978.

179. Woo, S.L., Ritter, M.A., Amiel, D., Sanders, T.M., Gomez, M.A., Kuei, S.C., Garfin, S.R., and Akeson, W.H. The biomechanical and biochemical properties of swine tendons—Long term effects of exercise on the digital extensors. Connect Tissue Res 7:177–183, 1980.

180. Wray, R.C., Jr., Holtmann, B., and Weeks, P.M. Clinical treatment of partial tendon lacerations without suturing and with early motion. Plast Reconstr Surg 59:231–234, 1977.

181. Wray, R.C., Jr., Moucharafieh, B., and Weeks, P.M. Experimental study of the optimal time for tenolysis. Plast Reconstr Surg 61:184–189, 1978.

182. Young, R.E.S., and Harmon, J.M. Repair of tendon injuries of the hand. Ann Surg 151:562–566, 1960.

CHAPTER 43

Tendon Transfers in the Hand and Forearm

Joseph P. Leddy and Eric D. Strauss

PRINCIPLES

"A tendon transfer is that procedure in which the tendon of insertion or of origin of the functioning muscle is mobilized, detached or divided, and reinserted into a bony part or into another tendon to supplement or substitute for the action of the recipient tendon."[6] These procedures are utilized in the upper extremity following irreparable nerve damage, loss of function of the musculotendinous unit through trauma or disease, and in certain nonprogressive or slowly progressive neurological disorders.

Stability of the wrist is essential for good hand function. The synergistic action of wrist flexion accompanies finger extension, whereas wrist extension accompanies finger flexion. These coordinated movements occur below the conscious level and facilitate balanced hand function.

Some authors feel it is easier to retrain synergistic muscles following their transfer.[2] Experience has shown that the use of synergistic transfers is not mandatory and that virtually any muscle in the forearm and hand can be transferred to perform a certain function provided that one adheres to the fundamental principles of tendon transfers.

Mayer,[46-49] Steindler,[76] Bunnell,[16-19] Boyes,[6] and others have described the essential principles of the tendon transfer operation.

1. *Correction of Contractures.* Prior to any tendon transfer operation, the joints must be freely movable because a transferred muscle-tendon unit cannot overcome a fixed-joint contracture. If splinting and therapy are not successful, capsulotomy may be necessary to release the contracture prior to the transfer.

   Likewise, the skin and soft tissues must be supple and free of scarring. The tendon transfer will not function well in a scarred bed, and, occasionally, a pedicle or a free flap will have to be done prior to the tendon transfer.

2. *Adequate Power in the Transfer.* If the muscle is too weak, the desired function will not be performed and the deformity might recur. If the muscle is too strong, the opposite deformity may result, limiting function in the hand.[73] The power of the muscle is determined by its cross-sectional area.[30] The transferred muscle will most likely lose some power; therefore, only muscles rated 4+ or better should be considered acceptable donor motors.[34]

3. *Sufficient Amplitude in the Transfer.* The amplitude of a muscle is a function of its sarcomere length.[4] This is a fixed value for any particular muscle. However, the effective amplitude of a muscle can be increased in two ways. The first is by freeing the muscle from its fascial attachments. The brachioradialis is a prime example since its amplitude may be increased by more than 100 percent in this manner.[31] The second method is by changing a muscle from monoarticular to biarticular. The effective amplitude is increased by movement of the joint which the transferred tendon now crosses. Since amplitude can be limited by scarring and by adhesions in the area through which the tendon passes, one should choose a donor with more-than-adequate amplitude for the desired action.

According to Boyes,[6] the following values may be used as a practical guideline for amplitude:

Wrist motors	33 mm
Finger extensors FPL	50 mm
Finger flexors	70 mm

The surgeon must be familiar with the excursion of these donor muscles so that an appropriate selection can be made. The work capacity of a muscle is determined by the product of its power and amplitude.[6] The work capacity of the forearm muscles in kilogram meters $(kg \cdot m)$ is listed below.

Flexor carpi radialis	0.8
Extensor carpi radialis longus	1.1
Extensor carpi radialis brevis	0.9
Extensor carpi ulnaris	1.1
Abductor pollicis longus	0.1
Flexor pollicis longus	1.2
Flexor digitorum profundus	4.5
Flexor digitorum sublimis (superficialis)	4.8
Brachioradialis	1.9
Flexor carpi ulnaris	2.0
Pronator teres	1.2
Palmaris longus	0.1
Extensor pollicis longus	0.1
Extensor digitorum communis	1.7

Although the flexor carpi ulnaris (FCU) has the greatest work capacity of the wrist motors, its use has been questioned in tendon transfers because of its great importance to wrist function.[6] The wrist works in radial dorsiflexion and ulnar volar flexion. The importance of the FCU can be appreciated if one tries to work with a hammer. Knowledge of the power, amplitude, and work capacity of a particular muscle is essential in planning appropriate transfers.[11]

4. *A Satisfactory Line of Pull Must Be Provided.* The best course for a tendon transfer is a straight line of pull through unscarred soft tissues. This will maximize the retained power and amplitude of the transferred muscle. Each turn or bend in the transferred tendon can set up a point of friction causing loss of effective power and amplitude. However, it is not always possible for a transferred tendon to pull in a straight line. For instance, the ring finger flexor digitorum superficialis is often used as a donor for an opponensplasty with a pulley created on the ulnar aspect of the wrist near the pisiform so that the transfer pulls in the proper direction.[18]

5. *Functional Integrity Must Be Preserved.* The transferred tendon cannot be expected to perform more than one function and to have separate amplitudes for different motions. If the tendon is split and inserted into different sites, the force of the transfer will be expended on the tighter of the two and only that function will be performed.[73] Also, the transferred muscle-tendon unit should be expendable. The remaining motors must be able to perform the function of the transferred tendon. For instance, if both the flexor carpi radialis and flexor carpi ulnaris tendons are transferred to the dorsum of the hand and wrist, active wrist flexion will be lost and a permanent dorsiflexion contracture may result.[34] If, as in combined palsies, there are not enough motors, then an alternative technique must be employed, such as arthrodesis, tenodesis, and capsulodesis—any of which may be used to create a simple, yet balanced and functional system.

SURGICAL CONSIDERATIONS

The timing of tendon transfers depends upon the cause of the problem, the prognosis for recovery, and, to some extent, the preference of the patient. If there is no chance for functional recovery, transfers should be performed as soon as the patient is ready. Nerves regenerate at approximately the rate of 1 mm/day. Following nerve injury and/or repair, the date of expected recovery can be calculated by measuring the distance from the lesion to the most proximal muscle innervated by the injured nerve. If reasonable return is not present 3 months after the date of expected recovery, then tendon transfer can be considered.[55] Nerve recovery can also be evaluated by serial EMG studies and by an advancing Tinel sign in mixed nerves.

Early tendon transfers are defined as those performed within approximately 12 weeks of injury. The relative indications for these procedures include (1) proximal nerve lesions, (2) irreparable nerve lesions, and (3) other lesions with a statistically poor chance for acceptable recovery. Prerequisites of early transfer, as expounded by Omer[58] and Burkhalter,[24]

are that the donor tendon be completely expendable and that no imbalance will be created by neural regeneration. The proponents of early tendon transfer feel that there are certain advantages to be gained by this technique. They claim that function is improved early on and that the use of external splints can be avoided. They feel that this technique minimizes the tendency to develop abnormal usage patterns which can complicate rehabilitation of the injured hand. They also point out that early function promotes sensory reeducation.

Careful planning is essential prior to any surgical procedure since each patient has different deficits and needs. The surgery must be individualized for the patient, and the surgeon should be aware both of the "standard" transfers and of the several alternative methods. The systematic approach is recommended.[73] First, a list of the deficient functions should be made. Then, opposite this, a list of available working donor muscles should be compiled. Then, utilizing these two lists, the surgeon can decide which functions need restoration and which available donors are most appropriate for the tasks. In complex lesions, multiple transfers may be necessary to both sides of the wrist. In general, flexor transfers should precede extensor transfers.[73]

Multiple, short transverse incisions may be preferable to extended longitudinal incisions for the mobilization of donor tendons. Minimizing scar in the surrounding tissue is of paramount importance, and the course of the transfer must be planned with this in mind.[10] The tendons should be handled carefully, and hemostasis should be obtained. There should be good soft tissue coverage over the tendon junctures. Direct end-to-end, end-to-side, side-to-side, or tendon weave sutures may be utilized.[8] These techniques are described in Chap. 42.

Finally, a word about achieving proper tension in tendon transfers is appropriate.[54] It is not possible to give one general rule covering all situations, and experience is often the best teacher for this particular problem. The surgeon may place the hand in the position that it will assume when the tendon transfer is functioning at its maximum and then suture the tendon without any tension. It is usually preferable to make the transfer a little tight rather than lax.

Prior to discussion of individual nerve palsies and specific tendon transfers, a list of abbreviations will be useful.

ECRL	Extensor carpi radialis longus
ECRB	Extensor carpi radialis brevis
ECU	Extensor carpi ulnaris
FCR	Flexor carpi radialis
FCU	Flexor carpi ulnaris
BR	Brachioradialis
PT	Pronator teres
PL	Palmaris longus
EDC	Extensor digitorum communis
EIP	Extensor indicis proprius
EDQP	Extensor digiti quinti proprius
EPL	Extensor pollicis longus
EPB	Extensor pollicis brevis
APL	Abductor pollicis longus
APB	Abductor pollicis brevis
FDS	Flexor digitorum superficialis
FDP	Flexor digitorum profundus

RADIAL NERVE PALSY

Anatomy[32]

The radial nerve descends into the arm as a branch of the posterior cord of the brachial plexus composed of fibers of predominantly C6, C7, and C8. It curves behind the humerus from medial to lateral and pierces the lateral intermuscular septum where it passes distally between the brachialis and brachioradialis into the forearm. Prior to splitting into its superficial and posterior interosseous branches in the proximal forearm, the radial nerve innervates the BR and ECRL. The superficial radial sensory nerve provides sensation to the dorsoradial aspect of the hand. The posterior interosseous nerve then innervates the ECRB, ECU, EDC, EIP, EDQP, EPL, EPB, and APL. There is some variation with the innervation of the ECRB.

In a posterior interosseous nerve palsy, at least one radial wrist extensor, the ECRL, is intact.[34] This will provide extension of the wrist with some radial deviation. In a radial nerve injury proximal to the elbow, there normally will be no active wrist extension.

Problem

Loss of radial nerve function is a significant deficit. There is loss of extension of the wrist and metacarpophalangeal (MP) joints of the fingers and loss of extension and abduction of the thumb[3] (Fig. 43-1). There is inability to stabilize the wrist in neutral or in extension, and therefore power grasp is severely impaired.[24] The fingers and thumb cannot be widely opened for prehension.[67]

Treatment

Great care must be taken to prevent the development of contractures in a patient with radial nerve palsy. This may require various forms of splinting (Fig. 43-2) and therapy, but a full passive range of motion of all the joints must be main-

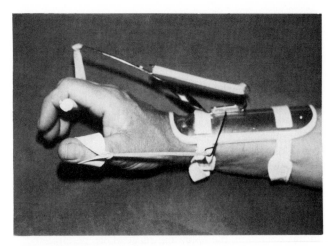

Figure 43-2 Thomas splint for radial nerve palsy to prevent contracture of the wrist, fingers, and thumb.

tained while awaiting nerve regeneration and before any surgery for tendon transfers.

Burkhalter is a strong advocate of early tendon transfer here since the tendon serves as an internal splint.[24] He transfers PT to ECRB in an end-to-side fashion as soon as possible after the injury. This stabilizes the wrist, allows some power grasp, and may make external splinting unnecessary. In its transferred state, the PT still functions as a pronator of the forearm. If there is inadequate motor return, further transfers can be done to provide MP joint extension and thumb extension and abduction. Early tendon transfer is not a universally accepted principle, but it does have some strong advocates.

The history of radial nerve transfers is long and complex and is well described by Boyes in his classic article.[5] Sir Robert Jones transferred the PT to ECRL and ECRB first, and this remains the procedure of choice today.[42] However, as Green points out, the "classic" Jones transfer is probably a misnomer since he described at least two different operations and neither one is widely used today.[34] In both these operations, he advocated transferring both FCU and FCR to the dorsum of the hand. Starr[75] (1922) and Zachary[80] (1946) emphasized the importance of retaining at least one wrist flexor for optimum function of the hand.

The patient with a radial nerve palsy needs wrist extension, MP joint extension, and extension and abduction of the thumb. Many donor motors are available. If there is a posterior interosseous nerve palsy, extension of the wrist may be intact because of a functioning ECRL and no transfer will be needed for wrist extension. The sensory deficit is usually not significant.

We prefer the transfers described by Boyes[6] in 1960. He described transferring

PT to ECRL and ECRB
FCR to EPB and APL
FDS long finger to EDC
FDS ring finger to EPL and EIP

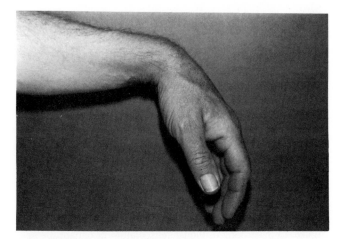

Figure 43-1 Radial nerve palsy. There is loss of active extension of the wrist and MP joints of the fingers and loss of abduction and extension of the thumb.

This set of transfers has several advantages. The FCU, which is the most important muscle in the wrist, is retained.[27] Because of the amplitude of the transferred superficialis tendons, simultaneous wrist and finger extension can be obtained. The FCR provides strong abduction for the thumb metacarpal. FDS of long finger provides extension of the fingers, and FDS of the ring finger gives independent extension to the thumb and index finger. FDS of long and ring fingers are passed through a large opening made in the interosseous membrane just proximal to the pronator quadratus muscle. The long finger FDS courses between the profundus mass and the flexor pollicis longus muscle, and that of the ring finger goes along the ulnar side of the profundus muscle. The transferred muscles are well-mobilized proximally so that muscle tissue rather than tendon is in the interosseous opening, thus lessening the chance for adherence of the transfer at this site.

One of the most common operations for radial nerve palsy is referred to as the *standard (FCU) transfer* by Green.[34] In this operation, the following transfers are performed:

PT to ECRB
FCU to EDC
PL to rerouted EPL

This operation has withstood the test of time and does have certain advantages. It does restore wrist and MP joint extension and also abduction and extension of the thumb. It is technically easier to perform than the Boyes transfers. However, in the opinion of the authors its major disadvantage is its use of the flexor carpi ulnaris as a donor motor. Since the wrist tends to work in radial dorsiflexion and ulnar volar flexion, this important motor should be retained if possible. Other authors[10] who agree with this concept have proposed a set of transfers which preserve the FCU:

PT to ECRB
FCR to EDC
PL to rerouted EPL

The reader is referred to the original texts for details of operative procedures and postoperative management. In general, the splints are removed 4 to 5 weeks postoperatively, and a supervised program of therapy is begun.

MEDIAN NERVE PALSY

With median nerve palsy, in sharp contrast to radial nerve palsy, the sensory deficit is very important.[20] There is loss of sensibility over the palmar aspect of the thumb and of the index, long, and radial half of the ring fingers, which are the most important contact areas in the hand. Every attempt at restoring this important function should be made.

Anatomy[32]

The median nerve arises from C6, C7, C8, and T1 and begins as a condensation of the lateral and medial cords of the brachial plexus. In the upper arm, it travels lateral to the brachial artery and then crosses to the medial side into the antecubital fossa entering the forearm between the two heads of the pronator teres. It proceeds distally in the forearm between the FDS and FDP musculotendinous units rising toward

the volar surface of the wrist as it enters the carpal tunnel between the PL and FCR. Because of their close proximity, injuries to the median nerve frequently involve injuries to the flexor tendons.

Treatment

The motor deficit in low median nerve injuries at the level of the distal forearm and wrist is paralysis of the abductor pollicis brevis, the opponens pollicis, and, to a varying extent, the flexor pollicis brevis.[40] There is great variability in the innervation of the thenar musculature and approximately one-third[28] of patients with low median nerve palsy will have sufficient power in the remaining flexor pollicis brevis muscle to obviate any type of opposition transfer[25] (Fig. 43-3). If opposition power is insufficient and cannot be returned by neurorrhaphy or nerve grafting, then tendon transfer should be considered. Good skin and supple joints are a prerequisite. There can be no fixed contracture of the first web space, or the operation will be a failure. Following nerve injury, appropriate splinting should be instituted to prevent the formation of a contracture. If a fixed contracture develops in the first web space, then surgical release with or without skin grafting, osteotomy of the metacarpal, or excision of the trapezium may be necessary to mobilize the web space prior to opponensplasty.

The history of tendon transfers for opposition of the thumb is long and complex.[44,51,53] Much of the early experience was gained from patients with poliomyelitis. There is no simple cookbook formula for opposition transfers in the thumb, and patients must be judged carefully regarding their specific needs and deficits. A strong motor will be necessary if the thumb adductor, the first dorsal interosseous, and the extensor pollicis longus are intact and functioning. If, however, these muscles are paralyzed owing to a combined nerve lesion or to some neurological disorder, then a weaker donor can be utilized. In isolated low median nerve palsy, Bunnell[18]

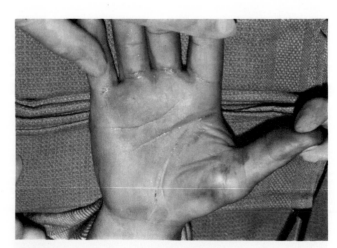

Figure 43-3 Atrophy of thenar musculature in patient undergoing carpal tunnel release. Deep head of the flexor brevis, innervated by the ulnar nerve, is visible.

taught us that the transfer should come from a fixed pulley near the pisiform, subcutaneously across the palm to the area of the MP joint of the thumb. If the pulley is made proximal to the pisiform, more abduction will be gained from the transfer. If the pulley is made distal to the pisiform, there will be more flexion and adduction resulting from the transferred tendon. This latter position is useful in a combined low median and ulnar nerve palsy.

There are many methods of insertion of the tendon transfer.[65,10,1] It may be sutured by a weave technique directly into the tendon of the abductor pollicis brevis muscle, simulating the action of this most important muscle of the thenar eminence. The tendon may also pass subcutaneously directly over the dorsum of the MP joint of the thumb to be attached to the dorsoulnar aspect of the base of the proximal phalanx.[18] This will allow the tendon to provide both abduction and pronation of the thumb. Extension of the interphalangeal joint of the thumb may be enhanced, if necessary, by suturing one slip of the transfer to the extensor hood and EPL.[66] If a tendon graft is needed to prolong the transfer, the EPB may be divided at its musculotendinous junction, leaving the insertion at the base of the proximal phalanx intact. The tendon is then passed subcutaneously across the palm toward the pisiform where it may be attached to the donor tendon.

In isolated low median nerve palsy, there is loss of the APB, opponens, and at least some portion of the flexor pollicis brevis. The antagonists are functioning and, therefore, a strong motor is necessary. There should be no contracture of the first web space. The line of pull of the transfer should be from the area of the pisiform. A loop is made in the FCU tendon at the level of the pisiform to act as a fixed pulley. One-half of the tendon is utilized just proximal to the pisiform to fashion this loop, and it is sutured to itself. The ring finger superficialis[68,69,77] can be used as a donor tendon unless it was damaged at the time of the injury to the median nerve. The superficialis tendon can be divided in the palm just proximal to the A1 metacarpal pulley. Through a separate incision, it is withdrawn into the proximal forearm, placed through the fixed FCU pulley at the level of the pisiform, and then tunneled subcutaneously across the palm to the level of the MP joint of the thumb. One slip can be sutured into the tendon of the abductor pollicis brevis and the other placed over the dorsum of the MP joint in a subcutaneous fashion to be attached to the dorsoulnar aspect of the base of the proximal phalanx. Alternatively, the tendon can be sutured, in toto, into the tendon of the abductor pollicis brevis or into the dorsoulnar aspect of the base of the proximal phalanx. If the FDS of the ring finger is not a suitable donor, other tendons such as the EIP, the EDQP, the ECU, and the abductor digiti minimi may be used.[21,39,41,45,63,64,70,79,82]

In long-standing cases of median nerve compression at the wrist with loss of thenar function, the Camitz[26] transfer has been advocated. At the time of carpal tunnel release, the palmaris longus tendon prolonged with a strip of palmar fascia is inserted into the tendon of the abductor pollicis brevis to provide palmar abduction of the thumb.

In high median nerve lesions, the loss is more serious. The sensory deficit remains the same as does the loss of thenar function. However, the entire FDS, the FDP of index

and long fingers, and the FPL are also lost (Fig. 43-4). The FCR is not functioning, but the FCU—innervated by the ulnar nerve—is working and provides adequate strength for wrist flexion. Therefore, the additional functional loss consists of loss of flexion at the interphalangeal joint of the thumb and loss of flexion of the index and long fingers. Since there is loss of FDS function, the ring finger superficialis cannot be utilized in the opponens transfer. Therefore, one of the alternatives mentioned above is carried out. FDP of index and long fingers can be attached side to side to the FDP of the ring and little fingers to produce flexion of the index and long fingers, although the power of grasp is not increased.[10] The BR, after being freed from its fascial attachments in the forearm, can be transferred to the FPL to provide flexion at the interphalangeal joint of the thumb and power and stability for pinch.[20] If more power is needed for flexion of the index and long fingers, the ECRL can be transferred to the FDP of the index and long fingers.[25]

Not all patients with high median nerve lesions will require extrinsic tendon transfers, since repair at this level will often result in return of adequate extrinsic function. It is rare to have good return of intrinsic thenar function in proximal median nerve lesions. If nerve repair is unsuccessful, if the lesion is irreparable, or if a large nerve graft is necessary, then consideration for these extrinsic transfers should be given.

THE ULNAR NERVE

Anatomy[32]

The ulnar nerve originates from C7, C8, and T1 and is formed from the medial cord and a portion of the lateral cord of the brachial plexus. It passes through the medial intermuscular

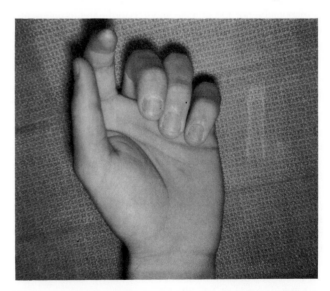

Figure 43-4 High median nerve palsy. There is loss of thenar function and loss of flexion at the IP joint of the thumb and at the DIP joint of index finger. Flexion at the DIP joint of the middle finger is weak but present.

septum in the midarm and down the medial side of the arm behind the medial epicondyle into the cubital tunnel. It enters the forearm between the two heads of origin of the flexor carpi ulnaris to lie anterior to the flexor digitorum profundus muscle mass. Distally, it becomes more superficial lying between the flexor digitorum superficialis and flexor carpi ulnaris tendons. It enters the hand through the canal of Guyon between the pisiform and the hook of the hamate medial to the ulnar artery. The motor branch then winds around the hook of the hamate into the palm and the sensory branch proceeds distally supplying sensation to the palmar aspect of the little finger and to the ulnar half of the ring finger.

The median and ulnar nerves may have anomalous communications in both the forearm and the hand. The Martin-Gruber anastomosis in the forearm transmits fibers from the median to the ulnar nerve in approximately 15 percent of patients. The Riche-Cannieu anastomosis occurs in the hand between the median and ulnar nerves.[59] Many different anatomical variations can be encountered, and, therefore, careful examination is important since not all ulnar nerve palsies present with the same clinical picture.

The intrinsic muscles of the thumb innervated by the ulnar nerve are the deep head of the flexor pollicis brevis, the adductor pollicis, and the first dorsal interosseous. The FPB is primarily a thumb metacarpal flexor.[1] The adductor pollicis flexes the MP joint slightly and moves the first metacarpal toward the second metacarpal. Since the adductor aponeurosis inserts into the dorsal extensor mechanism, the adductor pollicis also contributes to interphalangeal joint extension. The interossei and lumbricals are MP joint flexors and extensors of the proximal interphalangeal (PIP) and distal interphalangeal (DIP) joints. They are most effective as extensors when the MP joints are in slight flexion and least effective when the MP joints are in full flexion. The extrinsic extensors are most effective when the MP joints are flexed.[6] The extrinsic flexors and extensors provide prehension and power grasp. The ulnar-innervated intrinsic musculature in the hand is responsible for the precise, rapid, coordinated movements of the fingers and thumb which help make the hand such a marvelous organ.

Problems

There are multiple deficits in ulnar nerve palsy affecting almost all facets of hand function. Proper coordination of finger flexion requires initiation of flexion at the MP joints. With loss of function of the interossei and the ulnar two lumbricals, there is no independent flexion of the MP joints (Fig. 43-5). The sublimi and profundi act upon the DIP and PIP joints primarily and the MP joints secondarily. During grasp, therefore, the extrinsic muscles first flex the DIP and PIP joints curling the fingers into the hand. The MP joints flex last. Thus, the arc of flexion is shortened, and it is impossible to grasp large objects, which are actually pushed out of the palm during attempted flexion of the fingers.[78] Power grip is impaired, and the power and stability of pinch is severely compromised.[12,14,71,74] Froment described instability of key pinch with compensatory hyperflexion of the interphalangeal (IP) joint in 1915 (Fig. 43-6). The IP joint hyperflexes to increase

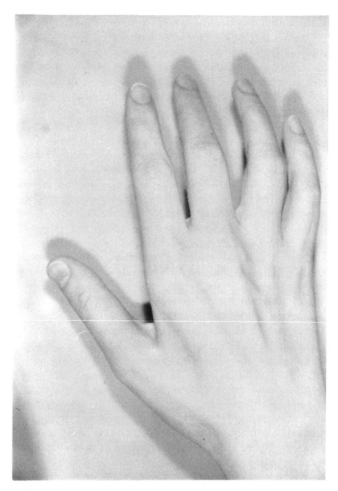

Figure 43-5 Ulnar nerve palsy with clawing of the ring and little fingers. There is obvious atrophy of the dorsal interosseous muscles.

the mechanical advantage of the extensor pollicis longus as a secondary adductor. Hyperextension at the MP joint occurs secondary to loss of the intrinsic musculature of the thumb. This IP joint hyperflexion and MP joint hyperextension gives the thumb a clawed appearance and disrupts the longitudinal arch of the thumb during key pinch. Loss of abduction and adduction of the fingers contributes to the impaired dexterity of the hand.

Clawing in ulnar nerve paralysis is most commonly seen in the ring and little fingers, although it may also be seen in the index and long fingers.[9] It is more common in loose-jointed individuals and may not be present in a person with very tight joints that cannot be passively hyperextended. Gradually, the extrinsic extensor tendons stretch out the volar plates of the MP joints which have lost their primary flexors. As the MP joints gradually hyperextend, complete extension of the PIP joints is not possible. As time goes on, if these joints are not properly exercised or splinted, fixed contractures develop with the MP joints in hyperextension and the PIP joints in flexion. Active and passive exercise programs and various forms of splinting are crucial factors in the prevention of these fixed deformities.

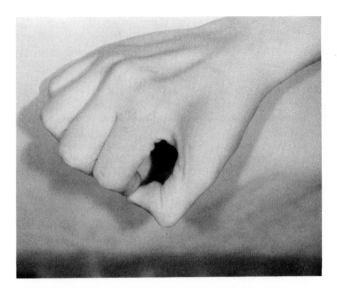

Figure 43-6 Froment's sign in ulnar nerve palsy. Weak and unstable pinch with hyperflexion at the IP joint.

In high ulnar nerve lesions, there is loss of the FCU at the wrist and FDP of the ring and little fingers. Loss of the ulnar two profundi further contributes to the loss of power grip. The importance of the FCU muscle has been discussed in the section on radial nerve lesions. In low ulnar nerve lesions, there is loss of sensation on the ulnar border of the hand, including the palmar surface of the little finger and the ulnar half of the ring finger. In high ulnar nerve lesions, the same loss is present along with absence of sensation on the dorsoulnar aspect of the hand. While the sensory deficit in an ulnar nerve lesion is significant, it is not nearly as important as loss of sensibility in the median nerve distribution.

Treatment

Every attempt should be made to repair an ulnar nerve laceration in the hope of regaining both sensibility and motor power.[13] Splinting and proper exercises are important in preventing the development of fixed contractures. Once it is obvious that there will be no recovery of motor function in an ulnar nerve lesion, then various procedures should be considered. In low ulnar nerve lesions, there is loss of intrinsic function of the fingers and thumb. If the longitudinal arch of the thumb collapses during key pinch, several options are available. Pinch strength may be diminished as much as 75 percent.[74] Restoration of pinch function in ulnar nerve palsy involves bringing the thumb metacarpal toward the index metacarpal with a strong motor. Maintenance of a stable thumb MP joint as a base upon which to pinch is important. Therefore, tendon transfers for pinch must provide balanced forces to the first metacarpal, the MP joint, and the index finger. Only a few of the more commonly used transfers will be discussed here, but a more complete listing is available in the bibliography.

A BR transfer can restore strong adduction to the thumb.[6] A free tendon graft is required and is attached by a pullout wire sutured to the base of the proximal phalanx of the thumb on the ulnar volar border. The graft is then passed along the surface of the paralyzed adductor muscle to the ulnar side of the third metacarpal where it is brought out to the dorsum of the hand between the long and ring finger metacarpals. Here, it is attached to the BR muscle which has been mobilized proximally to increase its excursion. Smith[74] used the ECRB prolonged with a free tendon graft placed between the bases of the index and long finger metacarpals going across the adductor muscle to be sutured into the base of the proximal phalanx of the thumb on its ulnar side near the adductor tubercle with a pullout wire and button. Among the other procedures available are the tendon loop operation, the tendon T operation, and transfer of the superficialis.[35,37] Some authors prefer fusion of either the MP or IP joint of the thumb[59] with or without an associated transfer to improve abduction of the index finger.[6,15,33,52,84]

Many different surgical procedures have been devised to compensate for the loss of active MP joint flexion. These procedures fall into two major categories: static and dynamic. If, when MP joint hyperextension is blocked passively, there is full DIP and PIP joint extension, then static procedures may be helpful in correcting the deformity. However, if fixed contractures are present, or if the extensor apparatus has stretched out over the dorsum of the PIP joint so that full extension here is not possible when MP joint hyperextension is blocked, then these techniques will not be successful. Some authors have used bone block techniques on the dorsum of the metacarpal head to prevent hyperextension of the proximal phalanx.[50] Others have suggested arthrodesis of the MP joints, but neither of these procedures is widely used at this point in time. Zancolli's volar plate capsulorrhaphy can limit MP hyperextension, but can stretch out in a person with strong extrinsic musculature.[12,81] Capsulodesis and pulley advancement is an effective procedure to limit MP joint hyperextension.[19,43] The volar plate is advanced proximally and inserted into bone in the metacarpal neck at the desired degree of flexion of the MP joint. The pulley advancement increases the moment of flexion across the MP joint, allowing more synchronous flexion of the fingers. This procedure will not add any strength to the grip. Other authors have used various tenodesis techniques to prevent the hyperextension at the metacarpophalangeal joints.[62,65,66] None of the static techniques increase the power of grasp.

Many different dynamic techniques have been advocated. These are basically designed to produce primary flexion at the MP joints,[83] thus providing synchronous finger flexion and, in some cases, adding to the power of grasp. Stiles advocated using superficialis tendons as transfers to provide MP joint flexion. His procedure has been modified by Bunnell,[19] Riordan,[65] and others.[7,56] Normally, the transfer is placed through the lumbrical canal beneath the transverse metacarpal ligament and then inserted into the lateral band of the finger. Because of the development of hyperextension at the PIP joint in some of these patients, many authors prefer to insert the tendon transfer into the A2 pulley or into the proximal phalanx instead of the lateral band.[22] A transfer of the flexor digitorum superficialis will not increase grip strength.[72] Other authors have transferred wrist extensors—the BR, EIP, and EDQP—to provide flexion at the MP joints.[10,23,65] These procedures can increase the power of grasp by adding a new motor unit to the flexor side of the hand. Other procedures have been devised to restore the flattened metacarpal arch and to correct an abduction deformity at the MP joint of the little finger.[6]

In high ulnar nerve palsy, there is loss of flexion at the DIP joints of the ring and little fingers and loss of the FCU. Some authors believe that in an isolated high ulnar nerve lesion, it is not necessary to correct these extrinsic losses.[10] However, if there is profound weakness in flexion of the ring and little fingers, the FDP of these two fingers can be attached side to side to the functioning FDP of the long finger to provide flexion. Since ulnar deviation is important in wrist flexion, one-half[59] or all of the FCR can be transferred to the FCU to provide ulnar volar flexion at the wrist.

COMBINED NERVE LESIONS

Combined nerve lesions are very difficult problems. They are often associated with injuries such as fractures and tendon or muscle damage. Without proper exercise and splinting, contractures often develop very quickly. The motors available for use in transfer are limited owing to the involvement of more than one nerve. All the basic principles discussed previously apply to the patient with combined nerve lesions. Goals for rehabilitation must be realistic since it is usually impossible to replace all of the lost function. Because of the limitation of available motors, static procedures, such as fusion, tenodesis, and capsulodesis must often be utilized. The reader is referred to other sources for a complete discussion of these intricate problems.[29,57,60,61]

REFERENCES

1. Adams, J., and Wood, V.E. Tendon transfers for irreparable nerve damage in the hand. Orthop Clin North Am 12:403, 1981.
2. Beasley, R.W. Principles of tendon transfer. Orthop Clin North Am 1:433, 1970.
3. Beasley, R.W. Tendon transfers for radial nerve palsy. Orthop Clin North Am 2:439, 1970.
4. Blix, M. Die lange und die spannung des muskels. Skand Arch F Physiol 3:295, 1891; 4:399, 1893; 5:150, 1894.
5. Boyes, J.H. Tendon transfers for radial palsy. Bull Hosp Jnt Dis 21:97, 1960.
6. Boyes, J.H. (ed): *Bunnell's Surgery of the Hand,* 5th ed. Philadelphia, Lippincott, 1970.
7. Brand, P.W. Paralytic clawhand with special reference to paralysis in leprosy and treatment by the sublimus transfer of Stiles and Bunnell. J Bone Joint Surg 40B:618, 1958.
8. Brand, P.W. Tendon grafting illustrated by a new operation for intrinsic paralysis of the fingers. J Bone Joint Surg 43B:444, 1961.
9. Brand, P.W. Tendon transfers for median and ulnar nerve paralysis. Orthop Clin North Am 1:447, 1970.
10. Brand, P.W. Tendon transfers in the forearm, in Flynn, J.F. (ed): *Hand Surgery,* 2d ed. Baltimore, Williams & Wilkins, 1975, pp 189–200.
11. Brand, P.W., and Beach, R. Relative tension and potential excursion of muscles in the forearm and hand. J Hand Surg 4:281, 1979.
12. Brown, P.W. Zancolli capsulorrhaphy for ulnar claw hand. J Bone Joint Surg 52A:868, 1970.
13. Brown, P.W. The time factor in surgery of upper extremity peripheral nerve injury. Clin Orthop 68:14–21, 1970.
14. Brown, P.W. Reconstruction of pinch in ulnar intrinsic palsy. Orthop Clin North Am 5:232, 1974.
15. Bruner, J.M. Tendon transfer to restore abduction of the index finger using the extensor pollicis brevis. Plast Reconstr Surg 3:197, 1948.
16. Bunnell, S. Repair of tendons in the fingers and description of two new instruments. Surg Gynecol Obstet 26:103, 1918.
17. Bunnell, S. Repair of tendons in the fingers. Surg Gynecol Obstet 35:88, 1922.
18. Bunnell, S. Opposition of the thumb. J Bone Joint Surg 20:269, 1938.
19. Bunnell, S. Surgery of the intrinsic muscles of the hand other than those producing opposition of the thumb. J Bone Joint Surg 24:1, 1942.
20. Burkhalter, W.E. Tendon transfers in median nerve palsy. Orthop Clin North Am 5:271, 1974.
21. Burkhalter, W.E., Christensen, R.C., and Brown, P. Extensor indicis proprius opponensplasty. J Bone Joint Surg 55A:725, 1973.
22. Burkhalter, W.E., and Strait, J.L. Metacarpophalangeal flexor replacement for intrinsic paralysis. J Bone Joint Surg 55A:1667, 1973.
23. Burkhalter, W.E. Restoration of power grip in ulnar nerve paralysis. Orthop Clin North Am 5:289, 1974.
24. Burkhalter, W.E. Early tendon transfer in upper extremity peripheral nerve injury. Clin Orthop 104:68, 1974.
25. Burkhalter, W.E. Median nerve palsy, in Green, D.P. (ed): *Operative Hand Surgery.* New York, Churchill Livingstone, 1982, pp 1029.
26. Camitz, H. Surgical treatment of paralysis of the opponens muscle of the thumb. Acta Clin Scand 65:77, 1929.
27. Chuinard, R.G., Boyes, J.H., Stark, H.H., and Ashworth, C.R. Tendon transfers for radial nerve palsy: Use of superficialis tendons for digital extension. J Hand Surg 6:561, 1978.
28. Curtis, R.M. Fundamental principles of tendon transfer. Orthop Clin North Am 5:231, 1974.
29. Edgerton, M.T., and Brand, P.W. Restoration of abduction and adduction to the unstable thumb in median and ulnar paralysis. Plast Reconstr Surg 36:150, 1965.
30. Elftman, H. Biomechanics of muscle. J Bone Joint Surg 48A:363, 1966.
31. Freehafer, A.A., Peckham, H., and Keith, M.W. Determination of muscle tendon unit properties during tendon transfer. J Hand Surg 4:331, 1979.
32. Gardner, E., Gray, D.J., and O'Rahilly, R. *Anatomy,* 4th ed. Philadelphia, Saunders, 1975.
33. Graham, W.C., and Riordan, D.C. Sublimis transplant to restore abduction of index finger. Plast Reconstr Surg 2:459–462, 1947.
34. Green, D.P. Radial nerve palsy, in Green, D.P. (ed): *Operative Hand Surgery.* New York, Churchill Livingstone, 1982, pp 1011–1027.
35. Goldner, J.L. Replacement of the function of the paralyzed adductor pollicis with the flexor digitorum sublimis—A ten year review. J Bone Joint Surg 49A:583, 1967.
36. Goldner, J.L. Tendon transfers in rheumatoid arthritis. Orthop Clin North Am 5:425, 1974.
37. Hamlin, C., and Littler, J.W. Restoration of power pinch. J Hand Surg 5:396, 1980.
38. Hamlin, C., and Littler, J.W. Segmental tendon graft restoration of extensor pollicis longus disruption. Proceedings of the American Society for Surgery of the Hand. J Bone Joint Surg 57A:792, 1975.
39. Henderson, E.D. Transfer of wrist extensors and brachioradialis to restore opposition of the thumb. J Bone Joint Surg 44A:513, 1962.
40. Highet, W.B. Innervation and function of the thenar muscles. Lancet 1:227, 1943.

41. Huber, E. Hilfsoperation bei medianuslahmung. Dtsch Z Chir 162:271, 1921.
42. Jones, R. Tendon transplantation in cases of musculospiral injuries not amenable to suture. Am J Surg 35:333, 1921.
43. Leddy, J.P., Stark, H.H., Ashworth, C.R., and Boyes, J.H. Capsulodesis and pulley advancement for the correction of claw finger deformity. J Bone Joint Surg 54A:1465, 1972.
44. Littler, J.W., and Cooley, S.G.S. Opposition of the thumb and its restoration by abductor digiti quinti transfer. J Bone Joint Surg 45A:1389, 1963.
45. Makin, M. Translocation of the flexor pollicis longus tendon to restore opposition. J Bone Joint Surg 49B:458, 1967.
46. Mayer, L. The physiological method of tendon transplantation. I. Historical: Anatomy and physiology of tendons. Surg Gynecol Obstet 22:182, 1916.
47. Mayer, L. The physiological method of tendon transplantation. II. Operative technique. Surg Gynecol Obstet 22:298, 1916.
48. Mayer, L. The physiological method of tendon transplantation. III. Experimental and clinical experiences. Surg Gynecol Obstet 22:422, 1916.
49. Mayer, L. The physiological method of tendon transplantation. Surg Gynecol Obstet 33:528, 1921.
50. Mikhail, I.K. Bone block operation for claw hand. Surg Gynecol Obstet 118:1077, 1964.
51. Minkow, F.V. Operations to restore thumb opposition. *Symposium on Tendon Surgery in the Hand.* St. Louis, 1975.
52. Neviaser, R.J., Wilson, J.N., and Gardner, M.M. Abductor pollicis longus transfer for replacement of first dorsal interosseous. J Hand Surg 5:53, 1980.
53. Ney, K.W. A tendon transplant for intrinsic hand muscle paralysis. Surg Gynecol Obstet 33:342, 1921.
54. Omer, G.E., Jr. Determination of physiological length of a reconstructed muscle tendon unit through muscle stimulation. J Bone Joint Surg 47A:304, 1965.
55. Omer, G.E., Jr. Evaluation and reconstruction of the forearm and hand after acute traumatic peripheral nerve injuries. J Bone Joint Surg 50A:1454–1478, 1968.
56. Omer, G.E., Jr. Restoring power grip in ulnar palsy. J Bone Joint Surg 53:814, 1971.
57. Omer, G.E., Jr. Tendon transfers in combined nerve injury. Orthop Clin North Am 5:377, 1974.
58. Omer, G.E., Jr. Tendon transfers as early internal splints following peripheral nerve injury in the upper extremity, in Hunter, J.M., Schneider, L.H., Mackin, E.J., and Bell, J.A. (eds): *Rehabilitation of the Hand.* St. Louis, Mosby, 1978, p 292.
59. Omer, G.E., Jr. Ulnar nerve palsy, in Green, D.P. (ed): *Operative Hand Surgery.* New York, Churchill Livingstone, 1982, p 1061.
60. Omer, G.E., Jr. Combined nerve palsy, in Green, D.P. (ed): *Operative Hand Surgery.* New York, Churchill Livingstone, 1982, p 1081.
61. Omer, G.E., Jr. The palsied hand, in Evarts, C.M. (ed): *Surgery of the Musculoskeletal System,* vol 2. New York, Churchill Livingstone, 1983, p 407.
62. Parkes, A.R. Paralytic claw fingers—A graft tenodesis operation. Hand 5:192, 1973.
63. Phalen, G.S., and Miller, R.C. The transfer of wrist extensor muscles to restore or reinforce flexion power of the fingers and opposition of the thumb. J Bone Joint Surg 29:993, 1947.
64. Riley, W.B., Mann, R.J., and Burkhalter, W.E. Extensor pollicis longus opponens plasty. J Hand Surg 5:217, 1980.
65. Riordan, D.C. Surgery of the paralytic hand. Instr Course Lect :79, 1959.
66. Riordan, D.C. Tendon transfers for nerve paralysis of the hand and wrist. Curr Pract Orthop Surg 2:17–40, 1964.
67. Riordan, D.C. Radial nerve paralysis Orthop Clin North Am 5:282, 1974.
68. Riordan, D.C. Tendon transfers in hand surgery. J Hand Surg 8(s):748, 1983.
69. Royle, N.D. An operation for paralysis of the intrinsic muscles of the thumb. JAMA 111:612, 1938.
70. Schneider, L.H. Opponensplasty using the extensor digiti minimi. J Bone Joint Surg 51A:1297–1302, 1969.
71. Smith, R.J. Balance and kinetics of the fingers under normal and pathological conditions. Clin Orthop 104:92, 1974.
72. Smith, R.J. Surgical treatment of the clawhand, in American Academy of Orthopaedic Surgeons: *Symposium on Tendon Surgery in the Hand.* St. Louis, Mosby, 1975, p 181.
73. Smith, R.J., and Hastings, H., II. Principles of tendon transfer. Instr Course Lect :129, 1980.
74. Smith, R.J. Extensor carpi radialis brevis tendon transfer for thumb adduction—A study of power pinch. J Hand Surg 8:4, 1983.
75. Starr, C.L. Army experiences with tendon transference. J Bone Joint Surg 4:3, 1922.
76. Steindler, A. Orthopaedic operations on the hand. JAMA 71:1288, 1918.
77. Thompson, T.C. A modified operation for opponens paralysis. J Bone Joint Surg 24:632, 1942.
78. Tubiana, R. Anatomic and physiologic basis for the surgical treatment of paralysis of the hand. J Bone Joint Surg 51A:643, 1969.
79. Wissinger, H.A., and Singsen, E.G. Abductor digiti quinti opponensplasty. J Bone Joint Surg 59:895, 1977.
80. Zachary, R.B. Tendon transplantation for radial paralysis. Br J Surg 23:350, 1946.
81. Zancolli, E.A. Claw hand caused by paralysis of the intrinsic muscles. J Bone Joint Surg 39A:1076, 1957.
82. Zancolli, E.A. Tendon transfers after ischemic contraction of the forearm. Am J Surg 109:356–360, 1965.
83. Zancolli, E.A. *Structural and Dynamic Basis of Hand Surgery.* Philadelphia, Lippincott, 1968.
84. Zweig, J., Rosenthal, S., and Burns, H. Transfer of the extensor digiti quinti to restore pinch in ulnar palsy of the hand. J Bone Joint Surg 54A:51, 1972.

CHAPTER 44

Traumatic Amputations and Replantation

John J. Leppard and M. Ather Mirza

SECTION A

Traumatic Amputations of the Hand and Wrist

John J. Leppard

CARPAL AND METACARPAL LEVEL

Disarticulations at the wrist level allow excellent pronation and supination of the forearm and hand unit. The difficulties of prosthetic fittings have been recently overcome, thus making amputations at this level a more attractive choice than previously thought.

Midpalmar or carpal amputations must be approached carefully. It is a serious mistake for the surgeon to prejudge what is and what is not worth saving in an injured or partially amputated palm.[15] An intact radiocarpal joint which allows wrist flexion and extension can be extremely useful to the patient. Replantation may be actively considered (see Chap. 39, Sect. B). A patient who has lost the fingers or even the thumb can remain extremely functional by utilizing the residual carpus and metacarpals as a broad terminal assist. Frequently, such a patient fitted with a terminal prosthesis discards it because the residual function is better without it. The primary reason for this residual function is the intact sensation in the remainder of the carpus hand unit. Thus, the surgeon should preserve as much of the midpalm and carpus as possible as long as it is sensate.

PROXIMAL PHALANX LEVEL

Amputations at the proximal phalanx level do not benefit from flexor power of the superficialis tendon. Intrinsic function allows only weak flexion at the metacarpophalangeal (MP) joint. Thus, serious consideration should be given in such circumstances to ray resection and reconstruction of the contiguous transverse carpal ligament (Figs. 44-1 and 44-2).[48] This procedure has been a longtime favorite of hand surgeons because it rectifies several predicaments all at once.

The obvious deformity of the stubby finger is immediately corrected. Small objects and coins thus no longer slip through the defect which would otherwise exist between the two normal fingers. In addition, the cosmetic influence and cascade of the contiguous digit is closely reapproximated by

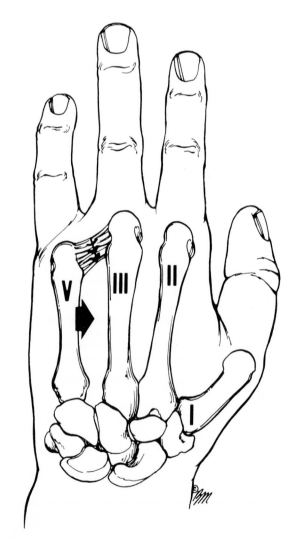

Figure 44-1 Reconstruction of the contiguous transverse metacarpal ligament can successfully narrow the defect that occurs after ray resection (in this case the fourth ray). *(From Green, David P., ed: Operative Hand Surgery. New York, Churchill Livingstone, 1982. Reprinted with permission.)*

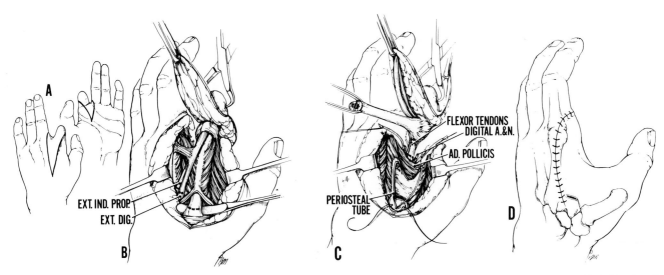

Figure 44-2 Ray resection should be carried out through a racket-type incision *(A, B)* with the metacarpal osteotomy being proximally placed *(C, D). (From Green, David P., ed: Operative* *Hand Surgery. New York, Churchill Livingstone, 1982. Reprinted with permission.)*

ray resection. This has significant functional ramifications because a finger that is left shorter than the proximal phalanx is frequently bypassed in daily use with the contiguous normal finger assuming most of the functional duties of its amputated neighbor. Exceptions do exist. For example, the problem is not so straightforward when two contiguous digits are amputated at the same short proximal phalangeal level. Resection of two contiguous rays would significantly narrow the breadth of such a palm and leave a three-fingered hand. Prosthetic replacement may be preferred.

Ray amputation of the index finger in an otherwise normal hand leads to a fairly satisfactory cosmetic result; nevertheless, a functional residual disability persists after such an amputation.[21,40] This disability is some weakness of pinch and grip. After ray resection of the long finger, the treating surgeon has two options. The first is reconstruction of the volar intermetacarpal ligament between the index and ring fingers, thus attempting to pull these two digits closer together. The second reconstructive alternative is the transposition of the index ray to the position of the long finger as originally described by Carroll.[16,54] This procedure immediately obliterates the dead space of the middle finger. However, the procedure has been associated with delayed union or nonunion of the osteotomy site in some cases. Similar choices exist for amputations through the ring or small finger.[27,28] In the case of the ring finger ray resection, transposition of the fifth ray to the ring position can be done. In amputation of the fifth ray, it is important to preserve the hypothenar musculature to serve as an adequate padding and cushioning of the ulnar side of the hand. Augmentation of existing interosseous musculature with that of the amputated digit should be discouraged, because intrinsic tightness can result.

MIDDLE PHALANX LEVEL

Amputations at the middle phalanx level can remain quite functional if the level is distal to the superficial flexor tendon

insertion.[17] In such cases, functional flexion of the proximal interphalangeal (PIP) joint can be maintained. Proximal to this insertion, however, flexion is less likely to be preserved. Consequently, a disarticulation through the PIP joint can be every bit as functional as a short middle phalangeal amputation.

DISTAL PHALANX LEVEL

In most cases consideration must be given to the type of fingertip that will result if greater than one-half of the distal phalanx is amputated. In such cases, very little supportive structure is left for the remaining nail and nail matrix. Often a "hook-nail" deformity or other such unattractive troublesome situations can result.[38] Thus, it is frequently advisable to remove not only the remainder of the injured nail but the proximal germinal matrix as well in order to prevent this deformity. If there is enough distal phalanx to support the nail, the hook-nail deformity will probably be prevented. The rule then is to preserve as much length and distal phalanx as possible, but the patient should be made aware of the continuing possibility of nail deformity. Such deformity can be surgically corrected later should the need arise. In distal digital amputations, one should properly identify each terminal digital nerve in carrying out the same careful neurectomy as for more proximal amputations. The bone should be rongeured to form a smooth contour that will not exert undue pressure on the soft tissues of the terminal portion of the amputation and produce a painful stump.

After division of the flexor digitorum profundus, a patient may be left with a so-called lumbrical-plus finger.[43] In this situation, flexion of the PIP joint is severely limited secondary to the additional tension exerted through the lumbrical. This muscle has had its origin moved proximally by the migration of the flexor profundus tendon, which no longer has an insertion into the distal phalanx. If a lumbrical-plus finger deformity is noted, it is frequently wise to section the proximal lumbrical as a delayed reconstructive procedure. This problem appears to be especially evident in tip amputations in the index finger.

FINGERTIP LEVEL

Of all amputations sustained traumatically, the one which presents most commonly is the fingertip amputation.[4,22]

In recent years, hand surgeons have become increasingly aware of the excellent regeneration and self-healing capacity of the finger pulp. This is not surprising given the rich vascular bed that is present in the finger pulp. With thorough and meticulous care, debridement, and proper regular dressing changes, the finger pulp amputation can shrink, granulate, and epithelize quite satisfactorily.[5] This "no-surgery technique" is especially indicated in the young child, in whom the ability to heal a distal amputation is most evident.[18,47] The initial tip discrepancy and cosmetic loss become less and less evident with each year of remaining growth.

This conservative treatment is also applicable to adult partial fingertip amputations. However, in adult patients other factors should be considered. Time loss from work can be a very real problem, and the period of such healing is frequently significant.[37] In addition, the hypersensitivity in such an escarified tip that has healed by secondary intention can often be so extreme as to necessitate a more proximal amputation at a later date. This can frequently occur after months of protracted waiting and loss of employment. Thus, the best interest of the manual laborer patient may be to carry out a slightly proximal amputation at the time of primary treatment. Such treatment allows primary closure of the wound and frequently the shortest recuperative period.

An alternative to amputation is the resurfacing of the distal pulp via advancement of more proximal undamaged tissue. This is the premise of the Atasoy (triangular volar advancement) and the Kutler (lateral tissue advancement) flap technique.[2,20,23,24,34,49]

Sometimes a full-thickness loss that has left the distal phalanx with some degree of soft tissue pulp can be repaired with a split-skin graft. The suggestion has been made that such treatment hastens the actual shrinkage of the defect in the tip by pulling the edges of the wound together. Whether or not this technique hastens the healing any more than treating by secondary intention granulation is conjectural at this point.[25,35,39]

When the skin loss extends to the volar surface of the flexor tendon, there is an additional problem. The surgeon is loath to amputate a large portion of the distal phalanx since the flexor sheath is still intact. However, the techniques so far described will not suffice. In such cases a cross finger flap is useful (Fig. 44-3).[10] In this procedure, the dorsal untraumatized skin and subcutaneous tissue are carefully dissected and elevated from an adjacent uninjured finger and attached to the traumatized defect in the contiguous injured finger.[29,30] This procedure resurfaces the volar surface that has been lost and allows adequate padding and soft tissue coverage of all the important volar surfaces of the finger. The dorsal aspect of the donor finger is then resurfaced with a free skin graft. This graft can be from the groin or from the flexor surface of the wrist. Detachment of such a pedicle graft is usually safely accomplished at 3 weeks after the attachment. Stiffness of the interphalangeal joints can often be a sequela of such a procedure, but gentle controlled range-of-motion exercises during the healing phase usually prevent this complication. In addition, the young patient has less of a tendency for such joint stiffness. The defect that is incurred on the dorsum of the donor digit does not result in functional disability since it is not on the tactile surface of the finger.

An alternative method to the cross finger flap is the thenar flap (Fig. 44-4). In this procedure the involved finger is flexed just enough to attach the damaged portion to a pedicle flap that is raised from the skin and subcutaneous tissues of

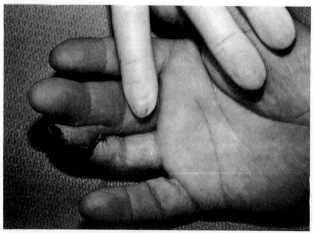

A

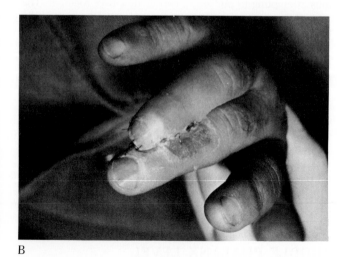

B

Figure 44-3 A. The cross finger flap provides fleshy pulp coverage. **B.** The donor defect is covered with skin graft to the dorsum of the long finger.

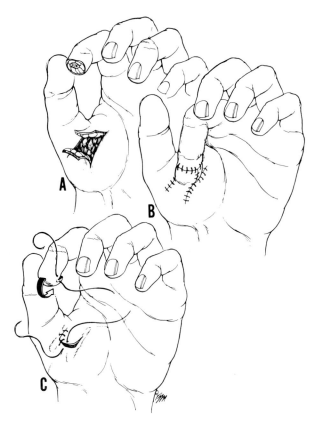

Figure 44-4 The thenar flap works well in the properly selected patient. Residual stiffness is minimized by proper positioning of the digit and aggressive therapy after "release." *(From Green, David P., ed: Operative Hand Surgery. New York, Churchill Livingstone, 1982. Reprinted with permission.)*

the thenar area. Some critics have warned against resultant stiffness of the damaged finger in this procedure, which is contraindicated in elderly or arthritic patients or in any condition that might predispose a patient to stiffness, including

Dupuytren's contracture and scleroderma. If the patient is not elderly or arthritic, the degree of flexion contracture can usually be kept to a minimum. The technique is useful, particularly in the index and long fingers. In order to minimize PIP joint stiffness, the flap should be disconnected from the thenar area at 12 to 14 days. It should not be immediately sutured tightly down at the junction of the proximal end of the flap and the proximal edge of the pulp defect but gently coaxed into place by progressively tightened adhesive Steri-Strips. Immediate tight suturing of the proximal end of the flap to the finger after disconnecting it from the thenar area causes under stress on the vascular supply of the flap from the tip of the finger and can result in flap loss.

THE THUMB

Amputations of the thumb can be managed somewhat differently than other digital amputations. The three joints of the thumb axis compose an arc of flexion that compensates for the loss of motion at any one of the individual joints. Such latitude allows the surgeon to consider alternative reconstructive modalities in the thumb that would not work in the finger. An amputated thumb can be expected to be quite functional as long as the distal portion of the remaining thumb reaches the MP joint level of the contiguous index finger. The distal pulp and tip amputation can often be treated in the same manner as fingertip amputations. More proximal levels, however, are matters of concern.

The thumb obviously functions more independently in the hand than other digits and thus is of greater functional importance, which indicates a need for greater effort in reconstruction and preservation of length than in the digits. Microsurgical replantation and repair probably have no greater use or indication than in the all-out attempts at preservation of an amputated thumb. In more distal levels (1 cm or less of thumb lost), where replantation may not be feasible, the volar advancement of Moberg can be utilized (Fig. 44-5).

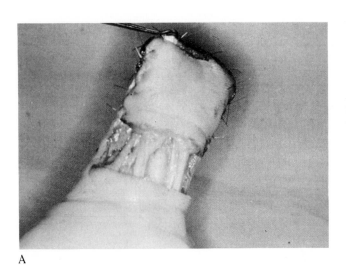

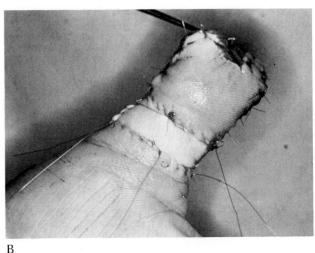

A   B

Figure 44-5 A. Volar advance flap: volar skin proximal to the deficiency is moved distally. **B.** Split skin graft fills the deficiency.

In such a procedure, the volarmost remaining tissue is incised laterally in the midaxial plane with preservation of both digital neurovascular bundles in the volar flap.[31] This incision must carefully preserve the circulation as well as the sensation to the flap. The flap itself must also be carefully dissected off the flexor sheath of the thumb. Next, the IP joint and the MP joint of the thumb are brought into as much flexion as is necessary to gain tip coverage with the flap. Resultant fixed flexion deformities of the thumb joints can occur after this procedure. However, the composite flexion of the joints of the thumb rarely makes this a functional disability. These contractures can also be minimized by aggressive hand therapy. Sutures which are used to attach the volar advancement flap in the thumb should be left in approximately 2 to 3 weeks to prevent proximal migration or wound dehiscence.

More proximal amputations in the thumb (greater than 1 cm of thumb length lost) require other management techniques. Despite the proliferation of more elaborate microsurgical transfers and reconstructions, the surgeon is probably best advised to pursue the most conservative and least risky procedures in thumb reconstruction. The distraction and augmentation techniques can provide a satisfactory thumb

(Fig. 44-6). These procedures are most applicable when the amputation level has left the remaining thumb just short of the contiguous index MP joint. In such a case, the thumb amputation should be cleaned and shortened only as much as necessary to allow primary closure after digital neurectomies and contouring of the remaining bone. At a later date, usually months, the technique and risks of distraction and augmentation procedures are explained to the patient in detail. When the tip of the thumb has healed completely with no signs of hyperemia, the first stage, a simple osteotomy in the thumb metacarpal, can be done. A distraction device such as a mini-Hoffman or Jaquet's device is attached via two distally placed pins and two proximally placed pins. Each pair of pins is separated by the osteotomy site through the thumb metacarpal. To further stabilize the osteotomy and in preparation for its distraction, one or two longitudinally placed Kirschner wires are also used. The wounds are primarily closed over the osteotomy. In the weeks after surgery, the patient is carefully supervised in the twice daily technique of lengthening the foreshortened thumb. About 1 to 2 mm of distraction per day can be tolerated by the patient. If the neurological or vascular compromise at the end of the digit occurs during the distrac-

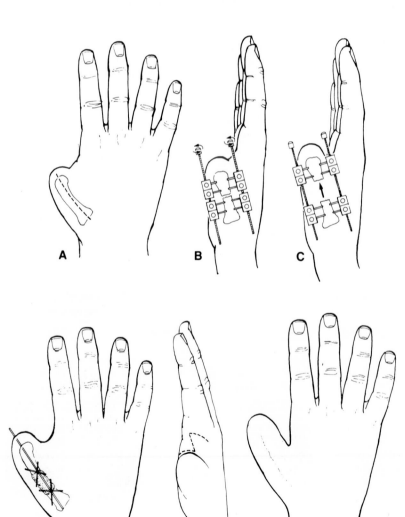

Figure 44-6 The distraction-augmentation staged reconstruction of the thumb is a relatively safe procedure (see text). First web space deepening *(E)* is often necessary. *(From Matev, I.B., J Hand Surg 5:43–46, 1973.)*

tion schedule, the surgeon should delay or curtail the distraction.

Once an appropriate length of the thumb has been achieved, usually when the distal portion of the thumb reaches the level of the index MP joint, the distraction of the thumb can be discontinued. At this state the second phase of the reconstruction is undertaken. The same dorsal incision utilized for the osteotomy is opened. The distracted attenuated periosteum should be incised longitudinally without disrupting these bone-forming tissues. Next, an autogenous iliac graft is obtained, shaped, and cut appropriately to fit neatly into the distraction space of the thumb metacarpal. The graft is usually fixed with percutaneously placed Kirschner wires. These wires can easily be removed in the office once the graft has sufficiently incorporated. Incorporation usually takes 3 to 6 weeks. Once fixation is achieved, the external fixation distraction device can be removed and hand therapy with dynamic and static splinting instituted. Frequently, Z-plasty and first web space deepening are necessary as a secondary procedure.

Amputations that occur at, or proximal to, the MP level are probably best treated at this time with microsurgical composite reconstruction. In one technique (the wrap-around) well-contoured portion of iliac graft is used as a structural extension to the remaining metacarpal of the thumb (Fig. 44-7). This is then covered by donor soft tissues which are dissected from the great toe. Microsurgical anastomoses of neurovascular structures in the soft tissue graft and the residual portions of the thumb are performed to complete the reconstruction. When successfully accomplished, this results in a functional thumb. The residual donor site in the great toe frequently can be treated by skin grafting or by creating a syndactyly to the second toe. A time-honored procedure which is extremely useful for treating patients with thumb amputation is pollicization of the index finger (Fig. 44-8).[36] This technique still remains the technique of choice in the younger patient. In pollicization after traumatic loss of the

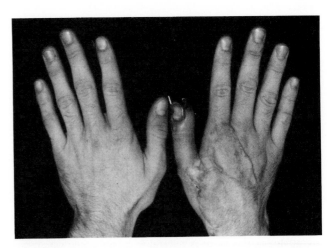

Figure 44-7 The "wrap-around" technique requires careful neurovascular dissection and microsurgical anastomosis to be successful. The cosmetic results can be quite gratifying.

thumb, careful assessment of the vasculature of the ray that is to be pollicized should be carried out preoperatively.

COMPLICATIONS
Painful Stumps, Scars, and Neuromas

Painful neuromas can usually be avoided by cutting each nerve cleanly while it is placed in maximal traction. This allows the cut nerve to retract into the remaining soft tissue cuff. Painful neuromas that persist months or years after amputation should be treated first with conservative techniques. These include alteration in the prosthesis, aggressive physical or occupational therapy with a specific desensitization program, localized infiltration with cortisone and long-acting

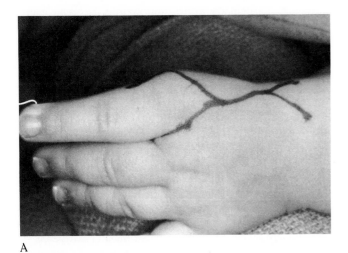

A

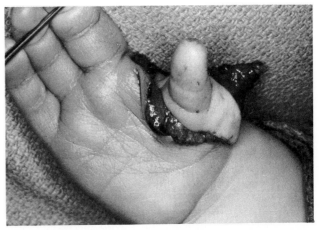

B

Figure 44-8 Pollicization of the index finger is still frequently considered the procedure of choice in thumb reconstruction. This is especially true in the child. **A.** The incision. **B.** The mobilized rotated digit prior to closure.

local anesthetics, and regular massage by the patients themselves. In this way sensitivity can frequently be minimized. In a recent series of Boswick,[9] phantom pain existed in almost all of 100 patients during the first month postinjury. Continuation of this pain was strongly associated with psychological perception and regressive disability.

One of the most resistant conditions is the neuroma of the superficial branch of the radial nerve. The sensitivity caused even by a neuroma-in-continuity can persist even when no complete laceration of this nerve has occurred during initial injury or surgery.

When a patient shows no improvement, other modalities should be pursued. Some of these are biofeedback, sympathetic blocks, regional Bier's blocks with guanethidine or reserpine, or even sympathectomies. Sometimes the appropriate advice at this point is referral to a pain clinic which has appropriate facilities and staff for administering these techniques.

Contractures which frequently occur in the amputated portion of the upper extremity can be minimized by early edema control. Bulky, well-padded, and mild compressive dressings are helpful adjutants to avoid edema and subsequent contractures. The range of motion of the remaining portions of the upper extremity can be maximized with early active, active assisted, and passive exercises supervised by a qualified physical therapist.

SECTION B

Replantation Surgery in the Upper Extremity

M. Ather Mirza

HISTORY

The first limb replantation attempts were made in the animal laboratory by pioneering vascular surgeons. In 1903 Hopfner successfully replanted the hind leg of several dogs and reported a survival of the limb of 1 to 10 days.[6] Carrel extended the postreplantation survival time to 22 days in 1906.[3] The work of Lapchinsky[11] and Snyder[21] showed that the toxic effects of ischemic tissues are greatly reduced by cooling the extremity and by perfusing the amputated limb with heparinized solutions. These two advances, which reduced the warm ischemia time, combined with improved anesthesia and the availability of antibiotics, microsutures, and specialized instruments have greatly contributed to the successful replantation of limbs in clinical practice.

In 1962 in Boston, Malt succeeded in replanting the amputated arm of a 12-year-old boy; he reported this case in 1964.[12] In 1963 a successful replantation of a severed forearm

in an adult was reported from China.[4] This ushered in the modern era of replantation surgery. In 1965 Kleinert reported successful anastomosis of digital vessels, with a loop used for magnification.[9] In 1966, Buncke successfully replanted rabbit ears and the thumbs of monkeys.[2] In 1968 Komatsu and Tamai reported successful replantation of a completely severed human thumb.[10]

Although replantation surgery had by 1968 become successful at the vascular level, the return of nerve function remained poor. Smith in 1963, however, reported fascicular nerve repair with the aid of an operative microscope.[20] In 1976 Millesi reported an 80 percent functional recovery with intrafascicular nerve grafting.[13] Despite multiple technical studies further improvement in the results of nerve repair has not been forthcoming.

DEFINITIONS

Microsurgery is any procedure that is performed with the help of magnification from an operative microscope. It is generally accepted that operating on structures of 1 mm or less requires magnification. However, the repair of larger structures is frequently facilitated by the use of magnification.

Replantation is the reattachment of severed anatomical components from any part of the body back to the same body. A total severance of any part of the body without any attachment is known as *complete amputation* (Fig. 44-9). An *incomplete amputation* is totally devoid of its functional circulation, and less than one-eighth of the normal skin is attached.[1,19]

Other terms are used to describe the mechanism of the amputation. A *guillotine amputation* is one produced by a sharp instrument. This type of amputation is ideal for replantation.[23] *Crush amputations* with localized crush do better than amputations with extensive crush, which are not ideal for replantation. However, any crush amputation is a poorer candidate for replantation than a guillotine amputation. An *avulsion amputation* is one in which the digit or the extremity is literally pulled out of the body. In avulsion amputations the neurovascular structures suffer extensive damage for various distances. Particularly in avulsion injuries a careful microscopic evaluation is necessary in order to determine the status of the vascular system within the amputated part. In the words of R. Daniel and J. Terzis: "It is far simpler to assess the quality of the digital artery by perfusion than by a failed anastomosis."[5]

GENERAL CONSIDERATIONS AND INDICATIONS FOR REPLANTATION

The replantation team consists of skilled microsurgeons as well as vascular, orthopaedic, thoracic, and general surgeons.[5,14,23] Each member of the team must know and be committed to the following philosophy if the procedures are to be functionally successful. Each member must (1) strive for expertise in his or her respective specialty areas of surgery; (2) have the personality traits necessary to work with demanding procedures, for long hours, and as part of a team; (3) be willing to maintain a high level of competence and technical

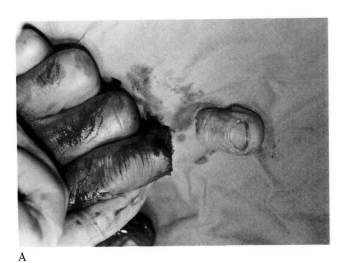

A

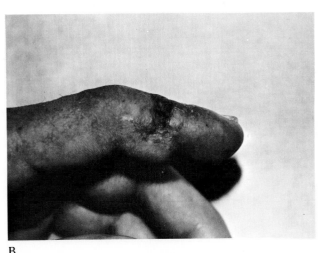

B

Figure 44-9 A. Complete amputation of left index finger by power saw at the level of the middle phalanx. **B.** Successful replantation of left index finger with a good functional and cosmetic result.

skills; and (4) accept the frequent disruption of schedules in order to perform these emergency procedures.[14]

Once the team has been selected, the next step is to teach all involved nursing staff the specialized care required by these patients. Then seminars, videotape, and lectures should be used to teach the police, fire, and fire ambulance personnel the emergency care of this type of patient and care of the amputated part. The police department, Air National Guard, fire department, and Coast Guard should be contacted and their cooperation sought for the transportation of these patients with special emphasis on transportation of the amputated part with proper wrapping and cooling procedures.[5,14,23]

The following are general indications for replantation: (1) All amputations at the level of the arm, forearm, carpus, and metacarpus should be replanted (Fig. 44-10). (2) All amputations involving the thumb at all levels except the midportion of the distal phalanx should be replanted (Fig. 44-11). (3) In case of multiple digits, an effort should be made to replant as many as possible. (4) Most digits amputated distal to the proximal phalanx should be replanted. (5) Index and/or small fingers amputated at the level of the metacarpal or proximal phalanx do not give satisfactory results after replantation and should be considered for the various revision/modification procedures available. (6) Children have great capacity for regeneration; thus all amputations in children should be replanted. (7) Avulsed digits and crushed digital amputations should be scrutinized for their salvage potential and functional prognosis.[5,14,23]

CARE OF THE AMPUTATED PART AND AMPUTATION SITE

Care of the amputated part is very critical to the success and survival of the replant. Lapchinsky[11] and Snyder[21] have effectively shown the beneficial effects of cooling in the survival of the replanted extremity in the experimental animal. Cooling

lowers the metabolic rate and thus the oxygen consumption of the tissues of the amputated part. Since muscles are one of the extremity tissues most sensitive to anoxia, the acceptable cooled ischemia time is, therefore, 6 h. In cases of digital amputations, the cooled ischemia time is much longer. Successful digital replantations after 12 to 20 h have been reported.[23]

The amputated part should be gently irrigated with copious amounts of Ringer's lactate or saline solution. The extremity then should be wrapped in a Ringer's lactate–soaked sterile towel in order to protect the tissues from desiccation. The wrapped extremity should be placed in a plastic bag, which is then placed in a container with crushed ice. The plastic bag and the sterile towel prevent the tissues from freezing. The bag should be appropriately labeled for proper identification. Dry ice must not be used! The tissue must not be put directly into ice!

Overzealous effort to achieve hemostasis by the use of clamps which damage the neurovascular bundles should be avoided. Most of the hemorrhage can effectively be controlled by local pressure. The stump should be irrigated with Ringer's lactate or saline solution and then wrapped in sterile compressive dressing. The first layer of dressing should also be soaked in Ringer's lactate.

CARE OF THE PATIENT

The survival of the replanted extremity is very dependent on the management of the amputated part prior to replantation. The overall management of the patient always takes precedence and becomes the primary responsibility of the peripheral hospital.[5,14,18,23]

Prehospital Care

Prehospital care consists of the following:[5,14,18,23]

1. Assess the general condition of the patient with primary concern on basic life support.

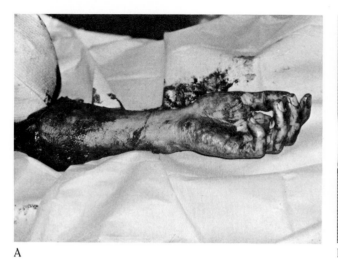

A

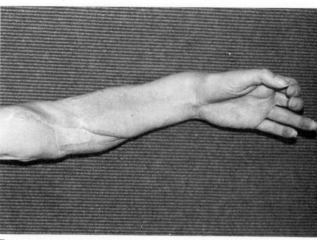

B

Figure 44-10 A. Proximal forearm amputation in a young male's dominant extremity. **B.** Successful replantation of the upper extremity. Some functional deficits remain because of the deficiencies in nerve regeneration.

2. Bandage the amputation stump and stop bleeding by direct pressure and elevation.
3. Collect, wrap, and cool the amputated parts.
4. Transport the patient to the nearest hospital expediently.[14]

Hospital Care

Care at the peripheral hospital consists of the following:[5,14,18,23]

1. Maintain patent airway.

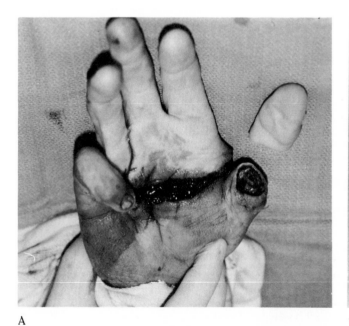

A

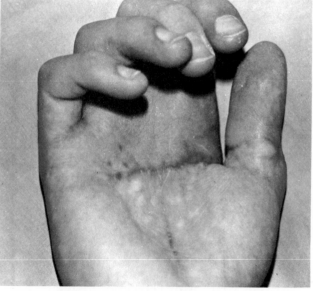

B

Figure 44-11 A. Thumb amputation secondary to power saw injury with associated partial amputation involving index and long fingers. All thumb amputations should be considered candidates for replantation if there are no other systemic medical contraindications to the long surgical procedure. **B.** Successful replantation of thumb and revascularizations of digits. Some restriction of finger flexion is noted.

2. Control and treat hemorrhage and shock.
3. Assess all systems of the patient.
4. Stabilize patient.
5. Insert peripheral intravenous line on the uninjured side.
6. Obtain pertinent history with special emphasis on allergies and tetanus inoculation.
7. Contact replant center and make arrangements for the transfer of the patient.
8. When patient is minor, attempt to have parent or guardian accompany the child.

Initial hospital care at the replant center consists of the following:[5,14,18,23]

1. Thoroughly assess the patient system by system.
2. Complete history and physical exam.
3. Check IV catheter for location and size; it should be large enough for blood transfusions.
4. Order appropriate baseline laboratory investigations.
5. Type and cross match 4 to 6 units of whole blood.
6. Obtain a 12-lead electrocardiogram.
7. Order appropriate x-ray studies including views of the amputated part and the amputation stump.
8. Insert urinary catheter and monitor urinary output.
9. Obtain necessary consents for the replant team surgery.
10. Assess the amputation site and the amputated part for feasibility of replantation.
11. Take cultures from the amputation site and then start appropriate prophylactic antibiotics.
12. Check tetanus toxoid immunization status and give a tetanus toxoid booster and/or tetanus immune globulin, if indicated.
13. Clean and shave the axilla on the injured side in the case of the upper extremity.
14. Obtain medical clearance if the patient is over 40 years of age or has a chronic or complicated medical history.
15. Document injury time, warm ischemia time, and cooled ischemia time.

Operating room protocol consists of the following:[5,14,18,23]

1. Have the operating microscope in the room with extra bulbs and fuses.
2. Have the operating table in place with the appropriate attachments.
3. Have pneumatic tourniquet ready for use.
4. Have all instrument trays prepared along with other supplies. (Appropriate instrumentation should always be ready at the replantation center.)
5. Have a microirrigation set-up ready.
6. Attach a 35-mm camera to the microscope, making sure the camera has fresh roll of film.
7. Prepare a warming blanket for the pediatric patient.[14]

GENERAL OPERATIVE MANAGEMENT

For most digital and wrist replants, regional anesthesia is preferred. This is usually brachial plexus block, either supraclavicular or infraclavicular. The long duration of surgery required for most of these cases makes general anesthesia less desirable, but for more proximal levels this is the best choice. For regional anesthesia we have used 0.25% bupivacaine HCl solution or 0.5% bupivacaine.[14]

Two operating teams working simultaneously, one on the amputation site and the other on the amputated part probably constitute the best method, especially in multiple digits.[5,23] Each team's main objective is to identify and tag arteries, veins, nerves, and tendons and prepare the bone for open reduction and internal fixation. The first step of any replantation is skeletal fixation, which should be expedient and stable. After bone fixation the next structure to repair in digital replantation is the extensor tendon and then the dorsal digital veins. The general rule is to anastomose two digital veins for each digital artery.[5,8,14,15,18,23] The digital artery is repaired next. This reestablishes the circulation to the digit. This is followed by repair of the flexor tendons and digital nerves. The skin closure should be very loose with a minimal number of sutures. The dressings should be soft, fluffy, and nonconstricting types.[5,8,14,15,18,23]

POSTOPERATIVE MANAGEMENT

Postoperative management is essential to the survival of the replant, and it is imperative to follow a strict regime (Table 44-1).[5,14,18,23] The most important of all the systems to watch is the circulation. This has to be monitored at intervals from the time the patient leaves the operating room until he or she reaches the tenth postoperative day. The various signs of failing circulation should be known to both the operating surgeon and the nursing staff. If there is venous compromise, the following will occur in the replanted member:

1. Capillary refill will be fast.
2. Color will be dark red to purple.
3. Turgor will be rapid.
4. Skin temperature will fall below 30°C.
5. If oxygen saturation is being measured it will fall below 80%.

If there is arterial compromise, the following will occur:

1. Capillary refill will be slow.
2. Color will be pale.
3. Turgor will be sluggish.
4. Skin temperature will drop dramatically below 30°C.
5. Oxygen saturation may drop precipitously.

The patient should be transferred from the recovery room to intensive care for the first 48 to 72 h. When future vascular problems may be anticipated, the patient should be given nothing by mouth.

The urinary catheter is left in place for 72 to 96 h after surgery. The extremity is elevated on pillows, and no hanging devices are used. The elevation is 15 cm above the level of the heart. If edema occurs, a higher elevation is indicated. The limb is lowered if cyanosis occurs.[5] The patient is given analgesics and sedatives. The intramuscular route is avoided. We have routinely used chlorpromazine (Thorazine), 25 mg tid. Chlorpromazine not only calms the patient down but also acts as a vasodilator. Intravenous antibiotics are continued for a period of 3 to 5 days. Anticoagulants are used fairly regularly at our institution. Heparin is the drug of choice and is given intravenously 20,000 units/24 h.[14] Enteric-coated aspirin, 650 mg bid, is given as an antiplatelet factor. The patient is well hydrated. The routine use of low-molecular-weight dextran (LMD), 2 units daily, is definitely indicated. It improves the microcirculation by preventing sludging of the red blood cells. It is very important to remember that once the LMD therapy is instituted, cross matching blood becomes very difficult; thus all cross matching should be completed before giving LMD.[14]

It is very important to emphasize to the patient the adverse effect of smoking upon the prognosis. The patient should be kept calm, and visitors should be limited. If the patient needs psychiatric help, it should be provided. Many times the patient can also be helped by talking to another patient who has gone through the replantation experience.

Frequent dressing changes should be avoided. The dressings should be changed only for good reasons, for example, blood-soaked dressings that are dried up and becoming constrictive should be changed. Before the patient is discharged, the bulk of the dressings is reduced so that the patient can start early therapy. If it is necessary to use plaster, only a splint on the palmar side should be used. If considerable edema follows major extremity replantations, skeletal (external) fixation may be used to achieve elevation without resorting to large casts which interfere with the circulation. We have successfully used transmetacarpal Steinmann pins for this purpose in a below-elbow replantation.

The patient is usually discharged on the tenth day. Specific instructions are given regarding elevation, smoking, observation for signs of circulatory compromise, and exposure to cold. Revisits should be scheduled every week for the next 4 weeks. The antibiotics are discontinued early, but aspirin and chlorpromazine are continued for the next 3 weeks. Physical therapy is started as soon as possible. There should be candid discussion with the patient regarding his or her ability to go back to work. If there are any questions about the patient's ability to perform a former occupation, arrangements for vocational rehabilitation should be made.

COMPLICATIONS

Good surgical judgment combined with technically competent microsurgery avoids most of the complications.

Intraoperative Complications

Intraoperatively, vascular complications are the most frequently encountered.

Arterial Complications

Spasm of the proximal segment is treated by trying to manipulate the segment by squeezing gently with jeweler's forceps, or by bathing the segment in 2% lidocaine solution. If all fails, one may try to strip the adventitia to reduce the neurogenic spasm.[5,14,23]

If the anastomotic site is clotted, the anastomosis should be checked and any suture which is questionable should be replaced. If this does not change the situation, the anastomosis should be taken down, a good proximal flow should be ascertained, and then the anastomosis should be repeated. Flushing the lumen out with a solution of heparin and xylocaine in Ringer's lactate is usually of great help.

The physician should make sure there is no excessive tension on the anastomosis because this has adverse effect on the flow of blood. In case of excessive tension on the suture line, either the bone should be shortened or an interposition vein graft should be considered.

Intimal damage or an intimal tag should be sought. If there is extensive intimal damage, the chances of the vessel remaining patent are very poor.

Venous Complications

Venous complications are encountered more frequently because of the low-pressure system and because of the greater technical difficulties in repairing the veins. One should make sure that a patency test was done on each of the vessels when the anastomosis was finished. Tension likewise must be avoided. Measures similar to those discussed with arterial anastomosis should be instituted to avoid tension.[5,8,15,23]

Postoperative Complications

Postoperatively the complications most frequently encountered are also vascular. If any vascular compromise exists, the first thing to do is to remove all the dressings, inspect thoroughly for any extrinsic pressure problems, and remove any tight sutures. One should make sure the patient is well-hydrated and normotensive. Next gentle local massage proximal to the anastomosis should be tried. If all fails, a stellate ganglion block, or even better an axillary block, should be tried. An axillary block not only acts as a ganglion block but also allows you to be ready to take the patient back to the operating room if this maneuver does not reestablish the blood supply. In the operating room, both the artery and the vein should be explored, and the measures already discussed should be instituted. Tsai reported 15 postoperative complications; a large number of them were venous.[22]

Bleeding

Bleeding could be a major problem if the patient were not closely observed. This is the reason for intensive care in the immediate postoperative period. Heparin is usually used in those patients in whom there is most concern for the patency of the blood vessels. These are the patients who have dual reasons to bleed: arterial leaks and/or venous compromise.

To stop arterial bleeding, first local measures such as topical application of hemostatic agents, elevation of the arm, and cessation of the anticoagulant therapy should be tried. If these do not work, the patient must be taken back to the operating room and the appropriate bleeding point ligated.

TABLE 44-1 Postoperative Regime

1. Prescribe complete bed rest.
2. Elevate the extremity on pillows.
3. Check circulatory status of the replanted extremity every 30 min for the first 24 h, every 60 min for the next 24 h, every 1 h for the next 48 h. Check
   a. Color (normal, cyanotic, or pale)
   b. Turgor (normal, rapid, or sluggish)
   c. Capillary refill (normal, slow, or fast)
   d. Temperature of amputated part and normal extremity, and the ambient temperature.
4. Give 500 ml of 5% dextrose in Ringer's lactate plus 5000 units of heparin IV every 6 h. Give low-molecular-weight dextran, 500 ml bid, run slowly.
5. Request laboratory investigations:
   Hematocrit and hemoglobin levels bid for 5 days.
   Prothrombin time and activated thromboplastin time bid until heparin is discontinued.
6. Prohibit smoking and coffee intake by the patient.
7. Prescribe analgesics and sedatives as required (see text).
8. Prescribe prophylactic antibiotics.
9. Limit visitors and keep patient environment quiet.

Sometimes excessive bleeding is an indication of venous compromise where the artery is still patent. In these cases there are signs of circulatory compromise. When the venous problem is corrected, the bleeding usually stops.

Later Complications

Infection

Fortunately, in spite of the severe nature of these injuries, the rate of infection is low. In our series there has not been any significant postoperative infection.[14] O'Brien and Morrison encountered a rate of infection less than 2 percent.[15]

Skin Slough

Although localized skin slough is frequently encountered at the skin edges, it is rarely of any great significance. If extensive, it may require skin grafting, or if the major structures are exposed, a pedicle graft may be necessary.

Fracture Union

Bone union is dependent to great extent on adequate rigid fixation. According to Urbaniak,[23] intramedullary Kirschner's wire is still the best and most expedient method of fixation. There is, however, an increased incidence of delayed union and nonunion[14] with Kirschner's wires. The author's own experience is that one should employ rigid internal fixation whenever time permits. The most expedient way to achieve this is through interosseous wiring, although the author does tend to agree with Urbaniak that Kirschner-wire fixation is appropriate in most instances, especially in multiple digital replantations.

Tendon Gliding Problems

If tendons are repaired primarily and early rehabilitation is started, the problems of tendon adhesions are minimized. There are occasional problems which have to be dealt with by tenolysis. In secondary repairs of the flexor tendons, one should consider the use of Silastic tendon prostheses.

Joint Stiffness

Stiffness can be prevented by early joint mobilization, which is why rigid internal fixation is so important.

Neural Complication

In the majority of cases the patient obtains protective sensibility.[5,8,15] The return of two-point discrimination is variable. The commonest complaint from our patients has been cold intolerance. The same was true in Urbaniak's series.[23]

REFERENCES

Section A: Traumatic Amputations of the Hand and Wrist

1. Abu-Jamra, F.N., and Khuri, S. The treatment of finger tip injuries. J Trauma 11:749–757, 1971.
2. Atasoy, E., Ioakimidis, E., Kasdan, M.L., Kutz, J.E., and Kleinert, H.E. Reconstruction of the amputated finger tip with a triangular volar flap. A new surgical procedure. J Bone Joint Surg 52A:921–926, 1970.
3. Bailey, R.W., and Stevens, D.B. Radical exarticulation of the extremities for the curative and palliative treatment of malignant neoplasms. J Bone Joint Surg 43A:845–854, 1961.
4. Barclay, T.L. The late results of finger tip injuries. Br J Plast Surg 8:38–43, 1955.

5. Bate, J.T. Second and third intention healing of finger tip amputations: A salvage procedure. Clin Orthop 47:151–155, 1966.
6. Beasley, R.W. Reconstruction of amputated finger tips. Plast Reconstr Surg 44:349–352, 1969.
7. Beasley, R.W. Local flaps for surgery of the hand. Orthop Clin North Am 1:219–225, 1970.
8. Blader, S., Gunterberg, B., and Markhede, G. Amputation for tumor of the upper arm. Acta Orthop Scand 54:226–229, April 1983.
9. Boswick, J.A. Neuroma formation following digital amputations. J Trauma 23:136–147, February 1983.
10. Brailliar, F., and Horner, R.L. Sensory cross-finger pedicle graft. J Bone Joint Surg 51A:1264–1268, 1969.
11. Brody, G.S., Cloutier, A.M., and Woolhouse, F.M. The finger tip injury—An assessment of management. Plast Reconstr Surg 26:80–90, 1960.
12. Burkhalter, W.E., Mayfield, G., and Carmona, L.S. The upper extremity amputee. Early and immediate post-surgical prosthetic fitting. J Bone Joint Surg 58A:46–51, 1976.
13. Byrne, H., and Clarkson, P. Traumatic amputations of the finger tips, in Flynn, J.E. (ed): *Hand Surgery.* Baltimore, Williams & Wilkins, 1966, p 543.
14. Carroll, R.E. Transposition of the index finger to replace the middle finger. Clin Orthop 15:27–34 1950.
15. Chase, R.A. Functional levels of amputation in the hand. Surg Clin North Am 40:415–423, 1960.
16. Childress, D.S., Hampton, F.L., Lambert, C.N., Thompson, R.G., and Schrodt, M.J. Myoelectric immediate post-surgical procedure: A concept for fitting the upper extremity amputee. Artif Limbs 13:55–60, 1969.
17. Clarkson, P. The care of open injuries of the hand and fingers with special reference to the treatment of traumatic amputations. J Bone Joint Surg 37A:521–526, 1955.
18. Douglas, B.S. Conservative management of guillotine amputation of the finger in children. Aust Paediatr J 8:86, 1972.
19. Elsahy, N.I. When to replant a finger tip after its complete amputation. Plast Reconstr Surg 60:14–21, 1977.
20. Fisher, R.H. The Kutler method of repair of finger tip amputations. J Bone Joint Surg 49A:317–321 1967.
21. Fisher, E.G., and Goldner, J.L. Index ray deletion—complications and sequel. J Bone Joint Surg 54A:898, 1972.
22. Flatt, A.E. *The Care of Minor Hand Injuries,* 3d ed. St. Louis, Mosby, 1972, p 137.
23. Frackelton, W.H., and Teasley, J.L. Neurovascular island pedicle—Extension in usage. J Bone Joint Surg 44A:1069–1072, 1962.
24. Freiberg, A., and Manktelow, R. The Kutler repair of finger tip amputations. Plast Reconstr Surg 50:371–375, 1972.
25. Graham, W.P. Incisions, amputations and skin grafting in the hand. Orthop Clin North Am 1:213–218, 1970.
26. Graham, W.P. Amputations, in Kilgore, E.S., and Graham, W.P. (eds): *The Hand, Surgical and Nonsurgical Management.* Philadelphia, Lea & Febiger, 1977, p 261.
27. Graham, W.C., Brown, J.B., Cannon, B., and Riordan, D.C. Transposition of fingers in severe injuries of the hand. J Bone Joint Surg 29:998–1004, 1947.
28. Harkins, P.D., and Rafferty, J.E. Digital transposition in the injured hand. J Bone Joint Surg 54A:1064–1067, 1972.
29. Hoskins, H.D. The versatile cross finger flap. A report on 26 cases. J Bone Joint Surg 42A:261–277, 1960.
30. Johnson, R.K., and Iverson, R.E. Cross finger pedicle flaps in the hand. J Bone Joint Surg 53A:913–919, 1971.
31. Keim, H.A., and Grantham, S.A. Volar flap advancement for thumb and finger tip injuries. Clin Orthop 66:109–112, 1969.
32. Kleinert, H.E. Finger tip injuries and their management. Am Surg 25:41–51, 1959.
33. Kritter, A.E. The bilateral upper extremity amputee. Symposium on amputation surgery and prosthetics. Orthop Clin North Am 3:419–433, 1972.

34. Lewin, M.L. Digital flaps in reconstructive and traumatic surgery. Clin Orthop 15:74–85, 1959.
35. Lie, K.K., Magargle, R.K., and Posch, J.L. Free full thickness skin grafts from the palm to cover defects of the fingers. J Bone Joint Surg 52A:559–561, 1970.
36. Littler, J.W. Principles of reconstructive surgery of the hand, in Converse, J.M. (ed): *Reconstructive Plastic Surgery,* vol IV. Philadelphia, Saunders, 1964, p 1612.
37. Metcalf, W., and Whalen, W. The surgical, social and economic aspects of a unit hand injury. J Bone Joint Surg 39A:317–324, 1957.
38. Metcalf, W., and Whalen, W.P. Salvage of the injured distal phalanx: Plan of care and analysis of 369 cases. Clin Orthop 13:114–123, 1959.
39. Micks, J.E., and Wilson, J.N. Full thickness of sole-skin grafts for resurfacing the hand. J Bone Joint Surg 49A:1128–1134, 1967.
40. Murray, J.F., Carman, W., and MacKenzie, J.K. Transmetacarpal amputation of the index finger: A clinical assessment of hand strength and complications. J Hand Surg 2:471–481, 1977.
41. Newmeyer, W.L., and Kilgore, E.S. Finger tip injuries: A simple, effective method of treatment. J Trauma 14:58–64, 1974.
42. Pack, G.T., and Crampton, R.S. The Tikhor-Linberg resection of the shoulder girdle. Clin Orthop 19:148–160, 1961.
43. Parkes, A. The "lumbrical-plus" finger. Hand 2:164–167, 1970.
44. Peizer, E., and Pirrello, T. Principles and practice in upper extremity prostheses. Orthop Clin North Am 3:397–417, 1972.
45. Porter, R.W. Functional assessment of transplanted skin in volar defects of the digits. A comparison between free grafts and flaps. J Bone Joint Surg 50A:955–963, 1968.
46. Robins, R.H.C. Finger tip injuries. Hand 2:119–125, 1970.
47. Sandzen, S.C. Management of the acute finger tip injury in the child. Hand 6:190–197, 1974.
48. Slocum, D.B., and Pratt, D.R. The principles of amputations of the fingers and hand. J Bone Joint Surg 26:535–546, 1944.
49. Snowe, J.W. The use of a volar flap for repair of finger tip amputations: A preliminary report. Plast Reconstr Surg 40:163–168, 1967.
50. Stein, R.B., and Walley, M. Functional comparison of upper extremity amputations using myoelectric and conventional prostheses. Arch Phys Med Rehabil 64:243–248, June 1983.
51. Thomas, A. Amputations of the upper extremity above the elbow. Surgical and prosthetic considerations. Instr Course Lect 8:242, 1951.
52. Tooms, R.E. Amputation surgery in the upper extremity. Orthop Clin North Am 3:383–395, 1972.
53. Tooms, R.E. Amputations through upper extremity, in Edmonson, A.S., and Crenshaw, A.H. (eds): *Campbell's Operative Orthopaedics,* 6th ed. St. Louis, Mosby, 1980, pp 857–867.
54. Tubiana, R., and Roux, J.P. Phalangization of the first and fifth metacarpals. Indications, operative technique and results. J Bone Joint Surg 56A:447–457, 1974.

Section B: Replantation Surgery in the Upper Extremity

1. American Replantation Mission to China. Replantation surgery in China. Plast Reconstr Surg 52:476–489, 1973.
2. Buncke, H.J., and Schultz, W.P. Total ear reimplantation in the rabbit utilizing microminiature vascular anastomosis. Br J Plast Surg 10:15, 1966.
3. Carrel, A., and Guthrie, C.C. Complete amputation of thigh with replantation. Am J Med Sci 131:297–301, 1906.
4. Chen, C.W., Chen, Y.C., and Pao, Y.S. Salvage of the forearm following complete traumatic amputation; report of a case. Chin Med J 82:632, 1963.
5. Daniel, R.K., and Terzis, J.K. *Reconstructive Microsurgery.* 1977.
6. Hopfner, E. Gefassnaht, Gefasstransplantation und Reimplantation an amputierten Extremitaten. Arch Klein Chir 70:417, 1903.
7. Jacobson, J.H., Suarez, E.L. Microsurgery in the anastomosis of small vessels. Surg Forum 11:243–245, 1960.

8. Kleinert, H.E., Juhala, C.A., Tsai, T.M., and Beek, A.V. Digital replantation—Selection technique, and results. Orthop Clin North Am 8(2):309–318, April 1977.
9. Kleinert, H.E., Kasdan, M.L., and Romero, J.L. Small blood-vessel anastomosis for salvage of severely injured upper extremity. J Bone Joint Surg [Am] 45:788–796, 1963.
10. Komatsu, S., and Tamai, S. Successful replantation of completely cut-off thumb: Case report. Plast Reconstr Surg 42:374, 1968.
11. Lapchinsky, A.G. Recent results of experimental transplantation of preserved limbs and kidneys and possible use of this technique in clinical practice. Ann NY Acad Sci 64:539, 1960.
12. Malt, R.A., and Harris, W.H. Replantation of severed arms. JAMA 189:716–722, 1964.
13. Millesi, H., Meissl, G., and Berger, A. Further experience with interfascicular grafting of the median, ulna and radial nerves. J Bone Joint Surg [Am] 58:209–218, 1976.
14. Mirza, M.A., and Krober, K.E. Organization and implementation of a community hospital microsurgical service for the management of amputation injuries. Microsurgery 5:136–139, 1984.
15. Morrison, W.A., O'Brien, B.M., and Macleod, A.M. Evaluation of

16. digital replantation—A review of 100 cases. Orthop Clin North Am 8(2):295–308, April 1977.
17. Nylen, C.O. The microscope in aural surgery, its first use and later development. Acta Otolaryngology 116(suppl):226–240, 1954.
18. Nylen, C.O. The otomicroscope and microsurgery 1921–1971. Acta Otolaryngol 73:453–454, 1972.
19. O'Brien, B. *Microvascular Reconstructive Surgery*. London, Churchill Livingstone, 1977.
20. O'Brien, B.M., and Miller, G.D.H. Digital reattachment and revascularization. J Bone Joint Surg [Am] 55:714–724, 1973.
21. Smith, J.W. Microsurgery of peripheral nerves. Plast Reconstr Surg 33:317, 1964.
22. Snyder, C.C., Knowles, R.P., Mayer, P.W., and Hobbs, J.C. Extremity replantation. Plast Reconstr Surg 26:251, 1951.
23. Tsai, T.M. Experimental and clinical application of microvascular surgery. Ann Surg 181:169–177, 1975.
24. Urbaniak, J.R. Replantation of amputated parts: Technique, results, and indications. Symposium on Microsurgery Practice in Orthopaedics. St. Louis, Mosby, September 1977 and May 1979.

CHAPTER 45

Infections in the Upper Extremity

Lawrence C. Hurst and Jay Nathan

Infections can turn a highly useful hand and upper extremity into a stiff and painful appendage. Amputation and even loss of life can result from a poorly treated hand infection.

The most common organism present in hand infections is *Staphylococcus aureus*.[33,37] *Streptococcus*, particularly group A, is the second most common organism in hand infections.

Streptococcus can also cause a necrotizing fasciitis. Anaerobic *Streptococcus* often infects burns and bite wounds. Anaerobic organisms are important agents in hand infections, and anaerobic cultures should always be obtained.[8,16] Clostridial organisms are a source of anaerobic infections which can result in tetanus and gas gangrene (clostridial myonecrosis).

Gram-negative bacteria also play a role in hand infections. The most common gram-negative organisms are *Escherichia coli*, *Proteus*, *Pseudomonas*, and *Klebsiella*. They are usually secondary invaders in wounds where the skin damage is great, or in immunocompromised patients. *Neisseria gonorrhoeae* is an important gram-negative organism to remember, particularly in sexually active young patients.

Viral lesions may occur in the hand. Cat-scratch fever produces a cutaneous pustule. It is presumed to be caused by the lymphogranuloma venereum group. The herpetic whitlow is a vesicular lesion seen with increased incidence in medical personnel. It is part of the differential diagnosis of a paronychia and must not be overlooked.

Fungal infections, though not common, may have serious consequences. They may contaminate a wound, especially in the debilitated, immunocompromised hospital patient. Appropriate antibiotics coupled with adequate surgical debridement are the cornerstone of treatment of these infections.

PATTERNS OF INFECTION IN THE HAND

The fascial spaces of the hand are closed anatomic compartments which when infected encourage abscess formation. Infection enters these spaces by direct puncture or by extension from an adjacent closed-space infection.[27] The most complete descriptions of the fascial compartments of the hand was the one done by Kanavel.[27] The predilection of the hand abscesses within its compartments renders treatment with systemic antibiotics alone ineffective. Surgical drainage is required. A thorough knowledge of the compartmental anatomy of the hand is necessary to understand the involvement of these spaces, where infection in these spaces can extend, and how they may best be drained.

CELLULITIS

This infection of the hand presents as a diffuse swelling, with erythema and ascending lymphangitis. A hemolytic streptococcus is often responsible. Fluctuation and pus are not found. Cellulitis is treated by elevation, splintage, and antibiotics. An attempt may be made to culture organisms by injecting a small amount of sterile nonbacterial static saline into the area of cellulitis and then withdrawing the fluid for culture.[30] X-ray films are taken to rule out a foreign body. Gout and/or tumor must always be considered in the differential diagnosis.

PARONYCHIA AND EPONYCHIA

Paronychia is the most common infection in the hand, with *Staphylococcus aureus* the usual offender. This infection can be initiated by foreign material lodging between the nail plate and paronychial tissue, by a hangnail which traumatizes the eponychial tissue, or even by the overuse of nail polish. A paronychia involves the radial and ulnar sides of the nail and surrounding tissue. If it involves the eponychium as well as the lateral fold, it is called an eponychia. Extension to the opposite side of the fingernail is termed a runaround.[38] Paronychias can be divided into two types, superficial and deep.

The superficial type is the easiest to treat. It presents as a small subcuticular abscess usually present at the epiparonychial junction. Incision of this small abscess without anesthesia combined with warm soaks and gauze dressing to keep the cavity open will overcome this infection.

The deep type of paronychial infection may start out as a cellulitis. In the cellulitis phase, the infection may be aborted by splints, warm soaks, and oral antibiotics. However, once an abscess forms, it must be drained. An important point is that the paronychia is swollen or compressed against the nail edge, thereby trapping the pus. To eradicate the infection, the paronychia must be separated from the nail. Most surgeons make a longitudinal incision paralleling the proximal nail and extending to its proximal eponychial border. The lateral quarter of the nail is removed to decompress the paronychia. If an eponychia is present, two longitudinal incisions are made. the eponychium is reflected proximally, and the proximal half of the nail is removed (Fig. 45-1). Incision and drainage of the abscess are completed and appropriate cultures taken (this includes fungal cultures). A petrolatum-impregnated dressing is then placed beneath the reflected skin. Antibiotics are recommended. Soaks are started 48 h after removal of the petrolatum-impregnated dressing. Splinting during the initial postoperative period promotes soft tissue healing. Range-of-motion exercises start when soaks are begun. The surgeon must not overlook a possible concomitant subungual abscess, apical abscess, or felon. In chronic paronychia, the possibility of tuberculosis, fungal infection, gout, or even carcinoma should be considered. Although rare, osteomyelitis of the distal phalanx can also complicate the seemingly trivial paronychia.

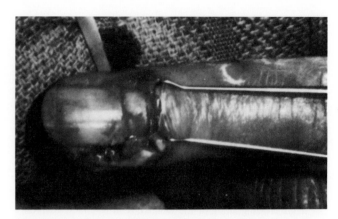

Figure 45-1 Surgical exposure after bilateral incisions and removal of proximal nail for eponychia.

SUBUNGUAL ABSCESS

Often subungual abscess results from extension of a deep paronychia under the nail. This can be distinguished by the presence of a "floating fingernail," or by pain elicited when pressure is applied to the center of the nail. Removal of the devitalized nail is mandatory. Most surgeons remove the proximal third of the nail, but the best overall results occur with total nail removal.[10] A petrolatum-impregnated gauze is placed over the exposed nail bed and under the eponychia. Cultures, soaks, splints, and antibiotics are employed as with an eponychia.

FELON

A felon involves the pulp space of the terminal phalanges of the fingers. It is a closed-space infection due to the fibrous septa in the pulp (Fig. 45-2). Although the most common cause of this infection is a puncture wound in the volar fat pad, it should be remembered that an overlooked or inadequately treated paronychia or subungual abscess may also result in a felon. The organism is invariably *Staphylococcus aureus*, coagulase-positive. Diagnosis is based on a careful

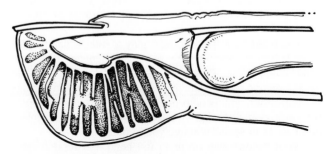

Figure 45-2 Cross-sectional anatomy of a felon. Note fibrous septa and collection of pus in the pulp abscess.

history and physical examination. The finger examination shows swelling volarly over the fat pad with exquisite tenderness secondary to increased tension in the closed space. Transillumination of the digit may reveal the abscess cavity and aid diagnosis.[43] One should be wary of an improvement in the level of discomfort since this may indicate necrosis. The abscess may expand and be complicated by a draining sinus volarly, osteomyelitis of the distal phalanx, and/or pyarthrosis of the distal interphalangeal joint. X-rays should always be used to rule out a foreign body or bony involvement.

The treatment of a felon is a combination of incision and drainage as well as systemic antibiotics. Antibiotics will not reach a closed-space infection but are effective against the associated cellulitis. The bulging fat pad distorts the local anatomy. Consequently, incisions used for drainage of a felon should be designed carefully. Slough of the volar fat pad is a serious complication which can be caused by too volar an incision. The dorsolateral hockey stick incision is the incision of choice. The incision is radially based in the thumb and little finger and ulnarly based in all the others. Small unilateral or bilateral lateral incisions are inadequate. Volar incisions may leave a tender scar but may be unavoidable, especially if the volar skin has already become necrotic. Fish mouth incisions should not be used because they are notorious for slough of the volar fat pad. After the fibrous septa are broken up and their attachment to the distal phalanx is released, the wound is packed open with sterile gauze. A culture is taken and antibiotics started. Dressing changes with wound repacking plus irrigation (or whirlpool) keep the wound open in the early postoperative period. Care must be taken not to violate an uninfected distal phalanx, joint space, or tendon sheath as this may result in iatrogenic spread of the infection.

WEB SPACE INFECTION

The web space is defined dorsally by the webbed skin, ulnarly and radially by the vertical septa, and volarly by the transverse palmar fascia. A sagittal section through a web space abscess shows that it consists of a volar and dorsal collection of pus with a communicating channel (Fig. 45-3). The infective process can originate from a fissure or puncture in the skin between the fingers, from an infected distal palmar callus, or from a septic subcutaneous lesion in the proximal finger. Physical examination reveals swelling volarly and dorsally. A sinus with purulent drainage may be present. The adjacent fingers assume an abducted posture. The important aspect with this type of infection is that the abscess cavity extends volarly and dorsally and that drainage of only one side leads to recurrent infection. The dumbbell-shaped abscess forms as the expanding abscess penetrates the palmar fascia near the superficial transverse metacarpal ligaments. Incisions must not be placed transversely across the web space, because this may lead to contracture. The volar incision curves ulnarly from the proximal flexor sheath of the involved digit proximally and ulnarly to the distal flexor crease of the palm. As the deeper section encounters the abscess cavity and is drained, dorsal pressure may cause in-

creased drainage. Dorsally a vertical incision starts out just proximal to the edge of the web space, continuing proximally to the diaphysis of the metacarpal (Fig. 45-3). The dorsal abscess is drained, and both wounds are irrigated. Both wounds are packed open with sterile gauze or drained, appropriate cultures taken, and empirical antibiotics started. Whirlpool baths, soaks, and active range-of-motion exercises are begun the next day.

TENDON SHEATH INFECTIONS

Tendon sheath infections are often the result of puncture wounds or lacerations. This closed-space infection can lead to severe limitation of motion as a result of destruction of the pulley system, adhesions, and liquefaction of tendon itself. Therefore, prompt recognition with immediate drainage is mandatory. Diagnosis is based on history of a wound and Kanavel's four signs: tenderness over the involved tendon sheath; pain on passive extension of the finger; flexed attitude of the finger; and fusiform swelling of the involved digit.[28] The ring, middle, and index fingers are the most commonly involved digits.[39] Coagulase-positive *Staphylococcus aureus* is

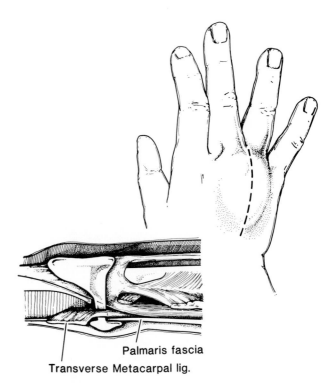

Palmaris fascia
Transverse Metacarpal lig.

Figure 45-3 A web space infection. The hand shows a dorsal swelling and incision. The insert shows the cross-sectional anatomy of a web space infection. Note the dorsal subcutaneous collection of pus communicating with a volar subcutaneous collection to form a dumbbell-shaped abscess. The metacarpophalangeal joint behind the abscess usually does not communicate with the web space infection.

the most common organism, but gram-negative bacteria may also be responsible for up to 20 percent of the cases.[36] Antibiotic therapy alone (after attempting to obtain culture by aspiration) may be curative if employed early in the infective process. However, if no improvement occurs in 24 h, incision and drainage should be performed. Postoperatively closed irrigation of the tendon sheath may be beneficial. Wounds should be left open and closed secondarily except if closed irrigation is used, in which case the wounds are closed primarily (Fig. 45-4). Whirlpool baths, soaks, and active range-of-motion exercises are started approximately 48 h postoperatively unless there has been some damage to the tendon. Possible extension of this infection into the other deep spaces and bursa of the hand should not be forgotten.

DEEP SPACE (THENAR AND MIDPALMAR) INFECTIONS

There are two major deep potential compartments in the hand: the thenar and the midpalmar space (Fig. 45-5). Infec-

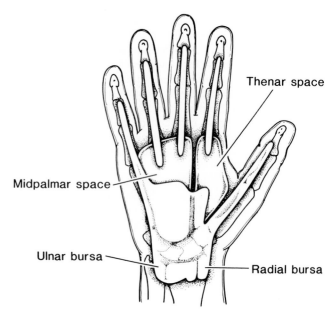

Figure 45-5 Deep spaces, bursae, and digital tendon sheaths of the hand.

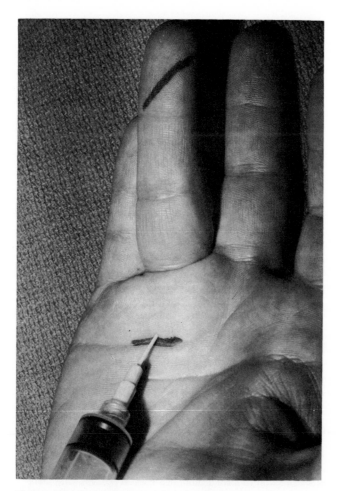

Figure 45-4 Incisions for tendon sheath drainage and closed irrigation.

tion in these spaces may occur through direct puncture wounds or by communications with an expanding abscess, i.e., an infective tenosynovitis. The midpalmar space is bounded dorsally by the third, fourth, and fifth metacarpals and volarly by the flexor tendons. Distally, the vertical septa of the palmar fascia serve as its endpoint and proximally midpalmar space is limited by a fascial layer at the end of the carpal tunnel. Radially and ulnarly the midpalmar and hypothenar septum are its boundaries. With infection of this space, the palm becomes flattened. The dorsum of the hand becomes swollen because the major lymphatics drain to the dorsum, and tenderness is present over the space. There may be fluctuation and erythema volarly over the space, and motion of the flexor tendons produces pain. Systemic signs of infection may also be present.

The treatment is incision and drainage. An incision along the distal palmar flexion crease allows a bloodless field and avoids the contracture of a vertical scar.[28] The abscess cavity is then copiously irrigated and left open with a drain in place. The drain is removed in 48 h and soaks and physical therapy begun. Antibiotics are started after wound cultures have been obtained. Specific antibiotic treatment is guided subsequently by the culture results.

The thenar space lies radial to the midpalmar septum and extends radially to the lateral edge of the adductor pollicis longus muscle. The thenar space is a potential space anterior to the adductor pollicis. Infection of this space leads to swelling volarly in the thenar region and pushes the thumb into abduction. This infection may arise from direct penetration from a puncture wound or from extension of a nearby infection in the midpalmar space, in the radial bursa, or in the flexor tendon sheaths of the thumb or infection finger. This infection is treated with incision and drainage. Possible communication of this abscess with other closed spaces should be The lesion may be approached dorsally and/or volarly. Incisions paralleling the contour of the web space should be avoided in order to prevent web contracture. Treatment protocol is as for midpalmar space infections.

RADIAL AND ULNAR BURSAL INFECTIONS

The radial and ulnar bursae represent fascial compartments that enclose the flexor tendons (Fig. 45-5). The radial bursa is a proximal extension of the flexor pollicis longus tendon sheath which extends through the carpal tunnel into the forearm. The ulnar bursa is a proximal extension of the flexor sheath of the flexor digitorum longus of the little finger. This bursa incorporates the other flexor tendons in the palm and extends to the distal forearm. Infection occurs through direct puncture or through extension of an infected tendon sheath. There is swelling, erythema, and tenderness over the anatomic boundaries of the respective bursa. One must not overlook the possibility of a communication between the two bursae which can result in a "horseshoe" abscess.[9] Extension into Parona's space in the distal forearm is also a possibility.[9] Treatment is by incision and drainage with packing retained for 48 h. Soaks and active range-of-motion exercises then commence with healing by secondary intention. Initially a parenteral antibiotic, usually a cephalosporin, is given parenterally as soon as cultures have been obtained. Subsequently, culture and sensitivity test results guide the choice of specific antibiotic therapy.

NECROTIZING FASCIITIS

Necrotizing fasciitis is a limb- and life-threatening soft tissue infection caused by a variety of aerobic and anaerobic bacteria.[54] The infective process may at first appear to be a benign, low-grade cellulitis, but bacterial enzymes promote rapid infection with concomitant soft tissue necrosis.[46] The infection at first involves the fascia but may spread to the skin, fat, and muscle.

Necrotizing fasciitis often involves substance abusers.[44] Many of these infections are caused by self-injection. Necrotizing fasciitis has several classic signs: skin bullae, crepitus, rapidly advancing cellulitis, skin necrosis, and high fever.[44] The white blood cell count is usually between 10,000 and 20,000.[44] Systemic bacteremia may produce several end-organ failures. Septic shock is commonly associated with upper extremity necrotizing fasciitis.

The cornerstone of therapy is early adequate surgical debridement with complete removal of all necrotic skin, fascia, fat, and muscle. With advancing cellulitis, it is important to debride the skin, fat, and fascia beyond the cellulitis to contain the infection,[44] because viable organisms can be present in the apparently normal tissue at the periphery of the cellulitis.[31] Delay or inadequate debridement leads to an increased potential for loss of limb or life. Antibiotics are an important adjunct to control systemic spread. Penicillin G in

high doses for the anaerobic organisms, and an antibiotic effective against penicillinase-producing *Staphylococcus aureus* as well as an aminoglycoside, should be used initially while awaiting culture results.[44] Careful surgical technique, adequate antibiotic regimens, and general medical support have achieved a 91 percent survival rate in these patients.[44]

TUBERCULOSIS

Treatment of tuberculosis lesions in the upper extremity includes open biopsy, drainage of all abscesses and sinus tracts, splinting, and chemotherapy with a three-drug regimen initially (isoniazid, rifampin, and ethambutol). Chemotherapy should continue for 2 years and/or for 1 year after the lesion has healed.[11] With failure of this regimen, fusion and/or excisional arthroplasty may be an alternative.

Tuberculous tenosynovitis appears mostly in the 20-to 50-year-old age group, affecting males more often than females. They tend to be older than patients with bony lesions.[32] Presenting symptoms are the same as those of other types of tenosynovitis. Early drainage before liquefaction of soft tissue structures occurs and leads to improved results. This combined with splinting, chemotherapy, and physical therapy is the key to treating this infection. Tuberculous dactylitis is dealt with in Chap. 22.

ATYPICAL MYCOBACTERIAL INFECTIONS

Nontuberculous mycobacterial infections rarely occur in the hand although *Mycobacterium kansasii*, *M. avium*, and *M. intracellulare* have all been documented in hand infections.[12,13,20,25] *M. marinum* remains the most common atypical mycobacterium.[19] Given the name *swimming pool granuloma*, *M. marinum* infection occurs as the result of exposure to fish bites or injuries, or contaminated pools or fish tanks. Patients usually have a preexisting wound or receive an inconsequential wound at the time of the inoculum.

There is no pathognomonic physical finding with *M. marinum* infections, although there is a prolonged nonpainful swelling of the finger, palm, wrist, or dorsum of the hand. There are three characteristic types: type 1, self-limited verrucal lesions; type 2, single or multiple subcutaneous granulomas with or without ulceration; and type 3, deep infections involving tenosynovium, bursae, or joints.[49]

The presumptive diagnosis of an *M. marinum* infection must be based on a history of exposure to a typical source, compatible physical examination, skin tests specific for *M. marinum*, and Gram stains of the purulent drainage. A definitive diagnosis rests on positive tissue culture and characteristic histological findings from an open biopsy (noncaseating granulomas). The medium for culture is Löwenstein-Jensen medium at 29 to 32°C. Differential diagnosis includes tuberculosis, gout, rheumatic synovitis, and fungal infection.[22]

There is controversy regarding the treatment for this lesion. Type 1 lesions may be treated with drug therapy alone.

Type 2 and type 3 lesions are most often treated by excisional biopsy and drug therapy started while awaiting culture results that may take as long as 6 weeks. The drug of choice for this infection is minocycline, 100 mg bid orally, continued for 4 to 6 months, although rifampin and ethambutol have also been recommended.[49] Recurrence has been noted and may be due to incomplete excision. However, with reexcision and continued drug therapy, these lesions are ablated. Intralesional steroids have not had a beneficial effect and may worsen the condition.

FUNGAL INFECTIONS

Fungal infections, though not as common as bacterial infections, may also have serious consequences. The diagnosis may be suspected by a typical fungal rash on the hand, but skin scrapings on 10% potassium hydroxide glass slides and fungal cultures on Sabouraud's or dermatophyte test media remain the basis for definitive diagnosis. Complement fixation tests may be helpful in the diagnosis of histoplasmosis and coccidioidomycosis. Skin tests may also prove useful if the patient is not anergic.[50] Fungal infections are found mostly in tropical climates. However, with the advent of iatrogenically produced immunocompromised patients through dialysis, steroids, and antibiotics, fungal infections have become increasingly common in the temperate zones. Antibiotics useful in treating fungal infections include miconazole, nystatin, amphotericin B, and griseofulvin. The dermatomycosis can often be treated solely with topical agents. Surgical drainage with debridement and adequate drug therapy is paramount in treating the deeper infections.

HERPETIC WHITLOW

Herpetic whitlow is a lesion of viral etiology, herpes simplex virus being the offending organism. It presents first as a painful digit with erythema and eventually vesicle formation. It is seen in dental and medical personnel, especially in those caring for patients with oral herpetic lesions. The course is usually self-limiting. The lesions become encrusted and desquamate with resolution in 7 to 21 days. Diagnosis is made from the typical history and physical examination with laboratory documentation. Oral scrapings or aspirated vesicular fluid show multinucleated giant cells. Laboratory evaluation may also show increased serum complement on initial and follow-up visits (3 weeks later), positive viral cultures, and normal or low white blood cell counts with increased lymphocytic and monocytic cells on the differential cell count.[47] The fluid within the vesicle is sterile and nonpurulent. Oral-digital contact is the mode of transmission. Symptomatic treatment is all that is needed in mild cases. In more established cases treatment with acyclovir for the virus and antibiotics for the secondary bacterial infection is warranted. This infection should not be confused with a paronychia or felon, because incising these lesions can lead to secondary infection.

PYOGENIC GRANULOMA

Pyogenic granuloma represents a mass of rapidly enlarging hyperactive granulation tissue at the location of an established chronic infection. It is a small raised area which is often beefy-red and bleeding (Fig. 45-6). Pyogenic granuloma may be mistaken for a cancerous lesion. The diagnosis is usually established by its typical appearance in accord with a history of an infectious process. Simple excision at its base with cauterization with silver nitrate is usually all that is necessary.

GONORRHEA

Although acute gonorrhea is widespread in the United States, chronic gonorrhea has decreased in incidence. Septicemic complications of gonorrhea infections include generalized dermatitis, arthritis, tenosynovitis, endocarditis, and meningitis.[29] The clinical picture commences with a bacteremic phase with fever, typical skin lesions, arthralgias, and tenosynovitis. Resolution of these symptoms occurs within a week, and a purulent arthritis may result. Septic arthritis is the most common complication of disseminated gonococcal infections.[41] Gonorrheal arthritis affects several joints initially, although severe symptoms rarely occur in more than one or two joints. Heat, tenderness, erythema, swelling, and severe pain with motion occur. The wrist and metacarpophalangeal joints are the most commonly affected.[51]

In young, sexually active patients without a history of trauma, there should be a high index of suspicion. Joint aspiration may reveal gram-positive diplococci on smear and culture; however, failure to recover the organism may occur in as many as 75 percent of the cases.[29] When the diagnosis is in doubt, the patient should be treated by incision and drainage along with empiric antibiotics. Observation alone of a closed-space or joint infection invites disaster. Penicillin is the drug of choice for gonorrheal infections, with tetracycline and erythromycin reserved for penicillin-sensitive patients.[51]

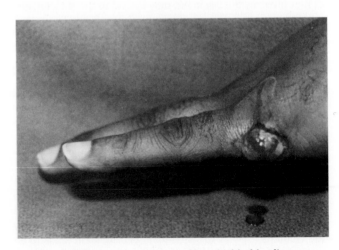

Figure 45-6 Pyogenic granuloma. Note friable bleeding surface.

BITES

Bite wounds are a major concern for the orthopaedic surgeon.[1] Depending on the inoculum, these wounds may result in stiffness, chronic osteomyelitis, necrotizing fasciitis, amputation, or even death. Every year 1 million people are bitten by animals or humans.[14] The majority of bite wounds are caused by dogs (70 percent), cats (10 percent) and humans (15 percent).[6] A far fewer number are caused by venomous creatures (i.e., snakes or spiders), but these can cause severe morbidity and mortality. The treating physician must always remember the catastrophic complications of tetanus and rabies.

Dog bites are the most common bite wound but involve the hand infrequently. They usually do not become infected unless there is significant soft tissue injury or joint involvement. Physical examination reveals puncture wound marks with erythema and cellulitis, and with or without purulent drainage and ascending lymphangitis. Culture often reveals a mixed infection of *Streptococcus*, *Staphylococcus aureus*, and *Pasteurella multocida*. A thorough irrigation and debridement with delayed primary closure is indicated. Penicillin and oxacillin alone can be used for these wounds, but when there is joint involvement, a second- or third-generation cephalosporin may be preferable.[3]

Although cat bites occur less often than human or dog bites, they become infected most frequently (30 to 50 percent).[55] The chief pathogens are *Streptococcus* (alpha and beta), and *P. multocida*. Given the high infection rate, antibiotic treatment seems appropriate after a thorough irrigation and debridement. Superficial wounds respond to oral penicillin, cefaclor, and doxycycline. Highly contaminated wounds require intramuscular penicillin G followed by oral penicillin VK. If *Staphylococcus aureus* is suspected (from the Gram stain), use of a penicillinase-resistant penicillin such as oxacillin is preferred. *Pasteurella multocida* (gram-negative rod) is responsible for 50 percent of infected dog bites and 80 percent of infected cat bites.[42] Within 48 h the wound infected with the organism becomes inflamed and may develop swelling and drainage. One-third of cases develop regional lymphadenopathy, and one-quarter develop low-grade fever.

Human bites also deserve special consideration. Although they account for approximately 15 percent of bite wounds, there is often a delay in diagnosis because these patients do not seek medical care immediately or do not volunteer the fact they were involved in an altercation. Despite this, fistfights probably account for 60 to 80 percent of all human bites.[19] The adult human mouth contains many anaerobes which can cause severe infections. The bites of children are relatively innocuous, probably due to the more aerobic nature of their oral microflora.[55]

Physical examination reveals findings similar to those of other bite wounds. Cultures usually grow an average of three organisms: *Staphylococcus aureus*, alpha and beta *Streptococcus*, and *Eikenella corrodens*. With the fingers extended, the wound may appear superficial and proximal to the joint; however, thorough irrigation and debridement with exploration for possible metacarpophalangeal joint involvement is mandatory (Fig. 45-7). Antibiotics are used for even the most superficial wounds. Penicillin for *E. corrodens* and oxacillin or a

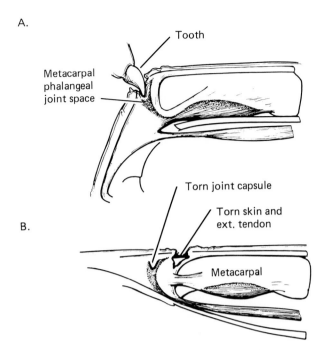

Figure 45-7 Mechanism of fistfight injury. **A.** Tooth piercing skin, extensor tendon, and joint capsule as patient strikes opponent in mouth. **B.** Patient releases fist by extending fingers. Hole in joint capsule now covered by intact tendon. Defect in skin and tendon now moves proximally and does not appear to communicate with joint.

second- or third-generation cephalosporin for *Streptococcus* and *S. aureus* are recommended until culture reports are available.

VENOMOUS BITES

Every year approximately 50 people die as a result of venomous bites. About 90 percent of these fatalities are caused by spiders, snakes, and insects.[23] Factors affecting the prognosis are age, size, and health of the patient; location of the bite; size of the animal or insect; presence of bacteria on animal or skin of the victim; and postbite exercise or exertion (Table 45-1).

TETANUS

Tetanus is caused by the anaerobic spore-forming organism *Clostridium tetani*, a slender gram-negative rod. The clinical manifestations of tetanus are due solely to the soluble exotoxin tetanospasmin, a neurotoxin thought to affect the motor end plates, spinal cord, brain, and sympathetic nervous system. *C. tetani* enters the body through soil and dirt present in wounds. It is introduced in its spore form and in a low-oxygen environment transforms to the toxin-forming vegetative form.

TABLE 45-1 Venomous Bites

Source	Symptoms	Lab findings	Treatment
Snakes Pit viper	*Local symptoms*: Sudden onset of severe burning pain; local swelling, bullae, edema, gangrene *Systemic symptoms*: Fever, N&V,* circulatory collapse, bleeding, miosis, delirium, convulsions	WBC 20–30 k; progressive anemia, thrombocytopenia, hypofibrinogenemia, increased PT and PTT, proteinemia, azotemia	Snakebite: *first aid*: Apply tourniquet to impede lymph flow, not venous return; rest extremity and patient; incision and suction of wound if farther than 15 min from hospital; *hospital care*: Antivenom, tetanus, respiratory support, fasciotomy as needed, surgical debridement near end of first week, antibiotics for gram-negative infections
Coral	*Local symptoms*: Little pain or swelling *Systemic symptoms*: Numbness and weakness in bite area, followed by ataxia, pupillary dilation, pharyngeal paralysis, N&V,* speech slurring, respiratory paralysis, seizures, death in 8–7 h	WBC 20–30 k; progressive anemia, thrombocytopenia, hypofibrinogenemia, increased PT and PTT, proteinemia, azotemia	
Spiders Black widow	Momentary pain, cramping in 15–60 min, boardlike abdomen, N&V,* diaphoresis, labored breathing; increased reflexes and blood pressure, tremor, occasionally death from cardiopulmonary failure	Fever and increased WBC	Put extremity in hot tub; one ampule of Ca gluconate (relieve cramps); cardiopulmonary support as needed
Recluse	Severe local pain in 2–8 h, bullae, erythema, ischemic necrosis resulting in deep ulcer and necrotic base		Local wound care, timely surgical debridement, treat secondary infection, possible use of steroids

*N&V, nausea and vomiting

Clinically the incubation period varies from 3 to 21 days with variation dependent on the distance the toxin must travel before reaching the central nervous system (location of the wound). The severity of the wound is not a determinant; 80 percent of the time the wound size is insignificant. The toxin produces rigidity of muscle groups. Trismus occurs in 50 percent.[52] Initial symptoms may progress to opisthotonos, seizures, cranial nerve palsies, diffuse sweating, and death. Laboratory evaluation is unrewarding: spinal fluid analysis is normal, and white blood cell count is normal or slightly increased. Diagnosis is by history and clinical evaluation. Unfortunately, the death rate is 45 to 50 percent so that proper tetanus prophylaxis as outlined in Table 45-2 is imperative. Patients in their second decade or older have an increased survival rate. A long incubation period also correlates with increased survival. Prophylactic antitoxin, when indicated, has dropped the fatality rate from 53 to 23 percent.[53] The cornerstone of treating established tetanus is appropriate antitoxin, wound care, nursing care, quiet environment, and adequate caloric intake. Usually 3000 to 6000 thousand units of antitoxin is adequate. Adequate wound care includes surgical irrigation and debridement. Penicillin, 1 million units intravenously every 6 h for 10 days, is employed to eradicate the vegetative forms of *C. tetani*. Tetracycline, 2 g/day, is used for penicillin-allergic patients. Muscle relaxants and sedatives may aid the patient as long as respiratory depression is avoided. An attack of clinical tetanus confers no immunity, and a survivor may still require immunization.

RABIES

Inherent to any discussion of bites is the need for rabies prophylaxis and treatment. The principal criterion is the likelihood of rabies in the biting animal.[26] Domestic dogs and cats have a low likelihood of being rabid. The wild animals most prone to rabies in the United States are bats, skunks, foxes,

TABLE 45-2 Tetanus Prophylaxis

Immunization history	Tetanus toxoid, ml	Tetanus immune G, units
Wound less than 24 h old; booster less than 1 year ago with prior full 3-dose immunization	None	None
Wound less than 24 h old; more than 1 year since booster; full previous immunization	0.5	None
Wound less than 24 h old; good likelihood of tetanus; full previous immunization	0.5	250
Wound greater than 24 h old or severe wound*	0.5	500
No history of prior immunization; clean minor wound	0.5	None
No history of prior immunization; severe wound*	0.5	500

*Consider prophylactic penicillin or tetracycline

TABLE 45-3 Rabies Treatment

Animal species	Condition of animal at time of attack	Treatment of exposed person
Dog and cat	Healthy and available for 10 days observation	None, unless animal develops rabies
	Rabid or suspected rabid	RIG* and HDVC**
	Unknown (escaped)	Consult public health officials. If treatment is indicated, give RIG* and HDCV**
Skunk, bat, fox, coyote, raccoon, bobcat, and other carnivores	Regarded as rabid unless proved negative by lab tests	RIG* and HDCV**
Livestock, rodents, and lagomorphs (rabbits and hares)		Consider individually. Local and state public officials should be consulted about the need for rabies prophylaxis. Bites of squirrels, hamsters, guinea pigs, gerbils, chipmunks, rats, mice, other rodents, rabbits, and hares almost never call for antirabies prophylaxis

*Rabies immune globulin.
**Human diploid cell vaccine.
Source: Centers for Disease Control, MMWR, 29:265, 1980. Data used with permission.

and raccoons. Rodents and rabbits are rarely infected with rabies. The human diploid cell vaccine (HDCV) is now the vaccine of choice for postexposure immunization and should always be given along with the rabies immune globulin. In deciding to treat a patient prophylactically, the guidelines from the Immunization Practices Advisory Committee of the Center for Disease Control (Table 45-3) should be followed.

GAS GANGRENE

Gas gangrene (clostridial myonecrosis) in the upper extremity is an infrequent occurrence but one that can lead to significant morbidity and mortality. It is caused by the gram-positive bacillus *Clostridium*, with *C. perfringens* the most common species. It is not true that gas gangrene occurs only with major trauma. It has even occurred following intravenous therapy[24] and after pinhole skin penetration from both-bone fracture of the forearm.[15]

Clostridium grows in tissues with low oxygen tension, the environment often encountered after significant trauma. However, any process that lowers the oxygen tension can result in clostridial infection if contamination with the organism occurs. The toxicity of this infection is due to the production of exotoxins. *Clostridium* produces nine exotoxins, of which the alpha toxin is the most lethal.[24] Intense edema follows infection with little or no inflammatory phase, further reducing the oxygen tension. The infection rapidly progresses and toxemia results.

Early diagnosis is the key to successful treatment. The earliest symptom is pain in the affected area, followed by chills, tachycardia, confusion, and toxemia. In the early stages the skin is cool and edematous. Later the wound develops a brownish discoloration with brown, foul-smelling drainage.[15] It is at this late stage that crepitance is present. The x-ray views will not reveal gas consistently in the early stages, and gas is not pathognomonic for gas gangrene.[40] Nonetheless, x-ray studies are mandatory and may aid in determining the extent of the infectious process. Gram stain of the drainage reveals a gram-positive bacillus, and treatment must begin before definitive cultures are available.

It cannot be emphasized enough that early diagnosis and treatment of this infection are paramount. Penicillin in dosages of 10 to 24 million units/day in combination with adequate surgical debridement (which may include amputation), and hyperbaric oxygen at 3 atm for 60- to 90-min intervals three times a day, provide optimal care. Tetracycline in dosages of 2 to 4 g/day may be used as an alternative in cases of penicillin allergy. Antitoxin is of questionable value.[45] Hyperbaric oxygen counteracts the hypoxic environment, thereby allowing peroxides to develop in the organism, inactivating it. Another benefit of hyperbaric oxygen is the inhibition of toxin production. With these regimens, mortality of this infection has decreased to 22 percent.[24]

REFERENCES

1. Aghababin, R.V., and Conte, J.E., Jr. Mammalian bite. Ann Emerg Med 9(2):79–83, 1980.
2. *American Medical Association—Drug Evaluations*, 5th ed. Chicago, American Medical Association, 1984.
3. Barrack, R.L., Mogabgab, W.J., Edmunds, J.O., and Skinner, H.B. Management of bite wounds. Orthop Rev 12(8):83–88, August 1983.
4. Brown, H. Fungus infections of the hand, in Flynn, J.E. (ed): *Hand Surgery*, 3d ed., chap. 14.7. Baltimore, Williams & Wilkins, 1981, pp 739–756.
5. Buchman, M.T., and Weis, E.P., Jr. Tetanus complicating an open trimalleolar fracture. J Bone Joint Surg 66A:139–141, January 1984.
6. Callahan, M. Dog bite wounds. JAMA 244(2):2327–2328, 1980.
7. Center for Disease Control. Rabies prevention. MMWR 29:265–280, 1080.
8. Citron, D.M., and Goldstein, E.J. Role of anaerobic bacteria in bite wound infections. Rev Infect Dis 6(suppl 1):March-April 1985.
9. Lampe, E.W. Surgical anatomy of the hand. Clin Symp 21(3):40.
10. Crandon, J.H. Lesser infections of the hand, in Flynn, J.E. (ed): *Hand Surgery*, 3d ed., chap 14.2. Baltimore, Williams & Wilkins, 1981, pp 680–687.
11. Daberies, R. Orthopaedic grand rounds. Orthopaedics 5(2):217–219, February 1982.
12. DeChairo, D.C., Kittredge, D., Meyers, A., and Corrales, J. Septic arthritis due to *Mycobacterium triviale*. Ann Rev Resp Dis 103:1224–1226, 1973.
13. Dixon, J. Non-tuberculous mycobacterial infections of the tendon sheaths in the hand. J Bone Joint Surg 23B(4):542–544, 1981.
14. Edlich, R.F., Spengler, and Rodeheaver, G.T. Bites. Compr Ther 9(12):41–47, 1983.
15. Fee, N.F., Dobranski, A., and Bisla, R.A. Gas gangrene complicating open forearm fractures. J Bone Joint Surg 59A(1):135–138, January 1977.
16. Finegold, S.M., and Murray, P.M. Anaerobes in burn wound infections. Rev Infect Dis 6(suppl 1) March-April 1985.
17. Fitzgerald, R.H., Jr., Cooney, W.P., III, Washington, J.A., II, VanScoy, R.E., Linscheid, R.L., and Dobyns, J.H. Bacterial colonization of mutilating hand injuries and its treatment. J Hand Surg 2:85–89, 1977.
18. Grossman, J.A.I., Adams, J.P., and Kunec, J. Prophylactic antibiotics in simple hand lacerations. JAMA 245:1055–1056, 1981.
19. Guba, A.M., Jr., Mulliken, J.B., and Hoopes, J.E. The selection of antibiotics for human bites of the hand. Plast Reconstr Surg 56(5):538–541, 1975.
20. Gunther, S.F., Elliot, R.C., and Brand, J.P. Experience with atypical mycobacterium infections in the deep structures of the hand. J Hand Surg 2:90–96, 1977.
21. Gunther, S.F. Nontuberculous mycobacterial infections of the hand, in Flynn, J.E. (ed): *Hand Surgery*, 3d ed., chap 14.1. Baltimore, Williams & Wilkins, 1981, pp 733–734.
22. Gunther, S.F., in Flynn, J.E. (ed): *Hand Surgery*, 3d ed., chap 14.1. Baltimore, Williams & Wilkins, 1981, pp 735–739.
23. *Harrison's Principles of Internal Medicine*, Petersdorf, R.G. et al (eds), 10th ed, sec 14. New York, McGraw-Hill, 1983, pp 1239–1248.
24. Hart, G.B., Lamb, R.C., and Strauss, M.B. Gas gangrene, a collective review. J Trauma 23(11):991–995, 1983.
25. Irwin, R.S., and Parker, M.D. *Mycobacterium kansasii* tendonitis and fascitis. J Bone Joint Surg 57A(4):557–559, 1975.
26. Jaffe, A.C. Animal bites. Pediatr Clin North Am 30(3):405–413, April 1983.
27. Kanavel, A.B. *Infections of the Hand*, 7th ed., chap 1. Philadelphia, Lea & Febiger, 1943.
28. Kanavel, A.B. *Infections of the Hand*, 7th ed. Philadelphia, Lea & Febiger, 1943, p 395.
29. Kraus, S.J. Complications of gonococcal infections. Med Clin North Am 56:1115–1125, 1972.
30. Kunin, C.M., and Oman, S.J. Needle aspiration in the diagnosis of soft tissue infections. Arch Intern Med 135:959–961, July 1975.
31. Ledingham, I., and Tehrani, M. Diagnosis/clinical course and treatment of acute dermal gangrene. Br J Surg 62:364–372, 1975.

32. Leffert, R.D., and Smith, R.J., Tuberculosis of the hand, in Flynn, J.E. (ed): *Hand Surgery*, 3d ed., chap 14.5. Baltimore, Williams & Wilkins, 1981, pp 719–730.

33. Lindberg, R.B., McManus, W.F., and Pruitt, B.A., Jr., in Flynn, J.E. (ed): *Hand Surgery*, 3d ed., chap 14.1. Baltimore, Williams & Wilkins, 1981, pp 636–639.

34. Lindberg, R.B., McManus, W.F., and Pruitt, B.A., Jr., in Flynn, J.E. (ed): *Hand Surgery*, 3d ed., chap 14.1. Baltimore, Williams & Wilkins, 1981, pp 636–676.

35. Lindberg, R.B., McManus, W.F., and Pruitt, B.A., Jr., in Flynn, J.E. (ed): *Hand Surgery*, 3d ed., chap 14.1. Baltimore, Williams & Wilkins, 1981, p 668.

36. Nevaiser, R.J. Closed tendon sheath irrigation for pyogenic flexor tenosynovitis. J Hand Surg 3:462–466, 1978.

37. Nevaiser, R.J., in Green, D.P. (ed): *Operative Hand Surgery*, chap 20. New York, Churchill Livingstone, 1982, p 771.

38. Nevaiser, R.J., in Green, D.P. (ed): *Operative Hand Surgery*, chap 20. New York, Churchill Livingstone, 1982, p 772.

39. Nevaiser, R.J., in Green, D.P. (ed): *Operative Hand Surgery*, Chap 20. New York, Churchill Livingstone, 1982, p 783.

40. Nichols, R.L., and Smith, J.W. Gas in the wound: What does it mean? Surg Clin North Am 55:1289–1296, 1975.

41. Ogiela, D.M., and Peimer, C.A. Acute gonococcal flexor tenosynovitis—Case report and literature review. J Hand Surg 6(5): September 1981, pp 470–472.

42. Peeples, E., et al: Wounds of the hand contaminated by human or animal saliva. J Trauma 20(5):383–389, 1980.

43. Samuel, E.P. Transillumination of whitlows of terminal phalanx. Lancet 1:763–765, 1950.

44. Schecter, W., Meyer, A., Schecter, G., Jiuliano, A., Newmeyer, W., and Kilgore, E. Necrotizing fasciitis of the upper extremity. J Hand Surg 7(1):15–20, January 1982.

45. Schurman, D.J., Uncommon infections in orthopaedic surgery in Evarts, C.M. (ed): *Surgery of the Musculoskeletal System*, vol 4, chap 10:223–10.242. New York, Churchill Livingstone, 1983.

46. Schwab, J.H. Biological properties of streptococcal cell particles, 1: Determination of the chronic nodular lesion of connective tissues. J Bacteriol 90:1405–1411, 1965.

47. Sehayik, R.J., and Bassett, F.H. Herpes simplex infections involved in the hand. Clin Orthop 166:138–140, June 1982.

48. The Medical Letter (issue 658) 26:36–38, March 30, 1984.

49. Wagner, R.F., Tawil, A.B., Colletta, A.J., Hurst, L.C., and Yecies, L.D. *Mycobacterium marinum* tenosynovitis in a Long Island fisherman. NY State J Med 81(7):1091–1094, June 1981.

50. *Washington Manual of Medical Therapeutics*, 23d ed., chap 10: Antibiotics and Infectious Disease, p 218.

51. Wehrbein, H.L. Gonococcus arthritis, a study of 610 cases. Surg Gynecol Obstet 49:105, 1929.

52. Weinstein, L. Current concepts, Tetanus. N Engl J Med 289:1293–1296, 1973.

53. Weinstein, L., in Flynn, J.E. (ed): *Hand Surgery*, 3d ed., chap 14.8. Baltimore, Williams & Wilkins, 1981, pp 756–764.

54. Wilson, B. Necrotizing fasciitis. Am Surg 18:416–431, 1952.

55. Winkler, W.G. Human deaths induced by dog bites in the United States fron 1974–1975. Public Health Department 92:425–429, 1977.

CHAPTER 46

Neoplasms Affecting the Upper Extremity

Martin M. Malawer and Harold M. Dick

SECTION A

Tumors of the Shoulder Girdle, Arm, and Forearm

Martin M. Malawer

The upper extremity is affected by bony and soft tissue neoplasms one-third as frequently as the lower extremity.[23] The tissues of the shoulder girdle are more often involved than the more distal arm or the forearm. The shoulder girdle is a common site for primary bony neoplasms. The proximal humerus is the third most common site for osteosarcomas, outranked only by the knee region.[4,5] Cartilage tumors, either benign or malignant, are more common in the shoulder girdle than in the lower extremity. In addition, the proximal humerus is the most common site for unicameral bone cysts (UBCs) and chondroblastomas.[12,22] Soft tissue tumors, though less common in the upper extremity than in the lower extremity, tend to favor the shoulder girdle. All soft tissue sarcomas may involve the periscapular or proximal humeral musculature, though lipomas and liposarcomas are the most common.[23]

In general, age is an important determinant of the type of tumor found. Ewing's sarcoma and osteosarcoma, the most common malignant bone tumors of the humerus, occur during adolescence; chondrosarcoma, in contrast, occurs during the third to seventh decades.[20] Characteristically UBCs and chondroblastomas occur prior to skeletal maturity. Metastatic tumors rarely occur below the age of 40 years. Although all carcinomas may involve the shoulder girdle, hypernephroma (renal cell carcinoma) has a unique propensity to involve the proximal humerus; conversely, metastatic lung carcinoma may involve bones distal to the elbow and wrist.

In this chapter, the specific anatomic site and its influence upon the clinical presentation and surgical management of both benign and malignant bone and soft tissue tumors are presented in detail. The surgical staging, indications, and management technique are emphasized.

SCAPULA AND PERISCAPULAR AREA
Clinical Characteristics

Tumors of the scapula present with pain, a mass, or both. They may become quite large before they are brought to the physician's attention. The most common malignant tumor of childhood is Ewing's sarcoma. During adulthood other primary round cell tumors may involve the scapula. Metastatic disease is most common over the age of 40 years. The most common benign lesions are solitary or multiple osteochondromas. If located on the inferior angle or against the chest wall, osteochondromas may present as a snapping scapula. Soft tissue sarcomas may involve either the suprascapular or the infraspinous musculature. Direct involvement of the underlying bone is infrequent. Radiation sarcomas of the scapula may develop secondary to radiotherapy for breast carcinoma; however, they are quite rare. Secondary chondrosarcomas may arise from an underlying osteochondroma. They are a common malignancy in the young adult.

Unique Considerations

Tumors arising within the body of the scapula are surrounded by a cuff of soft tissue in all dimensions during the early stages of development. As sarcomas enlarge they often produce a large axillary component that is not visible on plain radiographs. Lesions arising from the humeral neck or glenoid often involve the pericapsular tissue and/or the joint itself. This is especially true of malignant cartilage tumors, which may extend along all muscle tissues to the scapula. Important anatomic areas to evaluate for extension are the chest wall and the proximal humeral or pericapsular tissue (including the rotator cuff). The base of the axillary nodes also should be carefully examined.

Staging

Staging studies are similar to those used for evaluating tumors of the proximal humerus. Computed tomography (CT) is the most valuable means of determining the size and extent of local disease. It is especially useful in determining chest wall involvement. Arteriography is important in determining vascular involvement. Displacement is indicative of anterior (i.e., axillary) extension of tumor. Bone scan, although less helpful, may indicate rib involvement.

Biopsy

The biopsy site is a crucial factor in determining the final operative procedure for aggressive and malignant lesions of the scapula. Inadvertent contamination of the neurovascular structures or the chest wall must be avoided. In general, a posterior needle biopsy is recommended for tumors arising within the body of the scapula. If the lesion involves the scapula neck, a posterior approach directly through the deltoid and teres minor should be used. An anterior approach to the scapula neck should be avoided. If an open biopsy is required, it should be in line with the definitive incision. Most operative approaches (see below) involve an incision along the axillary border of the scapula. A small medial incision is recommended.

SURGICAL MANAGEMENT OF TUMORS OF THE SCAPULA

Malignant spindle cell sarcomas have traditionally been treated by forequarter amputation. In general, radical scapulectomy is a poor operation for stage IIB tumors because of extensive soft tissue extension. Scapulectomy with removal of adjacent normal muscle cuff (wide excision)(type IIIB; see Fig. 46-4) provides a curative margin for either stage IA or stage IB lesions as well as for aggressive lesions such as giant cell tumors and aneurysmal bone cysts. The Tikhoff-Linberg resection is an excellent operation for bony sarcomas of the scapula.[8,13,16] If the staging criteria are met, local control is equal to that of a forequarter amputation. Benign tumors are treated by simple excision or curettage.

Osteochondroma

Osteochondromas in children should be removed by simple excision. Many secondary chondrosarcomas develop from osteochondromas in this region. Care must be taken to avoid injuring the accessory nerve while removing a lesion arising from the upper border near the attachment of the levator scapulae. Osteochondromas from the inferior portion of the scapula may grow quite large and require a partial scapulectomy; this is often seen in multiple hereditary osteochondromas (Fig. 46-1). There is no functional loss if the osteotomy is done below the scapular spine. Soft tissue reconstruction is performed by reattaching the rhomboids to the teres major and trapezius. Active motion is begun within a few days. A sling is required for 5 to 7 days.

Chondrosarcoma

Benign osteochondromas may give rise to chondrosarcomas (Fig. 46-2);[10] thus, any large cartilaginous lesion of the scapula in an adult must be approached with a high index of suspicion. These lesions tend to be low-grade, stage IB.[24] Extreme caution must be taken in biopsy of a cartilaginous tumor; cartilage can easily be implanted within the soft tissues. Cartilage tumors approaching the glenohumeral joint may directly involve the joint space and readily implant on the articular cartilage. In such cases, an extraarticular resection is generally recommended. A Tikhoff-Linberg resection usually is curative.

Osteosarcoma

Osteosarcoma of the scapula is rare. Curative removal by Tikhoff-Linberg resection or forequarter amputation is required. The limiting factor in performing a limb-sparing procedure is the size of the extraosseous component. Neurovascular involvement requires a forequarter amputation. Chest wall involvement must be evaluated before surgery; if it is present, partial chest wall resection is required en bloc with ablation of the primary tumor.

Giant Cell Tumor or Aneurysmal Bone Cyst

Giant cell tumors and aneurysmal bone cysts often cause marked ballooning and destruction of the scapula. Small lesions may be treated by curettage, cyrosurgery, or both. If the neck of the scapula is not involved, a partial scapulectomy can be performed with minimal loss of function. Large lesions require a total scapulectomy. Reconstruction is accomplished by suspending the scapula (see below) from the clavicle by both a static and a dynamic reconstruction.

Ewing's Sarcoma

Ewing's sarcoma arising in the scapula is treated by radiation therapy in conjunction with chemotherapy. Functional results are excellent. Recently, partial scapulectomy has been recommended, on the theory that the scapula is an expendable

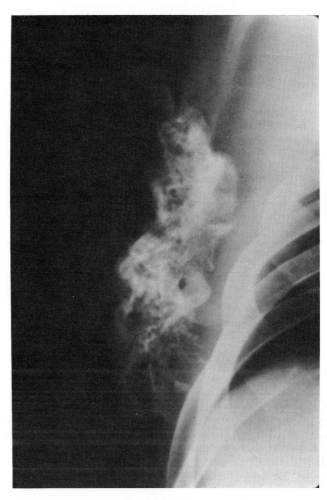

Figure 46-2 Secondary chondrosarcoma. A sessile osteochondroma of the scapula with malignant degeneration in a patient with multiple osteochondromatosis. A partial scapulectomy was performed. Secondary chondrosarcomas tend to be low-grade. (*From Malawer, M.M., Abelson, H.T., and Suit, H.D., in DeVita, Hellman, S., and Rosenberg, S.A., eds: Cancer, Principles and Practice of Oncology, 2nd ed. Philadelphia, Lippincott, 1985. Reproduced with permission.*)

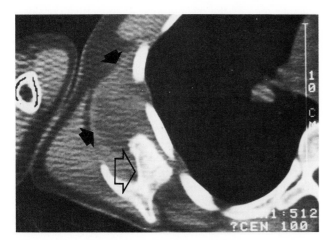

Figure 46-1 Osteochondroma of the scapula. CT of a large osteochondroma (*open arrow*) of the undersurface of the scapula adjacent to the chest wall. There is an associated soft tissue mass (*solid arrows*) suggesting malignant degeneration.

bone. However, total scapulectomy removes shoulder motion and so the scapula in that case cannot be considered an expendable bone. Scapulectomy can only be recommended if it effects a difference in local control of the tumor and thus has an impact on overall survival. This has not yet been demonstrated.

Periscapular Soft Tissue Sarcomas

Tissue sarcomas arising in the periscapular musculature usually can be treated satisfactorily by en bloc removal of the adjacent soft tissue and radiotherapy. Occasionally a soft tissue sarcoma arising from the deeper structures encases the scapula or extends directly into the bone. In these rare situations, scapulectomy is required. Appropriate staging studies indicate the best procedure. If the tumor is distal to the scap-

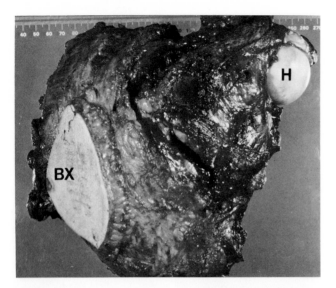

Figure 46-3 Posterior aspect of a gross specimen of a Tikhoff-Linberg resection. All muscles arising and attaching to the scapula are resected en bloc with the entire scapula, glenohumeral joint, and a portion of the distal clavicle. Note the humeral head H and the old biopsy site BX. The glenohumeral joint has been opened for demonstration purposes.

ular spine, a partial or total scapulectomy may be adequate. Involvement of the suprascapular musculature and/or rotators requires a Tikhoff-Linberg resection.

SURGICAL MANAGEMENT OF SHOULDER GIRDLE TUMORS

Tikhoff-Linberg Resection

The Tikhoff-Linberg resection is a limb-sparing procedure for sarcomas arising around the shoulder girdle.[9,13,16] The resection consists of en bloc removal of the scapula, clavicle, and proximal humerus with preservation of the arm (Fig. 46-3). Indications for the procedure are low- and high-grade sarcomas of the scapula and peri- and suprascapular soft tissue sarcomas. Conversely, bony sarcomas of the proximal humerus require resection of a large portion of the humerus with preservation of a portion of the scapula. This procedure has been termed a *modified Tikhoff-Linberg resection* and is discussed in detail in the following section.[13,16] A surgical classification of the shoulder girdle resections has recently been established (Fig. 46-4A).

Absolute contraindication to the Tikhoff-Linberg procedure is tumor involvement with the neurovascular bundle and/or chest wall; both types of involvement require a forequarter amputation. Relative contraindications include pathologic fracture, poorly planned biopsy with widespread tumor contamination, and lymph node involvement. Careful preoperative evaluation is required. CT is useful to determine possible chest wall involvement. Angiography is crucial to determine axillary vessel involvement. The interval between the tumor and vessels must be carefully evaluated. Venography

may be useful in evaluating possible intramural tumor thrombosis occasionally seen with tumors around the shoulder girdle. Bone scan is useful to determine bone and rib involvement.

Large skin flaps are required. The axillary vessels are first explored. If this interval is clear, resection then proceeds. One must be prepared to convert this limb-sparing attempt to a forequarter amputation if tumor is encountered. The most medial margin, the paraspinal muscles, and the base of the neck should be explored early if there is a question of involvement. These anatomic areas are poorly evaluated by all preoperative studies. It is important to realize that a forequarter amputation will not improve upon this margin. Resection includes all the muscles arising from the scapula and inserting on the proximal humerus, and an extraarticular resection of the glenohumeral joint. Occasionally the deltoid and the axillary nerve can be preserved. When possible, the deltoid muscle provides for a nice soft tissue reconstruction of the defect. Following resection, the reconstruction consists of suspension of the proximal humerus from the remaining clavicle by both Dacron tape and muscle transfers. Stabilization of the reconstructed "shoulder" is necessary to provide a fulcrum for elbow flexion. The long and the short head of the biceps and coracobrachialis are sutured through drill holes to the remaining clavicle. The pectoralis muscle is rotated to cover the defect and to give additional support. A similar maneuver is used following total scapulectomy.

In general, functional results are the same following a Tikhoff-Linberg resection and total scapulectomy. No active abduction is possible. Patients undergoing a Tikhoff-Linberg resection retain hand function and good elbow function. Appearance is improved by the use of a molded shoulder pad. The shoulder should be stable, and no external orthosis is required (Fig. 46-4B).

Total Scapulectomy

Total scapulectomy is indicated primarily for stage I or II tumors of the body of the scapula that do not involve the suprascapular area or the glenoid joint. Preoperative considerations are similar to those for a Tikhoff-Linberg resection. Both the neurovascular structures and the chest wall must be free of disease. If the tumor extends anteriorly and/or laterally and involves the rotator cuff or the glenoid, this procedure is not recommended. The skin flaps are similar to those obtained from the posterior limb during a Tikhoff-Linberg resection. All muscles are transected away from the bone, starting at the lowest point inferiorly. The neurovascular structures are approached from the back as the scapula is retracted away from the chest cephalad. Care must be taken to avoid injury to the musculocutaneous and axillary nerves near the coracoid and around the subscapularis muscle. One must be prepared to convert this approach to a formal Tikhoff-Linberg resection if the anterior or medial margins are questionable. Soft tissue reconstruction is mandatory to provide stability and to avoid a flail extremity. The author recommends a dual-suspension technique, utilizing Dacron tape from the clavicle for static support and reattaching the biceps and triceps through drill holes. Reattaching the deltoid to the pectoralis major and tra-

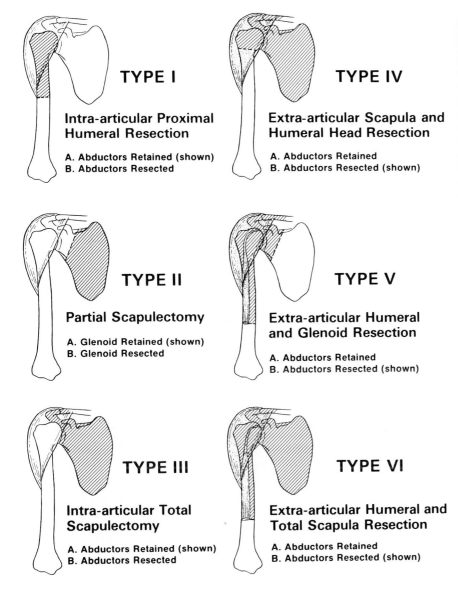

TYPE I

Intra-articular Proximal Humeral Resection

A. Abductors Retained (shown)
B. Abductors Resected

TYPE II

Partial Scapulectomy

A. Glenoid Retained (shown)
B. Glenoid Resected

TYPE III

Intra-articular Total Scapulectomy

A. Abductors Retained (shown)
B. Abductors Resected

TYPE IV

Extra-articular Scapula and Humeral Head Resection

A. Abductors Retained
B. Abductors Resected (shown)

TYPE V

Extra-articular Humeral and Glenoid Resection

A. Abductors Retained
B. Abductors Resected (shown)

TYPE VI

Extra-articular Humeral and Total Scapula Resection

A. Abductors Retained
B. Abductors Resected (shown)

Figure 46-4 A. Proposed classification of shoulder girdle resections for bone and soft tissue tumors. Types I to III are usually performed for low grade tumors, whereas types IV to VI are for high grade tumors. A and B relate to the status of the abductor mechanism: A = intact, B = resected. Types I to III are intraarticular resections and provide a marginal excision. Types IV to VI are extraarticular and accomplish a wide excision. The Tikhoff-Linberg resection is type IVB. (*Presented at the 4th International Symposium on Limb Salvage in Musculoskeletal Oncology, Kyoto, 1987.*)

pezius offers additional support. In general, the functional results are similar to those achieved by the standard Tikhoff-Linberg resection. The author has no experience with total scapula prosthesis as a mode of reconstruction.

Partial Scapulectomy

Removal of the scapula below the scapular spine leaves a functional shoulder joint. This procedure is indicated for low-grade lesions involving only the body of the scapula. A cuff of infraspinatus, subscapularis, and serratus anterior muscle usually can be preserved. Reconstruction consists of suturing these together to close the dead space and to reconstitute the points of origin and insertion of these muscles. Small tumors involving only the glenoid may be resected with preservation of the medial scapula. Reconstruction following glenoid resection is best accomplished by a primary arthrodesis of the

humerus to the remaining scapula. Functional results after partial scapulectomy are superior to those that follow total scapulectomy (Fig. 46-5).

TUMORS OF THE PROXIMAL HUMERUS
Clinical Characteristics

The proximal humerus is the second most common site for primary bony sarcomas.[4] In the adolescent such tumors are usually osteochondromas; in the adult they are primary and secondary chondrosarcomas.[10,11] The proximal humerus is the most frequent site for UBCs and chondroblastomas, two common benign bony lesions of childhood.[12,15,22] Bony metastases are common in the adult, and they may be confused with a primary sarcoma. Pain is the presenting symptom for most bony lesions. Pathologic fracture is rare except for the

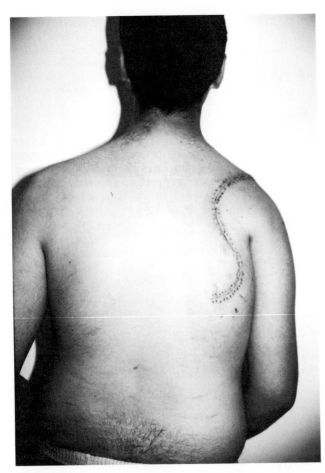

Figure 46-4 *(Continued)* **B.** Clinical appearance following a classical Tikhoff-Linberg resection. The entire scapula and an extraarticular resection of the proximal glenohumeral joint (type IV resection) was performed for a stage IIB osteosarcoma of the scapula. The shoulder remains stable following reconstruction with normal elbow and hand function.

UBCs. Hypernephromas may metastasize to the proximal humerus and may simulate a sarcoma. If the plain radiograph suggests a malignant lesion, staging studies should be performed prior to biopsy.

Unique Considerations

Tumors arising within the proximal humerus cause expansion of the head and greater tuberosity. The thin metaphyseal bone and the large metaphyseal vessels permit early extraosseous extension. Malignant tumors often present with large soft tissue components underneath the deltoid medially under the subscapularis and coracobrachialis muscles. Pericapsular and rotator cuff involvement occur early and must be evaluated. Figure 46-6 illustrates the various mechanisms of tumor spread from proximal humeral sarcomas. Careful physical examination of the axilla may demonstrate an unsuspected mass. The posterior deltoid and triceps area is another "quiet" area in which large extraosseous compo-

nents can hide. Large sarcomas may directly involve the chest wall. Neurological symptoms from brachial plexus displacement are rare.

Staging

Staging studies accurately predict resectability of lesions of the proximal humerus. CT is the most useful means of demonstrating extraosseous tumor extension and its relation to the underlying rib cage. Angiography can determine the relation of the brachial artery to the tumor and, by inference, of the major nerves to the tumor. Two views are required to determine if there is a clear interval between the lesion and the vessels. Angiography is the single most useful study in this region (Fig. 46-7). Preoperative embolization is not usually feasible for proximal humeral lesions because of the high risk of inadvertent distal embolization. Bone scintigraphy determines the intraosseous extent of tumor. Occasionally, a transauricular lesion is noted within the glenoid. Joint involvement is difficult to determine. Arthrography and ar-

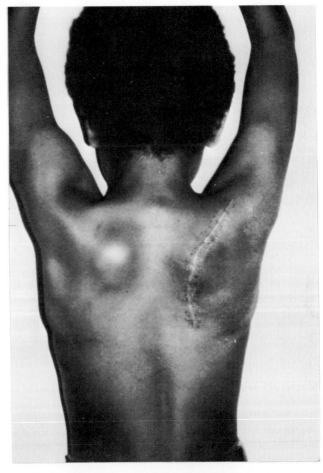

Figure 46-5 Partial scapula (infraspinal) resection. There is a full range of motion following partial scapula resection if the glenohumeral joint is preserved (by contrast, no active abduction follows total scapular Tikhoff-Linberg resection).

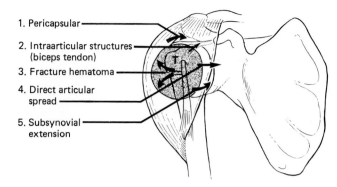

1. Pericapsular
2. Intraarticular structures (biceps tendon)
3. Fracture hematoma
4. Direct articular spread
5. Subsynovial extension

Figure 46-6 Mechanisms of tumor spread of proximal humeral tumors. There are five basic mechanisms. In general, articular involvement by tumor of the shoulder joint is more common than that of the knee joint.

the time of diagnosis. Curettage and bone graft were the treatments of choice until the 1970s. Local recurrence following curettage, with or without bone graft, ranged between 35 and 70 percent. In general, bone graft does not decrease the local recurrence rate. The belief that UBCs will disappear after fracture is misleading and only leads to unnecessary delays in treatment. Less than 1 percent of UBCs cure spontaneously following a fracture. Surgery is not indicated in the initial management of a UBC. Percutaneous high-pressure Renografin injection and intralesional methylprednisolone lead to clinical healing in over 90 percent of these patients (Fig. 46-8*A* and *B*). Biopsy is recommended only if diagnosis is uncertain. Reossification usually begins within 6 to 8 weeks (Fig. 46-8*C*). A second aspiration and injection are required in about 20 percent of patients.

throscopy should be avoided because of the possibility of tumor contamination.

Biopsy

The standard deltopectoral interval should not be utilized for tumors of the proximal humerus. This approach contaminates the subscapularis and pectoralis muscles and thereby potentially involves the neurovascular structures by extension along the deltopectoral and subscapularis fascia. All lesions of the proximal humerus are accessible to a well-placed Craig needle biopsy under fluoroscopic control through the anterior or the mid section of the deltoid. A small incisional biopsy can be performed through the same approach is necessary. Care should be taken not to involve the joint or the rotator cuff mechanism. It is important to remember the definitive incision for resection.

SURGICAL MANAGEMENT OF TUMORS OF THE PROXIMAL HUMERUS

Benign tumors of the proximal humerus are generally treated by curettage or excision. Low-grade (stage I) sarcomas have traditionally been treated by en bloc resection, while high-grade (stage II) sarcomas are treated by forequarter amputation. A modification of the Tikhoff-Linberg procedure (interscapulothoracic resection) has been utilized in select patients in order to accomplish a limb-sparing procedure. Shoulder joint disarticulation is a poor operative choice at this level. Cryosurgery has been successfully utilized for aggressive or recurrent giant cell tumor or chondroblastoma.

Unicameral Bone Cysts

The proximal humerus is the most common site of UBCs (Fig. 46-8). These lesions usually are asymptomatic until a fracture occurs. Two-thirds are active adjacent to the growth plate at

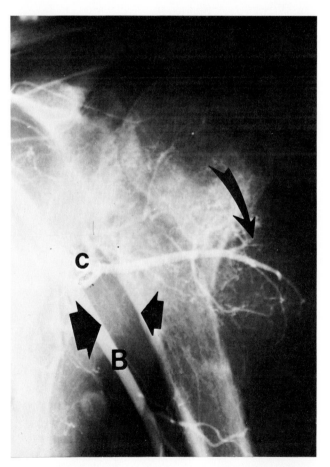

Figure 46-7 Angiography is the most useful staging study for determination of resectability of tumors of the proximal humerus. It demonstrates a lateral soft tissue component (*curved arrow*) with no evidence of tumor medially. If the interval (*solid arrows*) between the brachial artery *B* and the humerus is clear, resection is usually feasible. This patient underwent an extended Tikhoff-Linberg resection (see text for classification).

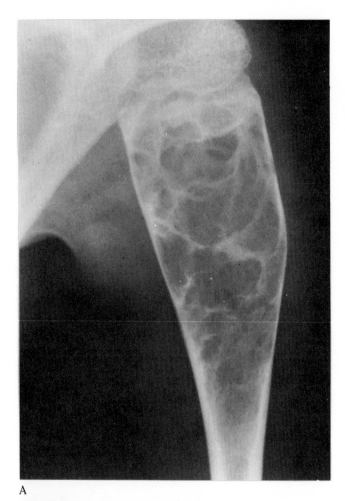

A

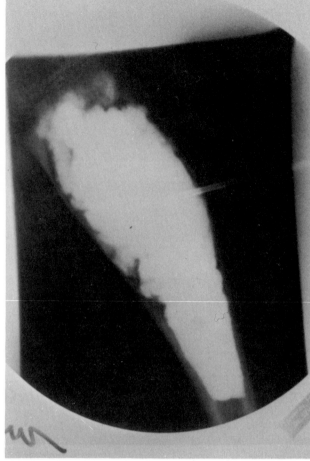

B

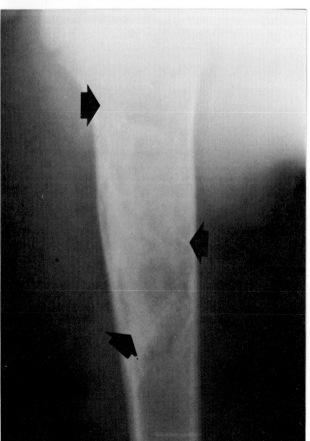

C

Figure 46-8 Unicameral bone cyst of the proximal humerus.
A. Plain radiograph showing a typical UBC with some expansion of the metaphysis and thinning of the cortices. **B.** The patient underwent aspiration, high-pressure Renografin injection, and intralesional methylprednisolone injection under fluoroscopic control. **C.** Ten months following percutaneous treatment, there is complete ossification of the defect (*solid arrows*). Aspiration and injection have replaced curettage as the main treatment of UBCs within the past decade.

Chondroblastoma (Codman's Tumor)

The proximal humerus is the most common site for this chondroblastoma.[7] Epiphyseal location is pathognomonic. Chondroblastomas lesions usually occur before skeletal maturity. Secondary aneurysmal bone cyst formation may confuse the diagnosis. Simple curettage has a recurrence rate of 35 to 50 percent. Cryosurgery is a reliable method of preventing local recurrence. Recurrent chondroblastoma may require a simple excision of the proximal humerus. Arthrodesis is recommended for the young patient.

Chondrosarcoma

The proximal humerus is a common site for central and peripheral chondrosarcomas. The peripheral lesions tend to be large but low-grade, whereas the central lesions tend to be of higher grade. Stage I tumors of the proximal humerus can be treated by wide excision with minimal functional deficit. High-grade sarcomas require a forequarter amputation or a

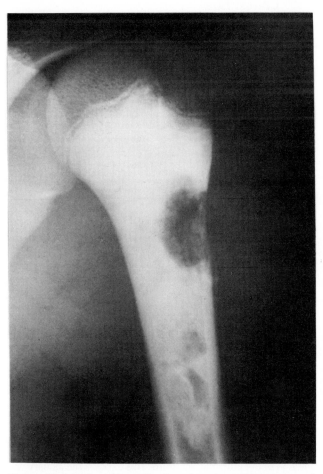

Figure 46-9 Plain radiograph of a sclerosing osteosarcoma of the proximal humerus. (*From Malawer, M.M., Abelson, H.T., and Suit, H.D., in DeVita, V.T., Hellman S., and Rosenberg, S.A; eds: Cancer, Principles and Practice of Oncology, 2nd ed. Philadelphia, Lippincott, 1985. Reproduced with permission.*)

modified Tikhoff-Linberg resection if the criteria are met. Intraarticular and synovial involvement seem to be more common with high-grade cartilaginous lesions in the proximal humerus location than with such lesions in other sites. Care must be taken not to contaminate the anterior structures when performing a biopsy. Reconstruction following a marginal resection for a low-grade lesion can be accomplished by prosthesis, allograft, or dual fibula autograft. A primary arthrodesis or an attempt at preserving a functional joint is possible in certain situations. If the rotator cuff and/or deltoid are removed, a primary arthrodesis usually is recommended. Following resection of a high-grade lesion (stage IIB), the aim is a stable shoulder with minimal motion in order to preserve function in the elbow and hand.

Osteosarcoma

The proximal humerus is the third most common site for osteosarcoma, following the distal femur and the proximal tibia (Fig. 46-9).[2,5] Osteosarcomas in the proximal humerus tend to have a poorer prognosis than those around the knee. Plain radiographs often suggest the correct diagnosis. All staging studies should be performed prior to biopsy. Most osteosarcomas of the proximal humerus have a significant extraosseous component. Biopsy is usually only confirmatory. If the axillary vessels are free of tumor, a limb-sparing procedure generally is indicated, although an extraarticular resection is preferred.[13,16] The majority of osteosarcomas of the proximal humerus can be treated by the modified Tikhoff-Linberg procedure. Contraindications are neurovascular, chest wall, or lymph node involvement.[13,16] Forequarter amputation is required if resection is not feasible (Fig. 46-10).

Metastatic Carcinoma

All carcinomas metastasize to the proximal humerus. Hypernephroma has a peculiar predilection for this location and may present a unique problem of uncontrollable bleeding. Hypernephromas are extremely vascular, reflecting their renal origin. Radiography reveals that hypernephromas cause marked destruction and ballooning, much like an aneurysmal bone cyst or a primary sarcoma. If one encounters a possible hypernephroma, angiography of the humerus and the kidneys is recommended prior to biopsy. Simple biopsy (even with a needle) may lead to severe hemorrhage. Angiography confirms the diagnosis of a renal lesion and at the same time allows embolization of the skeletal lesion. An alternative technique with biopsy is temporarily to occlude the axillary vessel with a balloon catheter during the surgical procedure. The author prefers to ligate the anterior and posterior circumflex vessels prior to biopsy. These vessels are easily identified at the inferior border of the subscapularis muscle. Care must be taken to identify the axillary nerve within the same interval. Treatment of metastatic carcinoma to the shoulder girdle generally involves radiation. A simple and reliable procedure is curettage and packing of the humeral head with polymethylmethacrylate and the insertion of intramedullary rods through a lateral incision. Prosthetic replacement is

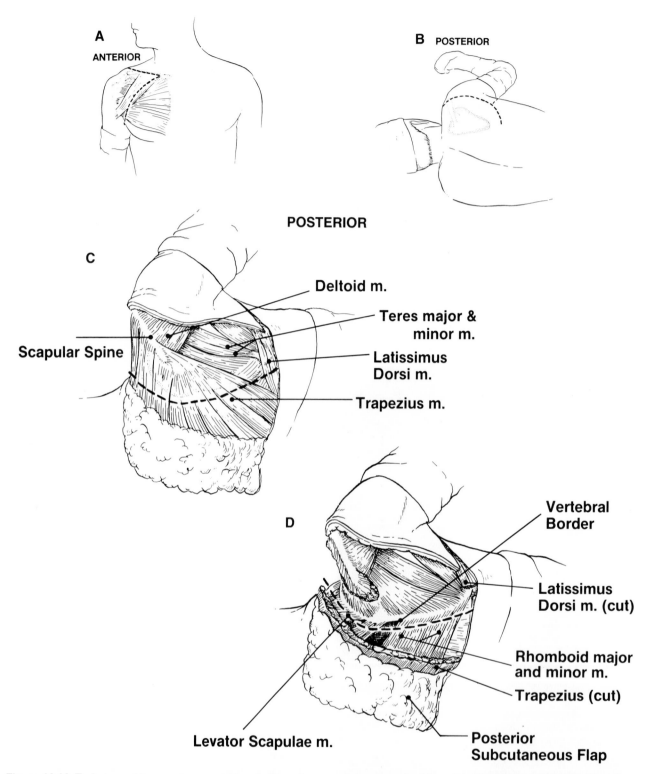

Figure 46-10 Technique of forequarter amputation. **A.** The anterior skin incision. **B.** The posterior skin incision. A lateral position is utilized. **C** and **D.** *Posterior dissection.* A large posterior, subcutaneous flap is developed. All muscles attaching to the axillary border of the scapula are transected with a cutting cautery including the levator scapulae and latissimus dorsi muscles. **E.** The serratus anterior muscle is transected and the entire scapula is anteriorly rotated. The axillary vessels can now be safely approached from this direction or alternately from the anterior approach. **F.** *Anterior dissection.* The pectoralis major and minor muscles are transected. The clavicle is transected at the junction of the proximal one-third. This exposes the axillary vessels and brachial plexus. These structures are now ligated and transected completing the amputation. **G.** The wound is closed over suction catheters.

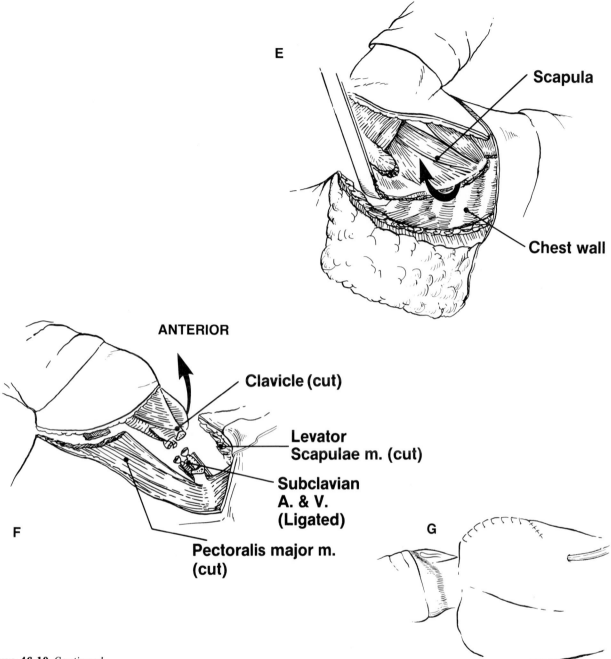

E

Scapula

Chest wall

ANTERIOR

Clavicle (cut)

Levator
Scapulae m. (cut)

Subclavian
A. & V.
(Ligated)

F

Pectoralis major m.
(cut)

G

Figure 46-10 *Continued*

rarely indicated. Cryosurgery combined with curettage has been reported to prevent bleeding at the time of surgery and to prevent tumor recurrence for nonradiosensitive tumors such as hypernephromas.

Surgical Procedures for Tumors of the Proximal Humerus

Forequarter Amputation (Interscapulothoracic Amputation)

Forequarter amputation entails removal of the entire upper extremity including the scapula and clavicle.[8] The surgical

technique is described in Fig. 46-10. The plane of dissection is between the scapula and clavicle and the chest wall. The main indications are high grade neoplasms involving the shoulder girdle and/or proximal humerus. Two surgical approaches are utilized. The anterior approach (Berger's technique) begins with ligation of the axillary vessels through an exposure made possible by removal of part of the clavicle. The second approach (Littlewood) is posterior and entails dividing the scapula from the chest wall. The axillary vessels are approached secondarily. The latter is favored because it facilitates vascular ligation and obviates operating through a small anterior incision. These procedures allow for development of a variety of skin flaps; the various sites of these tu-

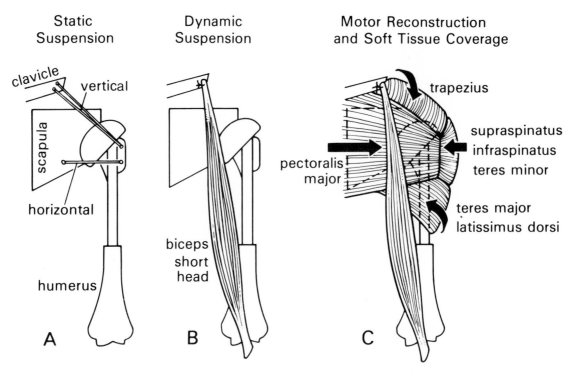

Figure 46-11 Technique of shoulder girdle suspension and reconstruction following resection (type V) for high-grade osteosarcoma. **A.** Static reconstruction is accomplished by the use of dual Dacron tapes. This protects the muscle transfers until healing occurs. **B.** The short head of the biceps is transferred to the outer edge of the remaining clavicle in order to restore the elbow flexors and to permit dynamic suspension. **C.** The entire shoulder girdle and the prosthesis (which act as a spacer) is covered and suspended by the transferred pectoralis major, trapezius, and latissimus dorsi muscles. Soft tissue reconstruction is mandatory to stabilize and to support the upper extremity following a major resection. External orthoses are rarely required.

mors make a choice necessary. Wound healing is rarely a problem. The necessity for forequarter amputation has decreased with the increasing popularity of a limb-sparing option, the Tikhoff-Linberg procedure, and its modifications.

Shoulder Girdle Resections (Limb-Sparing Procedures)

There are numerous types of shoulder girdle resections for neoplasms. There is no standard classification. Figure 46-4 summarizes the various types of procedures and a proposed classification.

Adequate resection of the proximal humerus for high grade bony sarcomas can be accomplished by a modified Tikhoff-Linberg procedure (type V).[13,16] This includes en bloc removal of 15 to 20 cm of the humerus and shoulder joint with the deltoid, rotator cuff, and portions of the biceps and triceps muscles. Reconstruction involves suspension of the arm, motor reconstruction, and provision of adequate soft tissue coverage (Fig. 46-11). Approximately 80 to 85 percent of proximal humeral sarcomas can be treated successfully by this limb-sparing option.

The angiogram is the most useful preoperative study. If the neurovascular bundle is clear, resection is feasible. All other structures can be removed. The length of bone resection is determined preoperatively from a bone scan. To avoid a positive margin at the site of humeral transection, the distal osteotomy is performed 6 cm distal to the area of abnormality. The major contraindications to local resection are tumor involvement of lymph nodes, chest wall involvement, pathological fracture, or massive soft tissue contamination.

Resectability is determined by early exploration of the neurovascular structures by division of the pectoralis major. This approach does not jeopardize formation of an anterior flap in patients who require forequarter amputation. Preservation of the musculocutaneous nerve is important. The short biceps muscle, responsible for elbow flexion, is the most important muscle left after resection. Extraarticular resection of the glenohumeral joint by medial scapulosteotomy is safer than intraarticular resection. In addition, scapular osteotomy not only removes the potential for tumor contamination of the operative field but also permits medialization of the prosthesis and thus a decrease in bulk in the area to be covered.[13,16] A custom prosthesis is used for reconstruction. Other options include dual fibula autografts with arthrodesis and allograft replacement. Irrespective of method of bony reconstruction, soft tissue reconstruction is required and is a main determinant of functional outcome. Proximal soft tissue reconstruction and suspension are essential to avoid postoperative pain, instability, and fatigueability. This is accomplished by a technique of "dual suspension" through static and dynamic reconstruction. Suspension by Dacron tape and muscle transfers of the pectoralis major, latissimus, and trapezius has proved effective. Hand and wrist function are normal following resection. Shoulder motion is minimal, but stable and scapulothoracic motion provides some internal and external rotation. Cosmesis is acceptable and can be enhanced with use of a shoulder pad.

BONY TUMORS OF THE ARM AND ELBOW

The humeral shaft is an uncommon site for primary malignant bone tumors. Common benign lesions are unicameral bone cysts (diaphyseal), fibrous dysplasia and enchondromas. All tend to occur during childhood and adolescence. The elbow is an uncommon site for bony neoplasms; there are no lesions peculiar to this joint. Benign humeral lesions may present

with a pathological fracture or as an incidental radiographic finding. Management of UBCs of the arm and elbow is similar to that of such lesions located elsewhere. Once the correct diagnosis is established, enchondromas and fibrous dysplasia are treated by simple curettage. Fracture through a benign lesion heals readily without the need of internal fixation. Metastatic carcinoma occasionally involves the humeral shaft and elbow and deserves special consideration.

Management of Pathological Fractures of the Humerus and Elbow

Most metastatic lesions of the humerus do not require surgery. Radiation therapy offers good relief from pain, and reossification often occurs. If, however, a patient also has metastatic disease of the lower extremities, the upper extremity should receive prompt surgical attention. This allows the patient to use crutches and to remain ambulatory.

Fixation of a pathological fracture is best performed by intramedullary fixation combined with PMMA. Plate and screw fixation usually is less reliable; furthermore, it requires more extensive surgical exposure. For lesions of the proximal two-thirds of the humerus, one small incision is made at the

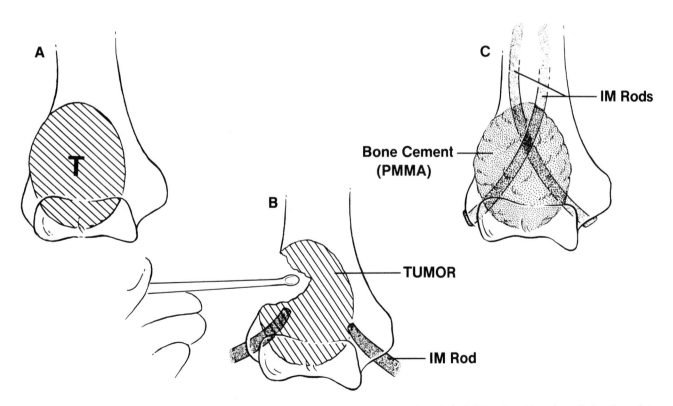

Figure 46-12 Technique of supracondylar reconstruction for metastatic tumor. Metastatic lesions of the distal one-third of the humerus are best treated by curettage of all gross tumor followed by the insertion of dual IM rods with polymethylmethacrylate (PMMA) fixation.

greater tuberosity for rod insertion, and another at the level of the fracture for PMMA insertion and reduction of the fracture. An anterior lateral incision along the humerus is recommended for exposure of the fracture site. The bicep is retracted medially and the brachialis is split anteriorly, in order to avoid exposure and possible damage to the radial nerve. The PMMA is cooled and an intramedullary rod is inserted antergrade. Lesions of the distal one-third require cross rods from the epicondyles (Fig. 46-12).

BONY TUMORS OF THE FOREARM AND WRIST

The distal radius is a common site for giant cell tumors. Osteosarcomas rarely occur in this location. The olecranon occasionally is the site of other lesions but none is specific for this area. Both tumors in this site present with pain and a mass, whereas pain usually is the sole presenting symptoms when these tumors occur around the knee. Tight anatomic constraints usually do not permit a limb-sparing procedure for stage IIB sarcomas of the distal radius. Thus the rare osteosarcoma requires a high trans-forearm amputation. In contrast, there are several surgical options for GCT at this site. Metastatic carcinoma occasionally occurs in the bones of the forearm. The lung is the most common source of metastasis of bones distal to the elbow.

Giant Cell Tumors of the Distal Radius

Clinical Aspects

The distal radius is the third most common site for giant cell tumors, following the distal femur and proximal tibia.[36] Ten percent of giant cell tumors occur in this location. Giant cell tumors of the distal radius often present early with cortical destruction and soft tissue extension due to thin cortices and the direct attachment of the pronator quadratus to the bone. CT accurately demonstrates the extraosseous extension and the relation of the tumor to the adjacent carpus and the distal ulna. Angiography is extremely useful in planning a surgical approach; the radial artery, and in some cases the ulnar artery, is markedly displaced and involved by tumor. In general, the distal radioulnar joint and the carpus must be closely evaluated before and during surgery to determine tumor involvement. Tumor usually is found within the pronator quadratus; this accounts for the significant rate of local recurrence. The articular cartilage may be contaminated by the carpus.

Surgical Management

The recurrence rate following simple curettage of a distal radial giant cell tumor does not significantly differ from that of a giant cell tumor at other sites, although one might as-

sume it would be lower since a more thorough curettage should be possible. Local recurrence is due to the biological aggressiveness of the tumor combined with microscopic extension into the adjacent soft tissues, specifically the pronator quadratus. If the tumor is small, curettage is recommended. The upper extremity is an ideal location for cryosurgery since the risk of pathologic fracture is slight.[14,18,19,21] Resection should include the distal radius en bloc with the distal ulna or proximal row of the carpus if either is involved in conjunction with the pronator quadratus, as well as a thin cuff of all muscles originating from the distal radius (Fig. 46-13). Resection and replacement by autogenous fibula is recommended for large lesions. Allograft replacements have had good results.[17] In general, a primary arthrodesis is recommended, although attempts at preservation of wrist motion following graft replacement also have yielded good short-term results. Alternatively, following resection, the carpus can be centralized onto the ulna and fused to create a one-bone forearm. This technique avoids the need for either an autogenous fibula or an allograft.

Metastatic Carcinoma

Metastatic cancer occasionally affects the radius and ulna. When this is the first sign, metastases may be confused with a primary sarcoma. The osteoblastic variants, lung and prostate most commonly mimic a bone-producing sarcoma. Biopsy is confirmatory. Radiation therapy offers good results. Surgery is rarely indicated; if necessary, intramedullary Steinmann pin fixation combined with PMMA gives good fixation.

SOFT TISSUE SARCOMAS OF THE ARM AND FOREARM

Between 15 and 25 percent of soft tissue sarcomas occur in the upper extremities.[23] The staging studies and principles of treatment are similar to those for such lesions in other sites. Unfortunately, most tumors in this area are treated as "benign," and the correct diagnosis established only after the final pathology returns. Soft tissue masses of the upper extremity should be assumed to be malignant until proved otherwise, and appropriate precautions should be taken regarding the site and timing of the biopsy. Because of anatomic constraints in this area there is less potential salvage following an inappropriate biopsy and/or "shell-out" procedure than in other anatomic sites. The type and grade of soft tissue sarcomas of the upper extremity do not differ from the general category of sarcomas. Surgical options often are limited because of previous treatment and anatomic considerations.

Anatomic Considerations

The arm and forearm consist of two well-defined anatomic compartments: in the arm there are the anterior compart-

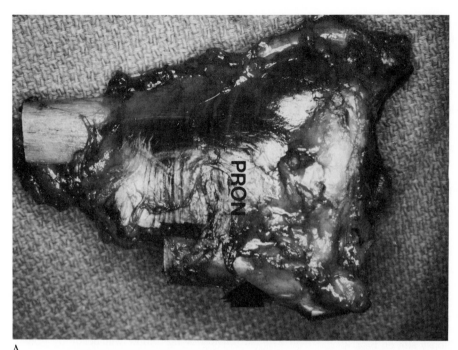

A

Figure 46-13 Giant cell tumor of the distal radius. **A.** Gross specimen following resection of the distal radius. The distal ulna (*solid arrow*) was also removed because of involvement by the tumor. Note that the pronator quadratus (*PRON*) covers the tumor. **B.** Bivalved gross specimen. Note the extraosseous component involving the pronator quadratus (*solid arrows*). This is a common finding which often makes primary resection mandatory. There was direct articular cartilage destruction (*hand*) with synovial involvement. This finding is less common. The proximal row of the carpus was partially resected.

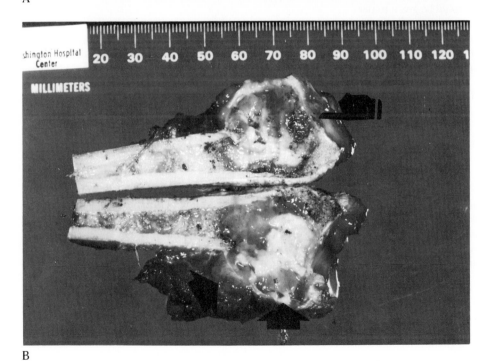

B

ment (biceps, brachialis) and the posterior compartment (triceps). The brachial artery and major nerves are within the anterior compartment, while the radial nerve and the profunda brachii artery are the main neurovascular structures of the posterior compartment. The ulnar nerve originates in an anterior location and then crosses posteriorly at the origin of the medial intermuscular septum. Similarly, the forearm con-

sists of a volar (anterior) and dorsal (posterior) compartment. In general, tumors in stage I or IIA remain confined to one compartment until they become quite large. Some lesions, however, originate extracompartmentally (stage I or IIB). Sarcomas of the arm can often be resected with minimal disability. The forearm offers more difficulty than the upper arm. Portions of muscle, or even entire muscles in each compartment, can be removed without loss of function. The main determinant of function is the degree of involvement of the major nerves.

Staging

Staging studies are similar to those used at other sites. In addition, the axillary area should be carefully examined, since sarcomas of the upper extremity may involve the regional lymph nodes. Lymph node involvement is most common with synovial and epithelioid sarcomas, which have a predilection for the forearm and hand.

Biopsy

Because of anatomic constraints in the arm and forearm, all biopsies must be planned with the intention of minimizing contamination and for removal of the biopsy site en bloc if the tumor is malignant. Consideration should be given to performing the biopsy with a frozen section and to proceeding with removal in one stage. Such a technique offers the best possibility of avoiding inadvertent contamination and the loss of a limb-sparing option. A small incisional biopsy or needle biopsy is recommended. The biopsy should be done under tourniquet control and be placed longitudinally.

Overall Management

Stage IA/B tumors can be treated safely with surgery alone if negative margins are obtained. Stage IIA/B tumors require surgical removal, chemotherapy, and radiotherapy if a marginal or wide excision has been performed. Radiotherapy to the upper extremity requires a high level of expertise to avoid serious sequelae such as fibrosis, contractures, lymphedema, pain, and local recurrence.

Surgical Management

Amputations are often required for sarcomas of the upper extremity: forequarter amputation for tumors of the proximal arm, and shoulder disarticulation and above-elbow amputation for lesions of the distal arm and forearm, respectively. Major neurovascular involvement is the most common reason for ablation. Limb-sparing surgery can be performed if a functional extremity can be salvaged. Function varies greatly following this surgery, depending on the location and combination of the nerves involved, and which of them have to be sacrificed. In general, sacrifice of the radial nerve is easily compensated for by secondary tendon transfers. Loss of the median or ulnar nerve leaves some function in the hand; how-

ever, sacrifice of both nerves results in serious loss of function.

SPECIFIC ANATOMIC COMPARTMENTS
Anterior (Biceps)

Angiography will accurately demonstrate the position of the brachial artery and the tumor. If the vessels are clear removal of the biceps and/or brachialis can be compensated for by a modified Steindler flexorplasty (proximal transfer of the forearm flexors).

Posterior (Triceps)

The triceps can be resected with minimal morbidity. If the radial nerve is involved it should be removed. Tendon transfers are performed secondarily. The triceps need not be reconstructed. Extension of the elbow will occur by gravity.

Volar (Forearm Flexors)

This is the most difficult compartment in which to perform a limb-sparing procedure. Deeply situated sarcomas that involve the radius and/or ulna and intermuscular septum may cross over to the extensor group, becoming extracompartmental. CT scanning is helpful in delineating the mass. Bone scintigraphy may determine osseous involvement. Osseous extension tends to be more common with forearm tumors than with lesions located elsewhere. Biplane angiography is essential to determine the vascular anatomy, which is often distorted. Either the radial or ulnar artery can be sacrificed if there is a patent deep palmar arch. If one artery is uninvolved a viable extremity is possible. Small tumors can be resected with negative margins. The superficial or deep flexors can be entirely removed if necessary. Each lesion must be carefully evaluated and a judgment concerning preservation of a useful extremity made. In general, a sensate hand with some function is far superior to a prosthesis.

Dorsum (Forearm Extensors)

The proximal extensors (mobile wad) are a favorite location for soft tissue sarcomas of the forearm. This entire group, along with the posterior interosseous nerve, can be resected without major loss of function; the only deficit is a wrist drop. If the underlying radius is involved it should be removed en bloc with the lesion. The remaining olecranon provides elbow stability. There is no need to reconstruct the resected proximal radius. An external orthosis is required. Tendon transfers are performed secondarily following radiotherapy. In general, tendon transfers following irradiation tend to function mainly as a tenodesis due to radiation fibrosis.

SECTION B

Tumors of the Hand and Wrist

Harold M. Dick

In the hand and upper limb occur the entire range of neoplasms possible in the musculoskeletal system. They are perhaps more dramatic and obvious in the hand because of their constant exposure and potential interference with hand function.

We will first consider the most frequent of these neoplasms, that is, the *benign* tumors of the hand and wrist.[14,24,27,28]

GANGLIA OF THE HAND AND WRIST

It is estimated that 50 to 70 percent of all soft tissue tumors of the hand and wrist are ganglion cysts (Fig. 46-14A). They appear to be more prevalent in women (3:1), and 70 percent occur between the second and fourth decade of life.

The cause is not known. However, there are various descriptions of etiologic factors including trauma, mucoid degeneration, and synovial herniation of the carpal capsule. Synovial rest cells have been described as well as de novo growths.

There are two common sites of occurrence. Dorsal carpal ganglion cysts, usually from the scapholunate ligament, occur in some 60 to 70 percent of some series; volar carpal ganglia are most commonly seen at the volar wrist crease between the flexor carpi radialis and the abductor pollicis longus (Fig. 46-14A).[2] The volar carpal ganglia appear to be from the scaphotrapezoid joint capsule.

Other variations of the ganglion include the volar retinacular ganglion and the mucoid cyst.

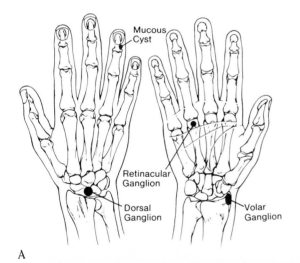

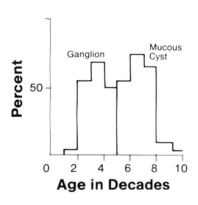

A

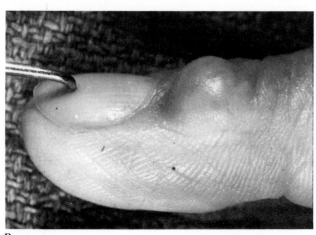

B

Figure 14-14 A. Incidence of ganglia in the hand and forearm. **B.** A 65-year-old woman with mucoid cyst at the dorsal distal interphalangeal joint of the right third finger.

The retinacular ganglion (10 to 20 percent) is the third most common ganglion of the hand. It appears only in the pulley areas of the flexor tendon retinacula, usually at the level of the A2 pulley of the digital flexor tendons. It rarely exceeds 1 cm in diameter and most often spontaneously subsides with time.

The mucoid cyst is a variant of the ganglion cyst (Fig. 46-14B).[21] It most commonly occurs on the dorsum of the digit at the level of the distal interphalangeal joint and invariably is associated with concurrent osteoarthritis and osteophyte formation known as Heberden's nodes.

In certain cases this ganglion may stretch the dorsal skin, groove the nail bed, and, infrequently, break the skin. Following resection, a skin graft and resection of the osteophytes of the distal phalanx may be required.

Most ganglion cysts are symptomatic, usually following acute or repetitive trauma. Some 30 to 35 percent of the ganglia are asymptomatic except for appearance.

On physical examination the ganglion cyst is found to be soft, transilluminates, and is 1 to 3 cm in diameter. It is often nonmobile.

Pathological examination shows a cystic cavity with viscous mucin of glucosamine, albumin, globulin, and a high concentration of hyaluronic acid. It is much more viscous than joint fluid.

The treatment of the ganglion cyst is usually reassurance for the nonsymptomatic lesions. When they are surgically excised, magnification and resection of a small portion of the wrist capsule is recommended. No closure of the defect is recommended.

There is a well-documented complication rate with surgery, including recurrence rates as high as 20 to 40 percent, and if the associated capsular tissue is not removed, sensory neuromas and keloid scar formation.

gives a clear radiolucency in comparison with the density of bone and other soft tissue. This is known as *Bufolini's sign.*

Morphological examination shows an encapsulated soft tissue mass, with characteristic yellow fat cells apparent microscopically. There is a very rare malignant counterpart.

The usual treatment is excision for diagnosis and cosmesis. The prognosis is excellent with a negligible recurrence rate.

BENIGN GIANT CELL TUMORS OF THE TENDON SHEATH

This category includes xanthofibroma, xanthoma, localized pigmented villonodular tenovagosynovitis, and benign fibrous histiocystomas.

Benign giant cell tumor of the tendon sheath is the second most common tumor of the hand after ganglia (Fig. 46-16A).[20,26,30] It occurs in the mature adult (40 to 60 years old). The tumor is commonly located on the index and middle digits on the volar and dorsal surfaces. It can envelop the neurovascular bundle and present problems in dissection.

These benign growths are usually painless, but when encroaching upon small joints they may restrict motion (Fig. 46-16B).[20,26]

On physical examination they are found to be firm, and nontender close to joints, and may be fixed in position. There are usually no roentgen findings.

Pathological examination shows variable-sized encapsulated yellow tissue with fatty areas. There are classic foam cells, and histological examination shows histiocytes and small nuclei. The cytoplasm is full of lipoid globules, and characteristic giant cells occur in various new beds.

The treatment of choice is resection, including portions of the tendon sheath or joint capsule if necessary. Recurrence

LIPOMAS OF THE HAND AND UPPER LIMB

Lipomas of the hand and upper limb are one of the commonest and most widely distributed tumors of the body.[18,25] There is an equal incidence in upper and lower limbs. They are more frequently proximal than distal. Ten to 20 percent of upper limb lipomas occur in the hand and wrist area.

There is a greater female incidence of (2:1), and the most frequent occurrence is in the third to sixth decades. The most frequent site is the thenar eminence; the tumors also occur at the level of the proximal phalanx in both the volar and the dorsal locations (Fig. 46-15). These growths are usually asymptomatic. They are often mistaken for ganglia. They occasionally cause nerve compression symptoms of the proximal volar forearm or the loge de Guyon.

The tumors are soft; they do not transilluminate as well as ganglia and are usually nontender and mobile. When the lipoma is located close to a cortical bone, it characteristically

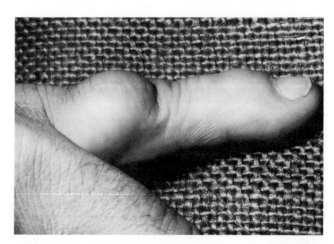

Figure 46-15 A 50-year-old woman with a lipoma of the fifth finger.

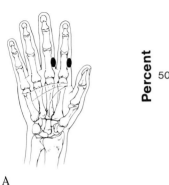
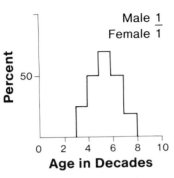
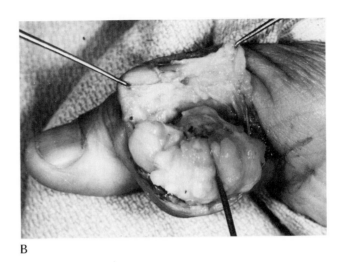

A
B

Figure 46-16 A. Incidence of xanthomas of the hand and forearm. **B.** Operative specimen of benign xanthoma of the flexor aspect of the thumb.

may be a problem if the tumor is not adequately excised. If a joint is involved, arthrodesis may be needed to prevent recurrence.

EPIDERMAL CYSTS (INCLUSION CYSTS)

The true incidence of epidermal cysts is not known.[3] The cause is thought to be microscopic trauma. There is a 2:1 male preponderance. The mean age is the third decade.

The most common site is the volar aspect of the distal phalanx of the index or middle finger.

Epidermal cysts present as a painless swelling with firm induration of the digital pad.

On x-ray examination there may be a smooth, round, radiolucent lesion centered in the volar aspect of the distal phalanx with thinning of the cortex. On histological examination, one finds a fibrous capsule with a keratin-filled space. Squamous epithelium may be present and is characteristic of the lesion.

The most effective treatment is surgical excision through a midlateral incision with curettage of the phalanx. Bone grafting may be necessary. There is a low recurrence rate.

GLOMUS TUMOR

Glomus tumor is one of the rarest of hand tumors.[4] Some series estimate that it constitutes 1 to 5 percent of all hand tumors. It occurs in the third to fifth decades of life. It is an unusual tumor of childhood and the elderly.

Over 50 percent of glomus tumors occur in the subungual location. However, they have been reported in a wide range of body surface sites including all the extremities and

the trunk. They usually present with a triad of severe pain, tenderness, and cold sensitivity.[4] Paroxysms of the triad are pathognomonic.

The physical findings often include ridging of the nail. The area is exquisitely sensitive to touch and temperature testing. A blue spot at the base of the nail is often present. The x-ray examination may show a well-defined radiolucent, eccentric lesion in the base of the distal phalanx.

The lesions are usually less than 1 cm in diameter. The histological examination shows polyhedral cells, fibrous stroma, and small blood vessels.

The most effective treatment utilizes magnification for the surgery. Nail removal is necessary to visualize the tumor. The lesion is usually well-encapsulated. The prognosis is excellent, and the relief spectacular, unless the glomus is not completely removed. There is a significant residual tumor incidence and/or recurrence rate with this surgery.

ENCHONDROMA

Enchondroma is the most common primary bone tumor of the hand (Fig. 46-17). It occurs in the second to fourth decades of life. The most common site is the proximal phalanx of the digits. Enchondroma is usually not symptomatic unless microfracture has taken place. Most of the physical findings of tenderness and swelling are usually due to fracture through the lesion. On x-ray films a diagnostic radiolucent lesion is present in the diaphyseal or metaphyseal portion of the phalanx with thinned cortex and flecks of calcification. The gross appearance is cartilaginous and ricelike. The histological examination shows benign cartilage.

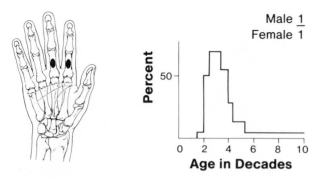

Figure 46-17 Incidence of enchondromas in the hand and forearm.

The definitive treatment is curettage with bone graft replacement. The prognosis is excellent with a minimal recurrence rate.[6,33]

OSTEOCHONDROMA

Osteochondroma is a rare occurrence as a solitary lesion in the hand (Fig. 46-18A).[16,19] It is frequently present, however, in many of the patients with multiple osteochondromas. There is a male preponderance. It is usually diagnosed in the first two decades of life. In the hand osteochondroma is usually most frequent in the metacarpals and proximal phalanges. It infrequently presents as a subungual lesion.

There is rarely pain associated with this tumor. It does, however, produce growth disturbances of shortening, angulation, hyperextension, and often loss of flexion.

The examination reveals bony prominences at the metaphyseal portions of the small tubular bones. The x-ray examination indicates projections of the cortex continuous with normal cortex (Fig. 46-18B).

Pathological examination often reveals normal bone cortex with a cartilaginous cap. The treatment is usually deferred until skeletal maturity. At that time osteotomy corrections for angulation and rotation may be required with excision.

The prognosis is excellent when the tumor is completely excised.

OSTEOID OSTEOMA

Osteoid osteoma is a very rare primary bone tumor (1 percent of all the bone tumors in the hand).[5,8] There is an equal incidence in males and females. The first two decades of life are the time of the most frequent occurrence. It is usually found in the phalanges, with only very rare findings in the carpus (Fig. 46-19).

The most diagnostic of findings is the characteristic

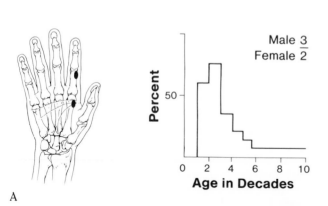

A

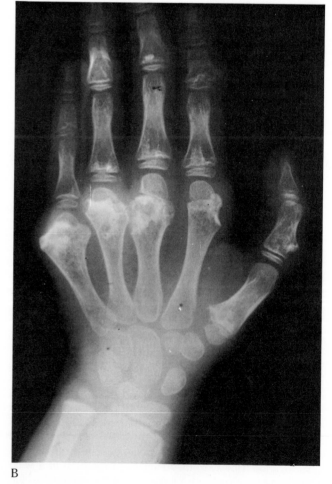

B

Figure 46-18 A. Incidence of osteochondroma in the hand and forearm. **B.** A 20-year-old man with multiple osteochondromas of the metacarpals and phalanges.

night pain dramatically relieved by aspirin in over 50 percent of the patients.

There is often localized tenderness when the osteoma is palpable. The classic x-ray view shows eccentric cortical sclerosis with a radiolucent nidus less than 1 cm in diameter. The bone scan and particularly the CT scan have been most helpful in confirming the diagnosis. The pathological examination is also very diagnostic, showing a soft tissue tumor within a sclerotic cavity. The histological examination shows vascularized osteoid tissue with abundant osteoblasts.

The treatment is curettage of the nidus, employing a dental drill and facilitated by x-ray control. The prognosis is dramatic and excellent with full removal.

JUVENILE APONEUROTIC FIBROMA

Juvenile aponeurotic fibroma is an uncommon soft tissue tumor, occurring in the first two decades of life; 50 percent occur in the hand and forearm.[11,29]

It is a painless growth that often has spotty calcification on soft tissue x-ray views and has the histological appearance of a cellular tumor with fat and muscle infiltration. There is dense collagenous tissue that also has evidence of infrequent calcification. The histological examination is very troublesome, leading many cases to be confused with malignancy.

There is a very high local recurrence rate without adequate resection.

MALIGNANT TUMORS OF THE HAND AND FOREARM

Primary malignant tumors of the upper limb below the elbow are fortunately very rare.[1,12,22,31] All tumors distal to the elbow in patients over 40 years of age should first be viewed as metastatic disease.

If the tumor is thought to be malignant on clinical and roentgenographic grounds, a careful evaluation should be performed prior to biopsy and/or surgery. This includes a complete blood cell count, determination of sedimentation rate, and determination of serum alkaline phosphatase and serum and urine protein levels when indicated for possible myeloma. Radioisotope scans and chest tomography should be performed for possible silent metastases when the tumor biopsy has been identified as malignant. CT and magnetic resonance imaging (MRI) are becoming more important in preoperative assessment and planning for reconstruction alternatives. Smith in 1977 outlined the objectives of treatment of malignant tumors of the hand.[28] (1) The goal of all malignant-tumor surgery is ablation of the tumor with a satisfactory tumor-free margin. (2) Functional reconstruction should rarely be performed at the same time as excision of the tumor. (3) All suspected malignancies should have incisional biopsies. (4) When the diagnosis is agreed upon, the decision

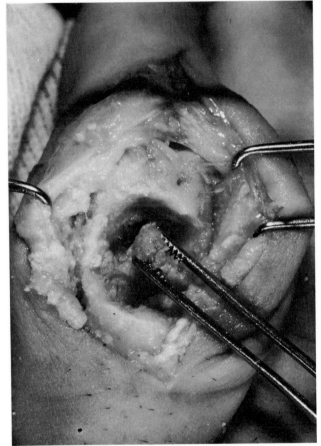

A

B

Figure 46-19 A. A 19-year-old man with osteoid osteoma (*arrow*) of the proximal phalanx of the right index finger. **B.** Nidus of the osteoid osteoma is exposed with the use of a dental drill.

for ablation versus preserved hand function requires great experience in oncology and in hand and upper limb reconstruction. (5) The use of adjuvant chemotherapy and/or radiation treatment has distinct advantages in the treatment, especially with the soft tissue malignancies.

The operative planning for reconstruction includes the following. (1) Assessment of final skin coverage needs, including possible interim split-thickness grafts or free tissue transfers, is almost mandatory. (2) The Esmarch bandage should be excluded to avoid tumor mobilization, but pneumatic tourniquet should be included for protection of normal structures. (3) Any elaborate reconstruction should be deferred until the pathologist has declared the actual specimen "margin free" of tumor.

We believe that the grading and staging of tumors should be done according to the method of Enneking and the Musculoskeletal Tumor Society.[12]

METASTATIC TUMORS OF THE HAND

In all patients over 40 years of age, especially if primary sites are already known (breast, lung, kidney), any painful radiolucent lesion of the upper limb skeleton should be suspected of being metastatic rather than a primary skeletal tumor.[34] The distal phalanx is the most common site. The carpus is the most unlikely site of metastases. The treatment choices are ablation or radiation therapy.

The prognosis at this stage is very poor, with the majority of patients in the end stage of their primary disease.

CHONDROSARCOMA

Cartilage tumors of the hand, especially enchondroma and multiple cartilage lesions of Ollier's disease, are well-discussed in the literature.[6,7,23,32,33] Some people believe these, especially the Ollier's lesion, may be precursors of malignant degeneration to chondrosarcoma. Chondrosarcoma is probably one of the most difficult diagnoses to confirm by histology because of the wide variation in mitotic and malignant cells. Much of the diagnosis rests upon the biological behavior of the tumor, i.e., rapid growth, pain pattern, and high recurrence rate, and the roentgen patterns of expansile growth with cortical destruction and extension to the soft tissues.

When the diagnosis is established, ablation by ray resection or amputation is the procedure of choice. The tumor is radioresistant and also not sensitive to chemotherapy protocols.

OSTEOGENIC SARCOMA

Osteogenic sarcoma is a truly rare primary bone malignancy occurring in the first two decades of life, usually in the distal radius, metacarpals, or phalanges.[13,15] It is usually a rapidly

progressive painful lesion that is most often a lytic destructive intramedullary lesion. Open biopsy and careful diagnosis are mandatory. The differential diagnosis with a benign osteoblastoma may be difficult.

The treatment should be surgical with ablation of the major site and often the next joint in proximity (Fig. 46-20). Lateral extension may require adjacent ray resections where indicated to add adequate margins. Adjuvant chemotherapy with doxorubicin hydrochloride (Adriamycin) and high-dose methotrexate is indicated for this tumor.

EWING'S SARCOMA

Ewing's sarcoma is an extremely rare tumor in the hand skeleton.[9,10,17] It usually occurs in the first two decades of life. The

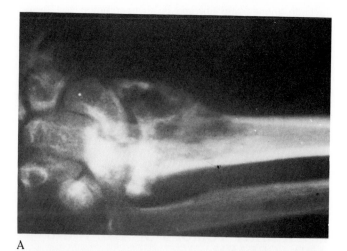

A

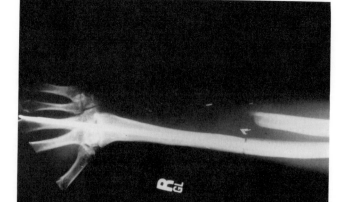

B

Figure 46-20 A. A 21-year-old white man with an osteosarcoma of the distal radius. **B.** The patient was treated by en bloc resection and allograft replacement with intramedullary rod fixation.

5-year survival rate has classically been 5 to 20 percent of patients. The reports of this tumor have been largely anectodal with no reports including more than two case descriptions.

The similarity in inflammatory presentation often suggests the diagnosis of osteomyelitis. The roentgen studies and even the histological examination often fail to facilitate differential diagnosis.

The treatment of choice is ablative surgery and adjuvant chemotherapy as well as radiation therapy if needed.

SOFT TISSUE MALIGNANT TUMORS

This area of oncology has a wide range of neoplasms including synovial sarcomas, epithelioid sarcomas, fibrosarcomas, malignant fibrous histiocytomas, and clear cell sarcomas. These tumors require careful review and often second opinions by expert pathologists to indicate the type of tumor. Careful staging, surgery, and radiation to the field plus chemotherapy have improved the prognosis. This group is the most difficult of limb tumors to diagnose, ablate, and treat for microscopic and distant disease.

The natural history of these tumors prior to radiation and chemotherapy was devastating, with an overall prognosis of 30 to 40 percent survival by 5 years. Recent preliminary studies have moved the prognosis to 50 to 70 percent.

REFERENCES

Section A: Tumors of the Forearm, Arm, and Shoulder Girdle

1. Biesecker, J.L., Marcove, R.C., Huvos, A.G., and Moke, V. Aneurysmal bone cysts: A clinicopathologic study of 66 cases.
2. Campanacci, M., Bacci, G., Bertoni, et al: The treatment of osteosarcoma of the extremity: Twenty years' experience at the Instituto Orthopedico Rizzoli. Cancer 48:1569–1581, 1981.
3. Campanacci, M., Giunti, A., and Olmi, R. Giant-cell tumors of bone: A study of 209 cases with long-term follow-up in 130. Ital J Orthop Traumatol 1:249–277, 1977.
4. Dahlin, D.C. *Bone tumors: General Aspects and Data on 6,221 Cases,* 3d ed. Springfield, IL, Thomas, 1978.
5. Dahlin, D.C., and Coventry, M.B. Osteosarcoma, a study of 600 cases. J Bone Joint Surg 49A:101–110, 1967.
6. Dahlin, D.C., Cupps, R.E., and Johnson, E.W., Jr. Giant cell tumor: A study of 195 cases. Cancer 25:1061–1070, 1970.
7. Dahlin, D.C., and Ivins, J.C. Benign chondroblastoma: A study of 125 cases. Cancer 30:401–413, 1972.
8. Francis, K.C. Radical amputations, in *Nora's Operative Surgery.* Philadelphia, Lea & Febiger, 1974, pp 1041–1051.
9. Francis, K.C., and Worcester, J.N., Jr. Radical resection for tumors of the shoulder with preservation of a functional extremity. J Bone Joint Surg 44A:1423–1429, 1962.
10. Garrison, R.C., Unni, K.K., Mcleod, R.A., et al: Chondrosarcoma arising in osteochondroma. Cancer 49:1890–1897, 1982.
11. Gitellis, S., Bertoni, F., Chieti, P.P., and Campanacci, M. Chondrosarcoma of bone. J Bone Joint Surg [Am] 1248–1256, 1981.
12. Malawer, M.M. The diagnosis, treatment and management of unicameral bone cysts by percutaneous aspiration, hemodynamic evaluation and intracavitary methylprednisolone acetate. Orthopedic Update Series vol. IV, Lesson 26, 1986.
13. Malawer, M.M. Surgical technique and results of limb-sparing surgery for high grade bone sarcomas of the knee and shoulder: Analysis of 33 consecutive case. Orthopedics 8:597–607, 1985.
14. Malawer, M.M., Dunham, W.K., Zaleski, T., and Zielinski, C.J. Cryosurgery in the management of benign (aggressive) and low grade malignant tumors of bone: Analysis of 40 consecutive cases. Presented at the American Academy of Orthopedic Surgeons (AAOS), New Orleans, February 1986.
15. Malawer, M.M., McKay, D.W., and Markle, B., et al: Analysis of 40 consecutive cases of unicameral bone cysts treated by high pressure renograffin injection and intracavitary methylprednisolone acetate: Prognostic factors and hemodynamic evaluation. 52nd Annual Meeting, Amer Acad Orthop Surg, Las Vegas, Nev., 1985.
16. Malawer, M.M., Sugarbaker, P.J., Lambert, P.T., et al: The Tikhoff-Linberg procedure: Report of ten patients and presentation of a modified technique for tumors of the proximal humerus. Surg 97:518–528, 1985.
17. Mankin, H.J., Fogelson, F.S., Thrasher, A.Z., et al: Massive resection and allograft transplantation in the treatment of malignant bone tumors. N Engl J Med 294:1247–1255, 1976.
18. Marcove, R.C.: A 17-year review of cryosurgery in the treatment of bone tumors. Clin Orthop 163:231–233, 1982.
19. Marcove, R.C., Lyden, J.P., Huvos, A.C., Bullough, P.B. Giant cell tumor treated by cryosurgery. A report of twenty-five cases. J Bone Joint Surg [Am] 55:1633–1644, 1973.
20. Marcove, R.C., Mike, V., Hutter, R.V.P., et al: Chondrosarcoma of the pelvis and upper end of femur. J Bone Joint Surg [Am] 54:561–572, 1972.
21. Marcove, R.C., Weiss, L., Vaghaiwall, M., and Pearson, R. Cryosurgery in the treatment of giant cell tumor of bone: A report of 52 consecutive cases. Clin Orthop 134:275–289, 1978.
22. Neer, C.S., Francis, K.C., Kiernan, H.A., et al: Current concepts in the treatment of solitary unicameral bone cysts. Clin Orthop 97:40–51, 1973.
23. Rosenberg, S.A., Suit, F.D., and Baker, L.H. Sarcomas of soft tissue, chap 36, in DeVita, V.T., Hellman, S., and Rosenberg, S.A. (eds): *Cancer, Principles and Practice of Oncology,* 2d ed. Philadelphia, Lippincott, 1985, pp 1243–1293.
24. Scaglietti, O., Marchetti, P.G., and Bartolozzi, P. The effects of methylprednisolone acetate in the treatment of bone cysts. Results of three years follow-up. J Bone Joint Surg [Br] 61:200–204, 1979.

Section B: Tumors of the Hand and Wrist

1. Andrew, T.A. Clear cell sarcoma of the hand. Hand 14:200–203, 1982.
2. Angelides, A.C., and Wallace, P.F. The dorsal ganglion of the wrist. J Hand Surg 1:228–235, 1976.
3. Byers, P., and Salm, R. Epidermal cysts of phalanges. J Bone Joint Surg 48B:577–581, 1966.
4. Carroll, R.E., and Berman, A.T. Glomus tumors of the hand. J Bone Joint Surg 54A:591–603, 1972.
5. Carroll, R.E. Osteoid osteoma in the hand. J Bone Joint Surg 35A:888–893, 1953.

6. Culver, J.E., Sweet, D.E., and McCue, F.C. Chondrosarcoma of the hand arising from pre-existent benign solitary enchondroma. Case report and pathological description. Clin Orthop 113:128–131, 1975.

7. Dahlin, D.C., and Salvador, A.H. Chondrosarcomas of bones of the hands and feet. A study of 30 cases. Cancer 34:755–760, 1974.

8. Doyle, L.K., Ruby, L.K., Nalebuff, E.G., and Belsky, M.R. Osteoid osteoma of the hand. J Hand Surg 10A:408–410, 1985.

9. Dreyfuss, U.Y., Auslander, L., Bialik, V., and Fishman, J. Ewing's sarcoma of the hand following recurrent trauma. A case report. Hand 12:300–303, 1980.

10. Dryer, R.F., Buckwalter, J.A., Flatt, A.E., and Bonfiglio, M. Ewing's sarcoma of the hand. J Hand Surg 4:372–374, 1979.

11. Eisenbaum, S.L., and Eversmann, W.W. Juvenile aponeurotic fibroma of the hand. J Hand Surg 10A:622–625, 1985.

12. Enneking, W.F. *Musculoskeletal Tumor Surgery.* New York, Churchill Livingstone, 1983.

13. Fleegler, E.J., Marks, K.E., Sebek, B.A., Groppe, C.W., and Belhobek, G. Osteosarcoma of the hand. Hand 12:316–322, 1980.

14. Fuhs, S.E., and Herndon, F.H. Aneurysmal bone cyst involving the hand. A review and report of two cases. J Hand Surg 4:152–159, 1979.

15. Goorin, A.M., Frei, E., and Abelson, H.T. Adjuvant chemotherapy for osteosarcoma. A decade of experience. Surg Clin North Am 61(6):1379–1389, 1981.

16. Green, D.P. (ed). *Operative Hand Surgery.* New York, Churchill Livingstone, 1982, pp 1636–1652.

17. Kedar, A., Bialik, V., and Fishman, J. Ewing sarcoma of the hand. Literature review and a case report of nonsurgical management. J Surg Oncol 25:25–27, 1984.

18. Leffert, R.D. Lipomas of the upper extremity. J Bone Joint Surg 54A:1262–1266, 1972.

19. Lucas, G.L. Hand tumors. A quick guide to types and treatment. Resident Staff Phys 25(12):85–92, 1979.

20. Merkow, R.L., Bansal, M., and Inglis, A.E. Giant cell reparative granuloma in the hand. Report of three cases and review of the literature. J Hand Surg 10A:733–739, 1985.

21. Newmeyer, W.L., Kilgore, E.S., and Graham, W.P. Mucous cysts. The dorsal distal interphalangeal joint ganglion. Plast Reconstr Surg 53:313–315, 1974.

22. Noellert, R.C., and Louis, D.S. Long-term follow-up nonvascularized fibular autografts for distal radial reconstruction. J Hand Surg 10A:335–340, 1985.

23. Palmieri, T.J. Chondrosarcoma of the hand. J Hand Surg 9A:332–338, 1984.

24. Phalen, G.S. Neurilemmomas of the forearm and hand. Clin Orthop 114:219–222, 1976.

25. Phalen, G.S. Lipomas of the upper extremity. J Bone Joint Surg 51A:1665–1666, 1969.

26. Phalen, G.S., McCormack, L.J., and Gazale, W.J. Giant cell tumor of tendon sheath in the hand. Clin Orthop 15:140–151, 1959.

27. Rinaldi, E. Neurilemomas and neurofibromas of the upper limb. J Hand Surg 8:590–593, 1983.

28. Smith, R.J. Tumors of the hand. Who is best qualified to treat tumors of the hand? J Hand Surg 2:251–252, 1977.

29. Specht, E.E., and Staheli, L.T. Juvenile aponeurotic fibroma. J Hand Surg 2:256–257, 1977.

30. Stevenson, T.W. Xanthoma and giant cell tumor of the hand. Plast Reconstr Surg 5:75–87, 1950.

31. Strickland, J.W., and Steichen, J.B. Nerve tumors of the hand and forearm. J Hand Surg 2:285–291, 1977.

32. Trias, A., Basora, J., Sanchez, G., and Madarnas, P. Chondrosarcoma of the hand. Clin Orthop 134:297–300, 1978.

33. Wu, K.K., Frost, H.M., and Guise, E.E. A chondrosarcoma of the hand arising from an asymptomatic benign solitary enchondroma of 40 years' duration. J Hand Surg 8:317–319, 1983.

34. Wu, K.K., and Guise, E.R. Metastatic tumors of the hand. A report of six cases. J Hand Surg 3:271–276, 1978.

CHAPTER 47

Dupuytren's Contracture

Lawrence C. Hurst and Marie A. Badalamente

Dupuytren's contracture is a debilitating fibromatosis which involves the palmar aponeurosis. Nodular thickenings form in the palmar fascia and may progress into the longitudinal bands resulting in fixed flexion contractures of the fingers (Fig. 47-1). The term *Dupuytren's diathesis* refers to the predisposition of some patients for multiple areas of involvement. Dupuytren's diathesis is associated with a positive family history and early onset of the disease. In patients with Dupuytren's diathesis, involvement may be present in the volar aspects of the hands, in the dorsum of the fingers in the form of knuckle pads, in the feet as plantar fibromatosis, and in the penis as Peyronie's disease.[16,69]

HISTORY

In 1614, Plater[56] described flexion deformities of the fingers which were probably Dupuytren's contracture.[61] Sir Ashley Cooper reported the condition in 1822.[7] Despite this, Baron Dupuytren's name appears to be the permanent eponym for this particular fibromatosis, because in 1830 he accurately described the condition in a dissected cadaver hand and correctly identified the palmar fascia as the predominantly involved tissue, and in 1831 presented a clinical case.

PATHOPHYSIOLOGY

Our understanding of the pathobiology of Dupuytren's contracture has progressed slowly in the past 150 years. However, the clinical features of the disorder are well-defined. As the fibromatosis slowly progresses over a period of years, flexion contractures of the fingers, web space contractures, and distal interphalangeal hyperextension contractures all contribute to a significant functional handicap. The normal palmar fascia has been well described.[26,29,30,48,62,70] The anatomic structures that become involved in Dupuytren's contracture are the longitudinal pretendinous bands, the spiral bands, the natatory ligaments, the lateral digital sheaths, Grayson's ligaments, and Cleland's ligaments (Fig. 47-2).[13,34,37,64] The ring and the little fingers are the most frequently involved digits in Dupuytren's contracture.[5,24] However, the radial digits and thumb-index web space may also become involved. In the first web, four separate pathological cords are possible: a radial longitudinal fibrous cord, a longitudinal cord secondary to the radial distal fibers of the

palmaris longus, a distal transverse interdigital cord secondary to Grapow's ligament involvement, and a transverse proximal web cord secondary to involvement of a proximal transverse commissural ligament. Involvement of any of these cords can result in interference with a web width and ultimately with grasp and pinch.[65]

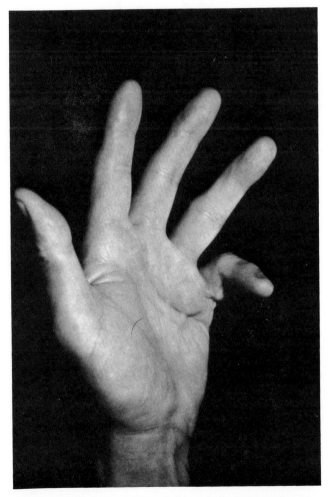

Figure 47-1 Fixed flexion contracture of the little finger in a patient with Dupuytren's disease. The characteristic nodular thickenings of the palmar fascia are evident at the metacarpophalangeal joint of the little finger.

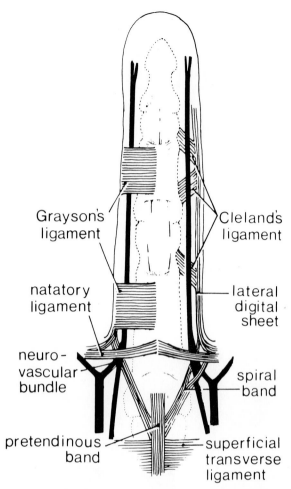

Figure 47-2 The normal structures of the finger that may be involved in Dupuytren's disease are the longitudinal pretendinous bands, spiral bands, natatory ligaments, lateral digital sheaths, and Grayson's and Cleland's ligaments. *(From McFarlane, R. M., Plast Reconstr Surg 54:31, 1974. Reprinted with permission.)*

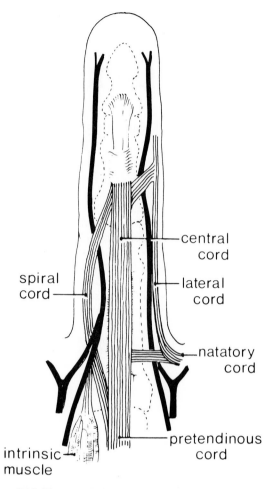

Figure 47-3 Three pathological cords may develop during the progressive palmar fibromatosis of Dupuytren's disease: the central, the spiral, and the lateral cords. *(From Chui, H. P. and McFarlane, R. M., J Hand Surg 3:1–10, 1978. Reprinted with permission.)*

As the fascial structures of the hand are progressively changed into pathological cords by the palmar fibromatosis, the fingers can develop a fixed flexion contracture. Three different pathological cords can develop in the palm and digits: the central cord, the spiral cord, and the lateral cord (Fig. 47-3).[34,37,38] The central cord develops when there is involvement of the pretendinous longitudinal bands and the fibrofatty tissues in the superficial fascia between the neurovascular bundles. The spiral cord develops when there is involvement of the pretendinous cords, the spiral bands, the lateral digital sheaths, and Grayson's ligament. At surgery, the spiral cord should be approached cautiously because it can medially and superficially displace the neurovascular bundles, particularly at the level of the first transverse finger crease.[37,60] The lateral cord develops in the lateral sheaths dorsal to the neurovascular bundles. This cord may also involve Cleland's ligaments. All three of these cords can cause fixed flexion contractures of the fingers. Natatory ligament involvement causes web contractures. Finally, the little finger may become contracted because of the cords or because of

the involvement of the abductor digiti minimi fascia and tendon.[29,37,70] Involvement of this intrinsic muscle may partially explain the increased frequency of the severe, persistent, and recurrent contracture in this digit.

The pathohistological characteristics of Dupuytren's contracture were first described in the now-classic work of Gabbiani and Majno.[12,35] These investigators correctly pointed out that the nodules in the affected palmar fascia are composed of smooth musclelike cells called myofibroblasts (Fig. 47-4). Myofibroblasts, which are best identified using the electron microscope, have distinct features compatible with contractile ability. These ultrastructural features are bundles of 4- to 8-nm fibrils within the cytoplasm that are oriented parallel to the long axis of the cell; deeply indented nuclei; and cell-to-cell and cell-to-stroma membrane attachment sites known as desmosomes and hemidesmosomes, respectively.[6,12,23,35,59,68] Fibril bundles also contain darkened areas known as dense bodies located beneath the cell membrane. Recently, the presence of a pH-dependent adenosine triphosphatase (ATPase) has been found to be associated with the fibril bundles in Dupuytren's myofibroblasts.[1] In muscle this enzyme is associated with cellular contraction.

Most authors adhere to the concept that the proliferation of myofibroblasts within the nodules of Dupuytren's contracture is a slowly progressive phenomenon. Luck's early report of the stages of cellular progression has since been substantiated.[34] The first occurrence is the proliferative stage of the disorder in which the myofibroblast cellularity in the palmar fascia increases with the collagen cords showing less cellularity. The second, residual stage, is characterized by a dense myofibroblast network and fewer cellular collagen cords. In the last, involutional stage, most nodular myofibroblasts have disappeared, but a fixed flexion contracture remains.

The origin of the myofibroblast is unknown. An extrinsic theory which states that the myofibroblasts originate subdermally has been proposed.[16,17] The puckering of the skin, so commonly seen in the disorder, is purported by this theory to reflect the contracture of the skin toward the underlying fascia because of subdermal involvement. Other investigators have proposed an intrinsic theory which states that fascial fibroblasts differentiate into myofibroblasts.[1,6,35,49,61]

The role that microvascular changes and secondary local hypoxia play in the stimulation of cellular changes in Dupuytren's contracture has also been investigated. It has been suggested that hypoxemia caused by excessive endothelial cells stimulates pericytes and/or vascular fibroblasts to differentiate into myofibroblasts.[8,17,27] This hypoxemia may also explain the presence of high levels of low-chain or volatile fatty acids in the palmar fascia of patients with Dupuytren's disease.[58] Despite this information on the vascular status in Dupuytren's disease, there is still no definite proof that the perivascular fibroblasts are the origin of the myofibroblasts.

There is increased metabolic activity in the diseased tissues from Dupuytren's contracture.[9] Despite the fact that the activity of lysosomal enzymes and of the enzymes involved in glucose catabolism is increased in Dupuytren's fascia,[15] it has not been possible to show conclusively that the increased metabolic rate is secondary to increased enzymatic activity. Rather, it is probable that the increased number of myofibroblasts,[9] which have an increased capacity to synthesize glycosaminoglycan and type III collagen, are responsible for the increased metabolic activity of the diseased tissue in Dupuytren's contracture.[2,4,9,10,44] Myofibroblasts and increased amounts of type III collagen coexist within a matrix of glycosaminoglycan.[1] Type III collagen undergoes a constant remodeling until the residual stage of the disease when an inextensible band has been produced.[21,22] Increased amounts of hydroxylysine, increased numbers of reducible cross-links, and the presence of hydroxylysinohydroxynorleucine have all been shown in Dupuytren's contracture.[2,4,9,10,21,22,44] In addition, collagen abnormalities have recently been shown to be more prevalent in the more grossly diseased fascia.[55] Despite these biochemical findings, a specific correlation between the development of the clinical contracture and the biochemical abnormalities has not been made.

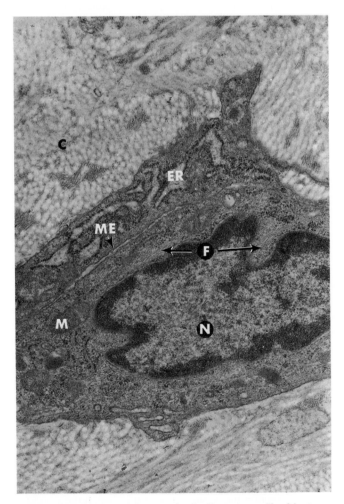

Figure 47-4 Electron micrograph of adjacent myofibroblasts from a nodule of Dupuytren's disease. The cells are separated by their respective membranes (*ME*). Myofibroblast ultrastructure includes a large indented nucleus (*N*), mitochondria (*M*), granular endoplasmic reticulum (*ER*), and intracellular filaments (*F*) oriented toward the long cell axis. Collagen fibrils (*C*) surround the cells. ×10,000.

INCIDENCE

The incidence of Dupuytren's disease is greater in northern European countries and in countries where a large part of the population is of northern European heritage.[39] The disease is rarely seen in non-Caucasians, but occasional cases have been reported.[43] The incidence of the disease steadily increases with age.[11,18] In one population study in Norway, 36.8 percent of the population between the age of 70 and 74 years showed evidence of Dupuytren's disease. Variable incidences have been reported in the sexes. Some reports suggest that the incidence is equal, particularly in older men and women,[39] while others report that the incidence is 2 to 10 times greater in men than in women.[45] The most commonly involved digits are the dominant ring and little fingers. The index finger has the lowest incidence of involvement.[47,65]

The relation between the incidence of Dupuytren's disease, occupation, and hand trauma remains unclear. Several reports emphatically state that there is no relation between occupation, injury, and the incidence of Dupuytren's contracture.[3,11,18] Others including Dupuytren himself stated that injury and/or heavy manual labor do play a role in increasing the incidence of Dupuytren's contracture.[31,61] Probably the best assessment is that trauma aggravates the pathological process in genetically predisposed individuals.[19,46]

The highest incidence of Dupuytren's contracture has been reported in patients with associated epilepsy, diabetes mellitus, chronic alcoholism, chronic pulmonary tuberculosis, and chronic lung disease.[11,18,25,53,57] These associated conditions may simply reflect the rising incidence of Dupuytren's disease in the elderly.

Ten percent of the patients with Dupuytren's contracture have a positive family history for this disorder. Dupuytren's disease is probably transmitted as a dominant gene with variable penetrance. This penetrance is almost complete in elderly men but not in women.[33] Despite a dominant gene transmission pattern, patients with Dupuytren's contracture do not show a specific pattern of HLA antigens.[25,63]

TREATMENT

The treatment of Dupuytren's contracture is presently surgical, although nonsurgical methods have been tried. Injections of enzymes, copper sulfate, cortisone, massage with vitamin E creams, physical therapy, therapeutic splinting, and radiation have all been ineffective.[16,39] Therefore, the treatment for Dupuytren's contracture remains surgical.

The aim of surgical treatment is to relieve the fixed flexion deformities by removal of the abnormal palmar fascia. Surgery does not cure Dupuytren's disease, but it may modify the progression and improve hand function. Potential surgical results can be predicted by the Legge and McFarlane outcome standard formula which estimates the residual postoperative contracture.[32] Surgery is indicated in patients with significant handicap who demonstrate a positive table top test.[20] In this test, the patient places the hand on a flat surface. When there are significant contractures of the metacarpophalangeal and/ or proximal interphalangeal (PIP) joints, the fingers and the palm cannot be placed simultaneously on the flat surface, thus constituting a positive table top test. Another indication for surgical treatment is a metacarpophalangeal contracture of greater than $30°$.[39] Palmar nodules alone are not an absolute indication for surgical treatment. Pain is also not an indication for surgery. In the proliferative stage, patients without contractures but with painful nodules would be advised that this may resolve as they move into the second, residual stage of the disorder. In patients with severe unrelenting pain, particularly if there is night pain, the possibility of an extremely rare condition, fibrosarcoma of the hand, should be considered.

Patients presenting with mild Dupuytren's disease who have painful associated trigger fingers should have their trigger fingers treated surgically; however, this should include a limited regional fasciectomy at the time of A-1 pulley release. Surgical treatment of the trigger finger without excision of the local fascia may result in an exacerbation of the Dupuytren's fibromatosis. In patients with Dupuytren's disease and coexisting carpal tunnel syndrome, the Dupuytren's contracture

should first be treated surgically while the carpal tunnel syndrome is treated nonoperatively. If after the Dupuytren's surgery, carpal tunnel syndrome symptoms continue, despite conservative therapy, then carpal tunnel release should be performed as a second procedure.[52]

Surgical treatment of Dupuytren's contracture is contraindicated when associated with advanced rheumatoid arthritis,[42] when the hand has trophic changes secondary to vascular insufficiency, and when the patient's general health is such that he or she will not be able to withstand the stress of surgery and anesthesia.[42,66]

The operative choices for Dupuytren's contracture include fasciotomy, regional fasciectomy, and total (radical) fasciectomy.[19,39] Closed fasciotomy is dangerous, particularly in the digit.[40,66] In the elderly patient, however, fasciotomy may be a useful treatment for a single palmar band or as a preliminary procedure.[19,39] However, fasciotomy should be done only by a surgeon who is experienced in this technique. Total fasciectomy has been abandoned because of significant surgical morbidity associated with this approach.[42,51,71] Regional fasciectomy with excision of grossly pathological fascia is the most popular current procedure.[19,39] However, Tubiana has warned that regional fasciectomy can lead to a higher recurrence rate in nonoperative areas.[66] The extensiveness of a procedure is determined by the evaluation of the individual case with special consideration being given to the patient's age, family history, alcohol history, epileptic history, sex, history of previous surgical treatment, and occupation, and the presence or absence of knuckle pads. No matter which operative procedure is employed, the prognosis is particularly poor in young patients with a strong family history, that is, those with Dupuytren's diathesis.[19]

Numerous incisions have been used for fasciectomies in Dupuytren's contracture. For example, Skoog and McCash popularized transverse incisions.[36,61] However, others have used midlateral and longitudinal incisions, longitudinal oblique incisions with Z-plasty, V-Y-plasty incisions, and zigzag incisions.[19,39,54,66]

Whatever incision is employed, it should provide exposure which allows proper identification of the neurovascular bundles while providing good access to the pathological tissues in the palm, fingers, and web spaces (Fig. 47-5). Skin flaps should be elevated with as much subcutaneous tissue as possible in order to maintain the subdermal vascular plexuses. Prior to closure, meticulous hemostasis should be achieved in order to prevent hematoma. A tourniquet should be used, but it is appropriate to lower the tourniquet and control any vigorous bleeding prior to reapplying the tourniquet and proceeding with surgical closure. Various adjunctive procedures such as volar PIP joint capsulotomy, skin grafts, arthrodeses, arthroplasties, and/or amputations are sometimes needed.[19,50,66]

Postoperative care begins in the operating room with the application of a bulky compressive dressing. If the wound is closed, a drain should be left in the wound for 24 to 48 h. Bulky dressings are removed at 3 to 5 days and smaller dressings applied. If an open-palm technique has been used, frequent early range-of-motion exercises and soaks are mandatory. McCash reports that these open incisions close in 2 to 5 weeks.[36] Our experience shows that this takes closer to

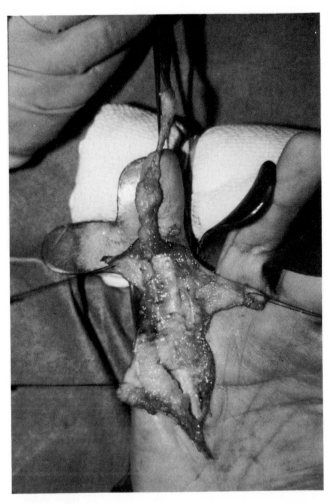

Figure 47-5 Operative exposure of affected tissue in the little finger of a patient with Dupuytren's disease. The affected palmar fascia is reflected distally to reveal the digital nerves and the flexor tendons.

2 months. With the closed-palm technique, at 3 to 5 days postoperatively, the bulky dressings are removed and hand therapy with static night extension splinting and daytime active range-of-motion exercises is begun under the supervision of the hand therapist.[41]

The overall postoperative complication rate in Dupuytren's surgery approaches 20 percent[39] with late sequelae in the range of 0.5 to 6 percent.[67] Common complications include hand edema, palmar hematoma, skin necrosis, infections, digital nerve laceration, digital artery laceration, joint stiffness, loss of grip strength secondary to loss of finger flexion, reflex sympathetic dystrophy, and digital loss secondary to vascular damage.[28,67] Hematoma often leads to skin necrosis and secondary infection. This sequence is so common that McFarlane has called this a complication triad.

The results of a 10-year follow-up study show 80 percent good results with patients demonstrating a normal-appearing palm, full extension, and full flexion.[40] However, Hakstian reported recurrence or extension of the disease in 50 percent of McIndoe's patients who were followed from 5 to 25 years, the

average follow-up being 11.1 years.[14] His data remind us that surgical treatment does not cure this disorder but only temporarily improves hand function. Since a large percentage of patients with Dupuytren's contracture are elderly, this improvement may last the rest of their lives. In young patients, however, recurrence, further functional loss, and additional surgery should be anticipated in a significant percentage of the operative cases.

REFERENCES

1. Badalamente, M.A., Stern, L., and Hurst, L.C. The pathogenesis of Dupuytren's contracture: Contractile mechanisms of the myofibroblasts. J Hand Surg 8:235–242, 1983.
2. Bazin, S., LeLous, M., Duance, V.C., Sims, T.J., Bailey, A.J., Gabbiani, G.D., Andiran, G., Pizzolato, G., Browski, A., Nicoletis, C., and Delaunay, A. Biochemistry and histology of the connective tissue of Dupuytren's disease lesions. Eur J Clin Invest 10:9–16, 1980.
3. Bell, R.C., and Furness, J.A. A study of the effect of recurrent trauma on the development of Dupuytren's contracture. Br J Plast Surg 30:149–150, 1977.
4. Brickley-Parsons, D., Glimcher, M.J., Smith, R.J., Albin, R., and Adams, J.P. Biochemical changes in the collagen of the palmar fascia in patients with Dupuytren's disease. J Bone Joint Surg 63A:787–797, 1981.
5. Brunner, J.M. The dynamics of Dupuytren's disease. Hand 2:172–176, 1970.
6. Chiu, H.F., and McFarlane, R.M. Pathogenesis of Dupuytren's contracture: A correlative clinical-pathological study. J Hand Surg 3:1–10, 1978.
7. Cooper, A. *A Treatise on Dislocations and Fractures of the Joints.* London, 1822.
8. Davis, J.E. On surgery of Dupuytren's contracture. Plast Reconstr Surg 36:277–314, 1965.
9. Delbruck, A., Reimers, E., and Schonborn, I. A comparative study of the activity of lysosomal and main metabolic pathway enzymes in tissue biopsies and cultured fibroblasts from Dupuytren's disease and palmar fascia. J Clin Chem Clin Biochem 19:931–941, 1981.
10. Delbruck, A., and Schroder, H. Metabolism and proliferation of cultured fibroblasts from specimens of human palmar fascia and Dupuytren's contracture. J Clin Chem Clin Biochem 21:11–17, 1983.
11. Early, P.F. Population studies in Dupuytren's contracture. J Bone Joint Surg 44B:602–613, 1962.
12. Gabbiani, G., and Majno, G. Dupuytren's contracture: Fibroblast contraction? An ultrastructural study. Am J Pathol 66:131–138, 1972.
13. Gosset, J. Dupuytren's disease and the anatomy of the palmodigital aponeurosis, in Hueston, J.T., and Tubiana, R. (eds): *Dupuytren's Disease,* 1st English ed. Edinburgh, Churchill Livingstone, 1974, pp 11–23.
14. Hakstian, R.W. Late results of extensive fasciectomy, in Hueston, J.T., and Tubiana, R. (eds): *Dupuytren's Disease.* New York, Grune and Stratton, 1974, pp 79–83.
15. Hoopes, J.E., Jabaley, M.E., Chi-Tsung, S., Wilgis, E.F.S., and Im, M.J.C. Enzymes of glucose metabolism in palmar fascia and Dupuytren's contracture. J Hand Surg 2:62–65, 1977.
16. Hueston, J.T. *Dupuytren's Contracture.* Edinburgh, Churchill Livingstone, 1963.
17. Hueston, J.T., and Tubiana, R. *Dupuytren's Disease.* GEM Monograph I. Edinburgh, Churchill Livingstone, 1974.
18. Hueston, J.T. The incidence of Dupuytren's contracture. Med J

Aust 2:999–1002, 1960.

19. Hueston, J.T. Current state of treatment of Dupuytren's disease. Ann Chir Main 3:81–92, 1984.

20. Hueston, J.T. Table top test. Med J Aust 18:189–190, 1976.

21. Hunter, J.A.A., Ogdon, C., and Norris, M.G. Dupuytren's contracture: I. Chemical pathology. Br J Plast Surg 28:10–18, 1975.

22. Hunter, J.A.A., and Ogdon, C. Dupuytren's contracture: II. Scanning electron microscopic evaluations 28:19–25, 1975.

23. Iwasaki, H., Muller, H., Stutte, H.J., and Brennscheidt, U. Palmar fibromatosis (Dupuytren's contracture): Ultrastructural and enzyme histochemical studies of 43 cases. Virchows Arch [Pathol Anat] 405:41–53, 1984.

24. James, J.I.P., and Tubiana, R. La Maladie de Dupuytren. Rev Clin Orthop 38:352, 1952.

25. James, H.I.P. The genetic pattern of Dupuytren's contracture and idiopathic epilepsy, in Hueston, J.T., and Tubiana, R. (eds): *Dupuytren's Disease.* New York, Grune and Stratton, 1974, pp 37–42.

26. Kaplan, E.B., and Milford, W. The retinacular system of the hand, in Spinner, M. (ed): *Kaplan's Functional and Surgical Anatomy of the Hand.* Philadelphia, Lippincott, 1984, pp 245–282.

27. Kischer, C.W., and Speer, D.P. Microvascular changes in Dupuytren's contracture. J Hand Surg 9A:58–62, 1984.

28. Kleinert, H.E., Leitch, I., Smith, D.J., and Lubbers, L.M. Problems in Dupuytren's contracture, in Strickland, J.W., and Steicher, J.B. (eds): *Difficult Problems in Hand Surgery.* St. Louis, Mosby, 1982, pp 402–408.

29. Lamb, D.W. Dupuytren's disease, in Lamb, D.W., and Kaczynski, K. (eds): *The Practice of Hand Surgery.* London, Blackwell Scientific, 1981, p. 476.

30. Landsmmer, J.F.M. Pathoanatomy of Dupuytren's contracture. *Atlas of Anatomy of the Hand.* Edinburgh, Churchill Livingstone, 1970.

31. Larsen, R.D., Takagishi, N., and Posh, J.L. The pathogenesis of Dupuytren's contracture. J Bone Joint Surg 42A:993–1007, 1960.

32. Legge, J.W.H., and McFarlane, R.M. Prediction of results of treatment of Dupuytren's disease. J Hand Surg 5:608–616, 1980.

33. Ling, R.S.M. The genetic factor in Dupuytren's disease. J Bone Joint Surg 45B:709–718, 1963.

34. Luck, J.V. Dupuytren's contracture: A new concept of the pathogenesis correlated with surgical management. J Bone Joint Surg 41A:635–664, 1959.

35. Majno, G., Gabbiani, G., Hirschel, H.J., Ryan, G.B., and Statkow, P.R. Contraction of granulation tissue in vitro: Similarity to smooth muscle. Science 173:548–550, 1971.

36. McCash, C.R. The open palm technique in Dupuytren's contracture. Br J Plast Surg 17:271–280, 1964.

37. McFarlane, R.M. Patterns of the diseased fascia in the fingers in Dupuytren's contracture. Plast Reconstr Surg 54:31–44, 1974.

38. McFarlane, R.M. Dupuytren's contracture, in Green, D. (ed): *Operative Hand Surgery.* London, Churchill Livingstone, 1982, chap 10, pp 463–497.

39. McFarlane, R.M. The current status of Dupuytren's disease. J Hand Surg 9A:103–708, 1984.

40. McFarlane, R.M., and Jamieson, W.G. Dupuytren's contracture: The management of one hundred patients. J Bone Joint Surg 48A:1095–1104, 1966.

41. McFarlane, R.M., Dupuytren's disease, in Hunter, J.M., Schneider, L.H., Mackin, E.J., Bell, J.A. (eds): *Rehabilitation of the Hand.* St. Louis, Mosby, 1978, pp 147–153.

42. McIndoe, A., and Beare, R.L.B. The surgical management of Dupuytren's contracture. Am J Surg 95:197–203, 1958.

43. Mennen, U., and Grabbe, R.P. Dupuytren's contracture in Negro: A case report. J Hand Surg 4:451, 1979.

44. Menzel, E.J., Piza, H., Zielinski, C., Endler, A.T., Steffen, C., and Millesi, H. Collagen types and anticollagen-antibodies in Dupuytren's disease. Hand 2:243–248, 1979.

45. Mikkelsen, O.A. The prevalence of Dupuytren's disease in Norway. Acta Chir Scand 138:695–700, 1972.

46. Mikkelsen, O.A. Dupuytren's disease—The influence of occupation and previous hand injuries. Hand 10:1–8, 1978.

47. Mikkelsen, O.A. Dupuytren's disease—A study of the pattern of distribution and stage of contracture in the hand. Hand 8:265–271, 1976.

48. Milford, L.W. *Retaining Ligaments of the Digits of the Hand.* Philadelphia, Saunders, 1968.

49. Millesi, H. Neve Gesichtspunkte in der pathogenese der Dupuytren' schen Kontracturn. Bruns Beitr Klin Chir 198:1–25, 1959.

50. Moberg, E. Three useful ways to avoid amputation in advanced Dupuytren's contracture. Orthop Clin North Am 4:1001–1005, 1978.

51. Neckesser, E.C. Results of wide excision of the palmar fascia for Dupuytren's contracture. Special reference to factors which adversely affect prognosis. Ann Surg 160:1007, 1964.

52. Nissenbaum, M., and Kleinert, H.E. Treatment considerations in CTS with co-existent Dupuytren's disease. J Hand Surg 5:544–547, 1980.

53. Noble, J., Heathcote, J.G., and Cohen, H. Diabetes mellitus in the aetiology of Dupuytren's disease. J Bone Joint Surg 66B:322–325, 1984.

54. Orlando, J.C., Smith, J.W., and Dorgon, D. Dupuytren's contracture: Review of 100 patients. Br J Plast Surg 27:211–217, 1974.

55. Parsons, D., Adams, S., Smith, R., and Glimcher, M.J. Collagen polymorphism in Dupuytren's disease. Trans ORS 10:116, 1985.

56. Plater, F. Observationum Liber 1:140, 1614; cited by Durel, L.

57. Pojer, J., Radivojeuie, M., and Williams, F. Dupuytren's disease: Its association with abnormal liver function in alcoholism and epilepsy. Arch Intern Med 129:561–566, 1972.

58. Rabinowitz, J.L., Osterman, A.L., Bora, F.W., and Staeffer, J. Lipid composition and de novo biosynthesis of human palmar fat in Dupuytren's disease. Lipids 18:371–379, 1983.

59. Seemayer, T.T.A., Lagace, R., Schurch, W., and Thelmo, W.L. The myofibroblast: Biologic, pathologic and theoretical considerations. Patho Annu 1:443–470, 1980.

60. Short, W.H., and Watson, H.K. Prediction of the spiral nerve in Dupuytren's contracture. J Hand Surg 7:84–86, 1982.

61. Skoog, T. Dupuytren's contracture with special reference to aetiology and improved surgical treatment; its occurrence in epileptics; note on knuckle pads. Acta Chir Scand 96(suppl 139):11–176, 1948.

62. Stack, H.G. *The Palmar Fascia.* Edinburgh, Churchill Livingstone, 1973.

63. Tait, B.D., and Mackay, I.R. HLA phenotypes in Dupuytren's contracture. Tissue Antigens 19:240–241, 1982.

64. Thomine, J.M. The development and anatomy of the digital fascia, in Hueston, J.T., and Tubiana, R. (eds): *Dupuytren's Disease,* 1st English edition. Edinburgh, Churchill Livingstone, 1974, pp 1–9.

65. Tubiana, R., Simmons, B.P., and DeFrenne, H.A.R. Location of Dupuytren's disease on the radial aspect of the hand. Clin Orthop Rel Res 168:222–229, 1982.

66. Tubiana, R. The principles of surgical treatment of Dupuytren's contracture, in Hueston, J.T., and Tubiana, R. (eds): *Dupuytren's Disease.* New York, Grune and Stratton, 1974, pp 71–77.

67. Tubiana, R., Fahrer, M., and McCullough, C.J. Recurrence and other complications in surgery of Dupuytren's contracture. Clin Plast Surg 8:45–50, 1981.

68. VandeBerg, J.S., Gelberman, R.H., Rudolph, R., Johnson, D., and Sicurello, P. Dupuytren's disease: Comparative growth dynamics and morphology between cultured myofibroblasts (nodule) and fibroblasts (cord). J Orthop Res 2:247–256, 1984.

69. Wheller, E.S., and Meals, R.A. Dupuytren's diathesis: A broad-spectrum disease. Plast Reconstr Surg 68(5)1:781–783.

70. White, S. Anatomy of the palmar fascia on the ulnar border of the hand. J Hand Surg 9B:50–56, 1984.

71. Zacharaie, L. Extensive vs. limited fasciectomy for Dupuytren's contracture. Scand J Plast Reconstr Surg 1:150–153, 1967.

CHAPTER 48

Avascular Necrosis in the Upper Extremity

Steven W. Margles

The term *aseptic necrosis* has been used to indicate that the necrosis of bone is not the result of infection. The designation *avascular necrosis* is preferable because it emphasizes the principal causative factor: a loss of adequate blood supply to all or a part of a bone. Various bones in the upper extremity may undergo avascular necrosis. The process is usually self-limiting because of spontaneous revascularization. However, during reparative healing the bone may undergo a degree of structural collapse. After an episode of avascular necrosis, the bone may take 2 years to reossify and regain its normal strength, and normal stresses on the bone may cause some loss of its normal bony architecture. This ranges anywhere from a small change to major collapse and fragmentation. In the larger bones, secondary osteoarthritis often develops. In the wrist, the arthritic process progresses not only because of the loss of congruity of the joints of the avascular bone but also because of the disorganization of the normal relation between the other intact carpal bones. To minimize the risk of this late complication of osteoarthritis, it is preferable to diagnose and treat the disease before the bone has undergone any appreciable change in shape. Treatments attempting to accomplish this have usually been designed to either increase the blood supply to the involved bone or decrease the stresses on it while the process undergoes its natural resolution.

Bone necrosis, fragmentation, fibrous proliferation, and new bone formation are the histological indicators of the avascular necrotic bone. In the earliest stages the radiographic appearance of the bone shows little or no change despite the clinical impression of an inflammatory process, but there is often synovitis in adjacent joints. With further progression, an apparent increase in the density of the involved bone occurs. This has been attributed to the relative decrease in density of the surrounding bone or bones, which may be responding to increased vascularity from the inflammatory response and addition of new bone on the necrotic bone that has not yet been resorbed. With progression, there is collapse of the bone with evidence of both fracture and fracture repair with changes of degenerative arthritis.

In the large bones of the upper extremity, the head of the humerus and the capitellum are the two areas most commonly affected. In the wrist and hand, the process is found, in order of decreasing frequency, in the lunate, scaphoid, capitate, and metacarpals. The disease has also been reported in the pisiform bone.[35] The vulnerable vascular supply of these bones and their susceptibility to trauma help to account for this order of frequency. In avascular necrosis associated with acute fractures, the scaphoid is most commonly affected.

Though frequently not recalled by the patient, some degree of trauma is involved in the initiation of most avascular disease in the wrist and hand. This may take the form of repeated minor injuries, such as may be sustained with the use of pneumatic tools.[26] Such trivial trauma may inexplicably lead to avascular necrosis in one person but not in another. In those bones with a greater amount of collateral circulation, the degree of trauma required to produce the avascularity of the bone seems to be greater.

The extraosseous or intraosseous blood supply to a bone may be lost secondary to vessel occlusion. Necrosis in carpal bones occurs in patients with systemic diseases requiring the use of prednisone[3,23,27] and in those receiving combination chemotherapy.[22] Steroid therapy apparently causes increased coagulability and viscosity of blood as well as systemic fat embolism. These changes are believed to be responsible for vessel occlusion and the development of avascular necrosis in the wrist, shoulder, and elbow. In patients with renal transplants and avascular processes of bone, Harrington et al found a positive correlation between the amount of prednisone used in postoperative management and the incidence of the avascular process.[23] Most commonly the changes were apparent approximately 6 months after the onset of treatment. The relatively high incidence of avascular necrosis associated with systemic lupus erythematosus is probably related to the use of prednisone in the treatment of this disorder.[21,60,65] Avascular necrosis of the lunate has been reported in association with sickle cell anemia.[30] In this patient, pathological studies showed sickling of red blood cells within the lunate vessels.

REGIONAL ETIOLOGIC CONSIDERATIONS

Carpal Vascular Anatomy

Excellent anatomic studies of both the intrinsic and the extrinsic vascular supply of the carpal bones have been carried out by Taleisnik and Kelly,[58] by Gelberman and co-workers,[15,17,18] and by Panagis et al.[45] A recent study[18] has shown that three main transverse arterial arches supply the carpal bones on the dorsal surface (Fig. 48-1) and that three others supply those on the volar surface (Fig. 48-2).

On the *dorsal* side, the three transverse arches are described as the radiocarpal arch, intercarpal arch, and distal metacarpal arch (Fig. 48-1). There are three arteries that with different frequencies contribute to all three transverse

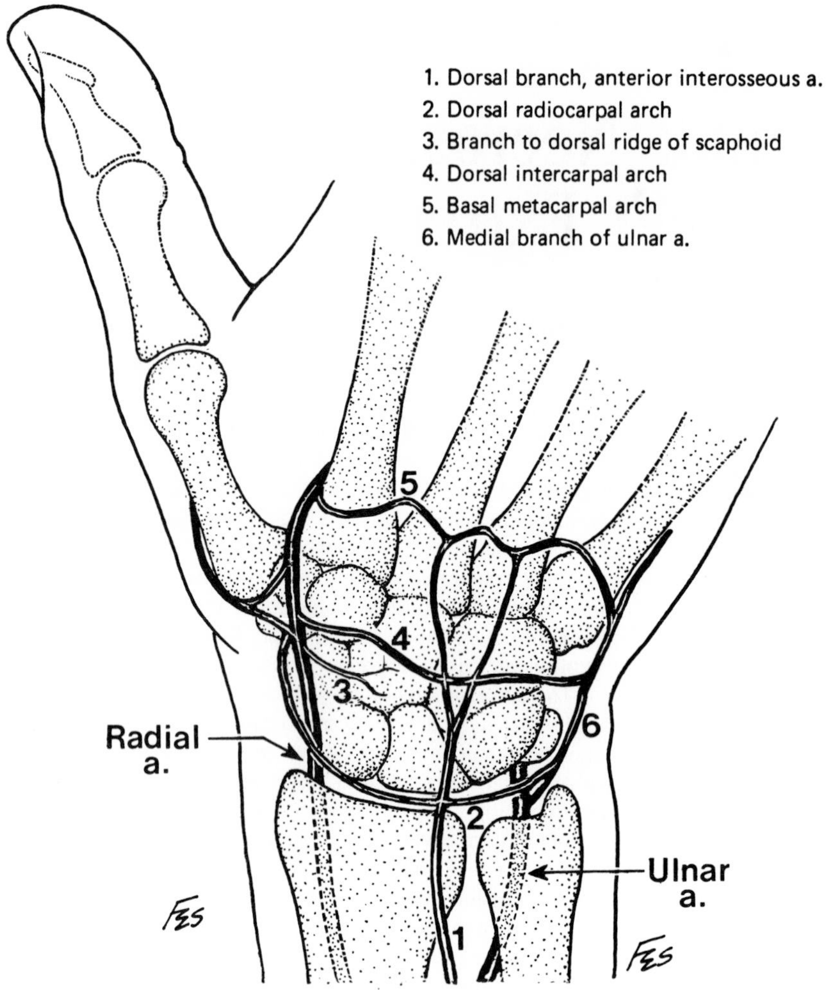

1. Dorsal branch, anterior interosseous a.
2. Dorsal radiocarpal arch
3. Branch to dorsal ridge of scaphoid
4. Dorsal intercarpal arch
5. Basal metacarpal arch
6. Medial branch of ulnar a.

Figure 48-1 Dorsal vascular anatomy. *(From Gelberman et al, J Hand Surg, 8:367,1983. Used with permission.)*

arches. These are the radial artery, ulnar artery, and dorsal branch of the anterior interosseous artery. The frequencies and combinations change with each arch. The dorsal radiocarpal transverse arch is supplied by the radial artery 100 percent of the time and by the other two arteries approximately 75 percent of the time. The most consistently present dorsal arch is the intercarpal arch. It is located between the proximal and distal carpal rows and is supplied by the same three arteries but with different frequencies. This arch is supplied by all three arteries 53 percent of the time, by the radial and ulnar arteries 20 percent of the time, by the radial artery and dorsal branch of the anterior interosseous artery 20 percent of the time, and by the ulnar artery and dorsal branch of the anterior interosseous artery 7 percent of the time. The most variable arch on the dorsal side is the distal metacarpal arch, which is complete in only 27 percent of patients and is totally absent in 27 percent of patients. In 46 percent of patients, it is found only on the radial side. It is supplied by perforating arteries, which come through the second, third, and fourth interosseous spaces.[18]

The *volar* side of the hand also has three transverse arches (Fig. 48-2). These are the radiocarpal arch, intercarpal arch, and deep palmar arch. They are supplied by the radial,

ulnar, anterior interosseous, and deep palmar recurrent arteries. The palmar radiocarpal arch is present 100 percent of the time, receiving contributions from the radial, anterior interosseous, and ulnar arteries in 87 percent of patients. In 13 percent of patients, there is no contribution from the anterior interosseous artery. The vessel runs approximately 8 mm proximal to the radiocarpal joint within the wrist capsule. The palmar intercarpal arch runs between the proximal and distal carpal rows and is the most variable, being present in only 53 percent of patients. It receives contributions from the radial, ulnar, and anterior interosseous arteries in 75 percent of patients studied. The anterior interosseous artery is absent in the remaining 25 percent. The palmar radiocarpal arch provides the predominant blood supply to the lunate and triquetrum.[18]

Most of the carpal bones receive their blood supply from these transverse arches, both dorsal and palmar. The dorsal intercarpal arch is the largest of the arches and provides the major supply to the distal carpal row. It also contributes to the lunate and triquetrum. The dorsal radiocarpal arch is the second largest, supplying the distal radial metaphysis, lunate, and triquetrum. The vessels to the scaphoid come directly from the radial artery. The pisiform has vessels coming di-

1. Palmar branch, anterior interosseous a.
2. Palmar radiocarpal arch
3. Palmar intercarpal arch
4. Deep palmar arch
5. Superficial palmar arch
6. Radial recurrent a.
7. Ulnar recurrent a.
8. Medial branch, ulnar a.
9. Branch off ulnar a. to dorsal intercarpal arch

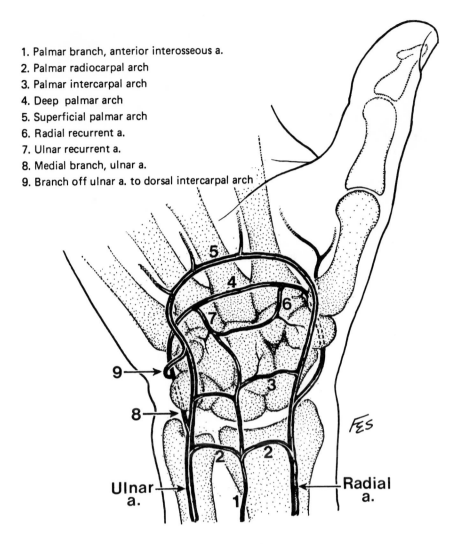

Figure 48-2 Volar vascular anatomy. *(From Gelberman et al, J Hand Surg, 8:367, 1983. Used with permission.)*

rectly from the ulnar artery. It should be noted from the preceding description that the posterior interosseous artery contributes little to the blood supply of the carpal bones.

The intraosseous blood supply of the carpal bones has been studied by Panagis et al.[45] They showed that the vessels supplying each bone enter through the noncartilaginous surfaces at sites of ligamentous attachments. It was found that 80 percent of the lunate bones had both a palmar and a dorsal blood supply, but 20 percent had only a palmar vessel.

In the *scaphoid,* the predominant blood supply is from the radial artery. Two major vessels, one dorsal and one volar, enter through the nonarticulating surface. The volar supply enters through the tubercle of the scaphoid and accounts for 20 to 30 percent of the intraosseous blood supply. The dorsal supply enters through the oblique ridge running from the radial articular surface to the trapezial trapezoid surface. Of this supply, 70 percent comes directly from the radial artery, 23 percent from the common stem of the intercarpal artery, and 7 percent from both intercarpal and radial arteries.[18] Panagis et al found no vessels entering through the scapholunate ligament. Both the dorsal and the volar supply occurred through the distal half of the scaphoid, with the proximal 70 to 80 percent of the scaphoid being supplied by the dorsal branch. There was no appreciable intraosseous

anastomosis between the dorsal and volar branches. This finding correlates well with the clinical experience of an increased incidence of avascular necrosis with more proximal scaphoid fractures. This limited blood supply probably accounts for the fact that avascular necrosis of the scaphoid secondary to fractures occurs with an incidence second only to the incidence found in the femoral head.

The *capitate* has four vessels that enter in its distal two-thirds on the dorsal aspect. There are on rare occasion small vessels entering proximally at the neck.[45] On the palmar surface, there are between one and three vessels entering more proximally than the dorsal vessels but still within the distal one-half of the bone. In one-third of patients studied, the entire head of the capitate was supplied from the palmar side without any dorsal contribution. Seventy percent of capitates were found to have no intraosseous anastomoses between the volar and dorsal vessels. The head of the capitate therefore is totally dependent on retrograde flow for its blood supply. This finding was confirmed by Vander Grend et al.[61] It has been observed that of the carpal bones, only the scaphoid, capitate, and 20 percent of the lunates have either a vessel entering only one surface or a large intraosseous area dependent on only one vessel.[45] These are also the carpal bones most commonly affected by avascular necrosis.

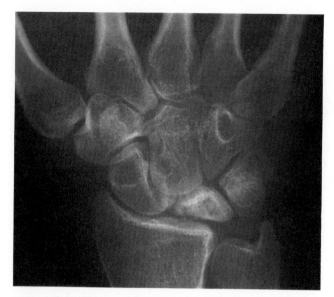

Figure 48-3 Negative ulnar variance; the distal end of the ulna is proximal to the distal end of the radius. With neutral variance, the two ends are equal. With positive variance, the distal end of the ulna is distal to the distal end of the radius.

Lunate Necrosis (Kienböck's Disease)

The correlation between negative ulnar variance and the increased incidence of avascular necrosis of the lunate was described by Hulten (Fig. 48-3).[25] A recent study[19] found the mean ulnar variance in the normal black population to be $+0.70$ mm, in the normal white population to be $+0.27$ mm, and in patients with Kienböck's disease to be -1.40 mm. The disease is rare in the black population. Also the ulnar variance was observed to be bilaterally symmetrical in normal patients but asymmetrical in 6 of 15 patients with avascular necrosis of the lunate. Overall, the incidence of negative ulnar variance in patients with avascular necrosis of the lunate was 87 percent. It has been hypothesized that the lunate receives its greatest shear stress when forced into an ulnar-deviating position. This may account for the increased evidence of Kienböck's disease noted in a population of patients with severe cerebral palsy causing wrist deviation.[52] In a wrist with a negative ulnar variance, there is increased shear in compression on the lunate, which may cause microfractures and avascular changes.

Palmer et al studied the relation between ulnar variance and the thickness of the triangular fibrocartilage complex.[44] They believed the triangular fibrocartilage functions as a stabilizer of the distal radioulnar joint, or as a cushion that transmits the axial loads between the ulnar carpus and the forearm. Although they reported an increase in the thickness of the thinnest portion of the disk in patients with negative ulnar variance, this was not found in all patients. It was thought that a thin disk in association with a negative ulnar variance put the patient at increased risk for development of avascular necrosis of the lunate. Procedures designed to re-

duce the variance to normal presumably provide a buttressing of the ulnar column, allowing more stress to pass through this column thereby decreasing the shearing stress.[2]

Transient radiographic changes consistent with a diagnosis of avascular necrosis of the lunate were seen in 3 of 24 patients after fracture-dislocation or dislocation of the carpus.[66] These all resolved spontaneously, and therefore expectant treatment is indicated in this situation.

Necrosis of the Scaphoid

Avascular necrosis of the scaphoid associated with a fracture is common. It has been reported to occur in 16 percent of patients in whom a scaphoid nonunion has developed.[13] Unassociated with a fracture it is known as *Preiser's disease*. This is in fact rare, and was first reported in the German literature in 1911. Additional reports have since been published.[1,3,8,14,27]

Necrosis of the Capitate

In the capitate, avascular necrosis has been associated most commonly with severe trauma.[42,61] It has also been linked with the use of tools producing extreme vibration.[26] When trauma has been suggested as the cause, it has most often been a dorsiflexion injury. A scaphocapitate syndrome consisting of avascular necrosis of the capitate after a transscaphoid-transcapitate-perilunate fracture-dislocation has been described.[61] Rarely, it has been reported unassociated with trauma.[6,28] As might be suspected from vascular studies of the capitate, it is the proximal pole of the bone that becomes avascular.

Necrosis of the Metacarpals

The rare cases of avascular necrosis of metacarpal bones have been associated with either trauma or systemic diseases.[3,10,32]

Necrosis of the Capitellum

Osteochondritis dissecans at the elbow mostly affects the capitellum, which is involved in 6 percent of patients with the disease. It usually occurs in the midteens, but a more acute form with fragmentation of the entire ossific nucleus of the capitellum is termed *Panner's disease*. The overlying hyaline cartilage remains normal histologically as it receives its nutrition from the synovial fluid. The underlying bone becomes infarcted. With the consequent softening of the underlying bone, the cartilage loses its support and may fracture. If it separates, it becomes an intraarticular loose body.

Repetitive trauma has been believed to be the major cause of osteochondritis dissecans of the capitellum.[29,53] Several authors have observed that the radial head is larger on the affected side. Smillie considered that repetitive compression between the radial head and capitellum accounts for the lesion.[53]

Necrosis of the Humeral Head

Trauma is the major cause of avascular necrosis of the proximal humerus. The vascular supply of the proximal humerus enters through the greater and lesser tuberosities. In a four-part fracture as described by Neer, the humeral diaphysis and the greater and lesser tuberosities are separated from the head.[40] With the loss of vascularization, the incidence of avascular necrosis is high. The vascular supply of the proximal humerus is also jeopardized by the use of prednisone. With the consequent softening of the bone, the articular surface loses its congruity, and osteoarthritis is the final result.

CLINICAL DIAGNOSIS

History

A history of systemic disease, particularly one for which prednisone or other corticosteroids were used, should alert the physician to the possibility of this diagnosis. Symptoms frequently arise several months after any trauma or use of medication. Patients usually complain of pain, stiffness, swelling, and weakness of the involved extremity.

A history of pain and swelling is most common when the elbow is affected. Heavy involvement in a throwing sport, particularly pitching, should suggest the possibility of osteochondritis dissecans of the capitellum. Maximum pain is noted with full extension. Once a fragment has become detached and is loose, locking may also occur. A painful arc of motion is the complaint in patients with shoulder involvement.

Physical Examination

On physical examination, the patient's wrist or elbow may demonstrate a mild swelling consistent with a synovitis that frequently accompanies the avascular process in the early stages. Palpation elicits tenderness in this area, which is usually localized to the diseased bone. Impairment of wrist motion is often in all planes. In patients with more advanced avascular necrosis of the lunate, evidence of scapholunate dislocation may be found. Moberg thinks that in many patients with Kienböck's disease, if symptoms of carpal tunnel syndrome are sought, they will be found.[36] Electrodiagnostic tests showed abnormalities in 50 percent of his patients examined. At the elbow, loss of extension is characteristic, and a painful limited range of motion is observed at the shoulder.

Diagnostic Aids

The diagnosis of avascular necrosis is usually confirmed by radiography. In the earliest stages the radiographs are normal, but in most patients a bone scan shows an increased uptake of contrast material in the area of disease.[5] Scan changes frequently precede radiographic changes by several months. Magnetic resonance imaging is capable of detecting areas of avascular necrosis.[50] Whether or not this test will become the best method of early diagnosis remains to be seen. The earliest radiographic change is a slight increase in

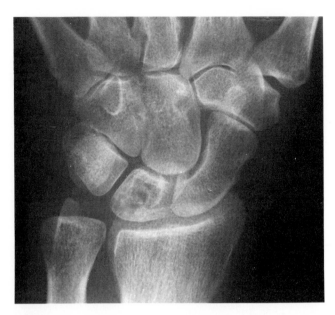

Figure 48-4 Stage 2 Kienböck's disease. Note cyst.

the relative density of the involved bone. Later, cystic changes (Fig. 48-4), fragmentation, and collapse of the diseased bone are seen. Tomography can be useful in identification of occult fractures in the earliest stages and for quantitation of fragmentation, which may be obscured on the plain films. For the lunate, the lateral projection is most useful (Fig. 48-5). As the process progresses in the wrist, collapse occurs with disorganization of the carpal relation. Eventually osteoarthritis becomes evident.

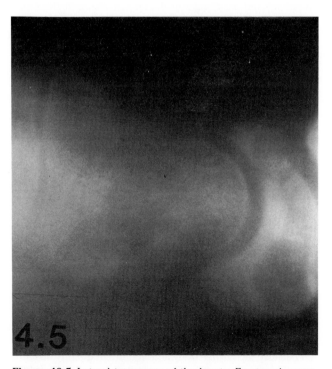

Figure 48-5 Lateral tomogram of the lunate. Fracture is more easily visible than on a plain radiograph.

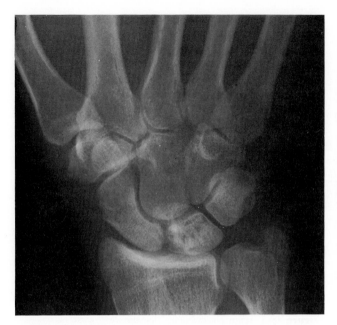

Figure 48-6 Stage 2 Kienböck's disease. Note increased density of lunate with maintenance of normal height.

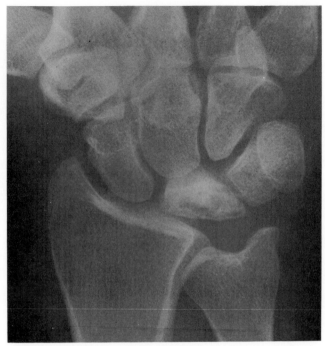

Figure 48-7 Stage 3 Kienböck's disease. The lunate is flattened with loss of carpal height.

Lichtman et al[31] have described four stages of Kienböck's disease, which may be useful in determining treatment. The first stage is characterized by acute symptoms of wrist sprain, normal radiographs, and sometimes fracture shown by tomography. In the second stage, radiographs show an increase in density but no change in the size or shape of the lunate (Fig. 48-6). Pain and evidence of synovitis are present. In the third stage, lunate collapse occurs with proximal migration of the capitate and loss of the normal carpal architecture (Fig. 48-7). The lunate may appear elongated on the lateral film, and stiffness in the wrist is increased. Finally, in the fourth stage, degenerative changes of osteoarthritis are present (Fig. 48-8).

At the elbow, the characteristic finding is an island of subchondral bone surrounded by a radiolucent zone. On the lateral view, cystic changes or flattening of the capitellum may be seen.

The radiographic changes at the proximal humerus are similar to those at the proximal femur. A crescent sign may be apparent. The appearance of radiodensities and cysts is followed by collapse of the articulating surface (Fig. 48-9).

The differential diagnoses include other painful pathological conditions of the joint: degenerative or posttraumatic arthritis, rheumatoid arthritis with synovitis, acute infection, metabolic inflammatory conditions, and ligamentous instabilities of the wrist. Although differentiation between these entities on the examination may be difficult, the bone scan, tomogram, and radiograph are usually quite definitive. An index of suspicion with respect to the capitellum is particularly helpful because the normal bony architecture frequently obscures the disease on the plain films. Similarly, an open epiphysis may make the bone scan much less useful. In these instances

tomography is especially valuable. Of importance in evaluating the radiographs is to look for evidence of degenerative changes. Their presence will considerably alter the treatment plan.

TREATMENT

Various treatments have been recommended for each of the bones of the upper extremities that may become involved in avascular necrosis (Table 48-1). Probably the largest variety

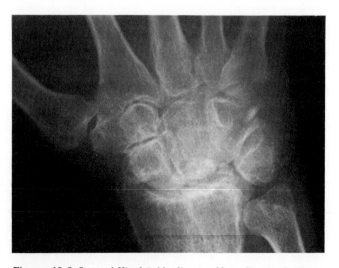

Figure 48-8 Stage 4 Kienböck's disease. Note disorganization of carpal bones and evidence of osteoarthritis.

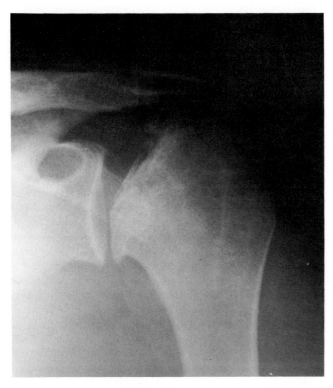

Figure 48-9 Avascular necrosis of the proximal humerus. Collapse of articulating surface with loss of congruity is illustrated.

of treatments have been recommended for the lunate. As in most areas of medicine, these large numbers of different methods of treatment reflect a lack of overwhelming success with any one of them.

Scaphoid

In the majority of patients, avascular necrosis of the scaphoid bone occurs secondary to fracture. This may or may not be associated with a nonunion. When nonunion is present, this aspect of the problem usually receives the attention, with the hope that its adequate healing will resolve the avascular process. Treatment of a nonunion in the scaphoid is discussed in another section of the text. Avascular necrosis has not been considered a contraindication to bone grafting techniques in the treatment of nonunion of the scaphoid. However, Green has found that if the proximal portion is totally avascular at the time of operation, none of the fractures will unite.[20] He also reported that only direct inspection at the time of operation, looking for punctate bleeding points, is useful in identifying the totally avascular bone.[20] Some persistence of the avascular process frequently occurs if the union does not become complete.[13] In those patients in whom avascular necrosis develops after a fracture of the scaphoid despite its adequate healing, prolonged immobilization is probably the best initial treatment. An alternative consideration is a vascularized pedicle bone graft using the pronator quadratus.[7]

TABLE 48-1 Described Treatments for Kienböck's Disease

Procedure	Reference	Advantages	Disadvantages	Comment
Immobilization	54	Avoids need for operation	Results not reproduced by others	Use for stage 1
Radial shortening	2	Leaves carpus alone	Does not address scapholunate dissociation	Use for stage 2
Ulnar lengthening	47, 59	Leaves carpus alone	Technically difficult with nonunion	
Dorsal flap arthroplasty	39	No foreign material	Poor support resulting in late carpal collapse	
Tendon interposition	48	No foreign material	Poor support for carpals	
Silastic interposition arthroplasty	55		Silicone synovitis, fractured or dislocated prosthesis	Use in conjunction with triscaphe fusion
Capitate-hamate fusion	12	Technically easy	Limited support	Use for stage 2
Triscaphe fusion	64	Excellent support, removes stress from lunate and reduces scapholunate dissociation	50% loss of wrist motion	Appropriate for stages 2 and 3
Vessel transplantation	7, 24	Increases blood supply to devascularized bone	Technically difficult	

In patients with Preiser's disease in whom no fracture has been noted, prolonged immobilization has not always been effective in preventing collapse of the proximal pole. Treatment in these cases, and in those in which collapses occurred after a fracture, has included resection of the proximal pole with interposition arthroplasty of tendon. Alternatively, Silastic and total silicone elastomer replacement of the scaphoid have been used by Swanson.[55] More recently, Swanson et al[57] have advocated adding a lunate-capitate fusion to minimize the stress loading on the silicone implant. The hope is that this will minimize breakdown of the implant and silicone synovitis. Several authors have pointed out the risk of these complications.[4,11,46,57] Silicone synovitis is most common when the silicone is required to bear a large stress load. The scaphoid and the lunate are the two most common replacements to result in a silicone synovitis. Although at one time Swanson[56] suggested stabilizing these implants with Kirschner's wires in the immediate postoperative period, this has now been found to be associated with an increased incidence of silicone synovitis.[11] For this reason, avoidance of Kirschner wire stabilization of the silicone implants is strongly recommended. Displacement or subluxation of the implants has been a consistent concern.[56]

In late cases in which arthritis has developed, not only in the joints of the scaphoid but also in the lunate-capitate joint, and there is advanced scapholunate collapse,[62] a combination of silicone replacement with lunate-capitate fusion or other fusion combination of the arthritic joints is mandatory. When several good joints still remain within the wrist, fusing only the affected joints seems worthwhile. Another option is a proximal row carpectomy with removal of the scaphoid and lunate if the articular surface of the capitate and lunar facet of the radius are intact. This procedure preserves a degree of motion and relieves pain in most patients. A total wrist arthrodesis remains an ultimate option.

Lunate

Treatment of avascular necrosis of the lunate is best considered in terms of the stages described by Lichtman et al (Table 48-1).[31] A reasonable consensus exists concerning the treatment of stages 1 and 4, but opinions concerning the treatment of stages 2 and 3 differ greatly. In patients with stage 1 disease with no appreciable radiographic changes, early cast immobilization with nonsteroidal anti-inflammatory drugs to minimize the synovitis is appropriate. Without the use of a bone scan or magnetic resonance imaging, it is not likely that the specific diagnosis would be made in these patients.

In stage 4 disease in which there is severe collapse and disorganization of the carpus with degenerative changes, a salvage procedure is indicated. As with the scaphoid, this may be a proximal row carpectomy, total wrist replacement, or partial or total wrist arthrodesis.

The prognosis for patients with stage 2 disease is better than for those with stage 3 disease. In stage 2, immobilization has been reported to give good results.[54] However, disappointments have also occurred.[16,31] For this reason, many physicians have turned to operation to protect the lunate from stress. In stage 2, when there has not been appreciable

collapse of the lunate, those procedures that do not require removal of the lunate and are designed to minimize the stress on the diseased lunate have a definite advantage. The hypothesis is that the unloaded lunate will not collapse and that with time the natural pathogenesis may result in revascularization of the lunate.

Based on observations of the relation between negative ulnar variance and the development of avascular necrosis of the lunate, procedures have been developed to minimize the discrepancy in length between these two bones.[2,36,47,59] In assessing negative ulnar variance, it is important to use standardized radiographs as described by Palmer et al[43] Differences in forearm rotation change the apparent ulnar variance. Thus, these authors suggest using a posteroanterior film of the wrist in neutral pronation and supination, which is obtained by abducting the shoulder 90°. The discrepancy between the two bones can be corrected by either lengthening the ulna or shortening the radius. The obvious advantage of this approach to the problem is that the bones of the wrist joint are left untouched, and when reconstitution of the lunate is successful an essentially normal wrist is preserved. It has the disadvantage, however, of being useful only in patients with a demonstrable negative ulnar variance. Because of the variation in the thickness of the triangular fibrocartilage,[44] it is hard to be certain on the basis of the radiograph alone of the amount of change required. The method also does not address the problem of scapholunate dissociation. Of the two possible procedures in this approach, radial shortening is probably the easier technically. Ulnar lengthening obviously requires bone grafting, and both procedures are probably best performed with meticulous rigid fixation techniques. The method has been used successfully for both stage 2 and stage 3 disease.[2,47,59] However, it was pointed out in the report of Almquist and Burns[2] that pain is not relieved completely, particularly if patients participate in strenuous activity. All patients obtain some increase in range of motion of the wrist postoperatively.

Procedures involving excision of the lunate bone have been reported widely. These include excision with replacement using various spacers, such as tendon,[48] Silastic rubber,[55] and dorsal flap arthroplasty.[39] All rely on the replacement to take the stresses previously passed through the lunate. Although successes have been reported with all the procedures, late carpal collapse and disorganization have been common. Therefore, additional procedures have been developed to maintain a better support of the carpus. In some patients, these have been used in combination with excision of the lunate. However, if the lunate is truly unloaded by these procedures, then it does not seem necessary to excise even a fragmented lunate when performing one of them. Specifically, two forms of intercarpal fusion have been described. Chuinard has suggested the capitate-hamate fusion.[12] He believes that once the hamate has united with the capitate, proximal migration of the capitate is prevented by a mass action effect. The central carpal pillar is supported by the stable ulnar hamate-triquetrum pillar, and the lunate is no longer forced by the descending capitate against the ulnar rim of the radius. The theory is not universally accepted. This fusion seems to provide only limited support to the lunate. Thus, the procedure should probably be reserved for patients

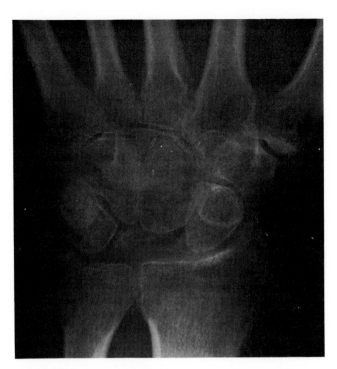

Figure 48-10 Loss of carpal height and organization after successful capitate-hamate fusion.

with stage 2 disease. When used in stage 3 disease, with excision of the lunate, additional collapse and carpal disorganization have been seen (Fig. 48-10).

Watson et al have reported the scaphotrapezial trapezoid (triscaphe) fusion.[63,64] With a triscaphe fusion, carpal collapse is prevented by fixing the scaphoid. Flexing and "shortening" of the scaphoid are consequently eliminated. A stable strut is produced maintaining the carpal height and decompressing the lunate during wrist motion. Although wrist motion is limited compared with the normal range, it frequently is better than the range of motion in a patient who has presented with acute avascular necrosis of the lunate. It is important in performing the triscaphe fusion not to straighten the scaphoid excessively but to place it at its normal angle of 45 degrees in relation to the articular axis of the lunate. Also, the outside dimensions of the bones involved in the fusion must be maintained. If the bones are forced together after resection of the cartilaginous surfaces, the carpal bones are immediately thrust into an abnormal pattern.

Use of revascularization procedures as described by Hori et al should probably be limited to those patients with stage 2 disease.[24]

Radiographically, the best method of quantitating the effectiveness of these procedures is to monitor the carpal height. McMurtry et al have described the most accepted method of recording this measurement.[34] Progression of carpal collapse is indicative of the degree of failure of treatment. Clinically, there seems to be good correlation between prevention of additional collapse and resolution of symptoms.

Capitate

In the early stages of avascular necrosis of the head of the capitate, particularly when associated with a fracture, treatment is best accomplished by bone grafting.[61] If this is unsuccessful or collapse has occurred, clinical improvement has been reported with resection of the proximal pole and interposition arthroplasty,[28] resection of diseased bone and drilling,[38] and cast immobilization.[49] However, the follow-up periods in these studies were short. Intercarpal fusion will probably give more reliable long-term results. Total wrist replacement and wrist arthrodesis remain as salvage procedures.

Metacarpals

The metacarpals may be affected in patients with severe systemic disease receiving prednisone,[32] and in this situation surgical intervention on the basis of the radiographic findings is usually not indicated. However, when the condition is secondary to isolated trauma and presents as a localized process, resection arthroplasty is probably the procedure of choice. This should only be performed after an adequate trial of appropriate rest and nonsteroidal anti-inflammatory medications.

Capitellum

Osteochondritis dissecans may frequently respond to conservative care.[33,51,53,67] Activity modification, splints, and nonsteroidal anti-inflammatory drugs are the mainstays of this form of treatment. If symptoms persist or there are signs of a loose body, then arthrotomy is indicated. In this non-weight-bearing joint, the simpler the procedure the better.

Removal of any loose fragments and drilling the base of the defect are recommended. Poorer results were found in the more complex bone-grafting procedures.[67] Drilling is thought to aid in the return of blood supply to the area and the production of cartilage. This cartilage may fill the defect, but its quality is not the same as that of normal hyaline cartilage.

Loss of elbow extension is the most common complication of procedures for osteochondritis dissecans.

Proximal Humerus

In patients with four-part fracture of the proximal humerus, the incidence of avascular necrosis is so high that primary hemiarthroplasty is usual.[41] Recently attempts at open reduction with internal fixation have been advocated.[37] Efforts to save the humeral head are particularly important in younger patients.[9] Among those in whom the condition is not secondary to trauma, a trial of conservative care in the form of rest and administration of nonsteroidal anti-inflammatory agents is indicated. When conservative care is not adequate in relieving the symptoms of avascular necrosis of the head of the humerus, total arthroplasty or hemiarthroplasty is indicated. These procedures are discussed elsewhere in this text.

REFERENCES

1. Allen, P.R. Idiopathic avascular necrosis of the scaphoid: A report of two cases. J Bone Joint Surg 65B:333–335, 1983.
2. Almquist, E.E., and Burns, J.F., Jr. Radial shortening for the treatment of Kienböck's disease—A 5- to 10-year follow-up. J Hand Surg 7:348–352, 1982.
3. Aptekar, R.G., Klippel, J.H., Becker, K.E., Carson, D.A., Seaman, W.E., and Decker, J.L. Avascular necrosis of the talus, scaphoid, and metatarsal head in systemic lupus erythematosus. Clin Orthop 101:127–128, 1974.
4. Atkinson, R.E., Smith, R.J., and Jupiter, J.B. Silicone synovitis of the wrist. Presented at the annual meeting of the American Society for Surgery of the Hand, Las Vegas, Nevada, 1985.
5. Bellmore, M.C., Cummine, J.L., Crocker, E.F., and Carseldine, D.B. The role of bone scans in the assessment of prognosis of scaphoid fractures. Aust NZ J Surg 53:133–137, 1983.
6. Bolton-Maggs, B.G., Helal, B.H., and Revell, P.A. Bilateral avascular necrosis of the capitate: A case report and a review of the literature. J Bone Joint Surg 66B:557–559, 1984.
7. Braun, R.M. Pronator pedicle bone grafting in the forearm and proximal carpal row. Orthop Trans 7:35, 1983.
8. Bray, T.J., and McCarroll, H.R., Jr. Preiser's disease: A case report. J Hand Surg 9A:730–732, 1984.
9. Bucholz, R.W. Orthopaedic trauma, in Bucholz, R.W., Lippert, F.G., III, Wenger, D.R., and Ezaki, M. (eds): *Orthopaedic Decision Making.* Philadelphia, Decker, 1984, pp 18–19.
10. Carstam, N., and Danielsson, L.G. Aseptic necrosis of the head of the fifth metacarpal. Acta Orthop Scand 37:297–300, 1966.
11. Carter, P.R., and Benton, L.J. Late osseous complications of carpal silastic implants. Presented at the annual meeting of the American Society for Surgery of the Hand, Las Vegas, Nevada, 1985.
12. Chuinard, R.G. Capitate-hamate fusion in the treatment of Kienböck's disease, in Tubiana, R. (ed): *The Hand.* Philadelphia, Saunders, 1985, pp 1117–1120.
13. Cooney, W.P., Linscheid, R.L., and Dobyns, J.H. Scaphoid fractures: Problems associated with nonunion and avascular necrosis. Orthop Clin North Am 15:381–391, 1984.
14. Ekerot, L., and Eiken, O. Idiopathic avascular necrosis of the scaphoid: Case report. Scand J Plast Surg 15:69–72, 1981.
15. Gelberman, R.H., and Menon, J. The vascularity of the scaphoid bone. J Hand Surg 5:508–513, 1980.
16. Gelberman, R.H., and Szabo, R.M. Kienböck's disease. Orthop Clin North Am 15:355–367, 1984.
17. Gelberman, R.H., Bauman, T.D., Menon, J., and Akeson, W.H. The vascularity of the lunate bone and Kienböck's disease. J Hand Surg 5:272–278, 1980.
18. Gelberman, R.H., Panagis, J.S., Taleisnik, J., and Baumgaertner, M. The arterial anatomy of the human carpus. Part I: The extraosseous vascularity. J Hand Surg 8:367–375, 1983.
19. Gelberman, R.H., Salamon, P.B., Jurist, J.M., and Posch, J.L. Ulnar variance in Kienböck's disease. J Bone Joint Surg 57A:674–676, 1975.
20. Green, D.P. The effect of avascular necrosis on Russe bone grafting for scaphoid nonunion. J Hand Surg 10A:597–605, 1985.
21. Griffiths, I.D., Maini, R.N., and Scott, J.T. Clinical and radiological features of osteonecrosis in systemic lupus erythematosus. Ann Rheum Dis 38:413–422, 1979.
22. Harper, P.G., Trash, C., and Souhami, R.I. Avascular necrosis of bone caused by combination chemotherapy without corticosteroids. Br Med J 288:267–268, 1984.
23. Harrington, K.D., Murray, W.R., Kountz, S.L., and Belzer, F.O. Avascular necrosis of bone after renal transplantation. J Bone Joint Surg 53A:203–215, 1971.
24. Hori, Y., Tamai, S., Okuda, H., Sakamoto, H., Takita, T., and Masuhara, K. Blood vessel transplantation to bone. J Hand Surg 4:23–33, 1979.
25. Hulten, O. Über anatomische Variationen der Handgelenkknochen: Ein Beitrag zur Kenntnis der Genese zwei verschiedener Mondbeinveränderungen. Acta Radiol 9:155–168, 1928.
26. James, E.T.R., and Burke, F.D. Vibration disease of the capitate. J Hand Surg 9B:169–170, 1984.
27. Kawai, H., Tsuyuguchi, Y., Yonenobu, K., Inoue, A., and Tada, K. Avascular necrosis of the carpal scaphoid associated with progressive systemic sclerosis. Hand 15:270–273, 1983.
28. Kimmel, R.B., and O'Brien, E.T. Surgical treatment of avascular necrosis of the proximal pole of the capitate—Case report. J Hand Surg 7:284–286, 1982.
29. King, J., Brelsford, H.J., and Tullos, H.S. Analysis of the pitching arm of the professional baseball pitcher. Clin Orthop 67:116–123, 1969.
30. Lanzer, W., Szabo, R., and Gelberman, R. Avascular necrosis of the lunate and sickle cell anemia: A case report. Clin Orthop 187:168–171, 1984.
31. Lichtman, D.M., Mack, G.R., MacDonald, R.I., Gunther, S.F., and Wilson, J.N. Kienböck's disease: The role of silicone replacement arthroplasty. J Bone Joint Surg 59A:899–908, 1977.
32. Lightfoot, R.W., Jr., and Lotke, P.A. Osteonecrosis of metacarpal heads in systemic lupus erythematosus: Value of radiostrontium scintimetry in differential diagnosis. Arthritis Rheum 15:486–492, 1972.
33. Lindholm, T.S., Osterman, K., and Vankka, E. Osteochondritis dissecans of elbow, ankle and hip: A comparison survey. Clin Orthop 148:245–253, 1980.
34. McMurtry, R.Y., Youm, Y., Flatt, A.E., and Gillespie, T.E. Kinematics of the wrist. II. Clinical applications. J Bone Joint Surg 60A:955–961, 1978.
35. Match, R.M. Nonspecific avascular necrosis of the pisiform bone: A case report. J Hand Surg 5:341–342, 1980.
36. Moberg, E. Treatment of Kienböck's disease by surgical correction of the length of the radius or ulna, in Tubiana, R. (ed): *The Hand.* Philadelphia, Saunders, 1985, pp 1117–1120.
37. Müller, M.E., Allgöwer, M., Schneider, R., and Willenegger, H. *Manual of Internal Fixation: Techniques Recommended by the AO Group,* 2d ed., Schatzker, J. (trans). New York, Springer-Verlag, 1979, pp 172–173.
38. Murakami, S., and Nakajima, H. Aseptic necrosis of the capitate bone in two gymnasts. Am J Sports Med 12:170–173, 1984.
39. Nahigian, C.S., Richey, D.G., and Shaw, D.T. The dorsal flap arthroplasty in the treatment of Kienböck's disease. J Bone Joint Surg 52A:245–252, 1970.
40. Neer, C.S., II. Displaced proximal humeral fractures. Part I. Classification and evaluation. J Bone Joint Surg 52A:1077–1089, 1970.
41. Neer, C.S., II. Displaced proximal humeral fractures. Part II. Treatment of three-part and four-part displacement. J Bone Joint Surg 52A:1090–1103, 1970.
42. Newman, J.H., and Watt, I. Avascular necrosis of the capitate and dorsal dorsi-flexion instability. Hand 12:176–178, 1980.
43. Palmer, A.K., Glisson, R.R., and Werner, F.W. Ulnar variance determination. J Hand Surg 7:376–379, 1982.
44. Palmer, A.K., Glisson, R.R., and Werner, F.W. Relationship between ulnar variance and triangular fibrocartilage complex thickness. J Hand Surg 9A:681–683, 1984.
45. Panagis, J.S., Gelberman, R.H., Taleisnik, J., and Baumgaertner, M. The arterial anatomy of the human carpus. Part II: The intraosseous vascularity. J Hand Surg 8:375–382, 1983.
46. Peimer, C.A., Medige, J., Eckert, B.S., and Wright, J.R. Invasive silicone synovitis of the wrist. Presented at the annual meeting of the American Society for Surgery of the Hand, Las Vegas, Nevada, 1985.

47. Persson, M. Causal treatment of lunatomalacia: Further experiences of operative ulnar lengthening. Acta Chir Scand 100:531–544, 1950.
48. Qvick, L.I., and Wilhelm, K.H. Tendon interposition arthroplasty after resection of necrotic carpal bone. Aust NZ J Surg 50:272–277, 1980.
49. Rahme, H. Idiopathic avascular necrosis of the capitate bone—Case report. Hand 15:274–275, 1983.
50. Reis, N.D., Lanir, A., Benmair, J., and Hadar, H. Magnetic resonance imaging in orthopaedic surgery: A glimpse into the future. J Bone Joint Surg 67B:659–664, 1985.
51. Roberts, N., and Hughes, R. Osteochondritis dissecans of the elbow joint: A clinical study. J Bone Joint Surg 32B:348–360, 1950.
52. Rooker, G.D., and Goodfellow, J.W. Kienböck's disease in cerebral palsy. J Bone Joint Surg 59B:363–365, 1977.
53. Smillie, I. *Osteochondritis Dissecans.* London, Livingstone, 1960.
54. Stahl, F. On lunatomalacia (Kienböck's disease): A clinical and roentgenological study, especially on its pathogenesis and the late results of immobilization treatment. Acta Chir Scand 95(suppl 126):1–133, 1947.
55. Swanson, A.B. Silicone rubber implants for the replacement of the carpal scaphoid and lunate bones. Orthop Clin North Am 1:299–309, 1970.
56. Swanson, A.B. Reconstructive surgery in the arthritic hand and foot. Clin Symp 31:22–28, 1979.
57. Swanson, A.B., Wilson, K.M., Mayhew, D.E., Page, B.J., II, Swanson, G. de G., and Maupin, B.K. Long-term bone response around carpal bone implants. Presentation and poster exhibit at the annual meeting of the American Society for Surgery of the Hand, Las Vegas, Nevada, 1985.
58. Taleisnik, J., and Kelly, P.J. The extraosseous and intraosseous blood supply of the scaphoid bone. J Bone Joint Surg 48A:1125–1137, 1966.
59. Tillberg, B. Kienböck's disease treated with osteotomy to lengthen ulna. Acta Orthop Scand 39:359–369, 1968.
60. Urman, J.D., Abeles, M., Houghton, A.N., and Rothfield, N.F. Aseptic necrosis presenting as wrist pain in SLE. Arthritis Rheum 20:825–828, 1977.
61. Vander Grend, R., Dell, P.C., Glowczewskie, F., Leslie, B., and Ruby, L.K. Intraosseous blood supply of the capitate and its correlation with aseptic necrosis. J Hand Surg 9A:677–680, 1984.
62. Watson, H.K., and Ballet, F.L. The SLAC wrist: Scapholunate advanced collapse pattern of degenerative arthritis. J Hand Surg 9:358–365, 1984.
63. Watson, H.K., and Hempton, R.F. Limited wrist arthrodeses. I. The triscaphoid joint. J Hand Surg 5:320–327, 1980.
64. Watson, H.K., Ryu, J., and DiBella, A. An approach to Kienböck's disease: Triscaphe arthrodesis. J Hand Surg 10A:179–187, 1985.
65. Weissman, B.N., Rappoport, A.S., Sosman, J.L., and Schur, P.H. Radiographic findings in the hands in patients with systemic lupus erythematosus. Diagn Radiol 126:313–317, 1978.
66. White, R.E., Jr., and Omer, G.E., Jr. Transient vascular compromise of the lunate after fracture-dislocation of the carpus. J Hand Surg 9A:181–184, 1984.
67. Woodward, A.H., and Bianco, A.J., Jr. Osteochondritis dissecans of the elbow. Clin Orthop 110:35–41, 1975.

CHAPTER 49

Specialized Rehabilitation Problems and Techniques in the Upper Extremity

Patricia Connolly, Ira Wolfe, Louis U. Bigliani, Meredith Cook Ferraro, and Joan Lehmann

SECTION A

Rehabilitation of the Shoulder

Patricia Connolly, Ira Wolfe, and Louis U. Bigliani

The exercise prescription for shoulder rehabilitation should specify the type of exercise, the amount of resistance, the number of times the exercise is to be performed, and the number of training sessions per week.

It is difficult to predict the amount of resistance necessary to stress the muscles and thus cause a training overload without injuring the patient. The severity of the injury, and the initial strength level, are necessary information in order to estimate the amount of work the patient will be able to do. The patient may begin with only the weight of the limb or 1 to 2 lb. If no other determinant can be found, 5 to 10 percent of body weight may be used in the initial phases, especially in the younger, stronger, or athletic patient.[11]

The number of times an exercise is performed is referred to as the *number of repetitions*. The number of times a given number of repetitions is performed is known as the *set*. The greater the number of repetitions performed, the lighter the resistance should be. Lightweight programs with multiple repetitions are for endurance and are therefore more aerobic. This type of program can be used to condition the muscle for heavier exercise. As the resistance increases, the repetitions decrease and the work becomes more anaerobic. There should be sufficient rest period between sets. Training sessions for strength should not be every day, but rather every other day, or three times a week.

BASIC SHOULDER PROGRAM

The basic principles of shoulder rehabilitation have been outlined by Hughes and Neer in a three-phase program of exercises proceeding in a step-by-step progression.[5] This program is geared primarily toward postoperative patients, but with appropriate modification it can also be utilized in many nonoperative patients.

Phase I Program

The first part of the phase I program consists of active assisted exercises which are illustrated in Fig. 49-1. They include the following:

1. *Pendulum exercises.* The patient stands bent over at the waist circling the arm outward with palm facing forward, and inward with palm facing backward. This can also be done with the upper extremity in a sling.
2. *Pulley exercises.* The patient stands or sits and grasps each end of the pulley cord. He or she uses the good arm to pull down and raise the injured arm and shoulder as high as possible.
3. *Assisted hyperextension.* Standing with a stick grasped in both hands behind the back, the patient raises the stick backward using the uninvolved arm to assist the involved arm.
4. *Assisted external rotation.* The patient lies in a supine position with the elbows flexed to 90° and gently rocks the involved forearm in and away from the body by holding a cane in both hands and using it to push the forearm out.
5. *Assisted forward flexion.* While lying on his or her back, the supine patient grasps the wrist of the injured arm with the free hand and gently raises the arms overhead.
6. *Full external rotation.* The supine patient raises the involved arm with contralateral assistance until the arm is

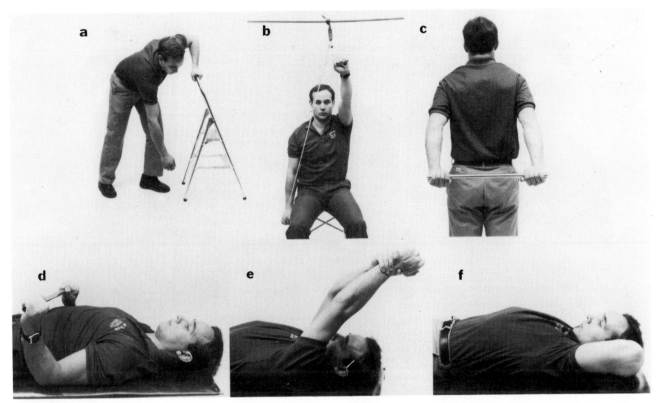

Figure 49-1 Basic shoulder program. Active assisted exercises. **a.** Pendulum exercises. **b.** Pulley exercises. **c.** Assisted hyperextension. **d.** Assisted external rotation. **e.** Assisted forward flexion. **f.** Full external rotation.

perpendicular to the table. Next the elbows are bent, bringing the hands behind the neck. The elbows are then gradually lowered out to the side, externally rotating the shoulder. The motion is then reversed.

There should be an order and time frame at which these exercises are started in the postoperative period. This depends on the specific surgery. For example, for glenohumeral joint replacement, pendulum exercises are started on the fourth postoperative day and followed by assorted external rotation exercises on the fifth day, pulley on the sixth day, and assisted hyperextension on the seventh day. The other exercises are then added later in the program. Each exercise should be done for 10 to 15 repetitions with three to four sets per day.

Isometric exercises constitute the second part of the phase I program. The goal here is to maintain strength and tone of all the noninvolved muscles while protecting any muscle involved in a surgical repair. With glenohumeral replacement, isometrics can be started between 17 and 21 days postoperatively.[5] These may be done first in a supine position with the affected arm at the side and the elbow flexed to 90°. The patient uses the opposite hand to give resistance to the inner forearm for internal rotation, and the outer forearm for external rotation (Fig. 49-2A). There should be a gradual buildup of muscle contraction while resistance is simultaneously increased so that no movement occurs. When the patient is competent in doing these, he or she can progress to doing the same exercises in a standing position, utilizing a

door jam for resistance. The same position is used, with the arm at the side and the elbow flexed to 90°. Isometric abduction can be performed by standing with the involved side facing a wall. With the arm at the patient's side and the elbow flexed to 90°, the patient simply pushes against the wall. Resistance to forward flexion can be done by standing with the arm in the same position, facing a wall, and pressing the fist against the wall.

Phase II Program

Phase II begins at 6 weeks and consists of active strengthening and stretching exercise. Active forward elevation is begun supine to help eliminate gravity. Using a stick, the involved arm is gently raised overhead with the uninvolved arm doing most of the work. As the operated shoulder gets stronger, the uninvolved arm does less and less work. The same gradual unweighting principle can be used with a pulley. Supine forward elevation can then be performed with a 1-lb weight which strengthens and stretches at the same time. Upright unassisted forward elevation with the elbow flexed can then be performed. A 1-lb weight may be added when tolerated by the patient.

Light resistance exercises with therapeutic elastic band or surgical tubing are also commenced. The material can be attached securely to a door knob for forward elevation, internal rotation, and extension exercises (Fig. 49-2B). For resisted

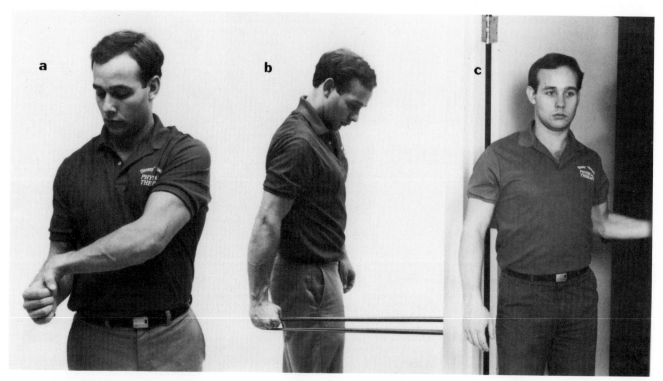

Figure 49-2 Basic shoulder program. Isometric exercises. **a.** Self-resisted isometric external rotation. **b.** Resisted shoulder extension with elastic band. **c.** Passive external rotation.

external rotation, it can be held in both hands or placed around the wrists with the arms at the side and elbow flexed to 90°.

Stretching exercises include forward elevation by holding onto the top of a door or other structure appropriate for the patient's height. Adjustments may be made by bending the knees slightly. External rotation can be obtained by standing with the affected arm in neutral and the elbow flexed to 90° and then placing the hand on the edge of a doorway and slowly rotating the body away (Fig. 49-2C). Internal rotation can be obtained by placing the involved hand behind the low back and grasping a towel between this hand and the opposite hand, which is reaching behind the head. The lower hand is gently pulled as high as possible using the towel. Phase II exercises should be done at least three times a day.

Phase III Program

Phase III is a continuation and progression of phase II. Resistance is increased by using a heavier grade of elastic band or rubber surgical tubing. Heavier weights may be used, but rarely does the weight exceed 5 lb. If the resistance is too great and/or pain occurs, then the weight should be decreased. Stretching is also intensified. The end of the door may be used to get more elevation, and the patient may also lean into the wall with an outstretched arm. Lying prone with the arm outstretched is also helpful. Exercises should be performed after a warm shower or massage. After 6 months, if full motion has been obtained, a maintenance program consisting of once-a-day stretching and strengthening exercises should be employed.

SPECIFIC APPLICATIONS

Rehabilitation following Insertion of a Shoulder Endoprosthesis

The preferred operative approach for total shoulder replacement is one which preserves the origin and insertion of the deltoid muscle. Since the only important muscle then incised is the subscapularis, active exercises can be started at 10 to 12 days. Where there is associated rotator cuff damage (e.g., in some cases of rheumatoid arthritis) and a cuff repair has been performed, then active exercises must be delayed for 6 weeks. Revision surgery must be dealt with on an individual basis.

When a prosthesis is used for a four-part fracture of the proximal humerus, repair of the tuberosities with suture or wire is necessary. In this instance, active exercises must be delayed until there is adequate bony union of the tuberosities. This should be checked with radiographs but normally takes at least 6 weeks. During this early period, it is important to prevent excessive internal rotation as this may displace the tuberosities. If for some reason the origin of the deltoid is removed, then active forward elevation must be delayed for 6 weeks. An abduction brace is rarely indicated in shoulder replacement but may have some use in severe rheumatoid patients who are stiff or to protect the deltoid if it has been advanced or transferred.

Rehabilitation following Surgery for Impingement Syndromes and Cuff Tears

When an anterior acromionoplasty for impingement without a rotator cuff tear is performed, 1 in. or less of the deltoid origin is detached from the acromion and distal clavicle. Therefore, active forward flexion should be delayed for approximately 6 weeks to protect the deltoid. All other active motion may be started earlier. When the rotator cuff has to be repaired, active external rotation and forward elevation are also delayed for 6 weeks. Isometrics for the posterior and middle deltoid may be started at 3 weeks. In cases of a large or massive rotator cuff tear, an abduction brace may be required to reduce the tension across the cuff repair. Depending on the quality of the cuff and the strength of the repair, passive exercises can be started on the fifth day in the brace without tension across the cuff repair. These exercises usually start with gentle external rotation followed by forward elevation as tolerated. The brace is usually removed at 6 weeks, but in stages. The arm is initially brought slowly down to 45°, and a pillow is placed beneath the arm for support. The patient returns the next day for removal of the pillow. Passive exercises are continued for another 2 to 3 weeks, and the arm is supported in a sling as needed. Active exercises are then started approximately 8 to 9 weeks after surgery.

Rehabilitation of the Unstable Shoulder

The goal of rehabilitation is to prevent or decrease the recurrence of shoulder dislocations and/or subluxation. Rowe found a recurrence rate of 94 percent in patients under 20 years of age and 74 percent in 20 to 40-year old patients with anterior dislocation.[13] These patients had been treated by immobilization, but the authors gave no specifics regarding their rehabilitation.

In a recent study from the U.S. Naval Academy, there was a recurrence rate of only 25 percent when a strict program of immobilization and strengthening exercises was employed.[1,2] Patients were immobilized for approximately 3 to 6 weeks. Isometric exercises, especially for internal rotators and adductors, were started at 2 weeks. Exercises then progressed from isometric to isotonic and isokinetic. Participants continued their rehabilitation until they had full strength, a negative apprehensive sign, and were able to return to all activities without incident. In posterior subluxation or dislocation the emphasis is on strength of the external rotations after a sufficient period of immobilization.[12]

Repairs for shoulder instability are usually protected for 6 weeks after surgery. For anterior instability, the arm is supported in internal rotation in a sling and swathe or shoulder immobilizer. In posterior instability, the arm is immobilized in external rotation by a cast or brace. In multidirectional instability, the arm is supported in a neutral position by a cast. Following removal of the immobilization device, passive assistive exercises to increase motion are started. Although the final goal of therapy is full motion, it is important not to get too much motion too fast as this may stretch out the repair. Isometrics to the deltoid and rotators can be started early.

Active exercises are usually begun in 2 to 3 weeks after some range of motion has been obtained. It is especially important to strengthen the anterior deltoid and internal rotators for anterior instability, and the posterior deltoid and external rotators for posterior instability. Strengthening exercises with free weights and/or weight machines are recommended.

Rehabilitation of the Frozen Shoulder

Gaining motion in a frozen shoulder can be one of the most difficult types of rehabilitation regardless of the cause. Precise measurements of starting ranges of motion should be made and serially recorded to document progress and, one hopes, to encourage the patient. Moist heat, an anti-inflammatory agent, and pain medication prior to therapy may all be necessary. The initial exercises must be gentle and should include pendulum, external rotation with a stick, and pulley exercises. The patient should be cautioned to use the pulley to bring the shoulder through a pain-free range of motion. As progress is made and confidence is gained, more stretching is added. The emphasis should be on stretching and not strengthening exercises. Passive mobilization techniques such as those described by Kaltenborn[7] and Mennell[9] may also be helpful. Peripheral nerve blocks, such as stellate ganglion block, just prior to therapy may also be helpful.[3] The patient must constantly be reassured that this is a long ongoing process that may take 6 months to a year to resolve.

Athletic Rehabilitation

The primary goal of a shoulder rehabilitation program for athletes should be a safe quick return to their primary sport. The injured shoulder should be protected from further injury while developing the shoulder's muscular strength. Cardiovascular fitness and other muscular strength levels should be maintained at an athletic level during rehabilitation. A positive psychological outlook can be promoted by maintenance of work levels equal to preinjury levels with the use of substitute activities. Also injury prevention should be stressed by continuing adequate warm-up and preseason stretching and strengthening exercises.

Maintenance of joint and muscle flexibility is vital in the total conditioning program for the athlete.[4] Conditioning as well as rehabilitation programs should include a minimum level of aerobic fitness for the entire body as well as the involved muscles. Aerobic resistive exercises for shoulder rehabilitation use high multiple repetitions, adequate rest, low resistance, and a moderate rate of motion. Once a solid aerobic base has been obtained, anaerobic strengthening can be started. Anaerobic training is characterized by low repetitions and high intensity. Examples of anaerobic work may be heavy-weight training, sprinting, rope jumping, and intensive bicycle riding.

In order to bring about positive physiological changes in strained muscle, as well as in the cardiac, respiratory, and circulatory systems of the body, a work overload must be applied. When the patient works at a level which exceeds the normal functioning capabilities of the body, various changes take place that cause the body to function with greater efficiency.[8] However, this must be done slowly and carefully in the injured athlete.

Stretching Exercises

The stretching program for the athlete depends on the type of injury, the healing time, and the sport. Healing or surgically repaired structures must be protected, and aggressive stretching may be delayed. Figure 49-1 illustrates the basic stretching exercises which may also be used in the athlete.[5] Contract-reflex and hold-relax techniques,[14] which allow contraction of the muscle, followed by relaxation and gentle stretching can be an effective means of increasing flexibility. These techniques can also be taught to athletes and used during body stretching before and after exercise or activity.

Strengthening Exercises

Strengthening exercises should work the muscles of the rotator cuff as well as the large muscles of the shoulder girdle. External rotation can be resisted by the opposite arm,[5] with surgical tubing,[1,2] or with weights. The arm is held at the side with the elbow flexed to 90°. The weight is then lifted up and into external rotation.[6,10] Internal rotation can also be resisted isometrically, with surgical tubing, or with weights. Using weights, the athlete lies supine with the arm at the side and elbow flexed to 90°. The hand with the weight is then moved into internal rotation.[6,10] The supraspinatus muscle can be isolated by bringing the shoulder into 90° abduction, 30° forward flexion, and internal rotation. A weight can be raised and lowered in this position.

These exercises must be chosen carefully and the patient monitored closely for any change in symptoms; as the patient progresses, advanced strengthening exercises which couple the action of the rotator cuff muscles with the shoulder girdle muscles are then added to the program.

SECTION B

Rehabilitation of the Hand

Meredith Cook Ferraro and Joan Lehmann

Close communication and teamwork between the surgeon, hand therapist, and patient is vital for successful rehabilitation.

HAND EXAMINATION

The therapist's examination of the hand should include observation of the normal resting attitude and recognition of any trophic and sudomotor changes associated with denervation.[23] Tendons should be examined for integrity, contracture, overstretching, and loss of tenodesis effect.

Fixed deformities or a tendency to assume positions of deformity are noted. Ligaments are evaluated for laxity, instability, or contracture. Vascular status is monitored by noting pulses, skin color, temperature, and edema.

Range of Motion

Motion of the entire upper extremity is measured when appropriate. Bilateral comparisons in joint mobility must be noted because limitations may be "normal" for a specific patient. Both active and passive measurements of the extremity range of motion should be taken. Discrepancies between these may indicate tendon excursion limitations or capsular tightness. Joint measurements may be taken on the lateral or dorsal aspect of the joint with the proximal joint stabilized. In the presence of dressings or moderate to severe edema, lateral measurements are preferred. Consistency in placement of the goniometer on either the lateral or the dorsal aspect of the joint is of prime importance in maintaining reliability. Specific positioning of the extremity for range of motion measurement is discussed by Fess and Moran.[53]

A more composite statement of integrated motion can be provided with total active motion (TAM) and total passive motion (TPM) measurements of a digit.[53] This method of recording the range of motion of a joint compares tendon excursion (TAM) to joint mobility (TPM). Total motion measurements provide the examiner with a single number which represents the summation of joint flexion measurements minus the summation of joint extension deficits for each digit. Measurements are taken with the digits in a fisted position to prevent external blocking.

Another method for determining finger motion is through measurement of the distance from the finger pulps to the distal palmar crease. The measurements are quickly and easily recorded. However, they lack the accuracy and the reliability of the total motion technique.

Muscle Function

Accurate manual muscle testing can define the extent of muscle function and supplement the surgeon's muscle-testing data. Manual muscle testing is used for defining peripheral nerve lesions. When testing is performed periodically, the data are used to monitor the status of nerve regeneration. Muscle testing is also mandatory in the preoperative evaluation of patients for potential tendon transfers. Muscle strength should be graded using the 0 to 5 system, which is defined in Chap. 40, on nerve injury.

Pinch and grip strength are measured with a commercially available gauge. Both grip and pinch strength should be measured with the patient seated, shoulder adducted and neutrally rotated, elbow flexed at 90°, and forearm and wrist in neutral position.[53] The clinical assessment committee of the American Society for Surgery of the Hand recommends that the second handle position of the adjustable handle dynamometer be used with three consecutive grip trials.[4] The results should be recorded in kilograms or pounds. Usually there is a 5 to 10 percent difference in readings between the dominant and nondominant hand.[11] If maximal force is used for each of the three trials, less than a 20 percent variation will exist between the readings of the tested hand.[11,165]Another method for measuring grip strength with the dynamometer involves testing strength on each of the five handle positions from smallest to largest. A normal bell curve should appear when kilograms (or pounds) of force are plotted for each of the five handle positions. The apex of the curve should appear at the middle of the handle positions, where gross grip strength is greatest.[11,50,51,121] Usually a flat curve appears when a patient applies less than maximal force.[5,50]

Three types of pinch strength are recorded. Lateral pinch, or key pinch, involves prehension of the thumb pulp to the lateral aspect of the index middle phalanx. Three-point pinch, or three-jaw chuck, requires force between the thumb pulp, index, and long fingers. Tip pinch involves prehension between thumb tip and tip of the index finger. Three successive trials should be performed for each pinch measured.[53] Strength measurements may vary according to the subject's sex, age, hand size, hand dominance, pain, occupation, and motivation, and the time of day tested.[165]

Sensibility

A hand with diminished or absent sensibility is poorly used, even if motor function is good. Without accurate sensory feedback, the hand is a blind, functionless unit.[117,118] When evaluating sensory function, the therapist seeks to define the sensory acuity and then relates it to the level of hand function. Administration of a battery of tests is preferred as there is no single, reliable, and consistent test available.[137] Selection of appropriate tests for an individual patient depends on the information desired, age, and concentration level of the patient. Other variables include the time of day tested, the environment, and the patient's attitude, mental status, and emotional status.

Tinel's sign may be used to follow the advancing terminations of the regenerating axons.[95] However, Seddon states that this sign is unreliable in the presence of partial unrepaired nerve lesions, when a positive sign can occur.[150] Henderson found that Tinel's sign becomes important in predicting regeneration approximately 4 months after injury.[62]

Sympathetic function including sudomotor, pilomotor, vasomotor, and trophic changes may be present. After nerve injury the area of loss of sympathetic function closely corresponds to the area of loss of sensory function because the cutaneous sympathetic fibers follow essentially the same pathway to the periphery as the cutaneous sensory fibers.[162] These sympathetic changes may resolve early but do not correlate with functional recovery.[38]

O'Riain observed that denervated skin does not wrinkle, and described a wrinkle test in 1973.[128] Phelps found that finger wrinkling does correlate with an absence of sensibility in complete lacerations. However, in nerve compressions, wrinkling does not indicate intact sensibility.[136] The Ninhydrin test identifies areas of disturbance of sweat secretion after peripheral nerve disruption.[118,134,136] These tests are considered objective because they require only passive cooperation of the patient. They may be especially helpful when evaluating children and those unwilling or unable to cooperate.

Dellon describes a method of testing and pattern of sensory recovery in the hand.[38] First to recover are pain and temperature senses, and then touch, beginning with sensibility to vibration of 30 Hz (cycles per second). Regeneration of the senses of moving touch, constant touch, and vibration of 256 Hz then follows. The order of return is primarily related to nerve fiber diameter and secondarily to reinnervation of the sensory receptor.[38]

The use of vibration is questioned because of a lack of stimulus specificity in a relatively small and confined space such as the hand.[44,90] In addition, if the tuning fork is placed other than perpendicular to the surface of application, the fine harmonic vibratory stimulus changes to a compressive stimulus.[116]

Two-point discrimination requires the patient to distinguish between two direct stimuli and detect each one as a separate entity. Discrimination requires finer reception acuity than does detection, which requires the patient to distinguish a single-point stimulus from normal background stimuli. The two-point discrimination test can be quickly administered using a blunt-tipped caliper. The static two-point discrimination test is commonly used because it is acknowledged to relate to the ability to use the hand for fine tasks.[119] Dellon refutes this correlation and describes the moving two-point discrimination test to assess fingertip sensibility, which is highly dependent upon motion.[39]

Light touch–deep pressure testing is utilized because pressure sensibility is a form of protective sensation since it warns of deep pressure or of low-grade repetitive pressure which may injure the skin. Light touch sensibility is a necessary component of fine discrimination.[23] The Semmes-Weinstein aesthesiometer[151] monofilament testing set is recommended. The test with the graded monofilament has been described as one of the most objective tests measuring cutaneous sensibility.[155,178] When this tool is used, a map of different thresholds of touch is obtained. The maps provide a visual picture of the sensation perceived by the patient. The maps can be predictors of the rate of neural return as well as the quality of return.[12] The aesthesiometer readings can be interpreted to project the patient's level of function.[12] Werner and Omer found that the presence of light touch sensibility does not correlate accurately with the presence of two-point discrimination.[178]

Recognition of common objects is the highest level of sensory function. Moberg used the term *tactile gnosis* to describe the hand's ability to see through performance of complex functions by feeling.[118] Moberg developed a pickup test which can be used for assessing median or combined median-ulnar lesions.[118] It is a timed observational test in which the patient is also the control. Observations of the prehension patterns used in task performance are made. Dellon took this test a step further by developing norms, standardizing the items, and requiring identification of them with the modified Moberg pickup test.[38]

Dexterity and Function

Dexterity and function of the patient's hand should be tested with standardized tests that measure precisely and accurately.[53] Commonly used tests include the Jebson hand function test,[72] Perdue pegboard,[167] Minnesota rate of manipulation test,[69] Crawford small parts dexterity test,[32] Valpar work sample,[170] Carroll quantitative test of upper extremity function,[27] and Bennett hand tool dexterity test.[13] These tests provide information about how the hand-injured patient functions in daily activities at home and at work.

HAND EDEMA

Edema is normally present in the extremity after injury or surgery. Edema causes pain, stiffness, and delayed healing.[65,138] With time, edematous soft tissues can become fibrosed by a foreign body type of tissue reaction.[111] If the edema remains, a serofibrinous exudate invades the area. Fibrin is deposited intraarticularly and around the tendons and ligaments, resulting in reduced mobility, flattening of the hand arches, tissue atrophy, and further loss of function.[67,101,111] Normal gliding of these tissues is eliminated, and a stiff, often painful, hand results. Scar adhesions form and further limit tissue mobility. If untreated, these losses may become permanent.[111]

Edema may be assessed with volumetric measurements. Brand and Wood developed this method of assessing composite mass.[19] The volumeter is based on the Archimedean principle of water displacement. When used properly the volumeter is accurate to within 10 ml.[176] Edema can also be assessed by taking circumferential measurements at specified anatomic landmarks; however, the accuracy of this technique depends upon consistency in placement[150] and in tension on the tape.[50] A Gulick tape[60] assists in maintaining consistency.

The therapist's and surgeon's role immediately after the injury is to prevent or minimize edema. In the first 3 to 5 days this may be achieved through bulky compressive dressings and elevation of the hand.[65] As the inflammatory process settles, active motion is begun to assist the return-flow dynamics. The return-flow circulation is to a large degree secondary to muscular activity.[10,67,87,111] Therefore, active exercises involving the full range of motion of the joint should be carried out as much as possible. Active motion can also be combined with the following edema-reducing techniques. Contrast baths, in which the hand is placed in warm and cool water, cause vasodilation and vasoconstriction, resulting in pumping of the edema. Retrograde massage to assist in return-flow dynamics is helpful when performed on a frequent basis.[65,67,111] Pressure wraps intermittently throughout the day with greater pressure distally than proximally assist with edema control.[65,67,73] These include string or Coban wrapping, Isotoner gloves, Jobst garment, tubular guards, finger stalls, or the Intermittent Compression Pump.[65] No one method of treating edema is universally superior to another. Selection of edema-reduction techniques depends on the therapist's preference and the individual patient's response.

NERVE INJURIES

Peripheral nerve injuries are challenging to the hand therapist. Whether the nerve injury is a neurapraxia, axonotmesis,

or neurotmesis, at some point there is sensory loss and weakness of the musculature innervated by the nerve. The therapeutic principles are the same for all classifications: to restore maximal motor power and sensibility to the hand.

After nerve repair or grafting, the hand is placed in a position of protection to prevent any tension on the newly repaired nerve for a period of 3 to 4 weeks.[9,73,79] Depending on the surgeon's preference, the therapist may, instead of a cast, fabricate a low-temperature thermoplastic splint to hold the extremity in the protected position several days postoperatively. The advantages are that the splint is rigid, lightweight, and easily molded to the hand and/or extremity. As wound healing progresses, the easily revised splint can be modified so that the range of the joints can gradually return to normal. Active range-of-motion exercises are encouraged at the available joints on the involved extremity including the shoulder. Active exercises activate the muscular pumps to stimulate the venous and lymphatic systems, which assist in control of edema.[65,73] Exercise also prevents disuse atrophy of the available muscles. The patient must also be instructed to elevate the hand in order to control postoperative edema by allowing gravity to assist the venous system.[65,73] Retrograde massage to the available digits is begun, the massage strokes always beginning distally and going proximally, thereby assisting the blood and lymph return.[86,174] The patient is given a home program of exercises and massage to be performed 4 to 6 times daily.

Once the period of immobilization has ended, the goals of the hand therapy program are to

1. Decrease residual edema.
2. Soften and desensitize the scar.
3. Restore range of motion and strength to the available joints and muscles.
4. Prevent deformity.
5. Promote visual protection of anesthetic areas.
6. Assure independence in activities of daily living.
7. Permit a return of the patient to work with adaptations or special equipment if necessary.

Various physical therapy modalities may be used, depending upon the individual patients and the problems they present. Full discussion of modalities is beyond the scope of this chapter, but if significant scarring is present, deep friction massage and Silastic elastomer[185] or Otoform[173] pressure should be utilized. Sensory evaluations are done monthly.

Dellon[35,36,37] describes the sensory nerve regeneration process as occurring in sequence as follows: regeneration of sudomotor activity (i.e., sweating), and then regeneration of sensitivity to pain, vibration at 30 Hz, moving touch, constant touch, and vibration at 256 Hz. Periodic sensory evaluations are indicated.

Sensory reeducation is the process of learning to interpret an altered profile of sensory impulses.[35,36,110] There are two phases of sensory reeducation: early and late. The early phase begins when detailed sensory evaluations of the proximal phalanx reveal regeneration of awareness of pain, light touch, light movement, and vibration at 30 and 256 Hz. Late-phase reeducation is begun when movement and constant touch are perceived by the fingertip. The timing for actual initiation of sensory reeducation is dependent on the level of nerve injury and repair and the progress of nerve regeneration. A quiet setting is necessary, and a highly motivated patient is recommended for successful sensory reeducation.[73]

The early phase of sensory reeducation consists of exercises of moving touch versus constant touch. The patient applies the stimulus of a pencil eraser either stroking or with various amounts of pressure proximally to distally along the digit. At first the patient does this with the eyes open; then the patient closes the eyes to perceive the stimulus and then repeats it while watching once again. The patient should follow through at home at least four to six times a day for 5 min.[35,79] Callahan has described a program to concentrate on localization in which the stimulus becomes smaller and lighter so that the final result is similar to stimulation with the Semmes-Weinstein monofilaments. This localization training is continued through the late phase of sensory reeducation.[24]

Late-phase sensory reeducation involves identification of objects to obtain tactile gnosis. The patients hold and manipulate objects with their eyes open and closed and concentrate on them but use different-shaped blocks, coins, nuts, and objects with variations in texture.[37] Tasks can be designed that require use of the hand such as picking out objects from a bowl of sand, rice, Styrofoam, and other materials.[24] The patient may also be asked to assemble different-sized nuts and bolts, both with vision and with vision occluded. Numerous activities have been devised for late-stage reeducation; all of them involve the use of the hand with continual sensory reevaluation and timing of tasks.[24] In clinical experience the patients who have incorporated and used their nerve-injured hands into their daily lives show the best results on periodic sensory reevaluations. Other clinicians report that continued use of the hand is necessary for maintaining sensory reeducation.[24,34,126,127]

Motor return in nerve injuries cannot be predicted. In recent years some have questioned whether motor point direct current (dc) stimulation to a paralyzed muscle is beneficial. Even with dc motor point stimulation by the patient five times a day with a home unit, muscle atrophy still occurs.[156] This is felt to be because of the tremendous frequency of stimulation necessary to maintain a muscle fiber and the number of motor units which have to be stimulated to get a full muscular contraction.[9,184] Proponents feel that direct current depolarizes the muscle fiber to maintain its integrity and prevent atrophy and connective tissue degeneration. Pachter and others studied the effect of electric stimulation on denervated muscle in rats and found greater muscle bulk and strength when stimulation was performed when electromyographic fibrillation potentials had decreased.[129] It has also been suggested that reinnervation may be retarded when stimulation is done too early.[122] Electric stimulation does play a part in reeducation of a muscle in the beginning stage of motor return.[184] If the muscle's optimal chronaxie value (minimal duration) of direct current with the negative pole is used in the pattern of functional motion or activity, the reinnervation is felt to be more effective.[122]

Splinting of the nerve-injured patient is necessary to prevent deformity while awaiting motor return.[73,79,81,102,103,133,184] For simplification, the splints for specific nerve injuries are discussed separately.

The median nerve–injured hand is often called the ape hand, because of the lack of opposition and palmar abduction of the thumb due to the lack of median-innervated thenar muscles. The index and long fingers may have a hyperextension tendency at the metacarpophalangeal joints due to the lack of lumbrical innervation. Splints are provided to position the thumb in palmar abduction and opposition. A C-bar opponens splint[73,133] or thumb post splint (Fig. 49-3)[133] is most frequently used. The hyperextension deformity of the index and long fingers usually does not have to be splinted once the thumb, index finger, and long finger are positioned to oppose one another. In a high median nerve injury, no additional splinting is necessary.[73,133]

With a low-level ulnar nerve injury, the hand tends to claw, with the ring and small fingers hyperextending at the metacarpophalangeal (MCP) joints and the interphalangeal (IP) joints flexing because of the paralysis of the lumbricals and interossei and unopposed long flexors of these digits. A positive Froment's sign is present because of the overpull of the flexor pollicis longus, which is attempting to stabilize the MCP joint in flexion. However, paralysis of the short thumb flexors and the adductor muscle results in MCP hyperextension and marked interphalangeal joint flexion.

The main principle for splinting the ulnar nerve–injured hand is to allow flexion while preventing hyperextension of the ring and small MCP joints and secondary overstretch of the lower joint capsules. In this way the splint assumes the function of the lumbricals and allows the extrinsic extensor, extensor digitorum communis, to function at the proximal interphalangeal (PIP) joints. Splints for this purpose are numerous. A molded plastic dorsal hyperextension MCP block with the metacarpophalangeal joints set in approximately 40° of flexion (Fig. 49-4), a wrist cuff with two flexion slings for the proximal phalanges of the ring and small finger,[133] and a Wynn Parry dynamic "lively" splint[184] are a few examples. In all of these the patient is able to function with full flexion of the ring and small fingers and almost full digital extension. With a high level of ulnar nerve injury, the flexor digitorum profundus of the ring and small fingers and the flexor carpi ulnaris are affected, but additional splinting is not needed.

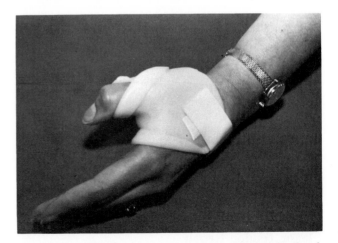

Figure 49-3 Median nerve injuries require splinting the thumb in a position of abduction and opposition, thereby substituting for the absent thenar musculature.

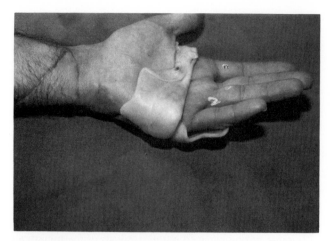

Figure 49-4 The ulnar nerve–injured hand assumes a claw hand deformity, in which the ring and small metacarpo phalangeal joints hyperextend and the proximal and distal interphalangeal joints flex. The claw deformity is corrected with a dorsal metacarpophalangeal extension blocking splint for the ring and small fingers which allows proximal and distal interphalangeal extension and total flexion of the digits.

The combined median and ulnar nerve–injured hand requires a splint to prevent hyperextension of the index long, ring, and small fingers as well as opposition and palmar abduction of the thumb due to total intrinsic paralysis. A dorsal thermoplastic hyperextension block with a thumb post can be fabricated, or a Wynn Parry splint for intrinsic paralysis can be utilized.[184]

If the radial nerve is injured, there is a wrist drop as well as a lack of extension of the digits at the metacarpophalangeal joints and a lack of extension of the thumb. Most have advocated the use of a dorsal outrigger which holds the wrist and the digits in extension and allows flexion.[79,102,184] Patient acceptance of this splint is not always good because of its size and the length of time they have to wear it while awaiting regeneration. A cockup splint is frequently used because the wrist is supported, giving strength, and patients are able to grasp and release by the use of their intrinsic musculature. Ideally, a "wrist control" splint[133] or dynamic wrist splint with an extension assist (Fig. 49-5) is utilized because it allows tenodesis function of the hand. In some instances, patients prefer to function in the position of wrist drop. The patient can be taught to grasp objects and then supinate the forearm to assist with holding the objects.[133]

Nerve-injured patients are a challenge to the surgeon and the therapist. If they regain functional sensation and use of the hand in their daily activities, the ultimate goal has been achieved.

REHABILITATION FOLLOWING TENDON INJURY

Flexor Tendon Repair

Historically results of flexor tendon surgery have been less than gratifying.[26,78,156] Today, primary repair of flexor ten-

dons, even if delayed 3 to 4 weeks, has taken precedence over secondary grafting.[157]

Early controlled motion (ECM), also called controlled passive motion, of flexor tendon repairs has been advocated by Duran and Houser[42,43] and by Kleinert[83,84,85] in order to minimize and control the postoperative formation of peritendinous adhesions. Strickland and Glogovac[161] compared the Duran technique of ECM to immobilization of flexor tendon repairs in zone II for 3½ weeks and concluded that ECM substantially improves the results by limiting adhesion formation. Lister, Kleinert, and Kutz[94] compared the Kleinert technique of ECM to immobilization of flexor tendon repairs in various zones. They found 75 percent of the tendons repaired in zone II, "no man's land," to have good to excellent results, while 84 percent of the tendons repaired in the other zones had good to excellent results in accordance with their established grading scale. (Zones are defined in Chap. 42.)

The rationale for the Duran method is that controlled passive range of motion protects the tendon juncture and allows for 3 to 5 mm of tendon excursion, therefore preventing adherence and allowing for differential gliding of the tendons (Fig. 49-6). The Kleinert method employs active extension of the involved digit and a return to a flexion posture by the use of a rubber band traction (Fig. 49-7). Electromyography during sustained contraction of the extensors (extensor digitorum communis) shows that there is no activity in the flexor digitorum profundis.[94] Therefore, this technique which keeps the flexor muscles relaxed still allows limited gliding of the tendon structure.

The Duran technique of controlled passive motion has been as reported in detail by Cannon and Strickland.[26]

Rehabilitation following Flexor Tendon Tenolysis

If adhesions have formed along the course of a muscle tendon unit following tendon repair, graft, fracture, or crushing injury, the limitation of gliding results in a decreased active range of motion. If this interferes with hand function, a tenolysis may be indicated.

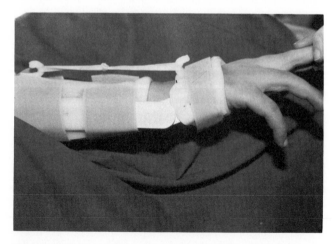

Figure 49-5 A dynamic wrist extension splint incorporates a wrist joint which allows flexion and extension, but controls radial and ulnar deviation by means of strong flexor musculature, and a rubberband assist for extensor musculature.

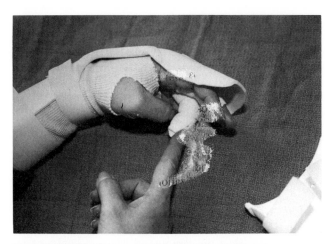

Figure 49-6 The Duran method of flexor tendon rehabilitation requires dorsal splinting of the wrist in 20° volar flexion, the metacarpophalangeal joints in 50° flexion, and the interphalangeal joints in neutral. The removable volar piece which prevents any flexion when not exercising has been removed to allow the performance of passive flexion exercises.

Preoperatively, the hand therapy program must achieve a maximal passive range of motion (ROM), provide supple skin and subcutaneous tissue, and strengthen the involved musculature. Postoperatively, the therapist must be told the active range of motion that was achieved in the operating room and the condition of the tendon and soft tissues. This way an immediate therapeutic goal of active ROM is set. The amount of soft tissue damage gives the therapist a guide to the tendency for additional new peritendinous adhesions to form and the amount of stress the tendon can endure.

In the past, motion following flexor tenolysis was started several days postoperatively or as soon as "soft tissue healing" permitted.[132,172] It is now felt that active exercises should begin on the first postoperative day.[26,66,147,148,179] In most cases the postoperative bulky dressing is removed and a lighter dressing is applied so that motion is minimally restricted. Total active flexion and extension exercises are begun. Flexion to the distal palmar crease is encouraged. Isolated active flexor digitorum profundus and flexor digitorum sublimis blocking exercises are begun as well as gentle passive flexion and extension of the interphalangeal joints. If forceful passive motions are done, edema and pain will increase. Gentle passive flexion, fist making with the patient actively holding the fist position with his or her own muscle power, and release exercises are begun.[26,147,148,158] Active wrist, elbow, and shoulder motions are encouraged, and elevation is stressed. The patient is instructed to complete the above-mentioned exercises for 5 to 10 min every waking hour.

If pain is a problem and the patient will not do the exercises, transcutaneous nerve stimulation is very effective in controlling pain.[25,74] Cannon and Strickland report utilizing sterile electrodes, which are placed on the patient in the operating room before the bulky dressing is applied. A continuous nerve block with a local anesthetic agent (bupivacaine) administered via an indwelling catheter has been successful in controlling pain.[22,66,148] Local nerve blocks given 30 min prior to therapy can also be utilized.

The approach to splinting of the postoperative tenolysis patient varies. Schneider and Mackin[148] recommend the use of a dorsal resting splint to rest the digits when they are not exercising and to maintain extension of the tenolysed tendon. Strickland splints the tenolysed digit in flexion in the postoperative dressing because he finds patients do not have a problem with extending the digit. The passive flexion effectively produces tendon glide of the lysed tendon when the patient actively extends the finger, while gliding is not ensured by passive flexion alone.[158] Splinting should be geared to correct any remaining joint or tendon tightness. If a joint flexion contracture is released, then the joint is statically splinted in extension for 2 weeks when it is not exercising. Many times buddy taping the operated digit to an adjacent normal digit during daily activities facilitates the rehabilitation.

After 2 postoperative weeks the patient is encouraged to begin light activities of daily living. Progressive strengthening exercises are begun at 3 to 4 postoperative weeks, depending upon the status of the tendon and soft tissues.

Two-Stage Flexor Tendon Reconstruction

If a patient has severely impaired functioning of the flexor tendons, two-stage flexor tendon reconstruction with silicon-rod insertion may be considered. The hand therapy program begins preoperatively to stage I (silicon rod) by obtaining maximal passive range of motion of the digital joints. This is done by maintaining strength of the proximal muscles by softening the scar with soft tissue massage, and by buddy taping the injured digit to the adjacent normal digit to encourage a normal range of motion.

The postoperative program after implantation of the silicon rod includes ROM, therapy, soft tissue softening, and edema control. If pulleys have been constructed, the surgeon may want them protected with the use of a ring over the pul-

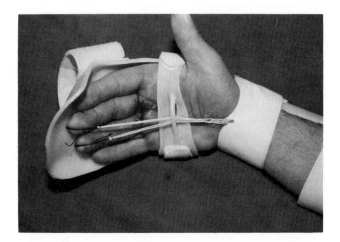

Figure 49-7 The Kleinert flexor tendon protocol provides a dorsal blocking splint with the wrist in 30 to 40° flexion with dynamic traction pulling the digits into flexion. Each hour, dynamic resistive extension, as shown here, is done to allow maximal interphalangeal extension. The pulley at the distal palmar crease allows more normal biomechanical splintage.

ley site.[26,99] The exercise program usually begins between 1 and 2 weeks postoperatively, and splinting for contractures may be necessary.

Stage II surgery usually takes place between 3 and 6 months after stage I. The postoperative therapy regime varies depending on the preference of the surgeon and therapist. Schneider and Mackin[99] and the authors utilize the Kleinert's traction protocol for zone II flexor tendon repairs. Some[26,79] utilize the Duran method of zone II flexor tendon rehabilitation, and others immobilize the digit for 3 to 4 weeks after grafting.[26,79,180] In the latter case, active and passive flexion exercises and active extension exercises are begun within the dorsal blocking splint at 3 postoperative weeks. Wilson begins passive flexion and active PIP motion at 4 weeks but does not allow active DIP flexion until 6 postoperative weeks.[180] The splint is discontinued at 6 weeks, and the flexor tendon protocol is followed.

Extensor Tendon Injuries

Extensor tendon repairs are treated more conservatively because of the inherent weakness of the muscle-tendon unit compared with that of the flexors. Timing of rehabilitation depends on the zone of injury (defined in Chap. 42) and the amount of soft tissue injury.

In zone V, extensor tendon repairs are immobilized for 3 to 4 weeks before active digital ROM exercise is begun.[92] A wrist cockup splint is used for 5 to 6 weeks and is then used only for protection, and active wrist motion is begun. Hand strengthening is begun at 8 weeks.

Extensor tendon repairs in zones III and IV are immobilized for 3 to 6 weeks,[41,73,79,92] and active remobilization of the wrist and digits begins. Protective splinting of the wrist in extension and the involved digit at the MCP level in mild flexion continues for the 3- to 6-week period when they are not exercising. Recently, early protected mobilization with dynamic extensor, splinting protecting the repair has been reported[2,54]; this allows forceful contraction of the antagonist (flexors) and therefore relaxation of the agonist (extensors).

In zone IIc, tendon injuries include the central tendon or the sagittal band injuries. Postoperatively, early controlled mobilization[2,54] or immobilization with the wrist extended and the MCP joint in 30 to 45° of flexion and the IP joint extension is important. At 4 weeks, active remobilization begins with protective splinting until 8 weeks.[92] Intrinsic tightness may occur; therefore, gentle passive stretching is indicated. Gentle strengthening of the flexors begins at 5 to 6 weeks, and strengthening of the extensor repair begins at 7 to 8 weeks.[92] Injuries in this zone have a good prognosis if there is no joint infection.[96]

In zone IIa and IIb, the extensors are the central tendon and the radial and ulnar intrinsics, or lateral bands. After repair, the tendons are immobilized with the metacarpophalangeal joint in flexion and PIP joint in extension.[15,96] In these zones if there is primary or delayed primary repair of the central tendon, the PIP joint is immobilized for 4 weeks and active DIP joint motion is begun at 2 postoperative weeks. This prevents the lateral bands from adherence, stiffness of the DIP joint is prevented, and the oblique retinacular ligament is stretched. If the surgical repair involves the lateral bands, then the DIP joint is not exercised until 4 postoperative weeks. Active proximal interphalangeal motion with night extension splinting begins at 4 to 6 weeks with careful monitoring of the development of an extension lag.[73,92,96] Full active extension should be maintained while flexion is gained. Dynamic extension splinting of the PIP joint is substituted for static PIP splinting at 4 to 6 weeks if the extensor is particularly adherent.[92] Buddy taping of the digit to a normal digit is also begun at this time.

Strengthening exercises are begun between 8 and 10 postoperative weeks depending on the range of motion present. If there is an extension lag at the PIP joint, then therapy is made more conservative by limiting dynamic flexion stretching and resisted extension exercises. If an extension contracture develops, then the therapy program concentrates on dynamic flexion and resisted flexion and extension. Closed boutonniere or extensor injuries in this zone are treated similarly.

Zone I injuries affect the DIP joint extension and may be open or closed with or without fracture. Open injuries are treated with immobilization of the DIP joint for 4 to 6 weeks, and active PIP joint motion is allowed. Active ROM exercises are begun for the DIP joint when immobilization is discontinued, and night extension splinting is continued until 8 weeks. If the injury is closed, the digital interphalangeal joint is splinted in extension or slight hyperextension continuously for 6 to 8 weeks.[1,31,92] Active flexion exercises are begun with protective night splinting for an additional 4 weeks.

In the digit the extensor tendons are extremely prone to adherence but if moved too early can attenuate. An experienced hand therapist must carefully assess this delicate balance in order to obtain optimal results.

Rehabilitation following Tendon Transfers

The hand therapist plays a significant role in the treatment of the patient who is to undergo tendon transfers. Preoperatively the therapist assists the surgeon in observing and assessing the function of the involved extremity. Nerve function is evaluated for sensory and motor performance, and manual muscle testing is completed. The range of motion of the joint is examined for contractures, functional use in activities of daily living, strength, and dexterity. This information is discussed with the surgeon, who decides which tendons are to be transferred. Preoperative therapy treatments involve restoring normal joint ROM by exercise and splinting, strengthening of the muscle to be transferred, and isolation of the muscle to be transferred.[88]

Postoperatively, the tendon transfer is immobilized in the range of 3 to 4 weeks depending on the type of transfer,[79,88,145] and active exercises are begun with protective splinting of the involved transfer. The goals of treatment are to increase ROM and strength, reeducate the transferred tendon, and encourage normal function of the hand. Electric stimulation[6,26,88] and biofeedback[26] are helpful in reeducating the transferred muscle. Strengthening exercises are begun at 6 weeks[73] with splinting only at night.[88] Progressive strengthening and normal use of the hand are encouraged as further wound healing progresses.

REHABILITATION IN RHEUMATOID ARTHRITIS

The chronic nature and degenerative course of rheumatoid arthritis necessitate development of a carefully planned treatment program to maintain the patient's physical, psychological, and functional abilities for as long as possible. Maintenance of hand function is important since the disabling nature of this disease may limit employment to the sedentary type for which good hand function is a necessity.[75] The therapy program plays an important role in attaining these goals. Hand therapy treatment is individualized and corresponds to the stage of the disease in the particular joint. Four phases of arthritis have been described:[106] the acute phase, the subacute phase, the chronic-active phase, and the chronic-inactive phase. Symptoms are most severe in the acute phase, and as the symptoms abate, the subacute phase of the disease begins. The chronic-active phase is defined as low-grade inflammatory levels for an extended period.[77] The chronic-inactive phase is the end stage, or burned-out stage of arthritis.

In the acute and subacute phases, adequate rest is emphasized.[112] Splinting is used to decrease inflammation and pain through immobilization. Immobilization supports the joint, reduces stress to the capsule, allows muscles to relax, and decreases inflammation.[45,56,130] Joint integrity and mobility are maintained through gentle passive or active range of motion exercises. These exercises are done to the point of discomfort.[112] In the subacute phase, muscle strength and endurance are maintained through performance of isometric or isotonic exercises. The less painful method is chosen since pain inhibits strength development.[77] Splinting may also be utilized for reducing muscle tightness. Median nerve compression may be alleviated by positioning the hand in a cock-up splint.[112] A joint-protection program is instituted to reduce stress and pain in the involved joints, consequently reducing inflammation and preserving the integrity of the joint structures.[28,112,168] Energy conservation and work simplification principles are incorporated into activities of daily living. The patient must learn to integrate these principles into everyday life and create a new habit repertoire. Patient education is emphasized. The arthritic disease process and its effects on the musculoskeletal system are discussed. The importance of rest and proper positioning is stressed. Group therapy to deal with issues of disturbance of self image, body image, job status, family relationships, and coping mechanisms may be helpful.[89]

THERAPY AFTER MP JOINT ARTHROPLASTY

The postoperative care and rehabilitation program are of great significance in the quality of the final result of the arthroplasty.[163] The purpose of treatment following MP joint arthroplasty is to obtain active functional MP joint flexion, prevent recurrent deformity, and protect repaired soft tissues.[29] Therefore, therapy is directed toward developing scar for stability and for allowing motion.[40] Treatment coincides with the biodynamics of scar formation. It is important to gain the desired active range of motion (0 to 70°) in the first 3 weeks.[163]

Between the third and fifth postoperative day, a dorsally based dynamic extension splint is fabricated to provide external stability and position the fingers in proper anatomic alignment with extension and slight radial deviation. The traction force is continually monitored for tension, rotation, and lateral pull. The splint is worn full-time for at least 3 weeks. Active and passive exercises in the flexion and extension planes are initiated to stress the scar and to remodel it dynamically. Immobilizing the IP joints in extension with removable dorsal splints may be helpful in gaining the active flexion of the MP joints. The therapist's goal in each session is to obtain 70° of active flexion and 90° of passive flexion.[40]

At 10 to 21 days postoperatively, dynamic flexion splinting may be started. Active extrinsic extensor exercises are begun in the intrinsic minus position to assist in activation of the muscle.[40]

At 4 postoperative weeks resistive extension exercises are begun in a dynamic flexion splint. The dorsally based dynamic extension splint is worn continuously for 4[163] to 6[40] weeks. The patient is then gradually weaned from the splint during the daytime. Nighttime splinting continues for at least 3 months postoperatively.

At 6 weeks postoperatively gentle resistive flexion exercises are begun. The patient is encouraged to use the hand for light activities and personal care[93,163] and to gradually incorporate the use of the hand in all activities. By 8 to 10 weeks postoperatively, normal use of the hand is encouraged. The exercise program is continued. The patient must understand that formal exercises may need to be practiced for up to 1 year to gain the best possible result. Further detailed therapeutic programs are also discussed in the literature.[93,163,164]

REHABILITATION FOLLOWING REPLANTATION

Rehabilitating the patient with a replanted part is a challenge to the surgeon and therapist. A continuum of communication must be maintained. The therapist must be aware of the medical status and surgical procedures performed on the patient as well as the surgeon's philosophy of treatment. The surgeon's long-term goals for the patient must be clarified so that appropriate therapeutic goals can be established. The timing of the therapeutic program depends largely on the level of replantation, extent and type of injury, presence of secondary complications, and surgeon's preference. Fess[52] has divided rehabilitation of the replanted part into five phases: stage 1, early healing; stage 2, active motion; stage 3, resistive motion; stage 4, maintenance and further surgical reconstruction; and stage 5, program assessment.

Stage 1, Early Healing

The early healing stage begins 1 day postoperatively. The therapist monitors the patient's physical and psychological condition. The patient is oriented to the various prospects of the rehabilitation program, and information provided by the surgeon is supplemented, in the hope that any unrealistic expectations for the replanted part after immobilization will be curbed. At 2 to 5 days postoperatively if the vascular status of the part is deemed stable by the surgeon, active and passive exercises to the uninjured joints which are immobilized may be initiated. Training in activities of daily living is initiated to enable the patient to function safely and as independently as possible. Early controlled mobilization may be instituted in this stage using techniques based on Kleinert[84] and Duran[43] for minimizing peritendinous adhesions of flexor tendon repairs in zones II and III. Traditionally, the replanted part was immobilized for 3 weeks with early passive mobilization avoided because of extensor and flexor tendon involvement.[155]

Stage 2, Active Motion

Active motion is initiated 10 to 21 days postoperatively.[21,109,155,166] The active motion program is carefully supervised as the repairs are vulnerable to rupture in the initial weeks. In addition, the patient is unable to determine the amount of stress placed on the repaired musculotendinous units when attempting to actively move the part since sensory feedback distal to the level of amputation is absent. The more pronounced the injury, the greater the difficulty the patient has identifying and using muscle groups. Visual cues are used. Biofeedback is of considerable value in helping to isolate and coordinate muscle groups.[52] Splinting is used to position the proximal joint, diminish tension on repairs, protect fracture stability, and protect the position of replanted part between exercise. Mobilization splints may be used to improve passive motion of the uninvolved joints adjacent to the replant that may develop stiffness during the initial period of immobilization.

Stage 3, Resistive Motion

Gentle resistive exercise can begin at the sixth postoperative week. The resistance is increased by graded increments over subsequent weeks. At 8 to 12 weeks the patient is permitted unrestricted use of the hand with precautions for the insensitive areas. Pinch, grip, and individual muscle strength may be measured at this time. Splinting is used to mobilize joints that have not responded favorably to exercise and more conservative splinting approaches. If necessary, sensory desensitization should be initiated. Sensibility evaluation may be performed to establish a baseline monitoring nerve regeneration. Sensibility evaluation is described earlier in this chapter.

Stage 4, Maintenance and Further Reconstruction

At this stage, a more realistic idea of the potential functional recovery of the part is apparent. The therapy program may be directed toward teaching a patient to use the extremity as an assist, and changing dominance if the dominant hand is involved. Plans to return to work or alternative employment are made. Returning to work can be stressful to the patient, especially if the injury occurred on the job. The therapist can assist in the patient's return to work with work-capacity training, performance of on-site job analysis, and communication with the employer.

Stage 5, Program Assessment

Program assessment involves a continuous effort to identify important variables and techniques that have provided consistently superior results so that the hand therapy program can be upgraded for future patients.

REHABILITATION OF THE RSD PATIENT

RSD (reflex sympathetic dystrophy) is a syndrome characterized by pain, swelling, stiffness, and discoloration.[91] The amount of original trauma does not necessarily correlate with the amount of pain and disability.[73] Waylett[175] surveyed normal patients as well as suspected and diagnosed RSD patients and found in RSD patients behavioral patterns with a trend for self-limiting behavior with conflicting goals. On clinical observation she found the RSD patient to need

1. Initial constant supervision.
2. A highly structured and simplified therapy program.
3. The motivation that he or she is an active participant in the therapy program.[175]

Early diagnosis of RSD or RSD tendency is important, since early treatment is more effective.[73,91,175] Medically, the abnormal sympathetic reflex can be eliminated, whether by sympatholytic drugs, local anesthetic blocks on somatic nerves or "trigger points," pharmacological or chemical blocks of the stellate ganglion and upper thoracic chain, or an upper thoracic sympathectomy.[91] The basis for hand therapy is patient education and a structured program of active exercises.[63,73,91,175] If active exercises are too aggressive or if passive exercises and manipulation are done with the patient, the sympathetic reactive process may increase and the patient will develop increased swelling, pain, and stiffness.[91]

The hand therapy program must be centered on reducing pain and edema and promoting motion and use of the involved hand. Therapeutically, pain can be controlled by transcutaneous nerve stimulation,[25,26,73,74,91] gentle active exercises and massage,[91] and, if necessary, stellate ganglion blocks, in conjunction with therapy. Heat modalities such as hot packs and paraffin frequently assist in reducing pain,[91,175] and this assists in promoting exercise for the patient and in decreasing edema if the heat is applied when the hand is elevated. Splinting is useful for resting the hand in order to relieve pain, with serial changes to improve ROM and for gentle dynamic forces to stretch and strengthen the hand.[91,175] Normal use of the hand must be encouraged to stimulate normal muscular activity. Functional activities and activities of daily living are utilized in the therapy program.

REFERENCES

Section A: Rehabilitation of the Shoulder

1. Aronen, J.G. Shoulder rehabilitation. Clin Sports Med 4:477–493, 1985.
2. Aronen, J.G., and Regan, K. Decreasing the incidence of recurrence of first time anterior shoulder dislocations with rehabilitation. Am J Sports Med 12:283–291, 1984.
3. Green, D.P. (ed). *Operative Hand Surgery.* New York, Churchill Livingstone, 1982.
4. Hatfield, F. *Powerlifting: A scientific approach.* Illinois, Contemporary Books, 1981.
5. Hughes, M., and Neer, C.S. Glenohumeral joint replacement and post operative rehabilitation. Phys Ther 55:850–858, 1975.
6. Jobe, F.W., and Moynes, D.R. Delineation of diagnostic criteria and a rehabilitation program for rotator cuff injuries. Am J Sports Med 10:336–339, 1982.
7. Kaltenborn, F.M. *Mobilization of the Extremity Joints.* Oslo, Olaf Norles Bokhandel, 1980, pp 92–113.
8. McArdle, W.D., Katch, F.I., and Katch, V.L. *Exercise Physiology.* Philadelphia, Lea & Febiger, 1981.
9. Mennell, J.M. *Joint Pain.* Boston, Little, Brown, 1964, pp 78–90.
10. Moynes, D.R. Prevention of injury to the shoulder through exercises and therapy. Clin Sports Med 2:413–422, 1983.
11. Narcessian, R.P. Personal communication.
12. Neer, C.S., and Welsh, R.P. The shoulder in sports. Orthop Clin North Am 8:583–591, 1977.
13. Rowe, C. Acute and recurrent anterior dislocation of the shoulder. Orthop Clin North Am 11:253–258, 1980.
14. Voss, D.E., Ionta, M.K., and Myers, B.J. *Proprioceptive Neuromuscular Facilitation.* Philadelphia, Harper & Row, 1985, pp 304–305.

Section B: Rehabilitation of the Hand

1. Abouna, J.M., and Brown, H. The treatment of mallet finger: The results in a series of 148 consecutive cases and a review of the literature. Br J Surg 55:653–667, 1968.
2. Allieu, Y., Asencio, G., Gomis, R., Teissier, J., and Rouzaud, J.C. Suture des tendons extenseurs de la main avec mobilisation assistee: A propos de 120 cas. Rev Chir Orthop 70(suppl)2:69–73, 1984.
3. Amadio, P.C., Jaeger, S.H., and Hunter, J.M. Nutritional aspects of tendon healing, in Hunter, J.M., et al (eds): *Rehabilitation of the Hand,* 2d ed. St Louis, Mosby, 1984, pp 255–260.
4. American Society for Surgery of the Hand. *The Hand: Examination and Diagnosis,* 2d ed. New York, Churchill Livingstone, 1983.
5. Aulicino, P.L., and DePuy, T.E. Clinical examination of the hand, in Hunter, J.M., et al (eds): *Rehabilitation of the Hand,* 2d ed. St. Louis, Mosby, 1984, pp 25–48.
6. Baker, L.L. *Functional Electrical Stimulation: A Practical Clinical Guide,* 2d ed. Rancho Los Amigos Hospital, Downey, California, 1981.
7. Barber, L.M. Occupational therapy for the treatment of reflex sympathetic dystrophy and posttraumatic hypersensitivity of the injured hand, in Fredericks, S., and Brody, G.S. (eds): *Symposium on the Neurologic Aspects of Plastic Surgery.* St. Louis, Mosby, 1978.
8. Baxter, P.L. Physical capacity evaluation and work therapy, in Hunter, J.M., et al (eds): *Rehabilitation of the Hand.* St. Louis, Mosby, 1978, pp 694–708.
9. Beasley, R.W. *Hand Injuries.* Philadelphia, Saunders, 1981.
10. Beasley, R.W. Principles of managing acute hand injuries, in Converse, J., McCarthy, J., and Littler, J.W. (ed): *Reconstructive Plastic Surgery,* 2d ed. Philadelphia, Saunders, 1977, vol 6, pp 3000–3102.
11. Bechtol, C. Grip test: The use of the dynamometer with adjusta-

ble handle spacings. J Bone Joint Surg 36A:820–824, 832, 1954.
12. Bell, J.A. Light touch-deep pressure testing using Semmes-Weinstein monofilaments, in Hunter, J.M., et al (eds): *Rehabilitation of the Hand,* 2d ed. St. Louis, Mosby, 1984, pp 399–406.
13. Bennett, G.K. *Hand-Tool Dexterity Test.* New York, Harcourt, Brace, Jovanovich, 1981.
14. Berkman, E., and Miles, G. Internal fixation of metacarpal fractures of the thumb. J Bone Joint Surg 25:816–821, 1943.
15. Blue, A.I., Spira, M., and Hardy, S.B. Repair of extensor tendon injuries of the hand. Am J Surg 132:128–132, 1976.
16. Bora, F.W. Nerve response to injury and repair, in Hunter, J.M., et al (eds): *Rehabilitation of the Hand.* St. Louis, Mosby, 1978.
17. Boscheinen-Morrin, J., Davey, V., and Connolly, W.B. *The Hand: Fundamentals of Therapy.* London, Butterworths, 1985.
18. Boyes, J.H. (ed): *Bunnell's Surgery of the Hand,* 5th ed. Philadelphia, Lippincott, 1970, pp 597–601.
19. Brand, P., and Wood, H. *Hand Volumeter Instruction Sheet.* U.S. Public Health Service Hospital, Carville, Louisiana.
20. Brand, Paul W. Hand rehabilitation—Management by objectives, in Hunter, J.M., et al (eds): *Rehabilitation of the Hand.* St. Louis, Mosby, 1984, pp 3–5.
21. Bright, D., and Wright, S. Postoperative management in replantation, in *American Academy of Orthopaedic Surgeons, Symposium on Microsurgery: Practical use in Orthopaedics,* St. Louis, Mosby, 1979, pp 83–95.
22. Brown, P.W. The assessment of phalangeal and metacarpal fractures. Surg Clin North Am 53(6):1393–1437, 1973.
23. Callahan, A.D. Sensibility testing: Clinical methods, in Hunter, J.M., et al (eds): *Rehabilitation of the Hand,* 2d ed. St. Louis, Mosby, 1984, pp 407–431.
24. Callahan, A.D. Methods of compensation and reeducation for sensory dysfunction, in Hunter, J.M., et al (eds): *Rehabilitation of the Hand,* 2d ed. St. Louis, Mosby, 1984, pp 432–442.
25. Cannon, N.M., et al.: Control of immediate postoperative pain following tenolysis and capsulectomies of the hand with TENS. J Hand Surg 8:625, 1983.
26. Cannon, N.M., and Strickland, J.W. Therapy following flexor tendon surgery. Hand Clin 1:147–165, February 1985.
27. Carroll, D. A quantitative test of upper extremity function. J Chronic Dis 18:479–491, 1965.
28. Carter, M.S. Joint protection program, in Hunter, J.M., et al (eds): *Rehabilitation of the Hand,* 2d ed. St. Louis, Mosby, 1984, pp 663–664.
29. Carter, M.S., and Wilson, R.L. Postsurgical management in rheumatoid arthritis, in Hunter, J.M., et al (eds): *Rehabilitation of the Hand.* St. Louis, Mosby, 1978, pp 496–502.
30. Charnley, J. *The Closed Treatment of Common Fractures,* 3d ed. Baltimore, Williams & Wilkins, 1972, pp 1–92.
31. Crawford, G.P. The molded polyethylene splint for mallet finger deformities. J Hand Surg [Am] 9:231–237, 1984.
32. Crawford, J.E., and Crawford, D.M. *Crawford Small Parts Dexterity Test Manual.* New York, Harcourt Brace Jovanovich, 1981.
33. Curtis, R.M., and Engalitcheff, J. A work simulator for rehabilitating the upper extremity: Preliminary report. J Hand Surg 6:499–501, 1981.
34. Davis, D.R. Some factors affecting the results of peripheral nerve injuries. Lancet 1:87, 1949.
35. Dellon, A.L. *Evaluation of Sensibility and Reeducation of Sensation in the Hand.* Baltimore, Williams & Wilkins, 1981.
36. Dellon, A.L., Curtis, R.M., and Edgerton, M.T. Reeducation of sensation in the hand after nerve injury and repair, Plast Reconstr Surg 53:297–305, 1974.
37. Dellon, A.L., and Jabaley, M.E. Reeducation of sensation in the hand following nerve suture. Clin Orthop 163:75–79, 1982.
38. Dellon, A.L. The M2PD Test: Clinical evaluation in the hand, in *Evaluation of Sensibility and Reeducation of Sensation in the*

Hand. Baltimore, Williams & Wilkins, 1981.

39. Dellon, A.L. The moving two point discrimination test: Clinical evaluation of the quickly adapting fiber/receptor system. J Hand Surg 3:474–481, 1978.

40. DeVore, G.L. Preoperative assessment and postoperative therapy and splinting in rheumatoid arthritis, in Hunter, J.M., et al (eds): *Rehabilitation of the Hand,* 2d ed. St. Louis, Mosby, 1984, pp 695–702.

41. Doyle, J.R. Extensor tendons—Acute injuries, in Green, D.P. (ed): *Operative Hand Surgery,* vol 2. New York, Churchill Livingstone, 1982, pp 1441–1464.

42. Duran, R.J., Houser, R.G., and Stover, NM.G. Management of flexor tendon lacerations in zone 2 using controlled passive motion postoperatively, in Hunter, J.M., Schneider, L.H., Mackin, E.J., and Bell, J. (eds): *Rehabilitation of the Hand.* St. Louis, Mosby, 1978, pp 217–224.

43. Duran, R.J., and Houser, R.G. Controlled passive motion following flexor tendon repair, in zones 2 and 3 in *AAOS Symposium on Tendon Surgery in the Hand,* St. Louis, Mosby, 1975, pp 105–114.

44. Dyck, P.J., O'Brien, P.C., Bushek, W., et al: Clinical vs. quantitative evaluation of cutaneous sensation. Arch Neurol 33(9):651–656, 1976.

45. Ehrlich, G.E. (ed): *Total Management of the Arthritic Patient.* Philadelphia, Lippincott, 1973.

46. Ejeskar, A. Finger flexion force and hand grip strength after tendon repair. J Hand Surg [Am] 7:61–65, 1982.

47. Ejeskar, A. Flexor tendon repair of no-man's land: Results of primary repair with controlled mobilization. J Hand Surg [Am] 9:171–177, 1984.

48. English, C.B., Rehm, R.A., and Petzoldt, R.L. Blocking splints to assist finger exercise, Am J Occup Ther 36:(4)259–262, 1983.

49. Ferraro, M.C., Coppola, A., Lippman, K., and Hurst, L.C. Closed functional bracing of metacarpal fractures. Orthop Rev 12:49–56, 1983.

50. Fess, E.E. Documentation: Essential elements of an upper extremity assessment battery, in Hunter, J.M., et al (eds): *Rehabilitation of the Hand,* 2d ed. St. Louis, Mosby, 1984, pp 49–78.

51. Fess, E.E. The effects of Jaymar dynamometer handle position and test protocol on normal grip strength. Proceedings of the ASHT. J Hand Surg 7:308, 1982.

52. Fess, E.E. Rehabilitation of the patient with an upper extremity replantation, in Hunter, J.M., et al (eds): *Rehabilitation of the Hand,* 2d ed. St. Louis, Mosby, 1984, pp 569–581.

53. Fess, E.E., Moran, C.A. *Clinical Assessment Recommendations.* American Society of Hand Therapists, 1981.

54. Frere, G., Moutet, F., Sarorius, Ch., and Vila, A. Controlled postoperative mobilization of sutured extension tendons of the longer fingers. Ann Chir Main 3:139–144, 1984.

55. Frykman, K., and Nelson, E.F. Fractures and traumatic conditions of the wrist, in Hunter, J.M., et al (eds): *Rehabilitation of the Hand,* 2d ed. St. Louis, Mosby, 1984, pp 165–179.

56. Gault, S.J., and Spyker, M.J. Beneficial effect of immobilization of joints in rheumatoid arthritis and related arthritides: A splint study using sequential analysis. Arthritis Rheum 12:34–44, 1969.

57. Gelberman, R.H., and Manske, P.R. Factors influencing flexor tendon adhesions. Hand Clinic 1:35–42, 1985.

58. Gelberman, R.H., Woo, S.L.Y., Lothringer, K., Akeson, W.H., and Amiel, D. Effects of early intermittent passive mobilization on healing canine flexor tendons. J Hand Surg [Am] 7:170–175, 1982.

59. Green, D.P. (ed). *Operative Hand Surgery.* New York, Churchill Livingstone, 1982.

60. Gulick Measurement Tape Product #1160, Best Priced Products, P.O. Box 1174, White Plains, New York 10602.

61. Harrand, G. The Harrand guide for developing physical capacity evaluations. Menomonie, Wisconsin, Stout Vocational Rehabilitation Institute, 1982.

62. Henderson, W.R. Clinical assessment of peripheral nerve injuries: Tinel's test. Lancet 2:801–805, 1948.

63. Hinterbuckner, C. Management of shoulder-hand syndrome, in Ruskin, A.P. (ed): *Current Therapy in Physiatry: Physical Medicine and Rehabilitation.* Philadelphia, Saunders, 1984, pp 263–266.

64. Holst-Nielson, F. Subcapital fractures of the four ulnar metacarpal bones. Hand 8:290–293, 1976.

65. Hunter, J.M., and Mackin, E. Edema and bandaging, in Hunter, J.M., et al (eds): *Rehabilitation of the Hand,* 2d ed. St. Louis, Mosby, 1984, 146–153.

66. Hunter, J.M., Sensheizer, F., and Mackin, E. Tenolysis, in Strickland, J.B., and Steichen, J.B. (eds): *Difficult Problems in Hand Surgery.* St. Louis, Mosby, 1982, pp 312–318.

67. Hunter, J.M., and Salisbury, R.E. Evaluation of oral trypsin-chymotrypsin for prevention of swelling after hand surgery. Plast Reconstr Surg 49(2):171–175, 1972.

68. Hunter, J.M., and Cowen, J. Fifth metacarpal fractures in a compensation clinic population. J Bone Joint Surg 52A:1159–1165, 1970.

69. Instructions for 32023 (4207) Minnesota Manual Dexterity Test, Lafayette Instrument Co., Sagamore and North 9th Street, Lafayette, Indiana.

70. Jaeger, S.H., and Mackin, E.J. Primary care of flexor tendon injuries, in Hunter, J.M., et al (eds): *Rehabilitation of the Hand,* 2d ed. St. Louis, Mosby, 1984, pp 261–271.

71. Jahss, S.A. Fractures of the metacarpals: A new method of reduction and immobilization. J Bone Joint Surg 20A:176–186, 1938.

72. Jebson, R., Taylor, N., Trieschmann, R., et al. An objective and standardized test of hand function. Arch Phys Med Rehabil 50:311–319, 1969.

73. Kasch, M. Acute hand injuries, in *Occupational Therapy: Practice Skills for Physical Dysfunctions,* 2d ed. pp 307–329.

74. Kasch, M.C., and Hester, L.A. Low-frequency TENS and the release of endorphins. J Hand Surg 8:626, 1983.

75. Kay, A.G.L. Management of the rheumatoid hand. Rheumatol Rehabil 18(suppl 1):76–81, 1979.

76. Kelsey, J.L., et al.: *Upper Extremity Disorders: A Survey of Their Frequency and Cost in the United States.* St. Louis, Mosby, 1980.

77. Kendall, P.H. Exercise for arthritis, in Licht, S. (ed): *Therapeutic Exercise,* 2d ed. New Haven, Connecticut, Elizabeth Licht, 1965.

78. Ketchum, L.D. Primary tendon healing: A review. J Hand Surg [Am] 2:428–435, 1977.

79. Ketchum, L.D., and Klug, M.S. A rational basis for post operative management of hand surgery problems, in Tubiana, R. (ed): *The Hand,* vol 2. Philadelphia, Saunders, 1985, 71–79.

80. Ketchum, L.D., Martin, N.L., and Kappel, D.A. Experimental evaluation of factors affecting the strength of tendon repairs. Plast Reconstr Surg 59:708–719, 1977.

81. Kiel, J.H. *Basic Hand Splinting: A Pattern Designing Approach.* Boston, Little, Brown, 1983.

82. Kilbourne, B.C., and Paul, E.G. The use of small bone screws in the treatment of metacarpal, metatarsal and phalangeal fractures. J Bone Joint Surg 40A:375–383, 1958.

83. Kleinert, H.E., et al: Primary repair of flexor tendons. Orthop Clin N Am 4:865–876, 1973.

84. Kleinert, H.E., Kutz, J.E., and Cohen, M.J. Primary repair of zone 2 flexor tendon lacerations, in *AAOS Symposium on Tendon Surgery in the Hand.* St. Louis, Mosby, 1975, 91–104.

85. Kleinert, H.E., and Verdan, C.: Report of the Committee on Tendon Injuries. J Hand Surg [Am] 8:794–798, 1983.

86. Knapp, M.E. Massage, in Krusen, F.H. (ed): *Handbook of Physical Medicine and Rehabilitation,* 3d ed. Philadelphia, Saunders, 1982, pp 386–388.

87. Knapp, M.E. Aftercare of fractures, in Krusen, F.H. (ed): *Hand-*

book of Physical Medicine and Rehabilitation, 2d ed. Philadelphia, Saunders, 1971, pp 579–582.

88. Kolumban, S.L. Preoperative and postoperative management of tendon transfers, in Hunter, J.M., et al (eds): Rehabilitation of the Hand, 2d ed. St. Louis, Mosby, 1984, pp 476–481.

89. Krawitz, M., and Wolman, T. Group therapy in rheumatoid arthritis. Penn Med 82(12):35–37, 1979.

90. LaMotle, R. Symposium: Assessment of Levels of Cutaneous Sensibility. United States Public Health Service Hospital, Carville, Louisiana, 1980.

91. Lankford, L.L. Reflex sympathetic dystrophy, in Hunter, J.M., et al (eds): Rehabilitation of the Hand, 2d ed. St. Louis, Mosby, 1984, pp 509–531.

92. Lee, V.H. Rehabilitation of extensor tendon injuries, in Hunter, J.M., et al (eds): Rehabilitation of the Hand, 2d ed. St. Louis, Mosby, 1984, pp 353–357.

93. Leonard, J., Swanson, A.B., and deGroot, and Swanson, G. Postoperative Care for Patients with Silastic Finger Joint Implants (Swanson's Design), 3d ed. Dow Corning Wright, 1984.

94. Lister, G.D., Kleinert, H.E., Kutz, J.E., and Atasoy, E. Primary flexor tendon repair followed by immediate controlled mobilization. Hand Surg [Am] 2:441–451, 1977.

95. Lister, G.L. The Hand: Diagnosis and Indications. London, Churchill Livingstone, 1977.

96. Lovett, W.L., and McCalla, M.A. Management and rehabilitation of extensor tendon injuries. Orthop Clin North Am 14:811–826, October, 1982.

97. Lundborg, G., Holm, S., and Myrbage, R. The rate of the synovial fluid and tendon sheath for flexor tendon nutrition: An experimental tracer study on diffusional pathways in dogs. Scand J Plast Reconstr Surg 14:99–197, 1980.

98. Lundborg, G., and Runk, F. Experimental intrinsic healing flexor tendons based upon synovial nutrition. J Hand Surg [Am] 3:21–23, 1978.

99. Mackin, E.J. Therapist's management of staged flexor tendon reconstruction, in Hunter, J.M., et al (eds): Rehabilitation of the Hand, 2d ed. St. Louis, Mosby, 1984, pp 314–323.

100. Mackin, E.J., and Maiorano, L. Postoperative therapy following staged flexor tendon reconstruction, in Hunter, J.M., Schneider, L.H., Mackin, E.J., and Bell, J. (eds): Rehabilitation of the Hand. St. Louis, Mosby, 1978, pp 247–261.

101. Madden, J.W. Wound healing: The biological basis of hand surgery, in Hunter, J.M., et al (eds): Rehabilitation of the Hand, 2d ed. St. Louis, Mosby, 1984, pp 140–145.

102. Malick, N.H. Manual on Dynamic Hand Splinting with Thermoplastic Materials. Pittsburgh, Harmarville Rehabilitation Center, 1974.

103. Malick, M.H. Manual on Static Hand Splinting, 2d ed. Pittsburgh, Harmarville Rehabilitation Center, 1972.

104. Manske, P.R., and Lesker, P.A. Comparative nutrient pathways to the flexor profundus tendons in zone II of various experimental animals. J Surg Res 34:83–93, 1983a.

105. Manske, P.R., Whiteside, L.A., and Lesker, P.A. Nutrient pathways to flexor tendons using hydrogen washout technique. J Hand Surg [Am] 3:32–36, 1978.

106. Manual for Allied Health Professionals. Arthritis Foundation, New York, 1973.

107. Matheson, L.N. Work Capacity Evaluation: A Training Manual for Occupational Therapists. Trabuco Canyon, California, Rehabilitation Institute of Southern California, 1982.

108. Matheson, L.N., and Ogden, L.D. Work Tolerance Screening, Trabuco Canyon, California, Rehabilitation Institute of Southern California, 1983.

109. May, J., Bryant, A., and Gardner, M. Digital replantation distal to the proximal interphalangeal joint, J Hand Surg 7:161–166, 1982.

110. Maynard, C.J. Sensory reeducation following peripheral nerve injury, in Hunter, J.M., et al (eds): Rehabilitation of the Hand. St. Louis, Mosby, 1978, pp 318–323.

111. McIntee, P.M. Therapist's management of the stiff hand, in Hunter, J.M., et al (eds): Rehabilitation of the Hand, 2d ed. St. Louis, Mosby, 1984, pp 216–230.

112. Melvin, J.L. Rheumatic Disease: Occupational Therapy and Rehabilitation, 2d ed. Philadelphia, Davis, 1982, 315–349, 351–371, 383–391.

113. Meyer, V.E., Chiu, D.T.W., and Beasley, R.W. The place of the internal skeletal fixation in surgery of the hand. Clin Plast Surg 8:51–64, 1981.

114. Milford, L. in Crenshaw, A.H. (ed): Campbell's Operative Orthopaedics, 5th ed. St. Louis, Mosby, 1978, pp 163–171.

115. Miller, W.R. Fractures of the metacarpals. Am J Orthop 7(7):105–108, 1965.

116. Mitchell, E. Symposium on Assessment of Levels of Cutaneous Sensibility. United States Public Health Service Hospital, Carville, Louisiana, 1980.

117. Moberg, E. Methods for examining sensibility in the hand, in Flynn, J.E. (ed): Hand Surgery. Baltimore, Williams & Wilkins, 1966, pp 435–439.

118. Moberg, E. Objective methods of determining functional value of sensibility in the hand. J Bone Joint Surg 40B:454–466, 1958.

119. Moberg, E. Objective tests for determining the functional value of sensibility in the hand. J Bone Joint Surg 40B:454–476, 1958.

120. Moberg, E. The shoulder hand finger syndrome. Surg Clin North Am 40:367, 1960, 367–373.

121. Murray, J. The patient with the injured hand. Presidential address. American Society for Surgery of the Hand. J Hand Surg 7:543–548, 1982.

122. Nelson, A.J. Implications of electromyographic examinations for hand therapy, in Hunter, J.M., et al (eds): Rehabilitation of the Hand, 2d ed. St. Louis, Mosby, pp 486–492.

123. Nichols, P.J.R. Rehabilitation Medicine: The Management of Physical Disabilities. London, Butterworth, 1976, pp 161–180.

124. Nunley, J.A., and Urbaniak, J.R. Treatment of extensor tendon injuries of the hand. Orthop Surg (Update Series) 2:2–8, 1982.

125. Omer, G. Management of pain syndromes in the upper extremity, in Hunter, J.M., et al (eds): Rehabilitation of the Hand, 2d ed. St. Louis, Mosby, 1984, pp 503–508.

126. Omer, G.E. Sensory evaluation by the pickup test, in Jewett, D.L., McCarroll, H.K., Jr., and Relton, H. (eds): Nerve Repair and Regeneration: Its Clinical and Experimental Basis. St. Louis, Mosby, 1980, pp 250–251.

127. Onne, L. Recovery of sensibility and psuedo-motor activity in the hand after nerve suture. Acta Chir Scand 300(suppl):1–69, 1962.

128. O'Riain, S. New and simple test of nerve function in the hand. Br Med J 3:615–616, 1973.

129. Pachter, B.R., Eberstein, A., and Goodgold, J.G. Electrical stimulation effect on denervated skeletal myofibrils in rats. Arch Phys Med Rehabil 63(9): 427–433, 1982.

130. Partridge, R.E.H., and Duthie, J.J.R. Controlled trial of the effect of complete immobilization of the joints in rheumatoid arthritis. Ann Rheum Dis 22:91–99, 1963.

131. Peacock, E.E., Madden, J.W., and Trier, W.C. Postoperative recovery of flexor tendon function. Am J Surg 122:686–692, 1971.

132. Peacock, E.E. and Van Winckle, W. Surgery and Biology of Wound Repair. Philadelphia, Saunders, 1970.

133. Pearson, S.O. Splinting the nerve injured hand, in Hunter, J.M., et al (eds): Rehabilitation of the Hand, 2d ed. Philadelphia, Mosby, 1984, pp 452–456.

134. Perry, J.F., Hamilton, G., Lachenbruce, P.A., et al. Protective sensation in the hand and its correlation to the ninhydrine sweat test following nerve laceration. Am J Phys Med 53:113–118, 1974.

135. Personal communication, Yasoma Challenor, M.D., Management of peripheral nerve injuries and sensory reeducation., *Harlem Hospital Center,* New York City, April 14, 1984.

136. Phelps, P., and Walker, E. Comparison of the finger wrinkling test results to established sensory tests in peripheral nerve injury. Am J Occup Ther 31:9 365–372, 1977.

137. Poppen, N.K. Clinical evaluation of epineural suture of digital nerves: Clinical evaluation of the von Frey and two-point discrimination tests and correlation with a dynamic test of sensibility, in Jewett, D.L., and McCarroll, H.K., Jr. (eds): *Nerve Repair and Regeneration: Its Clinical and Experimental Basis.* St. Louis, Mosby, 1980, pp 252–260, 277–278.

138. Prendergast, K.H. Therapist's management of the mutilated hand, in Hunter, J.M., et al (eds): *Rehabilitation of the Hand,* 2d ed. St. Louis, Mosby, 1984, pp 156–162.

139. Pulvertaft, R. Forward to first edition, in Hunter, J.M., et al (eds): *Rehabilitation of the Hand.* St. Louis, Mosby, 1978, p xi.

140. Rockwood, C.A., Jr., and Green, D.P. (eds): *Fractures in Adults,* 2d ed. Philadelphia, Lippincott, 1984, pp 313–409.

141. Rosenthal, E. A. The extensor tendons, in Hunter, J.M., et al (eds): *Rehabilitation of the Hand,* 2d ed. St. Louis, Mosby, 1984, pp 324–352.

142. Sarmiento, A., and Latta, L.L. *Closed Functional Treatment of Fractures.* New York, Springer-Verlag, 1981.

143. Sarmiento, A., Latto, L., and Sinclair, W.F. Functional bracing of fractures. Instr Course Lect 25:184–237, 1976.

144. Schneider, L.H. *Flexor Tendon Injuries.* Little, Brown, and Boston, 1984.

145. Schneider, L.H. Tendon transfers in the upper extremity, in Hunter, J.M., et al (eds): *Rehabilitation of the Hand,* 2d ed. St. Louis, Mosby, 1984, pp 470–475.

146. Schneider, L.H., Hunter, J.M., Norris, T.R., and Nadeau, P.O. Delayed flexor tendon repair in no man's land. J Hand Surg [Am] 2:452–455, 1977.

147. Schneider, L.H., and Hunter, J.M. Flexor tenolysis, in *AAOS Symposium on Tendon Surgery in the Hand,* St. Louis, Mosby, 1975, pp 157–162.

148. Schneider, L.H., and Mackin, E.J. Tenolysis, in Hunter, J.M., Schneider, L.H., Mackin, E.J., and Bell, J. (eds): *Rehabilitation of the Hand.* St. Louis, Mosby, 1978, pp 229–234.

149. Schneider, L.H., and Mackin, E.J. Tenolysis: A dynamic approach to surgery and therapy, in Hunter, J.M., et al (eds): *Rehabilitation of the Hand,* 2d ed. St. Louis, Mosby, 1984, pp 280–287.

150. Seddon, H. *Surgical Disorders of Peripheral Nerves,* 2d ed. New York, Churchill Livingstone, 1975.

151. Semmes-Weinstein Aesthesiometer. Research Designs, Inc., 7320 Ashcroft, Suite 103, Houston, Texas 77081.

152. Semmes, J., Weinstein, S., Ghent, L., and Teuber, H.L. *Somatosensory Changes After Penetrating Brain Wounds in Man.* Harvard University Press, Cambridge, Massachusetts, 1960.

153. Simonetta, C. The use of "AO" plates in the hand. Hand 2:43–45, 1970.

154. Smith, R.J., and Peimer, C.A. Injuries to the metacarpal bones and joints. Adv Surg 11:341–374, 1977.

155. Steichen, J.B., Harmon, K.S., Fess, E.E., and Strickland, J.W. Rehabilitation of the upper extremity replantation patient, in Hunter, J.M., et al (eds): *Rehabilitation of the Hand,* 2d ed. St. Louis, Mosby, 1978, pp 407–414.

156. Stillwell, G. Electrotherapy, in Kolthe, F., Stillwell, G., and Lehmann, J. (eds): *Krusen's Handbook of Physical Medicine and Rehabilitation,* 3d ed. Philadelphia, Saunders, 1982, 360–371.

157. Strickland, J.W. Flexor tendon repair. Hand Clinics 1(1):55, 1985, pp 55–68.

158. Strickland, J.W. Flexor tenolysis. Hand Clin 1(1):121–132, 1985.

159. Strickland, J.W. Opinions and preferences in flexor tendon surgery. Hand Clin 1:187–191, February 1985b.

160. Strickland, J.W. Results of flexor tendon surgery in zone II. Hand Clin 1:167–179, February 1985.

161. Strickland, J.W., and Glogovac, S.V. Digital function following flexor tendon repair in zone II: A comparison of immobilization and controlled passive motion techniques. J Hand Surg [Am] 5:537–543, 1980.

162. Sunderland, S. *Nerves and Nerve injuries,* 2d ed. New York, Churchill Livingstone, 1978.

163. Swanson, A.B., deGroot Swanson, G., and Leonard, J. Post operative rehabilitation programs in flexible implant arthroplasty of the digits, in Hunter, J.M., et al (eds): *Rehabilitation of the Hand,* 2d ed. St. Louis, Mosby, 1984, pp 665–680.

164. Swanson, A.B., and deGroot Swanson, G. Postoperative rehabilitation program for flexible implant arthroplasty of the fingers, in Inglis, A. (ed): *American Academy of Orthopaedic Surgeons: Symposium on Total Joint Replacement of the Upper Extremity.* St. Louis, Mosby, 1982, pp 238–254.

165. Swanson, A.B., Goran-Hagert, C., and deGroot Swanson, G. Evaluation of impairment of hand function, in Hunter, J.M., et al (eds): *Rehabilitation of the Hand,* 2d ed. St. Louis, Mosby, 1984, pp 101–132.

166. Tamai, S. Twenty year experience of limb replantation: Review of 293 upper extremity replants. J Hand Surg 6:311, 1981.

167. Tiffin, J., and Asher, E. The Perdue pegboard: Norms and studies of reliability and validity, J Appl Psychol 32:234, 1948.

168. Trombly, C.A. Arthritis, in Trombly, C.A. (ed): *Occupational Therapy for Physical Dysfunction,* 2d ed. Baltimore, Williams & Wilkins, 1983.

169. U.S. Department of Labor, Employment, and Training Administration: *Dictionary of Occupational Titles,* ed 4. Washington, D.C., U.S. Government Printing Office, 1977.

170. Valpar Corporation, 3801 East 34th St., Suite 105, Tucson, Arizona.

171. Verdan, C. Primary repair of flexor tendons. J Bone Joint Surg [Am], 42:647–656, 1960.

172. Verdan, C.E., Crawford, G.P., and Martini-Benked-dach, Y. The valuable role of tenolysis in the digits, in Cramer, L.M., and Chase, R.A. (eds): *Symposium on the Hand,* vol 3. St. Louis, Mosby, 1971.

173. WFR Corp., Ramsey, N.J.

174. Wakim, K.G. Physiological effects of massage, p 42; and Cyreax, J.H. Clinical applications of massage, p 130, in Licht, S.L. (ed): *Massage, Manipulation and Traction,* 3d ed. Baltimore, Waverly Press, 1971.

175. Waylett, J. Therapist's management of reflex sympathetic dystrophy, in Hunter, J.M., et al (eds): *Rehabilitation of the Hand.* St. Louis, Mosby, 1984, pp 533–537.

176. Waylett, J., Seibly, D. A study to determine the average deviation accuracy of a commercially available volumeter. J Hand Surg 6:300, 1981.

177. Weber, E.R., Harden, G., and Haynes, D. Synovial fluid nutrition on flexor tendons, paper presented at the 36th Annual Meeting of the American Society for Surgery of the Hand, Las Vegas, Nev, Feb. 23, 1981.

178. Werner, J.L., Omer, G.E. Evaluating cutaneous pressure sensation of the hand. Am J Occup Ther 24:5, 347–356, 1970.

179. Whitaker, J.H., Strickland, J.W., and Ellis, R.K. The role of flexor tenolysis in the palm and digits. J Hand Surg 2:462–470, 1977.

180. Wilson, R.L. Flexor tendon grafting, in Strickland, J.W. (ed): *Hand Clinics,* vol 1. Philadelphia, Saunders, 1985, pp 97–107.

181. Wilson, R.L., Carter, M.S. Management of hand fractures, in Hunter, J.M., et al (eds): *Rehabilitation of the Hand,* 2d ed. St. Louis, Mosby, 1984.

182. Wilson, R.L., Carter, M.S. Joint injuries in the hand: Preservation of proximal interphalangeal joint function, in Hunter, J.M., et al (eds): *Rehabilitation of the Hand,* 2d ed. St. Louis, Mosby, 1984, 195–205.

183. Wolfort, F.G. (ed): *Acute Hand Injuries—A Multispecialty Approach.* Boston, Little, Brown, 1980, pp 134–144.

184. Wynn Parry, C.B. *Rehabilitation of the Hand,* ed 4. London, Butterworth, 1981.

185. 382 Medical Grade Elastomer, Dow Corning Wright, Arlington, Tenn. 38002.

INDEX

CAMBA (calcaneal axis-metatarsal base angle), 1142
Cameron knee, 1381
Camitz transfer for median nerve palsy, 723
Campbell fascial arthroplasty, 637
Camper's chiasm, 701
Campomelic dysplasia, 481–482
Camptodactyly, 531, 533
Camurati-Eenelmann dysplasia, 487
Canadian type of prosthesis, 383, 384
Canaliculi of bone, 57
Cancellous bone, 56, 92, 136, 177
Cancellous screws, 564, 567, 1248, 1264
Candida, 314, 942, 947
CANP (calcium-activated neutral protease), 667
Cantilever failure, 1343
Capillary hemangioma, 328–329
Capital drop, 1353, 1354
Capitate, 547, 781, 783, 784, 789
Capitate-hamate fusion, 787, 788
Capitellum, 566–567, 781, 784, 789
CAPP (*see* Child Amputee Prosthetic Project)
CaPPi (*see* Calcium pyrophosphate dihydrate crystals)
Capsulitis, adhesive, 400–401, 407
Capsulorrhaphy, 448, 583, 584
Capsulotomy, 691, 1442
Caput ulnae syndrome, 647, 650
Carbenicillin, 306
Carbon fiber-polylactic acid-coated ligaments, 1294
Carbonic anhydrase deficiency, 487
Cardiomelic syndrome, 488
Carditis in juvenile rheumatoid arthritis, 213
Carpal bones, 555
  avascular necrosis of, 784
  carpal tunnel syndrome and, 674
  congenital anomaly of, 531, 534
  fractures and dislocations of, 544–547
  instability of, 555
  osteolysis of, 489
  replantation at level of, 735
  rheumatoid arthritis and, 648
  traumatic amputations and, 728
  vascular anatomy of, 781–783
Carpal height ratio, 526
Carpal ligaments, 554–556
Carpal tunnel syndrome (CTS), 673–676
  rheumatoid disorders and, 647, 651, 658–659
Carpectomy, 692, 695
Carpenter syndrome, 488
Carpometacarpal joint, 540
  carpal tunnel syndrome and, 674
  dislocation of, 543–544
  painful instability of, 662
  sprains of, 556–557
  surgical exposure of, 507
Carpus, 526, 527, 649, 652
  (*See also* Carpal bones)
Cartilage, articular (*see* Articular cartilage)
Cartilage hair hypoplasia, 20

Cartwheel injuries, 1267
Cast wedging, 164, 179
Cat bite, 747
Cat-scratch fever, 741
Catabolin, 28, 30, 35, 46
Cataracts, 476
Cathespin B, D, or G, 28, 35
Catterall classification of Perthes disease, 1117
Cauda equina syndrome, 1005, 1009, 1018
C-D (Cotrel-Dubousset) instrumentation, 876, 878
Cefamandole, 1340
Cefazolin, 313, 1340
Cefotaxime, 303
Cefoxitin, 306
Cefsulodin, 313
Ceftazidime, 313
Ceftizoxime, 303
Cell body, neuron, 121
Cellular envelope of bone, 55, 58
Cellular immunity, 1001
Cellular isoform, 3
Cellulitis, 169, 420, 742, 747
Cementless prostheses, 143, 1348–1349, 1381–1382
Center edge (CE) angle of Wrisberg, 463, 1090–1139, 1333, 1356–1357
Central cord syndrome, 776, 907, 932
Central core disease, 458
Central nervous system, 121
Central spinal stenosis, 1021, 1024
Central venous pressure (CVP), 150
Centrum, 6
Cephalexin, 298
Cephalosporins, 314
  bursal infection of hand and, 745
  cervical spine surgery and, 978
  Lyme disease and, 217
  open fracture and, 170
  osteomyelitis and, 298, 303
  septic arthritis and, 313
  total hip replacement and, 1340
Cephalothin, 298, 307, 1340
Ceramics, 141–142
Cerebellar tonsils and vermis, 440
Cerebral calcification, 487
Cerebral cortex somatosensory evoked potentials, 128
Cerebral palsy, 433–439, 690–693
  dislocations in, 1356–1357
  scoliosis in, 881–884
Cerebro-cerebrospinal fluid circulation disturbance, 838
Cerebrohepatorenal syndrome, 489
Cervical cord injury, 931
Cervical disc disease, 949, 970, 971, 973
Cervical discs, 970
Cervical laminectomy, 978
Cervical osteoplasty, 1106
Cervical osteotomy, 1039
Cervical plexus, 971
Cervical spine, 812
  ankylosing spondylitis and, 237
  biomechanics of, 832–833
  calcification and, 951

Cervical spine (*Cont.*):
  cock robin attitude of, 832, 915, 918
  compression flexion injury and, 917
  congenital anomalies of, 838–846
  degenerative diseases and disc disorders of, 969–990
    spondylosis and disc disease in, 969–981
    stenosis in, 982–987
  fractures and dislocations of, 150, 910–922
    (*See also* Fractures and dislocations, of spine)
    classification, 915–916
    fusion of, 845, 911, 918, 980
    hyperextension and, 913
    infection of, 949, 951
    instability of, 832, 911, 913–915, 919
    intrinsic innervation of, 817
    juvenile rheumatoid arthritis and, 216
    lateral approach to, 825
    lateral roentgenogram and, 951
    magnetic resonance imaging and, 424
    neurofibromatosis and, 489
    rheumatoid spondylitis and, 1039–1041
    rotatory subluxation, 832, 915
    soft tissue injury of, 908–909
    stenosis of, 982, 983
    surgical approaches to, 822–824, 978–982, 986–987
    vertical compression and, 918
    (*See also* Atlantoaxial joint; Ligaments, of spine)

Cervical spondylosis, 969–981, 1044
  diagnosis of, 970–977
  pain mechanisms in, 972–973
  treatment for, 977–981
Cervical stenosis, 970
Chamberlain line, 839
Chance fracture, 930
Charcot foot, 1452, 1453
Charcot joints, 37, 309, 472, 1044
Charcot-Marie-Tooth disease (CMT), 471, 472
Charcot shoulder, 580
Chauffeur's fractures, 551
Cheilotomy, 1440
Chemical shift imaging, 426
Chemical synovectomy, 653
Chemotherapy:
  allograft and autograft and, 77
  Ewing sarcoma and, 346
  Hodgkin's disease and, 354
  juvenile rheumatoid arthritis and, 215
  osteosarcoma and, 333, 334, 380, 1396
  pathological fracture and, 73
  soft tissue sarcoma and, 322–323
  tuberculous spondylitis and, 949
Chesterman lateral approach to thoracic disc, 994
Chevron arthrodesis, 1387–1388
Chevron osteotomy, 1436

Leukopenia in systemic lupus
  erythematosus, 230
Lhermitte's phenomenon, 972, 991
Libman and Sacks endocarditis, 230
Ligaments:
  of acromioclavicular joint, 498, 511, 573
  augmentation of, during repair, 1293
  biomechanical properties of, 49,
    138–139, 1290
  crimp of, 48, 49
  of elbow: capsule, 402
    lateral ligament complex, 550, 568
    lateral ulnar collateral ligament, 500
    medial ligament, 500, 559, 560, 563
  of foot and ankle: bifurcate, 1060, 1159,
    1162
    calcaneocuboid, 1060, 1061,
      1071–1072, 1152
    calcaneofibular, 412, 1059, 1060, 1153,
      1161, 1238, 1455–1456
    calcaneonavicular, 1060–1061, 1074,
      1143–1144, 1157
    deltoid, 1059, 1070, 1158, 1161, 1237
    interosseous talocalcaneal, 152, 1159
    intersesamoid, 144
    long and short plantar, 451,
      1060–1061, 1153, 1159
    metatarsal, 1062, 1391, 1433
    spring, 1060
      (*See also* Calcaneonavicular
        ligaments)
    talofibular, 412, 1059, 1158, 1237
    tibiofibular, 1237–1239
  of hand and wrist: carpus, 404, 553–556,
    649
    Cleland's, 505
    Grayson's, 775–776
    of interphalangeal joint, 557–559,
      656–657
    metacarpophalangeal: of fingers, 520,
      557–558, 655
      of thumb, 557, 668
    radioulnar, 404, 551, 556, 649
    ulnarcarpal, 554, 555
  healing of, 50–51
  of hip: Bigelow, 1049
    capsule, 406, 1087, 1096
    ligamentum capitis femoris (teres),
      406, 1049, 1095, 1338
    transverse, 1087, 1095
  immobilization and, 50, 1292
  of knee: anterior cruciate, 1057, 1286,
    1290–1295, 1308
    arcuate, 1056, 1301
    coronary (meniscotibial), 1056, 1305
    Humphrey, 1057
    lateral collateral, 1057, 1285, 1300, 1301
    medial collateral, 1056, 1285,
      1298–1300
    oblique popliteal, 525, 1056, 1057
    patellofemoral, 1056, 1316, 1317
    patellomeniscal, 1057
    posterior cruciate, 1057, 1287,
      1295–1298
    Wrisberg, 1056–1057
  laxity of, 15, 489, 1174, 1285–1288

Ligaments (*Cont.*):
  of sacroiliac joint, 1028
  of shoulder joint: capsular, 398–401, 514,
    577, 580, 583
    coracoacromial, 497, 576
    coracohumeral, 497, 576
    inferior glenohumeral, 497, 514, 576
    middle glenohumeral, 497, 514, 576
    superior glenohumeral, 497, 514, 515,
      576
  of spine: alar, 822, 843
    anterior longitudinal, 832, 925
    apical, 832
    capsular, 833–835, 908, 919, 926
    Hoffmann's, of dura, 1023
    interspinous, 825, 926
    ligamentum flavum, 833, 835, 969,
      1023
    posterior longitudinal, 832
    supraspinous, 835, 926, 1015
    transverse of atlas, 832, 843, 914–915
  (*See also* individual joints; individual
    ligaments)
Ligamentum capitis femoris, 406, 1049,
  1095, 1338
Ligamentum teres (*see* Ligamentum
  capitus femoris)
Light chain polypeptides, 110
Light touch-deep pressure testing, 797
Limb bud, 7
  medial rotation in, 1169
Limb girdle dystrophy, 457
Limb-sparing procedure, 333, 385, 762–763,
  1403
  (*See also* Neoplasms)
Limb viability studies, 373
Lincomycin, 307
Lindholm technique for Achilles tendon
  rupture, 1454
Line of acetabular roof, 1088
Linked prostheses for total knee
  replacement, 1376
Lin's technique for posterior lumbar
  interbody fusion, 1016–1017
Lipids, 59
Lipoblast, 324, 325
Lipocyte hypertrophy, 1358
Lipoma, 423, 424, 768, 847, 848
  simple, 326–327
Liposarcoma, 324–325
Lipscomb condylectomy, 1392
Liquid crystal thermography, 1425
Liquid nitrogen and tumor surgery, 1447
Lisch nodules in neurofibromatosis, 884
Lisfranc amputation, 365, 1452
Lisfranc dislocation, 1252
Lissauer's tract, 812
Lithium salts, 211
Little League elbow, 559
Littler digital exposure, 505
Liverpool prostheses for elbow, 639–640
LMD (low-molecular weight dextran), 738
Load, 72, 79, 81, 83, 84
  bearing of, menisci and, 1302
  characteristics of intervertebral disc,
    835, 1002–1003

Load (*Cont.*):
  response of, muskuloskeletal tissues, 28,
    49, 81–86, 134–139
  tendons and, 138
  (*See also* individual joints)
Lobster-claw deformity, 488, 1132
Locked back syndrome, 1026–1027
Locked dislocation of glenohumeral joint,
  577
Locked-in syndrome, 911
Locked knee, 1283, 1303
Long bone, 24, 481
  epiphysis of, growth plate and, 24
Long finger ray resection, 729
Longissimus muscles of spine, 819, 820
Longitudinal relaxation times in magnetic
  resonance imaging, 417–418
Loose bodies, 402, 403, 411, 413, 1309
Loose endoprosthesis, 89, 143, 392, 638,
  1342, 1382
  (*See also* Endoprostheses; Total hip
    replacement; Total knee replacement)
Looser's zones in osteomalacia, 264
Lordoscoliosis, 861
Lordosis, 861, 889–892
  classification of, 865
  lumbar, 455, 1024
  postlaminectomy and, 888
  (*See also* Hyperlordosis)
Losee tests, 1291
Lottes nails for tibial shaft fracture, 1236
Low back pain, 1025, 1028, 1029
Low-density polyethylene, 142
Low-modulus coatings, 144
Low-molecular-weight dextran (LMD), 738
Lower extremity:
  amputations, 364
  arthrography of, 405–413
    (*See also* Arthrography)
  arthrogryposis and, 469–470
  avascular necrosis of (*see* Avascular
    necrosis)
  biomechanics of, 1064–1076
    foot and ankle, 1070–1075
    hip, 1064–1066
    knee, 1066–1070
  cerebral palsy in, 434–438
  congenital and developmental
    abnormalities of: foot, 1138–1168
    hip, 1077–1128
    knee and leg, 1129–1137
  foot disorders, 1431–1460
  fractures and dislocations: in adults,
    1209–1260
    in children, 182, 1261–1282
    (*See also* Fractures and dislocations)
  juvenile rheumatoid arthritis and, 215–216
  leg length discrepancy, 1186–1208
  mylomeningocele in, 445–453
  neoplasms in, 1395–1419
  nerve injury and entrapment (*see* Nerve
    entrapment; Nerve injury)
  osteoarthritis of: ankle, 1385, 1393
    hip, 1263, 1333
    knee, 1371
  poliomyelitis and, 463–467